P9-DZA-122

Organization of the Text

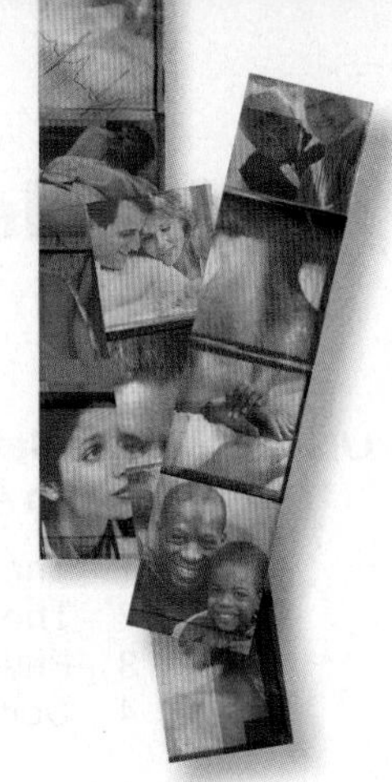

Case Study (woven throughout)

Presents a patient with a health concern corresponding to the chapter; ongoing related information, exercises, and details continue throughout the chapter.

Structure and Function

Reviews anatomy and physiology, with additional content on variations according to lifespan and culture.

Urgent Assessment

Summarizes emergency signs and symptoms to look for and immediate assessments and interventions.

Subjective Data

Focuses on areas for health promotion, risk factors, risk assessment, health goals, and health-related patient teaching. It also includes focused assessments for common symptoms. Questions for risk factors and symptoms are accompanied by rationales. Additional questions associated with older adult and cultural variations are included, as is sample documentation of findings.

Objective Data

Covers equipment, preparation, techniques, normal findings, abnormal findings, older adult and cultural adaptations, and sample documentation. Recurring checklists differentiate RN-level from APRN-level practice.

Critical Thinking

Discusses methods for organizing and prioritizing, key laboratory and diagnostic tests, and foundations for diagnostic reasoning.

Key Points

Key points of the chapter are summarized as reinforcement that the student has understood the most important information

Review Questions

These questions are consistent with the objectives at the beginning of the chapter and review important points.

Tables of Abnormal Findings

Cluster common abnormalities related to the assessment being explored, with compare-and-contrast information on key data points.

Brief Table of Contents

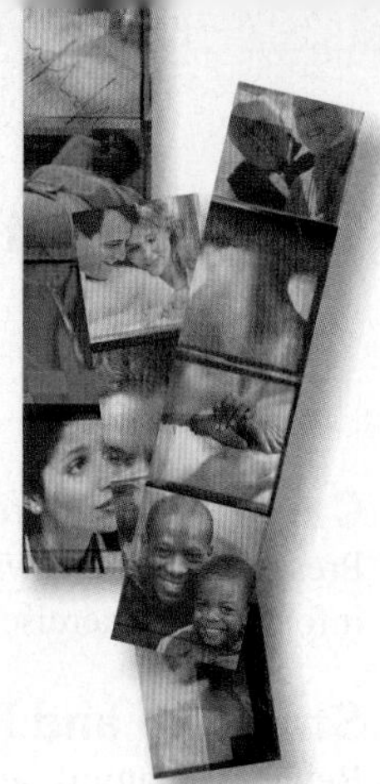

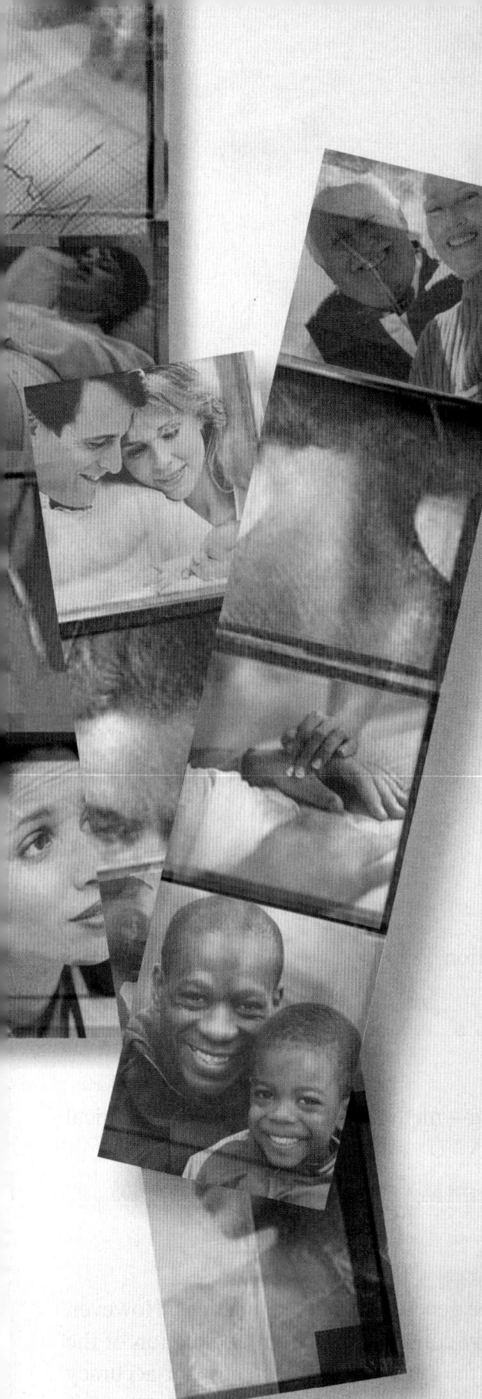

Nursing Health Assessment

A BEST PRACTICE APPROACH

Sharon Jensen, MN, RN
Instructor
School of Nursing & Dental Hygiene
University of Hawai'i at Manoa
Honolulu, Hawaii

EDITION 2

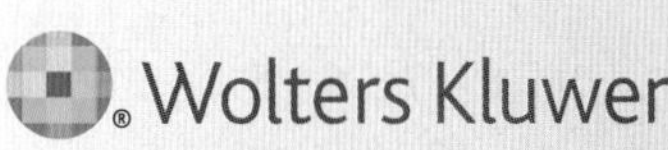

Philadelphia • Baltimore • New York • London
Buenos Aires • Hong Kong • Sydney • Tokyo

Acquisitions Editor: Chris Richardson
Product Development Editor: Annette Ferran
Developmental Editor: Rosanne Hallowell
Production Project Manager: Marian A. Bellus
Editorial Assistant: Zack Shapiro
Marketing Manager: Dean Karampelas
Design Coordinator: Joan Wendt
Illustration Coordinator: Jennifer Clements
Manufacturing Coordinator: Karin Duffield
Prepress Vendor: Absolute Service, Inc.

Printed in China

Library of Congress Cataloging-in-Publication Data

Jensen, Sharon, 1955- , author.
Nursing health assessment : a best practice approach / Sharon Jensen. — Second edition.
p. ; cm.
Includes bibliographical references and index.
ISBN 978-1-4511-9286-5 (alk. paper)
I. Title.
[DNLM: 1. Nursing Assessment--methods—Case Reports. 2. Medical History Taking—methods—Case Reports. 3. Physical Examination—methods—Case Reports. WY 100.4]
RT48
616.07'5—dc23

2014028217

LWW.com

9 8 7 6 5 4 3 2

RRS1507

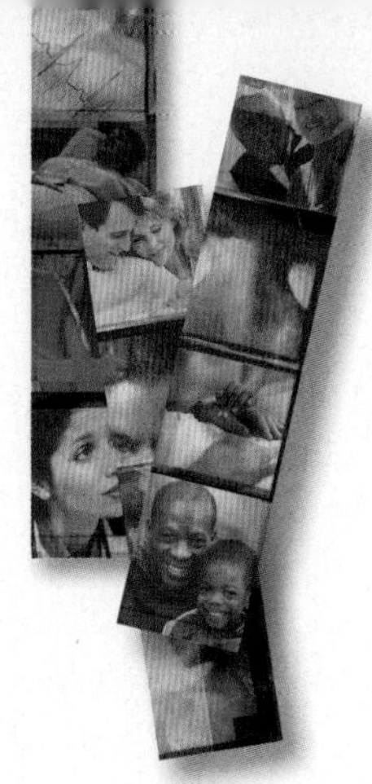

Acknowledgments

Sincere appreciation and warmest thanks are extended to the many people who were involved up front and behind the scenes.

- **The team at Wolters Kluwer Health** is truly invested in nursing and on the frontlines of health care. Annette Ferran, Rosanne Hallowell, Russ Hall, Corey Wolfe, Enrique Mares, Gwen Christensen, and the marketing team labor well beyond what is expected.
- **The contributors** worked diligently to revise the first edition manuscript and provide current evidence-based information in their specialty areas.
- **Nursing students in the United States, Canada, and internationally** are passionate about providing excellent care. Students do make a difference in the lives of educators, practicing nurses, and their patients.
- **Family, friends, and colleagues** provided support and encouragement to develop a text that shows how an assessment strongly supports high-quality outcomes.

We truly hope that this text lays out real-life situations so that nurses understand the importance of observation, with subjective and objective assessment as the process on which all nursing is based.

Inspiration

"The most important practical advice that can be given to nurses is to teach them what to observe."

(Florence Nightingale, Notes on nursing: What it is, and what it is not, *1860)*

Dedication

- To my parents, Jack and Gwen Erickson, who instilled in me my strong work ethic and understanding of community.
- Thank you to my siblings, Mike Erickson, Kathy Keithly, Alan Erickson, and their families who have supported me during this process.
- I honor and appreciate my children, Anna Jensen and Eric Jensen.
- To the students at Seattle University and the University of Hawaii, whose effort and ability allow me the privilege of serving as a guide and mentor during their education.

Contributors

Contributors to the Second Edition

Laura A. Blue, RN, MSN-Ed
Instructor
University of Hawai'i at Manoa, School of Nursing & Dental Hygiene
Honolulu, Hawaii
Chapter 3: Physical Examination Techniques and Equipment

Margie Bridges, MN, ARNP-BC, RNC-OB
Perinatal Clinical Nurse Specialist
University of Washington
Seattle, Washington
Chapter 26: Newborns and Infants

Ruth Chaplen, RN, DNP, ACNS-BC, AOCN
Associate Professor of Nursing
Rochester College, School of Nursing
Rochester Hills, Michigan
Chapter 16: Thorax and Lung Assessment

Yvonne D'Arcy, MS, CRNP, CNS
Pain Management and Palliative Care Nurse Practitioner
Suburban Hospital-Johns Hopkins Medicine
Bethesda, Maryland
Chapter 6: Pain Assessment

Jessica E. Gay, MSN, RNC-MNN
Clinical Instructor
University of Kansas Medical Center, KU School of Nursing
Kansas City, Kansas
Chapter 25: Pregnant Women

Nan Gaylord, PhD, RN, CPNP
Associate Professor
University of Tennessee, College of Nursing
Knoxville, Tennessee
Chapter 27: Children and Adolescents

Cynthia T. Greywolf, DNP-PMHNP, BC
Assistant Professor
AGNP Program Director
University of Hawai'i at Manoa, School of Nursing & Dental Hygiene
Honolulu, Hawaii
Chapter 22: Neurological and Assessment

Constance Hirnle, MN, RN-BC
Professional Development Specialist
Virginia Mason Medical Center
Seattle, Washington
Chapter 4: Documentation and Interdisciplinary Communication

Kathleen Kleefisch, DNP, FNP-BC
Assistant Professor of Nursing
Director, the Family Nurse Practitioner Program
Purdue University Calumet
Hammond, Indiana
Chapter 23: Male Genitalia and Rectal Assessment

Margaret Kramper, RN, FNP, CORLN
Allergy/Sinus Nurse Coordinator
Nurse Administrator
Department of Otolaryngology
Washington University School of Medicine
St. Louis, Missouri
Chapter 15: Nose, Sinuses, Mouth, and Throat

Jane Leach, PhD, RNC, IBCLC
Coordinator of Nurse Educator Program
Midwestern State University
Wichita Falls, Texas
Chapter 9: Mental Health and Violence Assessment

Janet Lohan, PhD, RN, CPN
Clinical Associate Professor
Washington State University, College of Nursing
Spokane, Washington
Chapter 8: Assessment of Developmental Stages

Jana McCallister, RN, MSN, PhD
Assistant Clinical Professor in Nursing
Director, Accelerated BSN Program
University of Texas at El Paso, School of Nursing
El Paso, Texas
Chapter 20: Abdominal Assessment

Amy Metteer-Storer, RN, BSN, MSN
Assistant Professor of Nursing
Cedar Crest College
Allentown, Pennsylvania
Chapter 2: The Health History and Interview
Chapter 18: Peripheral Vascular and Lymphatic Assessment

Jennifer R. Mussman, ARNP, CPNP, MN, DNP(c)
Senior Lecturer
Seattle University, College of Nursing
Seattle, Washington
Chapter14: Ears Assessment

Jessica Nishikawa, DNP, NP-C
Assistant Professor
University of Hawai'i at Manoa, School of Nursing & Dental Hygiene
Honolulu, Hawaii
Chapter 28: Older Adults

Heather O'Quinn, RN, MSN
Nursing Instructor
Simulation Lab Coordinator
Southside Virginia Community College
Chase City, Virginia
Chapter 7: Nutrition Assessment

Barbara Parker, RN, MS, APRN, FNP, CNM
Clinical Instructor
University of Kansas Medical Center, KU School of Nursing
Kansas City, Kansas
Chapter 25: Pregnant Women

Margaret S. Pierce, DNP, MPH, FNP-BC
Assistant Professor
University of Tennessee, College of Nursing
Knoxville, Tennessee
Chapter 12: Head and Neck, Including Lymph Nodes and Vessels

Julie Sabin, MSN, APRN, FNP-BC
Instructor
University of Hawai'i at Manoa, School of Nursing & Dental Hygiene
Honolulu, Hawaii
Chapter 1: The Nurse's Role in Health Assessment

Debra Lee Servello, DNP, ACNP
Assistant Professor of Nursing
ACNP Coordinator
Rhode Island College
Providence, Rhode Island
Chapter 5: Vital Signs and General Survey

Maureen Shannon, CNM, FNP, PhD, FAAN, FACNM
Associate Professor
Frances A. Matsuda Endowed Chair in Women's Health
University of Hawai'i at Manoa, School of Nursing & Dental Hygiene
Honolulu, Hawaii
Chapter 19: Breasts and Axillae Assessment

Mindy Stites, MSN, APRN, CCNS, ACNS-BC, CCRN
Critical Care Nurse Specialist
The University of Kansas Hospital
Kansas City, Kansas
Chapter 17: Heart and Neck Vessels Assessment

Danuta Wojnar, PhD, RN, FAAN, IBCLC
Associate Professor
Chair of Maternal/Child and Family Nursing
Seattle University, College of Nursing
Seattle, Washington
Chapter 10: Assessment of Social, Cultural, and Spiritual Health

Contributors to the First Edition

Yvonne D'Arcy, MS, CRNP, CNS
Pain Management and Palliative Care Nurse Practitioner
Suburban Hospital
Bethesda, Maryland
Pain Assessment

Karen S. Feldt, PhD, ARNP, GNP
Associate Professor
College of Nursing, Seattle University
Seattle, Washington
Older Adults

Cynthia Flynn, MSN, CNM, PhD, ARNP
General Director
Family Health and Birth Center
Washington, DC
Newborns and Infants

Nan Gaylord, PhD, RN, CPNP
Associate Professor
University of Tennessee, College of Nursing
Knoxville, Tennessee
Children and Adolescents

Nancy George, PhD, FNP-BC
Assistant Professor (Clinical)
Wayne State University
Detroit, Michigan
Eyes Assessment

Constance Hirnle, MN, RN, BC
Sr. Lecturer, SON, and Education Specialist
University of Washington Virginia Mason Medical Center
Seattle, Washington
Documentation and Interdisciplinary Communication

Kathleen Kleefisch, DNP, FNP-BC
Director of the Family Nurse Practitioner Program
Assistant Professor
Purdue University at Calumet
Hammond, Indiana
Male Genitalia and Rectal Assessment

N. Jayne Klossner, MSN, RNC
Director, Patient Care Improvement
Baptist Health System
San Antonio, Texas
Pregnant Women

Margaret Kramper, RN, FNP
Allergy Sinus Nurse Coordinator
Department of Otolaryngology/Head and Neck Surgery
Washington University
St. Louis, Missouri
Nose, Sinuses, Mouth, and Throat Assessment

Sharon Kumm, RN, MN, MS, CCRN
Clinical Associate Professor
University of Kansas
Kansas City, Kansas
Musculoskeletal Assessment

Janet Lohan, PhD, RN, CPN
Clinical Associate Professor
Washington State University
Spokane, Washington
Assessment of Developmental Stages

Amy Metteer-Storer, RN, BSN, MSN
Assistant Professor of Nursing
Cedar Crest College
Bethlehem, Pennsylvania
Peripheral Vascular and Lymphatic Assessment

Jennifer Mussman, RN, ARNP
Clinical Instructor
Seattle University
Seattle, Washington
Ears Assessment

Michelle Pardee, MS, FNP-BC
Lecturer
University of Michigan, School of Nursing
Ann Arbor, Michigan
Eyes Assessment

Debra A. Phillips, PhD, PMHNP
Associate Professor
Seattle University College of Nursing
Seattle, Washington
Assessment of Human Violence ("Mental Health and Violence Assessment" in 2nd edition)

Margaret S. Pierce, DNP, FNP-BC
Assistant Professor
University of Tennessee College of Nursing
Knoxville, Tennessee
Head and Neck with Lymphatics Assessment ("Head and Neck, Including Lymph Nodes and Vessels" in 2nd edition)

Barbara Rideout, MSN
Nurse Practitioner
Drexel University College of Medicine
Department of Family, Community, and Preventive Medicine
Philadelphia, Pennsylvania
Abdominal Assessment

Debra Lee Servello, RNP, MSN
Assistant Professor of Nursing
Rhode Island College School of Nursing
Providence, Rhode Island
General Survey and Vital Signs Assessment

Ann St. Germain, MSN, ANP-BC, WHNP-BC
Assistant Clinical Professor
Texas Woman's University, College of Nursing
Houston, Texas
Female Genitalia and Rectal Assessment

Karen Gahan Tarnow, RN, PhD
Clinical Associate Professor
University of Kansas School of Nursing
Kansas City, Kansas
Musculoskeletal Assessment

Lisa Trigg, PhD, PMHNP-BC
Instructor
University of Kansas
Kansas City, Kansas
Musculoskeletal Assessment

Joyce B. Vazzano, MS, APRN, BC, CRNP
Instructor
Johns Hopkins University School of Nursing
Baltimore, Maryland
Breasts and Axillae Assessment

Deborah Webb, RN (Deceased)
Neurological Clinical Nurse Specialist
Harborview Medical Center
Seattle, Washington
Neurological Assessment

Mary P. White, MSN, APRN, BC
Clinical Instructor
Director, Campus Health Center
Wayne State University College of Nursing
Detroit, Michigan
Skin, Hair, and Nails Assessment

Danuta Wojnar, PhD, RN
Assistant Professor
Seattle University, College of Nursing
Seattle, Washington
Assessment of Social, Cultural, and Spiritual Health

For a list of the contributors to the Student and Instructor Resources accompanying this book, please visit thePoint.

Reviewers

Ruth Chaplen, RN, DNP, ACNS-BC, AOCN
Associate Professor of Nursing
Rochester College, School of Nursing
Rochester Hills, Michigan

Diane Crayton, DNP, FNP, RN-BC
Assistant Professor
California State University, Stanislaus, School of Nursing
Turlock, California

Elaine Della Vecchia, PhD, RN, CCRN
Assistant Professor
New York Institute of Technology, Department of Nursing
New York, New York

Hobie Etta Feagai, EdD, MSN, FNP-BC, APRN-Rx
Professor, Course Coordinator
Hawai'i Pacific University, College of Nursing and Health Sciences
Kaneohe, Hawaii

Steve Glow, APRN-FNP
Associate Clinical Professor
Montana State University, College of Nursing
Missoula, Montana

Regina Hanchak, RN, MS
Professor of Nursing
Eerie Community College
Buffalo, New York

Jane Leach, PhD, RNC, IBCLC
Coordinator of Nurse Educator Program
Midwestern State University
Wichita Falls, Texas

Esther Levine Brill, PhD, APRN-BC, ANP
Professor
Long Island University, School of Nursing, Brooklyn Campus
Brooklyn, New York

Amy Ma, DNP, FNP-BC
Associate Professor
Director of Graduate Program
Long Island University
Brooklyn, New York

Judith McKenna, DNP, RN
Director, Nursing Education
Alma College
Alma, Michigan

Elizabeth Miller, DNP, MSN, BSN, RN, CCM, CMSRN
Assistant Professor of Nursing
Bowie State University
Bowie, Maryland

Kathy Moran, DNP, RN, CDE
Assistant Professor
University of Detroit Mercy, McAuley School of Nursing
Detroit, Michigan

Heather O'Quinn, RN, MSN
Nursing Instructor
Simulation Lab Coordinator
Southside Virginia Community College
Chase City, Virginia

Jennifer Richard, MSN, RN, CNE
Instructor of Nursing
University of Saint Francis
Fort Wayne, Indiana

Dina Rosenthal, MS, RN, CCRN
Clinical Nursing Instructor
Georgetown University, Medstar Washington Hospital Center
Washington, DC

Terri Summers, DNP, RN, MSN
Assistant Professor
Clayton State University
Morrow, Georgia

Karen Tarnow, RN, PhD
Clinical Associate Professor
University of Kansas Medical Center, KU School of Nursing
Kansas City, Kansas

Jennifer Wheeler, RN, MSN/Ed
Assistant Professor of Nursing
Jackson College
Jackson, Michigan

Samantha Wilson, AA, BSN, MSN
Associate Professor of Nursing
Germanna Community College
Fredericksburg, Virginia

For a list of the reviewers of the Test Generator accompanying this book, please visit thePoint.

Preface

Nursing Health Assessment: A Best Practice Approach reflects a progressive, modern approach to both nursing education and clinical nursing practice. The goal is to combine the most successful elements of "traditional" health assessment texts (e.g., two-column approach to physical examination and systems approach) with innovative elements to help students apply knowledge. The text not only includes thorough and comprehensive examinations for each specific topic but also presents features on safety integrating the QSEN competencies and clinical significance features that integrate clinical and theory (Benner's work on Transforming Nursing Education). It presents adequate information to teach and to reinforce knowledge.

Unique features assist students with application and analysis, enhancing their critical thinking skills and better preparing them for practice. It attempts to move students from beyond "noticing" to focused observation, recognizing deviation from expected, seeking information, making sense of data, and prioritizing (Tanner's work on Integrated Teaching). Case study features assist with application and analysis, enhancing critical thinking skills and better preparing all readers for active practice.

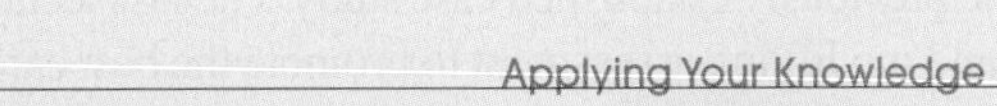

Applying Your Knowledge

You have reviewed how subjective and objective assessment data are used in developing a diagnosis, planning care, and evaluating progress toward established outcomes. Using the nursing process and your critical thinking skills, consider all the case study findings woven throughout this chapter. While answering the following questions, begin drawing conclusions to see how the pieces of assessment work together to create an environment for individualized, evidence-based, high-quality nursing care.

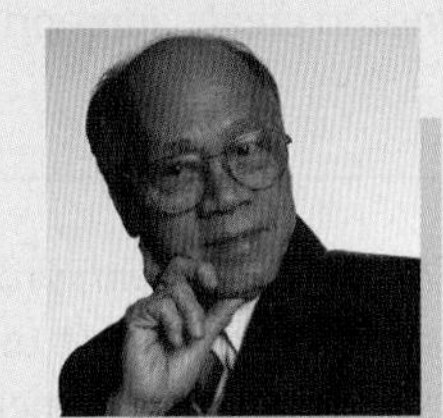

- Why is the sternal angle (angle of Louis) an important landmark for assessment of the thorax?
- What subjective data collected are cause for concern?
- What health promotion and teaching needs are identified for Mr. Lee?
- Is Mr. Lee's condition stable, urgent, or something requiring immediate attention?
- How will the nurse individualize assessment to meet Mr. Lee's specific needs, considering his condition, age, and culture?
- How will the nurse evaluate the success of patient teaching for Mr. Lee?

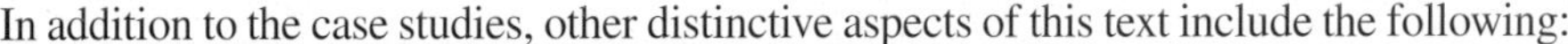

In addition to the case studies, other distinctive aspects of this text include the following:

- **Emphasis on health promotion, and risk factor reduction.** The emphasis is included in each "Subjective Data" section. Because history taking and risk assessment is so important to nursing practice, the history and risk factor questions are separated from assessment of the signs and symptoms.
- **Distinctions between common techniques and specialty or advanced practice skills.** A recurring table in the "Objective Data" section explains which techniques are more commonly performed in routine examinations to distinguish basic from specialty practice. This structure helps users prepare for actual patient interactions as well as to expect to modify techniques for individual situations.

TABLE 15.3 **Basic Versus Focused/Specialty or Advanced Techniques Related to Nose, Sinuses, Mouth, and Throat Assessment**

Technique	Purpose	Screening or Registered Nurse Assessment	Focused or Advance Practice Examination
Inspect the nose.	To gather information regarding the integrity of the nose	X	
Inspect the mouth.	To gather information regarding the integrity of the oral cavity	X	
Inspect the throat.	To gather information regarding the integrity of the throat	X	
Inspect the nose with otoscope and nasal speculum.	To gather information about inflammation, infection, and structure		X Inflammation, infection, structure

- **Focus on documentation and communication between health professionals.** There is a separate chapter on documentation and interdisciplinary communication. Each chapter includes samples of normal and abnormal documentation. Additionally, SOAP note and SBAR features show how assessment information is communicated both in writing and verbally.

Progress Note: Analyzing Findings

Remember Mr. Farhan, the patient with diabetes who was planning on fasting for Ramadan. Initial subjective and objective data collection is complete, and the nurse has spent time reviewing findings with the primary care provider. The following nursing note illustrates how subjective and objective data are collected and analyzed and nursing interventions are developed.

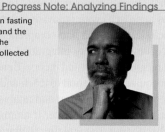

- **Emphasis on evidence-based critical thinking, diagnostic reasoning, knowledge application, and analysis.** End-of-chapter review sections contain questions and critical thinking challenges related to the previously established case study. The last section of each chapter focuses on prioritizing and modifying assessment to promote the best care possible and summarizing multiple findings to create appropriate plans for patient's health.

Organization of the Text

Unit 1, *Foundations of Nursing Health Assessment*, provides in-depth coverage of the basic components of nursing health assessment. The rest of the text builds on and expands the material in this first unit. The nurse's role in assessment, interview and health history, and techniques are included. The unit concludes with information on the important components of documenting findings and sharing them with other health care team members. Using the correct medical terminology and proper documenting is important, especially avoiding the use of "good" and "normal." A special icon notes documentation in the data collection column of the general examinations chapters.

Skin texture is firm, even, and elastic. Turgor is intact, as shown by rapid return of skin after pinching.

Unit 2, *General Examinations*, presents those assessments consistently applicable to all content areas. These topics reflect the holistic nature of nursing health assessment, as opposed to the traditional medical model that generally focuses on the physical domain and "body systems." Topics in Unit 2 include vital signs; pain; nutrition; developmental stages; mental health and violence; and social, cultural, and spiritual health.

Unit 3, *Regional Examinations*, presents individual chapters focusing on assessment of the key areas of the body, beginning with the skin and ending with the genital and rectal examinations. The material focuses primarily on adults to avoid overwhelming students with assessment of younger patients (usually presented at a later point in the curriculum). Older adult and cultural variations are highlighted at crucial points of review. Diversity is integrated to provide students with information and real-life situations.

Unit 4, *Special Populations and Foci*, presents content of assessments for pregnant women, newborns and infants, children and adolescents, and older adults.

Unit 5, *Putting It All Together*, reinforces the book's previous learning by outlining how to complete a full, comprehensive, head-to-toe examination for an adult. The hospitalized adult includes additional issues, such as focus on falls, skin breakdown, and sepsis. The head-toe-toe chapter includes a complete assessment that takes about an hour to complete, with over 100 points; this is a summary of the units previously studied in depth.

Chapter Organization and Features

Case Features

- Progressive case study material is woven throughout every chapter. From the beginning to the end of the content presentation, readers follow a patient's story and are challenged to apply their reading to the unfolding scenario. A recurring structure serves as a mechanism for supplying more information but also for reinforcing the core assessment foundations of critical thinking, therapeutic communication, documentation, findings analysis, application collaboration, and "pulling it all together." The case begins with a picture, reading, and bulleted list of three to five questions. These elements introduce the patient and generate beginning issues to consider.
- **Therapeutic Dialogue: Collecting Subjective Data** These displays provide examples of effective communication with patients in challenging situations, such as crying, cognitive impairment, or ethical issues. "Critical Thinking Challenges" offer an opportunity to consider how to collect subjective data in a holistic and challenging context.

Therapeutic Dialogue: Collecting Subjective Data

Remember Karen Pitoci, the 15-year-old girl receiving home care following hospitalization for anorexia nervosa. The home health nurse is collecting data to assess the patient's health. The nurse uses professional communication techniques to gather subjective data from Karen. The nurse is interviewing the patient to obtain a 24-hour diet recall.

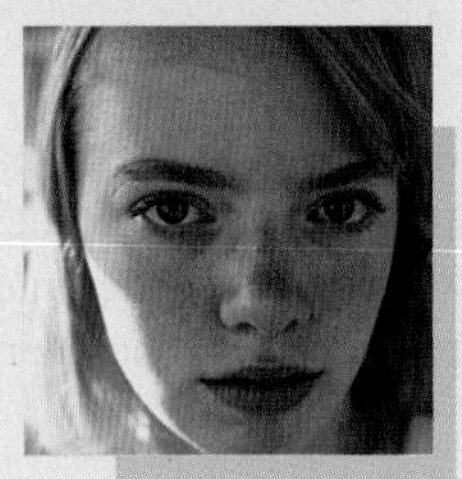

- **Progress Note: Analyzing Findings:** The feature focuses on documented summaries of findings related to the case in four areas: subjective data (S), objective data (O), analysis (A), and plan (P). The format follows the nursing process, with assessment as the first and most important step.
- **Documenting Case Study Findings:** The Documenting Case Study feature summarizes abnormal findings relevant to the case study patient in the physical examination: inspection, palpation, percussion, and auscultation.
- **Collaboration With the Interprofessional Team:** This unique feature describes scenarios in which the nurse in the case must coordinate referrals or other advocacy needs for the patient. The feature shows how to organize details using the SBAR framework: **S**ituation, **B**ackground, **A**nalysis (or **A**ssessment), and **R**ecommendations. A Critical Thinking Challenge ends the section, prompting the student to consider how the nurse might have better communicated findings and recommendations.

Collaborating With the Interprofessional Team

Both occupational and physical therapists work with patients to increase mobility and functional abilities for rehabilitation. Generally, physical therapists focus on larger motor groups, whereas occupational therapists focus on fine motor skills and the upper body. Nurses may consult occupational therapists for patients with difficulties involving bathing, dressing, grooming, home and money management, assistive technology, or increasing ROM, tone, sensation, or coordination.

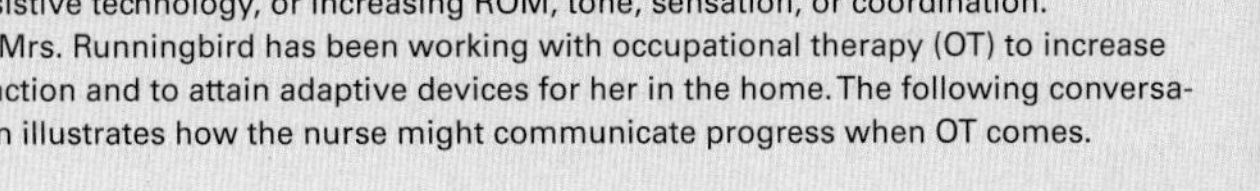

Mrs. Runningbird has been working with occupational therapy (OT) to increase function and to attain adaptive devices for her in the home. The following conversation illustrates how the nurse might communicate progress when OT comes.

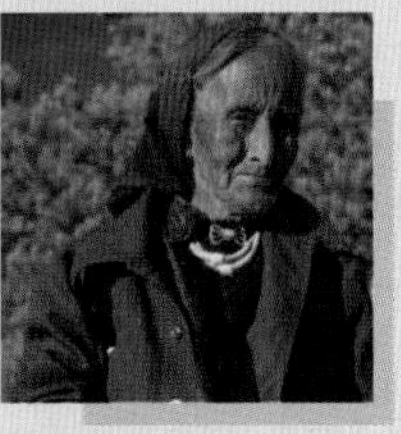

- **Laboratory and Diagnostic Testing:** Common tests are included to supplement the assessments and assist with critical thinking and diagnostic reasoning. For example, in the abdominal section, the labs for the liver and kidneys are included to trigger students to look up these findings as part of the critical thinking and diagnostic reasoning process.
- **Pulling It All Together:** A table shows how to bring all the elements of assessment together when arriving at a nursing diagnosis based on previous findings and beginning to develop goals, interventions, rationales, and evaluation criteria.

Pulling It All Together

The nurse uses assessment data to formulate a nursing care plan for Maria Ortiz. After these interventions are completed, the nurse will reevaluate the patient and document the findings in the chart to show critical thinking. This is often in the form of a care plan or case note similar to the one below.

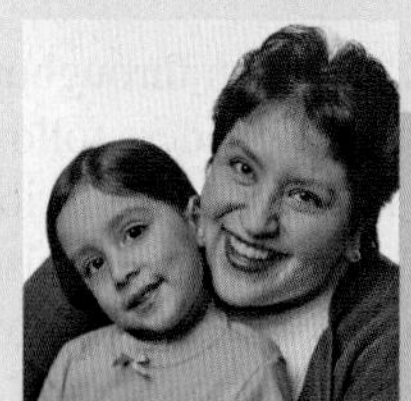

Nursing Diagnosis	Patient Outcomes	Nursing Interventions	Rationales	Evaluation
Knowledge deficit related to new diagnosis and medication	The patient states what to do for symptoms of hypoglycemia.	Discuss signs and symptoms of hypoglycemia. Discuss what to do if the patient is hypoglycemic, and provide a list of appropriate foods to increase blood glucose level.	Written information reinforces verbal information and can be used as a resource once the patient is at home.	Patient stated signs and symptoms of hypoglycemia. Patient named four foods that contain 10–15 g fast-acting carbohydrates. Patient will bring questions to next clinic visit.

- **Applying Your Knowledge:** This last case-related feature in the chapter includes summary text and repeats the bulleted questions found at the start of the chapter. This feature shows how assessment generates intervention, evaluation, and collaboration based on accurate and complete data to generate more effective care.

Other Features

- **Learning Objectives:** These objectives present the most important goals for learning by the time of completing the chapter.
- **Clinical Significance:** This feature highlights content critically related to a point of application. It may appear wherever applicable in the chapter.

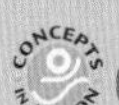

Clinical Significance

Reduced cardiac output is associated with the medical diagnosis of heart failure. In this clinical syndrome, reduced contractility causes preload to increase. Blood backs up, causing congestion. Congestion on the left backs blood into the lungs, whereas congestion on the right backs blood into the body, especially the legs and feet. Signs and symptoms of heart failure are shortness of breath, weight gain, and swollen ankles with decreased cardiac output.

- **Safety Alert:** These recurring boxes present important areas of concern or results that require immediate intervention or adjustments. Safety Alert features are placed wherever applicable in the chapter.

SAFETY ALERT

If a patient is experiencing chest pain, dyspnea, cyanosis, diaphoresis, or dizziness, focus assessment on collecting data to resolve the discomfort. Gather information while performing treatments (such as administration of oxygen and nitroglycerine tablets sublingually as ordered) and diagnostic tests (such as electrocardiography). If chest pain continues, ask for help because more than one clinician may be necessary to collect data and to intervene appropriately.

- **Equipment Needed:** This box reviews essential equipment that the nurse will want to identify, clean, and gather before entering the patient's room relative to each assessment.
- **Key Points:** Key points are summarized at the end of the chapter to reinforce the most important information.
- **Review Questions:** Each chapter has 10 test questions written as a summary. The case study and related critical thinking questions are a higher level of thinking. They should be discussed with the instructor.
- **Tables of Abnormal Findings:** Tables of abnormal findings are summarized at the end of the chapter. Art or tables of normal findings may be integrated into the chapter in the appropriate location, but comparative depictions of abnormal findings generally are found in groups at the end.

TABLE 20.2 **Abnormal Abdominal Findings**

Finding	Description
Common Sites of Referred Pain	Abdominal pain may present with pain directly over the organ involved or the pain may be referred to a site where the organ was located in fetal development because the human brain has no felt image for internal organs. During fetal development, the organs migrate to their final location, but the nerves persist in the former location, and the patient feels the referring sensation. Pain in referred areas without representative history or other physical findings may not have an abdominal origin.

Icons

This icon clues readers to visit thePoint to review a corresponding video asset.

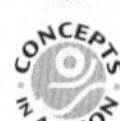

This icon clues readers to visit thePoint to review a corresponding animation.

A Comprehensive Package for Teaching and Learning

To further facilitate teaching and learning, a carefully designed package of instructor and student resources is available. In addition to the usual print resources, Wolters Kluwer Health is pleased to present multimedia tools that have been developed in conjunction with the text.

Resources for Students

thePoint Accessible through the access code in the inside front cover of the book, thePoint (thepoint.lww.com) offers a variety of resources for students that test knowledge and enhance understanding of health assessment. On thePoint, you will find the following:

- More than 500 self-study questions
- Concepts in Action™ Animations
- Watch and Learn™ Videos
- Journal Articles
- Spanish-English Dictionary with Pronunciation

Resources for Instructors

thePoint Instructors can access thePoint (thepoint.lww.com) using a code provided with each adoption. There they will find all of the student resources as well resources specifically designed to support instruction:

- A thoroughly revised Test Generator, containing more than 500 NCLEX-style questions
- Sample syllabus
- Strategies for effective teaching
- PowerPoint™ presentations, guided lecture notes, and prelecture quizzes

- An image bank
- Discussion topics and assignments
- Case studies

A Fully Integrated Course Experience

We are delighted to introduce an expanded suite of digital solutions and ancillaries to support instructors and students using Jensen's *Nursing Health Assesment: A Best Practice Approach,* 2nd edition. To learn more about any solution with the Jensen suite, please contact your local Wolters Kluwer representative.

Lippincott CoursePoint: An Adaptive Learning Experience

Lippincott
CoursePoint

Lippincott CoursePoint is a fully adaptive and integrated digital course solution for nursing education. CoursePoint synthesizes adaptive learning tools and content with an electronic version of the text and a wide array of integrated learning aids—all in one convenient location.

At the heart of CoursePoint is our adaptive learning system, powered by prepU. In numerous studies, prepU has demonstrated improved student performance in both nursing courses and on the NCLEX. CoursePoint extends prepU's adaptive tools by connecting students to the resources that will help them *understand* the correct answers, with quiz results linked to relevant sections of the *Nursing Health Assessment* integrated eBook as well as videos, animations, interactive tutorials, audio tutorials, and interactive case studies via SmartSense links

As the instructor, you have everything you need to develop your course, with easily accessible resources, organized by type or chapter, including the following:

- A thoroughly revised Test Generator, containing more than 500 NCLEX-style questions
- Sample syllabus
- Strategies for effective teaching
- PowerPoint™ presentations, guided lecture notes, and prelecture quizzes
- An image bank
- Discussion topics and assignments
- Case studies

CoursePoint's instructor reporting tools enable you to monitor individual student and class progress and strengths and weaknesses.

Lippincott
CoursePoint+

Available in Fall of 2015, Lippincott CoursePoint+ takes learning one step further by integrating additional skills and simulation tools within the CoursePoint platform. Specifically, CoursePoint+ integrates *vSim for Nursing: Assessment* to provide students with a complete skills experience.

Simulation and Innovative Resources

vSim for Nursing

- ***vSim for Nursing: Fundamentals*** **Lippincott's new computer simulation platform** *(available in Lippincott CoursePoint+ or via thePoint).* Codeveloped by Laerdal Medical and Wolters Kluwer, vSim for Nursing: Assessment helps students develop clinical competence and decision-making skills as they interact with virtual patients in a safe, realistic environment. vSim for Nursing records and assesses student decisions throughout the simulation, then provides a personalized feedback log highlighting areas needing improvement.

Lippincott
DocuCare

- **Lippincott DocuCare** *(available via thePoint)*. Lippincott DocuCare combines web-based electronic health record simulation software with clinical case scenarios that link directly to much of the material presented in Jensen's *Nursing Health Assessment*. Lippincott DocuCare's nonlinear solution works well in the classroom, simulation lab, and clinical practice.

Additional Media and Print Resources

A wide variety of resources are available to enhance the learning experience. Visit http://www.lww.com for purchasing options.

- ***Laboratory Manual for Jensen's Nursing Health Assessment: A Best Practice Approach*, 2nd edition**. Available at bookstores or at www.LWW.com, this student laboratory manual presents various exercises to reinforce textbook content and enhance learning. It is very helpful for students to complete these exercises before lab.
- ***Pocket Guide for Jensen's Nursing Health Assessment: A Best Practice Approach*, 2nd edition**. Available at bookstores or at www.LWW.com, this clinical reference presents need-to-know information in a concise, easy-to-use, highly visual format. If the course is condensed, this is a good resource.
- ***Lippincott's Nursing Health Assessment Video Series.*** Available at bookstores or at www.LWW.com, this engaging nursing-specific health assessment video series consists of 6 volumes and 23 topics. Volume 1 presents the basics of nursing health assessment and techniques of interviewing, performing the physical assessment, and collecting data. Volume 2 covers foundational assessments used for all clients. Volumes 3 to 6 systematically address assessment of all the body systems. Each topic introduces a client and a nurse and demonstrates the subjective and objective data collection methods relevant to the situation and body system. This video series can be used in conjunction with any nursing health assessment text for undergraduate nursing students and is available in student versions on thePoint or on DVD and in institutional versions on DVD or in streaming format.

prepU

- prepU for ***Nursing Health Assessment: A Best Practice Approach*, 2nd edition** includes personalized, adaptive quizzes linked to Jensen's textbook content that fosters formative assessment for students and instructors).
- Lippincott PassPoint for the NCLEX, powered by prepU, is an online, adaptive learning NCLEX preparation resource that allows students to take practice quizzes and comprehensive NCLEX-style exams.

Contents

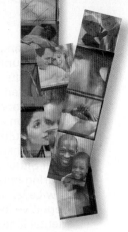

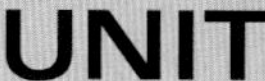

UNIT 1

Foundations of Nursing Health Assessment

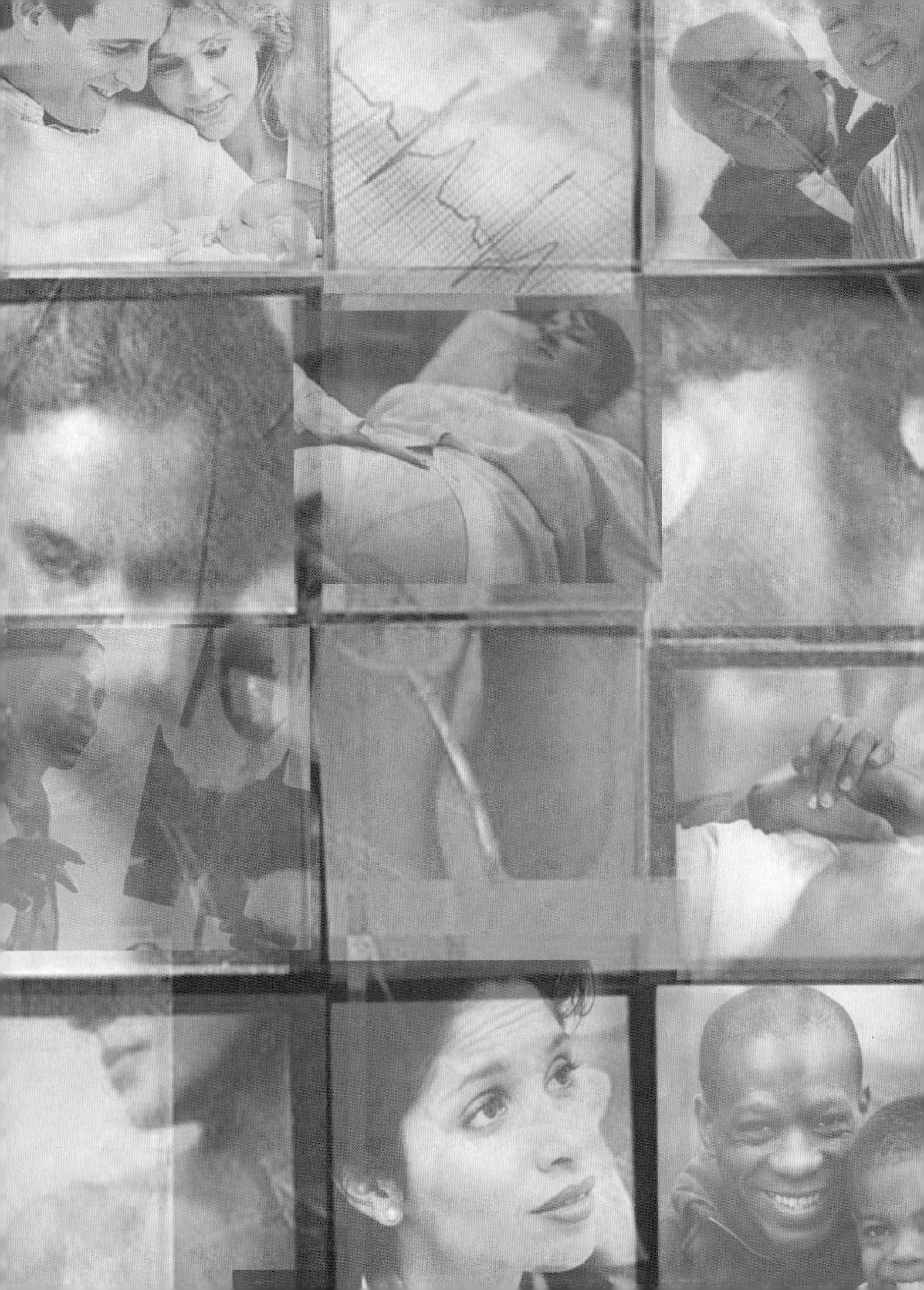

1

The Nurse's Role in Health Assessment

Learning Objectives

1. Describe the role of the professional nurse in health assessment.
2. Demonstrate knowledge of the purposes of health assessment.
3. Explain the relationship of health assessment to health promotion.
4. Explain the roles of the nursing process, critical thinking, and clinical reasoning in nursing care.
5. Demonstrate knowledge of the differences in the types and frequencies of assessments.
6. State the components of a comprehensive health assessment.
7. Describe organizing frameworks for collecting health assessment data.

Maria Ortiz, a 52-year-old Mexican American woman, has a follow-up appointment related to Type 2 diabetes mellitus, which was diagnosed 2 weeks ago during an annual physical assessment. Her primary language is Spanish; although her English skills are good, she has difficulty understanding complex medical terminology. Ms. Ortiz has been married for 30 years, and her three grown children live nearby.

Ms. Ortiz is 1.52 m (5 ft) tall, weighs 75 kg (165 lb), and has a body mass index (BMI) of 32.2; she eats a diet high in fats and starches. Her blood glucose levels at home have been elevated. She is otherwise healthy. Current vital signs are temperature 36.5°C (97.7°F) tympanic, pulse 82 beats/min, respirations 16 breaths/min, and blood pressure (BP) 138/78 mm Hg. Medications include an oral hypoglycemic and a daily vitamin.

You will gain more information about Ms. Ortiz as you progress through this chapter. As you study the content and features, consider the Ms. Ortiz's case and its relationship to what you are learning. Begin thinking about the following points:

- What are potential health promotion and teaching needs for Ms. Ortiz?
- How should the nurse approach a discussion of the patient's diet as related to her diabetes?
- How will the nurse individualize today's health assessment, considering the patient's gender, age, and culture?
- What is the role of the nurse in providing care for Ms. Ortiz at the next visit?
- On what areas of the physical examination will the nurse concentrate?
- How will the nurse evaluate the results of patient teaching with Ms. Ortiz?

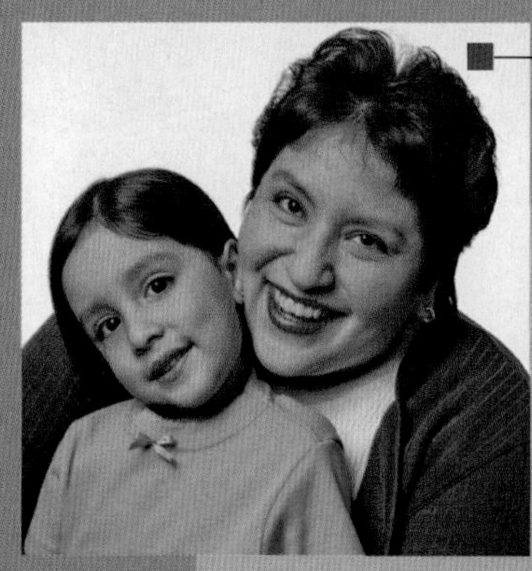

Nurses assess health on many levels, including psychosocial, physical, emotional, spiritual, and cultural. As a nurse, you will develop and use skills in communication to provide therapeutic responses to the concerns of patients. Wellness and health are concepts that influence the health beliefs and health behaviors of patients. You will explore factors related to such beliefs and behaviors in order to better understand how to promote health for patients and their families. You will use the nursing process to care for patients by assessing completely, making nursing diagnoses, developing outcomes, planning for care, performing interventions, evaluating effectiveness, and revising interventions as needed. The foundation of this collaborative process depends on having accurate and complete assessment data.

Role of the Professional Nurse

According to the American Nurses Association (American Nursing Association, 2013a), "Nursing is the protection, promotion, and optimization of health and abilities, prevention of illness and injury, alleviation of suffering through the diagnosis and treatment of human response, and **advocacy** in the care of individuals, families, communities, and populations." This definition serves as the basis on which the standards of the professional nursing practice and the scope of nursing practice are structured. Nursing has a focus comprising four main goals:

1. To promote health (state of optimal functioning or well-being with physical, social, and mental components)
2. To prevent illness (primary, secondary, tertiary)
3. To treat human responses to health or illness
4. To advocate for individuals, families, communities, and populations

The *Code of Ethics for Nurses with Interpretive Statements* (American Nurses Association, 2010a) and *Nursing: Scope and Standards of Practice* (American Nurses Association, 2010b) further describe nursing and its associated practice standards. The *Code of Ethics* focuses on the conscience of the nurse and respect for the individual and provides direction in the clinical setting. The *Scope and Standards of Practice* describes nursing duties and works in tandem with the nursing process, which consists of assessment, diagnosis, outcome identification, planning, implementation, and evaluation. This process is used to promote health and prevent illness, to reduce the risk of a disease, to reinforce good habits, and to maintain optimal functioning (Fig. 1.1). Examples of appropriate nursing interventions include implementation of educational programs, coordination of community resources, and patient and family teaching.

Roles for the baccalaureate generalist nurse are derived from the discipline of nursing: provider of care, designer/manager/coordinator of care, and member of a profession (American Association of Colleges of Nursing [AACN], 2011).

Care Responsibilities

Nurses provide direct care to help restore health for ill patients in hospitals, clinics, long-term care facilities, and schools. They work in rehabilitation centers and homes to help patients and their families cope with disability and in hospice to facilitate the most comfortable death for patients. Most registered nurses today work within a hospital setting.

Practitioners of medicine focus on the physical aspects of diseases and prescribe medications or other treatments. Nurses focus on how diseases are affecting activity levels and abilities to perform tasks as well as how patients are coping with their health issues and any related losses of

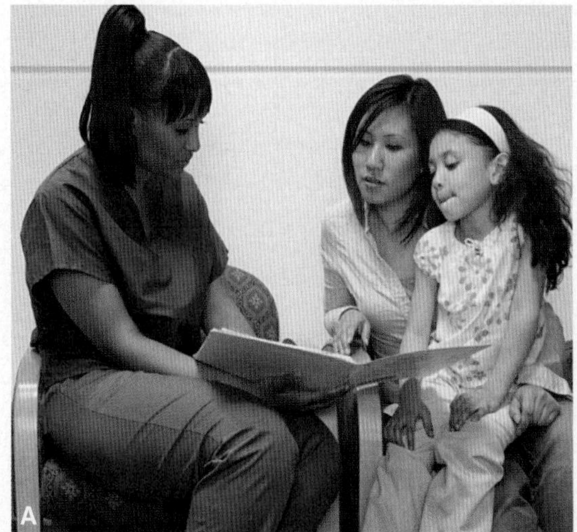

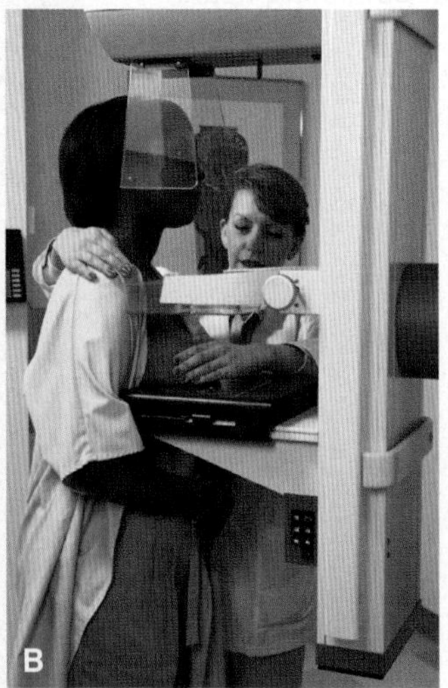

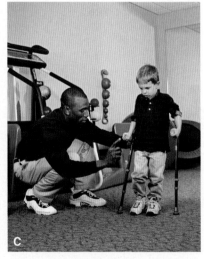

Figure 1.1 Nurses promote health and prevent illness in various ways. **A.** Family teaching during wellness visits reinforces positive habits and helps parents and children understand behaviors for optimal well-being. **B.** Conducting regular health screenings with patients, such as scheduled mammograms, is critical to reducing risks for disease. **C.** Assisting patients with long-term health challenges to restore or maintain optimal functioning is another essential nursing activity.

function. Nurses often work with primary care providers on medical diagnoses and collaborative problems. Independent nursing interventions include patient teaching, therapeutic communication, and physical procedures such as turning patients or assisting them with ambulation. Advance practice nurses may function autonomously and practice independently.

Managing Care

Nurses are constantly making treatment decisions to manage and coordinate care. Nurses often spend more time with patients and their families than other health care providers do and thus know their issues more completely. Nurses communicate findings to appropriate people and also document data to share information and identify trends. Referral of patients to other health care providers (e.g., dieticians or speech therapists) is discussed in this book in the feature entitled "Collaborating with Other Health Care Providers"; this feature uses the SBAR organization (*s*ituation, *b*ackground, *a*ssessment, *r*ecommendation). Documentation of care is described in the "Documenting Case Study Findings" feature, which uses a SOAP note organization (*s*ubjective, *o*bjective, *a*nalysis, *p*lan). Nurses use interprofessional communication and collaboration to improve patient health outcomes (AACN, 2011).

Member of a Profession

Nursing research and the underpinning of evidence-based practice can be traced back to Florence Nightingale in the middle 1800s. Today, nurses perform **scholarship** and **research** to provide care based on current evidence. Professional nursing practice is grounded in best practice, critical inquiry, and skilled questioning. Knowledge of patient care technologies and information systems is essential in the management of care. Nurses use systems to influence health care policy, finance, and regulatory agencies. Health promotion and disease prevention are necessary to improve health at both the individual and the population levels (American Nurses Association, 2010b).

In the professional role, nurses are **advocates** for the patient and the profession (AACN, 2011). As advocates, nurses take responsibility to protect the legal and ethical rights of patients. Values and ethical principles are beliefs or ideals to which a person is committed. Professional core values guide nurses to provide safe, humane care (AACN, 2011). Nursing values include the following:

- Respect
- Unity
- Diversity
- Integrity
- Excellence

Their roles as providers of care, managers, and members of a profession give nurses a unique advantage in understanding and acting on the patient's behalf in the most holistic way. Both registered nurses and advanced practice registered nurses fulfill the roles described.

The Registered Nurse

The **registered nurse (RN)** is licensed nationally and practices independently within the scope of nursing practice and diagnosis. Depending on the location of practice, the RN may be required to fulfill continuing education requirements and complete additional certificates. There are numerous employment opportunities for RNs; they practice wherever people need nursing care, including hospitals, homes, schools, workplaces, and community centers. More than 60% of RNs work in hospitals; other common areas of practice include community or public health, ambulatory care, nursing homes, and nursing education (American Nurses Association, 2010b).

RNs in hospitals develop assessment skills related to the speciality in which they practice. For example, in the emergency department (ED), nurses focus their assessment on life-threatening injuries and situations. In the intensive care setting, nurses assess patients using invasive monitoring equipment, such as an arterial line that goes into the patient's heart, or an intracranial pressure line that goes in to the patient's brain. On acute care units, nurses develop special skills such as cardiac and electrocardiogram monitoring or thorough neurological assessment skills. In these specialized settings, RN roles sometimes overlap with advanced practice roles.

The Advanced Practice Registered Nurse

There are many opportunities for RNs to advance their education and careers in a way that develops each individual's interests and uses his or her strengths and expertise. **Advanced practice registered nurse (APRN)** is an umbrella term given to an RN who has achieved a bachelor's degree in nursing science (BSN), which includes educational and clinical practice requirements, as well as a minimum of a master of science degree in nursing. The core curriculum for an MSN includes advanced health assessment, advanced pathophysiology, and advanced pharmacology combined with the specialty focused track, with a minimum of 500 clinical hours. According to the American Nurses Credentialing Center, by the year 2015, the current level of preparation necessary for the nurse clinician/APRN will move from a master's level to doctoral level (American Nurses Credentialing Center, 2013). The advancement to a doctoral level of study stems from an increasingly complex health care environment and the need to contribute with the greatest level of scientific knowledge through research.

APRNs are governed and monitored by professional organizations, state law, and the *Consensus Model for APRN Regulation: Licensure, Accreditation, Certification, & Education* (Advanced Practice Registered Nurse Joint Dialogue Group, 2008). The APRN roles include nurse practitioner (NP), certified nurse midwife (CNM), clinical nurse specialist (CNS), and certified registered nurse anesthetist (CRNA).

Nurse Practitioner

Through the core competencies of direct clinical practice, the **Nurse Practitioner (NP)** may care for patients throughout the patients' lifespan. The NP may also focus on primary care or acute care, with clinical track options in pediatrics, family practice, women's health, gerontology, acute care, and psychiatric/mental health care.

Certified Nurse Midwife

The practice of the **Certified Nurse Midwife (CNM)** has deep historical roots worldwide, with focus on gynecological care, pregnancy, birth, and contraceptive options. CNMs advocate for the woman to be an active participant in her health care choices.

Certified Registered Nurse Anesthetist

Certified Registered Nurse Anesthetist (CRNAs) are considered the oldest specialty within nursing practice. According to the American Association of Nurse Anesthetists (AANA, 2010), CRNAs have the authority to select, obtain, or administer the anesthetics, adjuvant drugs, accessory drugs, and fluids necessary to manage anesthesia, to maintain the airway, and to correct abnormal responses to anesthesia or surgery.

Clinical Nurse Specialist

The **Clinical Nurse Specialist (CNS)** is considered to be experienced and knowledgeable in a specific area. The American Nurses Association (1980, p. 23) defines the CNS as an RN "who, through study and supervised practice at a graduate level (masters or doctorate), has become expert in a defined area of knowledge and practice in a selected clinical area of nursing." Opportunities for the CNS can be found in critical care, cardiology, oncology, diabetic care, and psychiatry.

Registered Nurse Versus Advanced Practice Registered Nurse Assessments

The differences between the RN and the APRN assessments are included in each chapter of this text. At the beginning of each objective assessment section, there is a table that describes the usual scope of practice for each role. This is based on roles of the RNs and APRNs in the western hemisphere in developed countries, and each role will vary by the specialty. For example, the RN practicing in the neurological intensive care area may be an expert in extraocular movements, whereas an APRN in family practice has infrequent experience in this area. An RN practicing in rural health care or in a developing country may need to rely on percussion of the lungs because x-ray equipment is unavailable. Refer to your experts and faculty for the scope of practice in your area.

Nursing and Health Promotion

Health behaviors are influenced by a person's beliefs, culture, and perception of the benefits of such behaviors, as well as competing demands in the person's life. For example, a woman with a goal of weight loss may be influenced by family finances, family demands regarding food preparation, available time, and her previous success or failure losing weight. Health beliefs, factors, and experiences help determine who is likely to practice healthy behaviors and why. A nursing assessment that includes the patient's individual situation and experiences will help in the development of focused health promotion activities (Pender, Murdaugh, & Parsons, 2006).

As a nurse, you will assess patients for nutritional intake, activity and fitness levels, psychiatric status, safety and violence activities, and stress and coping measures. As you introduce screening questions, you will follow up with more in-depth questions in the higher risk areas. Rather than addressing all areas associated with healthy behaviors and overwhelming patients, you will collaborate with them to identify areas in which they are willing to make changes.

Wellness and Illness

Wellness is "an integrated method of functioning, which is oriented toward maximizing the potential of which the individual is capable" (Dunn, as cited in Zimmer, 2010, para. 4). The role of nurses is to facilitate this achievement through health promotion and teaching. Most people fall somewhere on a trajectory or continuum of wellness versus **illness**. The person who moves toward high-level wellness focuses on awareness, education, and growth. The person who moves toward illness and premature death develops signs and symptoms of disease or disabilities; unfortunately, this is when most treatment occurs in the current health care system. At the neutral point, there is no discernible illness or wellness.

Health is more than merely the absence of illness. Nurses collaborate with individuals, families, and communities to promote higher levels of wellness.

Risk Reduction: *Healthy People* Model

The U.S. Department of Health & Human Services (2013) has developed a national model for health promotion and **risk reduction** called ***Healthy People***. The goals of this project are to increase the length and quality of life for the population of the United States and to eliminate health disparities among different segments of that population. Every 10 years, progress is evaluated and the goals are restructured. The 10 leading areas of focus are as follows:

- Physical activity
- Overweight and obesity
- Tobacco use
- Substance abuse
- Responsible sexual behavior
- Mental health
- Injury and violence
- Environmental quality
- Immunization
- Access to health care

Each of these indicators has specific outcomes, such as "reduce the risk of development of hypertension and diabetes mellitus," "reduce exposure to secondhand smoke," and "reduce health disparities in children who are immunized." There are similar initiatives in countries around the world.

The three levels of interventions to promote healthy change are primary, secondary, and tertiary (Leavell & Clark, 1965):

- **Primary prevention** involves strategies aimed at preventing problems. Immunizations, health teaching, safety precautions, and nutrition counseling are examples.
- **Secondary prevention** includes the early diagnosis of health problems and prompts treatment to prevent complications. Vision screening, Pap smears, BP screening, hearing testing, scoliosis screening, and tuberculin skin testing are examples.
- **Tertiary prevention** focuses on preventing complications of an existing disease and promoting health to the highest level. Diet teaching for patients with diabetes, inhaler teaching for patients with lung disease, and exercise programs for those who have had myocardial infarction are examples.

What Is Health Assessment?

Health assessment is "gathering information about the health status of the patient, analyzing and synthesizing those data, making judgments about nursing interventions based on the findings, and evaluating patient care outcomes" (AACN, 2011). A health assessment includes both a health history and a physical assessment. According to the American Nurses Association (2013b), "An RN uses a systematic, dynamic way to collect and analyze data about a client, the first step in delivering nursing care. Assessment includes not only physiological data, but also psychological, sociocultural, spiritual, economic, and life-style factors as well. For example, a nurse's assessment of a hospitalized patient in pain includes not only the physical causes and manifestations of pain, but the patient's response—an inability to get out of bed, refusal to eat, withdrawal from family members, anger directed at hospital staff, fear, or request for more pain medication."

The **health history** includes interviewing to collect the patient's past medical and surgical histories, risk factors, and current symptoms. A comprehensive health history also includes nutrition; development; mental health; social, cultural, and spiritual dimensions; and safety issues. Data that you collect during the physical assessment vary depending on the seriousness of a patient's condition, health history, and current symptoms. In an emergency, you collect information that will help pinpoint the source of the issues and treat current conditions. For healthy patients seeking a wellness checkup, you focus the assessment on screening for high-risk conditions (e.g., overweight) and teaching and health promotion associated with common issues (e.g., nutrition and exercise).

You may also perform a health assessment to gain further insight into a patient's current condition and to establish a database against which subsequent assessments can be measured. You identify patterns and trends to determine whether a patient's condition is improving or worsening. Instead of using one piece of data in isolation, you think logically to analyze how data are related and what interventions may be indicated. You evaluate outcomes, and the assessment becomes a continuous part of the nursing process.

Nursing Process

The nursing process is a systematic problem-solving approach to identifying and treating human responses to actual or potential health difficulties (American Nurses Association, 2013b). It serves as a framework for providing individualized care not only to individuals but also to families and communities. It is patient centered, focusing on solving problems and enhancing strengths. The nursing process is applicable to patients in all stages of the lifespan and in all settings.

The parts of the nursing process include **assessing** the patient, analyzing data and making nursing **diagnoses**, determining patient **outcomes** or **planning** care, **implementing**, and then **evaluating** the patient's status to determine whether interventions were effective (Fig. 1.2). This evaluation is also an assessment of how well the patient is meeting the outcomes, while the patient's progress is continually assessed. From this evaluation, you may continue interventions or revise them depending on whether the patient is progressing toward the outcomes.

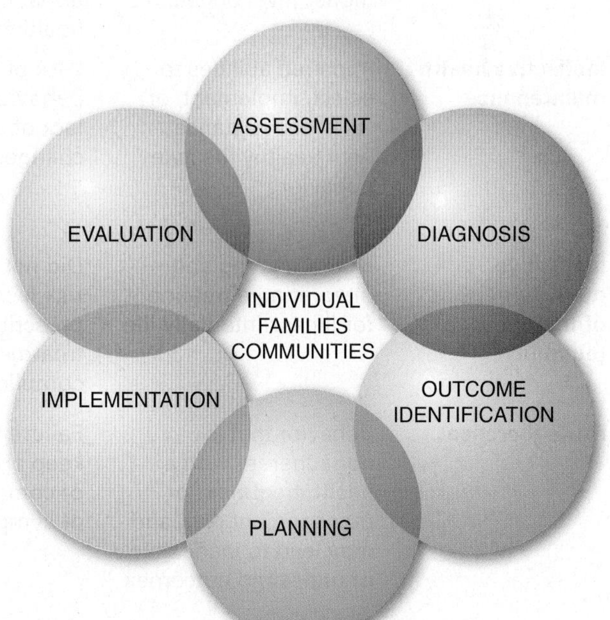

Figure 1.2 The phases of the nursing process are assessment, diagnosis, outcome identification or planning, implementation, and evaluation. Nurses apply these activities to the care of individuals, families, and communities.

Assess

The nursing process begins with a complete and accurate health assessment to promote health at the highest level. Because all future care is based on the health assessment, it is extremely important that health assessment data are complete and accurate. A health assessment is one of the most important activities of professional nurses.

The nursing process is not linear (i.e., progressing step by step). Rather, it is interactive and involves interrelated, sometimes overlapping, steps. As you collect assessment data, you simultaneously provide educational or emergency interventions. You also evaluate care during an assessment—for example, checking patients for adverse effects of medications. You set outcomes collaboratively with patients; established priorities guide not only the treatment plan but also the types of future assessments performed. For example, if a hospitalized patient's priority is sleep, you may decide to eliminate taking vital signs every 4 hours during the night if the patient's condition is stable.

Diagnose

Diagnosis is the clustering of data to make a judgment or statement about the patient's difficulty or condition. NANDA International (NANDA-I, 2012) defines nursing diagnosis as "a clinical judgment about individual, family or community responses to actual or potential health difficulties/life processes. A nursing diagnosis provides the basis for selection of nursing interventions to achieve outcomes for which the nurse is accountable."

NANDA-I has developed some common nursing diagnoses and interventions to provide a specific language and way of thinking. These are helpful for learning about the professional scope of practice. In clinical practice, nursing diagnoses are individualized to the patient or family, serving as a foundation for the identification of problems. You use diagnostic reasoning and critical thinking to formulate diagnostic statements. You use data clustering, cluster interpretation, and diagnostic validation to ensure accuracy in selecting the correct diagnosis. Diagnoses may identify actual problems, risks for developing the problems, and possible difficulties, or they may be wellness oriented.

You will find applicable nursing diagnoses throughout the chapters of this text. Common nursing diagnoses associated with health promotion are listed in Table 1.1.

Outcomes

Outcome identification includes the formulation of measurable, realistic, patient-centered goals. Goals are broader than

TABLE 1.1 Common Nursing Diagnoses Associated With Health Promotion

Diagnosis	Point of Differentiation	Assessment Characteristics	Nursing Interventions
Health-seeking behavior	Actively seeking ways to move toward a higher level of health	Expressed desire to seek higher level of wellness; concern about current conditions on health status	Prioritize learner needs based on patient preferences. Emphasize positive health benefits of positive lifestyle behaviors.
Ineffective health maintenance	Impaired abilities to select, implement, or look for assistance with healthy lifestyle behaviors	Lack of health-seeking behavior, lack of resources, lack of adaptive behaviors to changes	Assess feelings, values, and reasons for not following plan of care. Assess family, economic, and cultural patterns that influence plan of care.
Ineffective management of therapeutic regimen	Not regulating and integrating a treatment for illness into daily life	Did not take action to reduce risk factors; difficulty with prescribed regimen for treatment or prevention of complications	Encourage active participation. Review actions that are not therapeutic. Identify the reasons for nontherapeutic actions.
Nonadherence	Behavior that is nonadherent with a health treatment or management plan and may lead to ineffective or undesired outcomes	Failure to adhere to plan or keep appointments; evidence of complications; exacerbation of symptoms	Identify the cause of nonadherence. Monitor the ability to follow directions, solve issues, concentrate, and read. Identify cues that trigger healthy behaviors.

As part of the care planning for Ms. Ortiz, who was recently diagnosed with Type 2 diabetes, the nurse uses the diagnostic reasoning process to determine which nursing diagnoses best fit with her cluster of symptoms, including the patient's teaching needs. Because the patient has shown effective management of her treatment thus far, the best diagnosis is health-seeking behavior.

outcomes—for example, "Patient's pain is within acceptable limits." Goal identification provides for individualized care as you collaborate with patients. For example, when you give a patient in acute pain the prescribed pain medication, you assess the patient's pain level. You then collaborate with the patient to identify the patient's pain goal, determining what level of pain is acceptable and discuss if the patient's dose of medication should be increased.

Patient outcomes are more specific than goals; they are realistic and measurable (Alfaro-LeFevre, 2010). For example, it may not be realistic for a patient to be completely free of pain, but a level of 2 on a 0-to-10 scale (with 10 being the worst) may be acceptable to the patient. Because pain is subjective, you gather information from the patient about acceptable pain levels in addition to measurable and objective pain indicators, such as grimacing, elevated pulse and BP, or rubbing the affected body part. An example of an outcome is "patient states pain less than 2 on a 0-to-10 scale, without grimacing, pulse less than 80 beats/min, BP less than 120/80 mm Hg, and appears to be in comfortable position." Establishing outcomes also helps you set priorities for care, especially with complex issues (Moorhead, Johnson, Maas, & Swanson, 2013).

The most common nursing outcomes for each system are discussed in the system-specific chapters in this book.

Plan Care

Care **planning** activities include determining resources, targeting nursing interventions, and writing the plan of care. In addition to the standard care and physician orders, the nursing care plan requires that you analyze the individual patient and his or her needs in order to provide individualized and holistic care. You communicate the care plan verbally and also document it in the patient's chart so that the next care provider is aware of the plan. The agency or institution where you work will determine whether the plan of care is documented in a care plan format or in a care map, case note, clinical pathway, teaching plan, or discharge plan. Regardless of format, the care planning document incorporates the parts of the nursing process and critical thinking that nurses are incorporating into the patient care.

Implement

Nursing interventions are "any treatment, based upon clinical judgment and knowledge, that a nurse performs to enhance patient outcomes" (Bulechek, Butcher, Dochterman, & Wagner, 2013, p. xix). You use nursing interventions to monitor health status; prevent, resolve, or control a problem; assist with activities of daily living; or promote optimal health and independence (Alfaro-LeFevre, 2010). It is important for you to be aware of the standards of care within the agency where you work because these standards define normal activities (e.g., taking vital signs every 8 hours). Types of nursing interventions include assessment, education, supervision, coordination, referral, support, therapeutic communication, and technical skills.

You will find specific interventions in the case study for each system in the system-specific chapters in this text.

Evaluate

The **evaluation** of care is the judgment of the effectiveness of nursing care in meeting the patient's goals and outcomes based on the patient's responses to the interventions. The purpose of evaluation is to make judgments about the progress of the patient, analyze the effectiveness of nursing care, review potential areas for collaboration and referral to other health care professionals, and monitor the quality of nursing care and its effect on the patient (Alfaro-LeFevre, 2010). As a nurse, you will assess both the facilitators of and the barriers to goal attainment. Goals may be completely met, partially met, or completely unmet; additionally, new issues and nursing diagnoses may be developed (Alfaro-LeFevre, 2010).

To effectively evaluate, you must have knowledge of the standards of care, expected patient responses, and conceptual models and theories. With this basis of knowledge, and by using your interviewing skills for subjective data collection and your physical assessment skills for objective data collection, you can monitor the effectiveness of nursing interventions. It is also important for you to be aware of the most current research and use this evidence to direct care. You will use critical thinking throughout the nursing process to *a*ssess, *d*iagnose, *p*lan, *i*mplement, and *e*valuate care (ADPIE).

Critical Thinking

Critical thinking in nursing (Alfaro-LeFevre, 2010)

- Entails purposeful, outcome-directed (results-oriented) thinking
- Is driven by patient, family, and community needs
- Is based on the nursing process, evidence-based thinking, and the scientific method
- Requires specific knowledge, skills, and experience
- Is guided by professional standards and codes of ethics
- Is constantly reevaluating, self-correcting, and striving to improve

As a nurse, you are frequently involved in complex situations with multiple responsibilities. You are required to think through the analysis, develop alternatives, and implement the best interventions. Critical thinking is the key to resolving difficulties. If you do not think critically, you will deliver incomplete or misdirected care. Critical thinking is also essential to passing the National Council Licensure Examination (NCLEX). Accreditation visitors to colleges of nursing and health care facilities look for evidence of critical thinking ability.

Critical thinking is a required component of health assessment and nursing care (Alfaro-LeFevre, 2010). As a nurse, you use critical thinking to identify patterns and trends, consider missing or conflicting assessment information, and decide the type and frequency of future assessments.

Diagnostic Reasoning

The process of diagnostic reasoning is based on critical thinking (Fig. 1.3). **Diagnostic reasoning** includes gathering and clustering data to draw inferences and propose diagnoses.

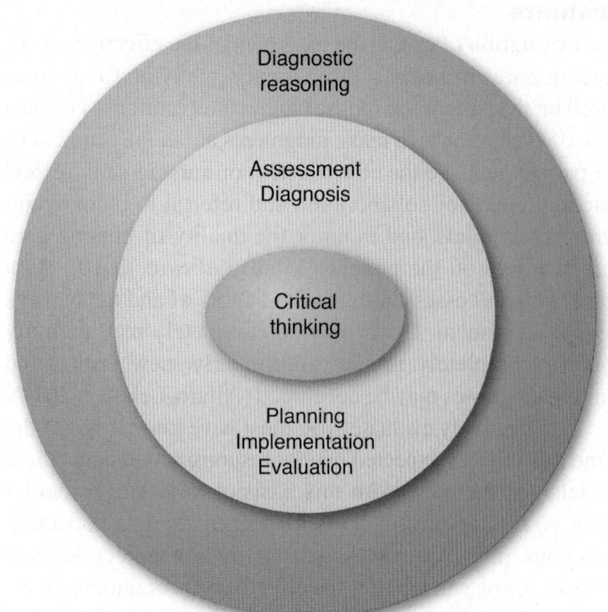

Figure 1.3 The diagnostic reasoning process.

A seven-step process for diagnostic reasoning can be used in the context of health assessment (Weber & Kelley, 2010):

1. Identify abnormal data and strengths
2. Cluster data
3. Draw inferences
4. Propose nursing diagnoses
5. Check for presence of defining characteristics
6. Confirm or rule out the nursing diagnosis
7. Document conclusions

Collaborative problems are those that you are monitoring that require the expertise of other health care providers for interventions. In the above example, the collaborative problem is written as "Potential Complication: Pneumonia." You monitor temperature, lung sounds, and sputum carefully for signs and symptoms of pneumonia and notify the primary care provider if they are present. Although pneumonia itself is not defined as a nursing diagnosis, the collaborative assessments and your nursing interventions in this situation are equally important. As a nurse, you also perform interventions in collaboration with other health care providers, such as diagnostic testing and medication administration (see Table 1.1).

Types of Nursing Assessments

Three types of nursing assessments are common: emergency, comprehensive, and focused. Emergency and focused assessments address focus on the immediate and highest priority problem. Comprehensive assessments are broad and wide ranging. The amount and type of information varies, however, for all types of assessment depending on the patient's needs, purpose of data collection, health care setting, and the nurse's role.

Emergency and Urgent Assessment

The **emergency assessment** involves a life-threatening or unstable situation, such as a patient in an ED who has experienced a traumatic injury. Staff members at the ED use triage to determine the level of urgency by considering assessments based on the mnemonic A, B, C, D, E:

- A—Airway (with cervical spine protection if an injury is suspected)
- B—Breathing—rate and depth, use of accessory muscles
- C—Circulation—pulse rate and rhythm, skin color
- D—Disability—level of consciousness, pupils, movement
- E—Exposure

All life-threatening problems identified during the initial assessment require the initiation of critical interventions:

- Provide assistance with circulation (cardiopulmonary resuscitation [CPR] if needed).
- Open the patient's airway.
- Assist the patient's breathing.
- Protect the cervical spine if the patient is injured.
- Ensure that the disoriented or suicidal patient is safe.
- Provide pain management and sedation.

You perform assessments and critical interventions simultaneously as life-threatening difficulties are treated. An urgent assessment includes C, A, B, and other events that are of particular concern. This is discussed in each chapter under the urgent assessment.

Comprehensive Assessment

The **comprehensive assessment** includes a complete health history and physical assessment. It is done annually on an outpatient basis, following admission to a hospital or long-term care facility, or every 8 hours for patients in intensive care.

In primary care, the history may be obtained by having the patient initially complete an in-depth form that includes a family and personal history of illness, medical treatment, and surgeries. You discuss the information with patients and clarify any incomplete or unclear areas. Note dates of diagnoses and treatments along with the rationale for taking medications—for example, if the patient is taking a beta-blocker, is it for high BP or for a history of myocardial infarction? A comprehensive history also includes a patient's perception of health, strengths to build upon, risk factors for illness, functional abilities, methods of coping, and support systems.

It is also important to reconcile the medication list with what the patient is actually taking to ensure that patients continue taking their normal medications (Institute for Healthcare Improvement [IHI], Medication Reconciliation, 2013a). If the patient is unable to participate in data collection because of the urgency of the problem, you may need to use secondary data sources for information, such as the history in the medical record or the patient's family members.

As part of the comprehensive assessment, you assess the patient's health beliefs and discuss health promotion measures. You conduct health screening according to national guidelines—for example, bowel cancer screening for a patient who has reached 50 years of age. You answer questions and provide patient teaching in preparation for diagnostic testing.

A comprehensive physical assessment includes all body systems and areas, usually in a head-to-toe format. This includes an assessment of the skin; head and neck; eyes; ears; nose, mouth, and throat; thorax and lungs; heart and neck blood vessels; arms and legs; breasts; abdomen; and musculoskeletal and neurological systems. Rectal and genital assessments are completed if necessary.

Comprehensive assessment is more in depth when performed by an NP. Differences between assessments performed by RNs and APRNs are discussed in each chapter.

Focused Assessment

A **focused assessment** is based on the patient's health issues. This type of assessment can occur in all settings, including the clinic, hospital, and home health setting. It usually involves one or two body systems and is smaller in scope than the comprehensive assessment but more in depth on the specific issue or issues. One example is a patient who presents to the clinic with a cough. The health history focuses on the duration of the cough, associated symptoms such as wheezing or shortness of breath, and factors that alleviate or worsen the cough. The physical assessment includes an assessment of the nose and throat, auscultation of the lungs, and inspection of sputum. You gather data to determine the cause of the cough so that the cough may be appropriately treated.

Priority Setting

Priority setting is an important skill in professional nursing practice. Its multidimensional nature and need for solid judgment make it challenging to learn. Priorities depend on the gravity of the patient's health care situation. You use clinical experience, knowledge, expertise, and judgment to determine priorities. Even expert nurses sometimes prioritize in different ways based on their experiences.

When prioritizing, you first address any life-threatening situation or any issue that needs immediate attention. If the patient is stable, then your priority is any issue that is very important to the patient, or something on which you are spending a lot of time. Life-threatening issues always take priority—for example, circulation, airway, and breathing would take priority over elevated temperature. Another example of a situation that requires immediate attention is a patient at risk for human violence or suicide.

An issue of top importance to a patient should also be considered high priority for you as the nurse. For example, a patient who is seen for an exacerbation of ulcerative colitis might indicate that a painful left knee is his highest priority. Often, however, priority setting is more subtle, such as deciding what to assess in a patient newly diagnosed with diabetes. Assessment information is used to direct care in all phases of the nursing process.

Frequency of Assessment

The frequency of assessment varies with the patient's needs, purpose of data collection, and health care setting. A patient in a long-term care setting may need a comprehensive assessment once a month, whereas a patient in an acute hospital setting may require an assessment once per shift (Fig. 1.4). Patients in intensive care settings have vital signs assessment and a focused assessment hourly. (A facility's standards of care often prescribe such time frames, so it is important for you to identify those standards for the unit and facility in which you are working.) Patients also have focused assessments following treatments to monitor their effectiveness. For example, if your patient who is short of breath is given an inhaler, listen to lung sounds after the treatment to see if there has been an improvement in wheezing. You also perform assessments to monitor for adverse effects from interventions—for example, assessing for pedal pulses after a cardiac catheterization in which the femoral artery is punctured. Use judgment to collect data at other times, based on a change in the patient's condition.

In the outpatient setting, the frequency of assessment depends on the course of illness and whether the disease process is improving or worsening. You also assess patients to evaluate the effectiveness of the treatment, such as follow-up for an infection, and for adverse effects of the treatment, such as immunosuppression from chemotherapy.

Well visits are also an important component of health assessment. Periodic health assessment focuses on the most common screening and prevention services for four age groups: (1) birth to 10 years, (2) 11 to 24 years, (3) 25 to 64 years, and (4) 65 years and older. Patients are seen more frequently in the youngest years to monitor growth and development and in later years for treatment of acute and chronic illnesses.

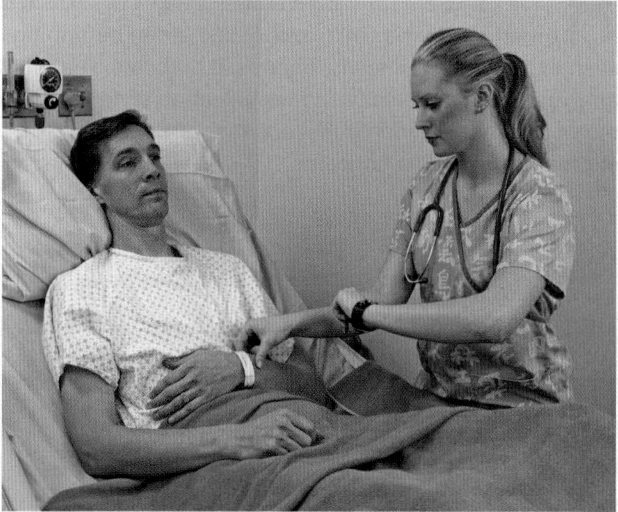

Figure 1.4 The frequency of assessment depends on the seriousness of the patient's condition, which is also related to the setting for care. Hospitalized patients may undergo assessments whenever there is a change of shift.

Lifespan Issues

A comprehensive assessment includes assessment of cognitive and emotional development in addition to physical growth. Your aim is to identify expected growth and development patterns, expected variations, and aberrations and deviations. From infancy through adolescence, growth and development are marked by rapid spurts. From adolescence through 25 years of age, growth and development proceed more slowly. Motor development occurs rapidly from birth through school age following maturation of the nervous system. Language skills develop rapidly in toddlers and preschool children as vocabulary increases and sentences become more grammatically complex. In this textbook, information on the older adult is included in each chapter; pregnant women and younger populations are covered in separate chapters.

Cultural Considerations

Knowledge of different cultures is essential for nurses working in all areas and settings of practice. **Cultural competence** refers to the complex combination of knowledge, attitudes, and skills that a health care provider uses to deliver care that considers the total context of the patient's situation across cultural boundaries (Purnell, 2009).

Culture is defined as the traits that a group of people share and pass from one generation to the next, including values, beliefs, attitudes, and customs (Spector, 2012). Subcultures exist within larger cultural groups, so it is important to learn what the patient's specific beliefs or needs are within the larger context. You need to recognize each patient's degree of assimilation into the dominant culture and the extent to which he or she identifies with the culture, considering such variables as dress, food, religion, and customs. An assessment for the effects of spirituality and religion on health is also important.

Components of the Health Assessment

During the interview, you use communication skills to gather data. In addition to speaking with the patient (verbal communication), you also observe the patient's body position, facial expression, and eye contact (nonverbal communication). Initially, you introduce yourself and explain the purpose of the interview. Confidentiality is important: you must obtain permission from the patient for other people to be present during the assessment or ask those people to step out for a few moments to allow some privacy. More information about the interview is found in Chapter 2.

The purpose of the health history is to collect family and personal histories of risk factors and past issues. Review the family history of medical difficulties or mental health issues with patients. Begin the personal history with biographical data on date of birth, primary language spoken, and allergies. A detailed history includes data on all systems, psychosocial and mental health, and functional status. Document the dates of problems along with treatments and treatment outcomes. More information on the health history is found in Chapter 2.

Subjective Data

The primary source in subjective data collection is the patient. **Subjective data** are based on patient experiences and perceptions. The individual describes the feelings, sensations, or

Therapeutic Dialogue: Collecting Subjective Data

Remember Maria Ortiz, introduced at the beginning of this chapter. She was seen in the clinic for newly diagnosed diabetes. The following conversation provides an example of an effective communication style for collecting subjective data. The nurse asks open-ended questions that provide Ms. Ortiz with an opportunity to express and validate concerns.

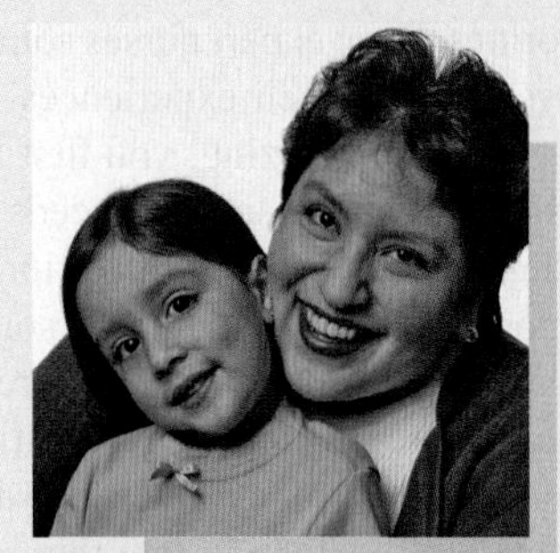

Nurse: Hello, Ms. Ortiz. How are you doing today?

Ms. Ortiz: Good.

Nurse: Tell me how things have been going for you.

Ms. Ortiz: Well, 2 weeks ago, they told me that I had sugar diabetes. It runs in my family, so I shouldn't be too surprised. I just haven't gotten used to this new diet.

(case study continues on page 13)

Nurse: Tell me more about your concerns.

Ms. Ortiz: Well, my mother was diabetic and she couldn't eat sugar. But they said that I can have a little dessert, just a little though. The dietician seemed to be more concerned about the cheese that I add to my refried beans.

Nurse: All food turns into sugar after you eat it, so having a little bit is OK. The dietician is thinking about the long-term effects of the fat in the cheese because it contains calories and cholesterol that can damage your blood vessels and lead to a heart attack, stroke, or kidney difficulties over time. It's a different way of thinking about it than it used to be.

Ms. Ortiz: Yes, it doesn't make sense to me. But things always change. Like this, I didn't think that I would end up with diabetes, too.

Nurse: Yes, it sounds like this is a little overwhelming to you.

Critical Thinking Challenge

- What clues is the nurse gathering about Ms. Ortiz's beliefs about her diabetes?
- What is the role of the nurse related to health promotion and teaching?
- What would you identify as the priority issue at this time?

expectations; you then document them as subjective data or put them in quotes. Your role relative to subjective data collection is to gather information to improve the patient's health status and to help determine the cause of the patient's current symptoms.

Objective Data

The physical assessment follows the history and focused interview, and includes **objective data**, which are measurable. You observe the patient's general appearance; assess vital signs; listen to the heart, lungs, and abdomen; and assess peripheral circulation. Chapters 11 through 24 include focused techniques specific to each body system. Because it is too overwhelming and time consuming to complete all focused techniques at once, only the most important screening assessments are included in the head-to-toe assessment. You use clinical judgment to decide which additional assessments to perform based on the individual patient.

Documentation and Communication

Documentation of both subjective and objective findings is essential for legal purposes and also to communicate findings to others. Accurate documentation provides a baseline so that changes are noted between assessments. Documentation may be in the form of flow sheets, case notes, or care planning. The Health Insurance Portability and Accountability Act of 1996 (Health Insurance Portability and Accountability Act, 2003) regulates the security and privacy of information. Confidentiality of documentation is essential, and only information that is pertinent to the care of the patient is shared. More information on documentation is found in Chapter 4. This textbook uses the SOAP note format, although other formats also document nursing thinking. Examples of SOAP documentation are included in Chapter 4 and also in each individual system chapter.

Communication of assessment data is also verbal. Care of the patient is collaborative, and nurses use an organized method when communicating with other health care providers. As the nurse, you describe the situation, background, and assessment data to make recommendations about the treatment that is indicated—a system known as SBAR communication (IHI, 2013b). You also use an organized method when giving a report between shifts or when transferring (handing off) patients to other departments, such as when a patient is sent to the operating room (Joint Commission on Accreditation of Healthcare Organizations, 2013). Examples of SBAR are included in Chapter 4 and also in each individual system chapter.

Progress Note: Analyzing Findings

The health-related issues of Maria Ortiz have been outlined throughout this chapter. The initial subjective and objective data collection is complete, and the nurse has spent time reviewing findings and results. This information now needs to be documented. The following nursing note illustrates how subjective and objective data are analyzed and communicated in the form of a SOAP note based on the nursing process.

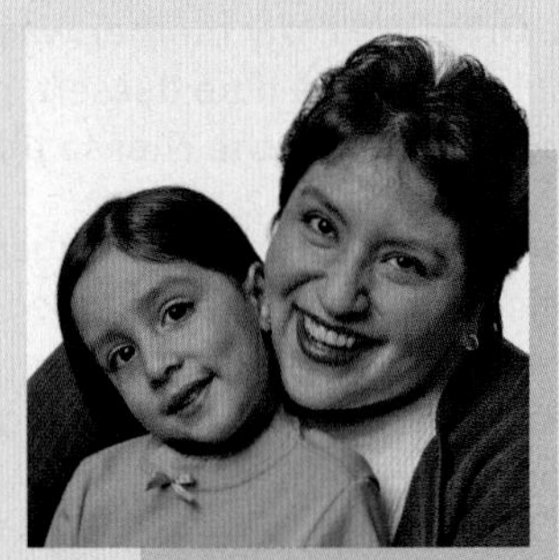

Subjective: "I just haven't gotten used to this new diet."

Objective: Alert and oriented. Skin pink, warm, and dry. Appears slightly overweight, good personal hygiene, appears stated age. BP 138/78 mm Hg, pulse 82 beats/min, and respirations 16 breaths/min. Current medications include an oral hypoglycemic medication and daily vitamin. Expressing concerns about diet and intake of sugar and fat. Typical diet is high in starch and fat and low in fresh fruits and vegetables.

Analysis: Health-seeking behaviors related to new diagnosis and medication.

Plan: Perform teaching on diet and safety related to potential hypoglycemia from oral hypoglycemic medication.

Critical Thinking Challenge

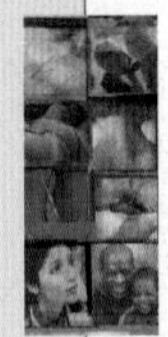

- What type of risk assessments will be performed at her next visit?
- What type of physical assessment might be performed at the next visit?
- How might the nurse consider Ms. Ortiz's culture, native language, and family in the assessment?

Frameworks for Health Assessment

There are three major frameworks for organizing assessment data: functional systems, head-to-toe system, and body systems (Table 1.2). All these methods provide an organizing framework so that nurses do not inadvertently forget any of the important assessment data. Each type begins with a general survey of the patient, vital signs, and level of distress. Developing a consistent and organized approach is more important than considering which system to use.

Functional Assessment

A **functional assessment** focuses on the functional patterns that all humans share: health perception and health management, activity and exercise, nutrition and metabolism, elimination, sleep and rest, cognition and perception, self-perception and self-concept, roles and relationships, coping and stress tolerance, sexuality and reproduction, and values and beliefs (Gordon, 1993). Often, nurses use the functional patterns to collect subjective data following a health history but a head-to-toe system for the physical assessment. Refer to Chapter 2 for more information.

Head-to-Toe Assessment

A **head-to-toe assessment** is the most organized system for gathering comprehensive physical data. Because data in one functional area are collected from different parts of the body, it is very inefficient to collect physical data by functional status. For example, peripheral circulation is assessed in both the arms and the legs. Rather than assess the arms and legs and come back to listen to the heart and lungs, it is more organized to proceed from head to toe. When exposing the chest, both the heart and the lungs are auscultated. The chest is covered, then the abdomen is assessed and covered, and the legs and feet are assessed last. This method is more efficient and provides more modesty for patients. See Chapters 29 and 30 for more information.

TABLE 1.2 Comparison of Assessment Frameworks

Functional Health Pattern	Head to Toe	Body System
Nutrition and metabolism	Head and neck	Neurological and cardiovascular
Cognitive perceptual	Eyes and ears	Neurological
Nutrition and metabolism	Nose, mouth, and throat	Gastrointestinal and respiratory
Activity exercise	Thorax and lungs	Respiratory
Activity exercise	Cardiac	Cardiovascular
Activity exercise	Peripheral vascular	Cardiovascular
Sexuality and reproductive	Breast	Reproductive
Nutrition and metabolism, sexuality and reproductive, elimination	Abdominal	Gastrointestinal, urinary, and reproductive
Activity exercise	Musculoskeletal	Musculoskeletal
Cognitive perceptual	Neurological	Neurological
Sexuality and reproductive	Male or female genitalia	Reproductive
Sexuality and reproductive, elimination	Anus, rectum, and prostate	Gastrointestinal and reproductive
Health perception, sleep, cognition, self-perception, roles, coping, sexuality, values	Functional health status	

Body Systems Approach

A **body systems assessment** approach is a logical tool for organizing data when documenting and communicating findings. This method promotes critical thinking and allows you to analyze findings as you cluster similar data. Data from the functional and head-to-toe assessments are reorganized. When reorganizing data related to the respiratory system, for example, you consider the patient's skin color with lung sounds and any shortness of breath to determine the seriousness of the issue and anticipate interventions. You also consider vital signs data,

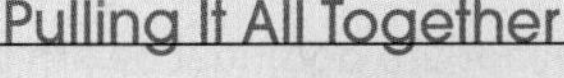

The nurse uses assessment data to formulate a nursing care plan for Maria Ortiz. After these interventions are completed, the nurse will reevaluate the patient and document the findings in the chart to show critical thinking. This is often in the form of a care plan or case note similar to the one below.

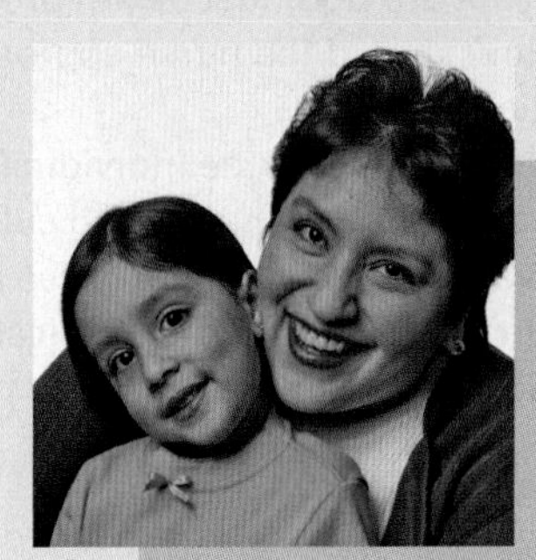

Nursing Diagnosis	Patient Outcomes	Nursing Interventions	Rationales	Evaluation
Knowledge deficit related to new diagnosis and medication	The patient states what to do for symptoms of hypoglycemia.	Discuss signs and symptoms of hypoglycemia. Discuss what to do if the patient is hypoglycemic, and provide a list of appropriate foods to increase blood glucose level.	Written information reinforces verbal information and can be used as a resource once the patient is at home.	Patient stated signs and symptoms of hypoglycemia. Patient named four foods that contain 10–15 g fast-acting carbohydrates. Patient will bring questions to next clinic visit.

including respiratory rate and oxygen saturation. In addition, you consider data from the general survey, such as posture, shortness of breath, and level of distress. If the patient with shortness of breath is also cyanotic and wheezing, you suspect a respiratory issue. If the condition is acute, you supply supplemental oxygen while contacting a primary care provider. Rather than identifying one piece of data in isolation, a systems approach allows you to cluster similar data to identify issues.

Evidence-Based Practice

Evidence-based practice is an approach to patient care that minimizes intuition and personal experience and instead relies on research findings and high-grade scientific support. **Evidence-based practice** helps you solve common problems through these four steps:

1. Clearly identify the issue or difficulties based on an accurate analysis of current nursing knowledge and practice.
2. Search the literature for relevant research.
3. Evaluate the research evidence using established criteria regarding scientific merit.
4. Choose interventions and justify the selection with the most valid evidence (Hoffman, Bennett, & Del Mar, 2013).

There are many ways to use research and evidence to provide holistic care to patients. The National Institute for Nursing Research (NINR; http://www.ninr.nih.gov/), formed in 1986, greatly increased the visibility and funding opportunities for nursing research. The International Honor Society for Nursing, Sigma Theta Tau (2009), has also increased its capacity to support and disseminate nursing scholarships for nursing research.

Some evidence is evaluated by performing clinical trials, such as measuring the accuracy of a new oral thermometer against core temperature. If there are several clinical trials, a systematic review of the quality trials becomes the standard criterion. The *Cochrane Database*, available in most medical libraries, is considered the most complete and accurate collection of systematic reviews. The National Clearinghouse Guidelines also have recommendations based on the clinical evidence. PubMed, a search engine which primarily accesses MEDLINE (Medical Literature Analysis and Retrieval System Online), is another Web site for obtaining the most current evidence. Many nursing facilities are implementing programs in which nurses develop a clinical question and find the best evidence to plan care. In this way, nurses base individual patient decisions on the best existing evidence rather than on their personal experience.

Applying Your Knowledge

Remember Ms. Ortiz, the 52-year-old patient who is being seen for a follow-up visit for her recently diagnosed diabetes. Consider responses to the questions introduced at the beginning of the chapter. Recognize how the knowledge gained in this chapter can be applied to her case using critical thinking.

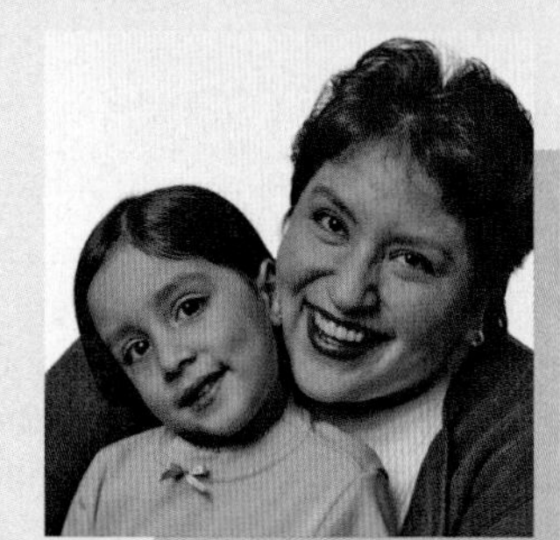

- What are potential health promotion and teaching needs for Ms. Ortiz?
- How should the nurse approach a discussion of the patient's diet as related to her diabetes?
- How will the nurse individualize today's health assessment, considering the patient's gender, age, and culture?
- What is the role of the nurse in providing care for Ms. Ortiz at the next visit?
- On what areas of the physical examination will the nurse concentrate?
- How will the nurse evaluate the results of patient teaching with Ms. Ortiz?

Key Points

- The role of the professional nurse is to promote health, prevent illness, treat human responses, and advocate for patients.
- Nurses are providers, designers, managers, and coordinators of care as well as advocates and educators.
- Nursing values include respect, unity, diversity, integrity, and excellence.
- Health can be conceptualized as a point between wellness and illness, either a high or low level of health.
- *Healthy People* is a U.S. government initiative to focus on health promotion and risk reduction strategies.
- The four main goals of nursing are to promote health, prevent illness, treat human responses to health and illness, and advocate for individuals, families, and communities.
- Steps of the nursing process include assessing, diagnosing, setting goals and outcomes, planning, intervening, and evaluating.
- Critical thinking is the key to resolving problems.
- Diagnostic reasoning is a process by which nurses use critical thinking to cluster the assessment information and to draw inferences and propose diagnoses.
- Types of assessments include emergency, comprehensive, and focused.
- Subjective data are based on the patient's experiences and perceptions.

- Objective data are measurable and usually collected as part of the physical assessment.
- Organizing frameworks for assessment include functional, head-to-toe, and body systems.
- Evidence-based nursing relies on research findings and high-grade scientific support.

Review Questions

1. A patient is having adverse effects resulting from a medication. The nurse calls the primary care provider to request a change to the medication order. The nurse is functioning as an/a
   A. educator.
   B. advocate.
   C. organizer.
   D. counselor.

2. Nurses advocate for underserved populations to reduce health disparities. This promotes
   A. autonomy.
   B. altruism.
   C. respect.
   D. human dignity.

3. Nurses belong to the American Nurses Association (ANA) as part of their
   A. ongoing professional responsibility.
   B. role as manager of care.
   C. wellness promotion for patients.
   D. cultural education activities.

4. The purpose of health assessment is to
   A. obtain subjective and objective data.
   B. intervene to correct difficulties.
   C. outline care that is appropriate.
   D. determine whether interventions are effective.

5. The nurse documents the following information in a patient's chart: "Cough and deep breathe every hour while awake." This is an example of
   A. evidence-based nursing.
   B. priority setting.
   C. comprehensive assessment.
   D. nursing interventions.

6. The nurse provides teaching about smoking cessation to a 20-year-old man. The nurse assesses that the patient is concerned because his father died from lung cancer. Which theory would the nurse most likely use when providing teaching to this patient?
   A. Health belief model
   B. Diagnostic reasoning model
   C. Cultural competence model
   D. Body systems model

7. Which of the following processes is the most important when providing nursing care to an ill patient?
   A. Writing outcomes
   B. Performing a focused assessment
   C. Collecting objective data
   D. Using critical thinking

8. A patient is admitted to a hospital for surgery for colon cancer. What type of assessment is the nurse most likely to perform upon admission?
   A. Emergency
   B. Focused
   C. Comprehensive
   D. Illness

9. Which of the following are components of a comprehensive health assessment?
   A. Nursing diagnoses
   B. Goals and outcomes
   C. Collaborative problems
   D. Examination of body systems

10. The nurse conducts the health history based on the patient's responses to the medical diagnosis. This type of framework is based on the
    A. functional framework.
    B. objective framework.
    C. coordinator framework.
    D. collaborative framework.

The Jensen suite offers these additional resources to enhance learning and facilitate understanding of this chapter:

- thePoint online resource, http://thepoint.lww.com/Jensen2e
- *Laboratory Manual for Nursing Health Assessment: A Best Practice Approach*
- *Pocket Guide for Nursing Health Assessment: A Best Practice Approach*
- *Lippincott DocuCare*, an electronic health record simulation software, http://thepoint.lww.com/docucare
- *Adaptive Learning | Powered by PrepU*, http://thepoint.lww.com/prepu

References

Advanced Practice Registered Nurse Joint Dialogue Group. (2008). *Consensus model for APRN regulation: Licensure, Accreditation, Certification & Education*. Based on the work of the APRN Consensus Work Group and the NCSBN APRN Advisory Committee. Washington, DC: Author.

Alfaro-LeFevre, R. (2010). *Applying nursing process: A tool for critical thinking* (7th ed.). Philadelphia, PA: Wolters Kluwer Health/Lippincott Williams & Wilkins.

American Association of Colleges of Nursing. (2011). *The essentials of baccalaureate education for professional nursing practice.* Retrieved from http://www.aacn.nche.edu/education-resources/baccessentials08.pdf.

American Association of Nurse Anesthetists. (2010). *Scope and standards for nurse anesthesia practice.* Retrieved from http://www.aana.com/resources2/professionalpractice/Documents/PPM%20Standards%20for%20Nurse%20Anesthesia%20Practice.pdf

American Nurses Association. (1980). *Nursing: A social policy statement.* Kansas City, MO: Author.
American Nurses Association. (2010a). *Code of ethics for nurses with interpretive statements*. Washington, DC: Author.
American Nurses Association. (2010b). *Nursing: Scope and standards of practice* (2nd ed.). Washington, DC: Author.
American Nurses Association. (2013a). *What is nursing?* Retrieved from http://www.nursingworld.org/EspeciallyForYou/What-is-Nursing
American Nurses Association. (2013b). *The nursing process*. Retrieved from http://www.nursingworld.org/EspeciallyForYou/What-is-Nursing/Tools-You-Need/Thenursingprocess.html
American Nurses Credentialing Center. (2013). *DNP fact sheet.* Retrieved from http://www.aacn.nche.edu/media-relations/fact-sheets/dnp
Bulechek, G. M., Butcher, H. K., Dochterman, J. M., & Wagner, C. M. (2013). *Nursing interventions classification (NIC)* (6th ed.). Philadelphia, PA: Elsevier.
Gordon, M. (1993). *Nursing diagnosis: Process and application* (3rd ed.). New York, NY: McGraw-Hill.
Health Insurance Portability and Accountability Act. (2003). *Standards for privacy of individually identifiable health information*. Retrieved from http://www.hhs.gov/ocr/privacy/
Hoffmann, T. Bennett, S., & Del Mar, S. C. (2013). *Evidence-Based Practice Across the Health Professions* (2nd ed.). Philadelphia, PA: Elsevier.
Institute for Healthcare Improvement (2013a). *Medication reconciliation to prevent adverse drug events.* Retrieved from http://www.ihi.org/explore/adesmedicationreconciliation/Pages/default.aspx
Institute for Healthcare Improvement. (2013b). *SBAR: Situation-background-assessment-recommendation*. Retrieved from http://www.ihi.org/explore/sbarcommunicationtechnique/pages/default.aspx
Joint Commission on Accreditation of Healthcare Organizations. (2013). *National patient safety goals*. Retrieved from http://www.jointcommission.org/PatientSafety/NationalPatientSafetyGoals/
Leavell, H. R., & Clark, E. G. (1965). *Preventive medicine for the doctor in his community: An epidemiologic approach*. New York, NY: McGraw-Hill.
Moorhead, S., Johnson, M., Maas, M. L., & Swanson, E. (2013). *Nursing outcomes classification (NOC): Measurement of health outcomes* (5th ed.). St. Louis, MO: Elsevier.
NANDA International. (2012). *Nursing diagnoses: Definitions and classification 2012-2014* (9th ed.). Oxford, United Kingdom: Wiley-Blackwell.
National Institute of Nursing Research. (2014). Retrieved from http://www.ninr.nih.gov/
Pender, N. J., Murdaugh, C. L., & Parsons, M. A. (2006). *Health promotion in nursing practice* (5th ed.). Upper Saddle River, NJ: Prentice Hall.
Purnell, L. D. (2009). *Guide to culturally competent health care* (2nd ed.). Philadelphia, PA: F. A. Davis.
Sigma Theta Tau. (2009). *Mission and vision*. Retrieved from http://www.nursingsociety.org/aboutus/mission/Pages/factsheet.aspx
Spector, R. E. (2012). *Cultural diversity in health and illness* (7th ed.). Upper Saddle River, NJ: Pearson Prentice Hall Health.
U.S. Department of Health & Human Services. (2013). *2020 Topics & objectives - Objectives A-Z.* Retrieved from http://www.healthypeople.gov/2020/topicsobjectives2020/
Weber, J., & Kelley, J. (2010). *Health assessment in nursing* (4th ed.). Philadelphia, PA: Wolters Kluwer Health/Lippincott Williams & Wilkins.
Zimmer, B. (2010). *Wellness*. Retrieved from http://www.nytimes.com/2010/04/18/magazine/18FOBonlanguage-t.html?_r=0

2

The Health History and Interview

Learning Objectives

1 Describe how nurses use active listening, restatement, reflection, elaboration, silence, focusing, clarification, and summarizing in verbal communication.

2 Differentiate the preinteraction, beginning, working, and closing phases of the interview process.

3 Describe sensitivity to intercultural communication, including working with patients who have limited knowledge of the English language, working with interpreters, and being sensitive to gender-related issues.

4 Differentiate primary from secondary data.

5 Compare and contrast emergency, focused, and comprehensive health histories.

6 Identify the components of the comprehensive health history and review of systems.

7 Complete a family history using a genogram to illustrate family patterns.

8 Perform a functional health assessment using Gordon's nursing framework.

Mr. Rowan, a 36-year-old Caucasian man, resides in an assisted living facility. He was diagnosed with AIDS 2 years ago. He has been nonadherent with his antiretroviral medication regimen because he dislikes taking "artificial substances" and believes that natural methods (e.g., nutrition) are more effective in managing his illness. He has been receiving meals and housekeeping as part of his services. The nurse has ongoing contact with him to encourage him to take his medications and also to assess his condition and needs.

You will gain more information about Mr. Rowan as you progress through this chapter. As you study the content and features, consider Mr. Rowan's case and its relationship to what you are learning. Begin thinking about the following points:

- Which techniques of therapeutic communication might the nurse need to use when talking with the patient?
- Is it important for the nurse to interview Mr. Rowan to assess how he contracted AIDS?
- What is the nurse's perceived risk of exposure to HIV/AIDS?
- What cultural, environmental, or developmental issues might the nurse anticipate for Mr. Rowan?
- How might the nurse's personal beliefs about AIDS and the use of alternative therapies affect communication with Mr. Rowan?
- How can the nurse know whether nonjudgmental care has been communicated, both verbally and nonverbally?

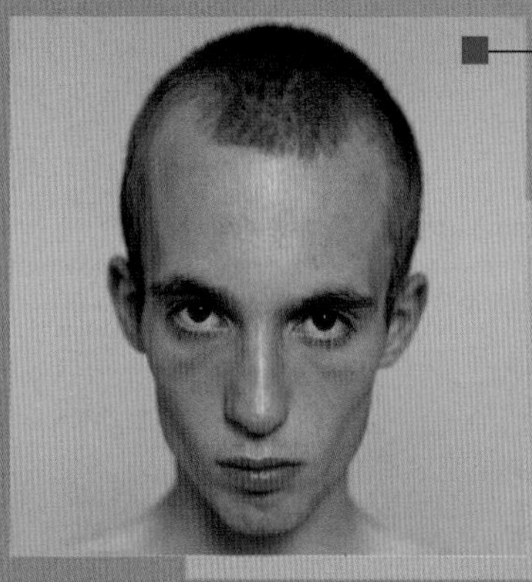

Through **therapeutic communication**, you and the patient work together to resolve problems by developing collaborative strategies and solutions. As you and the patient develop rapport with each other, the patient feels respected and understood. You perform health teaching based on each patient's needs and priorities and weave health promotion and disease prevention into care.

All nursing practice revolves around the **nurse–patient relationship**, which is built upon verbal and nonverbal communication within a specific setting. The nurse–patient relationship differs from personal and social relationships, because its foundation is the therapeutic use of self through verbal and nonverbal communication skills. As a nurse, you have a privileged role as a respected health care provider. Your relationships with patients are professionally intimate. In some situations, patients disclose information to their nurses that they do not even share with family members. Within the nurse–patient relationship, you learn wide-ranging things about patients, from minute physical details to deep-seated feelings about spirituality, culture, and psychosocial concerns.

During health history taking, you use special techniques and communication skills to gather complete and accurate data about the health state of patients. As you develop and refine your interviewing capabilities, conversation with patients becomes more comfortable, with smooth transitions from question to question. You develop a comfort level with periods of silence and an appreciation for its value in the interviewing process. You develop a style of communication that suits your personality and values, blending together the professional and the personal. Communication is one of the foundational components of the nurse–patient relationship; your ability to continually assess and build on communication skills is essential (Webster, 2013).

The purpose of taking the health history is to collect subjective data from patients. **Subjective data** are based on the signs and symptoms that the patient reports; they may not be perceived by observers. Additionally, you collect individual and family histories to obtain data about past and current medical problems, surgeries, and risks for disease. In your discussions with the patient and family, you also include information on health behaviors and activities that promote health. In many settings, patients complete comprehensive forms that you then review and ask questions about to add detail during the interview. This is all subjective information.

The Communication Process

Communication is a complex, ongoing, interactive process that forms the basis for building interpersonal relationships (American Association of Colleges of Nursing [AACN], 2008). It is a system of sending and receiving messages, forming a connection between sender and receiver (Fig. 2.1). This continuous and dynamic process is always subject to interpretation. The sender's purpose is translated into a code with verbal language cues. The receiver decodes the message, making meaning of the verbal and nonverbal messages. Subjective understanding, perceptions, and other variables greatly influence the actual decoding of the message, both correctly and incorrectly.

Additionally, culture can influence a person's understanding of communication. In many cultures, mental health disorders carry great stigma, so patients may describe psychosocial difficulties as a lack of sleep or as feeling tired. There are many other situations where culture affects communication. Americans of European descent typically speak loudly, whereas in Thailand, speaking loudly signifies ignorance (Balzer-Riley, 2012).

Both nurses and patients bring perceptions about the relationship with them. A patient who has had positive personal experiences with the health care system may be more open to developing a relationship with a nurse than one who has had negative experiences. Therefore, it is important that you assess the patient's perceptions of the health care system.

Therapeutic communication is a basic tool you use in a caring relationship with patients. In therapeutic communication, the interaction focuses on the patient and the patient's concerns. You assist patients to work through feelings and explore options related to the situation, outcomes, and treatments. This skill takes practice but can be learned with attention and awareness. It takes time to learn to listen for messages

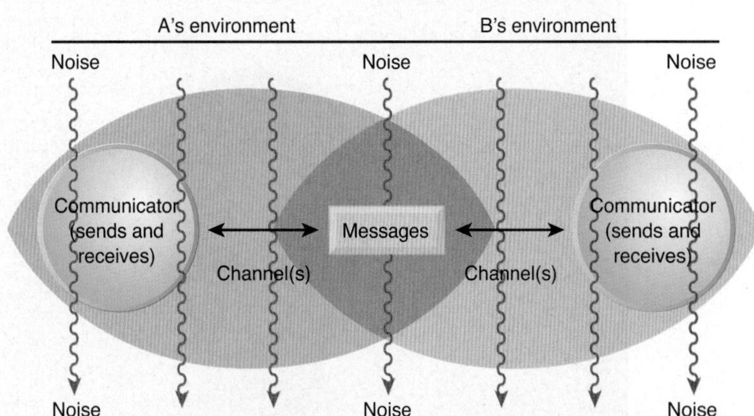

Figure 2.1 Communication is a system of sending and receiving messages, forming a connection between the sender and the receiver. (From Adler, R. B., & Proctor, R. F. [2013]. *Looking out/looking in* [14th ed., p.10]. Boston, MA: Wadsworth, Cengage Learning.)

BOX 2.1 Self-Assessment Tool: Communication—The Key to Patient Service

Instructions: **Rate yourself from 4 (very skilled) to 1 (not skilled).**

1. I feel good about my communication skills.	4	3	2	1
2. I smile at patients, families, and staff.	4	3	2	1
3. I make eye contact.	4	3	2	1
4. I introduce myself and wear my name badge.	4	3	2	1
5. I learn names and use the correct pronunciations.	4	3	2	1
6. If I don't understand, I seek clarification.	4	3	2	1
7. I take a moment to calm myself before interacting with patients.	4	3	2	1
8. I take responsibility for finding answers to questions.	4	3	2	1
9. I answer the telephone promptly and with a smile (that helps).	4	3	2	1
10. I explain procedures clearly.	4	3	2	1
11. I encourage patients and their families to ask questions.	4	3	2	1
12. I encourage feedback about my work.	4	3	2	1
13. I receive positive feedback about my work.	4	3	2	1
14. I thank a colleague who helps me.	4	3	2	1
15. I offer to help my colleagues.	4	3	2	1
16. I listen, knowing it is OK to be quiet and not have all the answers.	4	3	2	1
17. I respect the patient's confidentiality.	4	3	2	1
18. I apologize for delays.	4	3	2	1
19. When I touch a patient, I do it gently.	4	3	2	1
20. I dress professionally and pay attention to my grooming.	4	3	2	1
21. I try to do something extra for patients, families, and colleagues.	4	3	2	1
22. I am learning to deal with multiple demands on my time.	4	3	2	1
23. I give compliments to patients, family, and colleagues (yes, doctors, too!).	4	3	2	1
24. I understand that I am still learning and that it is impossible to be perfect.	4	3	2	1
25. I try to be myself, bringing my own special gifts to my nursing practice.	4	3	2	1

Scoring: Add the numbers you have selected. Remember that this is a self-assessment, and feedback from your instructor, peers, and patients adds more data.
77-100, High awareness of necessary skills.
53-76, Average awareness of skills. Review your lower scores and select areas for growth.
25-52, Low awareness of necessary skills. Pay more attention to skill development.
Adapted from Balzer-Riley, J. W. (2012). *Communication in nursing* (7th ed.). St. Louis, MO: Elsevier.

that might otherwise be unheard, but this careful listening contributes greatly to a therapeutic relationship. Caring and empathy are useful when communicating therapeutically. Balzer-Riley's (2012) Self-Assessment Tool (Box 2.1) is an excellent method for evaluating your developing communication skills and reflecting on your progress.

Caring encompasses your empathy for and connection with the patient. It also includes the ability to demonstrate emotional characteristics such as compassion, sensitivity, and patient-centered care (AACN, 2008). Your goal is to show warmth, care, interest, and respect and also to value patients unconditionally and nonjudgmentally. Patients will be more willing to discuss their health issues if they perceive you as caring, understanding, and nonjudgmental.

Empathy means the ability to perceive, reason, and communicate understanding of another person's feelings without criticism. It is being able to see and feel the situation from the patient's perspective rather than your own perspective. Being empathetic means asking questions that may help patients express how they are feeling and what they are thinking so that you understand the patient's point of view. You communicate to patients that you accurately appreciate their thoughts, feelings, and experiences. Empathy may be conveyed verbally or nonverbally. In some situations, such as death of a relative, you may exhibit empathy simply by holding a person's hand or offering a tissue. Empathy can be a complex process that is further challenged by many of our health care settings, which are often not optimal settings for dealing with things like death or accepting a poor prognosis (Bach & Grant, 2011). Through experience, you learn to communicate empathy in a variety of settings.

You need a comfortable **self-concept** to be aware of your own biases, values, personality, cultural background, and communication style. You build such awareness through self-reflection and through listening to and understanding feedback from others. Self-reflection increases your ability to be genuine and to connect with patients and to meet their needs. Having a comfortable sense of self allows you to work with patients of different personalities, cultures, and socioeconomic backgrounds. Self-awareness helps you identify what you do well and what your weaknesses are. When interviewing patients, self-awareness helps you recognize when you have communicated well and how you can improve your communication skills (Hurley & Linsley, 2012). Self-reflection will help you avoid the difficulties of ethnocentrism, in which your own biases may prevent you from developing a genuinely therapeutic relationship with patients (Balzer-Riley, 2012).

Nonverbal Communication Skills

Nonverbal communication is as important as—if not more important than—verbal communication. Physical appearance, facial expression, posture and positioning in relation to the patient, gestures, eye contact, tone of voice, and use of touch are all important components of nonverbal communication. For example, you should not assume that touch is culturally acceptable to a patient. Instead, be courteous and ask permission: "Is it OK if I feel your abdomen?"

Your physical appearance and demeanor send a message to patients. Thus, it is important to ensure that your dress and appearance are professional. Your facial expression should be relaxed, caring, and interested. Be aware that facial expressions common in certain social situations, such rolling the eyes, looking bored, or appearing disgusted, reduce trust and are thus inappropriate during interactions with patients. Your posture should be upright but relaxed and open; avoid "closed" positions, such as crossed arms, which may signal to patients that you are uninterested in them and their information. Use gestures intentionally to illustrate points, especially for patients who cannot communicate verbally. You may point with a finger or gesture an action, such as pretending to drink or pointing to the bathroom. Gestures should be purposeful rather than distracting from the communication.

To facilitate optimal eye contact, you need to be at eye level with the patient. If you stand while the patient is in bed, you will be taller than the patient, thus assuming a position of power. Conversely, if you sit on the patient's hospital bed or examining table, the patient may interpret this as getting too close or being unprofessional and even possibly as infringing on the patient's personal space. Moreover, considering principles of infection control, beds or tables may contain microorganisms or body secretions that you could transport from one room to another. For these reasons, sit in a chair at eye level with patients who are in bed during interviews (Fig. 2.2A). For patients seated on examination tables, you will be near eye level when standing (Fig. 2.2B). It is important to have a balance in eye contact during the interview. For some cultures, prolonged eye contact is considered threatening (Peate, 2012).

Touch is an essential and dominant component of the physical examination. During the initial interview, however, the patient may misinterpret touch from the nurse as being too casual. Instead of touching in this situation, use nonverbal skills to communicate messages to patients that facilitate a therapeutic relationship. If you are positioned near the patient's bed, speak carefully and maintain good eye contact, so that the patient will feel that he or she is being listened to.

Verbal Communication Skills

You learn effective interviewing skills through practice and repetition. You use these skills to encourage patients to further expand their initial brief answers and also to redirect patients when they wander from the topic.

Your speech should be of moderate pace and volume with clear articulation. A too-soft voice may indicate embarrassment or discomfort, whereas a too-loud voice may seem too powerful and controlling. Speech that is too fast indicates that you are rushed, whereas speech that is too slow might send a message that the nurse may think the patient is lacking in cognitive ability. For a patient with an untreated hearing impairment, you may need to speak louder and more slowly into the patient's better ear or position yourself so that patients can lip-read (Fig. 2.3).

For patients with limited knowledge of the English language, use simple and clear language but do not raise your voice. Instead of using complete sentences, you might speak in one or two words, such as "Pain?" Insert pauses in the conversation to allow patients an opportunity to speak; such pauses facilitate trust, respect, and sharing. They also give the patient the opportunity to consider the questions being asked.

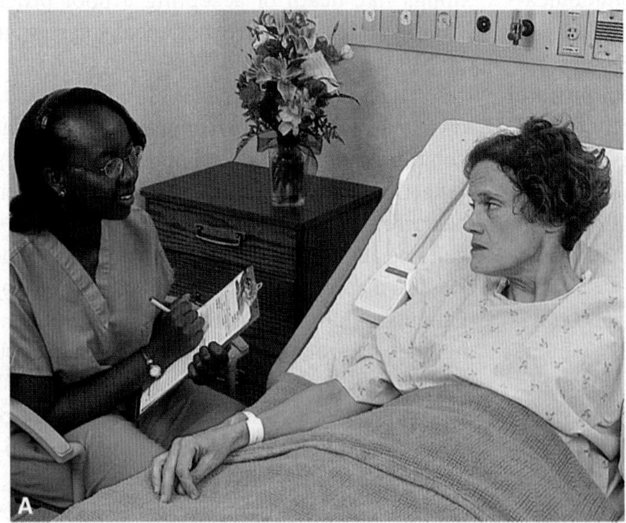

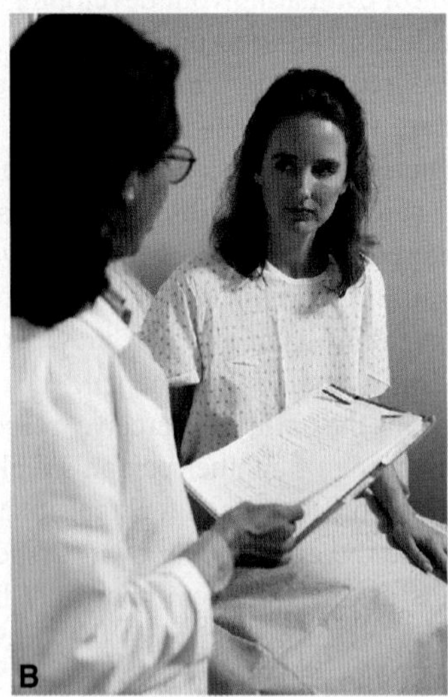

Figure 2.2 **A.** The nurse working with a patient who is in a hospital bed sits to be at eye level with the patient during the interview. **B.** The nurse stands to be at eye level with the patient on an examination table.

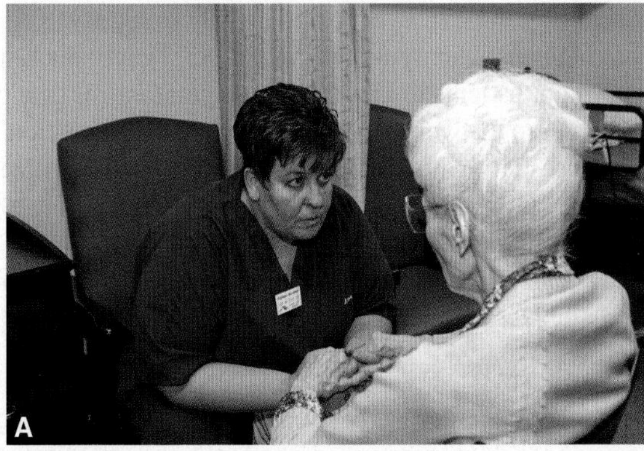

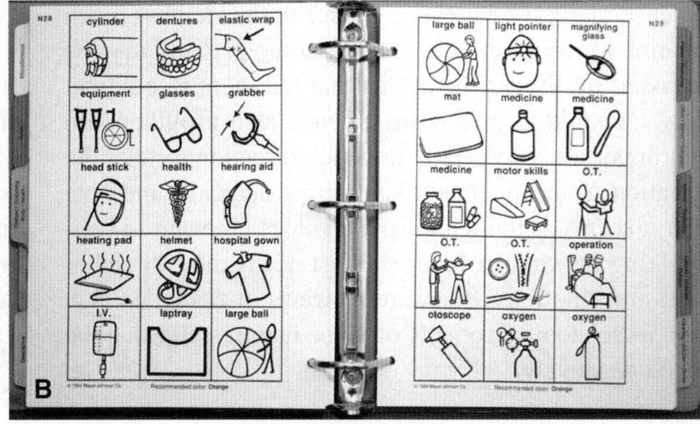

Figure 2.3 The nurse must be creative to communicate with patients who cannot fully interact verbally or who have sensory impairments. **A.** This nurse is making sure to sit directly in front of the patient with hearing difficulties and enunciate very clearly for the patient. **B.** Picture boards can be helpful for patients who cannot speak or who cannot communicate in the same language as the nurse.

Active Listening

Active listening is the ability to focus on patients and their perspectives. It requires that you constantly decode messages, including thoughts, words, opinions, and emotions. For example, if a patient is sad, it is appropriate for you to place your hand over the patient's hand and to show a facial expression of compassion. If a patient is angry, listen to the reason for the anger, such as treatment failure. Rather than respond in turn with anger, attend to the patient's feelings by pulling up a chair and taking the time to listen. Try to uncover the hidden message and show appropriate body language.

Talking about difficult feelings helps patients to heal. You are not expected to solve all the patient's difficulties but instead to therapeutically use the self to assist patients to deal with them.

> **SAFETY ALERT**
>
> *If talking about a situation seems to increase rather than diffuse a patient's anger, you may redirect the interview. If a patient is abusive or overly aggressive, it may be necessary to take a time-out by saying, "I understand that you're very angry right now. I am feeling a little defensive, so I can either have someone else come in to talk with you or come back in 15 minutes. Which would you prefer?"*

Restatement

Restatement relates to the content of the communication. You make a simple statement, usually using the patient's own words. The purpose is to ask the patient to elaborate. Restatement provides an opportunity for patients to further understand their communication. For example, you may repeat the patient's statement by saying, "So, you feel like there is a knot in your chest."

Reflection

Reflection is similar to restatement; however, instead of simply restating the patient's comments, you summarize the main themes of communication. The conversation may be longer, in which a patient discusses several elements related to a topic. Listen carefully to the different thoughts expressed and attempt to identify their relationship. With this technique, patients gain a better understanding of the issues that underlie their thoughts, which helps to identify their feelings. The following example illustrates how the nurse can use reflection.

> ***Patient:*** *I really hate getting shots. Do I really need to get a flu shot? My parents never had it, and they stayed healthy during the winter.*
> ***Nurse:*** *You sound a bit nervous about getting an injection. (Pause)*
> ***Patient:*** *The last shot that I had really hurt.*

In this situation, the patient was not questioning the need for the injection but was expressing anxiety about it because of previous experience. The nurse now knows to direct the conversation toward dealing with the anxiety rather than teaching about the risk for influenza.

Elaboration (Facilitation)

Encouraging **elaboration (facilitation)** is a technique that assists patients to more completely describe difficulties. You use responses that encourage patients to say more and continue the conversation. This shows patients that you are interested. You may nod your head, or say, "Um-hum," "Yes," or "Go on" to cue patients to keep talking. Another technique is to let patients know that their thoughts and feelings are common and to give them permission to discuss them. You might use a phrase such as, "Sometimes when patients are involved in a car accident, they have flashbacks or bad dreams."

Silence

You can use **silence** purposefully during the interview to allow patients time to gather their thoughts and provide accurate answers. You can also use silence therapeutically to communicate nonverbal concern. Silence can be difficult, especially for the novice interviewer who is just learning to use it as a communication tool. By using silence, you convey patience to the person being interviewed, indicating that you are interested in what the person is saying (Dart, 2011).

Silence may give patients a chance to decide how much information to disclose. For example, some patients may be embarrassed to discuss the events that led them to contract sexually transmitted infections. Silence also provides you with an opportunity to decide in which direction to take the conversation. You can attend to nonverbal language and note whether it seems as though the patient does not want to continue talking or whether he or she just needs time to gather thoughts and emotions. Be aware, however, that silence may not be appreciated by patients of some cultures and may be perceived negatively.

Focusing

Use **focusing** when patients are straying from a topic and need redirection. Focusing helps when you need to address areas of concern related to current difficulties. For example, you might say, "We were talking about the reaction that you had to the penicillin. Tell me more about that reaction." This response connects the patient's story to the initial need for information on the type of reaction, which is a safety issue needing further discussion. It keeps the conversation on track without changing the subject and conveys the message that you will assist the patient to provide important information.

Clarification

Clarification is important when the patient's word choice or ideas are unclear. For example, you may state, "Tell me what you mean by the evil eye." Another way to clarify is to ask, "What happens when you get low blood sugar?" Such questions prompt patients to identify other symptoms or give more information so that you can better understand the situation. You can also use clarification when the patient's history of illness is confusing. Putting data in chronological order or placing events in context can help make the story clearer. For example, you may ask, "When you had chest pain, first you took three nitroglycerin tablets and then you called 911—is that right?"

Summarizing

Summarizing happens at the end of the interview, during the closure phase. You review and condense important information into two or three of the most important findings. Doing so helps ensure that you have identified important information and lets the patient know that he or she has been heard accurately. It gives you and the patient future direction as you establish a therapeutic relationship.

Summarizing includes the progress made toward problem solving and things to think about later. It also gives patients an opportunity to add information they wish to be included in the interview or that they may have unintentionally omitted. For example, you may say, "It seems that you are most concerned about your appetite and lack of energy. We have talked about adding some low-cost and high-protein foods to your diet. When you come in for your next visit, we can talk about how that worked."

Therapeutic Dialogue: Collecting Subjective Data

A student nurse is visiting Mr. Rowan, introduced at the beginning of this chapter, to remind him to take his antiretroviral medications and to assess his current needs. The following conversations give two examples of interview styles. One style is more effective than the other.

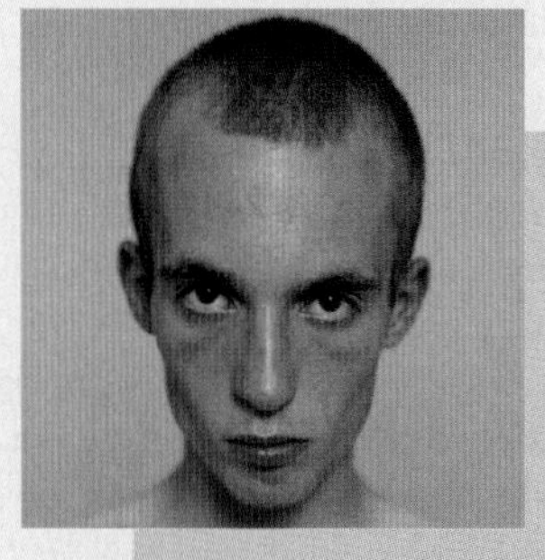

Less Effective

Nurse: Hi, Mr. Rowan. I'm Tom Fritz, a student who is working with your nurse. May I come in?

Mr. Rowan: OK. Do you want a glass of water?

Nurse: No, thanks. I just finished my lunch, and I'm full.

Mr. Rowan: So what do you want?

Nurse: I am here to check your medications by doing a pill count and also to see if you need anything.

Mr. Rowan: I already took my pills. You can count them if you want.

More Effective

Nurse: Hi, Mr. Rowan. I'm Tom Fritz, a student who is working with your nurse. Betsy said to let you know that she's available if you would rather talk with her.

Mr. Rowan: You're working with Betsy?

Nurse: Yes, she's seeing another patient but said that she could come and see you if you would prefer that.

Mr. Rowan: No, come on in. Would you like a glass of water?

Nurse: That would be great if it's not too inconvenient.

(case study continues on page 25)

Less Effective	More Effective
Nurse: That would be great. Do you have them nearby?	**Mr. Rowan:** (Gets water) You can sit down.
Mr. Rowan: They're right here. I don't like taking them, but if I don't, my nurse Betsy tells me that I need to take better care of myself. (Mr. Rowan gets medications.) You can sit down.	**Nurse:** Thank you so much. Tell me how you're doing today.
Nurse: No, thanks. I'm glad that you're taking the medications. The count is right. So it looks like you're doing okay.	**Mr. Rowan:** I'm OK—you're here to make sure that I took my medication, aren't you? I already took it—you can count the pills if you want.
Mr. Rowan: I'm feeling weak and tired. Is there anything else that you want?	**Nurse:** We can do that in a minute. I'd just like to talk for a little bit to see how you're feeling and if I can help in any way.
Nurse: No, I think that's it.	**Mr. Rowan:** Well, I'd rather be home, but I can't live by myself anymore. Every day I just seem to get weaker.

Critical Thinking Challenge

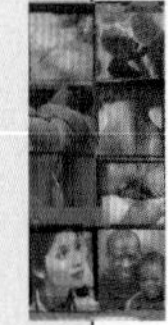

- Compare and contrast the data collected in the two dialogues. What therapeutic communication techniques were used in each?
- Can you identify any nontherapeutic responses?
- What was different in the way the two episodes started?
- What interactions occurred in both dialogues that might influence the student nurse's ability to establish trust with Mr. Rowan?
- What were the differences in outcomes at the end of each dialogue?

Nontherapeutic Responses

False Reassurance

Often in social situations, people use nontherapeutic casual responses. Probably the most common example is **false reassurance** to minimize uncomfortable feelings. In nurse–patient relationships, giving false reassurance can also minimize the amount of distressing information that the nurse has to handle. Nevertheless, such responses effectively end communication from the patient's perspective.

By providing false reassurance, you unconsciously indicate to patients that their concerns are not worth discussing. This situation enhances anxiety, which can increase a patient's urge to seek further reassurance and may diminish his or her trust. Examples of false reassurance are, "It won't hurt," or "Don't worry—it will be all right." It would be better instead to say, for example, "It will hurt a bit when I take off the bandage, but I'll do it quickly," or "It sounds like you're concerned that your cancer might have returned. I want you to know that I will be here when you get your test results tomorrow." This type of reassurance validates the patient's concerns and reassures him or her that you will be there to provide a therapeutic relationship.

Sympathy

Sympathy is feeling what a patient feels. When you are being sympathetic, you are not being therapeutic because you are interpreting the situation as *you* perceive it. In contrast, **empathy** is feeling what a patient feels from the *patient's* perspective. You keep the focus on the patient: this allows the patient to express himself or herself completely.

Unwanted Advice

Giving unwanted advice happens frequently in social situations. It is nontherapeutic in professional relationships because the advice is usually from your perspective, not the patient's. Because the advice is based on *your* experiences and opinions, it may not help the patient.

Giving advice differs from *providing information*. For example, if a patient asks, "How do I get rid of the lice in my son's hair?" you should answer based on your knowledge base as a nurse and the current evidence. A patient who asks, "Do you think that I should have my knee replaced? I don't really know what to do," requires a different type of response. In this situation, when you are using active listening, you understand that the patient is asking for an opportunity to discuss options rather than what you would want to do personally. Instead of responding to the request for an opinion, you might state, "Tell me what you know about the surgery," or "You sound concerned about having knee surgery." Such responses give patients an opportunity to explore choices more fully, clarify any confusing points, and weigh risks against benefits. They also incorporate the patient's perspective instead of adding potentially confusing or conflicting information or opinions. When you take time to focus on the concerns of patients, you help them through decisions by using active listening, reflection, and restatement. In this way, patients reach their own conclusions.

Biased Questions

Using leading or biased questions is often an unintentional nontherapeutic response. Biased questions carry judgment and lead patients to respond in a way that they think will be acceptable to you. Biased questions may also cause patients to feel guilty or inferior about unhealthy behaviors. An example of a biased question is, "You don't use drugs, do you?" To obtain a more honest response, ask objective questions such as, "It is important that we know what recreational drugs you are taking so that we avoid interactions with the medications that we are giving you. Do you use any recreational drugs?" In this way, you place the need for information within the context of health care. Patients will then understand that you want to provide the best care rather than to judge their unhealthy behaviors.

Changes of Subject

You may be tempted to change the subject when a situation is uncomfortable for you because of your personal experiences or coping mechanisms. For example, if you recently experienced the death of a parent, it may be challenging at this time for you to talk with a family about a patient who has terminal cancer. Avoiding the subject is not therapeutic for the patient; you need to recognize that you are using coping mechanisms to protect yourself from emotional distress. Self-reflection will help you become aware that you may be using less-than-therapeutic communication strategies; you can then seek to improve your approach. One strategy could be to control your emotions with patients and seek support from others. An alternate approach would be to choose to be honest with patients and families about your situation. If emotional control is too difficult, you should refer patients to other health care providers.

You also might find that you change the subject unconsciously when you are feeling rushed or stressed. In such cases, you may not take time to use active listening. For example, on a busy day, you want to complete the intake and output record at the end of your shift. When the patient says, "I'm feeling a bit nauseous," you may reply, "What did you have to drink?" instead of "How long have you been nauseous?" Although you may constantly strive to use active listening, some situations dictate the type of communication used. The goal is to prioritize and block out times to use active listening when patients need to talk. Part of the plan of care may be, "Allow 15 minutes of uninterrupted time every shift for therapeutic conversation."

Distractions

Distractions in the environment contribute to nontherapeutic communication. Hectic and rushed work environments abound across health care settings. This contributes to patient complaints about depersonalized care. Distractions come from various sources, such as equipment, other patients, colleagues, pagers, and cell phones. When equipment poses a potential source of distraction, silence any alarms and then resolve the problem before initiating conversation. An equipment alarm indicates an immediate problem that usually takes priority over therapeutic communication.

When a patient's roommate is asking for something, you must decide to either grant a simple request and then pull curtains and provide for privacy, or ask the roommate to wait by saying, "I'm listening to your roommate's lungs right now. I can get you some water in about 5 minutes." You prioritize the importance of answering a pager or cell phone based on the intensity of your conversation with the patient and the point in the interview. Answering a phone during the middle of a conversation is nontherapeutic; many patients may consider it rude. If answering a phone or pager is necessary, you should complete the topic being discussed and then ask for permission to answer by saying, for example, "I just received a call about a patient who needs pain medication. Would you mind if I stepped out for a moment to answer?"

Technical or Overwhelming Language

Using too many technical terms or providing too much information is another nontherapeutic response. As you develop medical vocabulary and knowledge, you must practice translating from medical terminology to lay language. For example, you document "dysphagia" but ask the patient about "trouble swallowing." It also is important to conduct the conversation at the knowledge level of your patient. You may use more technical descriptions with patients who work in health care than with patients who have limited medical knowledge. Complex concepts may best be presented through diagrams and pictures that illustrate points visually (Fig. 2.4). A patient's puzzled facial expression may be a nonverbal clue that the patient is not understanding the information being presented because you are using technical jargon or because of the way you are presenting the information.

Interrupting

Talking too much and interrupting are also examples of nontherapeutic communication. In order to exhibit caring behavior, you may need to be kinder, gentler, and less vocal than you may be in social situations. In your professional role as a nurse, you listen more than you talk. Those who are shy in social situations may exhibit excellent

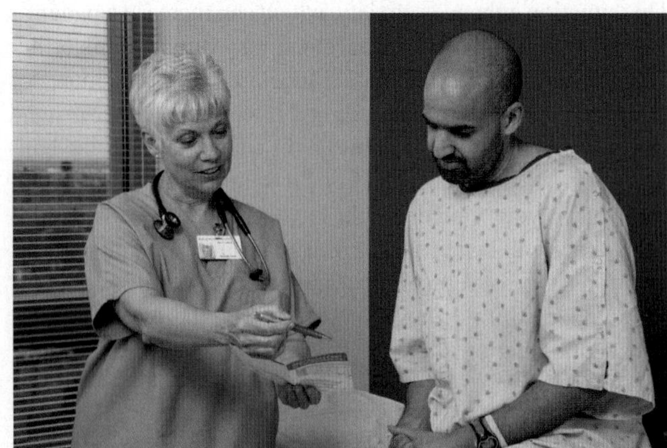

Figure 2.4 Diagrams, pictures, and other instructional materials can greatly assist with the processes of assessment and follow-up teaching related to findings.

therapeutic communication—not by talking but by communicating nonverbally through presence, facial expression, or touch. In health care settings, it is better to listen than to talk and to ask good questions rather than have all the right answers.

Professional Expectations

Learning when to use the various techniques of therapeutic communication is part of both the science and art of nursing. Because it is easy to identify too much with some patients, especially those who remind you of someone you know, it is important to establish clear professional boundaries. The nurse who becomes too involved with patients may experience burnout and decreased job satisfaction.

Nonprofessional involvement occurs when you cross the **professional boundary** relationship and establish social, personal, or economic ties with a patient. Although social chatting about the weather or current news may put patients at ease, too much personal conversation is unprofessional. Some disclosure may help establish a therapeutic relationship, but you should always present such information with a focus on the patient. For example, a nurse is working with parents of a child who was recently diagnosed with asthma. Coincidentally, the nurse's son also has asthma. The nurse may use that information to say, "I have a child with asthma, too. I noticed that the cough would get worse at night. What was the first thing that you noticed?" In this example, the nurse uses personal information to quickly redirect the conversation to focus on the patient and the family.

Sexual boundary violation is the clearest example of unprofessional involvement. Sexual contact is never acceptable within the therapeutic nurse–patient relationship. The American Nurses Association (2005) has established professional guidelines about behaviors such as dating or having outside contact with patients: "When acting within one's role as a professional, the nurse recognizes and maintains boundaries that establish appropriate limits to relationships."

Visiting patients beyond your role of the nurse or nursing student also breaks professional boundaries. You need to recognize that care continues with other health care professionals and trust that the health care system exists to meet ongoing needs. Although many times a nurse remembers and becomes attached to the first patients with whom he or she works, the nurse must not confuse the privileged intimacy associated with the nursing role with the intimacy involved in a social or personal relationship.

Intercultural Communication

During **intercultural communication**, the sender of an intended message belongs to one culture, whereas the receiver is from another. Cultural differences may relate to a group or ethnicity, region, age, degree of acculturation into Western society, or a combination of these factors (see Chapter 10). Differences in eye contact, facial expression, gestures, posture, timing, touch, and space needs are all culturally influenced. Language differences between you and the patient can compound cultural differences and prevent you from understanding the perspective of the patient. Voice volume, vocal tone, inflections, pronunciation, and accents also influence meaning. More than simple language translation, the cultural meanings of health, illness, and treatment are important factors to consider.

Communication etiquette refers to the code of conduct and good manners that show respect for others. Such etiquette varies between and within cultures. You must assess the degree to which each patient identifies with cultural norms. Additionally, many patients identify with multiple cultures. You should avoid assuming that patients follow cultural beliefs and assess the degree to which each individual perceives those beliefs.

Many cultures revere their elders, but in the U.S. culture, ageism can be a problem. It is not uncommon for the young to use patronizing terms to address the elderly, such as "honey" or "sweetie" (Balzer-Riley, 2012). This is demeaning to the older adult; you should take time to reflect on this. You can bridge cultural differences by being sensitive to variations and using caring communication techniques. Refer to Chapter 10 for more information.

Patients With Limited English Skills

Patients with limited English skills often identify language barriers as frustrating when navigating the U.S. health care system. When possible, use an interpreter; however, interpreters cannot be involved continuously throughout a patient's care. Thus, you must develop other communication tools. For example, you should cover one concept at a time instead of overwhelming the patient with several ideas at once. Use simple words or phrases to facilitate understanding. At times, you can pantomime questions, such as pretending to be in pain or having a questioning look on your face.

When communicating with patients who have limited English proficiency, remember the following principles:

- Limitations in English are not a reflection of intellectual functioning. A patient may be highly literate in another language but functionally illiterate in English.
- Patients tend to think in their native language and translate, thus delaying their responses.
- Patients interpret the message that reflects their cultural beliefs, often changing the speaker's intent.
- Written information in the native language supports verbal communication.

You can use a sheet with common phrases (e.g., "I am thirsty," "I need to use the bathroom") for patients who are literate in their native languages. Resources with pictures are helpful for patients who have good visual acuity but who cannot read. It is also helpful for the nurse to know a few key phrases in a patient's language to increase communication and trust.

Working With an Interpreter

You should establish the need for an interpreter during the patient's first contact with the health care agency. Even when a patient's language skills are fluent, a trained medical interpreter may be necessary for discussing sensitive topics, such as end-of-life care or permissions for consent to treat. In inpatient settings, interpreters may check in with patients daily. In such situations, it is helpful to maintain a list of questions and areas for patient teaching to cluster the most important information during the time that the translator is available (usually for a 30-minute period). Other occasions for using an interpreter are the admission assessment, complex treatments, patient education, informed consent, and discharge planning. U.S. federal law mandates the use of a trained interpreter according to standards established by The Joint Commission (2014). Interpreters are chosen based on language (e.g., Mandarin or Cantonese for a Chinese patient), dialect, gender for sensitive subjects, and social status if this is likely to be an issue.

Using children in the family, other relatives, or close friends as interpreters violates privacy laws because patients may not want to share personal information with relatives or friends. Additionally, friends and family who are unfamiliar with medical terminology may misinterpret information. When possible, a trained medical interpreter is preferred. Not only are medical interpreters knowledgeable in terminology but they also have a health care background. These interpreters also understand cultural health beliefs and practices and can help bridge the gap.

Interpreters are educated to remain neutral. Considering the natural communication process that involves the encoding and decoding of messages, however, interpreters still influence the content and context of communication. Issues can arise when interpreters add their opinion or bias to communication. You should pay attention to and look at patients during interviews to keep the focus on them rather than on the interpreter. In that way, you will be aware of nonverbal communication that seems inconsistent with the issues being discussed. See Box 2.2 for tips on communicating through interpreters.

BOX 2.2 Guidelines for Interpreter-Dependent Communication

- Take time to meet with the interpreter before meeting with the patient.
- Allow sufficient time. Working with an interpreter may take twice as long as a meeting in which a common language is spoken.
- Speak directly to the patient.
- Speak in short sentences then allow the interpreter to interpret.
- Develop alternatives to direct questions.
- Avoid difficult language, abstract concepts, and technical medical jargon.
- Speak slowly and clearly; use repetition as needed.
- Be aware of nonverbal messages.
- Avoid using family members as interpreters.

Gender and Sexual Orientation Issues

Communication styles vary between and within each gender group. Men commonly prefer more information and facts, whereas women often prefer more social and emotional interactions (Stewart, 2013). You may need to provide more information and structure for male patients and ask questions that focus more on emotional response, role adjustment, and coping mechanisms for female patients.

Gender also influences family roles, defined as a "set of beliefs about or expectations of male and female behavior and experiences within the family" (Wright & Leahey, 2012). Family roles can become involved in interviewing and history taking when cultural norms influence the nurse–patient relationship. For example, some cultures expect that the oldest male acts as the family leader and communicator. In other cultures, patients may prefer that the husband is spoken with to represent the family. Be aware of cultural norms and ask patients about their preferences.

You must also be aware of societal biases about sexual preference when working with gay, transgender, lesbian, and bisexual patients. Take care to treat all patients with respect and to provide pertinent information, such as safe-sex practices, for all patients. Issues related to sexual orientation often become prominent when patients have life-threatening or chronic illnesses. In many jurisdictions, the patient's life partner has no legal decision-making capacity. Sometimes, conflicts arise between life partners and other family members of patients. Because many companies do not recognize relationships outside of legal marriage, gay and lesbian partners may have limited health care insurance benefits, family leave, or bereavement leave.

Subtle heterosexual assumptions may arise in nursing communication. For example, the nurse may assume that a patient is heterosexual until the patient does or says something to disprove this. Consider the simple intake question, "Are you single, married, or divorced?" How would a patient with an unmarried partner respond? Some gays and lesbians may choose to hide their sexual orientations because of the heterosexual assumptions and fear of negative attitudes from health care providers or lack of confidentiality and family conflicts (The Joint Commission, 2012). A more inclusive, sensitive, and ultimately better question is, "Do you live alone or with someone?" because it provides a more direct avenue for finding out about support at home.

You may be afraid of behaving incorrectly with patients whose sexual orientation differs from your own. This fear can lead to insecurity and cause misunderstandings. Emotions such as uncertainty may lead to incongruent or "double" messages in communication. As a professional, you must be knowledgeable about gay patients, same-sex families, and gay culture in order to communicate naturally and to be aware of the assumptions communicated through language and behavior.

Phases of the Interview Process

As a nurse, you organize interviews to use time efficiently and help patients to feel that their needs are met. You are rewarded in the relationship by being able to help others.

Preinteraction Phase

Before meeting with the patient, you collect data from the medical record, including the previous history of medical illnesses or surgeries, current medication list, and problem list if these are available. You use this information to conduct the interview; it is helpful if you already know about some of the past situations and responses to treatments (Fig. 2.5). Review the record chronologically to detect patterns of illness such as declining functional status and to identify how things fit together. For example, a patient who was diagnosed with breast cancer had a mastectomy, developed postoperative infection and lung injury, and now is on oxygen. The record in this case assists in identifying why this patient with breast cancer has been placed on oxygen at home. The amount of information available in the preinteraction phase varies; for example, only a medical diagnosis may be available on the patient being admitted to the hospital for the first time.

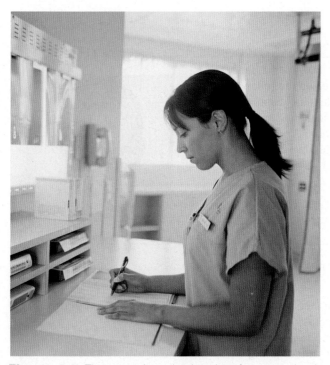

Figure 2.5 The nurse is reviewing data from a patient's medical record before meeting with the patient to conduct the initial interview.

Beginning Phase

Introduce yourself by name and state the purpose of the interview. An example is, "Hello, my name is Sam, and I am going to be your nurse this evening." At this moment, it is appropriate to ask the patient how he or she would like to be addressed. You can simply say, "What name would you prefer me to use?" Listen carefully for the correct pronunciation and, if necessary, ask the patient for confirmation that the pronunciation is correct. Shake hands if that seems comfortable for the patient and is appropriate for the setting.

To relax the patient, you may continue the beginning phase with a discussion of some neutral areas, such as the weather, especially if you note anxiety. Move through such discussion quickly, however, and introduce the purpose of the interview. For example, "Mrs. Lewis, I will need to ask you some questions about your personal and family history." You may also make some overall remarks based on the patient's record, such as "You have been in the nurse's office for a cold three times in the last 3 weeks. It doesn't seem like your cold is going away."

Privacy is essential, especially considering the Health Insurance Portability and Accountability Act (HIPAA) guidelines (U.S. Department of Health & Human Services [USDHHS], 2014) for confidentiality of information (see Chapter 4). Pull drapes around patients if conducting the interview in a hospital room or close the door if working in an examination room. In community settings where patients are disclosing personal information, identify an area where others cannot overhear the conversation before beginning.

Working Phase

During the working phase, you collect data by asking specific questions. Two types of questions used to collect information are closed-ended and open-ended questions. Each type has a purpose; you choose which type will better help elicit the appropriate information.

Closed-ended or **direct questions** are best for specific information that yields yes or no answers, such as, "Do you have a family history of heart disease?" In clinical settings, these questions commonly appear on forms that patients complete before meeting the nurse. During the interview, review completed forms with the patient, asking follow-up questions and clarifying information that the patient listed as problematic. You can also use closed-ended questions (e.g., "Is your pain sharp or dull?") to help cue patients who have had difficulty responding to an open-ended question. Closed-ended questions are also helpful for patients with communication challenges, such as those with dementia or limited knowledge of English.

Open-ended questions require patients to give more than yes or no answers. They are broad and yield responses in the patient's own words. Sometimes these answers are put in quotation marks in documentation. Examples of open-ended questions are, "What does your pain feel like?" and "How are you doing with the low-salt diet?"

You should avoid "why" questions because patients may find them difficult to answer and may view such inquiries as too interrogative or personal. Patients also may view such questions as accusatory and judgmental. For example, "Why haven't you stopped smoking?" is an example of a nontherapeutic leading or biased question as compared with the more therapeutic question, "Tell me about how difficult it is for you to stop smoking."

During the working phase, you also chart the patient's history and health problems. The goal is to achieve a balance between listening and documenting. Sometimes, documentation is on paper; at other times, you record on a computer. When using a computer, position yourself so that you can record data while maintaining eye contact with the patient and the patient's family (Fig. 2.6). If using paper to document, you may find that a clipboard placed in your lap allows you to record information without obstructing eye contact with the patient. Usually, you record unexpected findings during the interview and then return to the form later to note the absence of findings and other descriptions. This method allows you to maintain better eye contact with the patient during the interview. It takes practice to achieve a comfortable blend of recording assessments and listening.

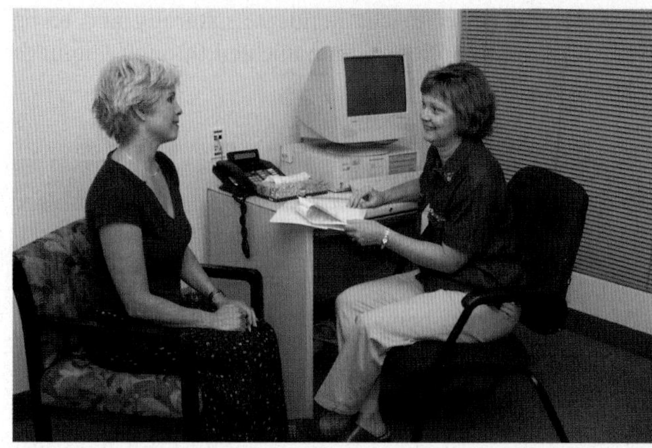

Figure 2.6 This nurse has situated herself so that she can talk and maintain eye contact with the patient while being able to record pertinent findings electronically.

Closing Phase

You end the interview by summarizing and stating what the two to three most important patterns or problems might be. For example, you might say, "It seems that you are most concerned about control of your pain. Would you agree?" Additionally, you can close the interview by letting the patient know the next steps, such as, "I'll make sure to put in your plan of care to ask about your pain level every hour." You also ask whether the patient would like to mention anything or needs anything else. Doing so gives the patient a final opportunity to express needs and feel that he or she has been heard. If you are using a checklist, the closing phase is a good time to review it for completeness and to make notes about future interventions. Thank the patient and family members for taking the time to provide information as you end the interview.

It is important to keep in mind that the initial meeting and interview with the patient are critical to the visit or hospital stay. It is the patient's initial perception of the setting and its care providers. In the acute care setting, the rapport that is developed may set the tone for the remainder of the patient's stay.

Progress Note: Analyzing Findings

After the initial interview, the student nurse assesses Mr. Rowan, the patient who has AIDS in the opening case study. The assessment revealed the following subjective and objective data. Begin to think about how the data are clustered and what additional data the nurse might want to collect. The nurse also uses critical thinking to analyze problems and anticipate nursing interventions. The following nursing note illustrates the use of diagnostic reasoning and nursing process.

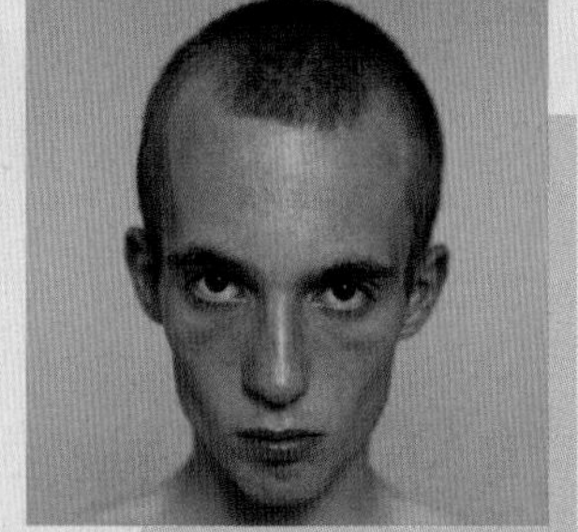

Subjective: "I'd rather be home, but I can't live by myself anymore. Every day I just seem to get weaker."

Objective: Appears slightly anxious and weak. Gait slow but steady. Can heat prepared meals in kitchen; housekeeping comes weekly for cleaning. Bathroom with grab bars by shower and toilet. No loose cords or rugs. Environment clean and without clutter. Pill count accurate. Dressing, grooming, and toileting independently.

(case study continues on page 31)

Analysis: Risk for impaired home maintenance and increasing weakness with disease progression.

Plan: Continue with meal and housekeeping services. Continue to assess for needs related to dressing, grooming, toileting, and meals. Further discuss nutrition and dietary supplements in addition to adherence to the medication regimen.

Critical Thinking Challenge

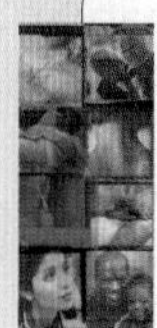

- What fears or concerns might the nurse have about visiting this setting or working with this patient?
- What elements should the nurse include when closing the interview process with Mr. Rowan?

SAFETY ALERT

If an interview reveals confidential material, disclose those things required to be reported by law, such as suicidal thoughts, violence at home, or rape. Inform the patient at the beginning of the interview that you must report harm to self or others to get needed assistance. You should notify authorities only after ensuring the victim's safety.

Health History Sources

Primary and Secondary Data Sources

The individual patient is considered the **primary data** source. Charts and information from family members are considered **secondary data** sources. When possible, patients provide subjective information regarding their health behaviors and situations. Subjective information is from the perspective of the patient. Secondary sources are all other sources of information.

Reliability of the Source

Record the person who provides the information as well as their reliability. A **reliable historian** provides information that is consistent with existing records and comprehensive in scope. If information differs from past descriptions, or if details change each time, the patient may be unreliable or considered an **inaccurate historian**. Note any discrepancies and identify other sources (i.e., previous records) to confirm the history.

Components of the Health History

Usually, you collect demographic data first and then elicit from the patient a complete description of the reason for seeking health care because that information usually is most important. How much additional data you collect depends on the reason for the visit, pertinence of the data, and time restrictions within the setting. Determine which data to collect beyond the minimum required.

Data may be collected in an emergency, during a visit for a specific problem (e.g., shoulder pain), or during a wellness visit. Refer to Table 2.1 to compare and contrast emergency, focused, and comprehensive health histories. The following sections explain the components of the comprehensive health history.

Demographic Data

Depending on the health care setting, personnel at a front desk or admissions department often collect demographic data from patients, including name, address, and billing information (Fig. 2.7). Occupation and insurance may be sensitive issues for some patients. In such cases, explain the reason for asking about them, such as, "Sometimes people are concerned about how they will pay for their care. Do you have any insurance or financial concerns with which you might like help?"

Demographic data include environmental data about exposure to contagious diseases, travel to high-risk areas, and concerns about exposure to pollution, hazards, and allergens. For hospitalized patients, assess housing information to identify the level of independence and support needed following discharge. Additional considerations for discharge planning and referral to home care services include number of stairs and concerns about structural barriers. Collect occupational information to evaluate the ability of patients to work safely and return to work if an illness is present. Assess any concerns about occupational hazards, personal protective equipment, handicapped access, and adaptive devices.

Reason for Seeking Care

The reason for seeking care is a brief statement, usually in the patient's own words, about why he or she is making the visit.

TABLE 2.1 Types of Health Histories

Type	Purpose	Components
Emergency	Nurses collect the most important information and defer obtaining details until patients are stable. They elicit the reason for seeking care along with current health problems, medications, and allergies.	Care focuses on gathering information so that interventions can resolve the immediate problem. Assessments and interventions are concurrent.
Focused	The focused health history involves questions that relate to the current situation.	An example is the patient visiting the primary care provider about a cough. In this case, the nurse asks about the length, severity, and timing of the cough and other related factors. During focused health histories, nurses do not perform a complete review of systems (discussed later).
Comprehensive	The comprehensive health history takes place during an annual physical examination, for sports participation screenings, and during a hospital admission.	It includes demographic data, a full description of the reason for seeking care, individual health history, family history, functional status, and a history in all physical and psychosocial areas.

You can ask, "Tell me why you came to the clinic today," or "What happened that brought you to the hospital?" Record this information in the subjective part of documentation; consider putting the statement in quotes. If a patient replies by giving a medical diagnosis, such as "heart attack," encourage the patient to describe symptoms, such as "shortness of breath and chest pain." When taking the health history, you record the **symptoms**, or subjective sensations or feelings of patients, versus the **signs**, or objective information that you will assess during the physical examination.

Date of Interview: __________

Patient Name: __________

Gender: ____ Date of Birth: __________ Age: ____

Primary Language: __________

Religious Preference: __________

Marital Status: S M W D Other

Address: __________

____

Type of Dwelling: __________ Transportation: __________

Emergency Contact: __________

____

Occupation: __________ Insurance: __________

Information obtained from: Patient __________ Other __________

Figure 2.7 A sample of a demographic data form completed during arrival at or admission to a health care facility.

History of Present Illness

Collect information about the present illness by beginning with open-ended questions and having the patient explain symptoms. A complete description of the present illness is essential to an accurate diagnosis. Additionally, you should ask questions about the symptoms in six to eight categories to assist the patient to be more specific and complete. For example, if a patient states, "I've been having some abdominal pain," ask questions to try to find out its source and associated symptoms.

Some providers use a mnemonic to remember the elements that are important to assess for the presenting symptom. Examples are as follows:

- OLDCARTS (*o*nset, *l*ocation, *d*uration, *c*haracter, *a*ssociated or aggravating factors, *r*elieving factors, *t*iming, *s*everity)
- PQRSTU (*p*rovocative or palliative, *q*uality, *r*egion, *s*everity, *t*iming, *u*nderstanding patient perception)
- COLDSPA (*c*haracter, *o*nset, *l*ocation, *d*uration, *s*everity, *p*attern, *a*ssociated factors/how it affects the patient)
- Location, duration, intensity, description, aggravating factors, alleviating factors, pain goal, and functional impairment (see Chapter 6)

Regardless of the order of the data, guide the conversation following the cues of the patient, and use a mental checklist to ensure that you have assessed all categories before the end of history taking.

Location

Ask, "Where does it hurt?" and observe the patient's nonverbal cues. If the patient has difficulty describing the location, you might ask, "Show me where it hurts," and note not only the location but also nonverbal responses. If a patient points to a location, the area of pain is more specific than if he or she circles with the palm of the hand over a broad area.

Duration

Duration refers to the timing and frequency of the problem. To establish duration, ask, "When did you first notice the pain?" and record the date and time specifically (month and year) instead of documenting "yesterday." In this way, future health care providers can easily identify the date. Duration also refers to whether the pain is constant or intermittent, how long it lasts, and whether it goes completely away or cycles off and on. There are differences in the assessment of acute, chronic, and neuropathic pain (see Chapter 6).

Intensity

Ask the patient, "How bad does it hurt?" To provide a quantifying measurement, ask the patient to rate his or her pain on a 0-to-10 scale, with 0 being no pain and 10 being the worst imaginable. Other pain scales use faces and descriptors (see Chapter 6).

Quality/Description

Ask the patient, "What does the pain/discomfort feel like?" If the patient cannot describe it, provide cues by asking, "Is it sharp or dull?" or "Is it stabbing or more achy?" A question for associated symptoms is, "Do you notice anything else when you have the pain?" If patients have difficulty understanding the question, you may ask, "When you have the pain, do you notice any sweating?" (which is common with chest pain) or "Do you notice a special feeling before you have a seizure?" to evaluate for an aura (common preceding a seizure).

Aggravating/Alleviating Factors

Ask the patient, "Is there anything that you notice that makes it worse?" regarding aggravating factors. "What were you doing when you noticed the pain?" A possible follow-up question would be, "Is there anything that you notice that consistently causes or happens with the pain?" Assess for relieving factors by asking, "What seems to make it better?" or "What have you tried to make it go away?"

Pain Goal

Ask the patient, "What is an acceptable level of pain?" or "What do you hope that we can get your pain down to?" A pain goal should be set to allow patients to perform the most important activities easily. Usually, a goal of zero to mild pain (0 to 3 on a 10-point scale) is acceptable.

Functional Goal

Pain can affect the ability to perform common movements and tasks. Assess the effects of pain on the patient's functional ability by questioning the patient about sitting, rising from a chair, standing for a while, climbing stairs, shopping, driving, and participating in sports. Pain is dynamic and increases with activity.

Past Health History

The past health history includes an assessment of medical and surgical problems along with the treatment and course. Some problems are acute, others resolve, and others are chronic. Document dates of initial diagnosis and surgeries—for example, "Appendectomy 2003; testicular cancer 1/2006; orchiectomy 2/2006; chemotherapy with cisplatin, etoposide, and bleomycin 3/2006; currently in remission." Also note any serious accidents and injuries. When documenting past medical and surgical history, it is important to note any sequelae or ongoing problems. Chart events chronologically when possible so that future readers can easily identify the sequence. Note current problems on the problem list.

For female patients, note the obstetric history, including number of pregnancies (gravida) and number of births (para). If any pregnancies are incomplete, document the reason (e.g., spontaneous abortion).

Include in the record any childhood illnesses with potentially lasting effects (e.g., polio, varicella). Also, record the date of the most recent immunizations for tetanus; pertussis; polio; measles; rubella; mumps; influenza; hepatitis A, B, and C; and pneumococcus. Also ask about screening tests and the results, such as tuberculin skin test, Pap smear, mammogram, colonoscopy, stool for occult blood, cholesterol, and blood pressure. Document the date of the last physical assessment.

Current Medications and Indications

Ask patients about current medications, including name, dose, route, and frequency. Identify the purpose of each medication because some drugs have more than one use. For example, one patient may take a beta-blocker for blood pressure control, whereas another may take the same drug to prevent a second myocardial infarction. Additionally, query the patient about any over-the-counter medications, supplements, or herbal remedies in use. If the patient is confused about any medication, ask the patient or family member to bring in the pill bottles to ensure accuracy (Fig. 2.8). For hospitalized patients, you must reconcile all medication lists with medications taken regularly at home so that patients continue using the correct drugs (The Joint Commission, 2014). It is important to explain to patients that any medications may interact with disease processes or with additional medications being given, for example, in the hospital.

Verify allergies with patients and compared those stated their medical records. When asking about allergies, it is essential to note the type of response, such as rash, throat swelling, difficulty breathing, or anaphylactic shock. Some patients may confuse an adverse effect or adverse reaction with an allergy; these should also be noted. For example, a patient may become nauseous when given opiates, but you should note this response as an adverse reaction. You would chart a response that includes throat swelling and difficulty breathing as an allergic reaction. It is critical to document both the medication and the patient's reaction to it for future reference. Allergies must be appropriately noted in the chart, and the hospitalized patient must have a name band applied noting the allergy.

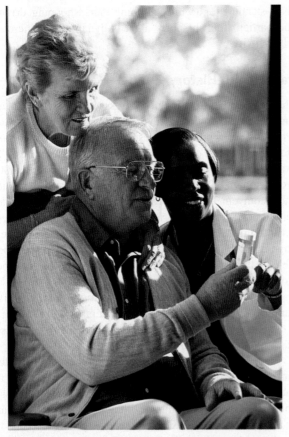

Figure 2.8 It can be helpful for patients who are taking multiple medications, supplements, and over-the-counter drugs to bring these with them to health assessment appointments.

Family History

Ask the patient about the health of close family members (i.e., parents, grandparents, siblings) to help identify those diseases for which the patient may be at risk and to provide counseling and health teaching. The following familial conditions are important to note: high blood pressure, coronary artery disease, high cholesterol, stroke, cancer, diabetes mellitus, obesity, alcoholism, drug addiction, and mental illness. Additionally, obtain the health history of children and identify patterns of disease that might be genetically transmitted. Ideally, the family history is recorded in a centralized area on a computer, and all health care providers can contribute.

A common tool used to understand family patterns is the genogram (Fig. 2.9). This graphic representation allows you to map family structures and compile a large amount of information visually. Genograms make it easier for you to identify the complexity of families and validate patterns pertinent to patients. A complete family history can take as little as 15 minutes or as long as 2 hours. Each family member is represented by a box (male) or circle (female). The patient is noted by using an arrow or doubling the line. Sometimes, the nuclear family is circled. Marriages are identified by lines between people; divorces are indicated by placing a double slash through the line. Deaths are noted by the use of an X inside the box or circle. Children are linked to parents through a vertical line, beginning with the eldest on the left. The medical history is listed below the symbol. A key is included to clarify the meaning of symbols. This graphic representation compiles information into a concise pattern of family history.

Functional Health Assessment

Functional health patterns (Table 2.2) are especially important to nursing because they focus on the effects of health or illness on a patient's quality of life. By using this approach, you can assess the strengths of patients as well as areas needing improvement (Gordon, 1987). Some of the questions are personal and difficult to answer, so it is best to thread the questions throughout the history and address the more personal questions toward the end of the conversation. As you give care, you can integrate these questions into other activities, such as giving a bath or chatting before the next appointment, instead of sitting down and asking the questions in a structured and sequenced order. Identify issues that may be potential problems for patients and prioritize to ask those first.

You also assess the patient's ability to perform self-care activities, or **activities of daily living (ADLs)**. These include behaviors such as eating, dressing, and grooming. You score

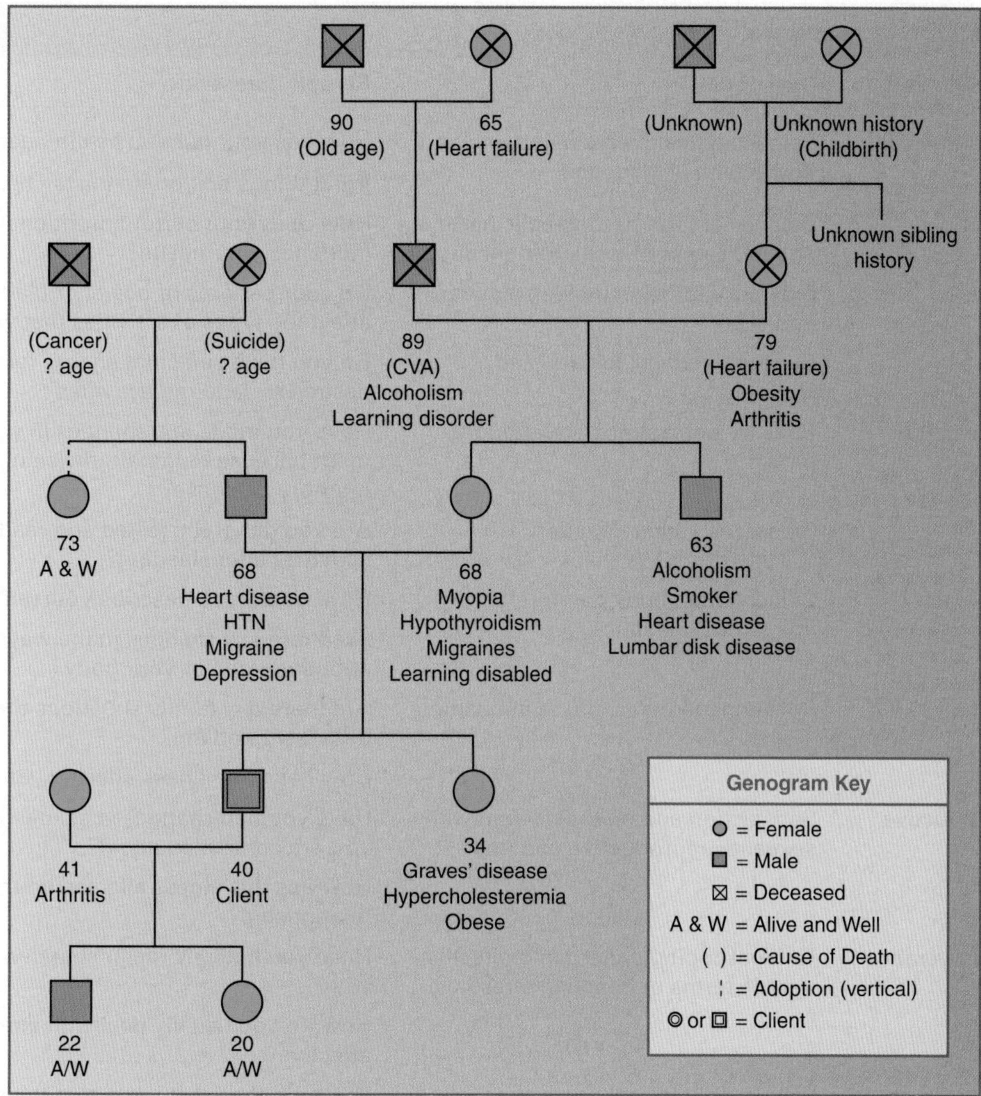

Figure 2.9 An example of a genogram.

these items based on whether the patient is totally independent, needs assistance from a person or device (e.g., a cane), or is dependent on others. See Box 2.3.

Growth and Development

During the health history with pediatric populations, observe growth to determine how children compare with peers. Assess physical activities, fine and gross motor skills, and speech. Developmental assessment of infants, children, and adolescents is especially important to determine the achievement of developmental milestones and to gain awareness of deficits to facilitate early intervention and management.

Psychosocial development is part of assessment for all age groups, because even some adults have delays and do not progress as expected. For example, abuse of drugs and alcohol can interfere with relationships, employment, and housing. A patient who has a drug or alcohol problem may not reach the generativity stage but instead remains self-absorbed. For all patients, you should also carefully evaluate the cognitive stage; this is especially pertinent for those at either end of the lifespan. Assess that younger patients are appropriately developing abstract thinking skills, and evaluate older patients for any signs of memory decline. Refer to Chapter 8 for more complete information on the assessment of growth and development.

Review of Systems

The **review of systems** is a series of questions about all body systems that helps to reveal concerns as part of a comprehensive health assessment. In a clinical setting, the patient usually fills out a form that asks for pertinent information; you then review the answers with the patient to obtain a more complete and accurate history. You may ask the patient about any symptoms related to each body system, such as a cough regarding the respiratory system. You may also integrate these questions during the physical examination of each region, such as asking about chest pain when listening to the heart. The systems review can vary in sequence and format based on the setting, the acuity or degree of illness (and thus urgency of the problem),

TABLE 2.2 Gordon's Functional Health Patterns

Functional Health Pattern	Description	Sample Questions
Health perception/health management	Perceived health and well-being and how health is managed	How has your general health been? What things do you do to stay healthy?
Nutrition/metabolic	Balance of food to metabolic need and indicators of local nutrient supply	How does your current nutritional status influence your health?
Elimination	Excretory function (bowel, bladder, and skin)	Do your patterns of bowel or bladder habits affect the types of activities that you do?
Activity/exercise	Exercise, activity, leisure, and recreation	Do you have sufficient energy for completing desired or required activities?
Cognition/perception	Sensory perceptions and thought patterns	Have you made any changes in your environment because of impaired vision, hearing, or memory decrease?
Sleep/rest	Sleep, rest, and relaxation	Are you generally rested and ready for activities after sleeping?
Self-perception/self-concept	Self-concept, body comfort, body image, feeling state	How would you describe yourself? Are there any changes in the way that you feel about yourself or your body?
Role/relationship	Role engagements and relationships	Are there any family situations that you have difficulty handling? How has your illness affected your family?
Sexuality/reproductive	Satisfaction and dissatisfaction with sexuality, reproductive patterns	Have you had changes in sexual relations that you are concerned about? How has this illness affected your sexual relationship?
Coping/stress tolerance	General coping pattern and effectiveness in terms of handling stress	Have you had any major changes in the past year? How do you usually deal with stress? Is it effective?
Values/beliefs	Values, beliefs (including spiritual), or goals that guide choices or decisions	What are the most important things to you in life? What gives you hope when times are troubled?

BOX 2.3 Activities of Daily Living

Self-Care Activities
Eating
Bathing
Dressing
Grooming
Toileting

Mobility
Walking: miles, blocks, across a room
Climbing stairs, up or down
Balance
Grasping small objects, opening jars
Reaching out, down, or overhead
Use of devices

Home Maintenance
Heavy housekeeping: vacuuming, scrubbing floors, making beds
Light housekeeping: dusting, wiping surfaces, dishes
Washing laundry
Cooking
Shopping
Managing finances
Driving

and the style of the nurse. In the review of systems, data collected is subjective information; **objective data**, or that completed in the physical assessment, is documented separately.

In addition to the problems covered in a review of systems, you also obtain information from the patient about health promotion practices and provide teaching about areas of interest or concern. Usually, you begin with a general question, such as, "How is your appetite?" and progress more specifically, such as, "Have you had any nausea, food intolerances or allergies, or gastric reflux?" For healthy behaviors, you may ask, "What types of foods do you eat to stay healthy?" In the review, you document not only the presence of findings but also the absence of problems or symptoms, such as "No nausea, constipation, or diarrhea."

It is good practice to logically organize your approach to the review. Most patients are unaware of the order you are following, however, so they also might remember other symptoms when talking about another topic. The conversation may be out of order from the usual body systems format. If a patient forgets to mention symptoms associated with the presenting problem, document those symptoms with the presenting situation. If the patient forgets to mention major health events, document them with the health history. When you arrive at the section of the review that includes the presenting situation, ask only those questions that have not yet been covered. Explain to the patient that, although the review is lengthy, it is an opportunity to double check for completeness and accuracy of past and current problems. When documenting findings, reorganize the information so that data regarding a problem is clustered together. For example, if a patient is nauseous and vomiting, you may cluster together findings from the nutrition—hydration, skin, and abdominal assessments.

Box 2.4 presents a list of topics covered during the review of systems; note that the questions are not mutually exclusive. For example, weight gain or loss is part of the general health state, but it also provides information about fluid

BOX 2.4 Review of Systems

- **General health state.** Weight gain or loss, fatigue, weakness, malaise, pain, usual activity, fever, chills.
- **Nutrition and hydration.** A history of conditions that increase the risk of malnutrition or obesity. Nausea, vomiting. Normal daily intake, weight and weight change noting if changes were intentional or not, dehydration, dry skin, fluid excess with shortness of breath, or edema in the feet and legs. Diet practices to promote health.
- **Skin, hair, and nails.** A history of skin, hair, or nail disease. Rash, itching, pigmentation or texture change, lesions, sweating, dry skin, hair loss or change in texture, brittle or thin nails, thick or yellow nails.
- **Head and neck.** A history of high or low thyroid hormone level. Headaches, syncope, dizziness, sinus pain.
- **Eyes.** A history of poor vision or vision problems, glaucoma, cataracts, hearing loss, ear infections. Use of contact lenses or glasses, change in vision, blurring, diplopia, light sensitivity, burning, redness, discharge. Last eye examination and any changes at that time.
- **Ears.** A history of ear or hearing problems. Ear pain, change in hearing, tinnitus, vertigo. Last hearing evaluation and results, ear protection.
- **Nose, mouth, and throat.** A history of mouth or throat cancer. Colds, sore throat, nasal obstruction, nosebleeds, cold sores, bleeding or swollen gums, tooth pain, tooth extractions, implants, dental caries, ulcers, enlarged tonsils, dry mouth or lips. Difficulty chewing or swallowing, change in voice. Last dental cleaning and exam, results.
- **Thorax and lungs.** A history of emphysema, asthma, or lung cancer. Wheezing, cough, sputum, dyspnea, last chest x-ray and results, last tuberculin skin test and results.
- **Heart and neck vessels.** A history of congenital heart problems, myocardial infarction, heart surgery, heart failure, arrhythmia, murmur. Chest pain or discomfort, palpitations, exercise tolerance. Any screening tests such as ECG or stress test, screening for cholesterol and triglycerides, and results for any of these tests.
- **Peripheral vascular.** A history of high blood pressure, peripheral vascular disease, thrombophlebitis, blood clots, peripheral edema, ulcers, circulation, claudication, redness, pain, tenderness. Any screening tests such as an ankle-brachial index and results.
- **Breasts.** A history of breast cancer or cystic breast condition. For adolescents, concerns about breast changes. Pain, tenderness, discharge, lumps, last mammogram and results, frequency and date of last self-examination.
- **Abdominal-gastrointestinal.** A history of colon cancer, gastrointestinal bleeding, cholelithiasis, liver failure, hepatitis, pancreatitis, colitis, ulcer, or gastric reflux. Appetite, nausea, vomiting, diarrhea. Food intolerance or allergy, constipation, diarrhea, change in stool color, blood in stool. Last sigmoidoscopy, colonoscopy, stool for occult blood and results.
- **Abdominal-urinary.** Renal failure, polycystic kidney disease, urinary tract infection, nephrolithiasis. Pain, change in urine, dysuria, urgency, frequency, nocturia, incontinence. For children, toilet training, bed-wetting.
- **Musculoskeletal.** A history of injury, arthritis. Joint stiffness, pain, swelling, restricted movement, deformity, change in gait or coordination, strength. Pain, cramps, weakness.
- **Neurological.** A history of head or brain injury, stroke, seizures. Tremors, memory loss, numbness or tingling, loss of sensation or coordination.
- **Male genitalia.** A history of undescended testicle, hernia, testicular cancer. Pain, burning, lesions, discharge, swelling. Change in penis or scrotum, protection against pregnancy and sexually transmitted infections. Testicular self-examination, frequency.
- **Female genitalia.** A history of ovarian or uterine cancer, ovarian cyst, endometriosis, number of pregnancies and children. Pain, burning, lesions, discharge, itching, rash. Menstrual and physical changes, protection against pregnancy and sexually transmitted infections. Last Pap smear and results.
- **Anus, rectum, and prostate.** A history of hemorrhoids; prostate cancer; benign prostatic hyperplasia; urinary incontinence, pain, burning, itching; for men, hesitancy, dribbling, loss in force of urine stream. Screening PSA test and result.
- **Endocrine and hematological system.** A history of diabetes mellitus, high or low thyroid levels, anemia. Polydipsia, polyuria, unexplained weight gain or loss, changes in body hair and body fat distribution, intolerance to heat or cold, excessive bruising, lymph node swelling. Result of last blood glucose test.

balance, edema, and appetite. Adapt topics to the patient and direct conversation in a way that is comfortable and logical. Omit topics that do not apply and add topics that seem pertinent. Although the list in Box 2.4 uses medical terminology, you should use common lay language so that the patient better understands the topics and questions. These questions are further explored in the individual chapters of this text.

Psychosocial and Lifestyle Factors

Psychosocial and lifestyle issues may naturally arise during the review of systems. Because many of these questions are personal, it is best to ask them at the end of the interview, after a rapport has developed and trust has been established. Some examples of areas that involve sensitive questions are sexual orientation, risk for domestic violence, and drug use (see Chapter 9).

Social, Cultural, and Spiritual Assessment

You assess overall psychosocial well-being as part of the screening of the functional health patterns, including self-perception/self-concept, role/relationships, and coping/stress tolerance. You obtain detailed information when patients have a history of psychosocial situations or indicators of current distress. You also assess cultural beliefs and health practices that may influence care.

You assess spirituality and belief systems during the functional health screening questions related to values or beliefs. Additionally, you evaluate specific spiritual beliefs, religious preferences (including whether it is an organized religion or independent), and the rituals and practices that may affect health status. You can use this information to support the patient during times when hope and guidance are needed. You also ask about religious preference so that referral to pastoral care can be initiated, if that is the patient's preference.

See Chapter 10 for more complete information on cultural, spiritual, and social assessment.

Mental Health Assessment

If the patient is anxious, depressed, or sounds illogical, or if an association exists between current physical status and psychiatric concerns, mental health requires a closer examination. You may ask the patient, "Describe any changes that you have had in your mood or feelings." and "Have you ever been treated for any problems with your mood or behavior?" Note medications during the initial history and ask follow-up questions regarding the purpose and effectiveness of any psychiatric drugs. Additionally, you may use specific techniques for psychiatric screening, such as a depression screening tool or a full mental status examination. When the primary concern is psychiatric, you perform a complete mental health assessment (see Chapter 9).

You assess alcohol and drug use by direct questioning and also observation of behaviors that indicate impairment, such as slurred speech, nodding off, and unstable gait. Although this may be an uncomfortable area for beginners to ask about, most patients recognize that you need information to avoid medication interactions, evaluate the effects of use on the current illness or injury, and refer to treatment programs to improve health. For example, you may ask, "How many alcoholic drinks are usual for you in a week?" or "Do you use any recreational drugs?" To normalize the response, you might say, "A lot of college students like to party. If you party, how much do you usually drink?" You also assess tobacco use directly by asking, "Have you ever smoked cigarettes, vaporizers, a pipe, cigars, or chewed tobacco?" If the patient answers yes to this question, ask how many packs of cigarettes, cigars, pouches or plugs of chewing tobacco per day and for how long.

For a complete assessment of drug and alcohol use, see Chapter 9.

Human Violence Assessment

Because of the high prevalence of physical abuse of children and women, especially during pregnancy, it is often the policy in health care agencies that nurses routinely question patients about this (Centers for Disease Control and Prevention, 2013). Because of the sensitive nature of the topic, you should pose questions so that the patient feels comfortable talking. Examples include, "Some women have experienced being hurt by someone. Within the past year, have you been hurt either physically or sexually by anyone?" and "Sometimes your mom or dad might get angry with you. What happens when your mom or dad gets mad?"

You should suspect abuse if injuries are inconsistent with explanations, if the story changes over time, if the patient has delayed getting treatment, if there is a past history of injuries or accidents, if there is associated drug or alcohol abuse, or if there is a history of mental illness. Commonly, the patient's abuser is overly protective, may refuse to leave the room, or dominates the interview. Abused children may be overly attentive in an attempt to please the parent or guardian. Refer to Chapter 9 for more information.

> *SAFETY ALERT*
> *When child or elder abuse is suspected, you are obligated to report it to a supervisor and obtain assistance from social work or case management for further assessment. In some states, permission is required of the victim of domestic abuse because of the increased risk when the abuser is aware. Document findings objectively in the medical record and avoid judgment (see Chapter 9).*

Sexual History and Orientation

The comprehensive history includes sexual history and sexual orientation to establish a baseline for health behaviors and identify the need for education. This may be another uncomfortable area for beginning nurses to ask about, but you need to recognize that these questions can provide information that allows for health teaching to prevent disease and illness. Consider sexual history and pattern as a topic for health promotion, especially in high-risk patients such as those with multiple partners or having unprotected sex. You can introduce these questions during discussions of reproductive function or healthy behaviors or during the personal and social histories.

You may say, "As part of your physical examination, we like to provide information on healthy sexual practices. Would you like information about safer sex?" Some other questions are, "Have you had intimate contact, oral sex, or intercourse in the past year?" "How many partners have you had in the past year?" and "What measures do you take to protect yourself from sexually transmitted infections?" Avoid bias about sexual orientation, sexual practices, culture, age, and marital status.

It is good to provide opportunities for younger children to ask questions about sexuality; this can increase patients' comfort level in discussing sexual topics with health care providers later in life. Conversely, do not omit the discussion of sexual history and orientation with members of the aging population, who may remain sexually active.

Lifespan Considerations

Parents, legal guardians, or other adult representatives serve as primary interview sources of health care information when patients are children. As they age and become more independent, children can participate more fully in interviews. Elderly patients may, in some cases, also have a legal guardian.

When obtaining information from a guardian, be sure to address the patient as well. For example, with a pediatric patient, address the child by name and make eye contact with the child as well as the guardian. In the case of an elderly patient who has a family member along, focus the interview on the patient rather than making the assumption that you should collect the information from the family member rather than the patient. Be sure to validate the roles of people bringing children to the attention of the health care facility. For example, a mother may be accompanied by a boyfriend who is not the child's father; a stepparent may bring in a child; or a child of gay parents may have two mothers or fathers. For the elderly, roles of others present during the interview should also be established.

It is important to address parents by the names they prefer. It in unprofessional to call parents "mom" or "dad." Address children by their first names. Nonverbal communication is very important with young children, who may have limited verbal skills. Toddlers and preschoolers are quick to notice anxiety, pain, distress, or discomfort in either a caregiver or a nurse. Health care settings may provoke anxiety in children because many have had immunizations and tests that involved pain or discomfort. Instead of the formality found in other settings, pediatric and family practice settings usually are colorful, and many health care providers there wear playful bright clothing as well. These environments are child proofed, so parents and providers need to worry less about supervising their child for safety and feel more comfortable and relaxed and thus are more likely to provide accurate assessment data.

You collect the health history for infants from parents (Fig. 2.10). As children move into adolescence, you may interview the parent and adolescent together. The relationship between the adolescent and the parent determines how you collect data. It may be more comfortable and reliable to ask questions regarding sexual activity and recreational drug use with the parent absent. You may ask parents to step out of the room for a moment.

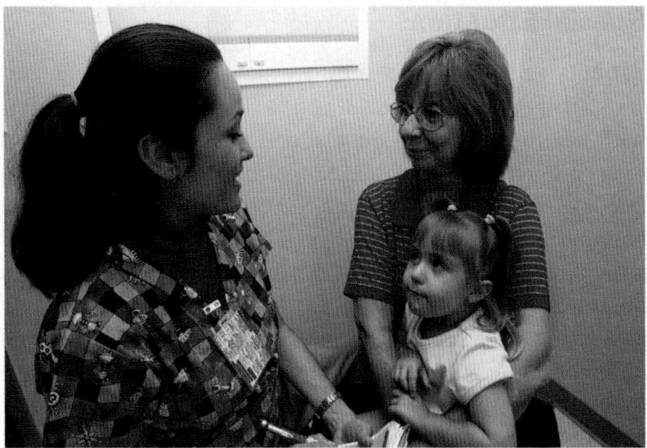

Figure 2.10 The nurse relies on parents and other caregivers to supply health history information for infants and children.

When taking the health history for a child, it is especially important to include the pregnancy, birth, and perinatal histories. Also ask about immunizations and growth and development. Assess family structure, function, and home environment. In addition, ask about dietary intake and practices because food choices change at each age (see Chapters 26 and 27).

Older Adults

With older adults, be aware of the increased risk for sensory deficits that might alter the history taking, such as loss of vision or hearing. Also, older adults may have more complex histories because of their increased prevalence of disease and may require some additional time to process information. It is important to identify the pattern of the illnesses and recognize how they might be related. In addition to the increased risk of illness because of family history, lifestyle choices also begin to influence health later in life (see Chapter 28).

Cultural Considerations

Cultural factors influence the beliefs of patients about their health status. As previously discussed, you should consider religious and spiritual, social, political, economic, and educational factors that influence beliefs and care decisions. You should also be aware of illnesses that are more common among certain groups of patients, such as diabetes or genetically inherited diseases. Questions about the patient's environment might include safety in the home, transportation issues, or community involvement. The environmental assessment is necessary to evaluate the risk of exposure to hazardous substances. An exposure history includes the agent, length of exposure, and type of exposure. You can use this information to make a referral for further evaluation and follow-up if necessary.

Special Situations

Patients in health care settings may have emotional responses. Fears about illness, results from tests, interactions with health care professionals, and other factors may lead to crying, anxiety, or anger. Sometimes, problems arise related to sexual aggression or the crossing of professional boundaries. Other patients have special situations that require altering the usual approach to interviewing. Examples include hearing impairment, reduced level of consciousness, and the influence of drugs or alcohol. You can adapt therapeutic techniques to complete the interview in these special cases.

Hearing Impairment

One in three adults older than 70 years of age has some type of hearing loss (National Institute on Deafness and Other Communication Disorders, 2014). If you suspect that a patient has a new or previously unsubstantiated hearing loss, ask, "Just to be sure that you understand, please repeat what I said." For patients using hearing aids, make sure that such devices are turned on and working. Gently touch or use visual signals with a hearing-impaired patient before speaking to him or her to verify that the patient is paying attention. Closing the door may help to limit background noise. To ensure patient understanding, give thorough explanations, provide diagrams and pictures, and supply written information. Have the patient validate understanding by asking open-ended questions.

Many deaf patients communicate through a combination of methods, such as signing, writing, using speech, and moving the lips. They may sign with larger, quicker, and more forceful motions when expressing urgency, fear, or frustration. They may pantomime or use facial expressions to communicate. To facilitate lip reading, sit closer to the patient. Use regular speech volume and lip movement, but speak more slowly. If the patient does not understand, use different wording because the sounds involved may be better decoded.

Low Level of Consciousness

Patients with a low level of consciousness may be unable to communicate to provide answers to interview questions. In such cases, you will need to rely on family members and previous documentation. Physical examination and circumstances surrounding the reduced level of consciousness assume more importance until you have obtained a complete history. Refer to Chapter 22 for more information.

Cognitive Impairment

Patients with dementia often have word-finding difficulties. As dementia increases, they may often substitute sound-alike words and sounds, making conversation difficult to track. It is important to allow these patients time to process as much as possible to avoid a one-sided conversation. Because it is easy to discount the communication as disordered or unreliable, many patients with dementia have unmet needs. Pain, hunger, thirst, and other basic needs that remain unaddressed may produce behaviors that others interpret as anxious or agitated (see Chapter 6). When these nonverbal behaviors are present, it is essential to perform assessments to help identify the source of the problem. Patients with closed-head injuries commonly have difficulties related to attention and social skills. They may need redirection and coaching on the organization and appropriateness of their communication.

Mental Illness

Patients with mental illnesses often have difficulty attending to and sequencing communication. Observe such patients for behaviors that indicate distraction, such as looking around the room or appearing to hear noises. Patients with mental illness may process communication better if it contains clear, short phrases that require one step in thinking rather than complex directions. It also may be helpful to use restatement, reflection, or focusing to redirect conversation to the health topic being assessed (see Chapter 9).

Anxiety

Health care issues can cause great anxiety, which is an expected response to a threat to well-being. Behaviors that indicate anxiety are nail-biting, foot-tapping, sweating, and pacing. A voice may quiver, speech may be rapid, and language or tone may be defensive. These behaviors are an attempt to relieve anxious feelings. A mild level of anxiety heightens awareness of the surroundings and fosters learning and decision making. High levels of anxiety decrease perceptual ability and can progress to panic and immobilizing behavior.

You can use active listening, honesty, and a calm and unhurried manner to reduce anxiety. If anxiety is severe, you can teach the patient breathing and relaxation exercises, use therapeutic touch, and provide structure so that the patient knows that he or she will remain safe.

Crying

Health issues are sensitive; they sometimes pose sad situations for both patients and the nurse. When sensitive issues arise, use therapeutic communication techniques rather than progressing with additional interview questions. If you notice that a patient is sad, you may say, "You look sad when talking about your prognosis" to show empathy for the patient. You can provide support through silence, acknowledging feelings, or offering a tissue (Fig. 2.11). Avoid giving false reassurance. Crying is therapeutic and patients usually feel better after having a chance to express the associated emotions. Grief is an expected part of illness; it is therapeutic to express feelings of grief. At times, you may also become emotional; in this case, it is acceptable to tear up. However, sobbing or frank expression of emotion by the nurse is not therapeutic.

Anger

When patients are angry, listen for the associated themes and avoid becoming defensive or personalizing the situation. As a beginning nurse, you may think you did something wrong and

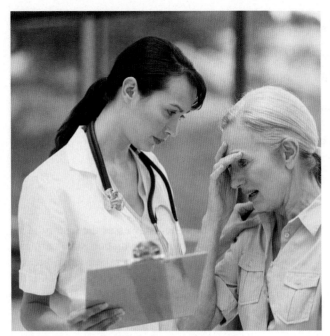

Figure 2.11 The nurse needs to be prepared for emotional reactions to health concerns and challenges from patients and use his or her judgment about the best ways to offer support and provide a caring presence.

feel bad, but usually, anger from a patient does not directly relate to you. Such emotion usually is a response to a situation in which the patient has lost control and feels anxious or helpless. Acknowledge the patient's feelings by saying, "I understand that you are upset about being asked this question another time" or "I'm sorry that you're so angry." The nurse validates and encourages patients to express their feelings. The purpose of talking the emotion through is to help patients connect their emotions with related events.

Alcohol or Drug Use

Patients with chemical impairment have difficulty answering complex questions; use direct and simple questions instead. Interview questions include the type of drug, amount ingested, and date and time of the last drink or use. Explain that this information is important to provide accurate data regarding withdrawal. Patients who have used drugs or alcohol may provide an unreliable history with a story which changes over time. Be aware that memory may be impaired and that drug use and withdrawal can cause confusion. As with patients who have reduced consciousness, you will rely more on the circumstances and physical assessment data with patients who have substance use disorders. As the patient becomes sober and family members are available, you can discuss details about length of use, pattern of use, and related injuries or illnesses.

Personal Questions

When interviewing patients, you ask questions within the nursing role. Some patients do not understand the boundaries that define the nurse–patient relationship and instead may ask you personal questions. This situation can be uncomfortable because you must choose how much (if anything) to disclose. You may briefly provide a response or choose simply to redirect the conversation, keeping it patient-centered. For example, you might say, "My husband is a teacher. Tell me more about the occupational hazards that *you* have," or simply, "I would rather talk about the occupational hazards in *your* workplace."

Sexual Aggression

Sexual aggression includes inappropriate jokes, flirtatious comments, sexual suggestions, or sexual advances. Patients with low self-esteem may flaunt their sexual prowess as a way to increase feelings of self-worth. Listen for these themes in an attempt to understand why the patient is acting this way and, most importantly, set limits on these behaviors. Although you may be shocked, embarrassed, or angry, you need to confront sexual innuendos and make clear that such behavior is not acceptable. You may say, for example, "It makes me very uncomfortable when you tell that type of joke. I would prefer that we talk about other things," or "Yes, I have a boyfriend. Tell me more about your support systems." If aggression is physical, it may be necessary to set limits, such as, "If you touch me there again, I will need to leave the room."

Applying Your Knowledge

Although assessment can be viewed in isolation, it is important to realize that you must be prepared to do something with this information. The reason for completing the assessment is to have data that are accurate and complete so that a plan can be developed with interventions that promote health. All pieces of the nursing process are interdependent and consider patients holistically.

Using the previous steps of diagnostic reasoning, organizing, and prioritizing, consider all the case study findings woven throughout this chapter. When answering the following questions, begin drawing conclusions and see how the pieces of assessment work together to create an environment for personalized, appropriate, and accurate care.

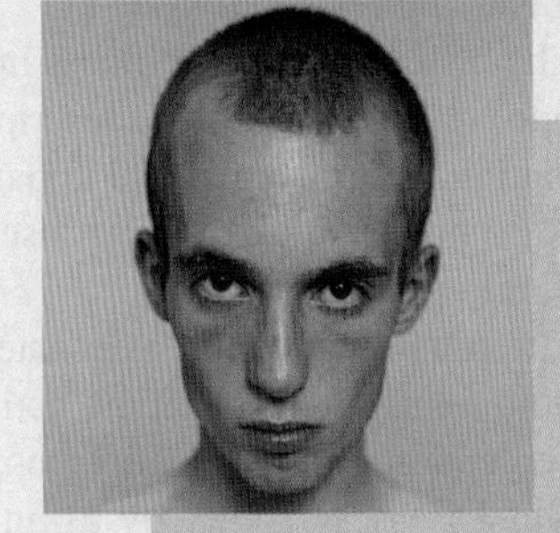

- Which techniques of therapeutic communication might the nurse need to use when talking with the patient?

(case study continues on page 42)

- Is it important for the nurse to interview Mr. Rowan to assess how he contracted AIDS?
- What is the nurse's perceived risk of exposure to HIV/AIDS?
- What cultural, environmental, or developmental issues might the nurse anticipate for Mr. Rowan?
- How might the nurse's personal beliefs about AIDS and alternative therapies affect communication with Mr. Rowan?
- How can the nurse know whether nonjudgmental care has been communicated, both verbally and nonverbally?

Key Points

- Nonverbal communication should be congruent with verbal communication.
- Active listening, restatement, reflection, elaboration, silence, focusing, clarification, and summarizing are techniques to facilitate therapeutic communication.
- Nontherapeutic responses include false reassurance, sympathy, unwanted advice, leading or biased questions, changes of subject, distractions, too many technical terms, and talking too much.
- The phases of the interview process include preinteraction phase, beginning phase, working phase, and closing phase.
- Intercultural communication requires sensitivity to and knowledge of specific cultures, including language challenges, health beliefs, and gender issues.
- Assessment of newborns, infants, and children includes the care provider and his or her relationship to the patient.
- Privacy and respect are essential when assessing adolescents.
- Nurses collect primary data from patients. They collect secondary data from other sources such as the chart or family members of the patient.
- An emergency assessment occurs when the patient's condition is unstable; a focused assessment is narrower and more specific to the presenting problem; a comprehensive assessment covers all body systems for screening and health promotion.
- Components of the comprehensive health history include the reason for seeking care, history of present illness, past health history, current medications and indications, family history, functional health assessment, growth and development, and review of systems.
- The history of present illness includes assessment of location, intensity, duration, description, aggravating and alleviating factors, functional impairment, and pain goal.
- A complete family history uses a genogram to illustrate family patterns.
- The functional health assessment includes health perception, nutrition, elimination, activity, sleep, cognition, self-perception, roles, sexuality, coping, and values.
- Nurses assess ADLs by asking about feeding, bathing, toileting, dressing, grooming, mobility, home maintenance, shopping, and cooking.
- A complete review of systems assesses the history of all body systems including nutrition/hydration, skin/hair/nails, head/neck, eyes/ears, heart, peripheral vascular, breasts, abdominal, musculoskeletal, neurological, genitalia, rectum, and endocrine/hematological. Any follow-up to problems or results to tests are included.

Review Questions

1. A patient says that she is having throbbing pain that she rates as 6 on a 10-point scale. This is referred to as
   A. subjective primary data.
   B. subjective secondary data.
   C. objective primary data.
   D. objective secondary data.

2. The nurse is gathering the health history data before performing the physical assessment. This phase of the interview process is the
   A. preinteraction phase.
   B. beginning phase.
   C. working phase.
   D. closing phase.

3. The patient is crying after being given a diagnosis with a poor prognosis. The best response from the nurse is
   A. "Don't cry. It will be OK."
   B. "My mother has the same thing."
   C. "I think that you should have surgery."
   D. "I'll stay with you." (gets a tissue)

4. When gathering the family history, the nurse draws a genogram
   A. using circles for males and squares for females.
   B. putting the patient on the left to show birth order.
   C. inserting lines between parents to show marriage.
   D. listing health problems above the symbol for the patient.

5. The mother of an infant with severe asthma is extremely anxious. The nurse is treating the patient in the emergency room. When collecting the history, the best response of the nurse is
   A. "You must be extremely worried."
   B. "I'd be in worse shape than you are if it was my baby."
   C. "Is there anyone here that you can talk to?"
   D. "You seem worried, but I need to ask a few questions."

6. The nurse asks, "What are the most important things to you in life?" to assess the functional pattern related to
   A. role.
   B. self-perception.
   C. coping.
   D. values.

7. To assess self-perception, the nurse asks
   A. "How would you describe yourself?"
   B. "Are you having difficulty handling any family problems?"
   C. "What gives you hope when times are troubled?"
   D. "How do you usually deal with stress? Is it effective?"

8. The nurse who asks about feeding, bathing, toileting, dressing, grooming, mobility, home maintenance, shopping, and cooking is assessing
   A. whether the patient is a reliable historian.
   B. functional health patterns.
   C. ADLs.
   D. review of systems.

9. The nurse assessing an older adult focuses the health history on
   A. previous pregnancies, obstetrical history, and psychosocial factors.
   B. birth history, immunizations, and growth and development.
   C. sensory deficits, illness history, and lifestyle factors.
   D. religion, spirituality, culture, and values.

10. The nurse performs patient teaching after assessing that the nutritional history reveals that the patient generally consumes a high-fat, high-calorie diet. This critical thinking
   A. uses subjective data to analyze findings and intervene.
   B. documents and communicates data using appropriate medical terminologies.
   C. individualizes health assessment considering the age, gender, and culture of the patient.
   D. uses assessment findings to identify medical and nursing diagnoses.

The Jensen suite offers these additional resources to enhance learning and facilitate understanding of this chapter:

- thePoint online resource, http://thepoint.lww.com/Jensen2e
- *Laboratory Manual for Nursing Health Assessment: A Best Practice Approach*
- *Pocket Guide for Nursing Health Assessment: A Best Practice Approach*
- *Lippincott DocuCare*, an electronic health record simulation software, http://thepoint.lww.com/docucare
- *Adaptive Learning | Powered by PrepU*, http://thepoint.lww.com/prepu

References

American Association of Colleges of Nursing. (2008). *The essentials of baccalaureate education for professional nursing practice*. Washington, DC: Author.

American Nurses Association. (2005). *Code of ethics for nurses with interpretive statements*. Washington, DC: Author.

Bach, S., & Grant, A. (2011). *Communication and interpersonal skills in nursing* (2nd ed.). London, United Kingdom: Learning Matters Ltd.

Balzer-Riley, J. W. (2012). *Communication in nursing* (7th ed.). St. Louis, MO: Elsevier

Centers for Disease Control and Prevention. (2013). *Intimate partner violence*. Retrieved from http://www.cdc.gov/ViolencePrevention/intimatepartnerviolence/index.html?source=govdelivery

Dart, M. A. (2011). *Motivational interviewing in nursing practice: Empowering the patient*. Sudbury, MA: Jones and Bartlett.

Gordon, M. (1987). *Nursing diagnosis: Process and application* (2nd ed.). New York, NY: McGraw-Hill.

Hurley, J., & Linsley, P. (2012). *Emotional intelligence in health and social care: A guide for improving human relationships*. London, United kingdom: Radcliffe Publishing Ltd.

National Institute on Deafness and other Communication Disorders. (2014). *Hearing loss and older adults*. Retrieved from http://www.nidcd.nih.gov/health/hearing/pages/older.aspx

Peate, I. (2012). *The student's guide to becoming a nurse* (2nd ed.). Oxford, United Kingdom: Wiley–Blackwell.

Stewart, M. (2013). *Male and female communication: Differences worth noting*. Retrieved from https://www.achievesolutions.net/achievesolutions/en/Content.do?contentId=10241

The Joint Commission. (2012). *Advancing effective communication, cultural competence, and patient- and family-centered care for the lesbian, gay, bisexual, and transgender (LGBT) community: A field guide*. Oak Brook, IL: Author.

The Joint Commission. (2014). *National patient safety goals*. Retrieved from http://www.jointcommission.org/standards_information/npsgs.aspx

Ulrich, C. M. (2012). *Nursing ethics in everyday practice*. Indianapolis, IN: Sigma Theta Tau International.

U.S. Department of Health & Human Services. (2014). *Medical privacy—National standards to protect the privacy of personal health information*. Retrieved from http://www.hhs.gov/ocr/hipaa/.

Webster, D. (2013). Promoting therapeutic communication and patient-centered care using standardized patients. *Journal of Nursing Education*, 52(11), 645–648.

Wright, L. M., & Leahey, M. (2012). *The nurse and families: A guide to family assessment and intervention* (6th ed.). Philadelphia, PA: F.A. Davis.

3

Physical Examination Techniques and Equipment

Learning Objectives

1 Demonstrate knowledge of routine practices and additional precautions for infection control and safety.

2 Demonstrate knowledge of anatomical positions and anatomical terms.

3 Describe inspection and the specific characteristics to be assessed.

4 Describe palpation and the specific characteristics to be assessed.

5 Explain the physical properties of sound and sound conduction.

6 Describe percussion and the specific characteristics to be assessed.

7 Describe auscultation and the specific characteristics to be assessed.

8 Demonstrate knowledge of the equipment used during the physical examination.

9 Document findings from the four basic examination modes of inspection, palpation, percussion, and auscultation.

Chris Chow is a 6-year-old boy visiting the clinic today with a fever and "stuffy nose." He came in with his mother who took the day off from work to stay home with him. His temperature is 38.6°C (101.5°F) tympanic, pulse 110 beats/min, respirations 20 breaths/min, and blood pressure 108/66 mmHg. Chris is healthy and meeting developmental milestones, as indicated on the documentation from his well-child visit 2 months ago. He is being seen by an advanced practice registered nurse practitioner (APRN).

You will gain more information about Chris as you progress through this chapter. As you study the content and features, consider Chris's case and its relationship to what you are learning. Begin thinking about the following points:

- What information does the nurse gain about patients during inspection, palpation, percussion, and auscultation?
- How does the nurse use safety and infection control principles during the assessment?
- What basic examination modes and equipment does the nurse practitioner use during the physical assessment?
- How might the nurse organize the assessment sequentially to include the different body systems in this focused assessment for the child?
- What factors might be contributing to Chris's illness?
- How will the nurse practitioner evaluate the outcome of her teaching?

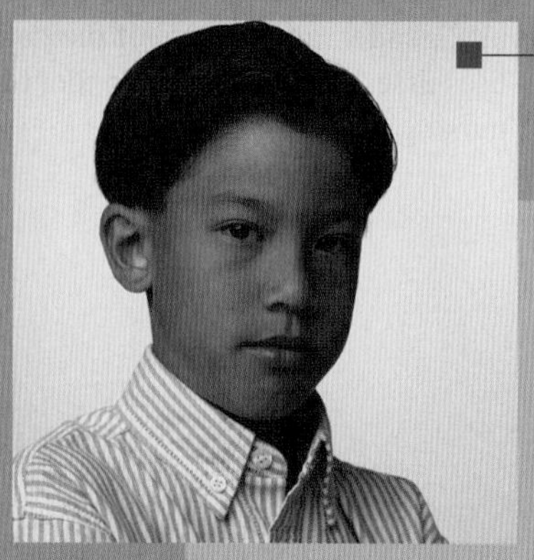

As discussed in Chapter 2, an accurate and complete health history provides information to guide the physical assessment. You will combine objective data from the physical assessment with subjective data from the health history to form a complete assessment database as well as to develop an impression of the underlying cause of health problems.

The four techniques of inspection, palpation, percussion, and auscultation form the basis of physical assessment. **Inspection** means observation of the patient for general appearance and specific details related to the body system, anatomical region, or condition under examination. With **palpation**, you use your hands to feel the firmness of body parts, such as the abdomen. With **percussion**, you use tapping motions with your hands to produce sounds that indicate solid or air-filled spaces over the lungs and other areas. You use the stethoscope to perform **auscultation**, in which movements of air or fluid are heard in the body over the lungs and abdomen.

Precautions to Prevent Infection

During assessment, you come into direct physical contact with the patient. Thus, it is essential that you follow infection control principles, including, but not limited to, diligent hand hygiene, use of gloves, and standard precautions (Fig. 3.1).

Health care environments contain a multitude of organisms that pose threats, especially for patients who are immunocompromised, those who have recently undergone surgery, and those who have indwelling medical devices (e.g., urinary catheters, endotracheal tubes, intravenous lines). Multidrug-resistant organisms, including methicillin-resistant *Staphylococcus aureus* (MRSA), vancomycin-resistant enterococci (VRE), and certain gram-negative bacilli are becoming more prevalent. Treatment of such pathogens is becoming increasingly difficult. Because of these threats, you must take special measures to prevent the spread of infection before, during, and after conducting assessments.

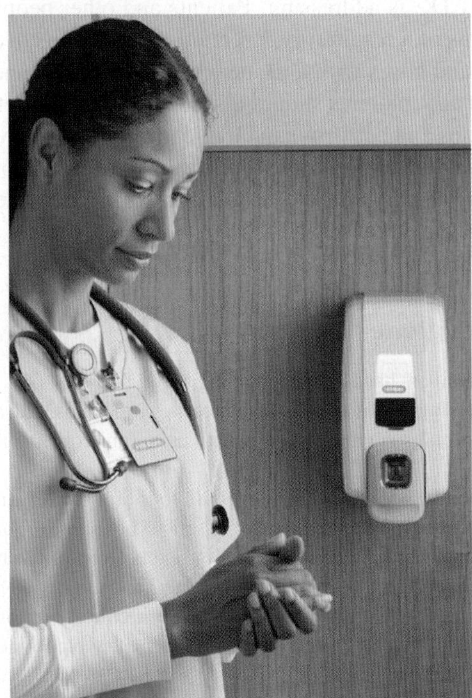

Figure 3.1 The nurse performs hand hygiene in preparation for conducting a physical examination.

Hand Hygiene

> ⚠ *SAFETY ALERT*
> *The single most important action to prevent an infection is* ***hand hygiene****. Contact transmission from the hands of health care providers to patients is the most common mode of transmission because microorganisms from one patient are then spread to others* (Centers for Disease Control and Prevention [CDC], 2013).

Patient-to-patient transmission of pathogens requires five sequential steps:

1. Organisms are present on a patient's skin or in the immediate environment.
2. Organisms are transferred from the patient to the nurse's hands.
3. Organisms survive on the nurse's hands for at least several minutes.
4. The nurse omits (or performs inadequate or inappropriate) hand hygiene.
5. The nurse's contaminated hands come into direct contact with another patient or environment in direct contact with the patient.

The CDC and the World Health Organization (WHO, 2013) recommend hand hygiene as a first line of defense to decrease nosocomial infections and to prevent transmission of microorganisms. Hand hygiene is implemented at specific occurrences for optimal effectiveness. Occurrences are as follows:

- Prior to contact with the patient
- After contact with the patient or environmental equipment
- After removal of gloves
- Prior to invasive procedures

Use of alcohol-based hand rubs during these occurrences is appropriate and preferred. Handwashing with soap and water is necessary when hands are visibly soiled with blood or body fluids.

Note also that health care providers' nails should be trimmed to ¼ in. or shorter. Artificial nails should not be worn.

Use of Gloves

The CDC (2013) has recommended that health care providers wear gloves (1) to reduce the risk of their acquiring infections from patients, (2) to prevent the transmission of flora from health care workers to patients, and (3) to reduce transient

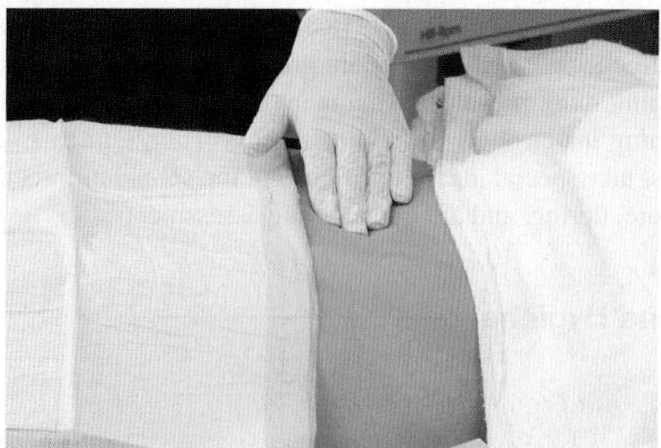

Figure 3.2 Use of gloves is important to protect against the spread of infection in cases in which the nurse could be exposed to a patient's body fluids. The nurse is wearing gloves while examining a patient with problems with urinary and fecal incontinence.

contamination of the hands of personnel by flora that can be transmitted from one patient to another.

Wear gloves when touching blood, body fluids, secretions, excretions, and contaminated items. Put on clean gloves just before touching the mucous membranes and nonintact skin of patients. Wear gloves when general contact with any "wet" body secretion is anticipated. For example, you do not need to wear gloves when taking an oral temperature, because only the thermometer cover comes into contact with the patient's oral secretions. However, you do need to wear gloves while assessing the back of a patient who has urinary incontinence to avoid potential contact with any urine that may be present. You wear gloves for personal protection and to avoid spreading organisms to other patients or from one body area to another (Fig. 3.2).

When to Change Gloves

Change gloves in the following circumstances:

- Between tasks and procedures on the same patient after contact with a material that contains a high concentration of microorganisms (such as a dressing changes or tracheostomy care)
- When going from a contaminated to a cleaner area

Glove Removal

Remove gloves promptly after use, before touching noncontaminated items and environmental surfaces, and before going to another patient. Remove gloves before touching the computer, supply drawers, and equipment. Perform hand hygiene immediately after glove removal to avoid transfer of microorganisms to other patients and environments.

> **Clinical Significance**
>
> Gloves should not be worn from the room out into the hallway. This increases risk of the transmission from a "dirty" to a "clean" area. Gloves also are removed when going from the bedside to the computer.

Hand hygiene is the single most important element of standard precautions. See Box 3.1 for a summary of the indications for hand hygiene.

Standard Precautions

Nurses use **standard precautions** with all patients to reduce the transmission of pathogens in both diagnosed and unknown infections. The intention of standard precautions is to prevent disease transmission during contact with nonintact skin, mucous membranes, body substances, and bloodborne contacts (e.g., needlestick injury). Because many patients are unaware of being infected, standard precautions serve to help ensure that health care providers treat all patients equally.

Respiratory hygiene/cough etiquette is another area that the CDC is addressing. Patients and other people with symptoms of a respiratory infection are asked to cover their mouths and noses with a tissue when coughing or sneezing. Additionally, patients should dispose of tissues directly into receptacles and perform hand hygiene after hands have been in contact with respiratory secretions. If a tissue is not available, cough etiquette encourages coughing into the inner aspect of the elbow (CDC, 2013).

BOX 3.1 Indications for Handwashing and Hand Hygiene

- When hands are visibly dirty or soiled, wash hands with either a nonantimicrobial soap and water or an antimicrobial soap and water.
- If hands are not visibly soiled, use an alcohol-based hand rub for routinely decontaminating hands in all other clinical situations.
- Decontaminate hands before having direct contact with patients and after contact with a patient's intact skin (e.g., taking a pulse or blood pressure, lifting a patient).
- Decontaminate hands if moving from a contaminated body site to a clean body site during patient care.
- Decontaminate hands after contact with inanimate objects (including medical equipment) in the immediate vicinity of the patient.
- Decontaminate hands after removing gloves.
- Before eating and after using a restroom, wash hands with a nonantimicrobial soap and water or with an antimicrobial soap and water.
- Wash hands with nonantimicrobial soap and water or with antimicrobial soap and water if an exposure to *Bacillus anthracis* or *Clostridium difficile* is suspected or proven. The physical action of washing and rinsing hands under such circumstances is recommended, because alcohols, chlorhexidine, iodophors, and other antiseptic agents have poor activity against spores.

From Centers for Disease Control and Prevention. (2011). *Hand hygiene in healthcare settings*. Retrieved from http://www.cdc.gov/handhygiene/Guidelines.html

TABLE 3.1 Recommendations for Standard Precautions

Mask, eye protection, face shield	Wear a mask and eye protection or a face shield to protect mucous membranes of the eyes, nose, and mouth during procedures and activities that are likely to generate splashes or sprays of blood, body fluids, secretions, and excretions.
Gown	Wear a gown (a clean, nonsterile gown is adequate) to protect skin and to prevent soiling of clothes during procedures and activities that are likely to generate splashes or sprays of blood, body fluids, secretions, or excretions. Remove a soiled gown as promptly as possible and wash hands to avoid transfer of microorganisms to other patients or environments.
Patient care equipment	Ensure that reusable equipment is not used for the care of another patient until it has been cleaned and reprocessed appropriately. Ensure the proper discarding of single-use items.
Environmental control	Ensure that the facility has adequate procedures for the routine care, cleaning, and disinfection of environmental surfaces, beds, bed rails, bedside equipment, and other frequently touched surfaces.
Linen	Handle, transport, and process used linen soiled with blood, body fluids, secretions, and excretions in a manner that prevents skin exposures and contamination of clothing and that avoids transfer of microorganisms to other patients and environments.
Occupational health and bloodborne pathogens	Never recap used needles. Do not remove used needles from disposable syringes by hand; do not bend, break, or otherwise manipulate used needles by hand. Place used disposable syringes and needles, scalpel blades, and other sharp items in appropriate puncture-resistant containers. Use mouthpieces, resuscitation bags, or other ventilation devices as an alternative to mouth-to-mouth resuscitation methods in areas where the need for resuscitation is predictable.
Patient placement	Place a patient who contaminates the environment or who does not (or cannot be expected to) assist in maintaining appropriate hygiene or environmental control in a private room.

From Siegel, J. D., Rhinehart, E., Jackson, M., & Chiarello, L. (n.d.). *2007 Guideline for isolation precautions: Preventing transmission of infectious agents in healthcare settings.* Retrieved from http://www.cdc.gov/ncidod/dhqp/pdf/isolation2007.pdf

The CDC has developed transmission-based precautions for airborne, droplet, and contact routes of transmission. Health care providers combine the use of these specific precautions with standard precautions. The general guideline is for health care providers to wear personal protective equipment whenever they are at risk for coming into contact with body secretions from patients, such as droplet exposure during patient's coughing while the health care provider is performing tracheal suctioning. Refer to Table 3.1 for a summary of standard precautions.

Latex Allergy

Latex allergy usually results from repeated exposures through skin contact or inhalation to proteins in natural rubber latex. Reactions usually begin within minutes of exposure to latex, but they can occur hours later and produce various symptoms. Nurses and other health care workers are more likely to have latex allergy than is the general population (8% to 12% among health care worker vs. 1% in the general population) (U.S. Department of Labor, Occupational Safety and Health Administration [OSHA], 2013). Patients can develop an allergy to latex at any time, especially those who are frequently admitted to the hospital.

The best preventive action is to avoid contact with latex when possible. Health care facilities can establish latex-free zones for patients and staff. Nurses should take care to avoid carrying any latex substances into such zones, including stethoscopes, urinary catheters, and vials with rubber stoppers. To avoid increasing exposure to latex (which can increase allergy rates), institutions are encouraged to use powder-free, low-allergen gloves and latex-free equipment such as catheters and IV tubing.

Skin Reactions

Nurses have a higher rate of skin reactions than the general population because of their higher frequency of hand hygiene. To minimize the adverse effects of hand hygiene and decrease transmission of pathogens, health care professionals should be encouraged to use alcohol-based rubs as the preferred method of hand hygiene, in accordance with WHO recommendations, to reduce the prevalence of hand eczema that can be caused by the use of soap and water.

Therapeutic Dialogue: Collecting Subjective Data

The nurse's role in subjective data collection is to gather information to improve the patient's health status and to help determine the cause of the patient's current symptoms. Remember Chris, the 6-year-old boy with a cold who is visiting the clinic with his mother. He is anxious about coming to the clinic because he received an immunization during his previous appointment. The nurse uses professional communication that is appropriate for the child's developmental level to gather subjective data.

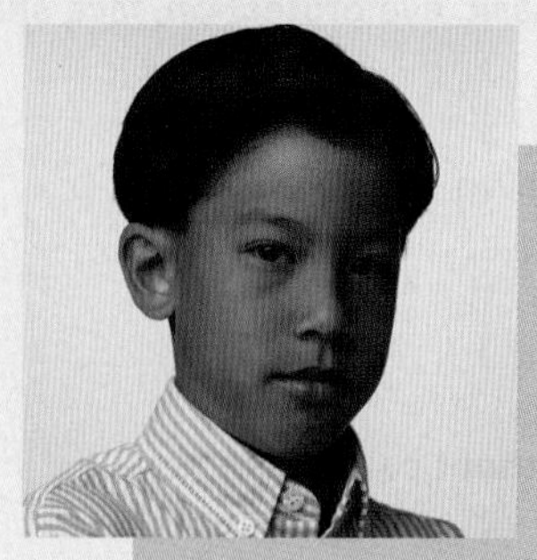

Nurse: Hi, Chris. How are you?

Chris: I feel sick. Am I going to have to get a shot today?

Nurse: No, you had your shots last time. Today, I want to listen to your lungs and look in your mouth and ears. Do you want me to listen or look first?

Chris: Mom, I don't want a shot.

Mother: You don't need one today. How about if you come and sit on my lap and Nurse Lesley can listen to your lungs?

Chris: OK. What does that thing do anyway? (points to the stethoscope)

Nurse: I can hear the air moving in your lungs and your heart beating. Would you like to listen first?

Chris: Sure. (The nurse positions the stethoscope for Chris, who smiles as he listens.)

Nurse: So he's had a fever?

Mother: Yes, it's been up to 102.5 (F; 39.2° C).

Nurse: Are there any other symptoms?

Mother: Yes, a runny nose and a bit of a cough, too.

Nurse: That's the air moving in and out as you breathe (smiles). Can I listen now?

Critical Thinking Challenge

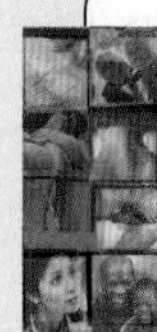

- What are the first things that the nurse considers during the interview and examination?
- Why did the nurse allow Chris to sit in his mother's lap?
- How might the nurse facilitate comfort and reduce anxiety when performing the other techniques and using other equipment such as an otoscope and ophthalmoscope?

Clinical Significance

As we proceed into the specific techniques of assessment, it may be helpful to practice these elements on yourself as you read along and then later on a willing peer, friend, or family member to increase your confidence and dexterity.

Inspection

Inspection is the first technique of the overall general survey and for each body part because it generally provides a wealth of information. Inspection is the one technique that is performed for every body part and body system.

Perform inspection by consciously observing the patient for physical characteristics and behaviors, noting any odors. Initially, observe the patient for overall characteristics including age, gender, level of alertness, body size and shape, skin color, hygiene, posture, and level of discomfort or anxiety. This overall observation, called the general survey, is intentional and conscious for beginners. With experience, gathering data from inspection becomes second nature, and this information is collected while performing other techniques or interventions. Inspection begins with the initial contact with each patient and continues through each individual body system.

The purpose of gathering data during this initial phase is to gain an overall impression of the patient and to assess the severity of the situation. Observe for cues that might indicate a situation that needs further assessment. Following the general survey, proceed to assess specific body areas and systems.

During inspection, adequate exposure of each body part is necessary. At the same time, you should take measures to maintain the comfort and privacy of the patient through appropriate draping, especially over the breasts in women and genitalia in both men and women (Fig. 3.3). Adequate lighting is essential to observe color, texture, and mobility. Inform patients of the need to look at the body part along with the rationale; ask patients for permission before doing so, especially when assessments involve compromising the patient's modesty. For example, "I need to look at your mastectomy incision to see how it is healing. Is it OK if I lift your gown?"

Sometimes devices limit visibility, such as a splint over a knee. When possible, loosen or remove such devices to adequately observe the skin for any red, inflamed, or infected areas and also to determine adequate circulation. Examine each body part and use specific descriptions. For example, when inspecting the abdomen, note the shape (whether it is flat or distended), size, skin color, texture, and any bruising, veins, or prominent movements. A common technique is to consider overall shape first and then compare the two sides for symmetry.

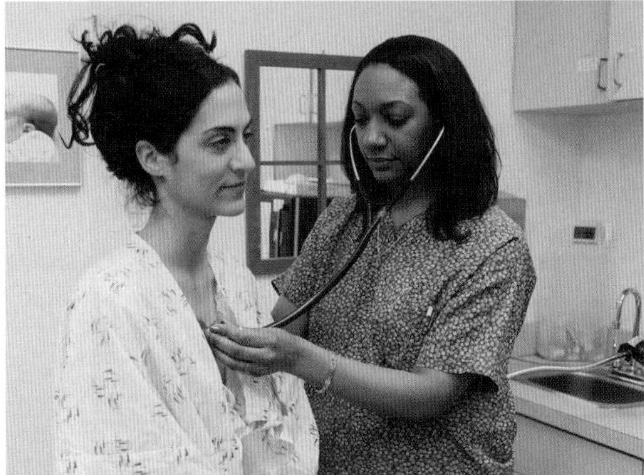

Figure 3.3 Proper draping and gowning are essential to preserve the patient's privacy and build trust. The nurse is careful to expose only those areas pertinent to the immediate examination and to redrape or re-cover the patient upon completion.

In addition to using the correct inspection techniques for each body system, it is important to label and document findings appropriately. One challenge that beginners face is identifying details and subtle differences. Accurate descriptions are essential for legal documentation and communication of findings. Upcoming chapters describe associated normal and abnormal findings for various body systems and regions, along with associated medical terminology.

Pay attention to individual details of inspection. Note whether verbal, nonverbal, and inspection data match, and then identify any preliminary patterns or clusters. If the patient appears anxious, note facial expression, nervous gestures, body position or pacing, and voice characteristics. Inspection provides objective physical data leading to accurate diagnoses and treatment and also allows for inclusion of the emotional state of the patient.

Palpation

Palpation is the use of touch to assess texture, temperature, moisture, size, shape, location, position, vibration, crepitus, tenderness, pain, and edema. Before performing this technique, inform the patient of the need to palpate the body part, along with the rationale, and ask for permission or consent to use touch. For example, during abdominal assessment, you might say, "I know that you're having some abdominal pain, but I would like to gently feel your abdomen to see if a particular area is sensitive. Would that be OK with you?" Begin with a gentle and slow technique while inspecting the patient's face for nonverbal indicators of discomfort, such as a furrowed brow or grimacing.

Use different parts of the hand depending on the data that you are gathering. The fingers are best for some techniques, whereas the palms are best for others. Use your finger pads for fine discrimination because they are the most mobile parts of the hand. Some examples of the need for fine discrimination include locating the pulses, lymph nodes, or small lumps and for assessing for skin texture and edema. The palmar surface of the fingers and finger joints are best for assessing firmness, contour, position, size, pain, and tenderness. The palm of the hand is best during abdominal assessment. The back of the hand (dorsal side) is most sensitive to temperature. If a patient complains of being hot, turn the hand over and use the dorsal side to evaluate temperature because the skin there is thinner and more sensitive. Vibratory tremors can sometimes be felt on the chest as the patient speaks; these are best palpated with the ulnar, or outside, surface of the hand.

Light Palpation

Begin with light palpation to allow the patient to become accustomed to the touch. If pain is present, you might say, "Let me know if this hurts you," to gain trust and increase comfort. Avoid any tender or painful areas until the end. Ensure privacy by draping and warm your hands before beginning. It may be necessary to warm your hands under running water or to gently rub them together. Short and smooth nails also are

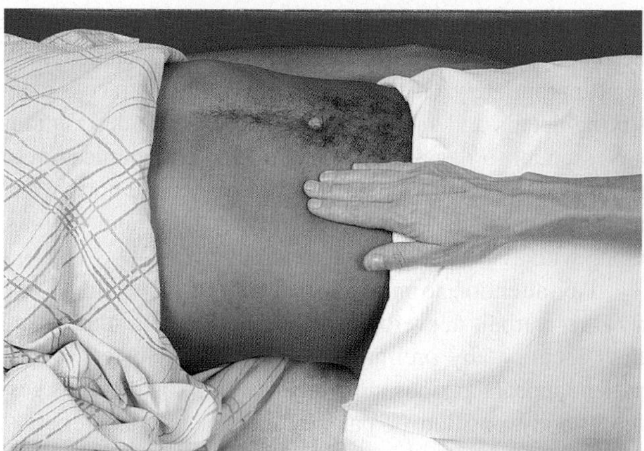

Figure 3.4 Technique for light palpation. The nurse would wear gloves in cases with contamination risk, but gloves are not required in every case..

necessary to avoid causing discomfort. Palpation is difficult when patients' muscles are tense, so use a gentle, calm, and easy touch to assist patients to relax.

Light palpation is appropriate for the assessment of surface characteristics, such as texture, surface lesions or lumps, or inflamed areas of skin (e.g., over an intravenous site). Place the finger pads of the dominant hand on the patient's skin and slowly move the fingers in circular areas of approximately 1 cm in depth (about ½ in.) (Fig. 3.4). Intermittent palpation using this technique is more effective than a single continuous palpation, because your fingers sense the movement of skin and tissue beneath the finger pads. Patients may perceive this gentle light palpation as a light massage in the absence of pain. Communicate concern for patients verbally with conversation during the procedure and nonverbally through this caring touch.

Moderate to Deep Palpation

Use moderate palpation to assess the size, shape, and consistency of abdominal organs. Additionally, note any unexpected findings of pain, tenderness, or pulsations. The same gentle circular motion of light palpation is appropriate, but instead of the finger pads, use the palmar surface of the fingers. Pressure is firm enough to depress approximately 1 to 2 cm. Observe the patient for any guarding, grimacing, or tension during moderate palpation.

During deep palpation, place the extended fingers of the nondominant hand over the dominant hand to use the pressure of both hands. Use the same circular motion to palpate 2 to 4 cm.

> ⚠ *SAFETY ALERT*
>
> *Deep palpation should not be used over areas that pose a risk of injuring patients, such as over an enlarged spleen or inflamed appendix.*

As with other types of palpation, explain the purpose, touch gently at first, and ask about uncomfortable feelings. With deep palpation, you might say, "I'm going to touch you and push down more deeply than before. Let me know if you feel pain or want me to stop." As palpation proceeds, continue conversation, asking the patient about pain, presenting symptoms, or contributing factors while observing for nonverbal signs of tenderness or discomfort.

As a beginner, you may initially be able to concentrate only on the technique. As you gain skill, you will be able to palpate, assess symptoms, and teach all at the same time.

Percussion

The third technique of physical assessment is **percussion** to produce sound or elicit tenderness. You will tap your fingers on the patient, similar to the tapping of a drumstick on a drum. The vibrations that the fingers produce create percussion tones conducted into the patient's body. If the vibrations travel through dense tissue, the percussion tones are quiet; if they travel through air or fluid, the tones are louder. The loudest tones are over the lungs and hollow stomach; the quietest are over bones. Two methods of percussion are direct and indirect.

Direct Percussion

With direct percussion, tap with your fingers directly on the patient's skin (Fig. 3.5). Examples include percussion of the sinuses in patients with sinus infections and percussion of the thorax in newborns to assess the air-filled lungs. Direct percussion is easier to learn than indirect percussion. For percussion of the sinuses with the hand, the nurse gently taps in the periorbital area for pain that may indicate allergies, congestion, or infection. Percussion that is too weak may not reveal important findings, whereas percussion that is too strong may elicit too much pain. Thus, moderate tapping is recommended.

Indirect Percussion

Rather than directly striking a patient, you can use your nondominant hand as a barrier between the dominant hand and

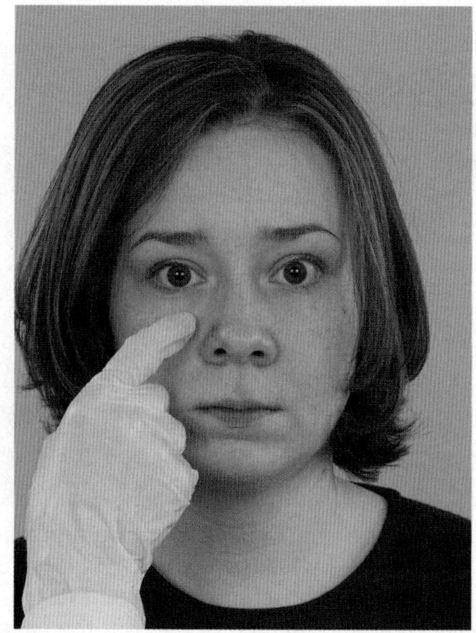

Figure 3.5 Direct percussion of the sinuses.

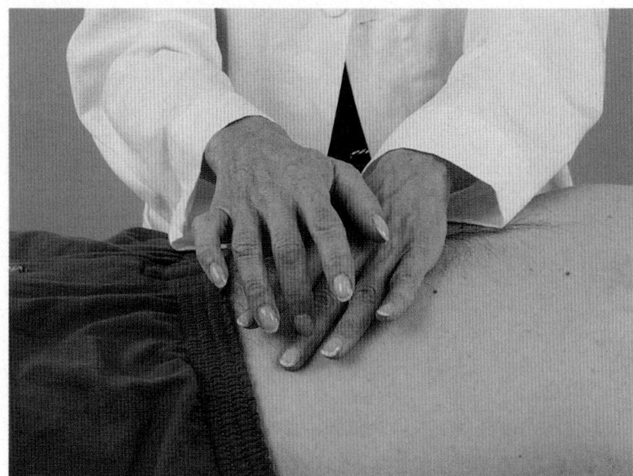

Figure 3.6 Indirect percussion.

the patient. This is known as indirect percussion. Place your nondominant palm on the patient and initiate a quick, moderately strong tap with the dominant hand. Use the ulnar surface of the fist to percuss the kidneys. As with direct percussion, you will practice until you demonstrate a comfortable strength.

The most common and also the most difficult sounds to elicit are the indirect sounds. You can best differentiate among the sounds by moving from area to area and listening to the changes in volume and pitch. It is also easier to hear the difference from resonant to dull. Thus, when you learn indirect percussion, it is easiest to go from the center of the abdomen with tympany and move upward to the liver where dullness is percussed.

Indirect percussion requires coordination of both hands. Place the hyperextended middle finger of your nondominant hand firmly over the area to be percussed. Lift the other fingers on that hand from the patient and spread them slightly to avoid contact with the patient, which can dampen the sound of the striking finger. Then position the slightly flexed middle finger of your dominant hand approximately 2 to 3 cm (about 1 in.) above the distal interphalangeal joint in contact with the patient. Using only the wrist of the dominant hand, raise the dominant finger 4 to 5 cm (about 2 in.) and quickly strike and raise the nondominant joint twice while listening for the elicited sound (Fig. 3.6). Then move the nondominant hand and strike twice in a new area.

As a beginning learner, you will need to practice first to elicit a sound loud enough to hear. After perfecting the technique, you will listen carefully and compare sounds to identify the types of note heard. Some helpful hints when learning percussion are as follows:

- Most of the nondominant finger should be touching the patient; otherwise, the sound transmission will be decreased.
- The motion of the striking finger should be quick, forceful, and snappy. The snapping finger must be brisk for a loud sound.
- Because you must use the tip of the finger, nails must be short and smooth to avoid causing discomfort to the patient and to facilitate good contact. Using the pad of the finger dampens the sound.
- The downward motion of the striking hand should be from the wrist, not the finger, elbow, or arm.
- To avoid dampening the sound, immediately withdraw the snapping finger once the nondominant finger is struck.
- The nurse who has small hands and fingers needs to strike more forcefully than the nurse who has large hands.

Percussion Sounds

There are four different percussion tones in the body: **flat**, **dull**, **resonant**, and **tympanic**. In addition to intensity or loudness, you will listen to the pitch, duration, and quality of sound.

Intensity or *loudness* refers to how soft or loud the sound is. The louder the sound, the louder the intensity and the easier it is to hear. If air fills the structure, there is more ability to vibrate and the sound is louder.

Pitch or *frequency* depends on how quickly the vibration oscillates. It is similar to music: if the frequency of the sound is fast, the pitch is high; if the frequency of the sound is slow, the pitch is low. Although both the lungs and the hollow stomach are loud, the lungs are low-pitched and the stomach is high-pitched. See Table 3.2 for a list of percussion tones and their characteristics.

Duration refers to how long the sounds last once elicited. A sound that is freer to vibrate, such as is found over air-filled spaces, has a longer duration.

Quality means the subjective description of the percussion sound, such as a low-pitched thud of short duration versus a drumlike sound with high pitch and long duration. The process might be compared to the listening skills of a musician: beginners listen to the sound of the overall orchestra, whereas advanced musicians identify the sounds of the

TABLE 3.2 **Percussion Sounds**

Tone	Intensity	Pitch	Duration	Quality	Location
Hyperresonant	Very loud	Low	Long	Booming	Emphysematous lungs
Resonant	Loud	Low	Long	Hollow	Healthy lungs
Tympanic	Loud	High	Moderate	Drumlike	Gastric bubble (stomach)
Dull	Moderate	High	Moderate	Thud	Liver
Flat	Soft	High	Short	Dull	Bone

trombone, bassoon, and violin. You will take time to first develop the technique, and then you will develop the listening skills to compare the different types of sounds.

Auscultation

During auscultation, you will listen for sounds produced by the body, usually from movement of organs and tissues. A stethoscope is used to transmit sounds that are normally unheard. Auscultation requires a quiet environment with minimal to no distractions.

Common assessments involving auscultation include blood pressure, lungs, heart, and abdomen. The blood pressure produces sounds that correlate with the bounding of the pulse. Air moving in and out with each breath generates soft and rustling sounds in the lungs. The heart produces the typical "lub-dub" with the snapping closure of the heart valves. Peristalsis in the abdomen produces typical gurgling or growling sounds.

Descriptors vary depending on the body part auscultated; this detail is provided in the individual chapters that follow. You will describe sounds in terms of intensity, pitch, duration, and quality. Descriptors for quality are similar to those used for percussion, although the sounds differ with auscultation—for example, crackles or gurgles (Table 3.3).

The Stethoscope

The stethoscope conducts sound from the patient's body to the listener and also blocks environmental noise to more clearly pinpoint the patient's body sounds. It does not amplify sounds—it only conducts them—so listen carefully to the minor differences between sounds that are often very soft.

The stethoscope includes the ear tips, earpiece, flexible tubing, and chestpiece. To be effective, the ear tips must fit into the ear canal snugly but comfortably. Ear tips come in different sizes and firmnesses, so nurses choose the type that works best depending on personal ear shape and size.

Clinical Significance

Earpieces are tilted slightly forward so that the angle on the earpiece is forward in the same direction as the nose (Fig. 3.7). This positioning directs the sound toward the tympanic membrane.

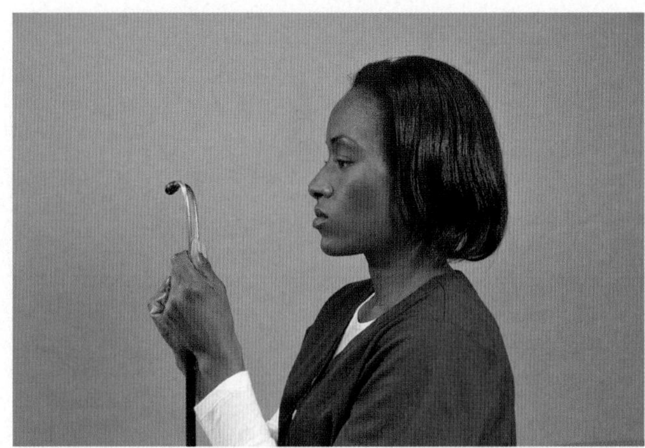

Figure 3.7 Correct positioning of the stethoscope to direct sound toward the tympanic membrane.

Tubing is thick to block environmental noise and short (55 to 69 cm [about 21 to 27 in.]) to increase transmission and reduce distortion of sound. Some pediatric nurses may cover their stethoscopes with colorful fabric or attach a small toy to distract children from touching the tubing during examination, which then needs to be cleaned between uses.

Most stethoscopes have a diaphragm and bell on the chestpiece (Fig. 3.8A). The bell is used with light skin contact to hear low-frequency sounds, whereas the diaphragm is used with firm skin contact to hear high-frequency sounds.

Clinical Significance

This chestpiece swivels back and forth between diaphragm and bell; when the chestpiece is turned to the bell, the diaphragm does not conduct sound. You may want to place the earpieces in the ears and gently touch the bell or diaphragm before auscultating to ascertain whether the chestpiece is turned toward the bell or diaphragm (Fig. 3.8B).

Other stethoscopes have only a diaphragm that changes between bell and diaphragm modes with pressure changes on the chestpiece. Use light contact to hear low-frequency sounds (similar to the bell) and press firmly for high-frequency sounds (similar to the diaphragm). The diaphragm is typically used for most sounds, such as lung and heart sounds, although the bell works best for detecting low-pitched heart murmurs. For

TABLE 3.3 Comparison of Auscultation Sounds

	Intensity	Pitch	Quality	Duration	Location
Blood pressure	Soft to loud	High	Swooshing or knocking	60–100/min	Arm
Abdominal sounds	Soft to loud	High	Gurgly, intermittent	5–35/min	Abdomen
Heart sounds	Moderate	Low	Lub-dub, rhythmic	60–100/min	Anterior thorax
Vesicular lung sounds	Soft	Low	Rustling, wispy	Inspiration greater than expiration, 12–20/min	Anterior and posterior thorax

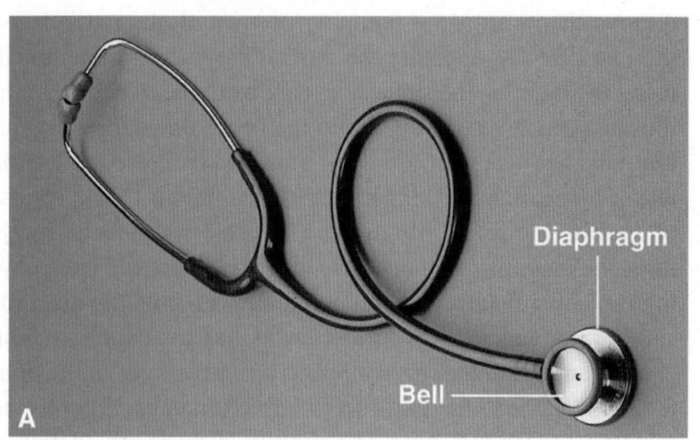

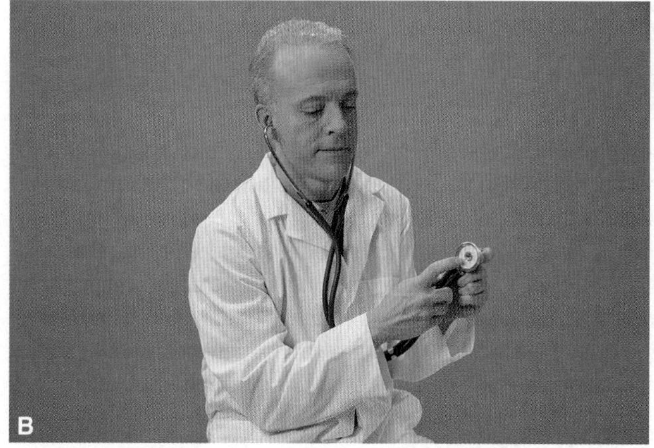

Figure 3.8 A. The stethoscope. **B.** Gently tap the bell or diaphragm after placing the stethoscope in the ears to check that the correct piece is on.

this reason, heart sounds are usually auscultated with both the diaphragm and the bell.

Make sure to disinfect the stethoscope between patients to avoid spreading pathogens (Schneider et al., 2011). Place the stethoscope directly on the patient's skin so that complete contact with the skin surface is made. If there is a gap, which is common when measuring blood pressure in the antecubital fossa, room noise is conducted and the blood pressure sounds are more difficult to hear. Have the patient straighten the arm to optimize contact. An appropriate-sized chestpiece also facilitates good skin contact; it is best to use a pediatric stethoscope with small children. When holding the chestpiece, place the endpiece between the index and the middle fingers, not on top of the stethoscope, which distorts the sound. Position the stethoscope so that tubing is away from objects that might brush against it, which produces extraneous noises that make it difficult for beginners to hear underlying body sounds. If the patient has a large amount of hair on the chest, it may be helpful to moisten the hair to avoid the crackly noises caused when the hair rubs against the stethoscope.

Documenting Case Study Findings

The nurse practitioner has just finished conducting a physical assessment of Chris, the 6-year-old boy with a cold. Review the following important findings revealed by each of the steps of objective data collection for Chris. Begin to think about how the data cluster together and what additional data the nurse might want to collect while thinking critically about the difficulties and anticipating nursing interventions.

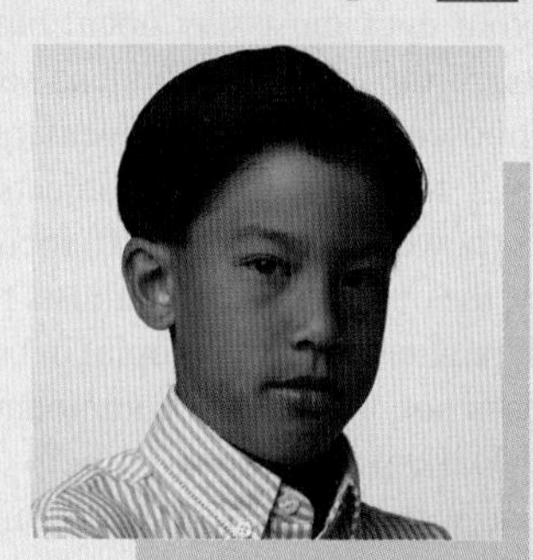

Inspection: Somewhat anxious boy, sitting in mother's lap. Face flushed, breathing easily, no shortness of breath. Dry, hacking cough. Oropharynx red without lesions or drainage. Tonsils slightly red and enlarged, graded 3+. Nares red with some clear thin drainage. External canals are clear. Tympanic membranes are pearl gray without perforation. Light reflex and landmarks intact. Hearing intact.

Palpation: No tenderness or swelling over sinuses.

Percussion: Thorax resonant.

Auscultation: Lungs clear, no wheezing or adventitious sounds.

Reflexes: Normoactive bilaterally.

Advanced Techniques and Special Equipment

Some physical assessment techniques require special equipment. Examples of such equipment include the ophthalmoscope, visual acuity chart, otoscope, tuning fork, percussion hammer, vaginal speculum, goniometer, and skinfold calipers. Because many of these tools relate specifically to one body system, they are discussed in the individual chapters of this book as relevant. Equipment discussed in the following paragraphs is included in more than one body system or has complicated instructions.

Using the Ophthalmoscope

The ophthalmoscope is a handheld system of lenses, lights, and mirrors that enables visualization of the interior structures of the eye (Fig. 3.9). The head of the ophthalmoscope attaches to the base, which is both a place to hold on to the ophthalmoscope and a power source with a rechargeable battery. The head contains the system of lights, lenses, and mirrors. When not in use, the base is plugged in for charging, while the head is stored to avoid damage.

Attach the head to the base by fitting the adapter of the base into the head and pushing down while turning the head clockwise. Turn on the ophthalmoscope by depressing the on/off switch. For routine use, the aperture commonly selected is the large full spot. Other choices include small light spot for small pupils, a green light to filter out red, a grid used to locate structures and lesions, and a slit used to determine the shape of lesions. Hold the ophthalmoscope firmly against your face, so that the eye looks directly through the viewing aperture. Both of your eyes must stay open, but your focus is on the view through the aperture. The lens selector dial focuses the ophthalmoscope, similar to binoculars. The black numbers (power of +20 to +140) focus on objects near, whereas the red numbers (power of −20 to −140) focus on objects far away. In this way, the ophthalmoscope adjusts for nearsightedness (myopia) or farsightedness (hyperopia) in both the nurse and the patient. It does not, however, accommodate for astigmatism.

Darken the room to help dilate the patient's pupils because the eye is visualized through the pupil. Eyeglasses obstruct visualization, so if you or the patient wears glasses, remove them. To avoid bumping noses with the patient, use the eye directly opposite the patient's eye being examined, using the hand on the same side. (For example, when examining the patient's right eye, hold the ophthalmoscope in your left hand and use your left eye.) Starting with zero, adjust the lenses using the index finger to bring the fundus (background) of the eye into focus. Moving the lens selector dial clockwise turns the magnification more positive, or closer, whereas moving the lens selector dial counterclockwise turns the magnification more negative, or further away. Ask the patient to look at a distant fixation point while you point the light of the ophthalmoscope into the pupil from approximately 25 to 30 cm (about 10 to 12 in.) away and slightly lateral to the patient's line of vision. Visualization of the red reflex is the first step in examination of the eye. See Chapter 13 for more details on this technique, use of the ophthalmoscope, and other topics.

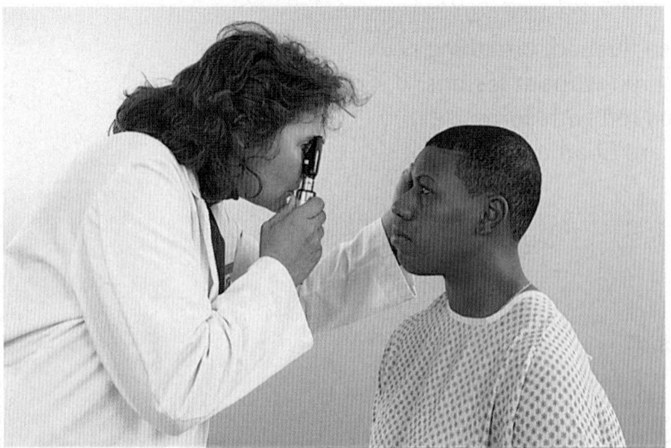

Figure 3.9 Positioning of the ophthalmoscope to visualize the interior structures of the eye.

Using the Otoscope

The otoscope directs light into the ear to visualize the ear canal and tympanic membrane. The otoscope's head and body connect and are activated in the same way as with the ophthalmoscope.

Select the proper-sized speculum, choosing the largest size that fits most comfortably into the patient's ear, and place it on the otoscope. Hold the otoscope's base between the thumb and the fingers upside down; brace the ulnar surface or fingers of the hand against the patient's cheek. This positioning allows you to move with the patient if the patient moves unexpectedly, as might happen with a child who has ear tenderness related to an infection.

While inserting the speculum, straighten the adult patient's ear canal by gently pulling the auricle up, back, and slightly away from the head (Fig. 3.10A). Insert the speculum gently into the ear canal, directing it slightly down and forward. You may also ask the patient to tilt the head toward the opposite shoulder to assist with visualization. With pediatric patients, pull the auricle down and back to straighten the ear canal; it may be easier to do this closer to the ear lobe (Fig. 3.10B). The technique and other findings are discussed in further detail in Chapter 14.

Using the Tuning Fork

The tuning fork is used in examinations of two anatomic regions: with a neuromuscular assessment, to determine vibration sense, and during assessment of hearing, to determine conductive versus sensorineural hearing loss. Depending on their design, tuning forks create vibrations that produce sound waves of low-pitched or high-pitched frequencies.

The tuning fork used to check for *hearing loss* produces a high-pitched tone of 512 to 1,024 Hz, within the range of human hearing (Fig. 3.11). While holding the fork at the base, activate it by briskly squeezing and stroking the outside of the tongs from base to tips or gently tapping the tongs against the knuckles to produce a soft ringing sound. Avoid touching the tongs once you have activated them, as this dampens the sound. If the fork is struck too harshly, the sound is too loud and

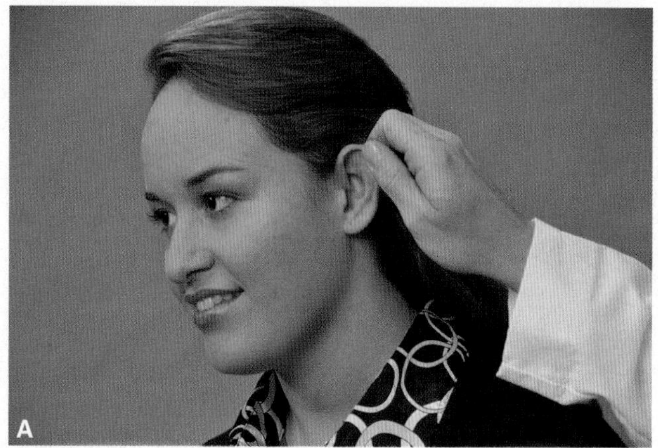

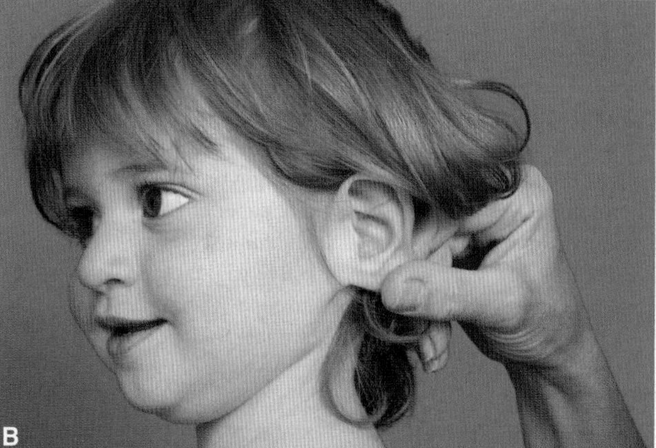

Figure 3.10 Placement of the ear for using the otoscope in **(A)** adults and **(B)** children.

takes too long to quiet to test the fine threshold of normal hearing. Gentle strokes or taps produce a softer sound for testing.

The tuning fork for determining *vibration sense* produces vibrations at a lower frequency of 128 to 256 Hz. Activate this lower pitched device by tapping it against the heel of the hand. Hold this fork at the base and apply the base to a bony prominence. The patient should feel a buzzing or tingling sensation.

Using the Reflex Hammer

The neurological reflex hammer is designed to test neurological responses of the deep tendons to assess for abnormalities of the central or peripheral nervous system. The most common uses during the physical examination includes assessment of the knee, ankle, brachial, elbow, and wrist tendons. There are several different types of reflex hammers. The Taylor hammer is used most commonly; it has a triangular rubber mallet attached to a metal handle. The pointy end of the hammer head is generally used on the upper body, whereas the flat end is used on the lower body. The hammer is gently swung using the wrist, in arclike fashion, to strike the tendon.

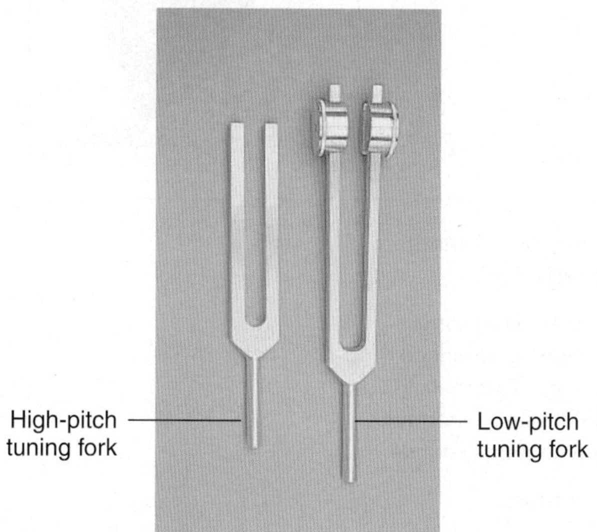

Figure 3.11 Tuning forks.

> **Clinical Significance**
>
> Hold the rounded part of the handle loosely and allow it to swing between the fingers, causing a brisk tap over the tendon. Practice the technique on yourself or a partner to gain expertise.

It may be more comfortable for the patient if you place your index finger over the tendon and strike midway between the tip and second joint of the finger, buffering the impact to the tendon. Use this technique when checking the smaller tendons of the wrist, ankle, and arm.

Responses are recorded as hypoactive, hyperactive, or normoactive.

Equipment for a Complete Physical Assessment

Gather all equipment needed for the physical assessment before entering the room to avoid interruption and to increase the patient's trust. Appropriate equipment depends on the type of examination. For example, if a patient has an appointment for a full physical assessment and Pap smear, lay out all the materials necessary for a complete physical assessment (Box 3.2), in addition to a speculum, gloves, material for cytology slide, lubricant, and fecal occult blood test materials.

For the general assessment in a hospital setting, you will need the following equipment: vital signs equipment (thermometer, alcohol, electronic or manual blood pressure machine, watch with second hand, stethoscope), scale, flashlight, and materials for recording findings.

Lifespan Considerations: Older Adults

Older adults may chill more easily than younger patients, so you should consider offering them an additional blanket or drape. These patients may also fatigue quickly, so it is important to perform the most important assessments in the

BOX 3.2 Equipment for Complete Physical Assessment

Platform scale with height measure	Clean gloves
Tongue depressor	Tuning fork: low pitched
Thermometer	Flashlight or penlight
Snellen chart	Coin, paper clip, key, or pen
Blood pressure cuff/machine	Ophthalmoscope
Tape measure	Bivalve vaginal speculum
Watch with second hand movement	Otoscope
Reflex hammer	Materials for cytological study
Stethoscope	Tuning fork: high pitched
Cotton swab	Lubricant
	Nasal speculum
	Fecal occult blood test materials

The equipment is listed in the order in which it is needed, and this order is also reflected in the order of the chapters in this textbook.

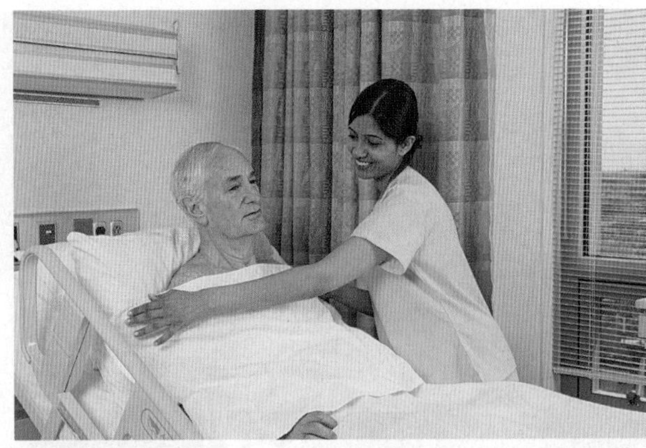

Figure 3.12 Slightly elevating the head of the bed or examination table may help facilitate breathing for older adults. Covering the patient to avoid chilling is another important consideration for patients in this age group.

beginning. When positioning older adults, slight elevation of the head of the bed or examination table may help facilitate breathing (Fig. 3.12).

Cultural Considerations

Each assessment must be individualized according to the patient's cultural, religious, and social beliefs. Many patients are anxious prior to physical assessment. Anxiety may be related to fear of disclosing private or uncomfortable information, embarrassment about being touched or looked at, or worry about unexpected findings. If there is a language barrier, arrange for a trained medical interpreter.

Before starting the examination, ask the patient about his or her preferences, such as having a family member in the room or having a same-gender examiner. Perform less invasive assessments first, such as taking vital signs, and save the most personal assessments for the end.

Progress Note: Analyzing Findings

Initial collection of subjective and objective data for Chris Chow has been completed by the nurse practitioner. The following nursing note documents the analysis of subjective and objective data and beginning development of nursing interventions.

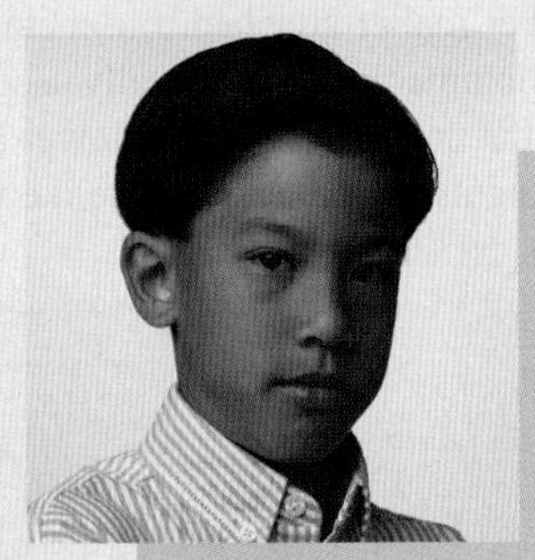

Subjective: A 6-year-old child seen for fever, sore throat, and "runny nose." Mother states that patient has had a fever for 2 days; symptoms are not resolving.

Objective: Face flushed, breathing easily, no shortness of breath. Dry, hacking cough. No tenderness or swelling over sinuses. Oropharynx red without lesions or drainage. Tonsils slightly red and enlarged, 1+. Nares red with clear, thin drainage. External canals clear. Tympanic membranes pearl gray without perforation. Light reflex, landmarks, and hearing intact. Thorax resonant. Lungs clear, no wheezing or adventitious sounds.

Analysis: Fever, viral rhinitis, and pharyngitis causing impaired comfort.

(case study continues on page 57)

Plan: Encouraged to drink at least 2 L of fluid a day. Frozen treats and Jell-O may be included in fluid intake. Take acetaminophen as needed for pain relief. Encouraged frequent rest, including naps during the day. Taught measures for infection control including disposal of tissues, covering mouth, and hand hygiene.

Critical Thinking Challenge

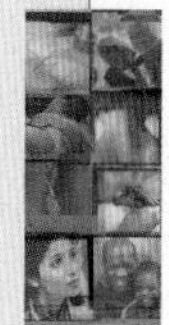

- What techniques and equipment did the nurse use during the physical assessment?
- How is the role of a nurse practitioner different from that of a registered nurse?
- How will you as a beginner learn, practice, and perfect these techniques used in assessment? How will you learn the finer distinctions in pitch, tone, and quality?

Applying Your Knowledge

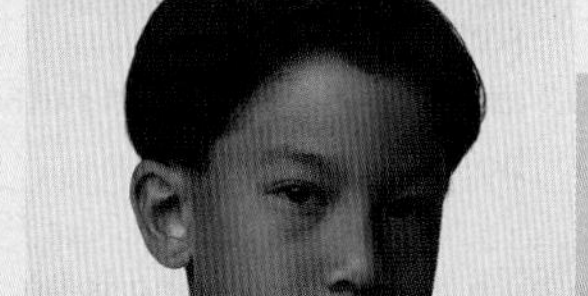

Using the steps of diagnostic reasoning, organizing, and prioritizing, consider all the case study findings woven throughout this chapter. When answering the following questions, begin drawing conclusions and see how the pieces of assessment must work together to create an environment for personalized, appropriate, and accurate care.

- What information does the nurse gain about patients during inspection, palpation, percussion, and auscultation?
- How does the nurse use safety and infection control principles during the assessment?
- What basic examination modes and equipment did the nurse practitioner use during the physical assessment?
- How might the nurse organize the assessment sequentially to include the different body systems in this focused assessment for the child?
- What factors might be contributing to Chris's illness?
- How will the nurse practitioner evaluate the outcome of her teaching?

Key Points

- Hand hygiene is the most important action to prevent nosocomial infections.
- Nurses and other health care providers use standard precautions with every patient because many patients may not be aware that they are infected.
- Latex allergies are more common in nurses and in patients frequently hospitalized than in the general public.
- Nurses wear gloves during anticipated contact with body secretions and remove them when going from contaminated to cleaner areas.
- Inspection, percussion, palpation, and auscultation are the four techniques of physical assessment.
- Inspection relies on vision and smell to assess general status as well as each body system.
- Nurses use light palpation to obtain an overall impression and deep palpation to assess pain, masses, and tumors.
- Percussion sounds vary based on tone, intensity, pitch, quality, duration, and location.
- Nurses commonly examine the heart, lungs, and abdomen with a stethoscope.
- An ophthalmoscope, visual acuity chart, otoscope, tuning fork, reflex hammer, vaginal speculum, goniometer, and skinfold calipers are equipment for advanced techniques used during the complete assessment.

Review Questions

1. Which of the following interventions is most important to prevent nosocomial infections?
   A. Proper glove use
   B. Hand hygiene
   C. Appropriate draping
   D. Quiet environment

2. Standard precautions
   A. are used on every patient because it is not always known whether a patient is infected.
   B. state that hand gel is used for infection with *Clostridium difficile*.
   C. include the use of gowns, gloves, and masks with all patients.
   D. recognize that transmission-based precautions are common.

3. Latex allergies
   A. always result in anaphylactic reactions and shock.
   B. can be reduced by moisturizing the hands after washing.
   C. cannot be caused by equipment such as a stethoscope.
   D. are more common in nurses and in frequently hospitalized patients.

4. Which of the following is an appropriate use of gloves?
   A. Gloves are worn during anticipated contact with intact skin.
   B. Gloves are removed when going from clean to contaminated areas.
   C. Gloves are worn during anticipated contact with body secretions.
   D. Gloves are removed when assessing the back of an incontinent patient.

5. Which of the following is an example of inspection?
   A. Heart rate and rhythm regular
   B. Lungs clear
   C. Abdomen tympanic
   D. Skin pink

6. The patient is complaining of abdominal pain. What technique is used to form an overall impression?
   A. Auscultation
   B. Light palpation
   C. Direct percussion
   D. Deep palpation

7. Tympany is a percussion sound commonly located in the
   A. thorax.
   B. upper arm.
   C. abdomen.
   D. lower leg.

8. Which organs or body areas does the nurse auscultate as part of the admitting assessment?
   A. Heart, lungs, and abdomen
   B. Kidneys, bladder, and ureters
   C. Abdomen, flank, and groin
   D. Neck, jaw, and clavicle

9. What technique facilitates accurate auscultation?
   A. Earpieces of the stethoscope are positioned to point toward the back.
   B. The tubing of the stethoscope is long and dark in color.
   C. The chestpiece of the stethoscope is sealed against the skin.
   D. The diaphragm of the stethoscope is used for low-frequency sounds.

10. When assessing the child, the nurse makes the following adaptation to the usual techniques:
    A. A pediatric stethoscope is used for better contact.
    B. The child is seated away from the parent.
    C. The room is full of toys for play.
    D. The child is undressed, including the diaper.

The Jensen suite offers these additional resources to enhance learning and facilitate understanding of this chapter:

- thePoint online resource, http://thepoint.lww.com/Jensen2e
- *Laboratory Manual for Nursing Health Assessment: A Best Practice Approach*
- *Pocket Guide for Nursing Health Assessment: A Best Practice Approach*
- *Lippincott DocuCare*, an electronic health record simulation software, http://thepoint.lww.com/docucare
- *Adaptive Learning | Powered by PrepU*, http://thepoint.lww.com/prepu

References

Centers for Disease Control and Prevention. (2014). *Healthcare-associated infections (HAI)*. Retrieved from http://www.cdc.gov/hai/

Schneider, A., Tschopp, C., Longtin, Y., Renzi, G., Gayet-Ageron, A., Schrenzel, J., & Pittet, D. (2011). *Predictors of stethoscope contamination following a standardized physical exam. BMC Proceedings*, 2011, 5(Suppl. 6), P304.

Siegel, J. D., Rhinehart, E., Jackson, M., & Chiarello, L. (n.d.). *2007 Guideline for isolation precautions: Preventing transmission of infectious agents in healthcare settings*. Retrieved from http://www.cdc.gov/ncidod/dhqp/pdf/isolation2007.pdf

U.S. Department of Labor, Occupational Safety and Health Administration. (2013). *Latex allergy*. Retrieved from http://www.osha.gov/SLTC/latexallergy/index.html

World Health Organization. (2013). *WHO guidelines on hand hygiene in healthcare*. Retrieved from http://whqlibdoc.who.int/publications/2009/9789241597906_eng.pdf

4

Documentation and Interdisciplinary Communication

Learning Objectives

1 Describe multiple purposes of the patient medical record.

2 Discuss the significance of accurate and timely documentation and the relationship between reporting patient assessment data and ensuring patient safety.

3 Compare and contrast various methods of documenting assessment data in the patient's record.

4 Provide a concise, clear handoff report using a template such as SBAR (*s*ituation, *b*ackground, *a*ssessment, and *r*ecommendation).

5 Discuss ethical and legal considerations when documenting and reporting assessment information into the patient record.

Mr. Chavez, 29 years old, was admitted to the hospital with a fractured humerus caused by a motor vehicle collision in which he was a passenger wearing his seat belt. His younger cousin, the driver, suffered a fractured tibia and fibula.

Mr. Chavez was born in Mexico; English is his second language, which he understands and speaks well. His temperature is 37.8°C (100°F) orally, pulse 110 beats/min, respirations 20 breaths/min, and blood pressure 122/66 mmHg. Current medications include patient-controlled analgesia with morphine for pain, an antibiotic, a multivitamin, a stool softener, and medications to be taken as needed for symptoms such as itching and nausea. Initial assessment was in the emergency department (ED); an admitting assessment occurred 4 hours earlier upon transfer to acute care. The nurse there is caring for him at the beginning of shift.

You will gain more information about Mr. Chavez as you progress through this chapter. As you study the content and features, consider Mr. Chavez's case and its relationship to what you are learning. Begin thinking about the following points:

- What is the importance of accurate and comprehensive documentation?
- Describe the difference between *recording* and *reporting*.
- What are important factors to consider when reporting?
- How do the patient's situation and urgent need for treatment influence the assessment, documentation, and communication of data?
- How does the collection of data fluctuate between a comprehensive and a focused assessment?
- Outline an example from the case study of Mr. Chavez that incorporates SBAR.
- How would you evaluate a successful handoff?

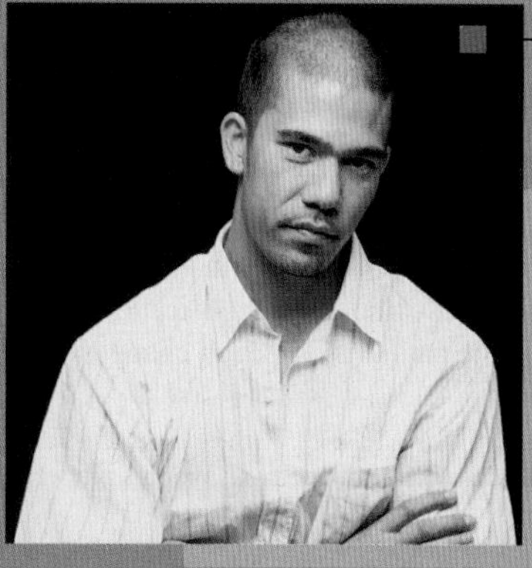

Prompt reporting and accurate recording of patient assessment data are essential to ensure safe and efficient delivery of care. In 2007, nearly 70% of all serious, often life-threatening, errors in health care (**sentinel events**) reported to The Joint Commission involved failures in communication as the root cause (The Joint Commission, 2013). Communication occurs both verbally and in writing. Documentation involves entering patient information into the written or computerized patient record. The patient clinical record contains recorded information from all health care encounters.

All health care team members document and retrieve information from the patient record as they plan and provide care. In the last decade, most health care agencies have transitioned the patient medical record from paper to a computerized, electronic form. Whether the patient record is paper or electronic, health care providers are responsible for always maintaining the confidentiality of all patient information.

Nurses use critical thinking and clinical judgment to determine when unexpected assessment data are significant, thus requiring verbal communication with other members of the health care team. Prompt accurate documentation and reporting help ensure safe delivery and individualization of patient care.

Patient Medical Record

Purposes of the Medical Record

The medical record serves multiple purposes. In addition to being a legal document, the medical record is used for communication among health team members, care planning, quality assurance, financial reimbursement by insurers, education, and research.

Legal Document

The patient record serves as a legal document recording the patient's health status and any care he or she receives. The patient record can be used in civil or criminal courts to provide evidence of wrongdoing. Health care agencies have policies and standards that govern documentation that staff members must follow. Documentation helps to ensure that patients pursuing litigation against nurses must demonstrate that nurses did not comply with agency standards and policies or did not act in a manner in which any prudent nurse would have acted under the same circumstances.

> **SAFETY ALERT**
>
> *The nurse must record normal assessment data, unexpected assessment data, and the time of the assessment. In the legal world, a typical saying is, "If it's not documented, it's not done." This reinforces the need to document not only unexpected findings but also normal findings. When listening to the lungs, it is important to note "lungs clear, no shortness of breath" to document that the assessments were performed and that the findings were normal to protect against false litigation. For significant unexpected findings, it is also important to document the name of the primary care provider who was notified, the time of notification, and any interventions. This provides evidence that the nurse communicated and acted on the assessment data to protect against negligence.*

Box 4.1 lists high-risk errors in documenting. Notice how many of these potential errors relate to the documentation of assessment data.

Communication and Care Planning

All members of the health care team access the assessment data documented in the patient's record to make care decisions. For example, a primary care provider reviews documentation from the patient's pain assessment to determine whether to increase, maintain, or decrease the amount of pain medication prescribed. A social worker reviews the record for evidence of family support or a description of the home environment to plan for discharge. Assessment data provide the basis for the plan of care (POC) that identifies problems, outcomes, and interventions for the patient. The POC helps caregivers coordinate and individualize care until discharge.

Quality Assurance

An **audit** occurs when an agency or outside group reviews the records of a health care facility to determine whether that facility is providing and documenting certain standards of care. During an *internal audit*, the goal is to evaluate the care provided for continual improvement. For example, an agency may audit the record to evaluate whether staff members are charting pain assessments in a timely manner on all patients. The audit might also include whether nurses are administering

BOX 4.1 High-Risk Errors in Documentation

- Falsifying patient records
- Failing to record changes in a patient's condition
- Failing to document the notification of the primary care provider when the patient's condition changes
- Performing an inadequate admission assessment
- Failing to document completely
- Failing to follow the agency's standards or policies on documentation
- Charting in advance

Adapted from Craven, R. C., Hirnle, C. J., and Jensen, S. (2013). *Fundamentals of nursing: Human health and function* (6th ed.). Philadelphia: Wolters Kluwer Health/Lippincott Williams & Wilkins.

PRN (i.e., *pro re nata*, or as-needed) pain medication for documented pain levels greater than 4 (on a 0-to-10 scale). Such an audit helps target interventions or education to improve pain management.

Accrediting agencies such as The Joint Commission or state agencies such as departments of health can establish standards and audit patient records to evaluate the quality of care provided. The Joint Commission accreditation is often required for facilities to obtain Medicare and Medicaid funding, so hospitals are motivated to comply with the standards in documentation and care that The Joint Commission sets.

The Joint Commission also requires each hospital to develop an ongoing objective review of patient records for continuous quality improvement and to demonstrate correction of any deficiencies noted during the review. For example, if the standard of care dictates that postoperative patients have a surgical site check and assessment of vital signs every 15 minutes after surgery, the team conducting the audit will review records to identify whether staff members are performing these assessments in a timely manner. Problem solving would occur at a systems level if the standard is not met, such as recommending an increase in unlicensed assistive personnel (UAP) to assist or scheduling surgeries more evenly.

Since the launching of the Sentinel Initiative in 2008, safety monitoring of medications and medical devices by the U.S. Food and Drug Administration (FDA) or other agencies is possible in real time by mining the electronic health record for significant data points (Sandhu, Weinstein, McKethan, & Jain, 2012). This will become easier and more productive as the electronic health record system becomes more robust.

Financial Reimbursement

Medicare, Medicaid, worker's compensation insurance, and third-party insurance companies depend on information in the patient's record to provide reimbursement for care. Documentation can support specific interventions that a primary care provider ordered (e.g., laboratory or diagnostic tests). Diagnosis-related groups (DRGs), a proactive payment system, have become the basis for hospital reimbursement. Detailed information in the patient record helps to support codable diagnoses that insurance companies use to determine the DRG (Fig. 4.1). Detailed charting of assessments and necessary interventions often can support approval for additional hospital days. Lack of appropriate charting can affect the authorization of financial payment. Insurance companies also audit patient records to ensure that billing is accurate and that no fraud has occurred.

Accurate assessments are needed to make accurate diagnoses. In 2008, Medicare and Medicaid stopped reimbursement for some hospital-acquired complications, referred to as **never events**, because they are preventable through the use of evidence-based guidelines and should never occur. Examples include foreign objects left in the body after surgery, catheter-associated urinary tract infections, stage 3 or 4 pressure ulcers, air emboli, infusion of incompatible blood, falls resulting in trauma, and air emboli. It is crucial for all nurses to document preexisting conditions and all assessment data related to "never events" to ensure proper hospital reimbursement.

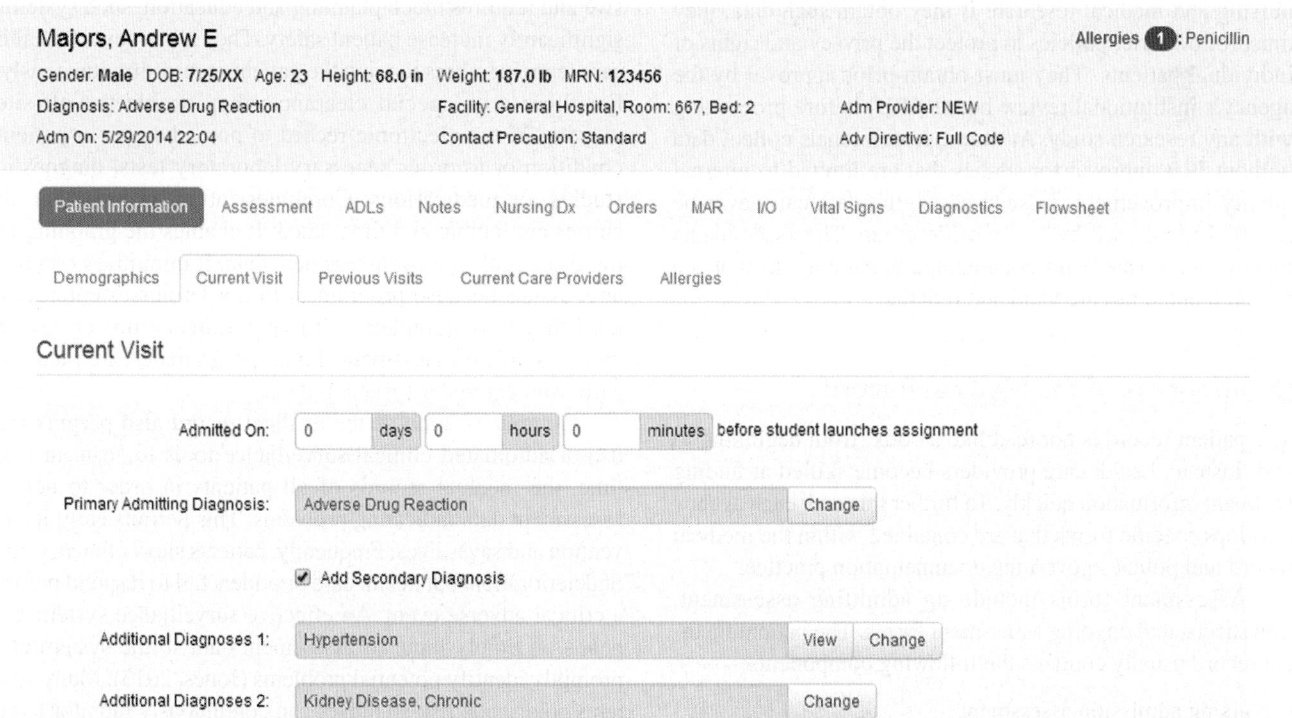

Figure 4.1 Nurses must take care to document accurately to support codable diagnoses used by insurance companies. (Courtesy of Lippincott DocuCare, http://thepoint.lww.com/docucare.)

In 2009, the Health Information Technology for Economic and Clinical Health (HITECH) Act established financial incentive programs from the Centers for Medicare and Medicaid Services to reward professional and agencies who demonstrate **"meaningful use"** of certified medical records. In this process, agencies demonstrate the ability to electronically transfer clinical information as the patient moves from one care provider to another or one health care system to another. Meaningful use also increases patients' electronic access to their own medical records (Wilson, Murphy, & Newhouse, 2012).

Education

Students in various health care disciplines review patient records to enhance clinical learning and to better understand complex clinical situations. They can access and review records during care delivery. At times, students come to the clinical area before their assigned shift to read the patient record and do the necessary research so that they can provide informed and individualized care.

Nursing grand rounds or classroom discussions can use specific patient situations to educate nurses and students. For example, an audit of charts from patients who experienced oversedation or respiratory depression from opioid administration may be collected and presented to staff members to help educate nurses about safe pain management. Assessment data are used to identify trends in respiratory rates and to detect early warning signs of clinical deterioration.

Research

Health care practitioners use patient records to obtain data for nursing and medical research. If they obtain such data, they must follow strict policies to protect the privacy and rights of individual patients. They must obtain prior approval by the agency's institutional review board (IRB) before proceeding with any research study. At times, professionals collect data without IRB approval for studies that are limited to internal quality improvement. In such cases, the data can never be reported to, or used by, any outside group. The assessments must be performed and documented accurately so that the research outcomes are valid and reliable.

Components of the Medical Record

The patient record is not read like a book, from beginning to end. Instead, health care providers become skilled at finding pertinent information quickly. To further this end, each agency develops specific forms that are contained within the medical record and policies governing documentation practice.

Assessment forms include an admitting assessment, flowsheets, and ongoing assessment forms. The patient medical record usually contains the following components:

- Nursing admission assessment
- History and physical examination (H&P) by the primary care provider
- Primary care provider's orders
- POC or clinical pathway
- Flowsheets documenting vital signs, intake and output (I&O), and routine assessments
- Focused assessment sheets (e.g., neurological or postoperative reassessment)
- Medication administration record (MAR)
- Laboratory and diagnostic test results
- Progress notes by different members of the health care team
- Consultations
- Discharge or transfer summary

Electronic Medical Record

Most clinical agencies have computerized part or all of the patient's medical record. Software programs allow nurses and other health care providers to enter assessment data quickly, usually by checking boxes and adding free text when appropriate. The electronic medication administration record (eMAR) interfaces medication orders with pharmacy dispensing and allows direct computer charting of medication administration (Fig. 4.2). Computerized provider order entry (CPOE) allows health care providers to enter all orders directly into the computer, electronically communicating orders to the laboratory, pharmacy, and nursing personnel (Arditi, Rège-Walther, Wyatt, Durieux, & Burnand, 2012). Appropriate staff members receive a computerized communication (i.e., task) when assessments, treatments, or medications are due during their assigned shifts. They also receive a message when the patient requires a reassessment (e.g., blood administration or restraint use).

Although implementing a computerized system is expensive and requires much planning and education, such systems significantly increase patient safety. They allow several health care team members to view the patient record simultaneously. For those with special clearance, they enable the off-site viewing of the electronic record to note changes in patient condition or to order necessary laboratory tests, diagnostic studies, or medications. Computerization ensures that all entries are legible and time dated. It enables the graphing of trends in vital signs or assessment data. It minimizes compliance issues because programs will not let nurses enter data until they have completed all required fields; this ensures a more complete assessment. Some programs create plans of care from entered assessment data.

Computerization of the medical record also permits the use of automated clinical surveillance tools to scan, in real time, the medical records of all patients in order to detect assessment data indicating problems. This permits early intervention and saves lives. Frequently, patients show clinical signs of deterioration, but health care providers fail to respond before a critical adverse event. An effective surveillance system depends on timely input of assessment data so the system can promptly identify potential problems (Jones, 2013). Many systems color-code risk so nurses can continuously monitor large groups of patients and quickly intervene for patients with a high-risk score. Some examples include tools for identifying the risk for skin breakdown and the risk for falling.

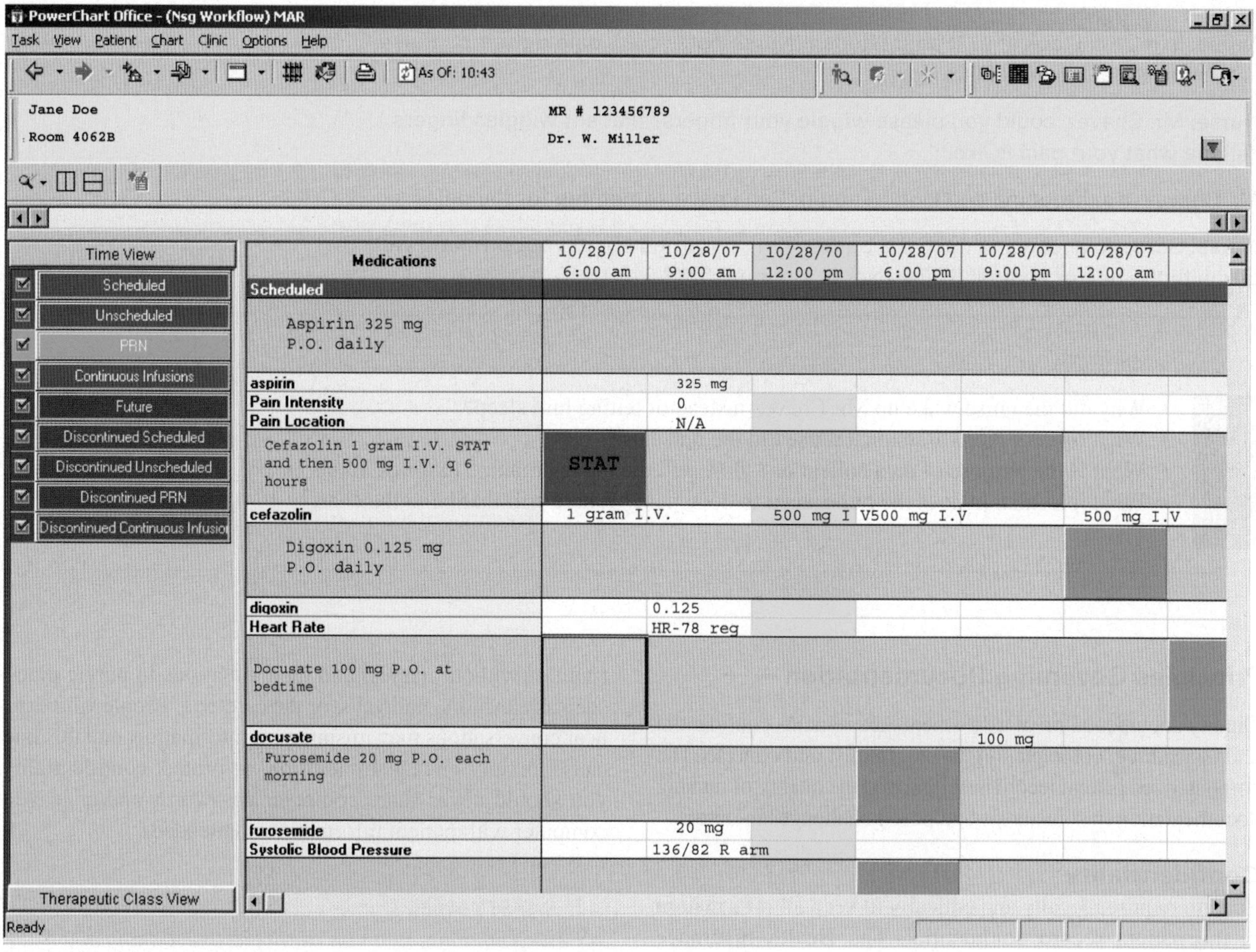

PowerChart Office - (Nsg Workflow) MAR

Task View Patient Chart Clinic Options Help

As Of: 10:43

Jane Doe MR # 123456789

Room 4062B Dr. W. Miller

Time View

- Scheduled
- Unscheduled
- PRN
- Continuous Infusions
- Future
- Discontinued Scheduled
- Discontinued Unscheduled
- Discontinued PRN
- Discontinued Continuous Infusio

Therapeutic Class View

Medications	10/28/07 6:00 am	10/28/07 9:00 am	10/28/70 12:00 pm	10/28/07 6:00 pm	10/28/07 9:00 pm	10/28/07 12:00 am
Scheduled						
Aspirin 325 mg P.O. daily						
aspirin		325 mg				
Pain Intensity		0				
Pain Location		N/A				
Cefazolin 1 gram I.V. STAT and then 500 mg I.V. q 6 hours	STAT					
cefazolin	1 gram I.V.		500 mg I	V500 mg I.V		500 mg I.V
Digoxin 0.125 mg P.O. daily						
digoxin		0.125				
Heart Rate		HR-78 reg				
Docusate 100 mg P.O. at bedtime						
docusate					100 mg	
Furosemide 20 mg P.O. each morning						
furosemide		20 mg				
Systolic Blood Pressure		136/82 R arm				

Ready

Figure 4.2 An electronic medication administration record improves safety.

Therapeutic Dialogue: Collecting Subjective Data

Remember Mr. Chavez, introduced at the beginning of this chapter. The nurse uses professional communication techniques to gather subjective data from Mr. Chavez at the beginning of the shift. As you read the conversation, consider the purpose of this data collection.

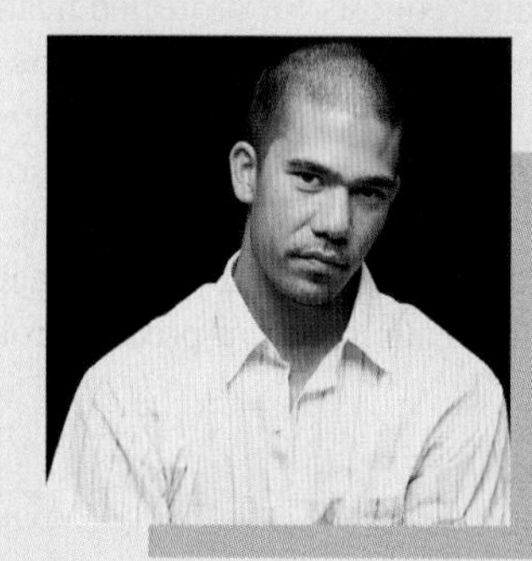

Nurse: Hi, Mr. Chavez. How are you feeling? (Waits 10 seconds.) (Touches patient.) Mr. Chavez, I'm Shannon, your nurse.

Mr. Chavez: Oh, sorry. I was sleepy. Let me sleep.

Nurse: OK, but first I need to look at your arm.

Mr. Chavez: OK (turns over). My arm hurts.

(case study continues on page 64)

Nurse: Is it OK if I look at it? (Patient nods.) (Nurse notes cool, pale right arm. Pulse is decreased. Capillary refill is slow.)

Nurse: Mr. Chavez, could you please wiggle your fingers? (Patient wiggles fingers.) Tell me what your pain is like.

Mr. Chavez: It's throbbing and kind of numb. Can I have something for the pain?

Nurse: Sure, go ahead and push the button. I'm concerned about your arm and will talk with the doctor about it. I'll be back in a minute. OK?

Critical Thinking Challenge

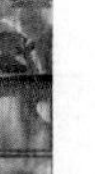

- Why did the nurse wake up Mr. Chavez instead of letting him sleep?
- What roles of the professional nurse did the nurse use?
- What is the purpose of data collection? How will the nurse organize findings in this case?
- What information does the nurse need to document? Where will that be in the chart?

Principles Governing Documentation

Quality documentation of assessment data remains confidential and is accurate, complete, organized, timely, and concise. The computerized patient record has improved the quality of nursing documentation in some areas and posed challenges in others.

Confidentiality

You are required legally and ethically to keep all information in the patient record confidential. The Health Insurance Portability and Accountability Act (HIPAA, 1996), which gives patients greater control over their medical records, became effective in 2003. HIPAA regulates all areas of information management, including reimbursement, coding, and security of records. The HIPAA Privacy Rule requires an agency to make reasonable efforts to limit use of, disclosure of, and requests for protected health information to the minimum necessary to accomplish the intended purpose.

Most agencies require students and employees to complete HIPAA training. HIPAA also provides for patient education on privacy protection, patient access to medical records, patient consent prior to disclosing information from the record, and patient recourse if privacy protections are violated.

> **SAFETY ALERT**
> *Health care providers who violate HIPAA may face fines of up to $250,000 or jail time (HIPAA, 1996). Employees have been terminated for breaching HIPAA laws concerning confidentiality.*

Confidentiality means keeping information private. This principle applies to computerized and written medical records and any information pertaining to health status or care received (Fig. 4.3). All patient information is confidential and may be discussed only with other health care professionals directly involved in the patient's care. You should never discuss patients (with or without names) and their situations in public places such as elevators, hallways, or the cafeteria. People who overhear conversations may misinterpret information, and this may cause anxiety or fear. In addition, to protect confidentiality, you should never share computer passwords and/or leave a computer with patient information unattended.

> **SAFETY ALERT**
> *Nursing students must be careful to de-indentify any patient information in written assignments in order to be HIPAA-compliant. Never take forms from the agency, even if the patient identification information is removed. Instead, copy information from the patient's chart into a notebook, without the patient's name.*

Privacy of the patient is additionally protected through de-identification or stripping away any individual identifiers (e.g., hospital or unit location, age) when patient data are exchanged for secondary use (Sandhu et al., 2012).

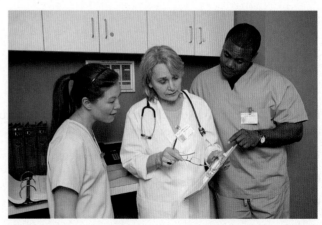

Figure 4.3 All providers strictly follow the HIPAA Privacy Rule.

TABLE 4.1 **Accurate Documentation Using Medical Terminology**

Ambiguous Documentation	Accurate Documentation
Vitals normal	T 37°C, P 80, R 12 breaths/min, BP 118/62 mmHg
Neuro status OK	Alert and oriented times 3, speech clear
Lung sounds good	Lung sounds clear
Heart sounds good	Heart rate and rhythm regular
Eating well	Ate 60% of regular diet
Voiding well	Voiding 700 ml of clear, yellow urine
No difficulties moving	Moves all extremities with full range of motion and 5/5 strength
Skin color good	Skin color pink
Family was here	Family visiting with appropriate interactions

T, temperature; P, pulse; R, respiration; BP, blood pressure.

Accuracy and Completeness

Assessment information that you enter into the patient's record must accurately reflect what you observe, hear, auscultate, palpate, percuss, or smell. Document subjective data using the patient's exact words whenever possible. Your descriptions should be as precise as possible. For example, you would document the size of a wound as "6 cm by 9 cm with a 1-cm depth" rather than as "large." Accuracy permits comparison of current findings with future data to detect changes in patient status. For this reason, avoid using the words "normal" or "good"; instead, use correct medical terminologies (e.g., "heart rate and rhythm regular," not "normal."). See Table 4.1.

To avoid potential errors, The Joint Commission discourages the use of certain abbreviations. It is important to be familiar with abbreviations and to use only those legally accepted. As you learn health assessment techniques, you also should focus on learning the language, labeling the findings, and identifying abbreviations.

Computerization of the patient medical record has greatly increased the legibility of its information. Nevertheless, handwritten entries still occur, and they must be clear and legible. This is especially true when recording numbers that can easily be confused. Black ink is usually required for written documentation to provide clarity when faxing documentation from the patient record.

On occasion, you will need to correct errors in documentation so that the record is accurate. In the written record, you make corrections by drawing a line through the error and placing your initials above the correction. The computerized record permits electronic correction of errors, retaining both the original entry and the correction (Fig. 4.4). Erasing, blacking out information, or using correction fluid is not permitted in paper records.

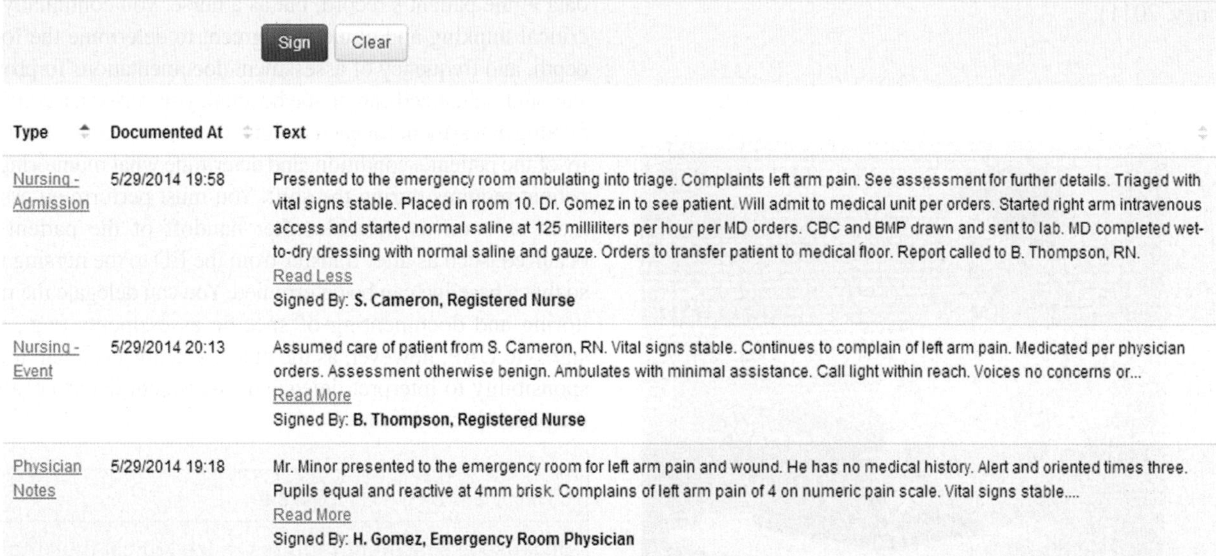

Figure 4.4 A sample of a corrected entry in a written patient record. (Courtesy of Lippincott DocuCare, http://thepoint.lww.com/docucare.)

Logical Organization

Organized entry of assessment data ensures a logical and systematic grouping of information. **Flowsheets** and documentation systems often cue you to a specific organizational structure. This encourages you to include all areas of assessment and provides an organized report so that other health care team members can use the information to make sound clinical decisions. You should also document entries concerning assessment chronologically so that a picture of that time certain assessments were made is clear. This is especially important if the patient record is used as evidence during litigation.

Timeliness

You must enter assessment data into the record in a timely manner. Most agencies have policies regarding the frequencies of assessments. For example, on a medical–surgical unit, a complete assessment may occur every 8 hours; in the intensive care unit, it may be every hour; and in the skilled nursing facility (SNF), it might be weekly. Computerized charting automatically reflects the time the entry is made, but you can change the documented time to reflect the time of the actual assessment. Paper charting should also reflect the specific time (e.g., 2:04 AM) rather than a shift designation (e.g., 7–3).

Batch charting (waiting until the end of shift or until all patients have been assessed to document) contributes to many potential errors. If you wait to record, you may forget important information or chart assessment data on the wrong patient. With **point-of-care documentation**, you document assessment information as you gather it, often using a portable computer (Fig. 4.5). You can do this during a home visit, a clinic visit, or in the patient's room during a hospital stay. Point-of-care documentation allows you to include the patient by verbalizing what is being entered into the record for verification; it provides more accurate, timely documentation and avoids the need for error-prone batch charting (Kenney, 2011).

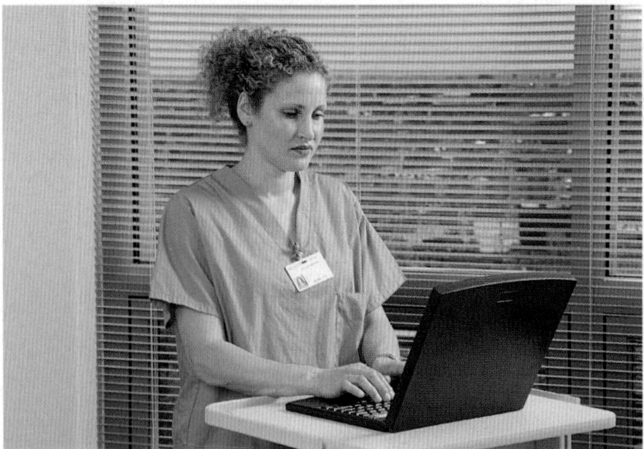

Figure 4.5 The nurse is using a portable computer on wheels to carry out point-of-care documentation.

Prompt documentation allows health care team members to use up-to-date assessment information to make clinical decisions. For example, a change in weight or vital signs might prompt a primary care provider to adjust a medication dosage. Computerized documentation systems allow other health care team members to review the patient record off-site and enables them to base decisions on the current record.

> **Clinical Significance**
>
> Clear documentation that reflects time sequencing is especially important for patients with unstable conditions. If litigation occurs, lawyers use documentation to reconstruct the sequence of events, the time of interventions, and the time that primary care providers were notified. In a code or emergency situation, the team should designate a single member to document so that entries are accurate and timely.

Conciseness

Good charting is complete, yet concise. Unnecessary elaboration confuses important issues. You should record the findings but not how you collected them. For example, you would document "BP (R) 124/78" instead of "BP was auscultated in the right arm at 124/78." Time is a precious health care resource; long rambling entries take more time to document and to read. In narrative notes, health care providers use sentence fragments (e.g., "alert and oriented") and approved abbreviations instead of complete sentences.

Generally, you chart information in one place and avoid "double charting." An exception is in the POC or progress note, in which you synthesize the most important information to show critical thinking about a problem.

Critical Thinking

Agency policy governs the precise documentation of assessment data in the patient's record, but as a nurse, you continually use critical thinking and clinical judgment to determine the focus, depth, and frequency of assessment documentation. To provide safe, individualized care in the hospital, you perform a complete nursing assessment for each assigned patient, evaluate the stability of the patient's condition, and determine what monitoring the patient requires during the shift. You must perform an assessment as soon as possible after handoff of the patient has occurred, such as after transfer from the ED to the nursing unit, so that a baseline can be determined. You can delegate the monitoring and documenting of specific assessments (e.g., vital signs) to UAP; however, as the nurse, you always retain the responsibility to interpret delegated assessment data to evaluate the patient's condition.

> **Clinical Significance**
>
> Because assessment requires much critical thinking and clinical judgment and is a professional responsibility, you cannot delegate it to UAPs.

Documenting Case Study Findings

The nurse has just finished a focused assessment of Mr. Chavez's fractured humerus. Review the following important findings that the relevant steps of objective data collection for Mr. Chavez revealed. Begin to think about how the data cluster together and what additional data the nurse might want to collect as he or she thinks critically and anticipates nursing interventions for the patient. Pay attention to how the nurse clusters data together to provide a more complete and accurate understanding of the condition.

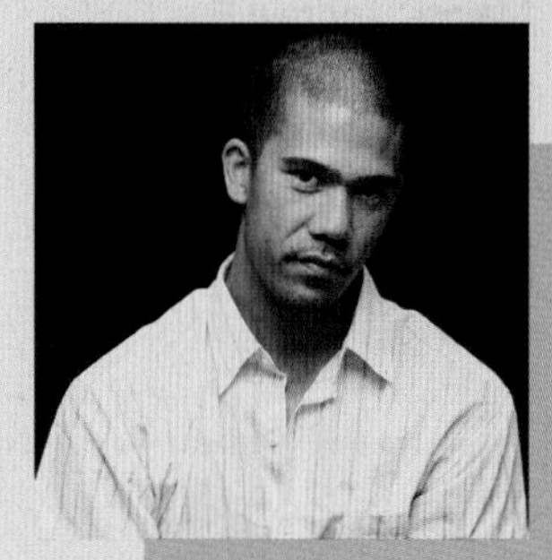

Inspection: Appears somewhat drowsy with grimacing caused by pain. Guarding right humerus. Wiggles fingers, states some numbness and tingling. States 8/10 pain throbbing from below elbow to fingers. Increasing since injury; particularly worse in the last 30 minutes. Movement increases pain. Given pain medication 2 hours ago for pain 4/10.

Palpation: Right radial artery 1+; limb pale and cool. Capillary refill 6 seconds. Sensation intact. Left arm pink, warm with 3+ pulse, no pain and intact sensation.

Based on knowledge and experience, nurses individualize assessments. For example, a middle-aged patient admitted for foot surgery may not require a comprehensive neurological assessment if he is alert and can answer questions appropriately. Conversely, an intoxicated patient with a head laceration who is admitted after an assault would definitely require a complete neurological assessment, including pupil checks, to promptly detect increased intracranial pressure or alcohol withdrawal (see Chap. 22). Although a primary care provider's order determines the minimum frequency of assessments, you would independently decide to increase the frequency and documentation of assessments if a patient's condition appears unstable or deteriorating. You would also use clinical judgment regarding when to notify the primary care provider regarding unexpected findings. You need to document such reporting, including the time of notification and the primary care provider's response.

Nursing Admission Assessment

You conduct the nursing admission assessment, sometimes referred to as the nursing history and physical, to obtain patient history and baseline data so that you can individualize care. In acute care facilities, policy usually requires the completion and documentation of the initial complete nursing assessment within 24 hours of admission. An SNF may require the completion of such an assessment within 3 days of the patient's admission. The agency usually provides separate forms to cue the assessment and standardize the documentation (Fig. 4.6).

The admission assessment provides all future care providers with comprehensive information about the patient's physical, psychological, functional, social, and spiritual abilities and forms the basis for an individualized POC. Care providers can refer to this initial assessment to obtain important baseline information and to detect changes in status.

Flowsheets

You usually document routine scheduled assessments on flowsheets. Flowsheets are efficient and standardize the collected information, permitting easy comparison among assessment data to detect trends or a sudden change in status. Common flowsheets in the patient's record include vital signs, I&O, routine assessments, and records involving diabetes care. More complex flowsheets are used in critical care, where frequent extensive physiological assessments are necessary to quickly detect and treat life-threatening problems.

Plan of Care and Clinical Pathway

An assessment of the patient allows for the development of a POC that individualizes the patient's goals, outcomes, and interventions. The POC is part of the permanent patient record, and nurses update it regularly and any time the patient's condition changes. A **clinical pathway** is a multidisciplinary tool that identifies a standard plan for a specific patient population (e.g., those undergoing total hip replacement). It includes patient problems, expected outcomes, and interventions within an established time frame. The POC or clinical pathway often provides the structure for shift report handoff.

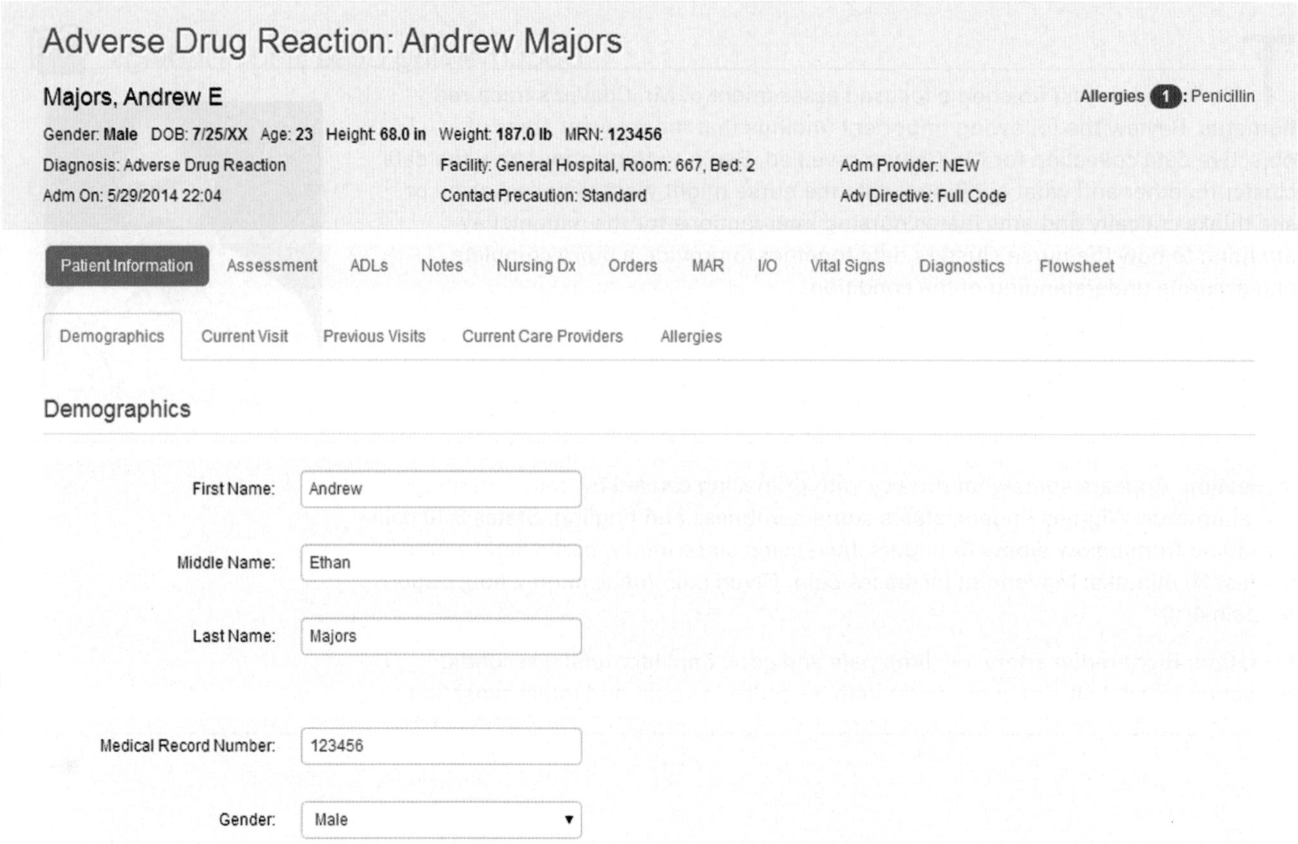

Adverse Drug Reaction: Andrew Majors

Majors, Andrew E

Allergies 1: Penicillin

Gender: **Male** DOB: **7/25/XX** Age: **23** Height: **68.0 in** Weight: **187.0 lb** MRN: **123456**

Diagnosis: Adverse Drug Reaction | Facility: General Hospital, Room: 667, Bed: 2 | Adm Provider: NEW

Adm On: 5/29/2014 22:04 | Contact Precaution: Standard | Adv Directive: Full Code

Patient Information | Assessment | ADLs | Notes | Nursing Dx | Orders | MAR | I/O | Vital Signs | Diagnostics | Flowsheet

Demographics | Current Visit | Previous Visits | Current Care Providers | Allergies

Demographics

First Name: Andrew

Middle Name: Ethan

Last Name: Majors

Medical Record Number: 123456

Gender: Male

Figure 4.6 A sample admission record. (Courtesy of Lippincott DocuCare, http://thepoint.lww.com/docucare.)

Progress Note (Case Note)

Multiple health team members (physician, physical therapist, respiratory therapist, social workers, and nurses) document in a **progress note** (sometimes called the case note) the patient's progress toward recovery. There has been a movement away from each team member documenting assessments in a discipline-specific section of the patient's record. The current trend is for personnel from different disciplines to consolidate all entries in one place. This permits all team members to quickly locate and read how the patient is progressing and meeting (or not meeting) goals.

Many nurses use progress notes to summarize how the patient is doing, but formats for this type of documentation can vary. Narrative, SOAP (*s*ubjective, *o*bjective, *a*nalysis, *p*lan), PIE (*p*roblems, *i*ntervention, *e*valuation), and DAR (*d*ata, *a*ction, *r*esponse) notes are common methods of recording assessments, interventions, and patient responses. Table 4.2 compares these formats of documentation.

Regardless of the format used, the progress note is an evaluative statement summarizing significant difficulties or improvements. Flowsheets record all collected assessment data, whereas progress notes allow nurses to use critical thinking to document and communicate priority issues to other health team members.

Narrative Notes

Using narrative notes, nurses record, in an unstructured paragraph, relevant assessments and nursing activities during a shift or visit. Usually, the organizing structure is time rather than an identified problem. Historically, narrative notes were very common, but most agencies are moving to more structured documentation formats. The more structured notes assist nurses to use assessment data to analyze findings, critically think about problems, and direct care at a higher level.

SOAP Notes

The SOAP format focuses on a single problem using the following presentation:

S: subjective assessment findings
O: objective assessment findings
A: analysis of the assessment data to identify a problem or indicate whether the problem is improving or worsening
P: plan for treating or improving the problem

Some agencies expand SOAP to SOAPIE, in which the *I* represents interventions to treat the problem and the *E* represents evaluation of the problem. This text uses the SOAP note format for documentation of unexpected findings in the case studies throughout.

Progress Note: Analyzing Findings

Remember Mr. Chavez, who was admitted to the hospital with a fractured right humerus. The nurse has performed a more complete assessment, clustered findings, and contacted the physician about concerns over inadequate tissue perfusion to the patient's arm. The following nursing note illustrates how the nurse collects and analyzes subjective and objective data and begins to develop nursing interventions.

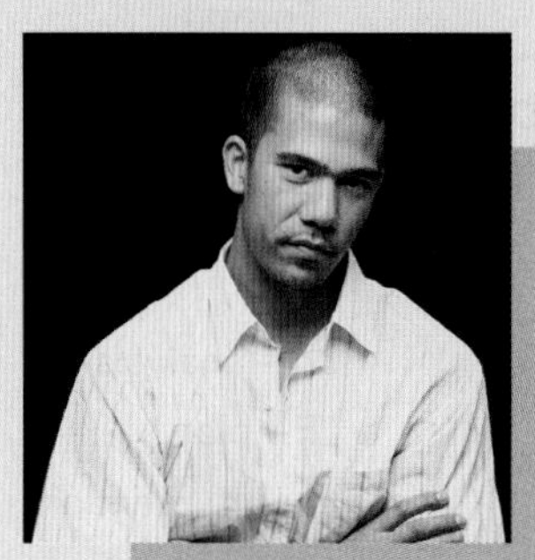

Subjective: States pain 8/10 from below elbow to fingertips. Characterized pain as numb and achy. Increased since admission, especially in the past 30 minutes. Morphine less effective now than earlier. Pain increased by movement.

Objective: Right radial artery 1+, limb pale and cool. Capillary refill 6 seconds. Sensation intact. Left arm pink, warm with 3+ pulse, no pain and intact sensation.

Analysis: Reduced tissue perfusion to right arm related to injury. Increasing pain.

Plan: Contacted Dr. Costa to evaluate limb. Patient seen at 19:30; primary care provider indicated that there was no change from baseline. Patient is on call for surgery for open reduction internal fixation (ORIF) this evening. Orders written to assess circulation, sensation, and movement (CSM) every hour. Morphine patient-controlled analgesia (PCA) orders increased—see orders. Reevaluate the effectiveness of morphine in 30 minutes.

Critical Thinking Challenge

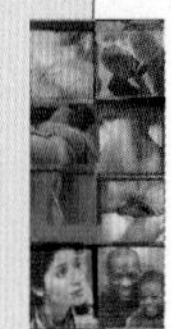

- How could you evaluate whether this assessment is a change from previous findings?
- How should the nurse organize information before contacting the primary care provider?
- What concepts of confidentiality should the nurse use if the patient asks about the status of his cousin or other people with injuries in the collision?
- What further assessments will be important for the nurse to perform and document? Where will the nurse document them?

TABLE 4.2 Comparison of Documentation Formats

	Format	Example	Advantages	Disadvantages
Narrative	Information written in phases, usually time sequenced	4/18/08, 15:00: 37°C, 98 beats/min, 22 breaths/min, 130/82 mmHg. Pt c/o pain 8/10; states he is using his PCA, but it doesn't help. Notified MD of pain level at 14:30. Pain is throbbing from fingers to elbow; has gotten worse over last 30 minutes. Pain increases with movement. Fingers of left hand pink, warm, able to move with strong pulse and no c/o of pain with movement. Right hand cool and pale with capillary refill 6 seconds. *S. Roberts, RN*	Easy to learn Easy to adjust length Can explain in detail	Time consuming Difficult to retrieve information May include irrelevant information Possibly unfocused and disorganized

(table continues on page 70)

TABLE 4.2 **Comparison of Documentation Formats** *(continued)*

	Format	Example	Advantages	Disadvantages
SOAP(IE)	S—subjective data O—objective data A—analysis P—plan I—intervention E—evaluation	4/18/08 15:00 S—States pain 8/10 from elbow to fingertips. Intensity increases with movement, especially over last 30 minutes. PCA does not seem to help. O—37°C, 98 beats/min, 22 breaths/min, 130/82 mmHg. Right radial artery 1+, limb pale and cool. Capillary refill 6 seconds. Sensation intact. Left arm pink, warm with 3+ pulse; no pain, intact sensation. A—Reduced tissue perfusion to right hand related to injury and inadequate pain control. P—Contact Dr. Cisco to evaluate patient. Saw patient at 14:30 and indicated no change from baseline; left orders for increased morphine dose. I—PCA morphine increase at 14:35, right hand elevated. E—Evaluate pain effectiveness in 30 minutes and increase CSM checks to hourly. *S. Roberts, RN*	All charting focuses on identified or new problems Interdisciplinary, so all team members chart on same progress note using same format Easy to track progress for identified problems Similar to steps in the nursing process	Specific focus, which makes charting general information difficult without identifying a problem Lengthy and time consuming Repeats assessment data on flowsheets
PIE	P—problem I—intervention E—evaluation	P—Inadequate tissue perfusion and inadequate pain control. I—Dr. Costa contacted at 14:30 to report pain 8/10 and cool, pale right hand with capillary refill of 6 seconds. He saw patient and left orders for increased PCA morphine. Right hand elevated. E—Dr. Costa reports circulation same as admission baseline. Continue hourly CSM checks; evaluate pain effectiveness after 30 minutes. *S. Roberts, RN*	Incorporates POC Includes outcomes, which increases quality assurance Less redundancy Easily adapted to computerized charting	May need to read progress note to determine POC if not on separate document Not multidisciplinary
DAR	D—data A—action R—response	D—37°C, 98 beats/min, 22 breaths/min, 130/82 mmHg. Right radial artery 1+, limb pale and cool. Capillary refill 6 seconds. Sensation intact. Left arm pink, warm with 3+ pulse, no pain, intact sensation. States pain 8/10 from elbow to fingertips. Intensity increases with movement; has increased especially over last 30 minutes; PCA does not seem to help. A—Dr. Costa contacted at 14:30 to report pain 8/10 and cool, pale right hand with capillary refill of 6 seconds. He saw patient and left orders for increased PCA morphine. Right hand elevated. R—Dr. Costa reports circulation is same as admission baseline. Continue hourly CMS checks and evaluate pain effectiveness after 30 minutes. *S. Roberts, RN*	Broad view, permitting charting on any significant area, not just problems Works well in ambulatory and long-term care	Not multidisciplinary May be difficult to identify chronological order May not relate to POC

(table continues on page 71)

TABLE 4.2 **Comparison of Documentation Formats** *(continued)*

	Format	Example	Advantages	Disadvantages
Charting by exception	Standards met—sign or check off Standards unmet—write narrative or SOAP note	Unexpected assessments require a note rather than signing off. See above for different note formats.	Efficient No duplicate charting because most assessments are charted on flowsheets Clearly outlines unexpected assessment	Expensive to develop and educate staff regarding standards Not prevention focused Not useful for ambulatory or long-term care May pose legal problems because details are often missing

Adapted from Craven, R. C., Hirnle, C. J., and Jensen, S. (2013). *Fundamentals of nursing: Human health and function* (6th ed., p. 212). Philadelphia: Wolters Kluwer Health/Lippincott Williams & Wilkins.

PIE Notes

The PIE format includes problem (**P**), interventions (**I**), and evaluation (**E**). Its goal is to incorporate the POC into the progress note. Patient assessments are not part of the PIE note but instead are charted on flowsheets. Some agencies adapt the PIE note to an APIE note, with *A* for assessment, so documentation reflects pertinent assessment data to support the problem (Craven, Hirnle, & Jensen, 2013).

DAR Note

The DAR system of documentation organizes entries by data (**D**), action (**A**), and response (**R**). Documentation can focus on areas of strengths as well as medical difficulties, family concerns, or nursing diagnoses. Using this chapter's case study as an example, data could include the phone conversation the nurse has with Mr. Chavez's mother, who is very worried and trying to get to the hospital to see her son, but she has younger children who cannot be left alone and no transportation. The data portion contains subjective and objective findings that support the focus of the note. The action section presents interventions and treatments, whereas the response section reviews how the patient responded or met outcomes (Craven et al., 2013).

Charting by Exception

Charting by exception (CBE) uses predetermined standards and norms to record only significant assessment data. Clearly identifying the standards and norms and educating all users take time and significant commitment from the agency using CBE. For example, a group may develop the standard of what it considers "normal" in each area of assessment (e.g., respiratory, mobility, psychosocial); these norms structure the patient assessment. Norms for respiratory function might include respiratory rate of 12 to 18 breaths/min, lungs clear to auscultation with no adventitious breath sounds, oxygen saturation above 93% on room air, and no dyspnea with activity. This cues nurses to assess respiratory rate, auscultate the lungs for adventitious sounds, assess oxygen saturation on room air, and assess whether an activity causes shortness of breath. If the patient's assessment matches the designated norms, the nurse checks a box. Any unexpected assessment findings require additional documentation.

Discharge Note

When a patient is discharged, you enter a discharge note in the chart. The note can be a computer-generated form, a hand-filled paper form, or narrative note in the progress notes. Your assessment of the patient should indicate that he or she is stable and has received teaching regarding medications and follow-up care. The discharge note should also contain patient discharge teaching, discharge medications, when to contact the primary care provider, condition at discharge, and time of discharge. Give a copy of the discharge summary with patient teaching and discharge medication to the patient.

The assessment information in the discharge note is used to identify necessary resources and strategies for successful home management. This information is useful for the social worker, physical and occupational therapists, and providers of follow-up care when the patient returns to the outpatient setting.

Home Care Documentation

In 2000, the federal government mandated that home care agencies use the *O*utcome and *As*sessment *I*nformation *S*et (OASIS) in the initial and ongoing assessments of all patients they care for in order to qualify for Medicare or Medicaid reimbursement. Assessment is performed initially to reassess the effectiveness of interventions and to measure whether the patient is meeting outcomes. The OASIS tool accurately measures the patient's status at various specified points during an episode of care (Centers for Medicare and Medicaid Services [CMS], 2013), thus providing the basis for measuring patient outcomes. OASIS data items include sociodemographic data, environmental information, support systems, health status, and functional status of all adult home care patients.

Because of the complexity of the OASIS system, additional education of nurses is necessary before using this system.

Long-Term Care Documentation

The Resident Assessment Instrument (RAI) governs documentation in long-term care settings. The RAI tracks goal achievement among long-term care residents and includes (1) minimum data set, (2) triggers, (3) resident assessment protocols, and (4) utilization guidelines. The goal of RAI is to coordinate the efforts of all members of the health care team to optimize the resident's quality of care and quality of life. The care team completes the assessment and planning, with participation from social work, physical therapy, and other disciplines. The RAI is a very comprehensive assessment tool.

Written Handoff Summary

Handoff, or transfer of care for a patient from one health care provider to another, significantly increases the risk of errors. Receiving staff must have up-to-date assessment data to safely care for the patient.

Traditionally, nurses think of handoff occurring during shift change, but handoff also occurs when a patient is transferred from one area of the hospital to another. For example, handoff occurs when a postoperative patient moves from the postanesthesia care unit (PACU) to the surgical floor or back to the medical unit after dialysis or an invasive diagnostic procedure. Transfers also occur when a patient is transferred from one health care facility to another (e.g., to a skilled nursing unit or a rehabilitation unit).

To minimize potential errors from lack of information, agencies often provide specific assessments on a written transfer summary in addition to a verbal report. Some agencies have created specific forms for this transfer of information, whereas others require documentation in the progress notes.

Verbal Communication

Verbal Handoff

A **handoff** occurs any time one health care provider transfers the responsibility for the care of a patient to another. Other industries such as aviation, power plants, and the National Aeronautics and Space Administration (NASA) Space Center have studied and standardized handoffs to prevent errors. Increasingly, the health care industry is paying attention to and standardizing handoffs. Effective communication at handoff is critically important to create a shared mental model around the patient's condition, which creates situational awareness and helps to minimize errors. The greater the number of handoffs and the more caregivers involved, the greater the risk for errors becomes.

In 2006, The Joint Commission developed its National Patient Safety Goal that required agencies to develop a standardized approach to handoff communications, including the opportunity to ask and respond to questions. Box 4.2 lists common handoff situations and strategies for effective handoff communication.

BOX 4.2 Handoff Reporting

Handoff

Occurs anytime the responsibility for care of a patient transfers from one care provider to another. Standardized reporting at handoffs promotes continuity of care and prevents errors.

Common Situation Handoffs

- At change of shift, when a new nurse is assigned to care for the patient
- When a nurse leaves for a meal or a break
- When a change in status requires transfer of the patient to another unit such as ICU
- When the surgical patient is transferred from the OR to the PACU or from the PACU to the surgical floor
- When the patient is admitted from the ED to a medical–surgical unit or to the ICU
- When the patient moves to or from a procedural care area for a diagnostic procedure or treatment (e.g., cath lab, GI lab, dialysis unit)
- When hospitalists or medical staff members change coverage

Strategies for Effective Handoff Communication

- Use a standardized format such as SBAR for handoffs so that all important information is presented in a predictable, clear manner.
- Communicate with face-to-face verbal update of current status and historical data with interactive questioning.
- Ensure limited interruptions.
- Use "read back" policies to ensure that both parties agree and comprehend.
- Use written documentation to supplement the verbal handoff.
- Cross monitor the handoffs of others with written and verbal communication.

ICU, intensive care unit; OR, operating room; GI, gastrointestinal.
Adapted from Clancy, C. (2006). Care transitions: A threat and opportunity for patient safety. *American Journal of Medical Quality*, *21*(6), 414–417.

Reporting

To provide safe patient care, nurses continually communicate with all members of the health care team. **Reporting** occurs at handoffs, during patient rounds, during patient and family care conferences, and when calling or texting a provider to report a change in status or provide requested information. Baseline assessment data or significant changes in patient status are crucial elements of most reporting.

In theory, effective communication seems like a simple task. In reality, it is very complex and often suboptimal. The Joint Commission (2013) reported 65% of sentinel events and 90% of root cause analyses conducted at a medical center in the Midwest included difficulties with communication as a contributing factor. Many barriers potentially contribute to difficulties in communication:

- Lack of structured format for communication
- Lack of standards and policies for communication
- Uncertainty about who is responsible and should be contacted
- Hierarchy of relationships
- Differences in ethnic background
- Poor clinical decision making regarding what needs to be reported
- Different communication styles of nurses and doctors

Qualities of Effective Reporting

To effectively communicate with members of the health care team, verbal communication must be organized, complete, accurate, concise, and respectful. An organizing framework, especially a tool such as SBAR, helps ensure complete and organized reporting. This textbook uses examples of SBAR to illustrate how nurses use and communicate assessment information in clinical settings.

Reporting, because it involves face-to-face communication, is influenced by nonverbal communication as well as the actual spoken words. It is important for you to maintain eye contact and to give your undivided attention during any reporting situation (Fig. 4.7). Negative nonverbal cues such as lack of respect, inattention, or irritation might negatively affect the quality or completeness of the report. Differences in communication style also influence reporting. Nurses are often instructed to be very descriptive and detailed in their communication, whereas physicians tend to be more concise and to focus on objective facts. Primary care providers may become impatient and inattentive with nurses who provide a rambling report. If a nurse, especially a student or a new graduate, experiences a hostile or disrespectful response when giving a report, he or she might hesitate or delay reporting significant information in the future.

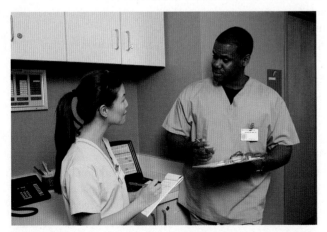

Figure 4.7 During reporting, the nurse should maintain attention, eye contact, and other positive nonverbal indicators.

Situation, Background, Assessment, and Recommendations (SBAR) Model

SBAR, first developed by Kaiser Permanente in Denver and supported by the Institute for Healthcare Improvement (IHI), is a shared mental model for improving communication between and among clinicians. Note that situation, background, and assessment are all based on the collection of complete and accurate assessment data. The last piece—recommendations—encompasses the nurse's suggestions for the next interventions using critical thinking and clinical judgment.

- **S**ituation: State concisely why you are communicating.
- **B**ackground: Describe the circumstances leading up to the current situation.
- **A**ssessment: Give objective and subjective data pertinent to the situation.
- **R**ecommendation: Make suggestions for what needs to be done to manage the difficulty.

Nurses most commonly use this model when contacting a provider regarding a patient issue. SBAR also can serve as a method for structuring communication during handoffs, when delegating care to nursing assistants, or when expressing concern regarding a patient's condition to the charge nurse or manager. Historically, nurses have always attempted to provide concise, organized verbal communication. The SBAR tool, however, gives a standardized format and provides clear articulation of what is desired. Refer to the case study collaboration example in this chapter as well as other case study collaboration features throughout this text.

Reporting to the Primary Health Care Provider

Reporting to the primary care provider can occur face to face, by telephone, by text messaging, or, in some settings (e.g., long term or home care), by fax. First, you need to identify the appropriate primary care provider to notify by checking the chart to ascertain the primary care provider, surgeon, or resident responsible for managing care. This becomes more complex in a teaching center, where multiple care providers are involved, or during nights or weekends when cross coverage occurs. In these situations, a call schedule helps to determine the appropriate person to contact. Valuable time can be lost if the process and schedule are unclear. You should use an organized framework such as SBAR to ensure that communications are clear and concise. Beginners learning this skill will be more organized and accurate if they write a draft of what they want to say before contacting the primary care provider.

Collaborating With the Interprofessional Team

At the change of shift, the nurse needs to organize information to provide a report on the patient. In this case, Mr. Chavez is still awaiting surgery, so staff members on the evening shift need to report to staff members on the night shift. After a brief introduction, the nurse reviews systems briefly. The nurse should organize pertinent items, including changes, so that the report is efficient and complete.

The following report illustrates how the nurse might organize the data and make recommendations about Mr. Chavez.

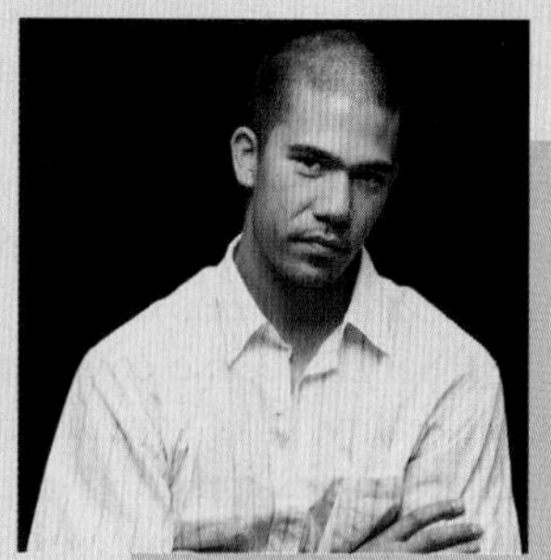

Situation: "I've been taking care of Mr. Chavez for the past 8 hours."

Background: "He was admitted with his cousin about 12 hours ago following a motor vehicle collision. His cousin is in Room 222 with a fractured tibia and fibula. Mr. Chavez fractured his right humerus and is waiting an ORIF tonight."

Assessment: "*Neuro:* He is drowsy from the pain medication but oriented. *CV:* His pulse is high at 122, R 20, BP 138/78. I think the BP is elevated because he's in pain. *Pulmonary:* His lungs are clear and oxygen saturation is 96%. *GI/GU:* Abdomen is soft with normal bowel tones. He's voiding in the urinal clear yellow urine, no stool. CSM is normal in both feet and left arm. However, his pulse is 1+ in his right hand, and it's cool and pale. His cap refill is also long at 6 seconds. I contacted the provider, who came and looked at the arm and said that there's no change, just to keep an eye on it. He's on hourly CSM checks now and there hasn't been a change. We also increased his dose of morphine because his pain was 8/10 but now is down to a 3, which is within his goal. The IV is infusing well with D5NS at 125/hr. It's a new IV from the ER, and I just changed the bag, so you have 1,000 ml hanging. *Psych/soc:* He doesn't have any family in the area and hasn't asked about his cousin yet."

Recommendations: "He's been using the PCA more frequently, so encourage him to do that before his pain gets too bad. We're basically just waiting for him to go to the OR to get the repair. He's on call and I think that he's next in line. He's NPO (nothing by mouth) because of scheduled surgery and his consent has been signed. Everything's in the chart and ready to go. His antibiotic is in the med room. Do you have any questions?"

Critical Thinking Challenge

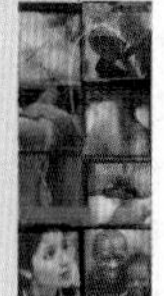

- What is the difference between what the nurse documents in the chart and shares in the report?
- What parts of the nursing process does the report include?
- How does the evening nurse use abbreviations to communicate and document data?
- What is the nurse's role in documenting the patient's immigration and insurance status in preparation for the surgery?

Telephone Communication

If a significant issue or problem occurs, you may need to phone or text the primary care provider to report this information. You may call the provider's office or page the provider to call back. When talking to a primary care provider on the phone, it is important to have the patient's record and other important information available for reference. It is important to document the call, including the time, who was called, what information you gave to the primary care provider, and what information you received. Most agencies now limit the use of telephone orders. For agencies that have CPOE, remote computer access allows providers to enter orders when they are off-site. If you are taking a telephone order, it is important to write the order and then read it back to the primary care provider to make sure it is correct.

> **SAFETY ALERT**
> *Students do not take telephone orders—only licensed nurses can do so. Nurses will always read back an order to the primary care provider to make sure that it is correct.*

Texting has become an increasingly common method of sharing a routine assessment update or reporting a sudden change in the patient's condition and requesting that the health care provider come to the bedside to assess the patient. Texting allows an interchange of information without waiting for a call back.

At times, you may need to elevate concerns regarding patient assessment data. CUS is a standardized Team STEPPS tool that uses standard terms: *C*oncerned, *U*ncomfortable, and *S*top: this is a safety risk. All staff are instructed to listen clearly to the words *concerned, uncomfortable,* and *stop: this is a safety risk*. For example, if Mr. Chavez's CMS checks suddenly revealed alterations in sensation and movement in his right hand, you could say, "I'm concerned that Mr. Chavez has decreased sensation and movement in his right hand that has changed from 1 hour ago. Could you come evaluate Mr. Chavez?" If this does not result in a health care provider visit, you could say, "I'm uncomfortable that Mr Chavez's circulation is severely impaired. Could you please come now to evaluate him?" If this does not get a positive response, elevate your concern to "This is a safety concern. If you do not come as requested, I will have the nursing supervisor evaluate Mr. Chavez." If your assessment data indicates an urgent problem, you can escalate to *this is a safety concern* immediately or call the medical emergency team (MET).

Voice communication badges, such as Vocera, have recently been developed to permit instant two-way voice communication with other team members. The system is activated by voice so hands are free to continue providing care or entering data into the medical record. These devices also include a text messaging system.

You may also communicate by telephone or text with other departments to provide or to obtain information. When patients are transferring from one setting to another (e.g., from ED or PACU), you may give the handoff report by phone. Nurses often receive laboratory data, especially critical values, by telephone. For any critical values, all health personnel must read back values obtained by telephone to ensure accuracy and avoid errors.

Patient Rounds and Conferences

Interdisciplinary rounds allow members of different disciplines to share assessment data in an effort to individualize and improve coordination of patient care. When rounds occur at the bedside and include the patient in the dialogue, your role as the nurse is to facilitate active participation to set goals and plan care. During rounds, you present assessment data on nursing issues such as mobility, fluid balance, pain management, and emotional or family issues. You can also help patients articulate questions or concerns. Shift handoffs are increasingly happening with the patient in the room to help communicate and plan the day (Fig. 4.8). Bedside shift reports have been found to increase patient participation and satisfaction, increase nursing teamwork and accountability, and improve communication among caregivers (Wakefield, Ragan, Brandt, & Tregnago, 2012).

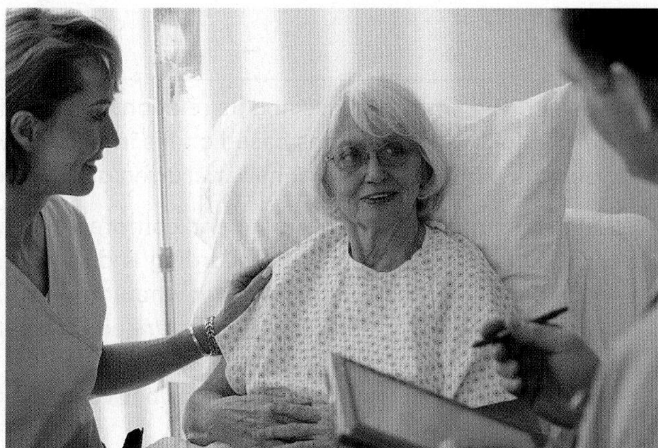

Figure 4.8 During a shift handoff in the patient's room, health care providers can communicate with each other and directly with the patient to plan the day effectively and to ensure that the patient can participate as much as he or she is able.

When working with patients who have complex health problems (e.g., end-of-life care), you may request or help facilitate a family care conference. Family members and all members of the health care team meet to discuss how best to provide and coordinate care in challenging situations. You need to plan these conferences in advance to coordinate schedules and to ensure that interpreters are present as needed.

Critical Thinking

You will use critical thinking and clinical judgment to determine what assessment data to include in a verbal report, how quickly to report the assessment, the proper team member to receive the information, and what method of reporting (e.g., face-to-face, telephone, text message) is most appropriate. Some reporting is scheduled at specific times—for example, shift change handoff. In other situations, you decide whether an assessment finding or a change in the patient's status requires immediate or routine notification of the primary care provider. For example, if you are the night nurse and a stable patient tells you that he has not had a bowel movement in 2 days, you would wait until the primary health care provider rounds in the morning to report the situation and get an order for a laxative. Conversely, if a patient's BP is low and she is NPO because of scheduled surgery, you would contact the provider for an IV order to prevent severe dehydration. If the situation is urgent and potentially life threatening, you may activate and report to a rapid response team. In this way, you use assessment information to take the next steps. Assessment information is never viewed in isolation from other parts of the nursing process.

Applying Your Knowledge

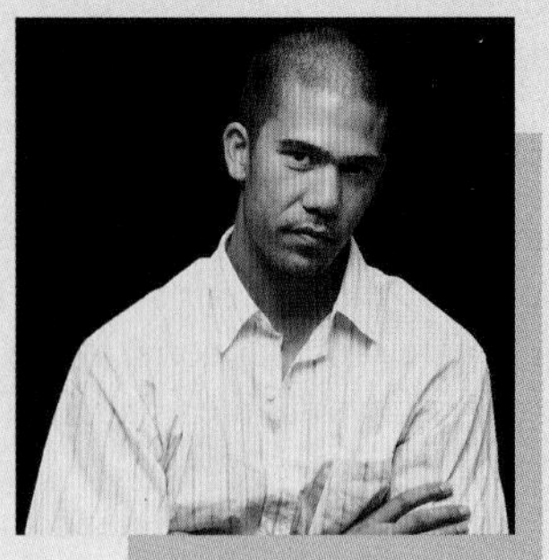

Consider Mr. Chavez's case and its relationship to what you are learning. Answer the following questions based on his initial injury, impaired tissue perfusion, pain, and the other changes that have occurred during the hours since admission.

- What is the importance of accurate and comprehensive documentation?
- Describe the difference between recording and reporting.
- What are important factors to consider when reporting?
- How do the patient's situation and urgent need for treatment influence the assessment, documentation, and communication of data?
- How does the collection of data fluctuate between a comprehensive and a focused assessment?
- Outline an example from the case study of Mr. Chavez that incorporates SBAR.
- How would you evaluate a successful handoff?

Key Points

- In addition to being a legal document, the patient record serves many purposes, namely, communication, care planning, quality assurance, financial reimbursement, education, and research.
- The computerized patient record helps ensure patient safety and enhances communication, because computerized documentation is legible and time dated, increases compliance, permits multiple simultaneous users, and permits surveillance of patient data to identify patients at risk.
- Critical thinking and clinical judgment are important in appropriately communicating and documenting assessment data to keep patients safe.
- Documentation should be accurate, objective, organized, concise, complete, and legible.
- Health care professionals must ensure confidentiality, governed by HIPAA, for all patient information, including what they document in the written or computerized record.
- Nurses can document assessment data in various forms in the patient's record (e.g., nursing admission assessment, flowsheets, progress notes, transfer or discharge summaries). Nurses working in home care and long-term care should follow the specific regulations governing documentation in those settings.
- Formats for nursing progress notes include narrative, SOAP, PIE, DAR, and CBE.
- Handoffs occur when one care provider transfers the responsibility for patient care to another care provider.
- SBAR is a mental model for organizing communication.
- Verbal communication of patient status occurs at handoff, over the telephone, via text message, and during rounds.
- Accurate and effective verbal communication and documentation are important to keep patients safe.

Review Questions

1. Which of the following are advantages of the electronic medical record? Select all that apply.
   A. Nurses can enter data by checking boxes and adding free full text.
   B. It is economical and easy to learn and implement.
   C. It allows primary care providers to directly order into the computer.
   D. It cannot be used as a legal document in case of a lawsuit.

2. Which of the following are high-risk assessments for liability? Select all that apply.
   A. Failure to document completely
   B. Inadequate admission assessment
   C. Charting in advance
   D. Bunch charting at the end of shift

3. Which of the following is the purpose of auditing charting?
   A. To enhance nurses' learning and understanding of complex clinical situations
   B. To identify staff members who document completely and counsel those who do not
   C. To determine if staff members are providing and documenting standards of care
   D. To locate data in the chart the evening before a morning clinical visit

4. Which of the following statements are acceptable under the HIPAA Privacy Rule? Select all that apply.
   A. Communicate report with the next nurse during change of shift.
   B. Communicate with the primary care provider about a patient's change in assessment.
   C. Consult in the hall with the instructor about the patient's unexpected findings.
   D. Describe patient assessment findings to a colleague in the cafeteria.

5. Which of the following is the proper technique for correcting written documentation?
   A. Use correction fluid and write over the error.
   B. Completely black out the error with a black marker.
   C. Write over the error in darker ink.
   D. Draw a single line through the error and initial.

6. What do the different formats of progress notes have in common?
   A. All use the nursing process in some form to show nursing thinking.
   B. All identify the patient outcomes or goals to evaluate.
   C. All include head-to-toe assessment data for completeness.
   D. All have a section for evaluation of care so that nurses may revise interventions.

7. What are some strategies for effective handoffs during change-of-shift report?
   A. Tape-record the report for efficiency.
   B. Vary the format to individualize to the patient.
   C. Allow an opportunity to ask and answer questions.
   D. Put report in writing so that the next shift care provider can get right to work.

8. In the SBAR reporting format, which of the following would be an example of data found in the assessment?
   A. Mrs. Kelly's diagnosis is Stage II breast cancer.
   B. Mr. Imami's lung sounds are decreased.
   C. Ms. Choi needs to have a social work consult.
   D. Mr. Jones was admitted at 10:30 this morning.

9. Nursing assessment of trends in an unconscious patient's neurological status over time is best recorded on
   A. an admission assessment.
   B. a POC.
   C. a progress note.
   D. a focused assessment flowsheet.

10. Your patient with a humerus fracture is stating pain of 5 on a 10-point scale. His hand is pale, cool, and swollen. His pain medication is ineffective, and he is at risk for compartment syndrome. What action will the nurse take first?
   A. Reassess the pain in 30 minutes and contact the provider if unresolved.
   B. Give additional pain medication and reassess the pain in 30 minutes.
   C. Document the unexpected findings and give an extra dose of pain medication now.
   D. Contact the primary care provider and document the findings now.

The Jensen suite offers these additional resources to enhance learning and facilitate understanding of this chapter:

- thePoint online resource, http://thepoint.lww.com/Jensen2e
- *Laboratory Manual for Nursing Health Assessment: A Best Practice Approach*
- *Pocket Guide for Nursing Health Assessment: A Best Practice Approach*
- *Lippincott DocuCare*, an electronic health record simulation software, http://thepoint.lww.com/docucare
- *Adaptive Learning | Powered by PrepU*, http://thepoint.lww.com/prepu

References

Arditi, C., Rège-Walther, M., Wyatt, J. C., Durieux, P., & Burnand, B. (2012). Computer-generated reminders delivered on paper to healthcare professionals; effects on professional practice and health care outcomes. *Cochrane Database of Systematic Reviews*, (12), CD001175. doi:10.1002/14651858.CD001175.pub3

Centers for Medicare and Medicaid Services. (2013). *Outcome and assessment information set (OASIS)*. Retrieved from http://www.cms.gov/Medicare/Quality-Initiatives-Patient-Assessment-Instruments/OASIS/index.html?redirect=/oasis/

Clancy, C. (2006). Care transitions: A threat and opportunity for patient safety. *American Journal of Medical Quality, 21*(6), 414–417.

Craven, R. C., Hirnle, C. J., & Jensen, S. (2013). *Fundamentals of nursing: Human health and function* (6th ed.). Philadelphia, PA: Lippincott Williams & Wilkins.

Health Insurance Portability and Accountability Act of 1996, Pub. L. No. 104–191, 110 Stat. 1936 (1996). Retrieved from http://www.hhs.gov/ocr/hipaa

Jones, B. (2013). Developing a vital signs alert system. *American Journal of Nursing, 113*(8), 36–44.

Kenney, C. (2011). *Transforming health care: Virginia Mason Medical Center's pursuit of the perfect patient experience.* New York, NY: Productive Press.

Sandhu, E., Weinstein, J. D., McKethan, A., & Jain, S. (2012). Secondary uses of electronic health record data: Benefits and barriers. *Joint Commission Journal on Quality and Patient Safety, 38*(1) 34–40.

The Joint Commission. (2013). *Sentinel event data.* Retrieved from http://www.jointcommission.org/topics/default.aspx?k=795

Wakefield, D., Ragan, R., Brandt, J., & Tregnago, M. (2012). Making the transition to bedside shift reports. *Joint Commission Journal on Quality and Patient Safety, 38*(6), 243–253

Wilson, M., Murphy, L., & Newhouse, R. (2012). Patients' access their health information: A meaningful-use mandate. *The Journal of Nursing Administration, 42*(11), 493–496.

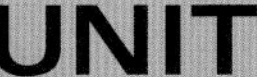

UNIT 2

General Examinations

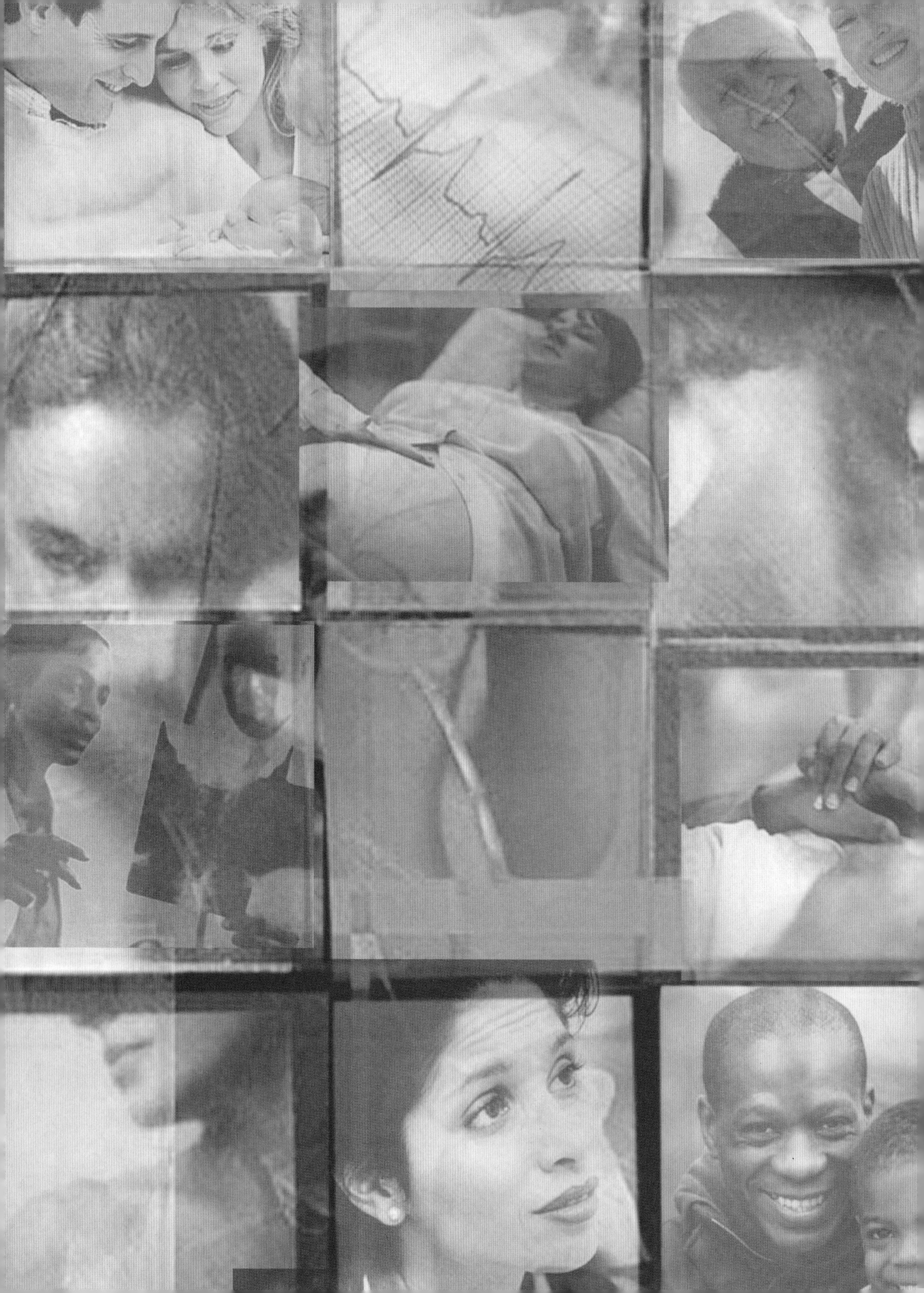

5

Vital Signs and General Survey

Learning Objectives

1. Describe the purpose of the general survey in the comprehensive physical examination.
2. Demonstrate knowledge of the importance of taking vital signs.
3. Describe factors that cause variations in vital signs and their measurement.
4. Identify risk factors for alterations in vital signs.
5. Critically assess, document, and report vital signs measurements.
6. Identify age-related variations in vital signs.
7. Identify cultural variations in vital signs.

Mr. Sanders is a 55-year-old Caucasian man who was admitted to the intensive care unit (ICU) following an episode of rapid heart rate and dizziness. He was monitored in the ICU for 2 days because he had atrial fibrillation (a cardiac arrhythmia, a fast and irregular heartbeat). He was placed on medication to decrease his heart rate; he also is taking an antihypertensive drug for high blood pressure. He was transferred in stable condition yesterday to the acute care medical unit.

You will gain more information about Mr. Sanders as you progress through this chapter. As you study the content and features, consider Mr. Sanders's case and its relationship to what you are learning. Begin thinking about the following points:

- Is Mr. Sanders' condition stable, urgent, or an emergency?
- What immediate health promotion and teaching needs are evident?
- What are the relationships among the patient's pulse, respirations, and blood pressure?
- How will a comprehensive general survey and vital signs measurement differ from a focused assessment for this patient?
- How will the nurse evaluate the effectiveness of the interventions performed for Mr. Sanders?

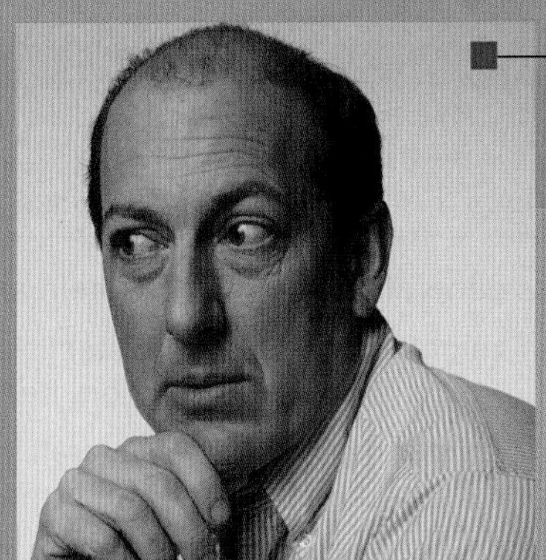

This chapter explores the assessment techniques required to perform the general survey and take vital signs.

The **general survey** begins upon first meeting the patient and is ongoing. While collecting the health history, nurses observe patients, develop initial impressions, and formulate plans for collecting objective data from the physical examination. An accurate and thorough physical examination requires keen observational skills.

Vital signs, encompassing temperature, pulse, respirations, and blood pressure (BP), are important indicators of the patient's physiological status and response to the environment. The fifth vital sign, pain, is covered in Chapter 6. Nurses assess vital signs frequently and use the findings as guidance for further physical assessment. Thus, being able to differentiate normal from unexpected results is crucial.

Urgent Assessment

Patient indicators of an urgent situation include extreme anxiety, acute distress, pallor, cyanosis, and a change in mental status. When such acute or urgent findings are present, the nurse begins interventions while continuing the assessment, including vital sign assessment of pulse, BP, and oxygen saturation.

> *SAFETY ALERT*
>
> *The nurse may call a rapid response team if he or she has an intuitive sense that something is going wrong with the patient or if the patient displays the following:*
>
> - *An acute change in mental status*
> - *Stridor*
> - *Respirations less than 10 breaths/min or greater than 32 breaths/min*
> - *Increased effort to breathe*
> - *Oxygen saturation less than 92%*
> - *Pulse less than 55 beats/min (bpm) or greater than 120 bpm*
> - *Systolic BP less than 90 or greater than 170 mm Hg*
> - *Temperature less than 35°C (95°F) or greater than 39.5°C (103.1°F)*
> - *New onset of chest pain*
> - *Agitation or restlessness*

Experienced nurses will assist beginners in determining the level of response needed.

Objective Data

Equipment

- Scale
- Height bar
- Stethoscope
- Thermometer
- Watch with second hand measurement
- Sphygmomanometer
- Pulse oximeter
- Tape measure (for infants)

Preparation

Make sure the room is warm, comfortable, and relaxing. Ensure a quiet, well-lit setting that provides privacy. Wash your hands, preferably in the presence of the patient, and cleanse the stethoscope with alcohol to prevent the transmission of bacteria or other pathogens. Have all necessary equipment in reach of the examination area.

Begin the general survey immediately upon meeting the patient and continue it throughout the assessment. Ask the patient to remove shoes and heavy outer garments before taking height and weight. Prior to assessment of vital signs, the patient should rest quietly for 5 minutes. Establish that the patient has not had anything to eat or drink and has not smoked for at least 30 minutes. The patient must remove constricting clothing to above the upper arm to provide access to the brachial artery for measurement of BP. The patient may be sitting or supine for vital signs (Joint National Commission VII, 2014).

Common and Specialty or Advanced Techniques

The routine screening assessment includes the most important and common techniques. The nurse may add focused or advanced techniques if there are concerns over a specific finding, such as an irregular pulse. The table summarizes the differences in techniques used in the screening and focused assessments.

Basic Versus Focused/Advanced Techniques in General Survey and Vital Signs

Technique	Purpose	Basic or Screening Assessment	Focused or Advanced Examination
Assess general survey.	Obtain an overall impression.	X	
Obtain height and weight.	Establish baseline; assess for changes from baseline.	X	
Obtain temperature, pulse, respirations, and BP.	Overall impression and screen for abnormal findings.	X	

(table continues on page 83)

Technique	Purpose	Basic or Screening Assessment	Focused or Advanced Examination
Obtain oxygen saturation.	Screen for low saturation in hospitalized and respiratory patients.	X	
Evaluate pulse deficit.	Gather information on peripheral perfusion.		X Irregular heart rate
Assess for orthostatic hypotension.	Identify volume deficit, impaired venous return, and risk for falling.		X Low fluid volume
Doppler pulse and BP	To measure pulse and BP when unable to obtain by manual methods		X Absent pulse or low BP

Basic Versus Focused/Advanced Techniques in General Survey and Vital Signs *(continued)*

General Survey

The general survey begins with the first moment of the encounter with the patient and continues throughout the health history, during the physical examination, and with each subsequent interaction. It is the first component of the assessment, when you make mental notes of overall behavior, physical appearance, and mobility. It helps to form a global impression of the patient. Physical appearance and mental status provide valuable clues to overall health. Assessment of these areas requires you to use your senses and observational skills to look, listen, and note any unexpected findings, sounds, or odors.

When you introduce yourself, you may touch the patient (not shake hands, as many times this is inappropriate). A touch not only portrays caring but also allows you to assess the patient. Note whether the patient makes eye contact, smiles, and speaks clearly. When you first meet the patient:

- What is your first impression? Are there any outstanding features?
- State the patient's name. Does the patient respond immediately?
- Is the patient's skin moist? Can the patient move the extremities completely? Assess the temperature and texture of the skin. Note muscle strength. Assess for edema, clubbing, malformations, or enlarged joints.
- Observe the patient interacting with others. Can he or she participate in conversation?
- Does the patient look healthy or ill?

As you proceed through the assessment, note the patient's physical appearance, body structure, mobility, and behavior. Because these characteristics are general overall indicators of health, consider how the data fit together with other body systems. Think about what other data you will want to collect to identify patterns. Begin the data collection as soon as you enter the room and continue until you leave.

Technique and Normal Findings	Abnormal Findings
Physical Appearance	
Overall Appearance. Does the patient appear the stated age? Is appearance consistent with chronological age? Are the face and body symmetrical? Are any deformities obvious? Does the patient look well, unhealthy, or in distress? The patient appears stated age. Facial features, movements, and body are symmetrical.	Deficiencies in growth hormones may cause patients to appear younger than they are. Severe illness, chronic disease, prolonged sun exposure, and various genetic syndromes may contribute to premature aging. Facial asymmetry may indicate Bell palsy or cerebrovascular ischemia. Obvious deformities may indicate fractures or displacements.
Hygiene and Dress. Note hygiene by observing clothing, hair, nails, and skin. What is the patient wearing? Is it appropriate for age, gender, culture, and weather? Is clothing clean and neat, or disheveled? Does it fit? Are any breath or body odors noted? Is there an odor of alcohol or urine? Is the patient's skin clean and dry? Are nails and hair well kept, neat, and clean? Dress is appropriate for age, gender, culture, and weather. The patient is clean and well-groomed. No odors are noted.	Poorly fitting clothes may indicate weight loss or gain. Bad breath can result from poor hygiene, allergic rhinitis, or infection (tonsillitis, sinusitis). Sweet-smelling breath may indicate diabetic ketoacidosis. Body odor may be from poor hygiene or increased sweat gland activity, which accompanies some hormonal disorders. Previously well-groomed patients who are now disheveled may suffer from depression. Eccentric makeup or dress may indicate mania. Worn or disheveled clothes may indicate inadequate finances or knowledge.

(table continues on page 84)

Technique and Normal Findings (continued)	Abnormal Findings (continued)
Skin Color. Observe for even skin tones and symmetry. Note any areas of increased redness, pallor, cyanosis, or jaundice. Observe for any lesions or variations in pigmentation. Note the amount, texture, quality, and distribution of hair. Skin color is even toned, with pigmentation appropriate for genetic background and no obvious lesions or variations in color. Hair is smooth, thick, and evenly distributed.	Pallor, erythema, cyanosis, jaundice, and lesions can indicate disease states (see Chapter 11).
Body Structure and Development. Is the patient's physical and sexual development consistent with expected findings for stated age? Is the patient obese or lean? Is the height appropriate for age and ethnicity? Are body parts symmetrical? Is the patient barrel-chested? Note the fingertips. Are there any joint abnormalities? Physical and sexual development is appropriate for age, culture, and gender. No joint abnormalities are noted.	Delayed puberty may indicate a deficiency of growth hormones. Altered growth hormones may lead to markedly short or tall stature. Disproportionate height and weight, obesity, or emaciation can indicate an eating disorder or hormonal dysfunction. Barrel chest may indicate long-standing respiratory disease.
Behavior. Note the patient's behavior. Is he or she cooperative or uncooperative? Is affect animated or flat? Does the patient appear anxious? The patient is cooperative and interacts pleasantly.	Uncooperative behavior, flat affect, or unusual elation may indicate a psychiatric disorder (see Chapter 9). Note that mild anxiety is common in people seeking health care.
Facial Expressions. Assess the face for symmetry. Note expressions while the patient is at rest and during speech and whether they seem appropriate. Are movements symmetrical? Does the patient maintain eye contact appropriate to culture? Facial expression is relaxed, symmetrical, and appropriate for the setting and circumstances. The patient maintains eye contact appropriate for age and culture.	Inappropriate affect, inattentiveness, impaired memory, and inability to perform activities of daily living (ADLs) may indicate dementia (e.g., Alzheimer disease) or another cognitive disorder. A flat or masklike expression may indicate Parkinson disease or depression. Drooping of one side of the face may indicate transient ischemic attack or cerebrovascular accident. Exophthalmos (protruding eyes) may indicate hyperthyroidism.
Level of Consciousness. Continually assess the patient's mental status throughout all encounters, but pay particular attention to it when gathering the health history. Can the patient state his or her name and location and the date, month, season, and time of day? Is the patient awake, alert, and oriented to person, place, and time? Note any confusion, agitation, lethargy, or inattentiveness. Is there a change in mental status? If the patient appears confused, ask him or her to respond to the following: • Tell me your full name. • Where are you now? • What is today's date? or What time of the day is it? The patient is awake, alert, and oriented to person, place, and time (abbreviated A&O × 3). He or she attends and responds to questions appropriately.	Confusion, agitation, drowsiness, or lethargy may indicate hypoxia, decreased cerebral perfusion, or a psychiatric disorder. Refer to Chapters 9 and 22. **SAFETY ALERT** *Change in level of consciousness often is the first indication of hypoxia.*
Speech. Listen to the speech pattern. Is the patient speaking very rapidly or very slowly? Is speech clear and articulate? Does the patient use words appropriately? Vocabulary and sentence structure may offer clues to educational level. Also, assess for fluency in language and the need for an interpreter. The patient responds to questions quickly and easily. Volume, pitch, and rate are appropriate to the situation. Speech is clear and articulate, flowing smoothly. Word choice is appropriate.	Slow, slurred speech may indicate alcohol intoxication or cerebrovascular ischemia. Rapid speech may indicate hyperthyroidism, anxiety, or mania. Difficulty finding words or using words inappropriately may indicate cerebrovascular ischemia or a psychiatric disorder. Loud speech may indicate hearing difficulties.

(table continues on page 85)

Technique and Normal Findings (continued)	Abnormal Findings (continued)
Mobility ***Posture.*** Note how the patient sits and stands. Is the patient sitting upright? When standing, is the body straight and aligned? Posture is upright while sitting, with the limbs and trunk proportional to the body height. The patient stands erect with no signs of discomfort and the arms relaxed at the sides.	Slumped or hunched posture may indicate depression, fatigue, pain, or osteoporosis. Long limbs may indicate Marfan syndrome. A tripod position when sitting can indicate respiratory disease (see Chapter 16). If the patient is in bed, note the position of the head of the bed or if the patient is lying on the left or right side.
Range of Motion. Can the patient move all limbs equally? Are there limitations? The patient moves freely in the environment.	Asymmetrical motion occurs in stroke; paralysis may accompany spinal cord injury. Limited range of motion might be present with injuries or degenerative disease.
Gait. If the patient is ambulatory, observe his or her movement around the room. Note whether movements are coordinated. Normally, a person ambulates with arms swinging freely at the sides. Note any tremors or involuntary movements as well as any body parts that do not move. Does the patient use assistive devices? Gait is steady and balanced, with even heel-to-toe foot placement and smooth movements. Other movements are also smooth, purposeful, effortless, and symmetrical.	Tics, paralysis, ataxia, tremors, or uncontrolled movements may indicate neurological disease. Patients with Parkinson disease may display a shuffling gait. Arthritis may result in a slow, unsteady gait. For patients in bed, note their ability to move and reposition themselves in bed, turn side to side, and sit up. Further evaluate any abnormalities when assessing the neurological and musculoskeletal systems during the comprehensive physical examination (see Chapters 21 and 22).

Anthropometric Measurements

Anthropometric measurements are the various measurements of the human body, including height and weight. Accurate measurements provide critical information about the adult's state of health and the child's growth pattern. They are important parameters for evaluating nutritional status, assessing fluid gain or loss, and calculating medication dosages.

Specific measurements can be compared with measurements on standardized charts. The first time a nurse meets a patient, he or she records height and weight as a baseline measurement. Afterward, the nurse takes measurements at regular intervals, depending on the patient's state of health and agency policy. A series of measurements provides more information than any single measurement. Baseline height and weight measurements provide a reference point for weight changes and for assessing body mass index (BMI). The BMI is considered a more reliable indicator of healthy weight than weight measurement alone (see Chapter 7). To obtain accurate height and weight, ask the patient to remove his or her shoes and heavy articles of clothing (e.g., winter coat). An accurate weight measurement is essential for nutrition assessment, dosing of medications, monitoring of fluid and nutritional status, and compliance with agency policies.

Technique and Normal Findings	Abnormal Findings
Height Measure patients older than 2 years of age with the patient standing. Ask the patient to place the heels up against a height bar. Feet should be together, with knees straight and the patient looking forward. Lower the horizontal bar until it touches the top of the patient's head. Read and record the measurement on the height bar (Fig. 5.1).	Chronic malnutrition may result in decreased height from lack of nutrients for proper growth. Decreased height also may result from osteoporosis. Hormonal abnormalities may cause excessive growth, as seen in gigantism and acromegaly, or deficiency in growth, as seen in dwarfism (see Table 5.9 at the end of the chapter).
Sometimes, patients cannot stand up straight for the measurement of height. In such cases, estimate the height by measuring "wingspan." Have the patient hold both arms straight from the sides of the body at right angles. Measure from the tip of one middle finger to the tip of the other middle finger. This distance is approximately the same as the patient's height and does not change with age.	The patient with muscle weakness, scoliosis, or a neurological disorder may not be able to stand.

(table continues on page 86)

Technique and Normal Findings (continued)	Abnormal Findings (continued)
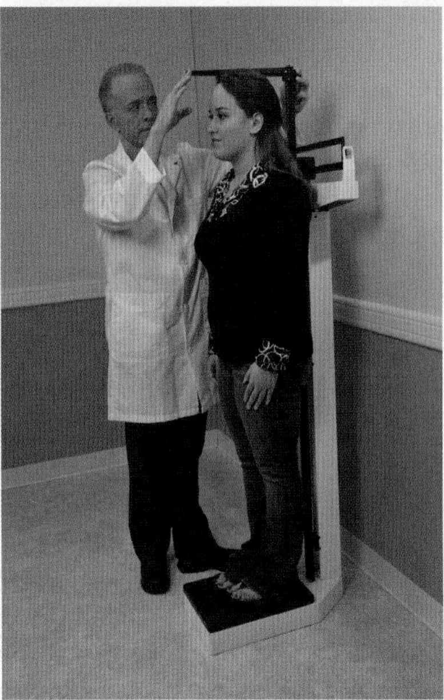 **Figure 5.1** Measuring height in an adult. A knee height may be used to measure stature in those unable to stand; there are equations to convert knee height to stature. *Height is recorded in centimeters or inches.*	
Weight Primary care facilities may use a calibrated balance beam scale for obtaining weights. Prior to weighing a patient, the nurse must balance the scale by sliding both weight bars to zero. The balancing arm should balance in the center of the gauge. Follow the manufacturer's instructions to balance if needed. Lock the scale if it is on wheels. Have the patient stand on the scale. Slide the lower weight bar to the right until the arm drops to the bottom of the gauge (Fig. 5.2). 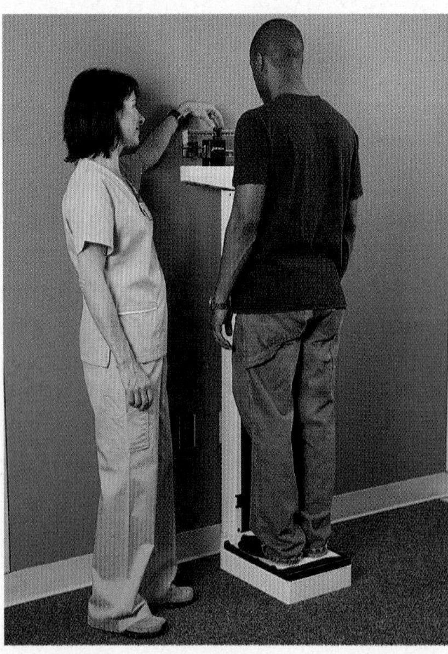 **Figure 5.2** Measuring weight in an adult.	Excessive unexplained weight loss may result from nutritional deficiencies, decreased intake, decreased absorption, increased metabolic needs, or a combination. Other causes may be endocrine, neoplastic, gastrointestinal, psychiatric, infectious, or neurological. Chronic disease also may contribute to weight loss. Excessive weight gain occurs when a person consumes more calories than his or her body requires. Overweight may result from endocrine disorders, genetics, or emotional factors such as stress, anxiety, depression, or guilt. Drug therapy, especially steroids, may contribute to weight gain. See Table 5.9 at the end of this chapter.

(table continues on page 87)

Technique and Normal Findings (continued)	Abnormal Findings (continued)
Slide the weight bar one notch back. Move the upper weight bar to the right until the arrow is balanced in the center of the gauge. The patient's weight is the total of these two readings. Record the weight. Many facilities use an electronic scale to weigh patients; hospitals may use a scale built into the bed or sling. These scales must be calibrated, or "zeroed," prior to use. Refer to a procedure manual for these instructions. *Weight is recorded in kilograms or pounds.* To obtain the most accurate readings when a series of weights is required, weigh the patient at the same time of the day in similar clothing each time. There are weight issues in some clinical settings especially hospitals, including the following: • The accuracy and reproducibility of weights taken on different scales and by different personnel • Weights of critically ill patients may be unavailable on admission; sometimes heights are also not measured • The fluid status varies with medications especially diuretics, diet, dialysis, and time of day • The accuracy of weight history data from patients and family members • Confounding factors such as wheelchairs, splints, casts, clothing, amputations, or spinal cord injuries	
Calculate BMI by dividing the weight in kilograms by the height in meters squared (or the weight in pounds divided by the height in inches squared and then multiplied by 703). *BMI is recorded as a single number.*	Underweight is BMI less than 18.5; overweight is BMI of 25–29.9; obesity is BMI greater than 30; extreme obesity is BMI greater than 40. Obesity poses risks for disease (National Heart, Lung, and Blood Institute, 2009). See Chapter 7 for more information.

Vital Signs

Temperature, *pulse*, *respirations*, and *blood pressure* make up the vital signs (commonly referred to as "vitals"). *Pain*, considered the fifth vital sign, is covered in Chapter 6. *Oxygen saturation* is also collected in hospitalized patients. Nurses must interpret the significance of vital signs within the context of other data from the patient assessment.

Vital signs reflect health status, cardiopulmonary function, and overall body function. They are called "vital signs" because of their importance as indicators of physiological state and response to physical, environmental, and psychological stressors. Changes in vital signs often indicate changes in health. Assessment of vital signs helps nurses to establish a baseline, monitor a patient's condition, evaluate responses to treatment, identify problems, and monitor risks for alterations in health.

Assessment of vital signs assists with the process of physical examination. Findings aid in determining which body systems need more thorough investigation. For example, if respiratory rate or rhythm is abnormal, the nurse auscultates the patient's lung sounds.

Before assessing vital signs, it is important to assess any medications the patient is currently taking. Be aware of the adverse effects of all medications administered because many medications alter vital signs. If a medication alters the patient's vital signs, the nurse assesses the effects and provides appropriate teaching to the patient.

The patient's physical condition, as well as the situation and agency policies, determine how often to assess vital signs (Box 5.1). Nurses are responsible for determining whether more frequent assessment of vital signs is warranted.

BOX 5.1 Frequency of Vital Signs

The nurse should take a patient's vital signs
- Upon admission to a facility
- Before and after any surgical procedure
- Before, during, and after administration of medications that affect vital signs
- Per the institution's policy or physician orders
- Any time the patient's condition changes
- Before and after any procedure affecting vital signs

The initial set of vital signs provides a baseline. A series of readings is more informative than a single value because the series can provide information about trends over time. Additionally, many variables may affect vital signs, including pain, stress, anxiety, and activity. It is imperative that nurses measure vital signs correctly and accurately, understand the data, and communicate appropriately.

Observe the patient for other findings to support your assessment. When encountering an unexpected value, obtain the vital sign(s) again to assess accuracy. Also look at the patient. Does he or she appear to be in distress? Note the color of the skin, respiratory effort, and behavior. Remember that normal readings vary according to age. Furthermore, a normal value for one patient may be unexpected for another. When assessing vital signs, compare the results to normal values for the patient's age and also to the patient's own baseline.

Occasionally, only one vital sign requires assessment. For example, when administering a cardiac medication, the nurse assesses heart rate, BP, or both, but not temperature. If fever is suspected, the nurse may take the temperature only. When administering an antipyretic for fever, the nurse reassesses the effect of the medication by measuring the temperature again.

> **Clinical Significance**
>
> When the condition of the patient is stable, the nurse may delegate the tasks of obtaining anthropometric measurements and vital signs to nursing assistants. In such cases, nurses retain legal responsibility for assessing findings and intervening when necessary. Principles of delegation are used.

Temperature

The *hypothalamus* is the body's thermostat; it functions to maintain a steady temperature throughout the day. This thermostat balances the heat produced from food digestion, exercise, and increased metabolism with the heat lost from evaporation of sweat and environmental exposure. This balancing act produces a steady state of temperature, which is required for cellular metabolism.

Body temperature is most commonly measured either in degrees Celsius (C) or degrees Fahrenheit (F) according to the agency's policy. Nurses should be familiar with both scales (Box 5.2).

Normal range of body temperature depends on the route used for measurement. Rectal and temporal artery measurements are higher than oral measurements. Axillary temperatures are lower than oral temperatures. No single temperature is normal for all adults. Body temperature varies with physical activity, age, gender, and state of health.

Temperature also varies with time of day because of the diurnal or circadian cycle. Body temperature is usually lowest in the early morning and typically peaks in the late afternoon. Temperature may vary as much as 0.5°C (1°F). Variation according to time of day is somewhat more pronounced in infants and children.

Moderate to hard exercise increases body temperature. In women of childbearing age, increased progesterone secretion that accompanies ovulation causes temperature to rise 0.3° to 0.5°C (0.5° to 1°F) and remain elevated until menses. Stress may elevate core (central) temperature as a result of increased production of epinephrine and norepinephrine. These neurotransmitters increase both metabolic activity and heat production.

To ensure accuracy, temperatures must be measured correctly using the appropriate device.

- *Electronic thermometers* are fast, safe, and convenient; they can accurately measure oral, rectal, and axillary temperatures (Fig. 5.3). These thermometers can measure temperatures in 2 to 60 seconds. Oral (blue tip) and rectal (red tip) probes are available; they come with disposable single-use covers. Equipment must be fully charged and correctly calibrated to ensure accuracy.

> **BOX 5.2 Conversion From Fahrenheit to Celsius and Celsius to Fahrenheit**
>
> C = (F − 32) × 5/9
> F = (C × 9/5) + 32

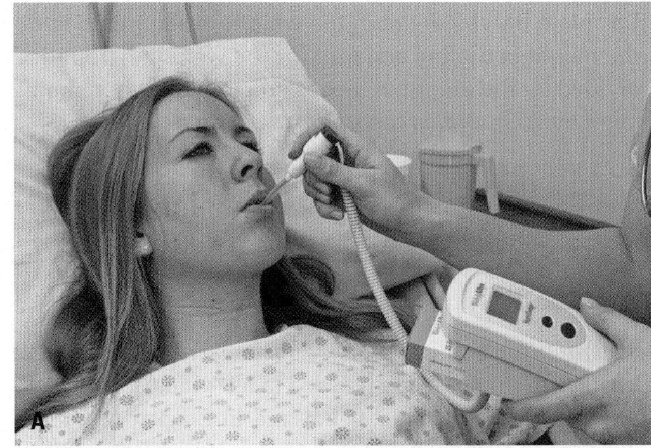

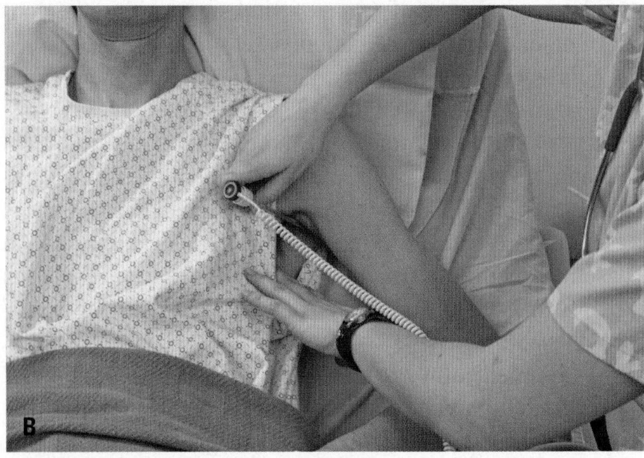

Figure 5.3 A. Oral temperature in sublingual pocket. **B.** Axillary temperature in axillar fold.

- *Disposable, single-use thermometers* can be used for oral and axillary temperature assessment. Readings are available within 1 minute. Disposable thermometers are effective in decreasing the spread of infection but are less accurate than electronic thermometers.
- *Tympanic thermometers* use infrared sensors to detect the heat that the tympanic membrane produces. The tympanic membrane thermometer is noninvasive, safe, efficient, and quick. Because the reading is so quick (2 to 3 seconds), it is commonly used in emergency departments and hospitals.
- *Temporal artery thermometers* are quick, safe, and convenient, and they do not require contact with mucous membranes. An infrared sensor measures body temperature by capturing the heat emitted from the skin over the temporal artery.

Determining Which Route to Use. The nurse uses critical thinking to decide on the correct route for temperature measurement. Factors such as age, level of consciousness, and the presence of medical equipment, such as endotracheal tubes, influence the choice of route for assessing temperature. Each site has advantages and disadvantages. The nurse determines the safest and most accurate site for assessment. Although agency policy and available equipment have an influence on site choice, the nurse is expected to select and use alternative methods when warranted by the patient's condition. The same site should be used when follow-up measurements are needed for comparisons. The nurse should keep in mind that the routes or devices that are easiest to use may not yield the most accurate results.

See Table 5.1 for a comparison of routes.

Oral Route. The oral route is common and comfortable for many patients, but it may be contraindicated for others. The sublingual pockets under the tongue are rich in blood supply that responds quickly to changes in the core temperature.

SAFETY ALERT

The oral route cannot be used to measure temperature in patients who are unconscious, orally intubated, confused, or in those who have a history of seizures. Taking oral temperatures is also contraindicated in cases of postoperative oral surgery or oral trauma. Oral thermometers are not recommended for children younger than 6 years of age.

TABLE 5.1 Advantages and Disadvantages of Various Temperature Routes

Route	Normal Temperature Range	Appropriate Use	Advantages	Disadvantages
Oral	36.5°–37.5°C (97.7°–99.5°F)	Older children and adults who are awake, alert, and oriented	Easily accessible and comfortable; provides accurate readings	Do not use with people who have altered mental status or recent oral surgery. Values may vary because of mouth breathing, oral intake, and smoking. Risk for body fluid exposure is increased.
Axillary	35.9°–36.9°C (96.7°–98.5°F)	Infants, young children, and patients with impaired immune systems	Easy to obtain	The nurse must hold the thermometer in place for longer time. Readings reflect temperature of the skin surface, which may be variable. This method may be less accurate than oral or rectal.
Rectal	37.1°–38.1°C (98.7°–100.5°F)	Adults requiring an accurate core temperature	Very accurate; more reflective of core temperature than other routes	This invasive method should not be used for people with rectal surgery, diarrhea, abscesses, or low white blood cell count. It is contraindicated for newborns and patients with cardiac disease. Risk is increased for exposure to body fluids.
Tympanic	36.8°–37.8°C (98.2°–100°F)	All patients except those with ear infection or ear pain	Easily accessible, quick, unaffected by oral intake or smoking	Studies have not proven accuracy. Thermometer is available only in one size. Positioning in children younger than 3 of age years is difficult.
Temporal	37.1°–38.1°C (98.7°–100.5°F)	All patients	Quick and easy to obtain	Diaphoresis or sweat can impair reading.

Axillary Route. The axillary route is less commonly used than the oral route. It can be used with infants and young children and also with patients of other ages who cannot have oral temperature assessed. Electronic or disposable thermometers may be used to measure axillary temperatures. Axillary temperatures are lower than oral temperatures by 0.3° to 0.5°C (0.5° to 1°F). One disadvantage of the axillary route is the need to wait for 30 minutes after washing the axilla. In addition, the axillary method measures skin surface temperature, which varies; therefore, the axillary temperature reading is less reliable than readings obtained using other methods (Lawson et al., 2007).

Tympanic Membrane. The tympanic thermometer should be avoided in patients with ear drainage, ear pain, suspected ear infection, or scarred tympanic membranes. One disadvantage of tympanic temperature measurement is that reports of accuracy are conflicting. Studies have shown as much as 0.5°C (1°F) variation between tympanic and core pulmonary artery temperatures. The positioning of the probe in the ear canal is inconsistent, which may account for falsely low readings and missed fevers (Sanderson et al., 2010).

Temporal Artery. Temporal thermometers are especially useful in confused or unconscious patients as well as children. Measurement on either the right or left side of the forehead is equally effective. If a patient is in the lateral position, the nondependent side of the forehead should be used.

Avoid moving the device too quickly across the forehead or breaking contact with the skin as this can cause inconsistent results. Another way to enhance accuracy is to keep the thermometer's infrared lens clean to avoid interference from buildup of skin oil (Lawson et al., 2007). As with tympanic thermometers, studies regarding accuracy of temporal thermometers have been conflicting (Carleton, Fry, Mulligan, Bell, & Brossart, 2012).

Rectal Route. Rectal temperature measurement, considered one of the most accurate methods, is used when other routes are not practical or when an accurate core reading is necessary. Although rectal temperatures accurately reflect core temperature changes, this route is inconvenient, causes discomfort to patients, and is disruptive to normal activity. Adults are usually uncomfortable having a rectal temperature taken.

> **SAFETY ALERT**
>
> *Rectal temperature measurement is contraindicated in newborns, infants, and young children; patients who are neutropenic; patients with rectal diseases; and those who have undergone rectal surgery. Patients with hemorrhoids and those with diarrhea should not have rectal temperatures assessed. The rectal route should also be avoided with patients who have cardiac conditions because insertion of the thermometer may cause vagal stimulation and reduced heart rate.*

In adults who cannot close their mouths because of intubation, surgery, change in mental status, or unresponsiveness, it may be necessary to use the rectal route if tympanic or temporal thermometers are unavailable.

Rectal temperatures are 0.4° to 0.5°C (0.7° to 1°F) higher than oral temperatures. Electronic and disposable thermometers are used to measure rectal temperatures. Rectal thermometers are differentiated from oral thermometers by color: rectal thermometers are red rather than blue.

Technique and Normal Findings	Abnormal Findings
Oral Temperature. To ensure accuracy, wait 15–30 minutes after a patient has smoked, had anything either hot or cold to eat or drink, or chewed gum. Turn the thermometer device on. Cover the tip of the probe with a protector. Gloves are unnecessary unless you expect contact with body secretions. Place the thermometer in the sublingual area at the base (back) of the tongue, which has a rich blood supply and corresponds with core temperature. Instruct the patient to keep the lips closed tightly and to breathe through the nose. Hold the probe until it beeps, then remove it. Note the reading and immediately dispose of the cover into a wastebasket. Electronic or disposable thermometers have replaced old glass thermometers containing mercury because of toxicity of mercury in the environment. *Average oral temperature is* 36.5°–37.5°C (97.7°–99.5°F). *If the patient has no fever, this is referred to as being* ***afebrile.***	**Hypothermia** is temperature less than 35°C (95°F). Prolonged exposure to cold may cause hypothermia. It may be induced purposefully during surgery to reduce the body's oxygen demands. **Hyperthermia**, also known as pyrexia or fever, is body temperature exceeding 38.6°C (101.5°F) orally. It occurs during infections caused by bacteria, viruses, and fungi. Another cause is tissue breakdown, as seen in trauma, surgery, myocardial infarction, and malignancy. Low-grade fever may occur with conditions that cause inflammation, such as in autoimmune disorders. Certain neurological disorders, such as cerebrovascular accident, cerebral edema, tumor, or cerebral trauma, can affect the thermoregulation of the brain. **SAFETY ALERT** *Fever above 39.5°C (103.1°F) in adults requires immediate assessment and rapid cooling measures. Monitor rectal temperature constantly during cooling measures to prevent a hypothermic response. Temperatures below 35°C (95°F) may require rewarming, according to established protocols.*

(table continues on page 91)

Technique and Normal Findings (continued)	Abnormal Findings (continued)
Axillary Temperature. Follow the procedure above, except place the electronic thermometer in the axillary fold and have the patient lower the arm. Hold it in place until it reads the temperature. Stay with the patient to ensure correct placement. *Average axillary temperature is* 35.9°–36.9°C (96.7°–98.5°F). *It is approximately 1°F lower than oral temperature.*	Axillary temperature is the least accurate, so if discrepancies are noted, recheck the temperature using another route.
Tympanic Temperature. Turn the unit on and wait for the ready signal. Place a disposable single-use cover on the probe tip. Then, place the tip gently in the patient's ear canal, angling the thermometer toward the patient's jaw. In an adult, pull the pinna up and back to straighten the ear (Fig. 5.4A). Take care not to force the probe or occlude the ear canal. Push the trigger and note the reading. Dispose of the cover directly into the wastebasket. Temperature readings are available in 2–3 seconds. *Average tympanic temperature is* 36.8°–37.8°C (98.2°–100°F). *It is approximately equal to oral temperature.*	Errors in temperature measurements using a tympanic thermometer have been attributed to user error. Proper positioning of the probe may decrease the incidence of error.
Temporal Temperature. Position the probe directly on the skin above the eyebrow in the center of the forehead. Activate the thermometer by depressing and holding the scan button. Move the probe slowly from the forehead, across the temporal artery to level with the top of the ear (Fig. 5.4B). Continue to hold the scan button while lifting and moving the probe to touch behind the earlobe. The process requires 5–7 seconds. *Temporal temperature is* 37.1°–38.1°C (98.7°–100.5°F). *It is approximately equal to oral temperature.*	Studies have shown that the temporal artery measurement using the forehead and behind the ear method is more accurate than temporal artery measurements using the forehead alone and is comparable with the oral temperature (Carleton et al., 2012).

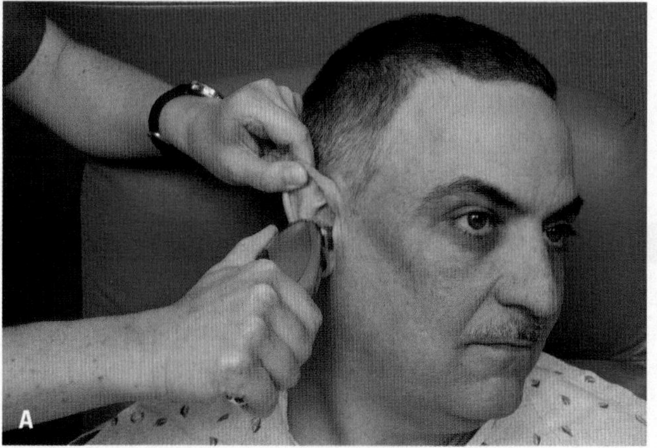

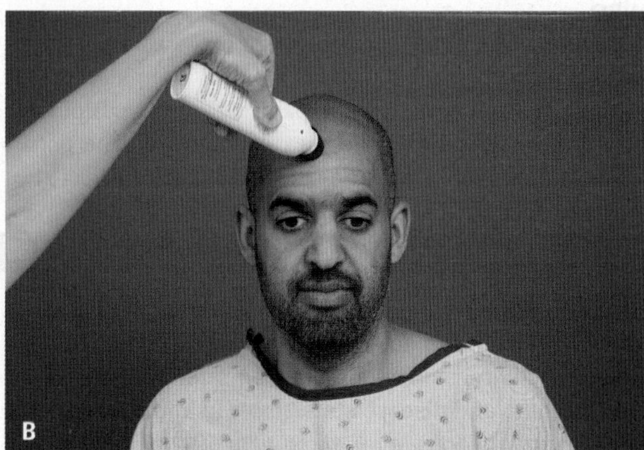

Figure 5.4 A. Tympanic temperature angling toward jaw. Pull pinna up and back. **B.** Slide temporal probe straight across forehead, lift, and then tap behind earlobe.

(table continues on page 92)

Technique and Normal Findings (continued)	Abnormal Findings (continued)
Rectal Temperature. To assess rectal temperature, ensure that the correct rectal tip is in place. Turn on the unit. Don gloves and cover the probe of the electronic thermometer with a protector. Lubricate the rectal thermometer, and insert the probe 2–3 cm (about 1 in.) into the adult rectum (Fig. 5.5). Hold the thermometer in place and stay with the patient until the temperature is read. Immediately dispose of the cover in the wastebasket. Using tissues, wipe off any lubricant remaining on the patient. Cover the patient and ensure that he or she is comfortable. *Average rectal temperature is* 37.1°–38.1°C (98.7°–100.5°F). *It is approximately 1°F warmer than oral temperature.* 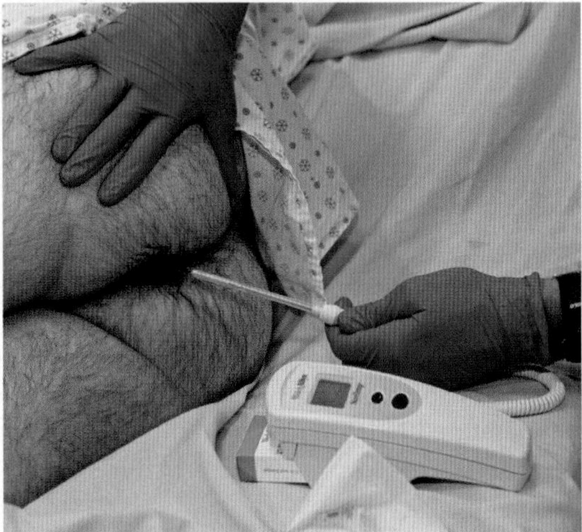 **Figure 5.5** Rectal temperature. Insert probe 2–3 cm into rectum.	Avoid placing the probe directly into stool, which may cause an inaccurate reading. The probe should be in contact with the rectal mucosa.

Pulse

Contraction of the heart causes blood to flow forward, which creates a pressure wave known as a pulse. The pulse is the throbbing sensation that can be palpated over a peripheral artery or auscultated over the apex of the heart. The pulse reflects the amount of blood ejected with each beat of the heart, which is the stroke volume. The number of pulsing sensations occurring in 1 minute is the heart (pulse) rate.

To assess the pulse, palpate one of the patient's arterial pulse points (usually the radial), noting the rate, rhythm, and strength (amplitude) of the pulse. Also note the elasticity of the vessel.

Technique and Normal Findings	Abnormal Findings
Rate. The normal range of heart rates varies with age. Infants and children have a faster heart rate than adults. Gender, activity, pain, stimulants, emotional state, medications, and disease state also can affect heart rate. *Normal heart rate for an adult is 60–100 bpm. See Table 5.2 for age-related variations.*	**Tachycardia** is a heart rate greater than 100 bpm in an adult. Trauma, anemia, blood loss, infection, fear, fever, pain, hyperthyroidism, shock, and anxiety can increase pulse rate as a result of increased metabolic demands or low blood volume. In patients with cardiac disease, tachycardia may indicate congestive heart failure, myocardial ischemia, or dysrhythmia. **Bradycardia** is a heart rate less than 60 bpm. Medications such as digoxin and beta-blockers decrease heart rate. Myocardial infarction, hypothyroidism, increased intracranial pressure, and eye surgery also can decrease heart rate. **Asystole** is the absence of a pulse. Cardiac arrest, hypovolemia, pneumothorax, cardiac tamponade, and acidosis can cause asystole.

(table continues on page 93)

TABLE 5.2 Age-Related Variations in Vital Signs (American Heart Association, 2013)				
Age	**Heart Rate** *Average (bpm)*	*Normal Range (bpm)*	**Respiration (breaths/min)**	**Blood Pressure (mm Hg)**
Newborn	120	70–190	30–40	73/55
Infant	120	80–160	20–40	85/37
Toddler	110	80–130	25–32	89/46
Child	95	70–115	20–26	95/57
Preteen	90	65–110	18–26	102/61
Teen	80	55–105	12–22	112/64
Adult	70–75	60–100	12–20	120/80
Well-conditioned athlete	May be 50–60	50–100	10–20	120/80

Technique and Normal Findings (continued)	Abnormal Findings (continued)
Rhythm. Pulse rhythm refers to the interval between beats. Pulses are described as regular or irregular. A regular pulse occurs at evenly spaced intervals. An irregular pulse has a varied interval between beats. If a pulse is irregular in rhythm, auscultate an apical pulse for 1 full minute.	Rhythm may vary with respirations, speeding up during inspiration and slowing with expiration. This is common in children and young adults and is called a sinus dysrhythmia or **sinus arrhythmia**.
A **pulse deficit** provides an indirect evaluation of the ability of each heart contraction to eject enough blood into the peripheral circulation to create a pulse.	
To assess for a pulse deficit, the beginner nurse and a colleague will at the same time assess the peripheral and the apical pulse rates and compare measurements (see Chapter 17). The more experienced nurse may be able to count the two simultaneously. The pulse deficit is the difference between the apical and radial pulse rates.	Pulse deficits are frequently associated with arrhythmias. It is essential to recognize a pulse deficit because it indicates the heart's ability to perfuse the body adequately. When cardiac contractions do not produce enough force or volume to perfuse, a difference exists between apical and peripheral pulses.
Strength. The strength of the pulse, or amplitude, indicates the volume of blood flowing through the vessel. It is described on a scale of 0–4+ (Table 5.3). *Normal strength is 2+.*	Heart failure, hypovolemia, shock, and arrhythmias can cause decreased pulse strength. Bounding pulses are noted with early stages of septic shock, exercise, fever, and anxiety.

TABLE 5.3 Scale for Measuring Pulse Strength

Scale	Description
0	Nonpalpable or absent
1+	Weak, diminished, and barely palpable
2+	Normal, expected
3+	Full, increased
4+	Bounding

Technique and Normal Findings (continued)	Abnormal Findings (continued)
Elasticity. The normal artery feels smooth, straight, and resilient. This is known as elasticity of the artery.	Vessels become less elastic with increasing age.

(table continues on page 94)

Technique and Normal Findings (continued)	Abnormal Findings (continued)

Any artery may be used to assess pulse rate, but the radial and apical arteries are the most common sites because of their accessibility (Fig. 5.6). Other peripheral sites are used to assess circulation to the extremities.

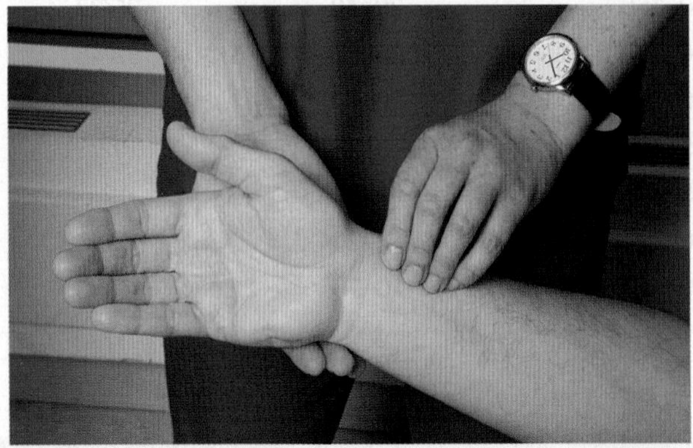

Figure 5.6 Taking a radial pulse.

In cardiac emergencies, the carotid and femoral pulses are assessed. These vessels are larger, closer to the heart, and more accurate in reflecting the heart's activity than are other pulse sites (Table 5.4).

Other sites used to assess circulation include the brachial, ulnar, popliteal, dorsalis pedis, and posterior tibial arteries (see Chapter 18).

The integrity of these peripheral pulses indicates the status of perfusion to the area distal to them.

⚠ SAFETY ALERT
The carotid pulse should be palpated only in the lower third of the neck to avoid stimulation of the carotid sinus. Never palpate both carotid pulses simultaneously. Palpating both together can significantly decrease cerebral blood flow and cause the patient to lose consciousness.

If a peripheral pulse is diminished or absent, the tissue below may have an inadequate blood supply. This finding indicates the need for further assessment (see Chapter 18).

⚠ SAFETY ALERT
Absent pulse indicates a need for further assessment. In combination with pain, pallor, or paresthesia, the viability of a limb may be threatened.

TABLE 5.4 Pulse Sites

Site	Location	Use
Temporal	Superior and lateral to the eye, anterior to the ear, over the temporal bone	Routinely in infants
Carotid	Medial edge of sternocleidomastoid muscle lateral to trachea	With infants and during shock and cardiac arrest in adults
Apical	Fifth intercostal space, left midclavicular line	To assess pulse deficit and auscultation of heart sounds
Brachial	Proximal to antecubital fossa, in the groove between the biceps and triceps muscles	With cardiac arrest in infants and to auscultate BP
Radial	Thumb side of forearm, at wrist	Routinely to assess heart rate in adults
Ulnar	Little finger side of forearm, at wrist	To assess ulnar circulation in hand and when performing Allen test (see Chapter 18)
Femoral	Inferior to the inguinal ligament in the groin	To assess circulation in lower extremities and during cardiac arrest
Popliteal	Behind the knee in popliteal fossa	To assess circulation in the lower extremities and to auscultate leg BP
Dorsalis pedis	Lateral to and parallel with the extensor tendon of the great toe	To assess circulation in the feet
Posterior tibial	Behind the medial malleolus	To assess circulation in the feet

(table continues on page 95)

Technique and Normal Findings (continued)	Abnormal Findings (continued)
Assessment. Use the pads of your index and middle fingers. Do not use the thumb, which itself has pulsations that may interfere with accuracy. Press the patient's artery gently against the underlying bone or muscle until you feel a pulsation. Do not press too hard because you may cut off the pulsation. If the pulse is regular in rhythm, count the beats for 30 seconds and then multiply by two to obtain the number of beats per minute. If the rhythm is irregular, auscultate the apical pulse for 1 full minute and assess for a pulse deficit (see Chapter 17). Assess the pulse for 1 full minute when obtaining a baseline on a patient. When counting, begin with "0" to avoid double-counting beats at both beginning and end. Right radial pulse is 68 beats/min, regular, and 2+/4+. To assess the apex of the heart, place the diaphragm of a stethoscope at the left, fifth intercostal space, midclavicular line, and auscultate for 1 full minute (see Chapter 16). On many patients, it may be easier to auscultate an apical pulse in the second or third intercostal space on the left, known as the Erb point. This avoids exposing the breast in women; also, the heart is closer to the chest wall, and usually the first and second sounds are heard equally well. Apical pulse is 60–100 bpm and regular.	*SAFETY ALERT* *Sudden changes in pulse rates or pulse rates greater than 120 bpm or less than 55 bpm may indicate life-threatening emergencies requiring immediate attention.*

Respirations

Respiration is the act of breathing, which supplies oxygen to the body and vital organs and eliminates carbon dioxide. Inspiration occurs when the intercostal muscles and diaphragm contract and expand the pleural cavity, creating a negative pressure for air to flow actively into the lungs. During expiration, the intercostal muscles and diaphragm relax, decreasing the space in the pleural cavity and passively pushing air out of the lungs.

Clinical Significance

Assess patients with **dyspnea** (difficulty breathing) in the position of greatest comfort to them. Repositioning may increase the work of breathing, which will alter the respiratory rate.

Rate and depth of respiration change with the demands of the body. Nurses assess for factors that influence respirations.

Technique and Normal Findings	Abnormal Findings
Observe both inspiration and expiration separately. Most patients are not aware of their breathing. Do not make the patient aware that you are assessing respirations. Increased awareness may alter normal respiratory pattern. One way to assess respirations is to maintain the position of fingers on the radial artery as if continuing to assess the pulse while counting respirations. *Normal respirations are relaxed, smooth, effortless, and silent.*	• **Exercise.** Respirations increase in rate and depth to meet additional oxygen demands. • **Anxiety/pain.** Sympathetic nervous system stimulation increases respiratory rate and depth. • **Smoking.** Chronic smoking alters pulmonary airways, increasing resting respiratory rate. • **Positioning.** Slouching impedes the ability of the lungs to fully expand, whereas standing or sitting erect promotes full expansion. • **Medications.** Narcotics, anesthesia, and sedatives decrease respiratory rate, whereas stimulants and bronchodilators increase it. • **Neurological injury.** Damage to the brainstem inhibits respiratory rate and rhythm. • **Hemoglobin levels.** Decreased levels of hemoglobin lower the oxygen-carrying capacity of the blood, which in turn increases respiratory rate to increase oxygen delivery.

(table continues on page 96)

Technique and Normal Findings (continued)	Abnormal Findings (continued)
	⚠ *SAFETY ALERT* *Further assessment is needed if the respiratory rate is less than 10 or greater than 32 breaths/min. Such findings may indicate acute distress and prompt the need for a rapid response.*
The respiratory rate is a count of each full inspiration and expiration cycle in 1 minute. Count for 30 seconds and multiply by two to obtain breaths per min. If any abnormalities are noted, assess respiratory rate for 1 full minute. *Normal respiratory rates for adults are 12–20 breaths/min, regular.*	**Tachypnea** is a rapid, persistent respiratory rate greater than 20 breaths/min in an adult. It may occur with fever, exercise, anemia, or anxiety. Persistent respiratory rate less than 12 breaths/min is **bradypnea.** It accompanies increased intracranial pressure, neurological disease, and sedation. **Dyspnea** is a term used for difficult breathing. Resting respiration that is deeper and more rapid than normal is known as **hyperpnea. Apnea** is the absence of spontaneous respirations for more than 10 seconds.
In addition to rate, observe for the rhythm, depth, and quality of respiration. Is the rhythm regular? As with the pulse, the rhythm refers to the interval between breaths. Regular respiratory rhythm has even intervals. Note the depth of respirations. Is the patient's breath shallow, moderate, or deep? Depth of respirations is a reflection of tidal volume. Also note if the patient uses any accessory muscles while breathing. Normal respiratory effort uses the diaphragm and intercostal muscles. Note the presence of retractions. *Normal respiratory rate, rhythm, and effort is called* ***eupnea****. Note that there are no retractions or use of accessory muscles.*	**Hyperventilation** is deep, rapid respiration, which may result from hypoxia, anxiety, exercise, or metabolic acidosis. **Hypoventilation** is shallow, slow respiration that may be related to sedation or increased intracranial pressure. Use of accessory muscles (e.g., abdominal or neck muscles) may indicate respiratory distress. Also note any cyanosis, retractions, or audible sounds such as wheezing or congestion. ⚠ *SAFETY ALERT* *High-pitched crowing sounds from tracheal or laryngeal spasm, called stridor, may indicate a life-threatening emergency. Any periods of apnea, tachypnea, bradypnea, or irregular respiratory pattern are indications of underlying disease and warrant further assessment.* Accessory muscles include the sternomastoid, rectus abdominis, and internal intercostals. Retractions, or a pulling inward of the soft tissue, are noted in the supraclavicular, intercostal, and costal margin area.

Examples include exercise, anxiety, pain, smoking, positioning, medications, neurological injury, and hemoglobin level.

Oxygen Saturation

Oxygen saturation is the percentage to which hemoglobin is filled with oxygen. Measurement of oxygen saturation does not replace measurement of arterial blood gases for assessment of abnormalities, but it does indicate abnormal gas exchange.

Pulse oximetry is a noninvasive technique to measure oxygen saturation of arterial blood.

⚠ *SAFETY ALERT*

Further assessment is required if the patient's oxygen saturation is less than 92%. This finding may require a rapid response. SpO_2 less than 85% indicates inadequate oxygenation to the tissues and may be an emergency.

Blood Pressure

Blood pressure (BP) is the measurement of the force exerted by the flow of blood against the arterial walls. The pressure in the arteries changes with contraction and relaxation of the heart. Maximum pressure is exerted on the walls of the arteries with contraction of the left ventricle at the beginning of systole. This is known as the **systolic blood pressure** (SBP). The lowest pressure, called the **diastolic blood pressure** (DBP), occurs when the left ventricle relaxes between beats. Five factors contribute to BP: (1) cardiac output, (2) peripheral vascular resistance, (3) circulating blood volume, (4) viscosity, and (5) elasticity of the vessel walls.

Millimeters of mercury (mm Hg) is the standard unit for measuring BP. BP is recorded as a fraction, with the SBP as the numerator and the DBP as the denominator. Average BP for adults is 120/80 mm Hg, with a range of 90 to 120 mm Hg

Technique and Normal Findings	Abnormal Findings
Assess capillary refill and strength of the pulse in the extremity to be used for measuring oxygen saturation. Typically, a finger is used to obtain a reading (Fig. 5.7).	
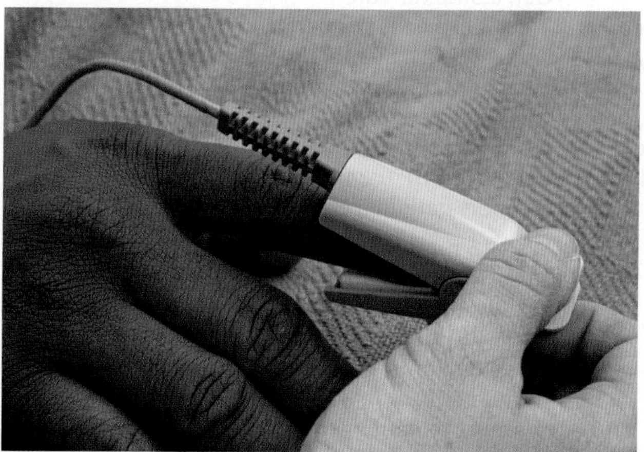 **Figure 5.7** Placement of the pulse oximeter for oxygen saturation.	
Nail polish may affect the accuracy of pulse oximetry readings so it should be removed. If patient's circulation is poor, consider using an earlobe or bridge of the nose.	
A newer oximeter sensor, which attaches to the forehead, has also been useful in patients with poor peripheral perfusion. When compared with arterial blood gases, the forehead sensor is more accurate than the finger probe (Smith, 2013).	
Potential errors in oximetry measurements may result from abnormal hemoglobin value, hypotension, hypothermia, patient movement, or skin breakdown. Falsely low measurements may be associated with cold extremities, hypothermia, and hypovolemia. Falsely high readings may be associated with carbon monoxide poisoning and anemia. *Normal pulse oximetry is SpO_2 from 92% to 99%. An SpO_2 of 85%–89% may be acceptable for patients with certain chronic conditions such as emphysema.*	Conditions that decrease arterial blood flow may compromise the accuracy of readings, such as peripheral vascular disease, edema, and hypotension. Patients with anemia may have a falsely elevated pulse oximetry reading from circulating hemoglobin containing sufficient oxygen but inadequate hemoglobin to carry adequate oxygen. Increased mortality is associated with both hypoxia and extreme hyperoxemia. Pulse oximetry readings of 100% may be an indication of hyperoxemia.

SBP and 60 to 80 mm Hg DBP. Variations occur normally and are influenced by many factors, including age, gender, ethnicity, weight, circadian cycle, position, exercise, emotions, stress, medications, and smoking.

- **Age.** BP increases gradually throughout childhood into the adult years.
- **Gender.** Before puberty, males and females show no discernible difference in BP. After puberty, males show a higher BP measurement than females, but this reverses after menopause, with BP tending to be higher in females than in males.
- **Ethnicity.** Compared with Caucasians, African Americans are 1.5 times more likely to have high BP. Native Americans, Alaska Natives, and Mexican Americans are 1.3 times more likely than Caucasians to have high BP (Centers for Disease Control and Prevention, 2013).
- **Weight.** For each 22 lb (10 kg) of extra weight, SBP elevates 2 to 3 mm Hg and DBP elevates 1 to 3 mm Hg.
- **Circadian (diurnal) cycle.** A daily cycle of BP occurs, with BP increasing late in the afternoon and decreasing in the early morning.
- **Position.** BP can drop as a patient moves from lying to sitting or standing. Lack of back support (as when a patient is sitting on an exam table) increases DPB by as much as 6 mm Hg. Crossing of the patient's legs may increase SBP by 2 to 8 mm Hg (Pickering et al., 2005).

TABLE 5.5 Common Errors in Blood Pressure Measurement

Error	Contributing Factors	Nursing Action
Falsely low reading	Noisy environment	Maintain a quiet environment during assessment.
	Too large cuff	Use a smaller cuff.
	Improper placement of earpieces of stethoscope	Place earpieces properly.
	Stethoscope not directly over brachial artery	Palpate brachial artery for stethoscope placement.
	Hearing deficit	Use amplified stethoscope.
	Deflating cuff too quickly	Decrease rate of deflation.
	Deflating cuff too slowly (false high diastolic)	Increase rate of deflation.
	Failing to palpate radial artery for estimated SBP	Estimate SBP using palpation.
	Arm position above level of heart	Support patient's arm at the level of the heart.
Falsely high reading	Assessing BP immediately after exercise	Wait 15 minutes after the patient has exercised to assess.
	Assessing anxious or angry patient	Wait until patient is calm.
	Cuff too small	Obtain larger cuff.
	Cuff wrapped too loosely	Wrap cuff snugly and smoothly.
	Reinflation of cuff during auscultation	Deflate cuff, wait 30 seconds, and reassess BP.
	Arm position below level of heart	Support patient's arm at the level of the heart.
	Patient supporting own arm	Support the patient's arm.
	Legs crossed	Uncross legs.
Inaccurate readings	Examiner's eyes not at level of the meniscus	Maintain eye level parallel with meniscus.
	Examiner bias	Do not anticipate or predict what BP should be.
	Defective or inaccurately calibrated equipment	Calibrate equipment regularly.
Other errors	Inflation of cuff too high, causing patient pain	Estimate SBP by palpation.

- **Exercise.** Increased activity increases BP, with a return to baseline within 5 minutes of stopping.
- **Emotions.** Fear, anger, and pain momentarily increase BP by stimulating the sympathetic nervous system.
- **Stress.** Patients under continuous tension will experience elevated BP.
- **Medications.** Many medications can lower BP, including antihypertensive agents, diuretics, narcotics, and general anesthesia.
- **Smoking.** Smoking causes increased vasoconstriction. BP returns to baseline in approximately 15 minutes after cessation of smoking.

A series of BP measurements provides more information than a single measurement. Elevated BP indicates a need for a series of follow-up readings to assess whether BP is consistently elevated.

BP is measured using a **sphygmomanometer** and stethoscope. The sphygmomanometer consists of an aneroid or mercury gauge and an inflatable rubber bladder in a cloth covering called the cuff. Many agencies have prohibited the use of mercury-containing devices and instead use electronic or automatic BP cuffs.

Cuffs are available in various sizes, ranging from very small for newborns to extra large arm cuffs for adults as well as thigh cuffs. It is important to choose the correct cuff size to obtain accurate readings (Table 5.5). The width of the cuff should equal 40% of the length of the patient's upper arm. The length of the bladder should equal 80% of the circumference of the limb (Fig. 5.8). If a large cuff is not available in a patient with morbid obesity, BP can be measured on the forearm; the cuff can be placed midway between the elbow and the wrist (Leblanc et al., 2013).

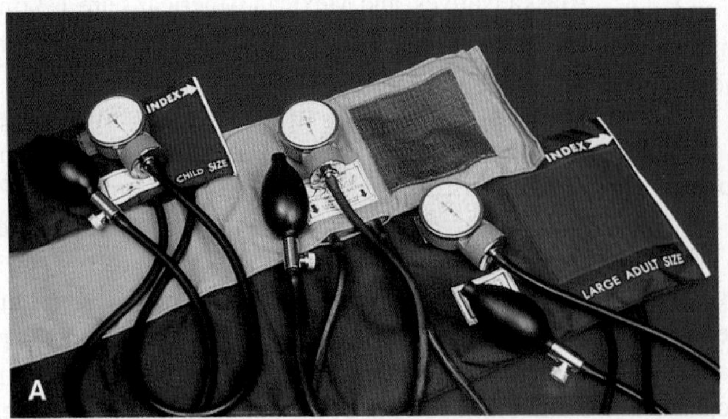

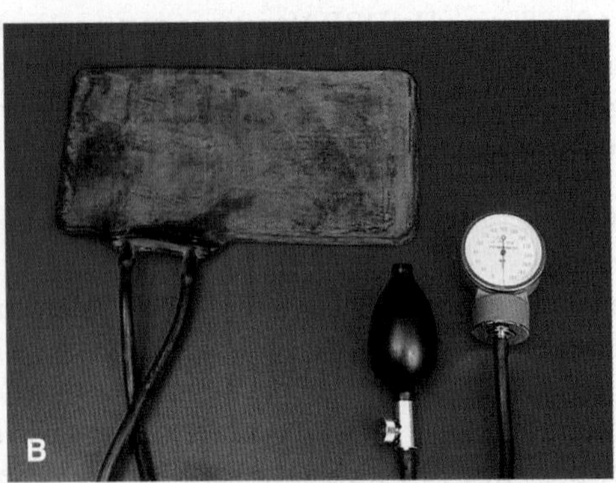

Figure 5.8 **A.** Three sizes of blood pressure cuffs. **B.** Bladder is inside the cuff.

Technique and Normal Findings	Abnormal Findings
Arm Blood Pressure. Before assessing BP in the arm, be sure the patient is calm and relaxed and has not eaten, smoked, or exercised for 30 minutes before the measurement. It is best to allow the patient to rest for at least 5 minutes before assessing BP (Joint National Committee on High Blood Pressure, 2014). Measure initial BP in both arms for comparison. A variation of 5–10 mm Hg between arms is normal. If the values are different, use the higher value but record both.	A difference of 10–15 mm Hg or more between the two arms may indicate arterial obstruction on the side with the lower value.
The patient may be supine or sitting. Support the bare arm at heart level with a table or pillow, with the palm upward (Van Velthoven, Thien, Holewijn, van der Wilt, & Deinum, 2010). If the patient is sitting, the patient's feet should be flat on the floor. Crossed legs may falsely elevate BP (Van Velthoven et al., 2010). The patient's back should be supported. Avoid having the patient talk, deep breathe, or move the head/neck or opposite arm during measurement as it will elevate the reading (Zheng, Giovannini, & Murray, 2012).	Do not allow the patient to hold up the arm because tension from muscle contraction can elevate SBP. Also make sure that the arm is at heart level. For each 5 cm change in arm position relative to the heart, there is a corresponding change in BP by 3–4 mm Hg. Elevating the arm above the heart may result in a false-low measurement and lowering it may result in a false-high measurement (Tomlinson, 2010).
Assess the extremity to be used for BP assessment. Do not use an extremity with a shunt, on the same side as a mastectomy, or with an intravenous (IV) infusion.	
Choose the correct cuff size. The cuff is 80% of the arm's circumference or 40% of its width.	⚠ *SAFETY ALERT* *Using a cuff that is too small causes a falsely high BP reading; using one that is too large causes a falsely low BP reading.*
Palpate the brachial artery above the antecubital fossa and medial to the biceps tendon. Center the deflated cuff approximately 2.5 cm (1 in.) above the brachial artery. Line up the arrow on the cuff with the brachial artery. Tuck the Velcro end of the cuff under so that the cuff is snuggly fastened around the arm.	
Estimate the SBP by palpating the brachial or radial artery and inflating the cuff until the pulsation disappears. Hold the bulb in your dominant hand. Close the valve on the bulb by turning it clockwise, but make sure that it will easily release. To control the bulb, it is easiest to brace your fingers against the metal of the valve. Squeeze the bulb to pump air into the bladder. Continue feeling the pulse, and identify when it disappears. Pump the cuff to 20–30 mm Hg above where the pulse stopped.	⚠ *SAFETY ALERT* *Estimating the SBP will prevent missing an* ***auscultatory gap****, a period in which there are no Korotkoff sounds during auscultation. An auscultatory gap occurs in approximately 5% of patients and up to 21% of patients with known vascular disease and hypertension (Aronow et al., 2011). Despite this high incidence, only about half of practicing nurses can identify an auscultatory gap (Bickley, 2013).*
Slowly open the valve by turning it counterclockwise to deflate the cuff 2–3 mm Hg per minute. Feel for the pulse, noting the number when the pulsation is palpable again, and then quickly deflate the cuff completely. This is the estimated SBP. Wait 15 to 30 seconds before reinflating the cuff to allow trapped blood in the veins to clear.	

(table continues on page 100)

Technique and Normal Findings (continued)	Abnormal Findings (continued)

Position the earpieces of the stethoscope in your ears with the earpieces pointed forward and check to make sure the chestpiece is turned so that you hear sound by tapping it lightly (Chap. 3). Place the diaphragm or bell of the stethoscope over the brachial artery, using a light touch (Fig. 5.9A). Most nurses use the diaphragm. Position yourself so that you can avoid bumping the tubing and can easily see the gauge. Note that you will not hear the tapping of the pulse until the cuff is inflated and the flow is partially obstructed.

The bell is designed to pick up low-pitched sounds, such as the turbulent blood flow caused by the BP cuff partially occluding the brachial artery. Although some texts recommend using the bell, the bell and diaphragm are equally effective in auscultating BP (American Heart Association, 2013).

Inflating the BP cuff around the extremity alters the flow of blood through the artery, which generates Korotkoff sounds (Fig. 5.9B). These sounds are audible with a stethoscope at a pulse site distal to the cuff.

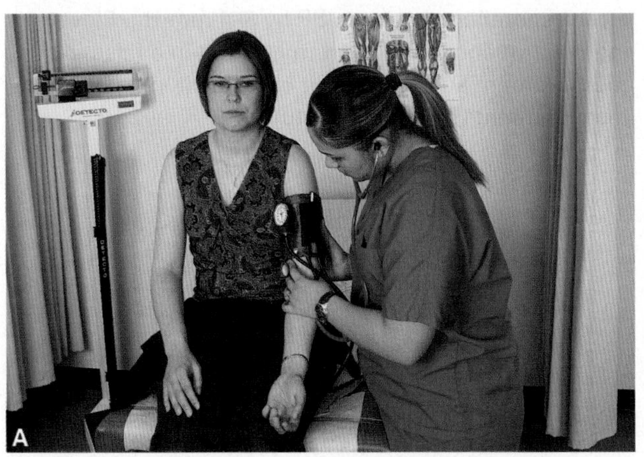

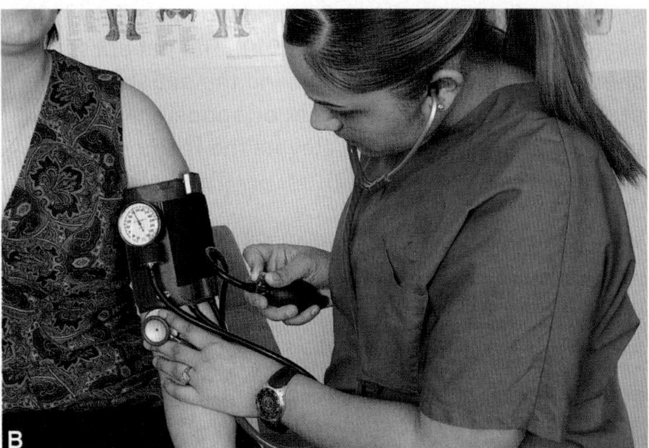

Figure 5.9 **A.** Arm blood pressure. Note placement of the earpieces of the stethoscope in the nurse's ears as she auscultates over the brachial artery. **B.** Inflating the blood pressure cuff around the arm alters arterial blood flow.

As pressure against the artery wall decreases from completely occluded blood flow to free flow, you can auscultate five distinct sounds (Table 5.6). You will hear sounds only during the period of partial occlusion and not when the artery is totally occluded or not occluded at all.

Quickly inflate the cuff to 20–30 mm Hg above the estimated SBP. Then deflate the cuff slowly, approximately 2–3 mm Hg, while listening for pulse sounds (Korotkoff sounds). Note the number when you hear the first Korotkoff sound, which coincides with the patient's SBP. A common tendency is to round to zero; be aware of this tendency so that you can avoid it. Make sure to read the gauge accurately (Pickering et al., 2005). Continue deflating the cuff, noting the point of the last pulse sound (Korotkoff IV) and when it disappears (Korotkoff V). Korotkoff V is used to define DBP (see Table 5.6).

Guidelines from the Joint National Committee on Prevention, Detection, Evaluation, and Treatment of High Blood Pressure (JNC 7) set the standards for diagnosis of high BP (Joint National Committee VII, 2014). See Table 5.7. **Hypertension** is not diagnosed on one BP reading alone but on an average of two or more readings taken on subsequent visits. **Hypotension** is SBP less than 90 mm Hg. Some adults have a normal low BP, but in most adults, low BP indicates illness.

Record BP in even numbers as a fraction, with SBP as the numerator and DBP as the denominator. Also record the patient's position, arm used, and cuff size if different from the standard cuff.

> ⚠ *SAFETY ALERT*
>
> *Any sudden change in BP may be an emergency. SBP less than 90, or 30 mm Hg below the patient's baseline, needs immediate attention. Sudden drop in BP can signify blood loss or a cardiovascular, respiratory, neurological, or metabolic disorder. Sudden, severe rise in BP (above 200/120 mm Hg) is a life-threatening hypertensive crisis.*

(table continues on page 101)

TABLE 5.6 Korotkoff Sounds

Phase	Description
I	Characterized by the first appearance of faint but clear tapping sounds that gradually increase in intensity; the first tapping sound is the systolic pressure
II	Characterized by muffled or swishing sounds; these sounds may temporarily disappear, especially in patients with hypertension; the disappearance of the sound during the latter part of phase I and during phase II is called the *auscultatory gap* and may cover a range of as much as 40 mm Hg; failing to recognize this gap may cause serious errors of underestimating systolic pressure or overestimating diastolic pressure
III	Characterized by distinct, loud sounds as the blood flows relatively freely through an increasingly open artery
IV	Characterized by a distinct, abrupt, muffling sound with a soft, blowing quality; in adults, onset of this phase is considered the first diastolic sound
V	The last sound heard before a period of continuous silence; the pressure at which the last sound is heard is the second diastolic measurement

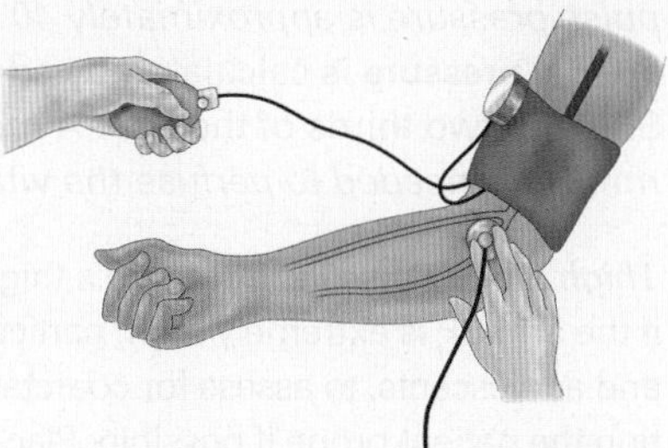

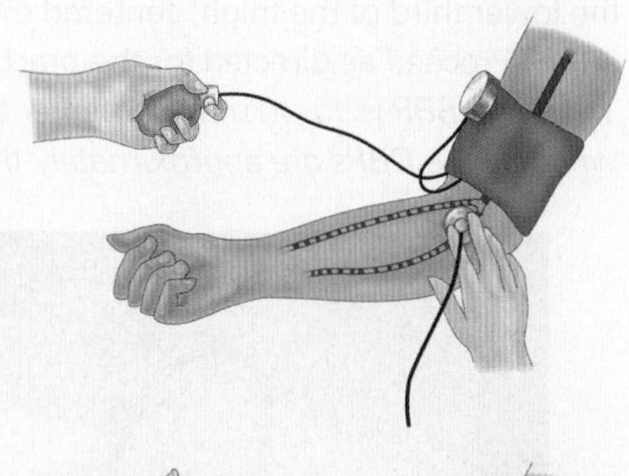

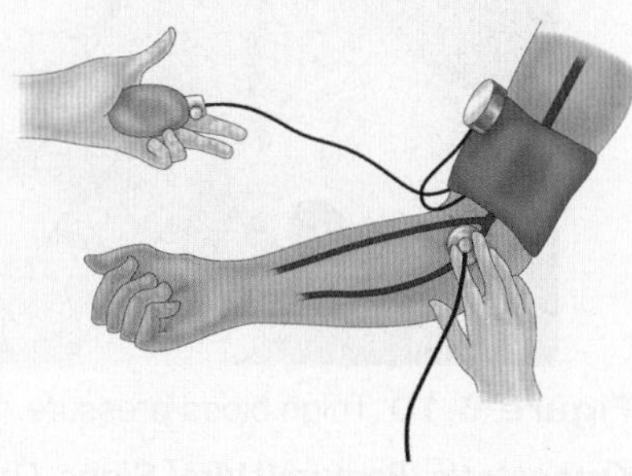

From Taylor, C., Lillis, C., LeMone, P., & Lynn, P. (2011). *Fundamentals of nursing: The art and science of nursing care* (7th ed.). Philadelphia, PA: Wolters Kluwer Health/Lippincott Williams & Wilkins.

TABLE 5.7 Classification of Blood Pressure in Adults

Blood Pressure Category	Systolic mm Hg (upper #)		Diastolic mm Hg (lower #)
Normal	Less than **120**	and	Less than **80**
Prehypertension	**120–139**	or	**80–89**
High blood pressure (hypertension) **stage 1**	**140–159**	or	**90–99**
High blood pressure (hypertension) **stage 2**	**160** or higher	or	**100** or higher
Hypertensive crisis (emergency care needed)	Higher than **180**	or	Higher than **110**

This chart reflects blood pressure categories defined by the American Heart Association.

Technique and Normal Findings (continued)	Abnormal Findings (continued)
Slow or frequent cuff inflations can cause venous congestion. Be sure to deflate the cuff completely after each measurement and wait at least 2 minutes between measurements.	

(table continues on page 102)

Technique and Normal Findings (continued)	Abnormal Findings (continued)
The **pulse pressure** is the difference between the SBP and the DBP and reflects the stroke volume. *Normal pulse pressure is approximately 40 mm Hg.* The **mean arterial pressure** is calculated by adding one third of the SBP and two thirds of the DBP. *A mean pressure of 60 mm Hg is needed to perfuse the vital organs.*	Decreased elasticity of the arterial blood vessel walls, as well as increased intracranial pressure, can cause the difference between SBP and DBP to increase. This is called a widened pulse pressure. Patients with hypovolemia, shock, or heart failure may exhibit a narrowed pulse pressure.
Thigh Blood Pressure. Compare a thigh BP with an arm BP if the arm BP is extremely high, particularly in young adults and adolescents, to assess for coarctation of the aorta. Position the patient prone if possible. Place a large cuff around the lower third of the thigh, centered over the popliteal artery. Proceed as directed for the brachial artery (Fig. 5.10). *The thigh SBP is 10–40 mm Hg higher than the arm SBP, whereas the DBPs are approximately the same in both sites.* 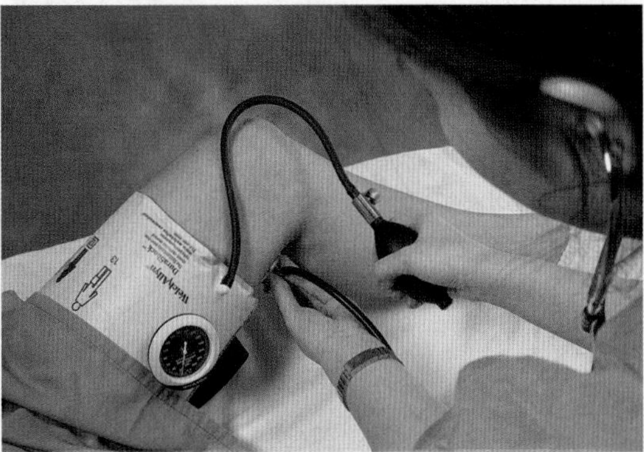 **Figure 5.10** Thigh blood pressure.	A thigh or calf may also be used if the patient's arms are unavailable, such as in those with bilateral burns or IV fluids. Coarctation of the aorta (congenital narrowing of the aorta) will produce high arm BP and lower thigh BP as a result of restricted blood supply below the narrowing.
Orthostatic (Postural) Vital Signs. Orthostatic vital signs are measured in patients to assess for a drop in BP and change in heart rate with position changes. When a healthy patient changes position, the peripheral blood vessels in the extremities constrict and the heart rate increases to maintain adequate BP for perfusion to the heart and brain. Orthostatic changes may indicate blood volume depletion. Some medications can have the adverse effect of causing orthostatic hypotension. Additionally, conditions that cause the arterial system to become less responsive, such as immobility or spinal cord injury, can cause orthostatic changes.	
Assess BP and heart rate with the patient supine, sitting, and then standing. The patient should rest supine for at least 2 minutes before the assessment of the baseline reading. Repeat measurements with the patient sitting and standing, waiting 1–2 minutes after each position change to assess the readings. *A drop in SBP of* less than *15 mm Hg may occur and is considered normal.*	Drop in SBP of 15 mm Hg or greater, drop in DBP of 10 mm Hg or greater, or increased heart rate indicates **orthostatic hypotension** and possibly intravascular volume depletion (Calkins & Zipes, 2011). Patients with orthostatic hypotension may exhibit dizziness, light-headedness, or syncope. Hypovolemia, certain medications, and prolonged bed rest may cause orthostatic hypotension. Autonomic dysregulation, as in Parkinson disease, interferes with the normal sympathetic response and may cause orthostasis. *SAFETY ALERT* *Patients with orthostatic hypotension are at risk for falling from dizziness, light-headedness, and syncope.*

(table continues on page 103)

Technique and Normal Findings (continued)	Abnormal Findings (continued)

Documenting Normal Findings

Parameters: Temperature and route; pulse rate, rhythm, strength, and site; respiratory rate, rhythm, quality, and depth; pulse oximetry; and BP are recorded on the vital sign flow sheet or other forms per agency policy. If a measurement was taken after administration of medications or other therapies, this should be documented in the nurse's notes. Strength of peripheral pulses can be documented either as a chart or diagram. When there is a distinct muffling of the Korotkoff sounds, record both readings (e.g., 138/92/72). Report abnormal findings to the primary care provider.

Normal Findings: T 37°C orally. R radial P 68 bpm, regular, elastic, 2+/4+. R—14 breaths/min, regular, no use of accessory muscles, no retractions. SpO_2—98%. BP 128/64 mm Hg, right arm, supine. T Roe, RN

Risk Reduction and Health Promotion

Teach patients to consistently weigh themselves at the same time of day, wearing clothing of similar weight. Educate patients about risk factors for hypothermia (i.e., frostbite; fatigue; malnutrition; hypoxemia; cold, wet clothing; alcohol intoxication) and hyperthermia (i.e., exercising in poorly ventilated areas and hot humid climate, sudden exposures to hot climates, tight-fitting clothing in hot environments, and poor fluid intake before, during, and after exercise).

Instruct patients who are taking cardiac medications, undergoing cardiac rehabilitation, or starting a new exercise regimen how to take their own pulse rates. Monitoring carotid pulse rate is the most common technique taught to patients. Teach coughing and deep-breathing exercises to patients who are undergoing surgery and those with decreased ventilation.

Educate patients about the risks of hypertension. Risk factors for hypertension include obesity, cigarette smoking, heavy alcohol consumption, prolonged stress, high cholesterol and triglyceride levels, family history, and renal disease. Primary prevention includes lifestyle modifications such as weight loss, regular exercise, dietary modifications, cessation of smoking, reduction of stress, and reduction of saturated fats and sodium in the diet.

Every interaction with a patient is a teaching opportunity. Even patients who are normotensive and have a body weight within normal limits can learn how to maintain a healthy body. The Joint National Committee on Blood Pressure VII (2014) published the following recommendations to help maintain controlled BP:

- If you are more than 10% above ideal body weight, lose weight.
- Limit alcohol to no more than 1 oz of ethanol per day.
- Exercise regularly.
- Limit sodium intake to less than 100 mmol/L/day.
- Quit smoking.
- Reduce dietary saturated fat and cholesterol.

Vital Signs Monitor

Many agencies use a monitor for all vital signs (Fig. 5.11). This portable device is usually on a stand that nurses can wheel from one room to another. It is plugged in when not in use to charge the battery. When taking vital signs with this machine, first unplug it and roll it next to the patient. Attach the cuff. (Because of infection control issues, each patient should have his or her own cuff; disinfect between patients if using the same cuff.) Place the cuff on the patient's arm and press the inflate button. After the display, remove the cuff. The monitor will display the pulse sensed during the BP or SpO_2 reading. Attach the finger clip for the SpO_2. Note the reading that the monitor displays. Load the probe cover on the thermometer. Place the thermometer for the appropriate mode. Note the reading after it is displayed. Eject the probe cover into the wastebasket using universal precautions. Wash your hands and disinfect the machine according to agency precautions before allowing it to come into contact with the next patient.

> **SAFETY ALERT**
> *When using automatic devices for serial readings, check the patient's cuffed limb frequently to ensure sufficient perfusion to areas distal to the cuff.*

Doppler Technique

Pulse and BP are difficult to auscultate or palpate in some patients, such as those in shock or with poor peripheral circulation. In such cases, health care providers use a handheld device called a **Doppler** transducer. This device senses and amplifies changes in sound frequency, which is audible as whooshing sounds similar to Korotkoff sounds. The

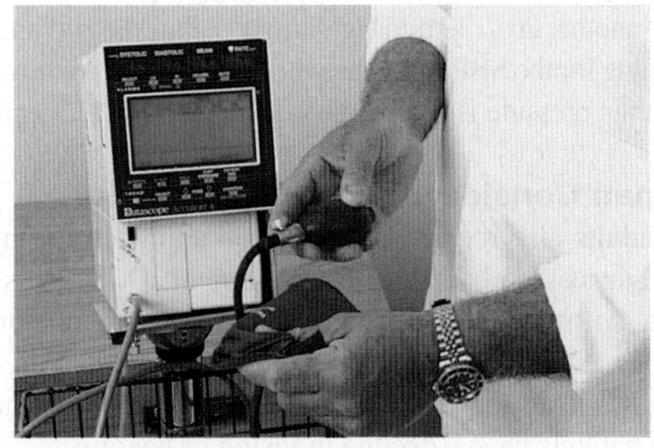

Figure 5.11 Vital signs monitoring device.

Documenting Case Study Findings

The nurse has just finished conducting a physical examination of Mr. Sanders, the 55-year-old man admitted to the hospital with an arrhythmia. Both normal and abnormal findings are documented, including the absence of positive findings. Review the following data that were collected during the general survey and vital signs. Begin to think about how the data are clustered and what additional data the nurse might want to collect while thinking critically about Mr. Sander's problems.

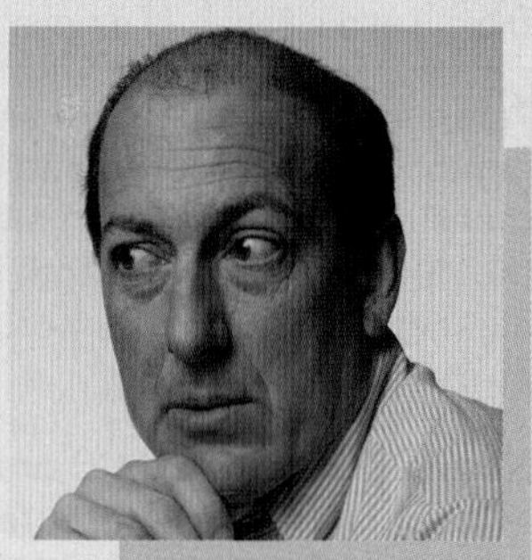

Inspection: A 55-year-old Caucasian man without obvious deformities, appears older than stated age; facial features and body structure symmetrical; wearing hospital gown, well-groomed. Skin even tone, pink, without lesions. Physical development appropriate for age and gender. Cooperative and interacts pleasantly. Facial expression relaxed, maintains eye contact. A&O × 3; responds appropriately to questions. Speech is clear and articulate. Sitting upright, posture erect, arms relaxed at the side. Gait steady, well-balanced. No signs of distress. T 36.9°C, po, R 14 breaths/min, regular, no use of accessory muscles. Height 1.62 m, weight 65 kg, BMI 24.8.

Palpation: Apical pulse 88 and irregular. Pulse deficit of 2 noted.

Auscultation: Blood pressure 142/66 right arm, sitting.

procedure for the assessment of the pulse using Doppler is as follows:

- Apply gel that is specifically for the Doppler to the transducer probe.
- Turn the Doppler on.
- Adjust the volume.
- Touch the probe lightly to the skin at the expected pulse site.
- Hold the probe perpendicular to the skin and move it slowly where you anticipate that the pulse should be until it is located.
- Wipe off the gel and mark the location of the loudest sound with indelible ink.
- Attempt to palpate the pulse in this location.

If you are taking a patient's BP using the Doppler transducer, put on the cuff first. After the pulse is located by Doppler, inflate the cuff until the sounds are no longer present. Pump up the cuff another 20 to 30 mm Hg. Slowly deflate the cuff and note the reading for the SBP when the whooshing sounds return. Only the systolic pressure is recorded by documenting 88/Doppler.

Lifespan Considerations: Older Adults

Older adults also require a specialized approach during the general survey and vital signs assessment. Do not rush the patient. Allow enough time for him or her to respond to questions and to ask questions. Do not assume that an older patient has a sensory deficit. For example, some but not all elderly patients have a decline in vision or hearing.

Cultural Variations

During the general survey of every patient, note any cultural influences such as dress, grooming, speech, and nonverbal communication. Some common cultural differences may include the following:

- Mexican American patients may expect nurses to show warmth to patients and family members—interactions should not be "strictly business." The nurse should be attentive, take some time, show respect, and, if possible, communicate in Spanish.
- In many Asian cultures, the spoken and written order of the name is last name then first name with no comma. This often creates confusion in the medical record. Care must be taken to use a consistent format.
- Southeast Asian patients use "krun" to describe a wide range of symptoms including "feeling ill," "feeling hot and cold," or "having a warm body." It may be translated as a fever, although a fever may not be present.
- Patients of Arab cultures may not disclose personal or sexual information.
- Some patients from East African countries apply skin decorations with henna. Black henna causes major errors in oxygen saturation readings, although red henna does not. Use of ear oximetry is recommended if patients have black henna applied to their fingertips (Ethnomed, 2013).

Technique and Normal Findings	Abnormal Findings
General Survey. By the eighth or ninth decade, physical appearance changes, with sharper body contours and more angular facial features. Posture tends to have a general flexion, and gait tends to have a wider base of support to compensate for diminished balance. Steps tend to be shorter and uneven. Patients may need to use the arms to help aid in balance. Observe normal changes of aging. Assess for any decreasing abilities to function and care for self. Note any changes in mental status.	Poor hygiene and inappropriate dress may indicate decreased functional ability, medication reactions, infection, dehydration, or malnutrition. Inappropriate affect, inattentiveness, impaired memory, and inability to perform ADLs may indicate dementia (e.g., Alzheimer disease). Changes in mental status may be from poor nutrition, medications, dehydration, underlying infection, or hypoxia.
Height and Weight. People in their 80s and 90s may be shorter than they were in their 70s as a result of thinning of the vertebral discs and postural changes (e.g., kyphosis or scoliosis), causing the spinal column to shorten. The proportions of the aging person tend to look different because the long bones do not shorten but the trunk does. The aging person tends to lose body weight during the eighth and ninth decades from muscle shrinkage and fat distribution changes. Subcutaneous fat is lost from the face and periphery, even with adequate nutrition.	**Kyphosis** is an exaggerated posterior curvature of the thoracic spine associated with aging.
Vital Signs	
Temperature. The temperature of older adults is at the lower end of the normal range. Because of changes in the body's temperature regulatory mechanism and decreased subcutaneous fat, aging adults are less likely to develop fevers but more likely are prone to hypothermia. *Mean body temperature for the older adult is 36°–36.8°C (96.9°–98.3°F).*	Temperatures considered normal for younger adults may constitute fever in older adults.
Pulse. Aging adults have a normal pulse range (60–100 bpm). Variation in rhythm may develop. The radial artery may stiffen from peripheral vascular disease; however, a rigid artery does not indicate vascular disease elsewhere in the body.	
The pulse rate of older adults takes longer to rise to meet sudden increases in demand and longer to return to resting state and tends to be lower than that of younger adults.	
Heart sounds may be more difficult to auscultate and the maximum impulse more difficult to palpate.	
Respirations. Aging causes rigidity of the costal cartilage, decreasing chest expansion and vital capacity. Decreased vital capacity and inspiratory volume can cause respirations to be shallower and more rapid than those of younger adults, with a normal respiratory rate of 16–25 breaths/min. Decreased efficiency of respiratory muscles results in breathlessness at lower activity levels.	

(table continues on page 106)

Technique and Normal Findings (continued)	Abnormal Findings (continued)
Pulse Oximetry. Placement of the pulse oximetry probe can present a challenge in older adults. Peripheral vascular disease, decreased carbon dioxide levels, cold-induced vasoconstriction, and anemia may complicate assessment of oxygen saturation on the fingers. Sensors designed for the forehead or bridge of nose may be a better choice.	
Blood Pressure. Pay special attention to proper cuff size when assessing BP in older adults because of loss of upper arm mass, obesity, and smaller arm size. BP tends to increase from atherosclerosis.	In older people, both SBP and DBP increase, but SBP more so, leading to a widened pulse pressure. Elevated BP in older adults is not a normal aspect of aging. Remind older adults to change positions slowly to avoid orthostatic hypotension, which increases the risk for falling.

Height varies little among racial groups as compared with other anthropometric measures. Height is affected by genetics, nutrition, and stressors. Mean height varies by gender. In men, Caucasians are tallest, followed by African Americans, and then Mexican Americans (Centers for Disease Control and Prevention, 2013). African American women are tallest, followed by Caucasian women, and then Mexican American women. Height is generally not a health concern unless more than a 20% deviation exists from the norm such as in gigantism or dwarfism (see Table 5.9 at the end of the chapter).

Overall weight of the U.S. population has increased by 24 lb in the past 40 years, whereas height has increased by only 1 in.; thus, BMI has increased by three units. This trend includes U.S. children and teenagers, whose BMI has increased by 4 units. In women 60 years of age and older, 61% of non-Hispanic black women are obese compared with 32% of Caucasian women and 37% of Mexican American women. The prevalence of obesity does not differ significantly by race or ethnic group in men (Ogden et al., 2007). Reduction of obesity is included in the goals for many developed nations.

Critical Thinking

Several nursing diagnoses can be addressed under vital signs assessment. Many are covered in the appropriate body systems chapters of this book. Table 5.8 provides some examples of

TABLE 5.8 Nursing Diagnoses Related to Vital Signs

Diagnosis	Point of Differentiation	Assessment Characteristics	Nursing Interventions
Hyperthermia	Temperature greater than 37.8°C (100°F)	Skin warm to touch, tachycardia, flushed skin, shivering, malaise, fatigue, and loss of appetite	Provide cooling measures, including fans, cooling blankets, fluid replacement, and cool baths (cold baths would cause shivering).
Hypothermia	Core temperature less than 35°C (95°F)	Tachycardia, peripheral vasoconstriction	Provide warming measures, including warming blankets and warmed IV fluids.*
Imbalanced nutrition, more than body requirements	Body weight greater than 20% over ideal	Eating response to external cues, sedentary activity level	Determine patient's motivation to lose weight. Observe nutritional intake. Assist with formulation of a food diary and plan for weight loss.
Imbalanced nutrition, less than body requirements	Body weight greater than 20% less than ideal	Weakness of muscles, inadequate food intake	Determine healthy body weight for age and height. Assess patient's ability to eat. Consider small frequent meals.
Impaired gas exchange	Changes in capillary refill and respiratory rate, rhythm, and effort	Decreased oxygen saturation, fatigue, confusion, tachypnea, tachycardia, and use of accessory muscles for breathing	Administer oxygen.* Teach coughing and deep breathing exercises. Instruct patient in use of incentive spirometer.
Ineffective breathing pattern	Changes in respiratory rhythm	Irregular respiratory rate and rhythm, periods of apnea	Encourage weight loss and smoking cessation. Apply continuous positive airway pressure (CPAP).*

*Collaborative intervention.

nursing diagnoses commonly seen in relation to vital signs and general survey. These diagnoses are based on vital signs measurements and supporting data. They are used to label the problem and plan care that is individualized to the patient.

Nurses learn the techniques for the general survey and vital signs assessment but use critical thinking to individualize assessments based on the patient. The nurse collects the data for an initial database, monitors trends in the baseline, and identifies patterns, such as a daily temperature spike in the late afternoon. Additionally, the nurse focuses the assessment on the patient situation and current symptoms.

Progress Note: Analyzing Findings

Consider the case of Mr. Sanders, the 55-year-old man admitted to the hospital with a cardiac arrhythmia. The initial collection of subjective and objective data is complete, and Mr. Sanders is stable. The plan of care includes patient teaching and planning for discharge tomorrow. Unfortunately, Mr. Sanders develops a new onset of symptoms. The following nursing note illustrates how the nurse focuses the assessment, analyzes subjective and objective data, and develops nursing interventions when he is having symptoms.

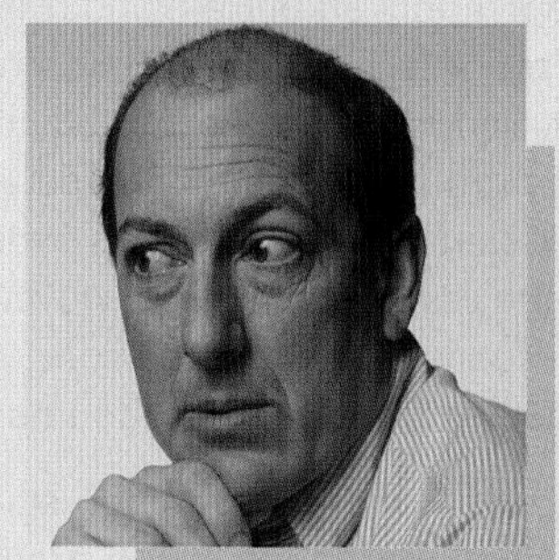

Subjective: "Every once in a while, I can feel my heart racing. It doesn't happen very often, but it feels like my heart's going to jump out of my chest. It's doing it right now." States no chest pain or pressure.

Objective: Skin color even and pink. Sitting upright, holding chest. Tense facial expression, maintains appropriate eye contact. Talking to his wife in complete sentences. Right radial pulse 122 bpm and irregular, strength 2+/4+; R 22 breaths/min and regular, no use of accessory muscles; BP 136/66 mm Hg right arm, sitting; oxygen saturation 96% on room air. Apical pulse 126 bpm and irregular.

Analysis: Subjective feeling of heart racing may be related to new onset of cardiac arrhythmia. Pulse deficit of 4 bpm indicates inadequate perfusion of some apical beats. BP lower than normal value may be related to decreased cardiac output with increased heart rate.

Plan: Contact primary care provider to inform of new onset of fast and irregular apical pulse. Reassess pulse and BP in 5 minutes. Take apical pulse for 1 full minute and assess for a pulse deficit. Stay with patient and his wife and assure them that the best care will be provided. Use touch and therapeutic communication to reduce anxiety. Primary care provider present and ordered STAT 12-lead electrocardiogram that indicated atrial fibrillation with a rate of 126 bpm. Consult with primary care provider on collaborative treatment.

Critical Thinking Challenge

- How is this focused assessment different from the previous health history documentation?
- Critique the objective data that the nurse documented. What patterns connect the general survey and vital signs with the focused findings?
- How are the subjective and objective issues similar or different?

Applying Your Knowledge

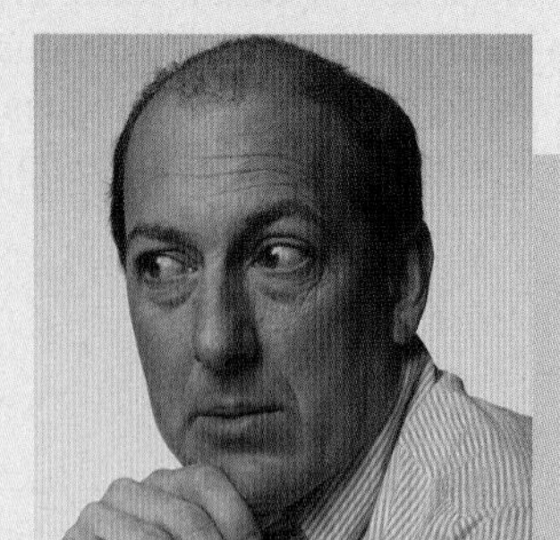

An accurate and complete general survey and vital signs measurement are the foundation for further assessment and interventions. At each encounter with the patient, perform a general survey. Take a complete set of vital signs at the beginning of each shift to establish a baseline. Additionally, assess pulse and BP before administration of medications to evaluate effectiveness and adverse effects, and hold the medications if the pulse or BP is too low. Continually collect assessment data and incorporate it into patient care.

You have been studying Mr. Sanders, who was initially admitted to the ICU following an episode of tachycardia and dizziness. He was started on antiarrhythmic medication, stabilized, and transferred to the acute care floor. He developed a new onset of tachycardia and was reassessed by the nurse. The nurse sought assistance; Mr. Sanders was successfully treated. He will need ongoing assessments related to his problems, including hypertension and arrhythmia.

Using the previous steps of diagnostic reasoning, organizing, and prioritizing, consider all the case study findings woven throughout this chapter. When answering the following questions, begin drawing conclusions and see how the pieces of assessment must work together to create an environment for personalized, appropriate, and accurate care.

- Is Mr. Sanders' condition stable, urgent, or an emergency?
- What immediate health promotion and teaching needs are evident?
- What are the relationships among the patient's pulse, respirations, and blood pressure?
- How will a comprehensive general survey and vital signs measurement differ from a focused assessment for this patient?
- How will the nurse evaluate the effectiveness of the interventions performed for Mr. Sanders?

Key Points

- The general survey begins with the first moments of patient encounter, progresses through the history and physical examination, and continues with each subsequent interaction.
- Extreme anxiety, acute distress, pallor, cyanosis, changes in mental status, and changes in vital signs may indicate the need for assistance and a rapid response.
- The general survey includes overall appearance, hygiene and dress, skin color, body structure and development, behavior, facial expression, level of consciousness, speech, mobility, posture, range of motion, and gait.
- Anthropometric measurements include height and weight.
- Vital signs reflect patient health status, cardiopulmonary function, and overall function of the body.
- The nurse assesses the appropriate route for temperature measurement: oral, axillary, tympanic, temporal artery, or rectal.
- The nurse assesses the pulse for rate, rhythm, amplitude, and elasticity.
- Smoking, positioning, medication, neurological injury, and hemoglobin levels affect the respiratory rate.
- The nurse assesses respirations for rate, rhythm, depth, and use of accessory muscles.
- An oxygen saturation level less than 92% indicates inadequate oxygenation to the tissues.
- Age, gender, ethnicity, weight, circadian cycle, position, exercise, emotions, stress, medications, and smoking affect BP.
- The brachial artery is commonly used to measure BP.
- Width of the BP cuff size should equal 40% of the length of the patient's upper arm, and length of the bladder should equal 80% of the circumference of the arm.
- Postural (orthostatic) vital signs are taken sitting, lying, and standing; orthostatic changes may indicate intravascular volume depletion.
- A vital signs monitor is commonly used in the hospital setting.
- The Doppler transducer is used if the pulse and BP are difficult to auscultate or palpate.
- Vital signs change in older adults because of physiological changes in the body.

Review Questions

1. The nurse assesses the following vital signs in a 78-year-old man: T 36.6°C, temporal; P 72 bpm, regular, 2+; R 18 breaths/minute, regular, no use of accessory muscles; BP 142/92 mm Hg. Which of the findings is abnormal?
   A. Pulse
   B. BP
   C. Respirations
   D. Temperature

2. What are the four characteristics of respirations?

3. The patient's radial pulse is weak and thready. The next action of the nurse is to
   A. transfer the patient to a critical care unit.
   B. notify the primary care provider.
   C. compare findings to previous findings and opposite extremity.
   D. assess vital signs every 15 minutes.

4. Which of the following patients should **not** have a temperature measured orally?
   A. An 84-year-old woman with diarrhea
   B. A 30-year-old patient with an earache
   C. A 45-year-old man with chest pain
   D. A 62-year-old woman who has had oral surgery

5. The nurse notes an irregular radial pulse in a patient. Further evaluation includes assessing
   A. for a pulse deficit.
   B. the carotid pulse.
   C. for diminished peripheral circulation.
   D. the brachial pulse.

6. Which actions will result in an **inaccurate** BP reading? Select all that apply.
   A. Obtaining a BP immediately after the patient has entered the room
   B. Using a BP cuff 80% of the arm circumference
   C. Asking the patient to hold out his or her arm above heart level
   D. Pumping the cuff 10 mm Hg above the palpated systolic BP

7. Adult patients may have variations in pulse rates with
   A. respirations.
   B. food intake.
   C. heat.
   D. exercise.

8. An unconscious 22-year-old man arrives at the hospital after experimenting with hallucinogenic substances. His vital signs are T 37.2°C, po; P 142 bpm; R 20 breaths/min; BP 100/64 mm Hg. The patient is experiencing
   A. tachycardia.
   B. eupnea.
   C. auscultatory gap.
   D. asystole.

9. An auscultatory gap is defined as
   A. a drop in the SBP of 15 mm Hg or more with position change.
   B. a period of silence heard between Korotkoff sounds.
   C. the difference between the apical and radial pulse.
   D. SBP minus the DBP.

10. Which of the following findings during the general survey may indicate a change in mental status? Select all that apply.
    A. Disheveled appearance
    B. Rapid speech
    C. Lethargy
    D. Asymmetrical movements

The Jensen suite offers these additional resources to enhance learning and facilitate understanding of this chapter:

- thePoint online resource, http://www.thepoint.lww.com/Jensen2e
- *Laboratory Manual for Nursing Health Assessment: A Best Practice Approach*
- *Pocket Guide for Nursing Health Assessment: A Best Practice Approach*
- *Lippincott DocuCare,* an electronic health record simulation software, http://www.thepoint.lww.com/docucare
- *Adaptive Learning | Powered by PrepU,* http://www.thepoint.lww.com/prepu

References

American Heart Association. (2013). *All about heart rate (pulse).* Retrieved from http://www.heart.org/HEARTORG/Conditions/More/MyHeartandStrokeNews/All-About-Heart-Rate-Pulse_UCM_438850_Article.jsp.

Aronow, W., Fleg, J., Pepine, C., Artinian, N., Bakris, G., Brown, A., . . . Harrington, R. A. (2011). ACCF/AHA 2011 expert consensus document on hypertension in the elderly: A report of the American College of Cardiology Foundation Task Force on clinical expert consensus documents. *Circulation, 123,* 2434–2506.

Bickley, L. (2013). *Bates' guide to physical examination and history taking.* Philadelphia, PA: Wolters Kluwer Health/Lippincott Williams & Wilkins.

Calkins, H., & Zipes, D. P. (2011). Hypotension and syncope. In R. O. Bonow, D. L. Mann, D. P. Zipes, & P. Libby (Eds.), *Braunwald's heart disease: A textbook of cardiovascular medicine* (9th ed., pp. 885–895). Philadelphia, PA: Elsevier.

Carleton, E., Fry, B., Mulligan, A., Bell, A., & Brossart, C. (2012). EM advances: Temporal artery thermometer use in the prehospital setting. *Canadian Journal of Emergency Medicine, 14*(1), 7–13. Retrieved from http://search.proquest.com/docview/1010360158?accountid=14752

Centers for Disease Control and Prevention (2013). Office of Minority Health. Racial and ethnic disparities. Retrieved from http://www.cdc.gov/minorityhealth/populations/REMP/definitions.html on October 26, 2013.

Centers for Disease Control and Prevention (2013). Adult Obesity Facts. Retrieved from http://www.cdc.gov/obesity/data/adult.html on October 27, 2013.

Ethnomed. (2013). *Clinical topics.* Retrieved October 27, 2013, from http://www.ethnomed.org/

James, P. A., Oparil, S., Carter, B. L., et al. (2014). 2014 Evidence-Based Guideline for the Management of High Blood Pressure in Adults: Report From the Panel Members Appointed to the Eighth Joint National Committee (JNC 8). *JAMA, 311*(5):507–520. doi:10.1001/jama.2013.284427.

Lawson, L., Bridges, E., Ballou, I., Eraker, R., Greco, S., Shively, J., & Sochulak, V. (2007). Accuracy and precision of noninvasive temperature measurement in adult intensive care patients. *American Journal of Critical Care, 16*(5), 485–496.

Leblanc, M. E., Croteau, S., Ferland, A., Bussières, J., Cloutier, L., Hould, F. S., . . . Poirier, P. (2013). Blood pressure assessment in severe obesity: Validation of a forearm approach. *Obesity (Silver Spring), 21,* E533–E541. doi: 10.1002/oby.20458.

National Heart, Lung, and Blood Institute. (2009). *Update: Clinical guidelines on the identification, evaluation, and treatment of overweight and obesity in adults.* Retrieved from http://www.nhlbi.nih.gov/guidelines/obesity/obesity2/index.htm.

Ogden, C. L., Yanovski, S. Z., Carroll, M. D., Flegal, K. M. (2007). The epidemiology of obesity. *Gastroenterology, 132*(6), 2087–2102.
Pickering, T., Hall, J., Appel, L., Falkner, B., Graves, J., Hill, M., . . . Rocella, E. (2005). Recommendations for blood pressure measurement in humans and experimental animals: Part 1: Blood pressure measurement in humans: A statement for professionals from the Subcommittee of Professional and Public Education of the American Heart Association Council on high blood pressure research. *Hypertension, 45*, 142–161.
Sanderson, B., Lim, L., Lei, K., Smith, J., Camporota, L., & Beale, R. (2010). A comparison of core and tympanic temperature measurement in the critically ill. *Critical Care, 14*(Suppl. 1), P329.
Stelfox, H. T., Straus, S. E., Ghali, W. A., Conly, J., Laupland, K., and Lewin, A. (2010). Temporal artery versus bladder thermometry during adult medical-surgical intensive care monitoring: An observational study. *BMC Anesthesiology, 10*(1), 13. doi:http://dx.doi.org/10.1186/1471-2253-10-13
Taylor, C., Lillis, C., LeMone, P., & Lynn, P. (2011). *Fundamentals of nursing: The art and science of nursing care* (7th ed.). Philadelphia, PA: Wolters Kluwer Health/Lippincott Williams & Wilkins.
Tomlinson, B. U. (2010). Accurately measuring blood pressure: Factors that contribute to false measurements. *Medsurg Nursing: Official Journal of the Academy of Medical-Surgical Nurses, 19*(2), 90–94.
Van Velthoven, M., Thien, T., Holewijn,. S, van der Wilt, G. J., & Deinum, J. (2010). The effect of crossing legs on blood pressure. *Journal of Hypertension, 25*(7), 1591–1592.
Zheng, D., Giovannini, R., & Murray, A. (2012). Effect of respiration, talking and small body movements on blood pressure measurement. *Journal of Human Hypertension, 26*, 458–462. doi:10.1038/jhh.2011.53

Tables of Abnormal Findings

TABLE 5.9 Abnormal Findings: Anthropometric Measurements

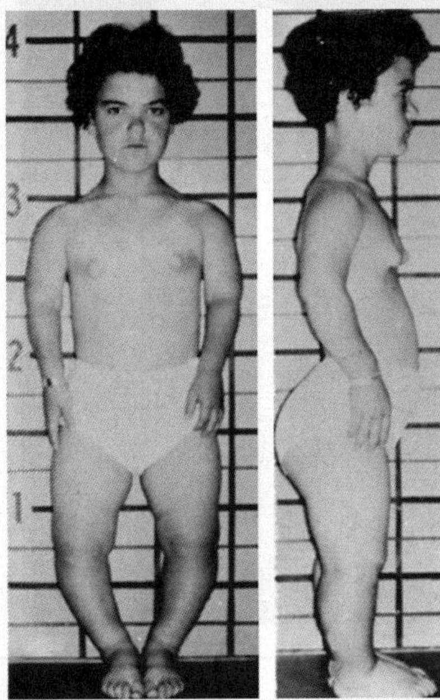

Achondroplastic Dwarfism. Characteristics of this genetic disorder include short stature, short limbs, and a relatively large head. Also note the thoracic kyphosis and lumbar lordosis.

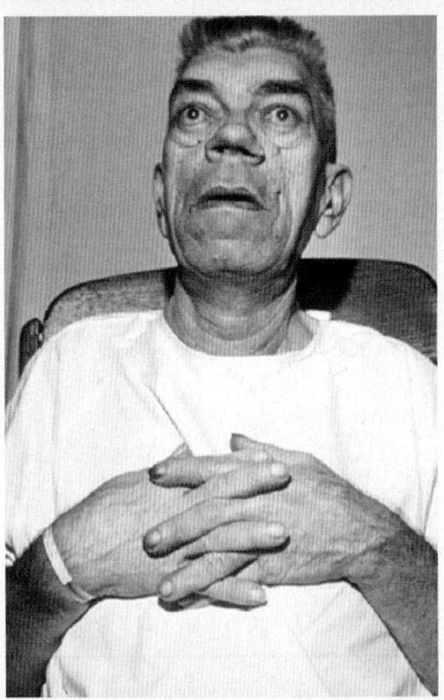

Acromegaly. This condition results from excessive growth hormone secretion during adulthood after normal body growth has been completed. Overgrowth of bone causes changes in the size of the head, face, hands, feet, and internal organs; height is not affected.

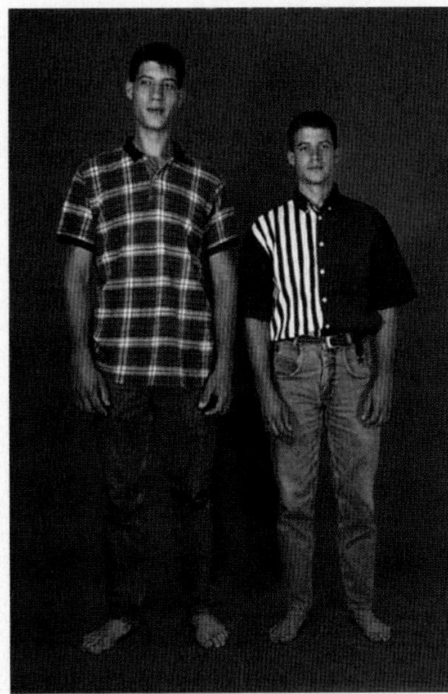

Gigantism. Excessive growth hormone secretion in childhood causes increased height and weight with delayed sexual development. Note the differences in these same-age individuals, one of whom has gigantism and the other whose anthropometric measurements are within expected limits.

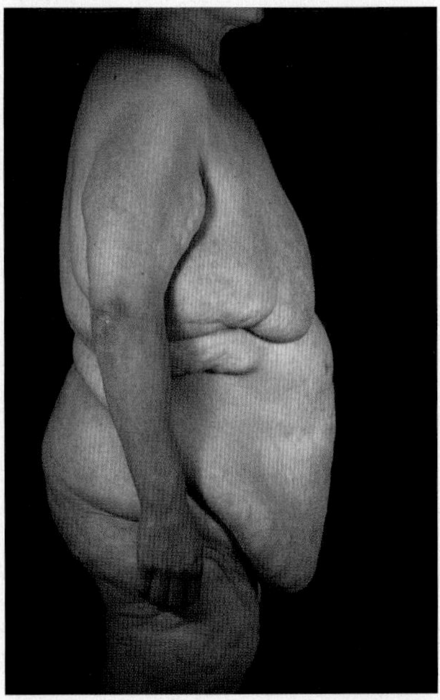

Obesity. Excessive body fat results when calories continually exceed body requirements. It can result from overeating, genetics, endocrine or hormonal disorders, lifestyle issues, or a combination of factors.

(table continues on page 112)

TABLE 5.9 Abnormal Findings: Anthropometric Measurements *(continued)*

Anorexia Nervosa. Severe restriction of caloric intake and disturbance in body image contribute to this psychiatric disorder. Affected patients are clearly emaciated and display other physical findings, such as brittle hair and nails, absent menstruation, delayed puberty, sunken eyes, dry skin, and other manifestations.

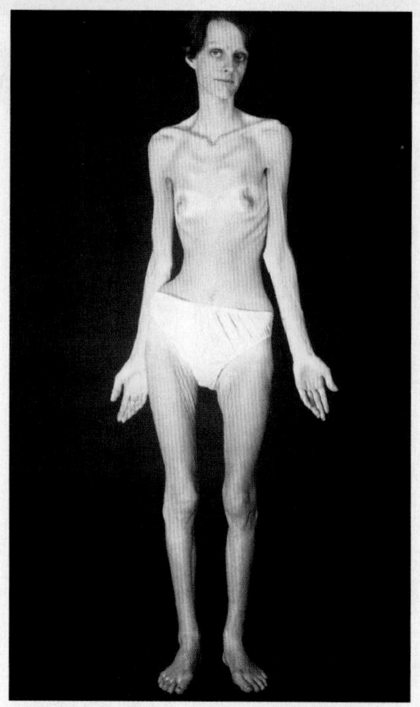

6

Pain Assessment

Learning Objectives

1 Discuss the basic theories of pain.

2 Identify the elements of pain transmission.

3 Determine the different types of pain.

4 Differentiate musculoskeletal pain from neuropathic pain.

5 Examine the one-dimensional, multidimensional, and behavioral pain tools for newborns, children, adults, and older adults.

6 Identify important topics for health promotion and risk reduction related to pain.

7 Collect subjective data related to pain.

8 Collect objective data related to pain using physical examination techniques.

9 Identify issues in assessing pain in special populations such as patients with opioid tolerance or difficulty talking about their pain.

10 Document and communicate data from the pain assessment using appropriate terminology and principles of recording.

11 Consider age, gender, condition, and culture of the patient to individualize the assessment of pain.

Mrs. Bond, 42 years old, is visiting the clinic for follow-up care for chronic widespread pain on both sides of her body related to fibromyalgia. She was diagnosed 5 months ago and still has not been able to control her pain at a desirable level. Her temperature is 37°C (98.6°F) orally, pulse 88 beats/min, respirations 16 breaths/min, and blood pressure 112/68 mmHg. Current medications include a selective serotonin reuptake inhibitor for depression, a benzodiazepine for muscle spasm, and an analgesic for pain. She had a comprehensive assessment documented 5 months ago and has been seen twice since for pain control.

You will gain more information about Mrs. Bond as you progress through this chapter. As you study the content and features, consider Mrs. Bond's case and its relationship to what you are learning. Begin thinking about the following points:

- How would you describe the mechanisms of pain?
- How would you differentiate between neuropathic and nociceptive pain?
- How would you assess pain if Mrs. Bond were a mentally challenged young adult? A cognitively impaired older adult?
- What factors might contribute to observations made during the pain assessment?
- What data would you use to plan patient education for the reduction of pain?
- How would you assess the effectiveness of health promotion strategies for the patient who experiences chronic pain?

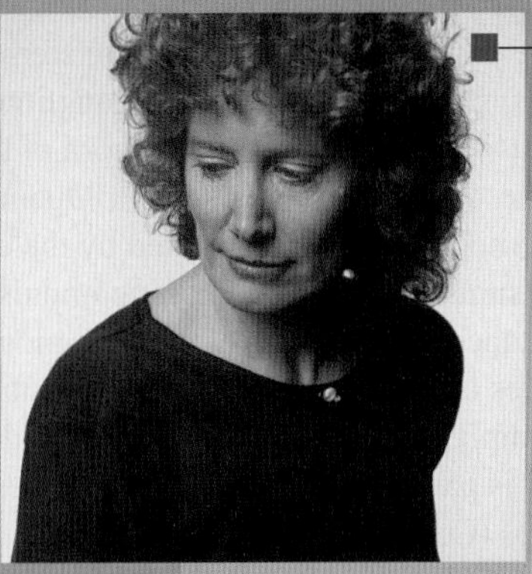

This chapter covers the assessment of pain using reliable and valid pain assessment scales. It presents the basic elements of pain assessment, as well as background information on pain, pain transmission, and assessing pain in difficult-to-assess populations.

Pain is one of the most common reasons patients seek help from health care professionals. Pain does not respect gender, age, or ethnicity. It can occur at any time, to anyone. Pain can profoundly affect quality of life, interactions with family and friends, sense of well-being and self-esteem, and financial resources. For many patients, pain is the result of injury or surgery, but for others pain has no identifiable cause.

Neuroanatomy of Pain

Peripheral Nervous System

Several different types of nerve fibers that transmit pain are located in the peripheral nervous system. The two main types of nerve fibers are as follows:

1. A-delta, large nerve fibers covered with myelin; they conduct pain impulses rapidly. Patients often describe the type of pain impulse that A-delta fibers conduct as sharp or stabbing (American Society for Pain Management Nursing, 2010).
2. C fibers, smaller unmyelinated nerve fibers; they conduct pain impulses more diffusely and slowly. Patients often describe the pain conducted by C fibers as achy and ongoing, even after the pain stimulus is removed (American Society for Pain Management Nursing, 2010).

C fibers release a pain-facilitating substance from nerve endings called substance P. The function of substance P is to quicken the transmission of the pain stimulus up the pain pathway. Bradykinin, another pain-facilitating substance, is released at the site of injury. It is a cellular chemical released from the damaged tissue. The function of bradykinin is to cause continued irritation at the injury site (American Society of Pain Management Nursing, 2010; D'Arcy, 2014).

These specialized peripheral A and C nerve fibers are referred to as **nociceptors**. They carry the pain signal to the central nervous system.

Central Nervous System

After the pain stimulus has been transferred into the central nervous system via the dorsal root ganglion, it synapses in the gelatinous substance in the dorsal horn of the spinal cord and enters the central nervous system. Opening or closing the "gate" to nociception is controlled by the combined effect of both the sum of the pain-facilitating impulse and the facilitating substances and the sum of the pain-blocking impulses and substances as they are received in the substantia gelatinosa. More simply, if facilitator impulses predominate, the pain stimulus is passed on; if blocking impulses predominate, the pain stops (Cervero, 2005).

If the pain is allowed to continue, the pain stimulus passes through the spinal cord into the lateral spinothalamic tracts, which lead directly to the thalamus, and then into the limbic system. In the limbic system, the emotions that control pain are produced; the stimulus is then passed to the cerebral cortex where the sensation is recognized as pain (Fig. 6.1). The whole process takes milliseconds (D'Arcy, 2014).

Two substances are very important to pain transmission at this level. Some nerves use substance P to fire at synaptic junctions. Glutamate is the neurotransmitter responsible for

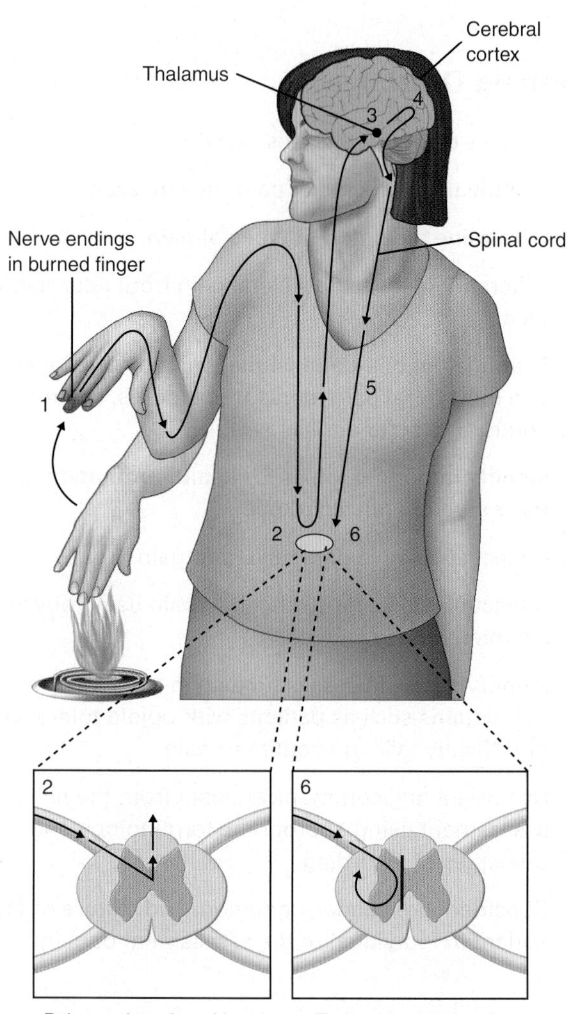

Figure 6.1 Pain transmission. (1) Pain begins as a message received by nerve endings, such as found in a burnt finger. (2) The release of substance P, bradykinin, and prostaglandins sensitizes the nerve endings, which helps to transmit the pain from the site of injury toward the brain. (3) The pain signal then travels as an electrochemical impulse along the length of the nerve to the dorsal horn on the spinal cord, a region that receives signals from all over the body. (4) The spinal cord then sends the message to the thalamus, and then to the cortex. (5) Pain relief starts with signals from the brain that descend by way of the spinal cord, where (6) chemicals such as endorphin S are released in the dorsal horn to diminish the pain message.

the communication of the peripheral nervous system with the central nervous system. An additional function of glutamate is thought to be activation of *N*-methyl D-aspartate (NMDA) receptors, which can help intensify and prolong persistent pain.

Clinical Significance

To treat some chronic pain conditions, health care providers may prescribe medications that increase serotonin levels, such as tricyclic antidepressants and selective serotonin reuptake inhibitors, to modulate incoming pain stimuli.

Descending nerve fibers from the locus ceruleus and periaqueductal gray matter transmit the response to the efferent nerve pathways. Substances that can modulate the pain response at this level include opiates, endorphins, and enkephalins. These substances can bind to the opiate receptors in the dorsal horn of the spine and block pain transmission. The calcitonin gene–related peptide (CGRP), located at the C-fiber nerve endings, produces local cutaneous vasodilation, plasma extravasation, and skin sensitization in collaboration with substance P production. Cytokines such as interleukins and tumor necrosis factor can sensitize C-fiber terminals and participate in the inflammatory and infection process involving mast cells (American Society of Pain Management Nursing, 2010; D'Arcy, 2014).

Clinical Significance

Opiates, antidepressants, and calcium channel blockers are pharmacological alternatives in the treatment of chronic pain.

Gate Control Theory

Currently, the theory of pain with the widest acceptance is the **gate control theory** (Melzack and Wall, 1975). This posits that the body responds to a painful stimulus by either opening a neural gate to allow pain to be produced or creating a blocking effect at the synaptic junction to stop the pain (Fig. 6.2). The steps for pain transmission in the gate control theory are as follows:

1. Continued painful stimulus on a peripheral neuron causes the "gate" to open through depolarization of the nerve fiber. This is accomplished by ion influx and outflow.
2. The pain stimulus then passes from the peripheral nervous system at a synaptic junction to the central nervous system up the afferent nerve pathways.
3. The pain stimulus passes up through and across the dorsal horn of the spine to the structures of the limbic system and the cerebral cortex.
4. In the cerebral cortex the stimulus is identified as pain and a response is created. The response, once generated, passes down the efferent pathways where reaction to the pain is created (D'Arcy, 2014).

Although this theory seems simple, proponents continue to expand and refine it. Recent data suggest that the degree of the stimulus can produce varied responses (Cervero, 2005).

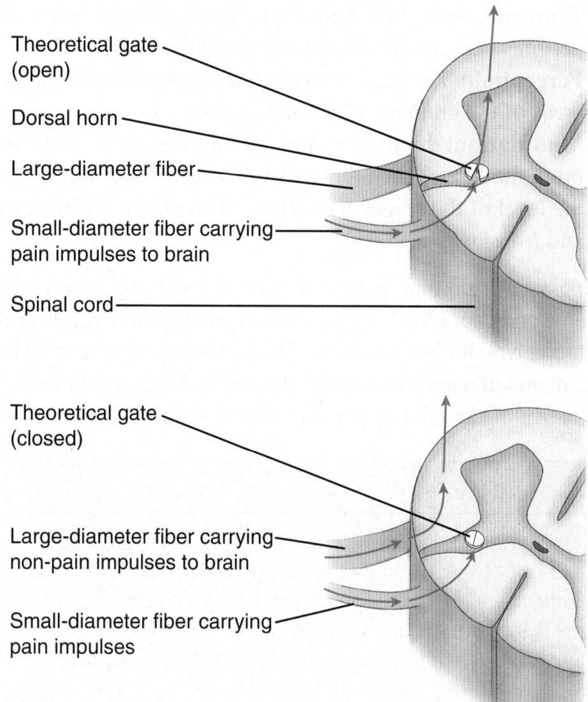

Figure 6.2 The gate control theory.

Current research focuses on those elements that can affect pain inhibition and stop the pain stimulus (Cervero, 2005). Additionally, pain-facilitating and pain-inhibiting substances that can either help or hinder pain processing have been discovered (Box 6.1).

Nociception

The most common clinical interpretation of pain transmission is a mechanism called nociception, which means the perception of pain by sensory receptors located throughout the body and called **nociceptors**. These nociceptors can produce pain resulting from heat, pressure, or noxious chemicals, such as those produced in the inflammatory process (D'Arcy, 2014). There are four steps in nociception:

1. **Transduction:** Noxious stimuli create enough of an energy potential to cause a nerve impulse perceived by nociceptors (i.e., free nerve endings).

BOX 6.1 Substances with a Role in Pain

Pain-facilitating substances
- Substance P
- Bradykinin
- Glutamate

Pain-blocking substances
- Serotonin
- Opioids (both natural and synthetic)
- Gamma-aminobutyric acid: gabapentin (Neurontin) and pregabalin (Lyrica)

2. **Transmission:** The neuronal signal moves from the periphery to the spinal cord and up to the brain.
3. **Perception:** The impulses being transmitted to the higher areas of the brain are identified as pain.
4. **Modulation:** Inhibitory and facilitating input from the brain modulates or influences the sensory transmission at the level of the spinal cord (Berry, Covington, Dahl, Katz, and Miaskowski, 2008).

Persistent or chronic pain can exist without any identifiable source and cause the body to adapt or change how it transmits or perceives the pain signal. These changes in transmission (**neuronal plasticity**) can cause the pain to become more severe by activating additional structures for facilitating transmission.

> **Clinical Significance**
>
> The transmission of a pain stimulus uses two separate but continuous systems: the peripheral nervous system and the central nervous system. Continued input from the peripheral nervous system can create a centrally mediated pain syndrome, in which pain occurs without a pain stimulus.

Types of Pain

Definitions of pain emphasize that it is an unpleasant experience (Box 6.2).Because pain is so damaging, it is important to understand just how this experience is created. Acute pain is meant to warn the body that some type of insult or injury has occurred. Chronic pain lasts beyond the normal healing period and has no useful role.

Acute Pain

Acute pain results from tissue damage, whether through injury or surgery. Acute pain is quite prevalent in hospital settings and primary care clinics. After the 73 million surgeries performed each year, 75% of postoperative patients report pain: 86% of them report pain ranging from extremely severe to moderate (Apfelbaum, Chen, Mehtam, and Tong, 2003).

> **BOX 6.2 Definitions of Pain**
>
> - **Pain:** "An unpleasant sensory and emotional experience associated with actual or potential tissue damage, or described in terms of such damage" (American Pain Society [APS], 2008). Pain is "whatever the experiencing person says it is, existing whenever he says it does" (McCaffery and Pasero, 1999).
> - **Acute pain:** Pain of a short duration that has an identifiable cause such as trauma, surgery, or injury (APS, 2008; American Society for Pain Management Nursing [ASPMN], 2002). Examples of acute pain are surgical pain and orthopedic injuries.
> - **Chronic pain:** Pain that lasts beyond the normal healing period of 3–6 months (American Society for Pain Management Nursing, 2002). There may be no identifiable cause. Examples of chronic pain are low back pain and sickle cell anemia pain.
> - **Neuropathic pain:** Pain that results from damage to nerves in the peripheral or central nervous system (Staats, et al., 2004). Examples of neuropathic pain include diabetic peripheral neuropathy, post herpetic neuralgia, and postmastectomy pain.

> **Clinical Significance**
>
> Untreated or undertreated acute pain may lead to chronic pain syndromes, such as **complex regional pain syndrome (CRPS)**, which are difficult to treat (D'Arcy, 2014).

Pain nociception has various locations. **Visceral pain** originates from abdominal organs; patients often describe this pain as crampy or gnawing. **Somatic pain** originates from skin, muscles, bones, and joints; patients usually describe somatic pain as sharp (D'Arcy, 2014). **Cutaneous pain** derives from the dermis, epidermis, and subcutaneous tissues. It is often burning or sharp, such as with a partial-thickness burn. **Referred pain** originates from a specific site, but the person experiencing it feels the pain at another site along the innervating spinal nerve (Fig. 6.3). An example is cardiac pain that a person experiences as indigestion, neck pain, or arm pain. Phantom pain is pain in an extremity or body part that is no longer there (e.g., a patient who experiences pain in a leg with an amputation).

Chronic Pain

Chronic pain is also prevalent in U.S. adults, with approximately 40% of adults experiencing it daily (Berry, Covington, Dahl, Katz, and Miaskowski, 2008; Cipher, Clifford, and Roper, 2006). Estimates of the costs of chronic pain, combining lost income, medical expenses, and worker nonproductivity, are $560 to 650 billion in U.S. dollars (Institute of Medicine, 2011). Because of the associated costs and loss of productivity, a stigma is associated with chronic pain and its treatment in the health care setting. It is also referred to as persistent pain in the health care setting because no cause or treatment can be determined.

Neuropathic Pain

After pain becomes a more constant stimulus, the nervous system can modify its function—an ability called **neuronal plasticity** (Rowbotham, 2006). This nervous system modification can lead to a phenomenon called **peripheral sensitization**, by which peripheral nociceptors are sensitized to **neuropathic** pain stimuli. As an example, inflammation can cause peripheral sensitization related to the continued release of inflammatory mediators (D'Arcy, 2014). This irritating process causes cytokines and growth factors to be recruited to the site of injury, prolonging the inflammatory response. Over time, this sensitization produces a condition in which nonpainful touch or pressure becomes painful.

Neuronal windup is produced when repeated assaults on the afferent neurons create enhanced response and increased activity in the central nervous system. Windup can cause

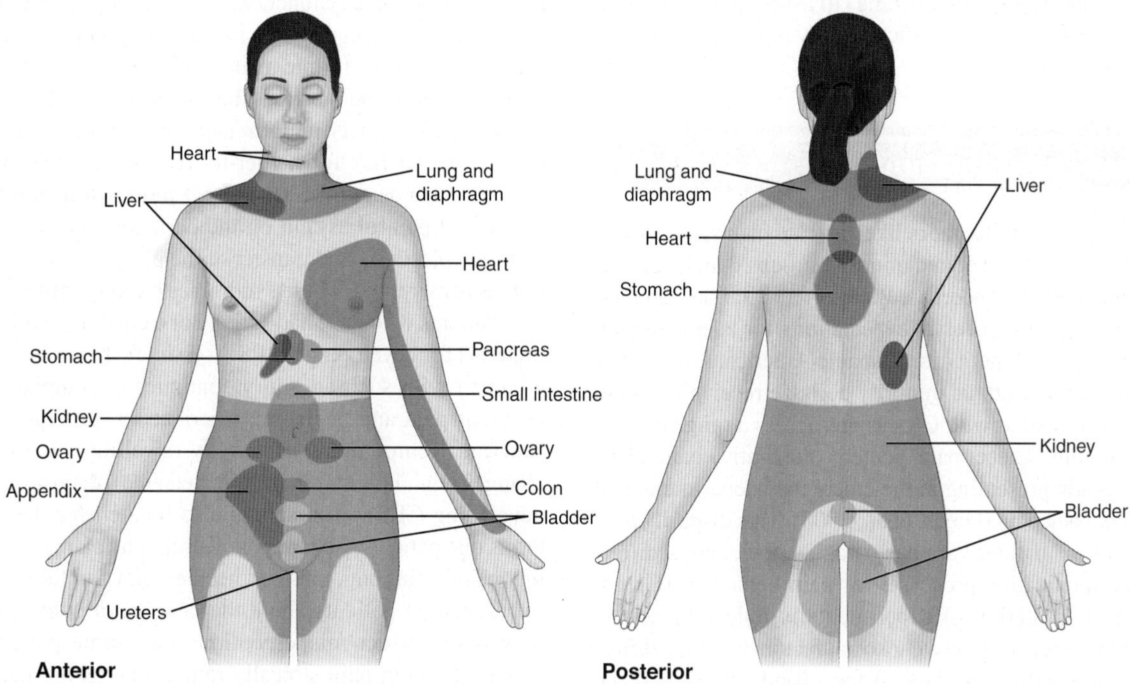

Figure 6.3 Common sites of referred pain.

tissues in the affected area to become extremely sensitive to pressure in areas not usually identified as painful. Examples of windup include rheumatoid arthritis and osteoarthritis (Rowbotham, 2006).

The following list includes some conditions resulting from physiologic responses to painful stimuli:

- **Neuronal plasticity:** Ability of the nervous system to change or alter its function
- **Windup:** Enhanced response to pain stimulus produced by prolonged pain production
- **Peripheral sensitization:** Result of inflammatory process that creates hypersensitivity to touch or pressure
- **Central sensitization:** Excitatory process involving spinal nerves produced by continued pain stimuli that can persist even after peripheral stimulation is no longer present (D'Arcy, 2007b)

Lifespan Considerations: Older Adults

Pain is prevalent in older adults, with 80% of all patients in long-term care facilities and 25% to 50% of community-dwelling elders reporting chronic daily pain (American Geriatric Society [AGS], 2002). Pain is not a normal consequence of aging. Chronic disease, such as osteoarthritis, peripheral vascular disease, or cancer, may affect accurate pain assessment. Patients who undergo surgical or diagnostic procedures may experience acute pain. They may be unable to distinguish whether their pain is surgically induced or chronic from pre-existing painful conditions. Because a larger segment of the U.S. population is aging, understanding how to assess pain in older patients is a critical skill for nurses.

Little is known about the effect of increased age on pain perception. No evidence suggests that pain sensation is diminished in older adults, which is a common misperception. Transmission along the A-delta and C fibers may become altered with aging, but it is not clear how this change affects the pain experience. Studies of sensitivity and pain tolerance have indicated that changes in pain perception are probably not clinically significant (American Geriatric Society, 2002; Reyes-Gibby, Aday, Todd, et al., 2007).

Health care provider issues also may affect the treatment of pain in older populations. Because older people are likely to experience more adverse effects from analgesia, especially from opiates, health care providers may undertreat pain in older adults.

When assessing the older patient for pain, determine whether the patient has any auditory impairment. If so, position your face in the patient's view, speak in a slow, normal tone of voice, reduce extraneous noises, and provide written instructions. If a patient has visual impairment, use simple lettering, at least 14-point type, adequate line spacing, and nonglare paper. The patient should wear eyeglasses or a functioning hearing aid if these devices are in normal use. Because older adults may process information more slowly than younger patients, allow adequate time for the patient to respond to questions (Herr, Coyne, Key, et al., 2006a).

Cognitive impairment, dementia, and delirium are more common in older adults (Linton and Lach, 2007). Accurately assessing pain is more challenging when patients have these conditions. Nevertheless, no evidence shows that patients with cognitive impairment experience less pain. Nurses should not consider pain reports from these patients any less valid than those from other patients. Health care providers may use behavioral observations of pain in patients (e.g., restlessness, guarding, pacing) to assess pain, but these observations are not pain specific and may represent responses to other conditions.

Cultural Considerations

Health care providers are more likely to rate pain scores lower in patients of racial and ethnic minority groups than in Caucasian patients (Green, Anderson, Baker, et al., 2003). There are also intergroup differences in expectations for adequate pain treatment. African Americans, Hispanic Americans, and other patients of racial or ethnic minority heritage receive less pain medication compared with Caucasians across a range of conditions, including cancer pain, acute postoperative pain, chest pain, acute pain presenting in the emergency department, and chronic low back pain (Green, et al., 2003). This disparity may be the result of patient variables such as nociceptive differences, communication processes, or pain behaviors (Green, et al., 2003). In studies of experimentally induced pain, no direct evidence relates biopsychosocial factors to ethnic differences in pain (Reyes-Gibby, Aday, Todd, et al., 2007). Ethnicity-related differences may exist, however, in willingness to communicate about pain to avoid being stereotyped.

Gender differences in pain exist. Conditions such as fibromyalgia, irritable bowel syndrome, migraines, and temporomandibular joint pain are more prevalent in women than in men (D'Arcy, 2014). Fibromyalgia-related pain is now classed as neuropathic pain with central amplification and dysregulation of the descending neural pain pathways (Smith and Barkin, 2010; Smith, Harris, Clauw, 2011). All patients show an increased physiological response to pain including heart rate and blood pressure increase. Conditions such as menstrual migraine have demonstrated the estrogenic effect of pain (Brandes, 2006). Although considerable attention has been devoted to biological variables such as hormonal influences and genetics, psychological and social factors might also account for gender differences in reporting pain. It is unknown whether fundamental, gender-specific differences in basic pain mechanisms exist. A better understanding of the physiological, social, and psychological issues that influence pain is needed.

As a nurse, you need to assess sociocultural variables such as ethnicity, acculturation, and gender that influence pain behavior and expression. You also need to identify social and contextual variables that may lead to pain disparities among racial and ethnic minorities. For example, you can work closely with the patient and his or her family to identify pain and functional goals that consider the patient's values, resources, and expectations (Green, et al., 2003).

Risk Reduction and Health Promotion

Pain can cause both physical and emotional harm. As a nurse caring for patients experiencing pain, it is crucial that you ensure adequate pain treatment. Acute pain that is not adequately treated can impair pulmonary function, decrease the immune response, and prolong the length of the patient's stay in the hospital. For the patient with chronic pain, adequate pain management decreases stress and increases the patient's ability to function.

If acute pain is undertreated or completely untreated, patients are at risk for harder-to-treat neuropathic pain syndromes, such as **complex regional pain syndrome** (CRPS). Continued painful assault on the peripheral nerves results in neuronal plasticity and transfer of the pain stimulus to the central nervous system. These syndromes are very difficult to treat.

Patients who have had surgery or a crush-type injury are at high risk for developing CRPS. You should be aware that when a patient with such an injury continues to complain of high levels of pain and begins to experience a subsequent loss of function, temperature sensitivity, swelling, or other skin changes (e.g., hair loss in the affected area), the patient may be developing CRPS. You should also be alert for the common terms that patients use to report neuropathic pain, such as burning, painful tingling, pins and needles, and painful numbness.

Teaching patients about the benefits of controlling pain may help correct misperceptions that some patients have about tolerating pain stoically rather than taking medication to relieve it. Pain has many negative consequences; it is important to help patients understand that reporting pain and treating pain are ways of maintaining a higher level of health and avoiding chronic pain syndromes. If the patient continues to refuse pain medication, you may consider asking the patient these questions:

- Do you have problems with taking pain medication?
- Can you afford the prescribed medication?
- Are unwanted adverse effects, such as constipation, nausea, or dizziness, causing you to refuse pain medications?

In some cases, patients can be given antiemetics, laxatives, or dosage adjustments that make it easier for them to tolerate pain medications. Above all, if a patient continues to refuse to take pain medication, it is extremely important to understand the root cause of this refusal so that appropriate treatment can take place.

Pain Is What the Patient Says It Is

Pain is what the patient says it is, and it exists whenever the patient says it does (McCaffery and Pasero, 1999). Pain assessment is always subjective (although there can be physiologic responses which are measurable). No right or wrong answer exists in pain assessment. For verbal patients, self-report is the standard criterion for assessing pain. As a nurse, you also assess additional pain behaviors, such as grimacing, rocking, or guarding. Increased heart rate and blood pressure are indicators of the physiological response to pain.

Subjective Data

In a basic pain assessment, ask the patient to rate pain intensity using a simple one-dimensional scale. An example is the numeric pain intensity (NPI) scale with 10 numbers ranked from 0 (no pain) to 10 (worst possible pain). The higher the number, the more severe the pain.

In addition to pain intensity, other basic elements of a pain assessment are discussed in the accompanying list of questions to assess symptoms.

After you have collected all data, the most important factor is to accept the patient's pain rating. It is incumbent upon professional nurses to respect the reports of pain as patients present them, and then act to help relieve the pain. Even if you question a patient's pain rating, you are obligated to accept the report of pain.

The use of in-depth questions to collect all the salient data from the pain assessment will be the biggest help in determining what types of interventions will be most beneficial for providing adequate pain relief to the patient. Using a reliable and valid pain assessment tool can help provide objective criteria for pain assessment. Some prefer to use mnemonics to remember the elements of pain assessment. One of these is **OPQRST**:

O: Onset
P: Provocative or palliative
Q: Quality
R: Region and radiation
S: Severity
T: Timing

Another mnemonic is **OLDCARTS**:

O: Onset
L: Location
D: Duration
C: Character
A: Alleviating/aggravating
R: Radiation
T: Timing
S: Severity

Whatever method you choose, be consistent and thorough with your assessments to better document findings and evaluation of the effectiveness of your interventions. This book uses a blend of assessments— location, duration, intensity, quality, aggravating and alleviating factors, pain goal, and functional goals—with a focus on how the pain affects the patient's life.

Signs/Symptoms	Rationale/Abnormal Findings
Location Where is your pain? (Ask the patient to point to the painful area. If more than one area is painful, have the patient rate each one separately, and note which area is the most painful.)	Note any pain that radiates from the affected area—for example, down the leg with a complaint of low back pain—because such radiation may affect treatment choices.
Duration How long have you had the pain? When did it start? When did it go away?	This question helps identify onset and duration. Pain for more than 6 months is chronic or persistent.
Intensity How much pain do you have on a 0 to 10 scale, with 0 being no pain and 10 being the worst possible that you can imagine? • Is the pain worse or better at different times of the day? • Does pain medication decrease the intensity?	If the patient cannot use a numerical rating scale, ask the patient if the pain is mild, moderate, or severe. The numbering scale assists in quantifying the pain that the patient is experiencing.
Quality/Description What does your pain feel like? • Describe the quality of the pain. (Allow the patient to describe the pain in his or her own words.) • Is it crampy, gnawing, burning, shooting, sharp, or dull? • Does it radiate or go anywhere?	Patient descriptors such as burning, painful numbness, or tingling may alert you to a neuropathic source for the pain.
Alleviating/Aggravating Factors • What makes the pain better? What makes it worse? • What methods have you used to manage the pain? • Does the application of heat have any effect? • Does a cold pack help relieve any of the pain? • Does activity increase the pain? • Does sitting down make the pain better?	Most patients will try to treat their own pain before they seek health care (DeLuca, 2008).

(table continues on page 120)

Signs/Symptoms	Rationale/Abnormal Findings
Pain Management Goal What would be an acceptable level of pain for you? (Setting a pain goal is helpful for all patients, but especially for those with chronic pain.)	Most patients do not expect to be pain free and are willing to tolerate some discomfort. Ask patients what pain level they think is acceptable, and then tailor interventions to achieve the patient's expectations.
Functional Goal What would you like to be able to do that you can't do because of the pain? (This question is most often used for patients with chronic persistent pain. Pain is dynamic and increases with activity [Falla, Farina, Dahl, and Graven-Nielsen, 2007].) • How does the pain interfere with your activities of daily living? • How far can you walk? • Can you care for yourself at home or do you require help? • What does the pain mean to you?	Setting a pain functionality goal with the patient allows you to measure the efficacy of pain interventions and adjust the treatment accordingly. Providing maximum pain relief and functionality is the goal of any pain-relief treatment for a patient with chronic pain (American Society of Pain Management Nursing, 2010; D'Arcy, 2007a; Joint Commission on Accreditation of Healthcare Organizations [JCAHO], 2001). Some patients believe that pain represents punishment or a worsening of disease.

Therapeutic Dialogue: Collecting Subjective Data

The nurse's role in subjective data collection is to gather complete information about the symptoms and to help determine the effectiveness of treatments. Remember Mrs. Bond, who was introduced at the beginning of this chapter. She is 42 years old and was diagnosed with fibromyalgia 5 months ago. Her pain control is less than desired; because this problem is her priority, the nurse will perform a complete assessment.

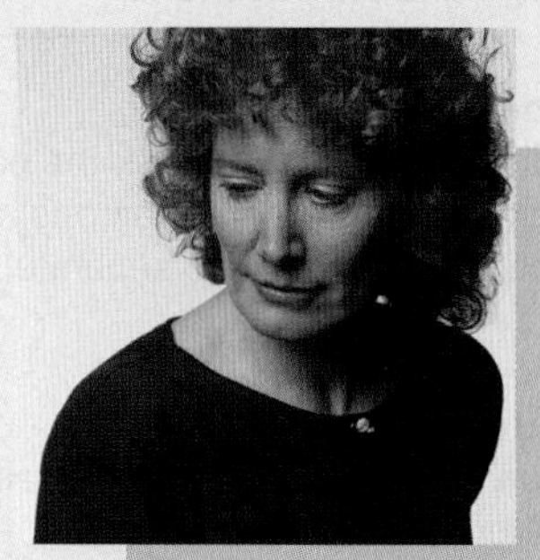

Nurse: Hi, Mrs. Bond. I see that you were here last month for continued pain. How is that for you today?

Mrs. Bond: It really seems like it's worse instead of better.

Nurse: That must be very frustrating for you. Let's talk a little bit about it. Can you show me where your pain is?

Mrs. Bond: (rubs lower back with her palm) It's here and then it goes down into my bottom and my legs.

Nurse: On a 0–10 scale with 10 being the worst and 0 no pain, how would you rate it?

Mrs. Bond: Probably about a 5.

Nurse: What level of pain would be acceptable to you?

Mrs. Bond: I would be happy with a 3.

Nurse: How would you describe it?

Mrs. Bond: It's an aching pain. In the morning, I'm so stiff that I can hardly get out of bed.

Nurse: Are there other things that you notice with it?

(case study continues on page 121)

Mrs. Bond: I have trouble sleeping and I just feel tired all of the time.

Nurse: What do you notice makes it worse?

Mrs. Bond: When I'm tired or stressed, it's worse.

Nurse: What makes it better?

Mrs. Bond: If I can get a good night's sleep, it seems better the next day.

Nurse: It seems that being tired is a big part of your pain. How has it influenced your usual activities?

Mrs. Bond: I used to love doing yard work, and I haven't been outside to work for 3 months. I miss that—not the housework, though (laughs)!

Critical Thinking Challenge

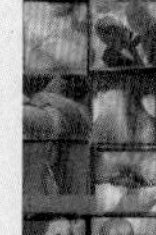

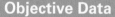

- What is the advantage of having Mrs. Bond point to where it hurts first?
- Why is it important to evaluate each item separately rather than combine them, as the less effective nurse did with the alleviating and aggravating factors?
- How does the more effective nurse use listening techniques to help Mrs. Bond to relax?

Objective Data

In addition to the subjective experience of pain, objective physiological effects exist (Table 6.1). Acute pain may activate a fight-or-flight stress response in patients. In such an event, blood pressure, pulse, and respirations may increase; the patient will feel the urge to move away from the painful stimulus. These commonly observed responses may not happen with chronic pain, however, because patients have adapted to its ongoing continued stress.

The stress response causes the release of epinephrine, norepinephrine, and cortisol. These hormones have neuroendocrine and metabolic functions. They use stored energy to facilitate the healing of injured tissues. Some effects of these hormones include increases in oxygen consumption, levels of blood glucose and lactate, metabolism, and ketones.

Muscle tension may increase with pain; the patient may respond by guarding, or protecting, the affected area. Although increased muscle tension helps to protect patients against further pain, chronic tension can contribute to impaired muscle metabolism, muscle atrophy, and delayed return of function.

Inadequately treated pain may contribute to nausea, diaphoresis, and vomiting. Providing pain medication will help alleviate these unwanted effects.

In addition to physiological responses, pain manifests with observable behavioral responses (see Table 6.1). Verbal reports are the most dependable. In patients who cannot verbalize, vocal responses may include moaning or crying. Six pain behaviors indicate pain in patients who cannot verbalize: (1) vocalizations, (2) facial grimacing, (3) bracing, (4) rubbing painful areas, (5) restlessness, and (6) vocal complaints (Feldt, 2000; Feldt, Ryden, and Miles, 1998). Many pain assessment tools incorporate the evaluation of these pain behaviors and facilitate accurate detection of pain in various patient populations.

Pain Assessment Tools

Pain assessment tools can be one-dimensional or multidimensional. One-dimensional tools rate only pain intensity, whereas multidimensional tools also include behavioral, affective, and functional domains. Some of the first multidimensional pain assessment tools were developed for assessing experimentally induced pain, chronic pain, and oncology pain they provide a more comprehensive pain assessment.

One-Dimensional Pain Scales

One-dimensional pain assessment tools measure one element of the pain experience—intensity. These tools seem simple, and the data they allow examiners to gather are limited; however, single-item ratings of pain intensity are valid and reliable indicators of pain intensity (Victor, Jensen, Gammaitoni, et al., 2008). These scales also help health care providers identify the effects of administered medications on pain intensity. A 2-point or 30% reduction in pain intensity on the Numeric Pain Intensity (NPI) scale is a clinically significant improvement in pain level (Farrar, Young, Lamoreaux, Werth, and Poole, 2001).

Visual Analogue Scale (VAS). The VAS is a 100-mm line with "no pain" at one end and "worst possible pain" at the other end. When using this scale, ask the patient to mark on the line the intensity of the pain he or she is experiencing. If the patient marks the line at 70 mm, you would note the pain level as 7/10.

TABLE 6.1 **Physiological and Behavioral Pain Indicators**

Pain Indicators	Findings
	Physiological Indicators
Neurological	Agitation, restlessness, stillness, irritability, fear, anxiety, fatigue
Cardiac	Tachycardia, increased blood pressure, increased oxygen demand, increased cardiac output
Pulmonary	Hyperventilation with anxiety or hypoventilation with pain, shallow respirations, hypoxia, depressed cough, atelectasis
Gastrointestinal	Nausea, vomiting, decreased bowel sounds, stress ulcer
Genitourinary	Reduced urine output, urinary retention
Musculoskeletal	Muscle tension, spasm, joint stiffness, immobility
Skin	Pallor, diaphoresis
Metabolic	Increased catabolism, increased glucose, increased lactate and ketones, impaired immune function, impaired wound healing
	Behavioral Indicators
Emotional	Depression, excessive sleeping, anxiety, fear, impaired individual or family coping
Social	Isolation, impaired role performance, impaired home maintenance, financial burden if unable to work
Vocalization	Moaning, groaning, grunting, sighing, gasping, crying, screaming
Verbalization	Stated pain, praying, counting, swearing, repeated phrases
Facial expression	Grimacing, clenching teeth, tightly shutting lips, staring, facial mask (flat affect), wrinkling forehead, tearing
Body actions	Thrashing, pounding, biting, rocking, rubbing, stretching, shrugging, rotating body part, shifting weight, massaging, immobilizing, guarding, bracing, applying pressure/heat/cold, assuming special position or posture, crossing legs

This tool is one of the simplest and most basic one-dimensional pain scales. One limitation of the VAS is that some older adults have difficulty marking on the line, and instead place the mark above or below 100 mm (D'Arcy, 2014; Herr and Mobily, 1993).

Verbal Descriptor Scale (VDS). The VDS uses words such as "mild," "moderate," and "severe" to measure pain intensity. It asks patients to select the word or phrase that best describes their pain. Some patients prefer to use words rather than a number to rate their pain. A limitation of the VDS is that the patient must be able to understand the meaning of the words.

Numeric Pain Intensity Scale. The NPI is the most commonly used one-dimensional pain scale (Fig. 6.4).In this 11-point Likert-type scale, 0 means "no pain" and 10 means "worst possible pain." The NPI asks patients to select the number that best fits their pain intensity—the higher the score, the more intense the pain. In general:

- Mild pain is considered to be in the 1 to 3 range.
- Moderate pain is considered to be in the 4 to 6 range.
- Severe pain is considered to be in the 7 to 10 range.

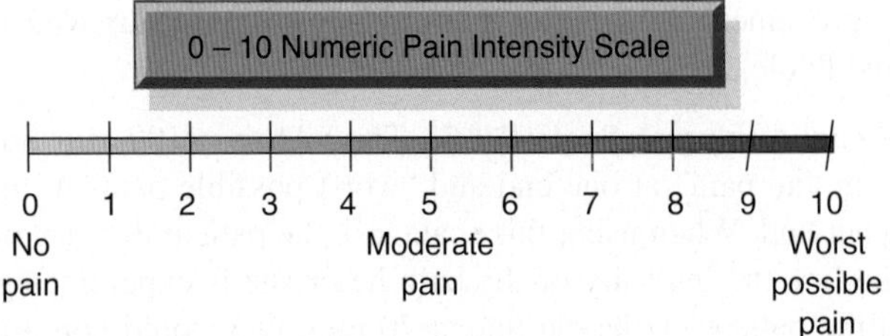

Figure 6.4 Numeric Pain Intensity Scale.

Clinical Significance

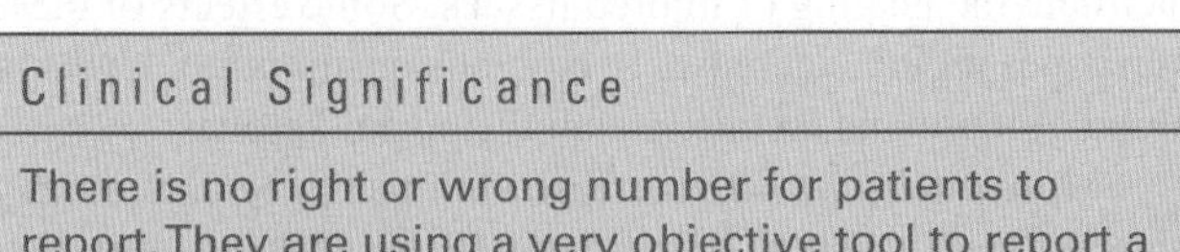
There is no right or wrong number for patients to report. They are using a very objective tool to report a subjective experience. Accept the pain rating the patient reports. Patient self-report is considered the standard criterion for pain assessment (American Pain Society [APS], 2008).

Combined Thermometer Scale. The combined thermometer scale, or pain distress intensity scale, combines the VDS and the NPI (Fig. 6.5). Some patients respond well to this scale and like its vertical orientation, with numbers that increase from the bottom up.

Multidimensional Pain Scales

Multidimensional scales are available for the assessment of chronic pain, malignant pain, or complex medical–surgical

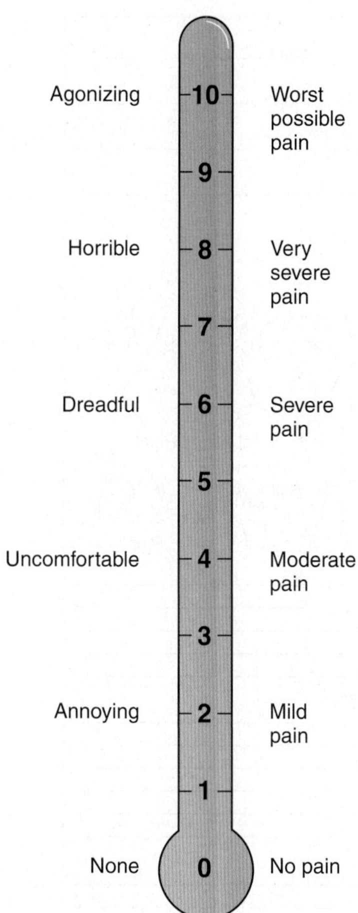

Figure 6.5 Pain distress intensity scale.

pain conditions. Figure 6.6 shows an example. Two commonly used scales are the McGill Pain Questionnaire (MPQ) and the Brief Pain Inventory (BPI). Both have a combination of indices that measure pain intensity, mood, pain location (using a body diagram), verbal descriptors, and questions about medication efficacy. They are most often used for research or with patients who are being actively treated for pain over an extended period.

McGill Pain Questionnaire. The MPQ was developed to measure pain in experimentally induced circumstances, following procedures, and with several medical–surgical conditions. It consists of a set of verbal descriptors used to capture the sensory aspect of pain, a VAS scale, and a present pain intensity rating made up of words and numbers. The tool has been found reliable and valid, and has been translated into several languages (McDonald and Weiskopf, 2001; Melzack, 1975, 1987; Mystakidou, Cleeland, Tsilika, et al., 2004). Limitations include scoring and weighting the verbal descriptor section and difficulty translating the verbal descriptor section into words that indicate syndromes.

Brief Pain Inventory. The BPI was first developed to measure pain in patients with cancer; however, it also has reliability and validity for assessing pain in patients with chronic nonmalignant pain (Daut, Cleeland, and Flannery, 1983; Raichle, Osborne, Jensen, and Cardenas, 2006; Tan, Jensen, Thornby, and Shanti, 2004; Williams, Smith, and Fehnel, 2006); it has been translated into various languages (Hølen, Lydersen, Klepstad, et al., 2008; Mystakidou et al., 2004). The tool can be administered either through an interview or in a self-report format completed by the patient. The BPI consists of a pain intensity scale, a body diagram to locate the pain, a functional assessment (general activity, mood, walking, employment, housework, relationships, sleep, and enjoyment of life), and questions about the efficacy of pain medications (Fig. 6.7). A limitations of the BPI is that the patient must be able to correlate the questions to his or her individual pain experience using the various scales.

Brief Pain Impact Questionnaire (BPIQ). Another way to assess pain quickly in patients with chronic pain is to use a set of structured questions, such as those in the BPIQ:

- How strong is your pain, right now, and at its worst or average over the past week?
- How many days over the past week have you been unable to do what you would like to do because of your pain?
- Over the past week, how often has pain interfered with your ability to take care of yourself, for example, with bathing, eating, dressing, and going to the toilet?
- Over the past week, how often has pain interfered with your ability to take care of your home-related chores such as grocery shopping, preparing meals, paying bills, and driving?
- How often do you participate in pleasurable activities such as hobbies, socializing with friends, and travel? Over the past week, how often has pain interfered with these activities?
- How often do you do some type of exercise? Over the past week, how often has pain interfered with your ability to exercise?
- Does pain interfere with your ability to think clearly?
- Does pain interfere with your appetite? Have you lost weight?
- Does pain interfere with your sleep? How often over the last week?
- Has pain interfered with your energy, mood, personality, or relationships with other people?
- Over the past week, have you taken pain medications?
- Has your use of alcohol or other drugs ever caused a difficulty for you or those close to you?
- How would you rate your health at the present time? (Weiner, Herr, and Rudy, 2002).

These questions capture the major elements of pain assessment for patients with chronic pain and are easy to use in the clinical setting. They assist in identifying the effects of pain on the patient's functional abilities and daily life so that you can fully formulate a holistic perspective on the patient's pain experience.

Lifespan Considerations

Pain assessment poses significant challenges in children and older adults. These patients have a need for adequate pain relief, yet assessing them for pain can be difficult.

Date ____________

Patient's name ____________ Age ________ Room ____________

Diagnosis ____________ Physician ____________

Nurse ____________

1. LOCATION: Patient or nurse marks drawing.

Right Left Right Left Left Right Right Left R L L R Left Right Left Right Right Left

2. INTENSITY: Patient rates the pain. Scale used ____________
   - Present: ____________
   - Worst pain gets: ____________
   - Best pain gets: ____________
   - Acceptable level of pain: ____________
3. QUALITY: (Use patient's own words, e.g., prick, ache, burn, throb, pull, sharp) ____________
4. ONSET, DURATION, VARIATION, RHYTHMS: ____________
5. MANNER OF EXPRESSING PAIN: ____________
6. WHAT RELIEVES THE PAIN? ____________
7. WHAT CAUSES OR INCREASES THE PAIN? ____________
8. EFFECTS OF PAIN: (Note decreased function, decreased quality of life.)
   - Accompanying symptoms (e.g., nausea) ____________
   - Sleep ____________
   - Appetite ____________
   - Physical activity ____________
   - Relationship with others (e.g., irritability) ____________
   - Emotions (e.g., anger, suicidal, crying) ____________
   - Concentration ____________
   - Other ____________
9. OTHER COMMENTS: ____________
10. PLAN: ____________

Figure 6.6 Sample multidimensional pain assessment tool.

Newborns, Infants, and Children

Assessment of pain in children is complex and challenging. The best practice is to consistently use a scale specific to the patient's age. Pain scales have been developed that are specific to infants and children. Infants in pain may exhibit brow bulge, eye squeeze, nasolabial fold, open lips, stretched mouth, lip pursing, taut tongue, chin quiver, and tongue protrusion (Grunau, Oberlander, Holsti, et al., 1998; Oakes, 2011). The difficulty with these behavioral measures is that they do not discriminate between pain behaviors and reactions from other sources of discomfort, such as hunger. You should assume that if a condition or procedure is painful for an adult, it is also painful for an infant or child.

Infants and children may exhibit physiological responses to pain, including increased heart rate, respiratory rate, blood pressure, palmar sweating, cortisone levels, oxygen, vagal tone, and endorphin levels. Because the preverbal infant cannot self-report pain, you must rely on these physiological and behavioral indicators.

The two most common tools used to assess pain in children are the Face, Legs, Activity, Cry, Consolability (FLACC) scale and the FACES pain scale. The FLACC scale was originally designed to measure acute postoperative pain in children 2 months to 7 years old. It uses the indicators of facial expression, leg movement, activity, crying, and ability to be consoled. Behaviors include frowning, kicking, arched back,

STUDY ID# ______________ HOSPITAL ID# ______________

DO NOT WRITE ABOVE THIS LINE

Brief Pain Inventory (Short Form)

Date: ____/____/____ Time: ________

Name: ______________ ______________ ______________
Last First Middle Initial

1. Throughout our lives, most of us have had pain from time to time (such as minor headaches, sprains, and toothaches). Have you had pain other than these everyday kinds of pain today?

1. Yes **2. No**

2. On the diagram, shade in the areas where you feel pain. Put an X on the area that hurts the most.

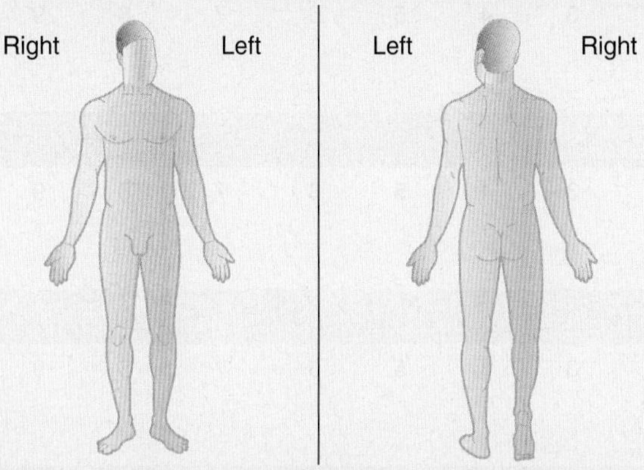

Right Left Left Right

3. Please rate your pain by circling the one number that best describes your pain at its **worst** in the last 24 hours.

0	1	2	3	4	5	6	7	8	9	10
No pain										Pain as bad as you can imagine

4. Please rate your pain by circling the one number that best describes your pain at its **least** in the last 24 hours.

0	1	2	3	4	5	6	7	8	9	10
No pain										Pain as bad as you can imagine

5. Please rate your pain by circling the one number that best describes your pain on the **average.**

0	1	2	3	4	5	6	7	8	9	10
No pain										Pain as bad as you can imagine

6. Please rate your pain by circling the one number that tells how much pain you have **right now.**

0	1	2	3	4	5	6	7	8	9	10
No pain										Pain as bad as you can imagine

Figure 6.7 Brief Pain Inventory.

(continued)

7. What treatments or medications are you receiving for your pain?

8. In the last 24 hours, how much relief have pain treatments or medications provided? Please circle the one percentage that most shows how much **relief** you have received.

0%	10%	20%	30%	40%	50%	60%	70%	80%	90%	100%
No relief										Complete relief

9. Circle the one number that describes how, during the past 24 hours, pain has interfered with your:

A. General Activity

0	1	2	3	4	5	6	7	8	9	10
Does not interfere										Completely interferes

B. Mood

0	1	2	3	4	5	6	7	8	9	10
Does not interfere										Completely interferes

C. Walking Ability

0	1	2	3	4	5	6	7	8	9	10
Does not interfere										Completely interferes

D. Normal Work (includes both work outside the home and housework)

0	1	2	3	4	5	6	7	8	9	10
Does not interfere										Completely interferes

E. Relations With Other People

0	1	2	3	4	5	6	7	8	9	10
Does not interfere										Completely interferes

F. Sleep

0	1	2	3	4	5	6	7	8	9	10
Does not interfere										Completely interferes

G. Enjoyment of Life

0	1	2	3	4	5	6	7	8	9	10
Does not interfere										Completely interferes

Figure 6.7 *(continued)*

crying, and difficulty being consoled. The tool has established reliability and validity.

Children 2 years and older can identify pain and point to its location. You can use a facial expression scale for children starting at approximately 3 years. The FACES scale (Fig. 6.8) uses six faces ranging from happy with a wide smile to sad with tears on the face. You ask the child to pick the face that best represents the pain he or she is experiencing. Face 0 is very happy because there is "no hurt"; Face 5 hurts "as bad as you can imagine." You point to each face, explain the pain intensity, ask the child to choose the face that best describes his or her own pain, and record the appropriate number. The young child's thinking is concrete and egocentric, so it is important to use vocabulary such as "no hurt" or "biggest hurt"

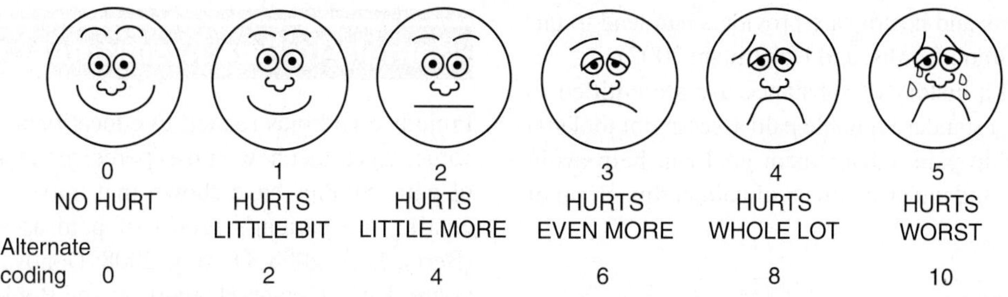

Figure 6.8 The FACES scale is used in children 2 months to 7 years old.

for the scale. You can also talk with the caregiver to learn vocabulary that the child uses at home to describe pain, such as "owie" or "ouchie." The FACES scale has been tested and validity has been established (Wong and DiVito-Thomas, 2006). The scale has also been used to measure pain intensity with children of different ethnicities and with cognitively impaired adults (Wong and DiVito-Thomas, 2006).

Starting between 7 and 10 years, children can use the numeric rating scales used with adults. Use of a color-coded scale, such as the combined thermometer, may be helpful (see Fig. 6.5). Additionally, with this scale the child can specify location and quality. He or she might describe the pain experience as horrible, terrible, terrifying, or stabbing.

Pain also affects children in the affective and sensory dimensions. Children may have reduced sleep, appetite, and fitness level, all of which can affect both school and play. Pain can disturb mood, leading to emotional distress, depression, and anxiety. It also can disrupt family functioning and make the child fearful for the future (Eccleston, Bruce, and Carter, 2006). An accurate assessment is essential for adequate treatment.

Older Adults

Older patients have some specific circumstances that can lead to problems with pain assessment. Pain is prevalent in older patients, and some see pain as just a natural part of aging. Many older patients have chronic illnesses that cause pain, such as osteoarthritis or diabetes. Older patients may fear uncontrolled pain, because it could result in hospitalization or affect their long-term ability to maintain independent living.

Older people may be stoic and conceal any expressions of pain or discomfort. They may be reluctant to report pain, because they want their providers to consider them "good patients," or they may fear that complaints of pain may lead to costly tests or expensive medications that they cannot afford. They also may fear dependence on others and thus avoid reporting or treating pain.

When assessing pain in an older adult, reassure the patient of your interest in the pain and your desire to help manage it. Be sure to also review the following:

- Question the patient about the effects of pain on diet, sleep, and mood. Unrelieved pain may lead to insomnia or depression and seriously affect the patient's quality of life.
- Ask about any comorbidities, such as osteoarthritis, which may cause pain or have an influence on medication choices.
- Review all medications that the patient is taking, including vitamins and herbal supplements. Older patients may not take medications as ordered or may refuse to take drugs that cause adverse effects such as sedation or constipation.

Assessment of pain leading to effective treatment can improve the quality of life for older adults. Providing adequate pain management for this population can occur through care and reassurance and by taking the time to assess pain accurately.

Special Situations

Patients Unable to Report Pain

The JCAHO instituted pain management guidelines in 2001 that mandated the assessment of pain for all patients (Joint Commission on Accreditation of Healthcare Organizations, 2001). Self-report is the most reliable indicator of pain, but many patients cannot communicate verbally. The development of behavioral tools for assessing pain in nonverbal patients is the newest area of pain assessment and a developing science.

When attempting to perform a pain assessment on a patient who cannot self-report pain, do the following:

- Attempt a self-report of pain.
- Try to identify any potential causes for pain.
- Observe patient behaviors.
- Ask the family or other caregivers if they have noticed any changes in behavior.
- Attempt an analgesic trial (Herr, Bjoro, and Decker, 2006b).

Patients with Opioid Tolerance

Patients with a history of opioid tolerance pose difficult challenges for pain assessment (D'Arcy, 2014). They have an altered physiologic response to the pain stimulus, and the repeated use of opioids causes their bodies to become more sensitive to pain. This sensitivity is called **opioid hyperalgesia** and can occur as soon as 1 month after opioid use begins.

Not only are patients with opioid tolerance more sensitive to pain, they face a high level of bias from health care providers. Because these patients are more sensitive to pain, they often report high levels of pain with little relief from usual doses of opioids. They are often labeled as drug seeking. Many health care providers fear that they will induce addiction in patients by providing them with opioids. Many patients with opioid dependence mistrust the health care system. These attitudes of patients and health care providers can lead to undertreated pain (Grant, Cordts, and Doberman, 2007).

Patients with a history of substance use are entitled to pain relief. Using a standard reliable pain assessment tool and setting a reasonable pain management goal can help avoid misunderstanding and undertreatment of pain in this group of patients.

> **SAFETY ALERT**
> *Some patients are at high risk when receiving pain medication. Be aware of common aberrant behaviors when reassessing patients, especially when opioids have been prescribed to treat pain: purposeful oversedation; negative mood changes, appearing intoxicated; increasingly unkempt or impaired appearance; involvement in car or other accidents; increased doses without authorization; reports of lost or stolen prescriptions; use of pain medication to ease situational stressors; abuse of alcohol or illicit drugs; or record of arrests.*

Reassessing and Documenting Pain

The JCAHO has set a standard that states that nurses must assess and reassess pain regularly. Most hospitals set their own standards for assessment, such as every shift or every 4 or 6 hours, depending on the specific practice area and needs of the patient. When pain is present, it is always reassessed to make sure that the treatments have been effective. This reassessment is always documented in the chart.

Reassessing pain is similar to reassessing a patient taking blood pressure medication or a patient with diabetes who needs regular blood glucose level testing. For patients taking pain medication, reassessment provides a reliable measure of the drug's efficacy. It allows you to determine whether pain intensity has decreased since administration, much as blood pressure should be lower once a patient takes blood pressure medication. Most hospitals have a standard timeframe for reassessment, such as 1 hour for oral medication and 30 minutes for pain medication given intravenously. They base these timeframes on the time it takes a pain medication to provide a noticeable decrease in pain intensity.

> **SAFETY ALERT**
> *Health care providers often write orders on an "as needed" (PRN) basis for hospitalized patients. You must use critical thinking and nursing judgment about administration, dose, route, and frequency. It is essential to accurately assess, document, and reassess the pain level and response to treatment.*

Figure 6.9 shows examples of documentation of pain intensity for (A) shift assessment and (B) medication administration reassessment. As a nurse, you are legally accountable for the quality of their pain management, including assessment, treatment, and reassessment (Camp and O'Sullivan, 1987).

Barriers to Pain Assessment

Prejudice and bias related to educational, family, or cultural values can affect how nurses perceive the patient's self-report of pain. Studies have shown that nurses have difficulty accepting the patient's report of pain as valid and credible (Berry, et al., 2008; D'Arcy, 2008; Donovan, Dillon, and McGuire, 1987; Drayer, Henderson, and Reidenberg, 1999). It is important to recognize the issues surrounding bias and prejudice and work to minimize their effect on pain management.

When a pain assessment is inaccurate or poor, patients suffer because of incorrect medication and treatment choices. Fear of respiratory depression and addiction affect pain assessment and management (Apfelbaum, et al., 2003; Donovan, et al., 1987). Focusing on pain relief as the primary end to the assessment process and treatment selection will help control fears and bias that can negatively affect patient care.

> **SAFETY ALERT**
> *Respiratory depression is an adverse effect of opioid administration. It is essential to observe for adverse effects and hold the medication if evidence indicates respiratory depression and increasing sedation.*

Critical Thinking

As a nurse, you are responsible for assessing pain and negotiating pain and functional goals with patients. Based upon those goals, you implement pharmacological and nonpharmacological interventions. You document the assessment, analysis, interventions, and reassessment in the patient record. Additionally, you may identify pain as a priority problem and consider its broader effects on sleep, activities, and mood. You can analyze and document this information in a SOAP (*s*ubjective, *o*bjective, *a*nalysis, *p*lan) note that shows this critical thinking.

Pain is a complex syndrome that involves an accurate and complete assessment. Pain is often a subjective symptom, although there are objective signs of its presence. Many pain tools have been developed for different populations. Pain assessment and its treatment is primarily within the role of nursing practice.

Nursing Diagnoses, Outcomes, and Interventions

Assess the patient's pain level in the initial pain assessment: use specialized pain tools if indicated. Using the assessment data, incorporate critical thinking to establish a nursing problem or diagnosis list.

Table 6.2 compares two nursing diagnoses, assessment characteristics, and interventions commonly related to pain (Moorehead, Johnson, Maas, and Swanson, 2013). The assessment data are the basis for the care provided to relieve acute or chronic pain.

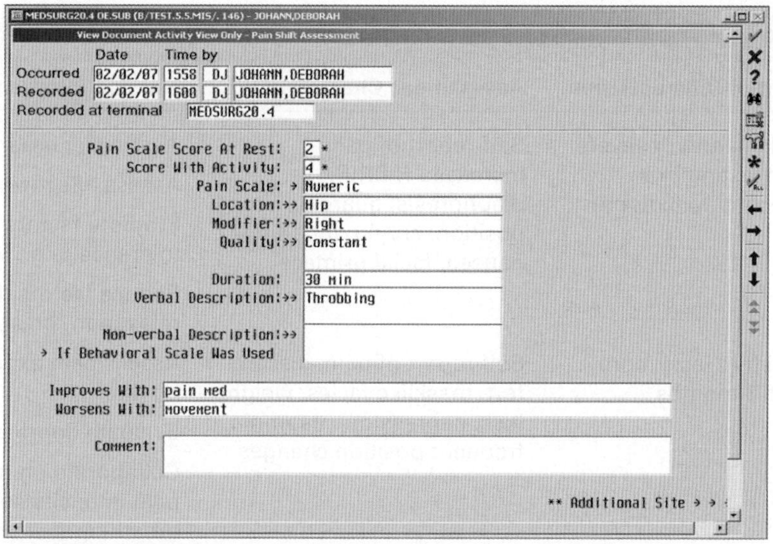

MEDSURG20.4 OE.SUB (B/TEST.5.5.MIS/. 146) - JOHANN,DEBORAH

View Document Activity View Only - Pain Shift Assessment

	Date	Time	by	
Occurred	02/02/07	1558	DJ	JOHANN,DEBORAH
Recorded	02/02/07	1600	DJ	JOHANN,DEBORAH

Recorded at terminal MEDSURG20.4

Pain Scale Score At Rest: 2 *
Score With Activity: 4 *
Pain Scale: → Numeric
Location:→→ Hip
Modifier:→→ Right
Quality:→→ Constant
Duration: 30 min
Verbal Description:→→ Throbbing
Non-verbal Description:→→
→ If Behavioral Scale Was Used
Improves With: pain med
Worsens With: movement
Comment:

** Additional Site → →

A

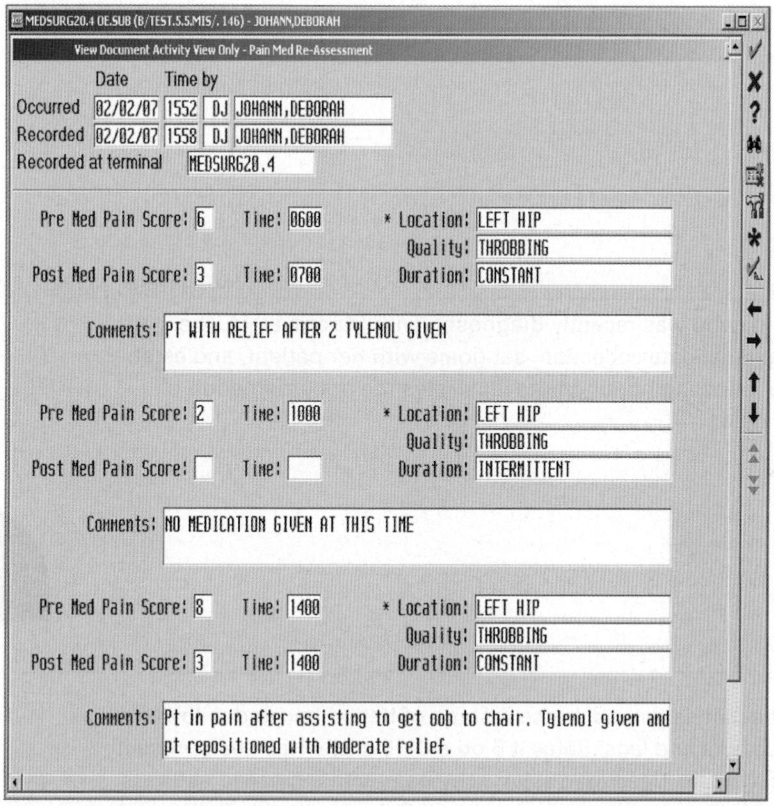

MEDSURG20.4 OE.SUB (B/TEST.5.5.MIS/. 146) - JOHANN,DEBORAH

View Document Activity View Only - Pain Med Re-Assessment

	Date	Time	by	
Occurred	02/02/07	1552	DJ	JOHANN,DEBORAH
Recorded	02/02/07	1558	DJ	JOHANN,DEBORAH

Recorded at terminal MEDSURG20.4

Pre Med Pain Score: 6 Time: 0600 * Location: LEFT HIP
Quality: THROBBING
Post Med Pain Score: 3 Time: 0700 Duration: CONSTANT
Comments: PT WITH RELIEF AFTER 2 TYLENOL GIVEN

Pre Med Pain Score: 2 Time: 1000 * Location: LEFT HIP
Quality: THROBBING
Post Med Pain Score: Time: Duration: INTERMITTENT
Comments: NO MEDICATION GIVEN AT THIS TIME

Pre Med Pain Score: 8 Time: 1400 * Location: LEFT HIP
Quality: THROBBING
Post Med Pain Score: 3 Time: 1400 Duration: CONSTANT
Comments: Pt in pain after assisting to get oob to chair. Tylenol given and pt repositioned with moderate relief.

B

Key:

- Questions with (→) indicate a group reponse is available.
- (→ →) indicates group response with option to write in.
- Questions without an arrow are free text.
- If pain score at rest is elevated, a consult is sent to the Pain Nurse and a care plan is Query linked
- A second page of this intervention is the same as the first, just allowing the RN to document to a site.

Figure 6.9 **A.** Example of an electronic shift pain assessment (i.e., done every shift). **B.** Example of a post pain medication assessment, completed after medication is given; can have multiple entries.

TABLE 6.2 Common Nursing Diagnoses Associated with Pain			
Diagnosis	**Point of Differentiation**	**Assessment Characteristics**	**Nursing Interventions**
Acute pain	Sudden and/or severe pain lasting from 1 second to 6 months	Self-report of pain; increased P, BP, R; diaphoresis; guarded position; crying; moaning; nausea; facial grimace	Administer ordered pain medication.* Assess effectiveness of medication. Promote factors that increase pain tolerance (e.g., music, distraction). Reduce factors that increase pain, relaxation, breathing, distraction.
Chronic pain	Pain that lasts more than 6 months	Self-report of pain, discomfort, masklike facies, weight loss, depression, insomnia, frequent position changes	Assess pain experience and effect on life. Evaluate depression. Collaborate on methods to reduce pain intensity such as relaxation and breathing, pain medication.* Evaluate adverse effects of medications.

*Collaborative interventions.

Progress Note: Analyzing Findings

Remember Mrs. Bond, who was recently diagnosed with fibromyalgia. The nurse has completed the initial data collection, set goals with her patient, and established a plan of care. The following nursing note illustrates the documentation of subjective and objective data.

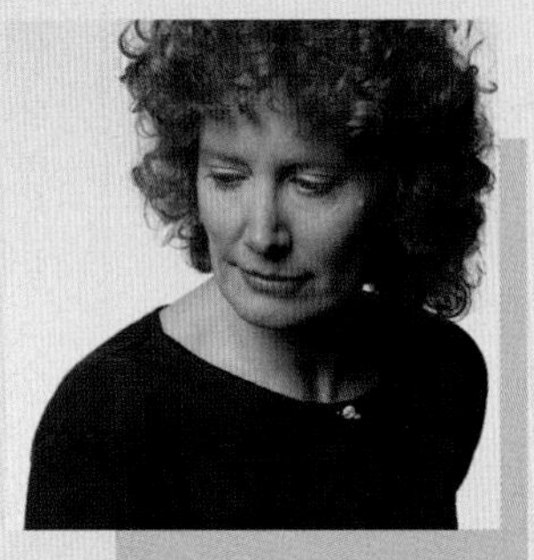

Subjective: States that the pain is getting worse instead of better. Located in lower back and radiates into buttocks and legs. Rates it 5 on a 0–10 scale. Has been present for 5 months since her diagnosis. Described as an achy pain with increased stiffness in the morning. Being tired or stressed out aggravates it. Being well rested alleviates pain. Able to perform functional activities with more effort except that she has not done yard work. Pain goal stated at 3.

Objective: Slightly overweight, appears older than her age. Facial expression: fatigued with dark circles under her eyes. Posture slightly slouched in chair, shifting from side to side frequently. Affect flat. Dress appropriate to weather, well groomed. T 37°C, P 112 beats/min, R 20 breaths/min, BP 142/88 mmHg.

Analysis: Chronic pain related to fibromyalgia.

Plan: Communicate findings to primary care provider. Provide patient education on medications and adverse effects. Discuss ways that patient can get some mild exercise 3 to 5 times weekly. Evaluate sleep hygiene and recommend routines that

(case study continues on page 131)

promote sleep. Discuss ways that she can do household tasks more efficiently to save her energy for enjoyable activities, possibly including some light gardening. Provide information about support group for patients with fibromyalgia.

Critical Thinking Challenge

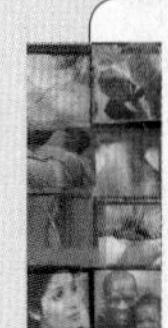

- Is subjective or objective data collection the higher priority when assessing Mrs. Bond's pain?
- What techniques of physical assessment might the nurse use when assessing Mrs. Bond?
- How do assessments from the general survey cluster with the pain assessment?

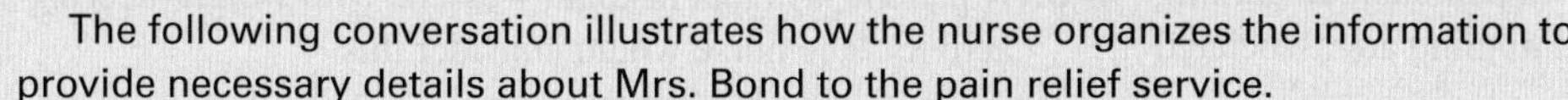

Collaborating with the Interprofessional Team

In many health care facilities, nurses initiate referrals based on assessment findings. In this case, the health care provider ordered a referral to the pain clinic because Mrs. Bond's pain is not responsive to traditional medical treatment. The nurse communicates the reason for the consult using the situation background assessment recommendation (SBAR) format. Other results that might trigger a pain consult include history of chronic pain, regular use of opioids for more than 3 months, substance abuse, difficult pain management, patient dissatisfaction with pain relief, high dose requirements, or significant adverse effects related to pain management.

The following conversation illustrates how the nurse organizes the information to provide necessary details about Mrs. Bond to the pain relief service.

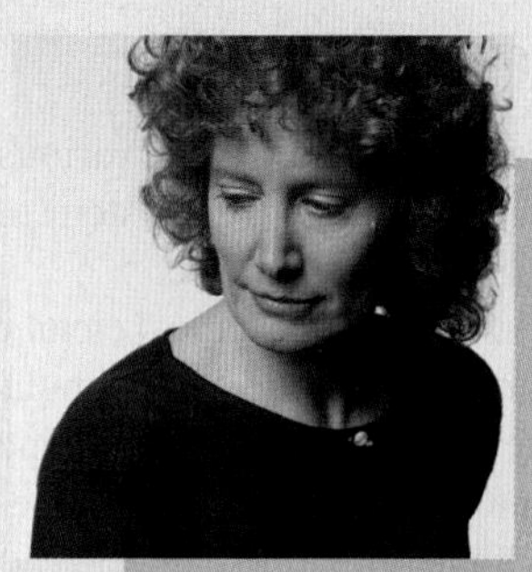

Situation: Hi, this is Belinda and I've been talking with Mrs. Bond about her pain management in the clinic today.

Background: She's 42 years old and was diagnosed with fibromyalgia about 5 months ago. We've been seeing her to help manage her pain. She is currently taking a selective serotonin reuptake inhibitor for depression, benzodiazepine for muscle spasm, and a central nervous system analgesic for pain.

Assessment: She's reporting a pain level of 5 and really would like to be down to about a 3. Mostly, it's an achy pain that is in her lower back on both sides of her body, upper shoulder pain, and pain that radiates into her buttocks and legs, the fairly typical type of fibromyalgia pain. She appears to be fatigued and a little depressed and is having difficulty sleeping.

Recommendations: We would like you to see her to see if you have any suggestions about a different medication dose or combination. She's been very patient in working with us on this and we would like to get something that works for her. She said that she could wait about a half an hour now, or come back to see you for another appointment.

Critical Thinking Challenge

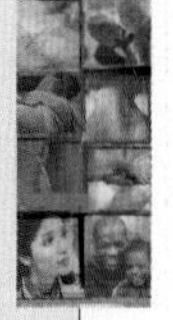

- At what point would you decide to contact other health care providers for more pain medication?
- What is the role of the nurse in working with the pain consult team?
- What parts of the pain treatment are within the nursing domain? Which are within collaborative practice?

Applying Your Knowledge

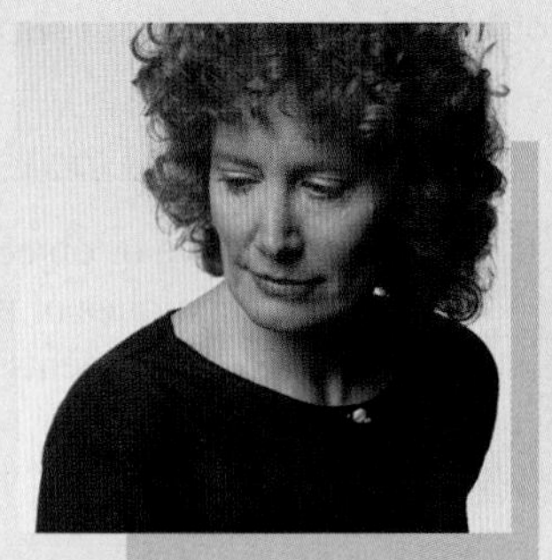

Now that you have completed the reading and case features for this chapter, consider Mrs. Bond's case and its relationship to what you are learning. Answer the following questions.

- How would you describe the mechanisms of pain?
- How would you differentiate between neuropathic and nociceptive pain?
- How would you assess pain if Mrs. Bond were a mentally challenged young adult? A cognitively impaired older adult?
- What factors might contribute to observations made during the pain assessment?
- What data would you use to plan patient education for the reduction of pain?
- How would you assess the effectiveness of health promotion strategies for the patient who experiences chronic pain?

Key Points

- Pain can result from various stimuli transmitted via the peripheral nervous system to the central nervous system where it is processed.
- Pain can be musculoskeletal or neuropathic, depending on the source of the pain stimulus.
- Verbal descriptors that patients use for pain include burning and tingling. Painful numbness and tingling are associated with neuropathic pain.
- A decrease of two points on the Numeric Pain Intensity scale is considered clinically significant.
- When assessing pain, you should use scales designed for the specific population to which the patient belongs (e.g., FACES scale for children).
- Patients with chronic pain need more than just a pain intensity rating; they require use of a multidimensional scale such as the BPI.
- You must believe the patient's report of pain.
- Avoidance of labeling and stigmatization is important for patients who are dependent on pain medications to control their pain.
- You should always assess a patient's pain. If the patient is nonverbal, you can use a behavioral pain scale designed to identify pain in that population.
- You must be aware of the legal implications of pain assessment. Not documenting an assessment means it has not been done.
- Reassessing pain can provide a means of determining the efficacy of an administered pain medication.

Review Questions

1. The patient has pain of a short duration with an identifiable cause. This is referred to as
   A. acute pain.
   B. chronic pain.
   C. neuropathic pain.
   D. complex pain.

2. To identify the location of pain, the nurse asks the patient
   A. how long he or she has had the pain.
   B. to rate the intensity of the pain on a scale from 0 to 10.
   C. to point to the painful area.
   D. to describe the quality of pain.

3. A patient says that his pain worsens with weight-bearing activity. The nurse would consider this
   A. an alleviating factor.
   B. a functional pain goal.
   C. quality/description.
   D. an aggravating factor.

4. Which of the following tools would a nurse use to perform a multidimensional pain assessment?
   A. Visual analogue scale
   B. Brief Pain Inventory
   C. Numeric Pain Intensity
   D. Verbal descriptor

5. For what circumstance would the nurse be most likely to assess pain using the McGill Pain Questionnaire?
   A. Verbal description
   B. Alleviating factors
   C. Functional status goal
   D. Pain goal

6. Which of the following indicators would be most likely to signify to the nurse that a patient is having pain?
   A. Falling asleep
   B. Rubbing a body part
   C. Relaxed body position
   D. Facial relaxation

7. A patient reports pain, depression, and insomnia. The nurse observes a masklike facial expression and frequent position changes. Which of the following is the nurse most likely to use to describe the patient's findings?
   A. Acute pain
   B. Chronic pain
   C. Neuropathic pain
   D. Chronic regional pain syndrome

8. With which of the following types of patients is the nurse most likely to use the FACES pain scale?
   A. Children
   B. Patients with dementia
   C. Older adults
   D. Unconscious patients

9. Which of the following is the rationale for the nurse to reassess the patient's pain after treatment?
   A. To pinpoint the pain's location
   B. To measure the pain's duration
   C. To establish the efficacy of medication
   D. To make changes to the patient's pain goal

10. Which of the following is a barrier to pain assessment?
   A. The nurse believes that patients suffer if under medicated.
   B. The nurse focuses on pain relief as a primary end to the assessment process.
   C. The nurse chooses treatment that will positively affect the patient's care.
   D. The nurse has difficulty accepting the patient's self-report as valid.

The Jensen suite offers these additional resources to enhance learning and facilitate understanding of this chapter:

- thePoint online resources, http//thepoint.lww.com/Jensen2e
- *Laboratory Manual for Nursing Health Assessment: A Best-Practice Approach*
- *Pocket Guide for Nursing Health Assessment: A Best-Practice Approach*
- *Lippincott DocuCare*, an Electronic Health Record simulation software, http://thepoint.lww.com/docucare
- *Adaptive Learning | Powered by PrepU*, http://thepoint.lww.com/prepu

References

American Geriatric Society. (2002). The management of persistent pain in older persons—The American Geriatric Society Panel on Persistent Pain in Older Persons. *Journal of the American Geriatrics Society, 50* (6), 205–224.

American Pain Society. (2008). *Principles of analgesic use in the treatment of acute and cancer pain* (5th ed.). Glenview, IL: Author.

American Society of Pain Management Nursing (ASPMN) (2010) Core Curriculum for Pain Management Nursing (2nd Ed.): Dubuque, IA: Kendall Hunt Publishing Co.

Apfelbaum, J., Chen, C., Mehtam, S., and Tong, G. (2003). Postoperative pain experience: Results from a national survey suggest postoperative pain continues to be undermanaged. *Anesthesia and Analgesia, 97* (2), 534–540.

Berry, P. H., Covington, E., Dahl, J., Katz, J., and Miaskowski, C. (2008). *Pain: Current understanding of assessment, management, and treatments*. Reston, VA: National Pharmaceutical Council, Inc and the Joint Commission on Accreditation of Healthcare Organizations.

Brandes, J. L. (2006). The influence of estrogen on migraine. *JAMA, 295* (15), 1824–1830.

Camp, L. D., and O'Sullivan, P. (1987). Comparison of medical, surgical, and oncology patients' descriptions of pain and nurses' documentation of pain assessments. *Journal of Advanced Nursing, 12*, 593–598.

Cervero, F. (2005). The gate control theory, then and now in the paths of pain. In H. Mersky, J. Loeser, and R. Dubner (Eds.), *The paths of pain*. Seattle, WA: IASP Press.

Cipher, D. J., Clifford, P. A., and Roper, K. D. (2006). Behavioral manifestations of pain in the demented elderly. *Journal of the American Medical Directors Association, 7* (6), 355–365.

D'Arcy, Y. M. (2003). Pain assessment. In P. Iyer (Ed.), *Medical-legal aspects of pain and suffering*. Tucson, AZ: Lawyers and Judges Publishing Company.

D'Arcy, Y. (2007a). *Pain management: Evidence-based tools and techniques for nursing professionals*. Marblehead, MA: HcPro.

D'Arcy, Y. (2007b). What's the diagnosis? *The American Nurse Today, 1* (4), 29–30.

D'Arcy, Y. (2008). Pain management survey report. *Nursing, 38* (6), 42–49; quiz 49–51.

D'Arcy Y. (2014) *A compact clinical guide to women's pain management*. Springer Publishing: New York.

Daut, R. L., Cleeland, C. S., and Flannery, R. (1983). Development of the Wisconsin Brief Pain Questionnaire to assess pain in cancer or other diseases. *Pain, 17*, 197–210.

DeLuca, A. (2008). Why chronic pain is a medical emergency. Retrieved May 17, 2010, from http://doctordeluca.com/wordpress/archive/chronic-pain-is-a-medical-emergency/

Donovan, M., Dillon, P., and McGuire, L. (1987). Incidence and characteristics of pain in a sample of medical, surgical inpatients. *Pain, 30*, 69–78.

Drayer, R. A., Henderson, J., and Reidenberg, M. (1999). Barriers to better pain control in hospitalized patients. *Journal of Pain and Symptom Management, 17* (6), 434–440.

Eccleston, C., Bruce, E., and Carter, B. (2006). Chronic pain in children and adolescents. *Paediatric Nursing, 18* (10), 30–33.

Falla, D., Farina, D., Dahl, M. K., and Graven-Nielsen, T. (2007). Muscle pain induces task-dependent changes in cervical agonist/antagonist activity. *Journal of Applied Physiology, 102* (2), 601–609.

Farrar, J. T., Young, J. P., Lamoreaux, L., Werth, J. L., and Poole, R. M. (2001). Clinical importance of changes in chronic pain intensity measured on an 11 point numerical pain rating scale. *Pain, 94*, 149–158.

Feldt, K. S. (2000). The checklist of non-verbal pain indicators (CNPI). *Pain Management Nursing, 1* (1), 13–21.

Feldt, K. S., Ryden, M. B., and Miles, S. (1998). Treatment of pain in cognitively impaired compared with cognitively intact older patients with hip fractures. *Journal of the American Geriatrics Society, 46*, 1079–1085.

Grant, M. S., Cordts, G. A., and Doberman, D. J. (2007). Acute pain management in hospitalized patients with current opioid abuse. *Topics in Advanced Practice Nursing*. Retrieved August 6, 2008, from http://www.medscape.com/viewarticle/557043

Green, C. R., Anderson, K. O., Baker, T. A., et al. (2003). The unequal burden of pain: Confronting racial and ethnic disparities in pain. *Pain Medicine, 4* (3), 277–294.

Grunau, R. V. E., Oberlander, T. F., Holsti, L., et al. (1998). Bedside application of the Neonatal Facial Coding System in pain assessment of premature neonates. *Pain, 76*, 277–286.

Herr, K., Bjoro, K., and Decker, S. (2006b). Tools for assessment of pain in nonverbal older adults with dementia: A state-of-the-science review. *Journal of Pain and Symptom Management, 31* (2), 170–192.

Herr, K., Coyne, P., Key, T., et al. (2006a). Pain assessment in the nonverbal patient: Position statement with clinical practice recommendations. *Pain Management Nursing, 7* (2), 44–52.

Herr, K. A. and Mobily, P. (1993). Comparison of selected pain assessment tools for use with the elderly. *Applied Nursing Research, 6* (1), 39–46.

Hølen, J. C., Lydersen, S., Klepstad, P., et al. (2008). The Brief Pain Inventory: Pain's interference with functions is different in cancer pain compared with noncancer chronic pain. *Clinical Journal of Pain, 24* (3), 219–225.

Institute of Medicine. (2011). *Relieving pain in America: A blueprint for transforming prevention, care, education, and research.* Washington, DC: The National Academies Press.

Joint Commission on Accreditation of Healthcare Organizations. (2001). *Pain assessment and management: An organizational approach.* Oakbrook Terrace, IL: Author.

Linton, A. and Lach, H. (2007). *Matteson and McConnells' gerontological nursing concepts and practice* (3rd ed.). St. Louis: Saunders.

McDonald, D. D. and Weiskopf, C. S. A. (2001). Adult patients' postoperative pain descriptions and responses to the Short Form McGill Pain Questionnaire. *Clinical Nursing Research, 10* (4), 442–452.

Melzack, R. (1975). The McGill Pain Questionnaire: Major properties and scoring methods. *Pain, 1*, 277–299.

Melzack, R. (1987). The short form McGill Pain Questionnaire. *Pain, 30*, 191–197.

Melzack, R. and Wall, P. (1975). Pain mechanisms: A new theory. *Science, 150* (699), 971–979.

Mystakidou, K., Cleeland, C., Tsilika, E., et al. (2004). Greek M.D. Anderson Symptom Inventory: Validation and utility in cancer patients. *Oncology, 67* (3–4), 203–210.

Oakes, L. L., (2011). *Compact clinical guide to infant and child pain management: An evidence-based approach for nurses.* New York: Springer.

Raichle, K. A., Osborne, T. L., Jensen, M. P., and Cardenas, D. (2006). The reliability and validity of pain interference measures in persons with spinal cord injury. *Journal of Pain, 7* (3), 179–186.

Reyes-Gibby, C. C., Aday, L. A., Todd, K. H., et al. (2007). Pain in aging community-dwelling adults in the United States: Non-Hispanic Whites, Non-Hispanic Blacks, and Hispanics. *Journal of Pain, 8* (1), 75–84.

Rowbotham, M. (2006). Pharmacologic management of complex regional pain syndrome. *Clinical Journal of Pain, 22 (5), 425–429.*

Smith H.S., and Barkin R.L. (2010). Fibromyalgia syndrome: a discussion of the syndrome and pharmacotherapy. *American Journal of Therapeutics*. 17(4):418-39. doi: 10.1097/MJT.0b013e3181df8e1b.

Smith, H.S., Harris, R., Clauw, D. (2011). Fibromyalgia: an afferent processing disorder leading to a complex pain generalized syndrome. *Pain Physician*, 2011 Mar-Apr;14(2):E217-45.

Staats, P. S., Argoff, C., Brewer, R., D'Arcy, Y., Gallagher, R., McCarberg, W., et al. (2004). Neuropathic pain: Incorporating new consensus guidelines into the reality of clinical practice. *Advanced Studies in Medicine, 4* (7B), S542–S582.

Tan, G., Jensen, M. P., Thornby, J. I., and Shanti, B. F. (2004) Validation of the Brief Pain Inventory for chronic nonmalignant pain. *Journal of Pain, 5* (2), 133–137.

Victor, T. W., Jensen, M. P., Gammaitoni, A. R., et al. (2008). The dimensions of pain quality: Factor analysis of the Pain Quality Assessment Scale. *Clinical Journal of Pain, 24* (6), 550–555.

Weiner, D. K., Herr, K., and Rudy, T. (2002). *Persistent pain in older adults: An interdisciplinary guide for treatment.* New York: Springer Publishing Company.

Williams, V. S., Smith, M. Y., and Fehnel, S. E. (2006). The validity and utility of the BPI interference measures for evaluating the impact of osteoarthritic pain. *Journal of Pain Symptom Management, 31* (1), 48–57.

Wong, D. and DiVito-Thomas, P. (2006). *The validity, reliability, and preference of the Wong Baker FACES Pain Rating Scale among Chinese, Japanese, and Thai children.* Philadelphia, Elsevier.

7

Nutrition Assessment

Learning Objectives

1 Discuss the role of primary nutrients in maintaining health.

2 Outline dietary choices based on the USDA MyPlate guidelines.

3 Discuss developmental, social, cultural, and religious factors affecting the nutritional status of patients.

4 Describe the nurse's role in nutritional assessment.

5 Evaluate the potential effects of medications and nutritional supplements on nutrient intake, absorption, utilization, and excretion.

6 Identify physical signs and symptoms of malnutrition.

7 Differentiate normal from abnormal findings in patients based on the calculation of body mass index (BMI) and ideal body weight, in addition to the consideration of muscle mass and fat distribution.

8 Consider age, condition, gender, and culture to individualize nutritional assessments for infants, children, adolescents, women who are pregnant, women who are lactating, and older adults.

9 Document and communicate data from nutritional assessments using appropriate terminology.

10 Use nutritional assessment findings to identify nursing diagnoses and initiate a plan of care.

Karen Pitoci, 15 years old, 170.2 cm (67 inches) tall, and weighing 39 kg (88 lb), was recently discharged from the hospital with a diagnosis of anorexia nervosa. This hospital stay was the most recent of three in the past year. Her mother, a full-time homemaker, is very involved in Karen's school and social activities.

The family is being visited today by a home health nurse for a follow-up assessment. The role of the home health nurse is to assess Karen's nutritional status and ability to care for herself at home.

You will gain more information about Karen as you progress through this chapter. As you study the content and features, consider Karen's case and its relationship to what you are learning. Begin thinking about the following points:

- What subjective and psychosocial data will the nurse collect from Karen and her mother?
- How might the nurse's previous experiences with patients who have eating disorders influence the assessment of Karen?
- What adaptations will the nurse make to the assessment based on Karen's condition?
- What factors are contributing to Karen's current nutritional status?
- What recommendations for further assessment of Karen by the interprofessional team would the nurse suggest?
- How will the nurse evaluate the success of the interventions of the interprofessional team with Karen?

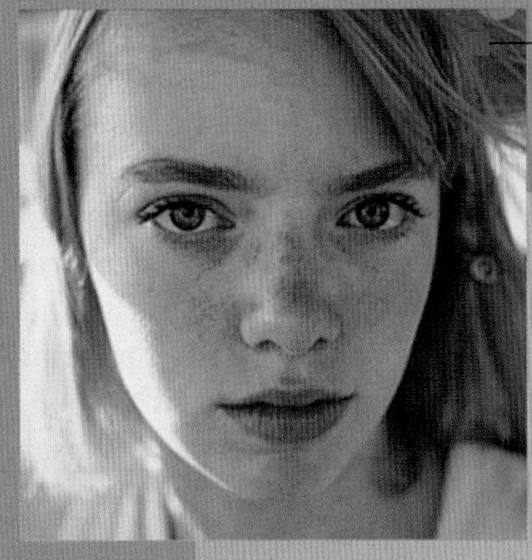

As a frontline provider of health care, the nurse is involved intimately in all aspects of assessing nutritional status for patients. The nurse determines whether caloric and nutrient intake is adequate and appropriate by analyzing data to identify existing and potential nutritional problems. Because foods, rather than nutrients, make up the building blocks of a wholesome diet, the nurse must be aware of nutrients in whole foods to accurately complete a nutritional assessment.

When completing a nutritional assessment, the nurse considers a broad range of influences on the patient's food choices. A complete nutrition assessment includes a history of food intake, weight and height calculations, laboratory data, and the use of specific nutritional tools when indicated.

Nutritional Concepts

Primary Nutrients

Primary nutrients, essential for optimal body function, include carbohydrates, proteins, fats, vitamins, minerals, water, and major electrolytes. Nutrients are the building blocks for tissue maintenance and repair. Furthermore, carbohydrates, proteins, and fats are sources of energy for the body. Fats yield 9 cal/g, whereas proteins and carbohydrates yield 4 cal/g. Vitamins and minerals also play key roles in cellular function. Water makes up more than half of adult body weight and is essential to supporting life, serving many vital functions within the body.

Carbohydrates

Carbohydrates provide the body's main source of energy. Sugars, which are simple carbohydrates, include glucose, dextrose, fructose, galactose, sucrose, maltose, and lactose. These simple carbohydrates are absorbed as basic units without undergoing digestion and hence provide a quick source of energy. Complex carbohydrates, also known as polysaccharides, include starch, glycogen, and fiber.

Primary sources of carbohydrates are natural and added sugars, starches, fiber, grains, fruits, and vegetables. The recommended daily allowance for carbohydrates varies depending on the activity level; the distribution range in a normal healthy diet is 45% to 65% of calories (U.S. Department of Health & Human Services [USDHHS] & U.S. Department of Agriculture [USDA], 2010).

Proteins

Proteins serve important functions in cell structure and tissue maintenance. Amino acids are the building blocks of all proteins. Amino acids—and thus proteins—are involved in many essential body functions, such as regulating fluid and electrolyte balance and transporting molecules and other substances through the blood. Body tissues such as muscles, bones, teeth, skin, and hair primarily consist of protein. Although the body can synthesize most amino acids from nonprotein dietary sources, eight essential amino acids must be obtained through dietary sources.

Lipids

Lipids, or fats, include triglycerides (fats and oils), sterols (e.g., cholesterol), and phospholipids (e.g., lecithin). Fats help to maintain body functions by providing essential fatty acids (linoleic and linoleic acids) and promoting the absorption of fat-soluble vitamins A, D, E, and K.

Triglycerides. Saturated fats (solid at room temperature) and hydrogenated fats raise levels of low-density lipoprotein (LDL) cholesterol. Saturated fats include those found in animal products such as butter, cheese, and fatty meats. **Hydrogenation** refers to the chemical processing of animal fats used by food manufacturers to extend the shelf life of products susceptible to rancidity, such as cookies and crackers.

> **Clinical Significance**
>
> Foods made with hydrogenated fats are particularly harmful to the diet because they are the largest contributors of trans fats. Empirical evidence suggests that trans fats are as damaging to the heart and blood vessels as saturated fats (Mente, de Koning, Shannon, & Anand, 2009).

Unsaturated fats (those that are liquid at room temperature) are known to reduce LDL levels as well as triglycerides (high levels of which are a major cause of coronary heart disease). Unsaturated fats come in two forms. They are either *omega-3 oils*, found primarily in fish oils and some plant oils such as canola, flaxseed, walnut, and hazelnut, or *omega-6 oils*, found in plant oils such as safflower, sunflower, corn, soybean, and cottonseed (Tangney, Rosenson, Freeman, & Rind, 2009). Monounsaturated fats such as canola and olive oils may lower cholesterol if consumed in place of saturated fats.

Cholesterol. Cholesterol is essential to cellular maintenance and repair; however, the body can synthesize sufficient cholesterol to meet its daily requirements. Cholesterol ingested in excess of daily requirements contributes to atherosclerosis, stroke, and myocardial infarction (heart attack). In the typical North American diet, cholesterol primarily comes from meat and egg yolks.

> **Clinical Significance**
>
> Because of the substantial rise in obesity throughout North America and the subsequent increase in incidence of diabetes and heart disease directly attributable to dietary triglycerides and cholesterol, the U.S. Department of Agriculture (2008) and the American Heart Association recommend that daily fat intake for adults should not exceed 20% to 35% of total calories (USDHHS & USDA, 2010). In addition, because saturated fats contribute heavily to elevated serum triglyceride and cholesterol levels, they should not exceed 10% of daily calories.

Phospholipids. Phospholipids are emulsifiers that occur naturally in many foods. They are also used extensively by the food industry. Phospholipids serve many vital functions such as transporting fat-soluble substances across cell membranes. Lecithin, the best known phospholipid, is a popular food supplement. Powdered soy lecithin lowers cholesterol absorption and LDL levels.

Vitamins and Minerals

Vitamins play a key role in the metabolism of most nutrients. Light-skinned people obtain vitamin D—also known as the "sunshine vitamin"—through exposure to sunlight. People living more than 37 degrees south or north of the equator (roughly above Washington, DC) cannot make adequate vitamin D from sun exposure during winter months, even with sun exposure on the face, hands, and arms (Hemmelgarn, 2009). Additionally, people who use sunscreens in sunny climates and dark-skinned people may require a dietary source to meet daily requirements. Older adults and those who smoke also need added vitamin D because aging and smoking tend to impair vitamin D synthesis.

> *SAFETY ALERT*
>
> *Low levels of vitamin D may contribute to falls and fractures; cardiovascular, autoimmune, and infectious diseases; some cancers; Type 1 and Type 2 diabetes; and reduced muscle strength. Conversely, excessive intake of fat-soluble vitamins (vitamins A, E, D, and K) may result in toxicity because these vitamins are stored in adipose tissue (Hemmelgarn, 2009).*

Another important vitamin is folate, a B vitamin considered essential to metabolism and cell synthesis. Dietary sources of folate include leafy greens, lentils, seeds, liver, orange juice, grains, cereals, and breads fortified with folic acid. Groups at risk for folate deficiency include patients with alcoholism, older adults, those who follow popular diets, and people of low socioeconomic status.

> *SAFETY ALERT*
>
> *Adequate maternal intake of folate before conception and in the first trimester of pregnancy reduces the incidence of neural tube defects (e.g., spina bifida). The U.S. Public Health Service recommends that all women of childbearing age and capable of pregnancy consume 400 mg of synthetic folic acid daily from either foods or supplements (Centers for Disease Control [CDC], 2014).*

Vitamin B_{12} and folate need each other to be activated (Dudek, 2010). Vitamin B_{12} is the only water-soluble vitamin not found in plants. In addition to being involved in DNA synthesis and maintaining red blood cells, vitamin B_{12} plays an important role in maintaining the myelin sheath around nerves. Sources of vitamin B_{12} include beef, lamb, organ meats, shellfish, sardines, salmon, canned tuna, catfish, pike, whiting, milk, and other dairy products such as yogurt and cheese.

Three minerals deserve special consideration in a healthy diet, particularly for vegetarians: iron, zinc (trace element), and calcium (Craig, 2009). Iron and zinc are best absorbed from animal sources; therefore, vegetarians may need to increase their intake of iron and zinc from plant sources, eggs, and dairy products. Vitamin C is required for proper absorption of iron and to meet daily requirements for calcium. Vegetarian food guides recommend eight servings of calcium-rich foods daily, such as calcium-fortified orange juice or breakfast cereals and legumes or leafy greens.

Supplements

Patients may not mention taking food supplements, such as vitamins and herbal remedies, when questioned during a nutritional assessment. It is important for the nurse to ask the patient about food supplements because certain drug–herb interactions may be serious and life threatening (Woo, 2008).

Herbs and foods beginning with the letter "g" (e.g., garlic, ginger, ginkgo, grapefruit) are most commonly involved in herb–drug interactions. Drugs with anticoagulant/antiplatelet activity (e.g., warfarin, aspirin) are also frequently involved in herb–drug interactions, causing excessive bleeding. Because many herbs adversely affect the liver, a potential exists for interaction with hepatotoxic medications (e.g., acetaminophen). St. John's wort (*Hypericum perforatum*) reduces the effectiveness of many medications prescribed for heart disease, depression, seizures, some cancers, organ transplant rejection, and oral contraceptives. Fatalities (although rare) have occurred with concurrent ephedra (*Ephedra equisetina*) (also known as ma-huang) and caffeine use (Woo, 2008).

Fluid and Electrolytes

Water is essential to life. The adult body loses 1,500 to 2,800 ml/day of water through perspiration, exhalation, and excretion of urine and feces. The body requires a minimum fluid intake of 1,500 ml/day to maintain the excretion of metabolic wastes through urine and feces. However, extreme environmental temperatures, high altitude, low humidity, fever, and exercise increase water loss. Therefore, the recommended **adequate intake** of water varies depending on gender, age, air temperature, physical activity level, and state of health. Careful monitoring of intake and output is necessary in infants and older adults, particularly when vomiting, diarrhea, or fever is present, or when the patient has other disease processes that require close monitoring of intake and output. Other conditions characterized by high water losses include burns, fistulas, hemorrhage, uncontrolled diabetes, and some renal disorders (Dudek, 2010). Nurses caring for anyone requiring fluid and electrolyte adjustments are advised to seek additional evidence-based information to guide practice.

Sodium and potassium are major electrolytes. Sodium regulates fluid balance and cell permeability and thus the movement of fluid, electrolytes, glucose, insulin, and amino acids across cellular membranes. Sodium serves to regulate acid–base balance, nerve transmission, and muscular irritability (Dudek, 2010). Although there is no recommended daily intake for sodium, and wide variation exists between individuals and among cultures, an average North American consumes far more sodium than required for health. As people age, they become more "salt sensitive," and their risk of developing high blood pressure, coronary heart disease, and renal failure increases. Limiting salt intake can be difficult because approximately 75% of sodium consumed in the average diet comes from salt added by food manufacturers (Dudek, 2010).

Potassium is also implicated in regulating fluid and acid–base balance. In addition, it functions in the regulation of nerve impulse transmission, carbohydrate metabolism, protein synthesis, and skeletal muscle contractility. The recommended potassium intake for the average adult is 4.7 g/day; however, on average, North Americans consume only 2.1 to 3.2 g/day (Dudek, 2010). African Americans have a lower-than-average potassium intake, a high salt sensitivity, and an increased rate of hypertension. As a rule, an inverse relationship exists between sodium and potassium in food: processed foods, which are typically low in potassium, tend to be high in sodium, whereas fresh, unprocessed foods are typically low in sodium and high in potassium.

> **⚠ SAFETY ALERT**
>
> *Potassium levels must be maintained within a very narrow range. A potassium level outside of the normal range needs immediate correction. A potassium level that is too high or too low may cause cardiac rhythm changes or potentially fatal cardiac dysrhythmias.*

Many drugs commonly prescribed for people with chronic illnesses, such as cardiovascular disease or renal failure, interfere with electrolyte balance. Low-sodium or high-potassium foods (or the opposite) may be desirable for patients taking these medications. The nurse should consult reliable sources of information on food and drug interactions.

Food Safety and Food Security

Food-Borne Pathogens. Food safety has gained importance in the past decade. *Salmonella* in peanuts and *Listeria* in cheeses and processed meats are contemporary examples of food-borne pathogens affecting the health of large segments of the population. **Food pathogens** sometimes travel huge distances, making them difficult to trace, and thus compromising the health and safety of many people in a matter of days. Despite the best efforts of regulatory bodies and food inspection agencies striving to maintain food safety, food-borne pathogens are becoming increasingly problematic.

Organic Food. Amid a growing body of evidence showing the link between herbicide and pesticide use in agriculture and certain cancers, many people are seeking organic food sources. Furthermore, the public has also questioned the use of antibiotics and hormones in raising cattle, pork, and poultry. Increased production of genetically modified foods has also contributed to a move toward consuming organically grown foods from plant sources (Magana-Gomez & Calderon de la Barca, 2008).

Food Security. Similarly, public awareness of the issue of food security is increasing. Food sources have become highly centralized. Modern urban lifestyles discourage people from growing and processing their own food. Food sources are sometimes continents away from where foods are consumed, occasionally resulting in sudden unexpected food shortages. Global climatic and catastrophic events may interfere with water and food production and distribution. Under such circumstances, nurses may be called on to assist in reestablishing food security within communities. Nurses are sometimes also engaged in triage and advocacy to ensure that the most vulnerable segments of society are not forgotten.

Nutritional Guidelines

The USDHHS and the USDA jointly publish guidelines for healthy eating. These agencies revise the guidelines every 5 years to address emerging health issues based on current research pertaining to optimal nutrition. For example, the 2010 guidelines, for the first time, considered gender, age, and activity levels in dietary recommendations. Changes in recommendations are also aimed at promoting healthy eating habits and reducing obesity, hypertension, heart disease, cancer, and diabetes.

MyPlate emphasizes the need to select foods from each of the five food groups to meet individual requirements for health while reducing fats, sugars, and sodium (Fig. 7.1). The overall aim is to encourage individuals to make wiser food choices and control portion sizes.

Lifespan Considerations

Women Who Are Pregnant

Pregnant women and lactating women require special nutritional considerations for healthy outcomes for themselves and their infants. They need an additional 300 to 500 cal/day, with an emphasis on protein sources, such as milk and meat, to boost tissue building. Whole foods offer the best bioavailable sources of vitamins and minerals and should always be the first choice; however, under certain circumstances, vitamin and mineral supplementation may be required, especially to ensure that daily needs are met for vitamins A and C, folate, iron, calcium, and zinc.

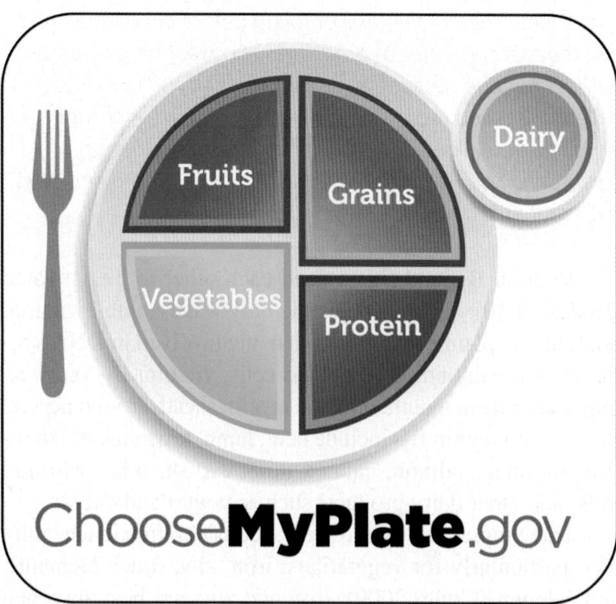

Figure 7.1 MyPlate reminds Americans to eat healthfully.

⚠ *SAFETY ALERT*

Women who do not meet nutritional requirements of pregnancy are at risk for having premature, low-birth-weight, or small-for-gestational-age infants. Their infants are also at higher risk for disabilities and congenital anomalies, including anencephaly, myelomeningocele, meningocele, oral facial cleft, structural heart disease, limb defect, urinary tract anomaly, and hydrocephalus (Dudek, 2010).

Infants, Children, and Adolescents

Ensuring dietary sources of essential amino acids from protein is critical for children because of their rapid growth (Pencharz, 2010). Additional protein is needed for tissue building in periods of rapid growth, such as adolescence. This is also the case when tissue damage occurs or during prolonged illness.

Infants, children, and adolescents require different nutrients based on developmental and growth factors. For example, fat intake is crucial to brain development in infants and young toddlers. Therefore, whole milk is recommended for children younger than 2 years of age.

Older Adults

Older adults also require special consideration during assessments of dietary requirements. Because of a diminished taste of sweet and salty foods, older adults may add sugar and salt to their diet at a time when they are at increased risk for diabetes, hypertension, and heart disease. Basal metabolic rate declines in older adults at the same time that their physical activity is reduced. When this occurs, caloric needs are significantly lower. Older adults are also at increased risk for malnutrition as a result of social isolation and depression related to loss of a companion or absence of family.

In addition, older adults may need vitamin D supplementation because of changes in nutrient metabolism, particularly when exposure to sunlight is reduced. Older people are advised to ensure adequate intake of vitamin D through dietary sources such as fortified milk and dairy products, fatty fish, and fortified cereals. Other nutrients not likely to be consumed in adequate amounts by older adults include calcium, folate, vitamin B_{12}, and riboflavin (Dudek, 2010).

Older adults may also experience a reduced sense of thirst, thereby increasing their risk for dehydration. They are also at increased risk for osteoarthritis, osteoporosis, dementia, and obesity. The diseases and disorders of older adulthood may increase the older adult's susceptibility to dubious claims made by manufacturers of pharmaceutical and nutritional supplements. Social isolation may further compound nutritional problems associated with aging.

Maintaining adequate nutrition is particularly problematic for people with reduced mobility and those receiving social assistance. These adults may lack the resources required to maintain a nutritious and appealing diet. Poor dentition may also be an issue. Missing teeth, gum disease, and poor-fitting dentures can detract from enjoyment of meals. Community programs such as Meals on Wheels offer food services to people with disabilities or chronic illnesses who live in social isolation.

Malnutrition and dehydration are also common among residents of long-term care facilities. Commercial supplements aimed at providing added protein and calories are not advisable over the long term (Dudek, 2010). Rather, the nurse should strive to make mealtimes as enjoyable as possible by encouraging both independent eating and family involvement. It is also advisable to adhere to the older adult's food preferences as much as possible and to maintain adequate hydration. Other recommendations for maintaining adequate nutrition among long-term care residents include providing clean, comfortable, pleasant surroundings; offering water; providing small, frequent meals; and minimizing distractions during meals. Refer to Box 7.1.

BOX 7.1 Factors That Affect Nutrition in the Older Adult

- Illness or chronic disease, including depression or dementia, which may alter nutrient needs or intake
- Excessive or inadequate intake of a limited variety of foods, with missing food groups, or compromised by alcohol
- Dental problems (e.g., missing or decayed teeth, poorly fitting dentures), which may lead to the avoidance of foods that are difficult to chew (e.g., fruits, vegetables, whole grains)
- Low economic status, which can compromise a food budget
- Social isolation. Older adults living alone are more likely to experience hunger than those in households with more than one older adult member.
- Use of three or more prescribed or over-the-counter daily medications. Drugs may affect nutritional status by altering appetite; ability to taste and smell; or digestion, absorption, metabolism, and excretion of nutrients. In addition, if a large percentage of a fixed income is spent on medications, less money is available for food.
- Significant unintentional weight loss (defined as 5% or more in 30 days, 10% or more in 180 days)
- Self-care deficits that may complicate food purchasing, food preparation, and eating
- Age older than 80 years

Adapted from Dudek, S. G. (2010). *Nutrition essentials for nursing practice* (6th ed.). Philadelphia, PA: Wolters Kluwer Health/Lippincott Williams & Wilkins.

Cultural Considerations

Food preferences are learned, and they vary depending on tradition, geography, education, income, and employment outside the home. Some cultural groups believe in the healing properties of foods, whereas others follow food restrictions during illness. It is important for nurses working with patients from different cultures to assess dietary habits. Box 7.2 outlines some items to consider.

Major U.S. cultural subgroups include Hispanics, African Americans, Asians, and Middle Easterners. Although each group shares certain eating practices, food choices vary widely within cultural subgroups. The nurse who recognizes that each culture has its own food standards— what is edible and what is not, how foods are prepared and when they are eaten, what role foods play in treating illness—is likely to avoid being ethnocentric when assessing nutritional status.

Additionally, food practices may be based on religious beliefs, such as fasting or abstaining from eating certain

BOX 7.2 Cultural Influences on Nutrition

- What foods are eaten during stress, trauma, or illness? To prevent illness?
- What are the common food preferences? Likes or dislikes?
- In what context is the food purchased, prepared, served, and eaten?
- What are the food nutrients, and what are acceptable versus prohibited foods?
- What are the accepted food combinations (e.g., hot and cold or milk and meat together)?
- How do foods facilitate communication and relationships within cultures?
- What geographic or environmental influences exist?

From Leininger, M. M., & McFarland, M. R. (2002). *Transcultural nursing: Concepts, theories, research, and practice* (3rd ed.). New York, NY: McGraw-Hill Professional.

foods. Some common restrictions include the following (Dudek, 2010):

- *Roman Catholic*: Avoid meat on Fridays, mainly during Lent (6 weeks preceding Easter).
- *Hindu*: Avoid beef, pork, and alcohol. Many are vegetarians.
- *Mormon*: Avoid coffee, tea, alcohol, and tobacco.
- *Seventh Day Adventist*: Many are lacto-ovo-vegetarians.
- *Judaism*: Eat only kosher meat and no shellfish; avoid consuming milk and meat in the same meal.
- *Islam*: Avoid pork and birds of prey. Fast during Ramadan.
- *Buddhism*: Many are lacto-ovo-vegetarians.

Collecting Nutritional Data

Collecting nutritional data is an ongoing process, partly because nutritional intake is an everyday activity. A patient may be seen in the primary care center or may enter hospital care with short- or long-term nutritional deficiencies (e.g., a person experiencing complications from cirrhosis). At least some malnutrition has been reported in up to 40% of hospitalized adults (Barker, Gout, & Crowe, 2011). Additionally, nutritional status seldom improves during hospitalization. Malnutrition may be generalized (targeted to specific nutrients), or it may exist in combination with obesity, cachexia, trauma, or aging.

The responsibility for screening patients to assess their level of nutritional risk and for reinforcing dietary counseling is often delegated to the nurse. The nurse's role in the nutritional assessment of patients is complex because of developmental, social, economic, and cultural factors. Nevertheless, nutrition screening is noninvasive, inexpensive, and easy to perform. Many examples of nutrition screening tools can be found through a simple internet search.

Parameters for a complete nutrition screening assessment include a risk assessment, focused history of common symptoms, comprehensive nutritional history, physical examination, calculated measurements, and serial laboratory values (especially during times of high metabolic demand, such as fever, pain, or infection, or during limited nutritional intake).

Urgent Assessment

Nutritional deficits are rarely acute; most of them develop over time. During trauma or stress, calorie needs increase. Stress factors that increase the risk for nutritional deficit include surgery, trauma, infection, head injury, and burns. Additionally, the patient may have reduced consciousness or injuries that make it difficult to take in nutrients. In acute illnesses, nutrition assessment and appropriate interventions should be addressed within days of the diagnosis.

Subjective Data

Areas for Health Promotion

Box 7.3 includes pertinent topics and interventions based on the World Health Organization's policy for countries with high levels of obesity. Prevention of obesity and promotion of healthy eating habits are the main focal areas for improving the health of people in developed nations. Children in developed countries are often at high risk for obesity, whereas many older adults are at high risk for poor nutrition.

Assessment of Risk Factors

An assessment of risk factors includes questions about past medical and surgical histories, medication and supplement use, family history, food and fluid intake patterns, and the patient's psychosocial profile (Dudek, 2010). If indicated, the nurse may follow up with a tested and valid tool for screening a specific population for risk factors.

BOX 7.3 World Health Organization Policy for Countries With High Obesity

- Promotion of breastfeeding
- Behavior change, communication, and/or counselling for improved complementary feeding
- Any supplementation to children
- Any supplementation to women or pregnant women
- Promotion of healthy nutrition through media (e.g., television, radio, newspapers, posters, websites)
- Measures to promote fruit and vegetable intakes
- Marketing of high-fat, energy dense, and/or micronutrient-poor foods
- Measures/initiatives to remove/reduce the salt content of processed foods
- Workplace-based intervention programs
- Measures/initiatives to remove/reduce trans fatty acids from processed foods
- Measures to affect food prices (e.g., high fat, salt, sugary products)
- Vending machines not allowed on school premises

From World Health Organization. (2014). *Nutrition*. Retrieved from http://www.who.int/nutrition/en/

History and Risk Factors	Rationale
Medical History Do you have a medical condition such as diabetes or hypertension?	Medical conditions such as diabetes and hypertension increase the risk of nutritional deficits. Patients with these conditions may benefit from nutrition therapy.
Do you have, or have you recently had, fever, sepsis, thermal injuries, skin breakdown, cancer, AIDS, major surgery, or trauma?	These conditions increase nutritional needs.
Do you have, or have you recently had, malabsorption or certain renal diseases?	These conditions lead to loss of nutrients; special attention to increased nutritional requirements is necessary.
Weight History Do you have a history of any concerns related to nutrition or weight?	Being underweight, overweight, or obese influences self-perception related to health. Asking about the patient's self-perception can be challenging, particularly when the body is visibly outside expected limits (e.g., if the patient is anorexic or obese). If the patient's self-perception is distorted or inaccurate, it is important to know that in order to address the issue. The main causes of malnutrition in the United States are poverty, alcoholism, hospitalization, aging, and eating disorders. Other risk factors for malnutrition are poor dentition, chronic illness, multiple medications, social isolation, severe burns, and lack of knowledge. Risk factors commonly associated with overweight and obesity include excessive intake of high-calorie foods, typically high in fat and sugar; not enough exercise; alcohol abuse; and lack of knowledge.
Appetite and Taste Changes • Have you noticed any changes in your ability to smell? In the taste of food? If so, what are the changes? • How would you rate your appetite? • How does food taste to you?	Senses of taste and smell decrease with aging. Additionally, some medications alter taste and smell. For example, amiodarone, a medication to regulate the heart rhythm, causes food to taste like garlic.
Gastrointestinal Symptoms. Have you ever been diagnosed with a gastrointestinal or other disease that affects nutrition, such as anorexia, heartburn, nausea, diarrhea, vomiting, or pain?	Gastrointestinal diseases may impair appetite and also reduce the absorption of nutrients.
Food Allergy or Intolerance. Have you ever been diagnosed with a food intolerance or allergy?	Be aware of the difference between food intolerance (symptoms include nausea, bloating, and flatulence) and food allergy (symptoms include hives, wheezing, and anaphylaxis). Food allergies and intolerances must also be considered when evaluating risk factors for malnutrition because they affect food choices. Patients intolerant to lactose, for example, need sources other than dairy products for calcium. Common food allergens include milk, eggs, soy, peanuts, other nuts (e.g., cashews, almonds), wheat, fish, and shellfish (Dudek, 2010).
Family History Do you have a family history of gastrointestinal or other diseases that influence your nutrition? • Who had the illness? • What was the illness? • When did the person have it? • How was the illness treated? • What were the outcomes?	Determine whether there is a family history of problems such as Crohn disease, Type 2 diabetes, cystic fibrosis, or anemia. Be respectful of cultural food patterns and preferences. Gather information on the patient's family history of obesity, cancer, heart disease, and atherosclerosis, which may be useful in developing a nutrition plan.

(table continues on page 142)

History and Risk Factors	Rationale
Food and Fluid Intake Patterns ***Eating Patterns.*** Describe a typical day's eating (include content and amount of meals, meal times, and snacking patterns). • Are you on a special diet? If so, please describe it. • Are there times of the day when you feel hungry? If so, when? What is satisfying? Are there particular foods that you like? Dislike? If so, please describe them. • Are any foods or food habits important to you? If so, please describe them. • Who shares your mealtimes?	Food habits and intake patterns may vary according to culture, religion, and region. Because variation is wide, it is important to obtain a history for the individual patient.
Fluid Intake Patterns • How much fluid do you drink each day? (How many glasses and approximate size of glass?) • Are there particular fluids that you like? Dislike? • Are there certain times of the day when you drink or refrain from drinking fluids?	Fluid intake may be in excess of needs, causing fluid volume excess. Low fluid intake may cause a fluid volume deficit, or dehydration.
• How much coffee, tea, and chocolate- or caffeine-containing beverages do you usually drink in a day? If you do not have any caffeine for a few days, how do you feel (e.g., headache, nausea, other sensations)?	Consumption of a large amount of unfiltered coffee, such as using a French press, may increase LDL levels and the risk for miscarriage (van Dam, 2008).
Psychosocial Profile ***Habits*** • Does stress affect your eating or drinking habits? If so, please describe. • Does smoking affect your appetite? If so, describe.	Some patients gain weight with stress, whereas others lose weight. Smoking impairs senses of smell and taste.
Cooking Ability • Who does your food shopping? • Do you have a food budget? If so, could you describe it? • How often do you eat out? Who prepares your food? • Does food preparation provide a source of enjoyment for you? • Could you describe your food preparation facilities?	Functional limitations influence the ability to obtain or prepare food. The nutrition–metabolic pattern involves more than just the nutrients ingested each day. It encompasses aspects such as culture, religion, and geography; food and fluid preferences and dislikes; patterns of eating, digestion, and allergies; shopping resources and skills; kitchen facilities and food preparation; the meaning of food and feeding; social patterns at meals; and gastrointestinal structures, including dentition. Such information aids in individualizing actions, assisting patients to modify current eating practices and adopting new eating patterns in everyday life. Knowing what roles a patient plays in groups can aid in prioritizing health problems that relate to the gastrointestinal system. For example, if a patient has primary food preparation responsibilities, he or she may need to relinquish them temporarily or permanently. Should major roles change, the patient will need to be able to assume other roles deemed equally important to maintain a contributing role with the group.
Dietary Lifestyle Changes • Do environmental or social factors affect your ability to make dietary changes? • Do you feel that you have sufficient resources to support healthy nutritional intake?	Many social functions revolve around food. If a patient's signs, symptoms, or treatments disrupt these social functions, social isolation can occur. Asking about such possibilities can be important when assessing a patient's overall health.
Medications and Supplements ***Medication Schedule*** • What system or systems have you developed to ensure an accurate schedule for your medications? • Are there particular reminders or methods that are helpful for you? If so, please describe them.	A medication history is included because diet and food intake affect medications. For example, dark green leafy foods can decrease the effect of some anticoagulants.

(table continues on page 143)

History and Risk Factors	Rationale
Barriers to Accuracy. Have you experienced any difficulty in getting or taking your medicines as they have been prescribed? If so, please describe.	Remembering to take medications requires intact memory and cognitive skills. If there is any difficulty, the nurse may obtain a Medi-Set pill organizer, which has small compartments for medications labeled with times of the day.
Adverse Effects. When do you tend to report any adverse effects of your medicines? As soon as you notice? When things get really bad for you? Only when they interfere with what you need to do? Never?	Patterns of health-seeking behavior vary widely. Some patients visit the provider for health promotion, whereas others defer care until a medical emergency occurs or when critically ill.
Resources for Medication-Related Information • From whom have you received most of your medication information? TV, relatives, neighbors, books, magazines, pharmacist, health store personnel, doctor, nurse, nurse practitioner, others? • Do you ask questions about your medicines? Do you expect that people helping you with medicines will give you needed information?	Nurses can provide patients with resources for medication information. It is important to teach patients to inform their providers of adverse effects, financial concerns, or other health beliefs that affect the ability to take medications as prescribed. An alternative plan can then be developed collaboratively with patients.
Supplements. Do you take any vitamin, mineral, or other nutritional supplements? If so, describe the substance, amount, and frequency.	Approximately one third of patients use some type of supplement; it is important to monitor for adverse effects and drug–supplement interactions.
Alcohol and Drug Use • How much alcohol do you drink? • Do you feel that you are a "normal" drinker? (By normal, I mean that you drink less than, or as much as, most other people.) • *If the patient does drink:* How much did you drink yesterday? Is that about usual for you? When did you take your last drink (date and hour)? What is your usual pattern for alcohol intake? If you do not have a drink for a few days, how do you feel? Have you ever gone through alcohol withdrawal? If so, when, and describe the circumstances. Do you go into delirium tremens (DT) if you do not drink for a few days? (See Chapter 9 for the CAGE questionnaire.) • Could you tell me about your drug use? (Ask about the substance and quantity after each question.) Do you smoke marijuana? Do you use, or have you used, other's prescription drugs? Sleeping pills? Downers? Uppers? Speed? Ritalin? Cocaine? Meth? Do you use, or have you ever used, hallucinogens? (Have you ever "tripped"?)	Alcohol can adversely affect the liver and its multiple functions, including protein synthesis. In addition, chronic alcohol exposure can injure the stomach and pancreas. Lack of the digestive enzymes produced by the pancreas can impair the absorption of nutrients, including fats. Alcohol intake can affect the metabolism of nutrients as well as alter the overall nutrient density of the diet. It is common for patients with a high alcohol intake to be deficient in the B vitamins and vitamin K.

Risk Assessment and Health-Related Patient Teaching

Nurses promote healthy nutrition in all settings including health fairs, schools, clinics, and hospitals. Patients often are interested in nutrition as a way to improve their health. Nurses can teach about the MyPlate guidelines for increasing the intake of fruits and vegetables and decreasing the intake of foods with low nutrient density. Patients can be taught to read food labels, especially when the intake of a nutrient needs to be limited because of dietary restrictions, such as a low-salt diet. When patients are placed on restricted diets, teaching must be performed. Many organizations, such as the American Diabetes Association, have helpful written materials to reinforce such teaching.

Focused Health History Related to Common Symptoms

Common Symptoms of Altered Nutrition

- Sudden or gradual changes in body weight
- Changes in eating habits
- Changes in skin, hair, or nails
- Decreased energy level

Signs/Symptoms	Rationale/Abnormal Findings
Changes in Body Weight What is your present height and weight? How do these compare with your height and weight 5 years ago? Have there been any changes in your weight over the past year? If so, please describe. How do you feel about your present weight?	Weight can change or remain stable with illness. A patient taking steroids may gain weight, whereas a patient undergoing cancer treatment may lose weight if nauseous or anorexic. Eating disorders, such as anorexia nervosa and bulimia nervosa, can profoundly affect nutritional health. Typically, patients with anorexia nervosa are preoccupied with distorted perceptions of themselves as fat when they are emaciated. They feel "fat" despite being underweight.
Change in Eating Habits Have you experienced a change in a regular diet pattern (number, size, and contents of meals)?	If yes, investigate potential causes (e.g., change in appetite, mental status, or mood; ability to prepare meals; ability to chew or swallow; nausea or vomiting). Patients with eating disorders reduce the size and content of meals or may binge and then purge.
Symptoms of Malnutrition • Have you noticed any changes in your hair, nails, and skin? If so, describe. • Would you say that you heal well? Poorly? Otherwise? Do you have any difficulty tolerating hot or cold weather?	Skin, hair, and nails are indicators of nutritional status because those cells turn over rapidly. Thin or brittle hair, thin skin, skin that bruises easily or flakes, and weak or brittle nails are typical symptoms of malnutrition.
• How much energy would you say that you have? • Has your energy level changed recently—for example, during the past year? If so, describe. See Box 7.4 for other symptoms of malnutrition.	A malnourished person lacks energy.

Comprehensive Nutritional History

If, after assessing risk factors and common symptoms, data reveal the patient to be at risk for altered nutrition, the nurse takes a comprehensive nutritional history. Commonly used tools include food records, food frequency questionnaires, and direct observations.

Food Records

Food records are integral to nutritional assessment. To ensure accurate and complete data collection, records ought to include all food supplements and drinks consumed over a specified period, including the amount and times they were consumed.

24-Hour Recall. A 24-hour recall consists of asking the patient what he or she had to eat and drink within a **24-hour** period. The nurse collects information from patients and their families without appearing judgmental (Fig. 7.2). He or she uses open-ended questions such as, "Tell me the first thing that you ate yesterday," or "When was the first time you ate or drank anything yesterday?" The nurse continues by asking,

BOX 7.4 Physical Signs and Symptoms Suggestive of Malnutrition

- Hair that is dull, brittle, dry, or falls out easily
- Swollen glands of the neck and cheeks
- Dry, rough, or spotty skin that may have a sandpaper feel
- Poor or delayed wound healing or sores
- Thin appearance with lack of subcutaneous fat
- Muscle wasting (decreased size and strength)
- Edema of the lower limbs
- Weakened hand grasp
- Depressed mood
- Abnormal heart rate, heart rhythm, or blood pressure
- Enlarged liver or spleen
- Loss of balance and coordination

From Dudek, S. G. (2010). *Nutrition essentials for nursing practice* (6th ed.). Philadelphia, PA: Wolters Kluwer Health/Lippincott Williams & Wilkins.

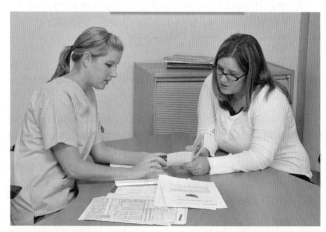

Figure 7.2 The nurse is reviewing a patient's food intake using the 24-hour recall method.

"Did you have anything else to eat or drink at the time?" and then "What was the next thing you had to eat or drink?"

With this method, the patient tends to overestimate low intakes and underestimate high intakes. To control this tendency, it is important for the nurse to use prompts such as "golf ball size" or "the size of your fist or thumb." Life-size models and digital images of various foods can also be useful in eliciting accurate portion estimates. Also, the nurse cues the patient to include beverages or condiments (e.g., "Did you have anything on the toast?"). It is important for the nurse to remember to ask about fortified foods, such as fruit juices and cereals fortified with calcium; other food supplements; and alcohol.

The 24-hour recall is reliable only if the patient or family can recall the type and amount of food eaten. Additionally, the intake over the past 24 hours may not be typical; for example, foods eaten on a weekend may differ from those eaten during the week. Therefore, the 24-hour recall is usually most complete and accurate when the nurse obtains a recall for both a weekday and a weekend day.

Three-Day Food Diary. To increase accuracy, the nurse may repeat diet recalls, stagger them through several health assessments, or have the patient keep a **3-day food diary**. The diary shifts most of the responsibility for data collection from the nurse to the patient. It is best for the patient to write down the intake immediately after eating. This record does not rely on memory, but the patient may consciously alter the diet during recording. It also is time consuming. For at-risk patients, an analysis of dietary intake is carried out in combination with weight, observation of signs and symptoms of poor nutrition, and consideration of laboratory values that reflect malnutrition.

Food Frequency Questionnaires. **Food frequency questionnaires** help assess the intake of certain required foods for special situations (e.g., calcium or folate in pregnancy). Nurses use these questionnaires to track the frequency of intake of a certain food or foods over time, such as each day, week, or month. Food frequency questionnaires are quick and are often combined with the 24-hour recall. They require accurate reporting and intact memory (Fig. 7.3).

Direct Observation

With hospitalized patients, it is possible to directly observe the amount and types of food they eat. Commonly, nurses describe intake as a percentage of the meal eaten, such as 50% of breakfast or 75% of dinner. When inadequate intake is suspected, the nurse can count the calories. The nurse records the percentage of each food eaten and the dietician performs a **calorie count** based on what is consumed. If intake is inadequate, the patient may need supplements such as high-calorie shakes.

Intake and Output. Documentation of **intake and output** is required to assess the adequacy of food and fluid intake and to comply with agency recommendations. In particular, documentation is required for nutrition support patients, including those on strict intake and output orders. Additionally, the nurse monitors the fluid intake and output for patients receiving intravenous fluids or for those at risk for fluid volume excess or deficit.

The nurse totals all the fluids taken in, both orally and intravenously. Some patients, such as those with fluid overload or renal disease, may have a fluid restriction. It is necessary to know how much each cup or container holds in order to document the totals.

The nurse totals the output by measuring urine output, drainage from tubes or drains, and emesis (vomiting). Many medical containers—such as emesis basins, urinals, and urinary containers (known as "hats") that are inserted into the toilet—are premarked with milliliter indications. Patients with drains, wounds, burns, or severe diarrhea need to have outputs closely monitored.

Calorie Count. Calorie count must be monitored for some patients, such as those on tube feeding or those weaning off of nutrition support, in order to determine the need for additional nutrition support. The nurse records the percentage of each food item eaten. This includes food provided by others or eaten off of the unit, any supplements, and any snacks or items removed from the patient's tray to be eaten at a later time. A physician's or registered dietician's order is typically required for a calorie count; the nurse's role is the documentation of the intake. A dietician uses this information to calculate intake versus estimated needs.

Nutrition Questionnaire

During the past 4 weeks, how often did you eat a serving of the foods listed here?

Mark only one ✗ for each food

	Last 4 weeks		Each week			Each day			
Number of times	0	1–3	1	2–4	5–6	1	2–3	4–5	6+
Milk						✗			
Hot chocolate	✗								
Cheese, plain or in sandwiches				✗					
Yogurt	✗								
Ice cream		✗							
	0	1	2	3	4	5	6	7	8

Figure 7.3 An example of a food frequency questionnaire.

Additional Questions	Rationale/Abnormal Findings
Older Adults What medications are you taking?	Patients taking medications or those with diseases that create less saliva or have xerostomia (dry mouth) are more likely to have problems with taste.
Use a screening tool to evaluate the risk of malnutrition in the older adult (Table 7.1).	Financial and transportation issues can limit access to nutritional foods. Functional abilities or sensory losses can affect the ability to physically prepare nutritious foods. Early cognitive losses that impair judgment, planning, foresight, or sequencing of complex tasks may reduce the ability to follow recipes or prepare complete meals. Recent weight loss can cause dentures to fit poorly and interfere with chewing.

Therapeutic Dialogue: Collecting Subjective Data

Remember Karen Pitoci, the 15-year-old girl receiving home care following hospitalization for anorexia nervosa. The home health nurse is collecting data to assess the patient's health. The nurse uses professional communication techniques to gather subjective data from Karen. The nurse is interviewing the patient to obtain a 24-hour diet recall.

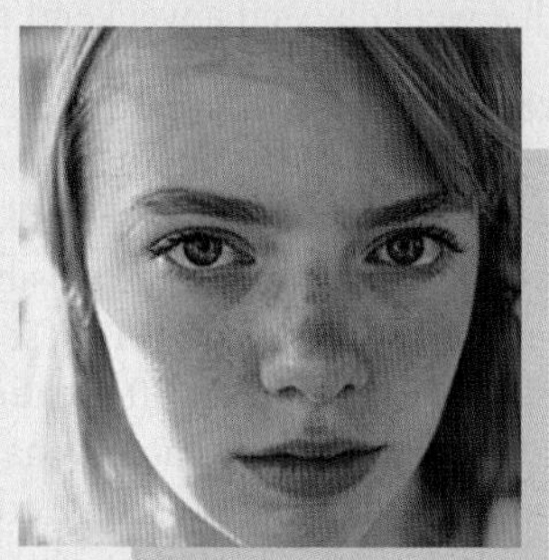

Nurse: So, Karen, tell me the first thing that you ate yesterday.

Karen: Some fruit.

Nurse: What kind of fruit was it?

Karen: A grapefruit.

Nurse: And did you have anything else with the grapefruit?

Karen: I had a yogurt.

Nurse: And was it the light yogurt or regular?

Karen: Light.

Nurse: How much of the yogurt did you eat?

Karen: (Silent, looks at mother)

Mrs. Pitoci: She only ate half of it.

Nurse: And did you have anything to drink with it?

Karen: Some water.

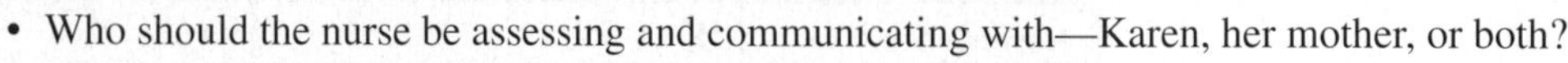

Critical Thinking Challenge

- Who should the nurse be assessing and communicating with—Karen, her mother, or both?
- What subjective and psychosocial data will the nurse collect?
- How will the nurse assess Karen's current nutritional status using objective data?
- What adaptations will the nurse make to the assessment based on the patient's condition?

TABLE 7.1 Tools to Evaluate Risk of Malnutrition in the Older Adult

Tool	Description	Validity and Reliability
Mininutritional assessment	Perception of health, global assessment, questions about diet, and anthropometric measurements	Widely validated, predictive of poor outcomes
Simplified nutrition assessment questionnaire	Four-item screening tool	Highly sensitive and specific for those at risk for greater than 10% weight loss
Screen II	Seventeen-item tool that evaluates food intake, chewing, swallowing, weight change, and social or functional barriers	High sensitivity and specificity, interrater reliability, and test–retest reliability
Malnutrition universal screening tool	Includes anorexia, disease, body mass index, and percentage of weight loss	Particularly sensitive for undernutrition in hospitalized patients
Determine	Ten-item checklist to increase the awareness of nutritional risk	Commonly used but criticized for lack of validity; more useful to promote nutrition awareness than to detect malnutrition

From Ritchie, C., Schmader, K. E., Lipman, T. O., & Sokol, N. (2009). *Geriatric nutrition: Nutritional issues in older adults.* Retrieved from http://www.uptodateonline.com.proxy.seattleu.edu/online/content/topic.do?topicKey=geri_med/8473&selectedTitle=1~150&source=search_result

Objective Data

Collecting objective data for a mininutritional assessment includes calculating body mass index (BMI) and percentage of weight change. Findings will determine the need for further anthropometric measurements and laboratory tests.

Equipment Needed

- Scale
- Measuring tape
- Growth charts (for children)
- Skin calipers

Preparation

Completing a physical assessment in a hospital, nursing home, or community setting may be embarrassing, especially for overweight or underweight patients. The nurse should reassure the patient of confidentiality and proceed with the examination in a straightforward, nonjudgmental manner while ensuring patient privacy and dignity. The table lists common versus specialty techniques for nurses related to nutritional assessment.

Common and Specialty Techniques

Objective assessment of the nutritional status of the patient is a multidisciplinary effort. The registered nurse (RN) assesses the patient's physical status, including skin color and texture,

Basic Versus Focused/Advanced Techniques in Nutrition

Technique	Purpose	Basic or Screening Assessment	Focused or Advanced Examination
Inspect physical status.	To take a general survey	X	
Look for signs and symptoms of malnutrition.	To assess if the patient appears well or poorly nourished	X	
Review for any weight change.	To determine if weight loss is significant	X	
Measure body mass index.	To compare weight to height to determine underweight or overweight status	X	
Take weight-for-height calculations.	To compare weight against national standards	X	
Measure waist circumference.	To determine cardiovascular risk with central obesity		X Cardiovascular risk
Measure triceps skinfold.	To calculate fat stores		X Fat stores
Measure MAMC.	To calculate fat and muscle stores		X Fat and muscle stores

hair color and texture, nail beds, and overall physical appearance. The RN also assesses the patient for signs and symptoms of malnutrition. In addition, the RN assesses the patient for any recent intentional or unintentional weight loss and calculates the BMI based on height and weight calculations gained throughout the collection of data.

The advanced practice registered nurse (APRN) continues the assessment of the patient's nutritional status by measuring waist circumference, triceps skinfold, and mid upper arm muscle circumference (MAMC).

These same measurements may also be taken by a registered dietician (RD), thus making this assessment a multidisciplinary effort. If the assessment is completed solely by the RN and APRN, referral to a nutritionist or an RD may be warranted based on the findings.

Technique and Normal Findings	Abnormal Findings
Body Type Observe body type, which is noted as small build, average build, or large build. *A wide variety of body types fall within the normal range.*	Morbidity and mortality are linked to poor diet and sedentary lifestyle with associated obesity. Obesity is a growing concern. Malnutrition is an issue in developing countries.
Note that muscle tone and mass decrease with age. *Aging also causes fat distribution to change: fat is lost from the face and neck, whereas it tends to increase in the arms, abdomen, and hips.*	Lack of subcutaneous fat with prominent bones, abdominal ascites, and pitting edema are abnormal findings. Amenorrhea is a cardinal symptom of eating disorders. Other physical consequences of eating disorders, such as cardiac failure or muscle wasting, can be fatal. **Cachexia** is a highly catabolic state with accelerated muscle loss and a chronic inflammatory response. In this syndrome, which is distinct from anorexia nervosa, production of proinflammatory cytokines contribute to the breakdown of fat and muscle protein, causing loss of both muscle mass and fat stores (Jatoi, Loprinzi, Hesketh, & Savarese, 2009). These inflammatory mediators accelerate inflammation, increase the production of C-reactive protein, and reduce albumin levels. Cachexia is common with cancer, hyperthyroidism, and AIDS and is difficult to treat.
General Appearance Observe general appearance. *A healthy adult appears energetic and alert, with erect stature. Skin, hair, and nails look healthy.*	Clinical findings of malnutrition can occur in many places throughout the body (see Table 7.4). Visible signs include muscle wasting, particularly in the temporal area, and muscle weakness; tongue atrophy; and bleeding or changes in the integrity or hydration status of the skin, hair, teeth, gums, lips, tongue, eyes, and, in men, genitalia (Bellini, Parsons, Lipman, & Wilson, 2009). See also Box 7.4. Malnutrition is less common than obesity in developed countries, but it can lead to poor health outcomes, including growth retardation, compromised immunity, poor wound healing and muscle loss, and physical and functional decline.
Swallowing Observe the patient's ability to swallow. *Swallowing is smooth, with no problems with the ingestion of food.* Observe if the patient has any of the following: • Difficulty staying awake for 15 minutes • Difficulty sitting upright for 15 minutes • Weak voice and cough (hoarse, strained, breathy, or wet) • Drooling • Slurred/unclear speech • Difficulty swallowing • Facial or tongue weakness/deviation • Prolonged intubation (more than 48 hours), or difficult intubation or extubation	Difficulty swallowing, known as **dysphagia**, is common in stroke and neuromuscular diseases. *SAFETY ALERT* *The patient is at risk for aspiration of secretions into the lungs and potential pneumonia. He or she should be placed on aspiration precautions, kept on nothing by mouth, and swallowing evaluations should be performed.*

(table continues on page 149)

Technique and Normal Findings (continued)	Abnormal Findings (continued)
Elimination Inspect urine, emesis, and stool. See Chapter 20.	Emesis refers to vomited contents from the gastrointestinal tract. The amount should be described and measured.
Body Mass Index **Body mass index (BMI)** is a guide for maintaining ideal **weight for height**. It is also used as a benchmark for obesity or protein–caloric malnutrition. BMI calculation is nonthreatening, noninvasive, and inexpensive. It has one major limitation: BMI can be elevated from large muscles or edema rather than from excess fat. Calculate BMI as follows: BMI = weight in kilograms OR weight in pounds ÷ height in meters squared (m^2) OR height in inches squared (in^2) × 703. BMI of 18.5–24.9 is healthy or normal.	BMI less than 18.5 or greater than 24.9 is abnormal and a health risk (Table 7.2). Adults with a BMI less than 17.5 or children and adolescents with a BMI less than the 5th percentile meet the criteria for an eating disorder.
Weight Calculations Among the most commonly used reference standards for height and weight are the Metropolitan Life Insurance Tables (Build Study, 1979). These were made available in 1959 and have not yet been revised. They are still used, although BMI is a preferred measure.	In theory, elbow width or wrist width correlates fairly well with muscle and bone mass.
Percentage of Ideal Body Weight. The **percentage of ideal body** weight is based on the ideal and current weight: Percentage of ideal body weight = current weight/ideal weight × 100. This calculation is valuable for assessing underweight but not overweight.	Mild malnutrition: 80%–90% of ideal weight Moderate malnutrition: 70%–80% of ideal weight Severe malnutrition: Less than 70% of ideal weight

TABLE 7.2 Classification of Overweight and Obesity by Body Mass Index, Waist Circumference, and Associated Disease Risks

			Disease Risk* Relative to Normal Weight and Waist Circumference†	
	BMI (kg/m^2)	Obesity Class	*Men 102 cm (40 in.) or Less Women 88 cm (35 in.) or Less*	*Men Greater Than 102 cm (40 in.) Women Greater Than 88 cm (35 in.)*
Underweight	Less than 18.5	—	—	
Normal	18.5–24.9	—	—	
Overweight	25.0–29.9		Increased	High
Obesity	30.0–34.9	I	High	Very high
	35.0–39.9	II	Very high	Very high
Extreme obesity	40.0+	III	Extremely high	Extremely high

*Disease risk for Type 2 diabetes, hypertension, and cardiovascular disease.
†Increased waist circumference can also be a marker for increased risk even in patients of normal weight.
From National Heart, Lung, and Blood Institute. (2009). *Classification of overweight and obesity by BMI, waist circumference, and associated disease risks.* Retrieved from http://www.nhlbi.nih.gov/health/public/heart/obesity/lose_wt/bmi_dis.htm

(table continues on page 150)

Technique and Normal Findings (continued)	Abnormal Findings (continued)
Percentage of Weight Change. Carefully assess the circumstances surrounding any change in weight to determine the cause. Cluster weight change data with other data to analyze whether the weight change is related to fluid, muscle mass, or fat stores. After collecting the usual weight from the history and current weight on a scale (see Chapter 5), calculate the **percent weight change** (percentage loss of usual weight) as follows: (usual weight – present weight) ÷ usual weight × 100 This calculation is valuable for assessing weight loss and malnutrition.	The following guidelines indicate significant weight loss: • 1%–2% in 1 week • 5% in 1 month • 7.5% in 3 months • 10% in 6 months (Dudek, 2010) Unintentional weight gain or loss is a significant finding. It may be caused by a change in fluid volume, such as in heart or kidney failure, or by a change in nutritional status. Weight gain may result from metabolic issues, such as hypothyroidism.
Percentage of Usual Body Weight Another calculation can be made based on the current and usual weight. The **percentage of usual weight** is calculated as follows: Percentage of usual body weight = current weight/usual weight × 100 This calculation is valuable for assessing weight loss and malnutrition.	Mild malnutrition: 85%–95% of usual body weight Moderate malnutrition: 75%–84% of usual body weight Severe malnutrition: Less than 75% of usual body weight
Waist Circumference Where fat is deposited on the body is a more reliable indicator of disease risk than the amount of fat deposited in the body. Use **waist circumference** to evaluate the amount of abdominal fat in men and women.	Waist circumference greater than 40 in. (102 cm) in men or greater than 35 in. (89 cm) in women increases the risk for chronic illness associated with adiposity (National Heart, Lungs, and Blood Institute [NHLBI], 2009). See Table 7.2.
The patient should stand straight with the feet together and arms hanging at the sides. Place the tape measure around the waist at the umbilicus. Have the patient take a normal breath and record the measurement when the patient breathes out (Fig. 7.4). 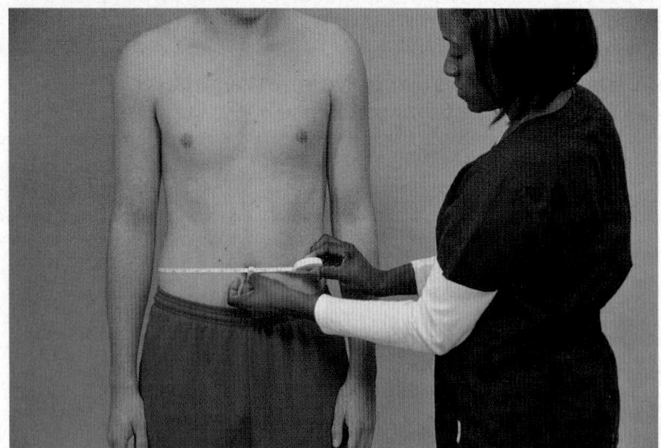 **Figure 7.4** Measuring the waist circumference.	The accumulation of abdominal body fat significantly increases the risk for Type 2 diabetes, hypertension, and cardiovascular disease. Waist measurement provides information about morbidity and relative risk of disease (NHLBI, 2009).

(table continues on page 151)

Technique and Normal Findings (continued)	Abnormal Findings (continued)
Waist-to-Hip Ratio Assess waist-to-hip ratio to determine body fat distribution as an indicator of risk to health. The waist-to-hip ratio is calculated as follows: Waist-to-hip ratio = waist circumference ÷ hip circumference (largest point). Note: Waist circumference measurement has largely replaced waist-to-hip ratio because it is easier and more accurate to measure (Bray, Xavier-Pi-Sunyer, & Martin, 2009).	A waist-to-hip ratio greater than or equal to 1.0 in men or greater than 0.8 in women indicates upper body (android) obesity, which puts the patient at risk for increased mortality and heart attack (NHLBI, 2009).
Skinfold Thickness Skinfold thickness is a measurement used to indicate subcutaneous fat reserves. It requires an experienced person using a reliable caliper at the correct standardized locations on the body. If this measurement is inaccurate, data will be misleading. Measurements of skinfold thickness are much less accurate than measurements of height or weight, especially in obese patients. Thus, it has little practical clinical value unless performed by the same person over a period of time to evaluate trends (Bray, et al., 2009). An RD usually takes this measurement. Measure the skinfold thickness at the triceps, subscapular, biceps, and suprailiac areas. Although the triceps is the most common area used, it does not accurately represent the adipose tissue of the entire body. For the **triceps skinfold** (TSF) measurement: • Locate the mid upper arm point with the arm at 90 degrees. • Use the fingers to gently grasp and pull away a vertical fold of the skin from the muscle (Fig. 7.5A). • Apply the calipers at a right angle to the midpoint. • Apply pressure on the calipers until the spring-loaded level is depressed completely (see Fig. 7.5B). • Take three readings 3 seconds apart and average the values. Normal findings are according to standardized tables that adjust for age and gender (Frisancho, 1981).	Patients above the 95th or below the 5th percentile are at risk for altered nutritional status.

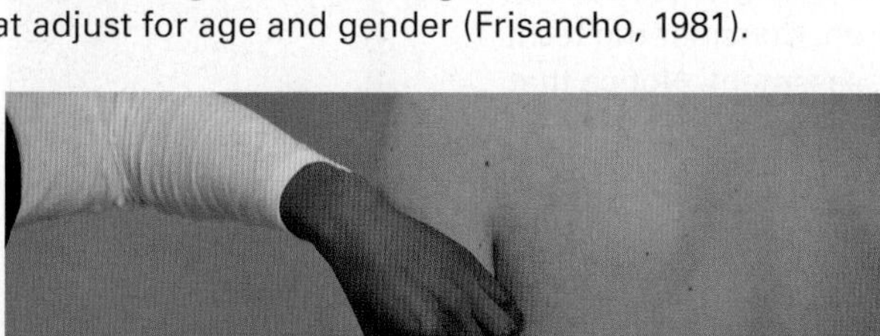

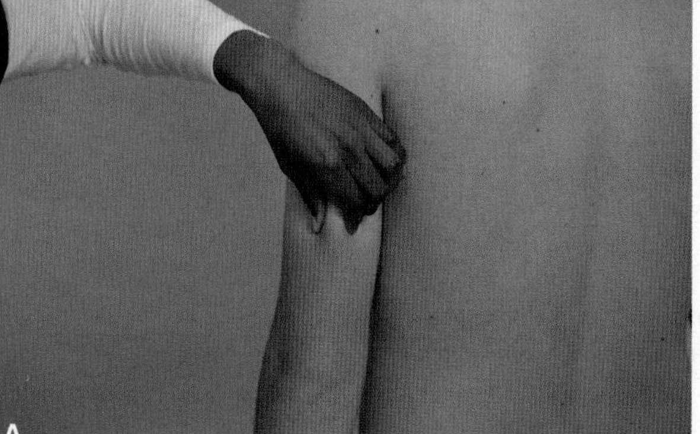

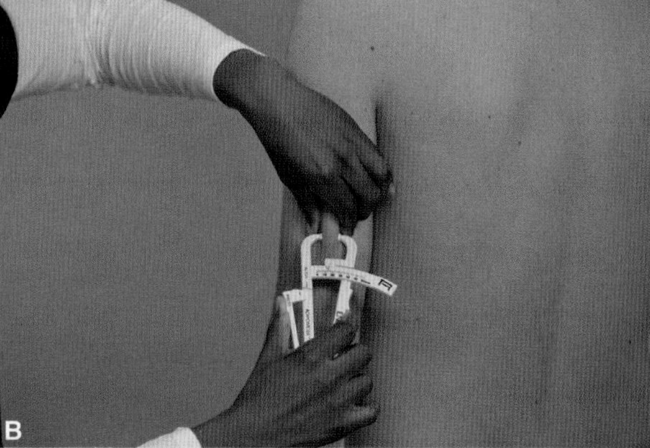

Figure 7.5 Measuring the skinfold thickness. **A.** Gently grasp and pull away a vertical fold of the skin from the muscle. **B.** With the calipers at a right angle to midpoint, apply pressure on the calipers until the spring-loaded level is depressed completely.

(table continues on page 152)

Technique and Normal Findings (continued)	Abnormal Findings (continued)
Mid Upper Arm Muscle Circumference The **MAMC** is an indirect measurement of bone, muscle area, and fat reserves. Measure around the arm, midway between the elbow and the shoulder (Fig. 7.6). 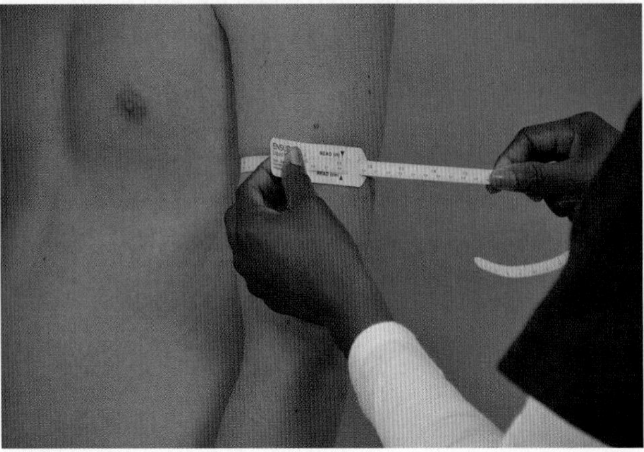 **Figure 7.6** Measuring the mid upper arm muscle circumference around the arm, midway between the elbow and the shoulder.	Findings below the 10th percentile are abnormal, indicating loss of muscle. Trends that decrease over time are also significant.
Derived Measures (using MAMC and TSF) The **MAMC and the mid upper arm muscle area (MAMA)** are indicators of muscle and body protein reserves. MAMC = Mid arm circumference (MAC) − ($\pi \times$ TSF) MAMA = (MAC − MAMC)$^2 \div 4\pi$ A higher number indicates more muscle. These findings are compared to charts with normal values.	Findings below the 10th percentile are abnormal, indicating loss of muscle. Trends that decrease over time are also significant.

Progress Note: Analyzing Findings

The home health nurse has just completed the physical examination of Karen Pitoci, the 15-year-old girl with anorexia nervosa. Review the following important findings revealed in each of the steps of data collection for Karen. Consider the techniques of subjective and objective data collected during the assessment. Notice that the objective data include findings from several body systems.

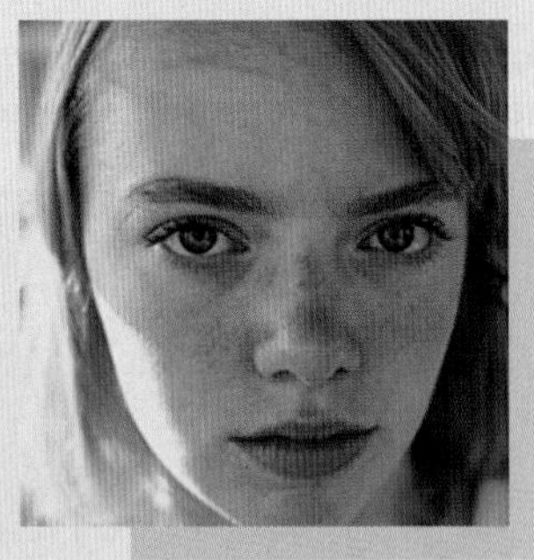

Subjective: "I'm still fat. I don't want to eat because I won't fit into my clothes anymore." 24-hour diet recall: one serving of fruit, half yogurt, half sandwich with pickle, celery, carrots, salad, diet soda.

Objective: The 15-year-old female is thin and appears older than her age. Height 170.2 cm (67 inches). T 36°C oral, P 88 beats/min, R 20 breaths/min, BP 108/66 mmHg. Taking

(case study continues on page 153)

fewer than 500 cal/day orally. Weight increased 1.1 lb, BMI 14.8, which is underweight. Ideal weight 125 lb, weighs 71% of ideal weight, moderate malnutrition. Skin pale and dry with some flaking. Appears distressed about eating. No edema, peripheral pulses strong. Nails brittle, skin very thin and dull. Wearing bandana, hair appears dull and thin. Eyes sunken with dark circles. Upper and lower extremities with full range of motion, muscle strength 5/5. Abdomen soft, concave, nondistended, nontender. Heart rate and rhythm regular. Lung sounds clear.

Analysis: Nutrition, less than body requirements related to low calorie intake.

Plan: Continue to encourage nutritious foods with adequate calories and protein. Schedule a visit next week to evaluate weight. Refer to a dietician for further counseling on food choices.

Lifespan Considerations: Older Adults

In older adults, measuring BMI and assessing for weight change are the simplest screening measures. It may be difficult to obtain an accurate weight in an older adult. A chair or bed scale that is regularly calibrated may be needed for patients who cannot stand on a scale.

Weight loss in older adults, especially unintentional, is associated with an increased risk of death. Low body weight is defined as less than 80% of ideal body weight (Ritchie, Schmader, Lipman, & Sokol, 2009). Interestingly, among older adults living in the community, loss of as little as 5% of weight over a 3-year period is associated with increased mortality. Residents of nursing homes have meaningful weight loss if they have lost 5% of usual body weight in 30 days or 10% in 6 months. Valid and reliable tools have been developed to screen for malnutrition in older adults (see Table 7.1).

Critical Thinking

Nurses usually complete nutrition assessments in collaboration with dieticians. Often, however, nurses are the first health care providers to identify patients at nutritional risk. Nutritional issues can affect all body systems, fluid balance, and **electrolytes**. Undernourished patients may have electrolyte imbalances, delayed healing, and slowed recovery from illness.

Common Laboratory and Diagnostic Testing

No single laboratory test is nutritionally specific. Health-related conditions or treatments can affect each measure. For example, with protracted illness or hospitalization, circulating proteins and nutrient storage pools shift, depending on resources and demands; body stores of macronutrients and micronutrients may decline to dangerously low levels. Most biochemical measures detect only circulating levels of nutrients; thus, reported values can lead to an incomplete nutritional picture because there is no indication of how much of a measured nutrient is still stored in the body. Therefore, serial tests should be used rather than a single value to achieve greater accuracy and to discover nutritional trends. Additionally, it is useful to cluster a group of tests and data together to analyze nutritional status.

Serum Proteins

The liver synthesizes several serum proteins. **Albumin** is a prime ingredient of blood oncotic pressure and a carrier protein for many body and pharmacological substances. The serum protein albumin level is low with liver cell damage, malnutrition, and renal disease. With a low albumin level, interstitial fluid is not drawn back into the vascular system, causing fluid to accumulate in the tissues. Because of the long half-life of albumin (18 to 30 days), this value is not the best indicator of current nutritional status, although it is often used. Another circulating protein, **prealbumin,** has a half-life of 2 days. Although less commonly ordered than albumin, prealbumin level is a better indicator of current nutritional status because of its shorter half-life. **Transferrin** has a half-life of 9 days; thus, the usefulness of measuring transferrin levels falls between that of prealbumin and albumin. Another serum protein is **creatinine;** however, because the kidneys excrete creatinine, it is more reflective of renal function. Total protein levels measure all circulating body proteins and provide an overview of protein stores.

Hemoglobin and Hematocrit

Low hemoglobin and hematocrit counts may indicate poor iron intake or absorption. Other factors such as bleeding, fluid excess, or low intake of vitamin B_{12} and folate may also decrease these values.

Lymphocyte Count

Severe malnutrition may compromise inflammatory response. An indicator of the ability to mount an immune response is the total leukocyte (white blood cell) count.

Creatinine Excretion

Creatinine excretion reflects muscle mass, but individual variations are wide. Creatinine in the urine is measured according to the patient's height. A 24-hour urine collection is needed; many potential sources of error may arise.

Nitrogen Balance

Nitrogen balance reflects total protein mass, but laboratory testing is expensive and time consuming. Three consecutive 24-hour measurements of urine are needed because of large variations; many potential sources of error may arise.

Skin Testing

Delayed-type hypersensitivity testing is performed by skin testing with common irritants. Theoretically, the immune response will be reduced in the malnourished patient. Skin testing is not commonly performed because it is uncomfortable; the immune response can be depressed during an acute illness even in the absence of malnutrition (Olendzki, Lipman, & Rind, 2009).

Lipid Measurements

Lipid measurements are used to assess the status of cardiovascular health and include total cholesterol, high-density lipoprotein, LDL, and triglyceride levels. Elevated levels are associated with risks for atherosclerosis, heart attack, and stroke.

Other Laboratory Tests

Anemias are associated with iron, vitamin B_{12}, and folate deficiencies. Sodium, potassium, magnesium, calcium, and phosphate are serum electrolytes associated with nutritional status. Because of other factors that can influence these values, they must be considered within a cluster of data rather than independently as a reflection of nutritional status (Olendzki et al., 2009).

Diagnostic Reasoning

Nursing Diagnosis, Outcomes, and Interventions

Patients may be at risk for fluid volume or nutritional imbalance as listed in the NANDA International (NANDA-I, 2012) nursing diagnoses. North Americans are at most risk for *Imbalanced nutrition: more than body requirements*, given that more than two thirds of the population is overweight or obese. The World Health Organization states that obesity is a much neglected public health warning sign, and that the world's population is becoming either obese or undernourished (Murray, Zentner, Pangman, & Pangman, 2009). North Americans with a lower socioeconomic background, minimal education, or eating disorders are at greatest risk for malnutrition today.

The risk of excess fluid volume exists. Accordingly, patients on intravenous therapy may experience fluid overload if fluid replacement is not closely monitored, particularly in cases of cardiac or renal failure. Older adults in care homes run the highest risk of deficient fluid volume. Other possible nursing diagnoses pertaining to nutrition include adult failure to thrive, risk for delayed development, and deficient knowledge. Adult failure to thrive may be linked to an endocrine or metabolic imbalance, whereas delayed development may be related to nutritional deficiencies in pregnancy.

Deficient knowledge is the most pervasive cause of nutritional imbalances. Hence, nurses have a significant role in patient education and follow-up regarding optimal nutrition for people from all sectors and age groups of society (Box 7.5). The ongoing proliferation of nutrition information means that nurses must access evidence-based sources of nutrition information regularly to maintain a credible body of knowledge. Table 7.3 compares and contrasts nursing diagnoses, abnormal findings, and interventions related to nutritional care (NANDA-I, 2012).

Nurses use assessment information to identify patient outcomes. Some outcomes related to nutrition include the following:

- *Imbalanced nutrition: less than body requirements*: The patient will show progressive weight gain toward the desired goal.
- *Imbalanced nutrition: more than body requirements*: The patient will state pertinent factors contributing to weight gain (Moorhead, Johnson, Maas, & Swanson, 2013).

After outcomes are established, the nurse implements care to improve the patient's status. The nurse uses critical thinking and evidence-based practice to develop interventions. He or she evaluates the patient to determine the effectiveness of those interventions and revises the plan as needed.

BOX 7.5 The Nurse's Role in Facilitating Nutritional Care

- Communicate with the registered dietician.
- Serve as a liaison between the physician and the dietician.
- Identify patients who may benefit from programs such as Meals on Wheels.
- Request a referral to a speech therapist.
- Confer with the discharge planner, social services worker, and physical or occupational therapist.

From Dudek, S. G. (2010). *Nutrition essentials for nursing practice* (6th ed.). Philadelphia, PA: Wolters Kluwer Health/Lippincott Williams & Wilkins.

TABLE 7.3 Common Nursing Diagnoses Associated With Nutrition

Diagnosis	Point of Differentiation	Assessment Characteristics	Nursing Interventions
Imbalanced nutrition: less than body requirements	Nutrient intake that fails to meet metabolic needs	Body weight 20% or more below ideal, body mass index (BMI) less than 20, lack of interest in food, nausea, vomiting, diarrhea	Weigh the patient daily. Monitor the intake. Provide nutritional supplements. Offer food frequently.
Imbalanced nutrition: more than body requirements	Nutrient intake that exceeds metabolic needs	Body weight more than 20% above ideal, BMI greater than 30, eating in response to cues other than hunger, triceps skinfold greater than 25 mm in women or greater than 15 mm in men	Have patient keep a food diary and record every item of food and drink. Teach reading of food labels. Weigh twice a week. Teach an increased intake of vegetables and fruits.
Excess fluid volume	Increased retention of isotonic fluid	Altered electrolytes, elevated creatinine, decreased hematocrit and hemoglobin, weight gain	Monitor intake and output. Weigh daily at the same time of the day. Evaluate serum sodium, creatinine, and hematocrit.
Deficient fluid volume	Decreased intravascular, interstitial, or intracellular fluid; dehydration	Decreased blood pressure, increased pulse, orthostatic blood pressure changes, thirst, dry skin, sunken eyeballs	Monitor intake and output. Weigh daily. Provide fluids every 2 hours. Treat causes including nausea, vomiting, or diarrhea.*

*Collaborative interventions.

Collaborating With the Interprofessional Team

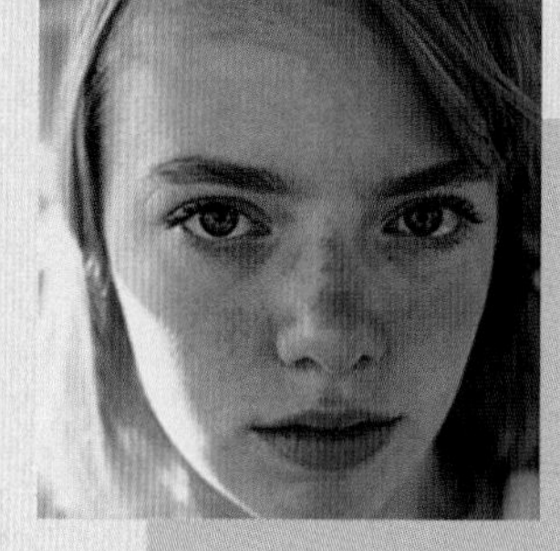

In addition to completing a nutritional assessment, the nurse facilitates the patient's nutritional care by serving as a liaison between the primary care provider and the RD. The nurse also confers with colleagues in social work and physical or occupational therapy during discharge planning to ensure that the patient benefits from community programs to provide easy-to-prepare food (see Box 7.5).

Patients with eating disorders respond best to a highly individualized, multidisciplinary approach to outpatient treatment consisting of nutrition counseling, psychotherapy, and family or group counseling. Treatment plans are designed to foster slow, gradual behavioral changes aimed at maintaining normal eating patterns and promoting long-term maintenance of ideal weight. This can be achieved only by involving the patient in establishing an individualized plan with realistic goals. Patients with eating disorders must be reassessed over time because they often experience chronic problems with eating and exercise as well as weight maintenance.

In many facilities, nurses initiate referrals for nutritional issues. Situations that might trigger a nutrition consult include patients who are food or housing insecure, those who have not eaten in several days, and those who have wasting syndrome. Additionally, patients with more than three nutrition risk factors or diagnoses who could improve with counseling can be referred to a dietician.

Karen has more than three nutrition risk factors, and her health state would improve if she ate more protein and calories. The following conversation illustrates how the nurse might organize data and make recommendations to the RD.

Situation: "Hi, I'm Frances Welly, a home health nurse working with Karen Pitoci, a 15-year-old female. She was recently hospitalized for anorexia. I saw her at home today."

Background: "She is eating only about 500 cal/day, and I think that she would benefit from a nutrition consult. Although her weight increased 1.1 lb, her BMI is 14.8 and

(case study continues on page 156)

she weighs 71% of ideal weight. She gets distressed about eating and increasing her calorie intake."

Assessment: "I am hoping that you might be able to negotiate some food choices that would be good for her."

Recommendations: "Would you be able to see her in the next week? Her mother may also want to participate, but I think that you might want to ask Karen for her permission. Thanks so much."

Critical Thinking Challenge

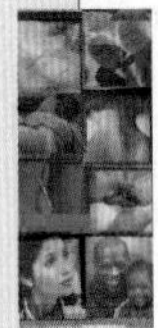

- Why did the nurse leave out most of the physical assessment data?
- How does the nurse use assessment data to make the recommendations?
- How does the assessment performed by the nurse compare to that performed by the dietician?

Pulling It All Together

The nurse uses assessment data to formulate a nursing care plan for Karen Pitoci. After completing the interventions, the nurse will reevaluate Karen and document the findings in the chart to show critical thinking. This is often in the form of a care plan or case note similar to the one below.

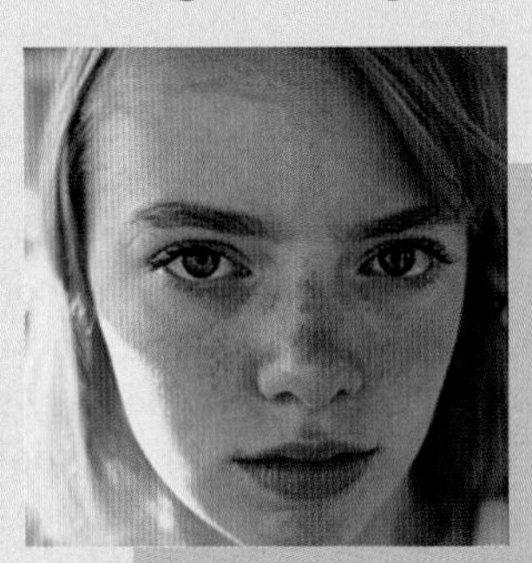

Nursing Diagnosis	Patient Outcomes	Nursing Interventions	Rationale	Evaluation
Imbalanced nutrition: less than body requirements	Gain 10% of body weight, or 9 lb, in the next 2 months.	Continue home visits. Assess weight at each weekly visit. Discuss the use of 30 ml of nutritional shake each hour.	Develop a relationship with family. Follow trends of weight over time. Small amounts of intake may be more acceptable.	The patient talks more about anorexia. Weight increased 9 lb. The patient declined the use of a supplement and will continue to increase the intake.

Applying Your Knowledge

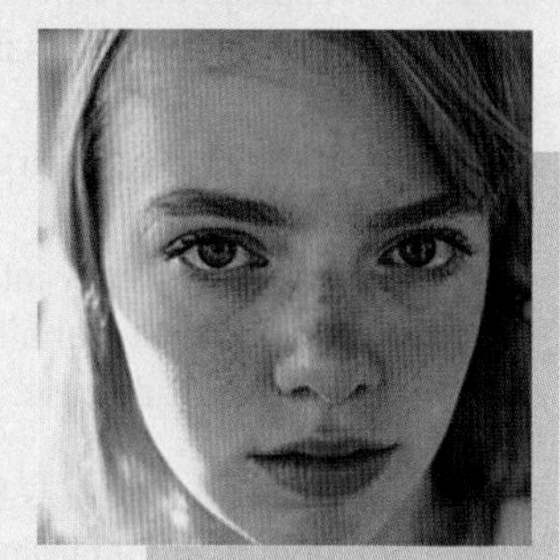

Using the previous steps of diagnostic reasoning, organizing, and prioritizing, consider all the case study findings woven throughout this chapter. When answering the following questions, begin drawing conclusions and see how the pieces of assessment must work together to create an environment for personalized, appropriate, and accurate care.

- What subjective and psychosocial data will the nurse collect from Karen and her mother?
- How might the nurse's previous experiences with patients who have eating disorders influence the assessment of Karen?
- What adaptations will the nurse make to the assessment based on Karen's condition?
- What factors are contributing to Karen's current nutritional status?
- What recommendations for further assessment of Karen by the interprofessional team would the nurse suggest?
- How will the nurse evaluate the success of the interventions of the interprofessional team with Karen?

Key Points

- Primary nutrients essential for optimal body function include carbohydrates, proteins, fats, vitamins, minerals, water, and major electrolytes.
- Vitamin D, folate, and B vitamin levels have important health implications.
- Drug–herb interactions may be serious—even life threatening.
- Three important minerals in a healthy diet are iron, zinc, and calcium.
- Water, sodium, and potassium need to be kept in balance for proper fluid and electrolyte functions.
- Inadequate intake of folic acid during pregnancy is linked to neural tube defects in newborns.
- MyPlate emphasizes the need to select foods from each of the five food groups while paying attention to portion size.
- Risk factors to review in a nutritional assessment include: medical history, abnormal weight history, appetite or taste changes, gastrointestinal symptoms, food allergies or intolerances, changes in eating or fluid patterns, poor food habits, inability to cook, poor lifestyle, multiple medications, inappropriate supplements or lack of supplements, and alcohol or drug use.
- Common symptoms that indicate potential nutritional problems include sudden or gradual changes in body weight, eating habits, skin, hair, nails, and energy level.
- Older adults at risk for malnutrition are those who take multiple medications; are socially isolated; or cannot shop, cook, or eat independently.
- The nurse recognizes that each culture has its own food standards, which determine what is edible, how foods are prepared, and special foods to eat when ill.
- Comprehensive nutritional screening tools include 24-hour recall, 3-day diet history, and food frequency questionnaire.
- BMI is calculated as weight in kilograms divided by height in meters squared (m^2). BMI of 18.5 to 24.9 is healthy, less than 18.5 is underweight, 25 to 29.9 is overweight, and 30 or greater represents obesity.
- Waist circumference is an indicator of accumulated body fat in the abdomen; a high circumference places the person at increased risk of obesity-related diseases and early mortality.
- Laboratory values related to nutrition include serum albumin, prealbumin, transferrin, total protein, creatinine, sodium, potassium, hemoglobin, hematocrit, total lymphocyte count, and hypersensitivity reaction.
- Nursing diagnoses related to nutrition include *Imbalanced nutrition: less than body requirements*; *Imbalanced nutrition: more than body requirements*; *Excess fluid volume*; and *Deficient fluid volume*.

Review Questions

1. The patient has serum values that are abnormal for sodium and potassium. The nurse recognizes that these values are important to maintain in normal range for proper
   A. tissue oxygenation.
   B. tensile strength in the hair.
   C. oil production in the skin.
   D. fluid and electrolyte function.

2. Primary nutrients essential for optimal body function include
   A. carbohydrates, proteins, and fats.
   B. folate, vitamin B_{12}, and iron.
   C. vitamins A, D, E, and K.
   D. iron, zinc, and calcium.

3. A patient reports taking St. John's wort along with a medication prescribed for heart disease. Which of the following is the most appropriate response from the nurse?
   A. Never take supplements in addition to prescribed medications.
   B. Supplements act in a very different way from prescribed medications.
   C. Some supplements may interact with your medications.
   D. It is known that St. John's wort interacts with medications for heart disease.

4. A woman who is pregnant is being screened for adequate intake of calcium and vitamin D. Which of the following tools is most appropriate for the nurse to administer?
   A. 24-hour recall
   B. 3-day diet history
   C. Food frequency questionnaire
   D. Comprehensive nutrition assessment

5. Which of the following is the healthiest eating plan?
   A. An eating plan that excludes lean meats, poultry, and fish
   B. An eating plan that allows for moderate intake of salt and sugars
   C. An eating plan that emphasizes low-fat milk and dairy products
   D. An eating plan that emphasizes fruits, vegetables, and whole grains

6. A patient has a BMI of 14. Which nursing intervention is indicated?
   A. Provide additional high protein and calorie shakes.
   B. Reduce total fat and calorie intake.
   C. Increase the intake of green leafy vegetables.
   D. Eat complete meals twice a day.

7. The nurse is caring for a patient with a BMI of 33. Which nursing diagnosis is most appropriate?
   A. Imbalanced nutrition: less than body requirements
   B. Imbalanced nutrition: more than body requirements
   C. Fluid volume excess
   D. Fluid volume deficit

8. From the list below, select the older adult at greatest risk for malnutrition.
   A. A 67-year-old married man with poor dentition
   B. A 73-year-old woman in a nursing home
   C. An 80-year-old widow who lives alone
   D. A 78-year-old widower who receives food from Meals on Wheels

9. A patient is admitted to the hospital with multiple trauma from an automobile accident 5 days ago. Which of the following is the best indicator of current nutritional status?
   A. Transferrin
   B. Total protein
   C. Albumin
   D. Prealbumin

10. Which of the following patients is at highest risk for complications related to folate deficiency?
    A. A 3-year-old boy who is developmentally delayed
    B. A 15-year-old girl who just started her menses
    C. A 24-year-old woman who is attempting pregnancy
    D. An 82-year-old man living in a nursing home

The Jensen suite offers these additional resources to enhance learning and facilitate understanding of this chapter:

- thePoint online resource, http://thepoint.lww.com/Jensen2e
- *Laboratory Manual for Nursing Health Assessment: A Best Practice Approach*
- *Pocket Guide for Nursing Health Assessment: A Best Practice Approach*
- *Lippincott DocuCare*, an electronic health record simulation software, http://thepoint.lww.com/docucare
- *Adaptive Learning | Powered by PrepU*, http://thepoint.lww.com/prepu

References

Barker, L. A., Gout, B. S., & Crowe, T. C. (2011). Hospital malnutrition: Prevalence, identification and impact on patients and the healthcare system. *International Journal of Environmental Research and Public Health, 8*(2), 514–527. doi:10.3390/ijerph8020514

Bellini, L. M., Parsons, P. E., Lipman, T. O., & Wilson, K. C. (2009). *Assessment of nutrition in the critically ill*. Retrieved from http://www.uptodateonline.com.proxy.seattleu.edu/online/content/topic.do?topicKey=cc_medi/17912&selectedTitle=6~150&source=search_result

Bernard, M. A., Jacobs, D. O., & Rombeau, J. L. (1986). *Nutrition and metabolic support of hospitalized patients*. Philadelphia, PA: W. B. Saunders.

Bray, G. A., Xavier Pi-Sunyer, F., & Martin, K. A. (2009). *Determining body composition in adults*. Retrieved from http://www.uptodateonline.com.proxy.seattleu.edu/online/content/topic.do?topicKey=obesity/7584&selectedTitle=2~150&source=search_result

Build Study (1979). Society of Actuaries and Association of Life Insurance Medical Directors of America, 1980.

Centers for Disease Control and Prevention. (2009). *Overweight and obesity*. Retrieved from http://www.cdc.gov/nccdphp/dnpa/obesity/index.htm

Centers for Disease Control and Prevention. (2014). *Folic acid helps prevent neural tube defects*. Retrieved from http://www.cdc.gov/features/folicacidbenefits/

Craig, W. J. (2009). Health effects of vegan diets. *American Journal of Clinical Nutrition, 89*(5), 1627S–1633S.

Dudek, S. G. (2010). *Nutrition essentials for nursing practice* (6th ed.). Philadelphia, PA: Wolters Kluwer Health/Lippincott Williams & Wilkins.

Frisancho, A. R. (1981). New norms of upper limb fat and muscle areas for assessment of nutritional status. *American Journal of Clinical Nutrition 34*, 2540–2545.

Hemmelgarn, M. (2009). Shedding light on vitamin D. *American Journal of Nursing, 109*(4), 19–20.

Jatoi, A., Loprinzi, C. L., Hesketh, P. J., & Savarese, D. M. F. (2009). *Clinical features and pathogenesis of cancer cachexia*. Retrieved from http://www.uptodateonline.com.proxy.seattleu.edu/online/content/topic.do?topicKey=genl_onc/4404&selectedTitle=1~77&source=search_result

Kirkland, R. T., Drutz, J. E., Augustyn, M., Motl, K. J., & Torchia, M. M. (2009). *Etiology and evaluation of failure to thrive (undernutrition) in children younger than two years*. Retrieved, from http://www.uptodateonline.com.proxy.seattleu.edu/online/content/topic.do?topicKey=gen_pedi/2884&linkTitle=EVALUATION&source=preview&selectedTitle=10~150&anchor=14#14

Leininger, M. M., & McFarland, M. R. (2002). *Transcultural nursing: Concepts, theories, research, and practice* (3rd ed.). New York, NY: McGraw-Hill Professional.

Magana-Gomez, J. A., & Calderon de la Barca, A. M. (2008). Risk assessment of genetically modified crops for nutrition and health. *Nutrition Reviews, 67*(1), 1–16.

Mente, A., de Koning, L., Shannon, H. S., & Anand, S. S. (2009). A systematic review of the evidence supporting a causal link between dietary factors and coronary heart disease. *Archives of Internal Medicine, 169*(7), 659–669.

Moorhead, S., Johnson, M., Maas, M. L., & Swanson, E., (2013). *Nursing outcomes classification (NOC): Measurement of health outcomes* (5th ed.). St. Louis, MO: Elsevier.

Murray, R. B., Zentner, J. P., Pangman, V., & Pangman, C. (2009). *Health promotion strategies through the lifespan* (2nd Canadian ed.). Toronto, ON: Prentice Hall.

NANDA International. (2012). *Nursing diagnoses: Definitions and classification 2012-2014* (9th ed). Oxford, United Kingdom: Wiley-Blackwell.

National Heart, Lung, and Blood Institute. (2009). *Classification of overweight and obesity by BMI, waist circumference, and associated disease risks*. Retrieved from http://www.nhlbi.nih.gov/health/public/heart/obesity/lose_wt/bmi_dis.htm

Olendzki, B., Lipman, T. O., & Rind, D. M. (2009). *Dietary and nutritional assessment in adults*. Retrieved from http://www.uptodateonline.com.proxy.seattleu.edu/online/content/topic.do?topicKey=nutritio/4489&selectedTitle=8~150&source=search_result

Pencharz, P. B. (2010). Protein and energy requirements for optimal catch-up growth. *European Journal of Clinical Nutrition*, 64, 55–57.

Phillips, S. M., Jensen, C., Motil, K. J., & Hoppin, A. G. (2009). *Indications for nutritional assessment in childhood.* Retrieved from http://www.uptodateonline.com.proxy.seattleu.edu/online/content/topic.do?topicKey=nutri_ch/5413&selectedTitle=10~150&source=search_result

Ritchie, C., Schmader, K. E., Lipman, T. O., & Sokol, N. (2009). *Geriatric nutrition: Nutritional issues in older adults*. Retrieved from http://www.uptodateonline.com.proxy.seattleu.edu/online/content/topic.do?topicKey=geri_med/8473&selectedTitle=1~150&source=search_result

Snyder, P. J., Matsumoto, A. M., O'Leary, M. P., & Martin, K. A. (2009). *Use of androgens and other drugs by athletes*. Retrieved from http://www.uptodateonline.com.proxy.seattleu.edu/online/content/topic.do?topicKey=r_endo_m/9455&selectedTitle=4~150&source=search_result

Tangney, C. C., Rosenson, R. S., Freeman, M. W., & Rind, D. M. (2009). *Lipid lowering with diet or dietary supplements*. Retrieved from http://www.uptodateonline.com.proxy.seattleu.edu/online/content/topic.do?topicKey=lipiddis/6831&selectedTitle=17~51&source=search_result.

U.S. Department of Agriculture. (2008). *Infant nutrition and feeding resource list.*

U.S. Department of Health & Human Services & U.S. Department of Agriculture. (2010). *Dietary guidelines for Americans* (7th ed.). Washington, DC: U.S. Government Printing Office.

van Dam, R. M. (2008). Coffee consumption and risk of type 2 diabetes, cardiovascular diseases, and cancer. *Applied Physiology of Nutrition and Metabolism, 33*(6), 1269–1283.

World Health Organization. (2014). *Nutrition*. Retrieved from http://www.who.int/nutrition/en/

Woo, T. M. (2008).When nature and pharmacy collide: Drug interactions with commonly used herbs. *Advanced Nurse Practitioner, 16*(7), 69–72.

Tables of Abnormal Findings

TABLE 7.4 Physical Signs of Nutritional Deficiency

	Signs	Deficiencies
Hair 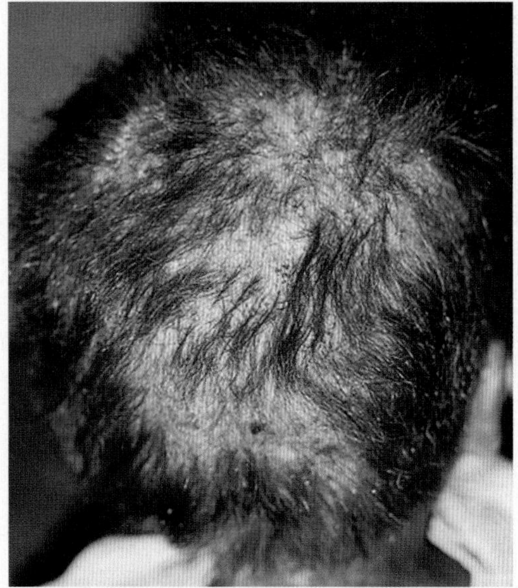 **Alopecia (hair loss)**	Alopecia Brittleness Color change Dryness Easy to pluck	Protein–calorie malnutrition Biotin Zinc Vitamins E and A
Skin 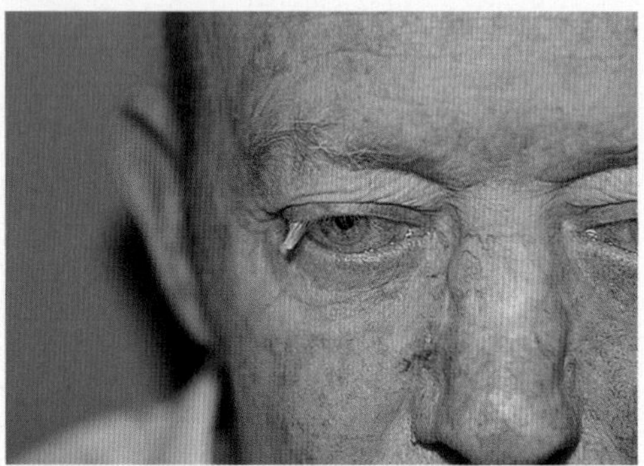 **Follicular keratosis**	Acneiform lesions Follicular keratosis Xerosis (dry skin) Ecchymosis Intradermal petechia Erythema Scrotal dermatitis Angular palpebritis	Vitamin A
Eyes 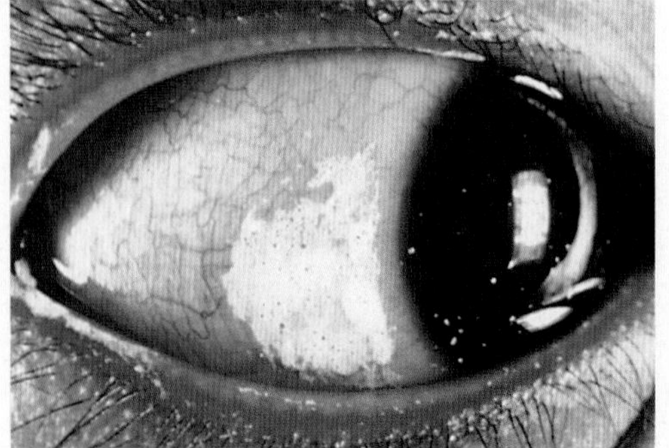 **Bitot spots**	Bitot spots Conjunctival xerosis	Vitamin A

(table continues on page 161)

TABLE 7.4 Physical Signs of Nutritional Deficiency *(continued)*

	Signs	Deficiencies
Mouth	Angular stomatitis	Vitamin B_{12}
	Atrophic papillae	Niacin
	Bleeding gums	Vitamin C
	Cheilosis	Vitamin B_2
	Glossitis	Niacin, folate, vitamin B_{12}
	Magenta tongue	Vitamin B_2
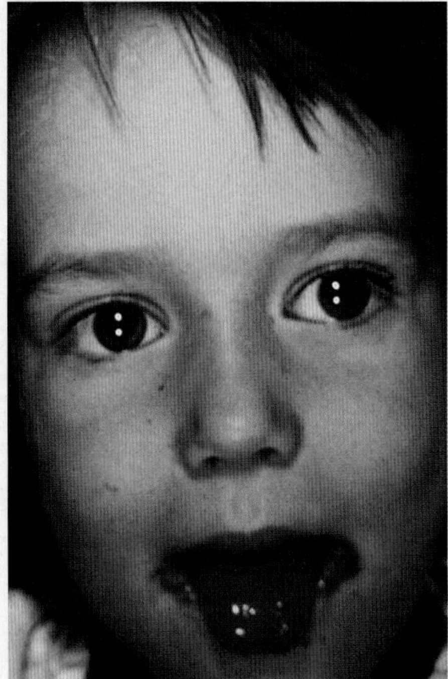 **Magenta tongue**		
Extremities	Genu valgum or varum	Vitamin D
	Loss of deep tendon reflexes of the lower extremities	Vitamins B_1 and B_{12}
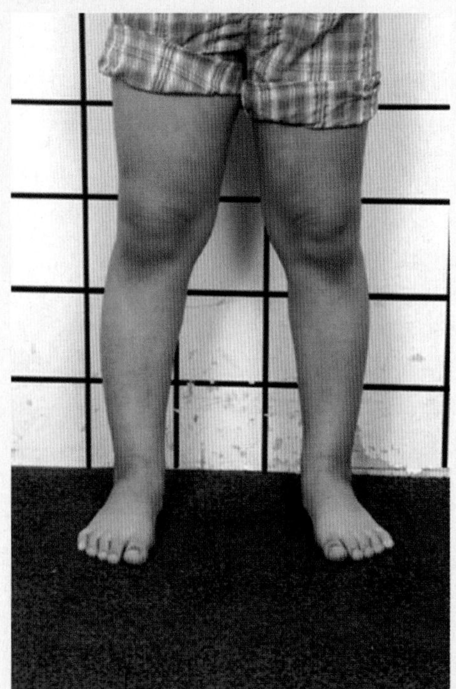 **Genu varum**		

Adapted from Bernard, M. A., Jacobs, D. O., & Rombeau, J. L. (1986). *Nutrition and metabolic support of hospitalized patients.* Philadelphia, PA: W. B. Saunders.

8

Assessment of Developmental Stages

Learning Objectives

1 Demonstrate knowledge of physical, psychosocial, and cognitive changes across the lifespan.

2 Describe both individual and family developmental tasks across the lifespan.

3 Identify important topics for health promotion and risk reduction across the lifespan.

4 Consider the patient's age, condition, gender, and culture to individualize health promotion interventions.

5 Collect subjective and objective data about the patient's adaptation to expected developmental tasks and the patient's relationship to health and wellness.

6 Collect subjective and objective data about alterations in the patient's adaptation to developmental tasks and the wellness risks of those alterations.

7 Analyze subjective and objective data and plan interventions to promote health and wellness across the lifespan.

8 Document and communicate data from the assessment of growth and development using appropriate terminology and principles of recording.

9 Identify nursing diagnosis and initiate a plan of care based on assessment findings.

Amber and Michael Carr have just become first-time adoptive parents to three biological siblings: Emily, 2 months old; Jacob, 2 years old; and Madeline, 5 years old. Amber, a 31-year-old real estate broker, will be leaving her job to care for the children. Michael, a 35-year-old tax accountant, is enthusiastic about fatherhood but worries about providing for the family's needs on only one income. Both Amber's and Michael's parents, who are in their late 50s and early 60s, are thrilled. They look forward to spending time with their grandchildren and teaching them about outdoor activities, such as camping and hiking.

You will gain more information about the Carrs as you progress through this chapter. As you study the content, consider this family's case and its relationship to what you are learning. Begin thinking about the following points:

- How much weight should 2-year-old Jacob have gained since birth?
- Why do Madeline and Jacob require supervision in the kitchen and bathroom?
- In what stage of psychosocial development is each member of the Carr family?
- In what stage of Piaget's cognitive thought is each member of the Carr family?
- What nursing diagnoses might be appropriate for members of the Carr family?
- How will the nurse individualize assessments of Emily, Jacob, and Madeline, considering their ages and that they are newly adopted?
- How will the nurse evaluate the success of health teaching with Amber and Michael about home hazards?

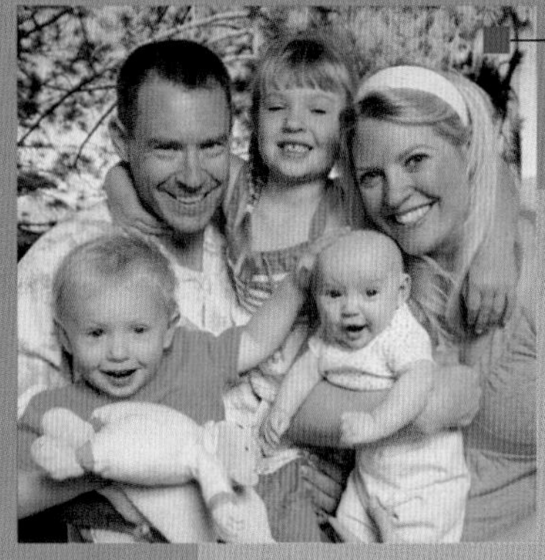

Each unique human experiences physical growth, psychosocial development, and cognitive development as he or she progresses from infancy through old age. Furthermore, each particular life journey varies in unique ways, depending on the person's environment and interaction with the world. Understanding the processes of growth and development is essential for nurses. It enables them to provide care and support as patients make inevitable transitions from one life stage to another, become more complex in their thinking and interactivity, and seek to maintain their health.

This chapter summarizes important information about growth and development across the lifespan. The content serves as a foundation for assessing patients of all age groups and their families. Nurses provide information, anticipatory guidance, role modeling, and protection to individuals, families, and communities to enable optimal, healthy growth and development for children and adults across the lifespan.

Subjective Data

Psychosocial, cognitive, and language **development** involves qualitative changes in an individual over time. Language acquisition and relationships with others are two examples of types of development (Leifer & Fleck, 2013). Developmental changes are not easily measured with universal tools. Therefore, this chapter covers such material within this section on "Subjective Data Collection."

Areas for Health Promotion

The Healthy People 2020 organization contains several goals associated with growth and development. See Table 8.1.

Psychosocial Development

Bronfenbrenner's Systems Model of Psychosocial Development

Uri Bronfenbrenner (1979) proposed a frequently cited systems model of **psychosocial development**, which describes the individual's development in interaction with the immediate environment. In this approach, development is continuous, important at all ages, and an active rather than a passive process.

Nested Ecological Systems. The environment in Bronfenbrenner's model consists of nested ecological systems—the microsystem, the mesosystem, the exosystem, the macrosystem, and the chronosystem. These ecological systems are involved in shaping, and being shaped by, the interactions of the individuals within those systems.

The individual interacts primarily within the *microsystem*: the close, consistent, and immediate setting, such as the immediate family, school, spiritual community, and peers (Bronfenbrenner, 1977, 1979).

In turn, the set of microsystems relate to each other and to the individual as the *mesosystem*: relationships between the family and a parent's work colleagues, or between the family and a child's school friends, happen at particular points along the person's developmental time frame (Bronfenbrenner, 1977, 1979).

The *exosystem* consists of contexts that do not directly involve the individual but that still have an effect on the person's behavior and development. For example, a school district sets the times that schools within that district begin and end the school day. These times may not fit well within a particular family's unique needs, such as the case of a single parent who works a night shift. The family has little say in the school district's scheduling decision, but the parent is expected to get the children to school on time while also following his or her own work schedule.

TABLE 8.1 Goals Related to Development

Goals	Patient Education Topics
Reduce air toxic emissions to decrease the risk of adverse health effects caused by airborne toxins.	Teach patients to avoid using a stove or heater without ventilation.
Reduce or eliminate indigenous cases of vaccine-preventable diseases.	Encourage timely immunizations.
Reduce the occurrence of developmental disabilities.	Screen for genetically transmitted diseases.
Reduce the occurrence of spina bifida and other neural tube defects.	Provide information on taking folic acid during pregnancy.
Increase abstinence from alcohol, cigarettes, and illicit drugs among pregnant women.	Provide information on the hazards of alcohol, cigarettes, and illicit drugs in pregnancy.
Improve the system for recording and referring infants and children with cleft lips, cleft palates, and other craniofacial anomalies to craniofacial anomaly rehabilitative teams.	Health care providers report and refer infants and children with cleft lips, cleft palates, and other craniofacial anomalies.

From *Healthy people 2020: What are its goals?* (n.d.). Retrieved from http://www.healthypeople.gov/About/goals.htm

The next level in Bronfenbrenner's model is the *macrosystem*, which is the level that includes culture, beliefs, values, faith-based beliefs, macroinstitutions such as the federal government and health services, and public policy and laws. The individual is affected by all of these components of the macrosystem, as are all of the interactions within the other levels of the model (Bronfenbrenner, 1977, 1979). For example, cultural standards about the relative value of education for boys versus girls in a society, or the types of socially acceptable work options for men and women within a culture, as well as roles for older adults within a society, have important influences on the individual choices open to a developing person.

The outer level of the Bronfenbrenner model is the *chronosystem*, or the time period during which the individual grows up and develops. For example, children growing up in the Great Depression of the 1930s had very different experiences than did their children, the baby boomer generation growing up in the 1950s and 1960s. Children who experience war, famine, or serious disease outbreaks during their childhoods find the environment much more hostile and less supportive than do children who do not have these same experiences. Traumatic experiences, nutritional deprivation, or disease may affect the development of such children all of their lives.

The Process-Person-Context-Time Model. For Bronfenbrenner, four interrelated components are important for nurses to consider as they examine development (Bronfenbrenner, 2005): (1) the developmental p*rocess*, the relationship between the person and the context; (2) the p*erson*, with his or her unique biological, cognitive, emotional, and behavioral characteristics; (3) the c*ontext* of the nested systems of the ecology within which the development of the individual proceeds; and (4) t*ime*, which moderates change across the person's life course. This *process-person-context-time* (PPCT) model gives the nurse a way to conceptualize the developmental system and the way the person interacts with that system.

Erikson's Model of Individual Development

Erik Erikson (1963) provided another valuable model for viewing individual development over time. His model divides the lifespan into eight stages, with different psychosocial tasks to complete at each stage (Fig. 8.1). Even if the person does not complete the task, according to Erikson, he or she still must move on to the next stage—which will, in turn, be more difficult because the basis for the new stage has not been established during a previous one.

Infant: Trust Versus Mistrust. The first task for the infant is **trust versus mistrust**. The infant learns that physiological regulation is linked to a caregiver's provision of comfort. This task depends on consistency, continuity, and sameness of experience; the infant learns that when he or she is uncomfortable, the caregiver comes and provides the appropriate soothing measure. Erikson also says that, by learning to cope with discomfort, the infant learns to trust himself or herself as well. Things that the infant does to get the attention of a caregiver so that his or her needs are met tells the infant that what he or she does matters; the infant develops a sense of self-efficacy in this way.

Toddler: Autonomy Versus Shame and Doubt. The task for the toddler is **autonomy versus shame and doubt**. The toddler learns about "two simultaneous sets of social modalities: holding on and letting go" (Erikson, 1963, p. 251). In situations that require a choice, toddlers are unable to determine which choice is appropriate. They may make choices that are unsafe such as crossing a road when a car is coming. Caregivers must help toddlers learn how to discriminate and choose appropriately. Otherwise, toddlers will doubt their senses of self and the environment and become reluctant to explore. Toddlers are learning to become independent and feed themselves, wash and dress themselves, and use the bathroom.

Preschooler: Initiative Versus Guilt. The preschooler's task is **initiative versus guilt**. According to Erikson, this task has "the quality of undertaking, planning, and 'attacking' a task for the sake of being active and on the move" (Erikson, 1963, p. 255). The preschooler is actively engaged in making plans, setting goals, and accomplishing them. Erikson describes the preschooler as "eager and able to make things cooperatively, to combine with other children for the purpose of constructing and planning" (Erikson, 1963, p. 258). The child learns to work with others and can share ideas and plans with peers. Learning to work with others helps the child continue to develop the sense of self-efficacy ("I am an important person in the group") that began in infancy.

School-Age Child: Industry Versus Inferiority. The life of the school-age child is, for Erikson, naturally centered on school. His or her task is **industry versus inferiority**. School prepares the child to become "a worker and potential provider" (Erikson, 1963). The child must learn to use the tools that adults commonly use within the specific society or environment. At the same time, the school in a literate society has its own culture "with its own goals and limits, its achievements and disappointments" (Erikson, 1963, pp. 258–259). As the child spends more time in the school culture, being prepared by teachers for the literate world, the influence of other adults dilutes the role of parents in the child's life. The danger in this stage is that the child will not be able to learn to use the adult tools and will feel a sense of inferiority and inadequacy. It is difficult for the child to be admitted to an adult role in society without the tools to deal with the technology and economy of the culture. If the family has not prepared the child for school, or school does not support the promises of earlier stages of development, the child suffers.

Adolescent: Identity Versus Role Confusion. In Erikson's model, puberty signals the end of childhood. The task for the adolescent becomes **identity versus role confusion**. With the somatic growth and genital maturity that accompany adolescence, the teen revisits some battles from earlier stages. Adult tasks and roles are now close at hand; adolescents are "concerned with what they appear to be in the eyes of others as compared with what they feel they are, and with the question of

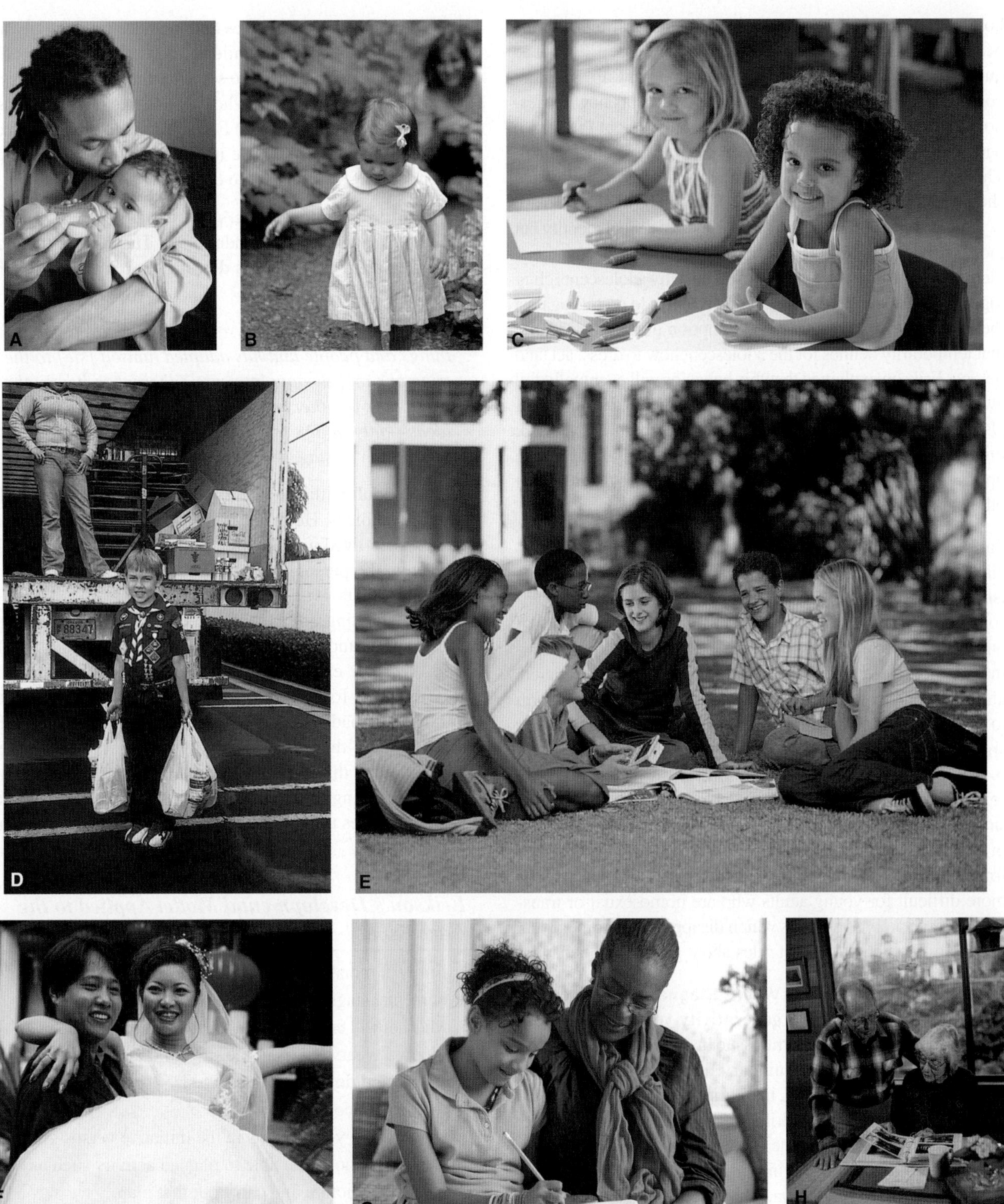

Figure 8.1 Erikson's psychosocial model involves the attainment of different qualities in each of eight life stages. **A.** Infants gain **trust** when caregivers consistently meet their needs. **B.** Toddlers develop **autonomy** as they make simple choices and exert some independent control. **C.** Preschoolers learn **initiative** by engaging in cooperative projects with others. **D.** School-age children develop **industry** by acquiring skills that will assist them in adult roles and responsibilities. **E.** Adolescents achieve **identity** by establishing their own opinions, views, and ideas apart from parents, peers, and other influences. **F.** Young adults achieve **intimacy** by fusing their identity with others. **G.** Middle adults attain **generativity** by sharing their knowledge with younger generations. **H.** Older adults achieve **ego integrity** through acceptance and pride in their life histories.

how to connect the roles and skills cultivated earlier with the occupational prototypes" available (Erikson, 1963, p. 261). The question, "What do you want to be when you grow up?" is more complex for the adolescent than for the child. It is now a question not only about a potential career but also about the sort of person the teen wishes to become and his or her social values. This interacts with cultural expectations of what the individual should do as an adult in the society of which he or she is a part.

Role confusion in this stage may involve sexual identity but more often involves the teen's struggle to choose an occupational identity. This confusion partially explains why adolescents cling together in cliques and crowds. Doing so helps to protect against the loss of identity through the assumption of a group identity that temporarily defines for the adolescent how to dress, act, and belong. Erikson explained that this behavior will eventually fall away as the individual defines his or her own identity. Individuals may decide not to take on roles that are culturally expected; this might mean preparing for a job traditionally held by the opposite sex or adopting dress, appearance, or behaviors that others may frown upon within a given culture.

Early Adult: Intimacy Versus Isolation. The sixth psychosocial task, occurring in early adulthood, is **intimacy versus isolation**. After the person has navigated the search for personal identity, he or she is willing to fuse with the identity of others. As Erikson expressed it, the person is "ready for intimacy, that is, the capacity to commit himself [sic] to concrete affiliations and partnerships and to develop the ethical strength to abide by such commitments, even though they may call for significant sacrifices and compromises" (Erikson, 1963, p. 263). By intimate relationships, Erikson meant not only sexual unions but also close friendships and physical expressions. Failure to accomplish this developmental task may result in isolation, in which the person separates himself or herself from others to avoid commitment to intimacy. This task may be more difficult for young adults who are homosexual or transgender, especially in cultures which disapprove of homosexual behavior or which have strict rules about gender and behavior.

Middle Adult: Generativity Versus Stagnation. The seventh stage in Erikson's model is **generativity versus stagnation**, which he described as a central issue in adulthood. Generativity "encompasses the evolutionary development which has made man [sic] the teaching, instituting, and learning animal" (Erikson, 1963, p. 266). Erikson argued that when adults focus too exclusively on the dependence of their children, they may forget about the importance of their own dependence on the next generation. The essence of generativity is that "mature man [sic] needs to be needed, and maturity needs guidance as well as encouragement from what has been produced and must be taken care of. Generativity, then, is primarily the concern in establishing and guiding the next generation" (Erikson, 1963, pp. 266–267).

Part of generativity involves letting the next generation go to walk their own path in life. Fearing what might happen to a child if he or she is let go, and clinging to the child, contributes both to the stagnation of the parent and stifles the intimacy necessary for the young adult as well.

Generativity also involves and includes productivity and creativity. Simply having children does not make an adult generative. In fact, adults who seem to think of themselves as their own "spoiled child" or who demonstrate physical or psychological invalidism have, in Erikson's model, fallen into the trap of stagnation. They have nothing to offer the next generation, even if they wished to contribute something.

Late Adult: Ego Integrity Versus Despair. Erikson's eighth and last stage applies to late adulthood. The task for the older adult is **ego integrity versus despair**. Ego integrity is difficult to achieve:

> *Only in him [sic] who in some way has taken care of things and people and has adapted himself [sic] to the triumphs and disappointments adherent to being, the originator of others or the generator of products and ideas—only in him [sic] may gradually ripen the fruit of these seven stages.* (Erikson, 1963, p. 268)

The older adult with ego integrity has come to terms with his or her life choices. He or she comes to recognize that the life that has been lived was the only possible one. If successfully completed, the person is ready to defend against physical or economic threats. If unsuccessful, the person will not come to this understanding of "the one and only life cycle" (Erikson, 1963, p. 269) and will then fear death, which results in despair. "Despair expresses the feeling that the time is now short, too short for the attempt to start another life and to try out alternate roads to integrity" (Erikson, 1963, p. 269). By late adulthood, there is no way to go back and try different paths; choices that were made in life are permanent now. However, coming to accept the life path chosen and the life lived contributes to integrity and combats feelings of despair.

Erikson's Developmental Model Applied to the Carr Family

- Emily, 2 months old, is in the trust versus mistrust developmental stage. She must learn to trust that Amber and Michael will care for her and that her needs will be met.
- Jacob, 2 years old, is in the stage of autonomy versus shame and doubt. His task is to learn self-control and independence.
- Madeline, 5 years old, is in the initiative versus guilt stage; she should be able to plan an activity such as painting a picture and carry out that plan.
- Amber and Michael are in early adulthood. Certainly, the addition of three children to their household will call for significant sacrifices and compromises in their marital relationship.
- Amber's and Michael's parents are committing themselves to being grandparents to Madeline, Jacob, and Emily. They want to demonstrate their generativity by teaching the new generation the things they previously taught their children.

Erikson finished his developmental stage model by relating the circular fashion of the stages. "Trust (the first of our ego values) is here defined as 'the assured reliance on another's integrity,' the last of our values" (Erikson, 1963, p. 269). Erikson further linked the circularity of the relationship between childhood and adulthood in the statement "healthy children will not fear life if their elders have integrity enough not to fear death" (Erikson, 1963, p. 269).

Cognitive Development

Jean Piaget (1952) formulated a theory of **cognitive development** that begins at birth and continues until adulthood. Like Erikson's model, Piaget's theory describes stages of development. Piaget claimed that the person uses experience to move from stage to stage as thinking becomes more sophisticated and complex in interaction with the environment.

Infant: Sensorimotor Stage

The first stage of cognition, the **sensorimotor** stage, is divided into six substages (Table 8.2).

Toddler and Preschooler: Preoperational Stage

The second stage of Piaget's cognitive model is the **preoperational** stage, which lasts from approximately ages 2 to 7 years (Piaget, 1952). The preoperational child is forming stable concepts. Mental reasoning begins, and the child constructs magical beliefs (Santrock, 2012). The child is highly egocentric at the beginning of the preoperational stage but begins, by the end, to be able to consider the perspectives of others. The preoperational child cannot yet think in a well-organized way, but during this period, the child moves from using primitive to more sophisticated symbols (Piaget, 1952).

Piaget divided the preoperational stage into two substages: (1) symbolic function and (2) intuitive thought. The child in the symbolic function substage, which lasts roughly from ages 2 to 4 years, can now mentally represent an absent object. For example, he or she can talk about a grandparent's house for many days after a visit. Scribbled designs represent people, houses, cars, clouds, and other objects (Santrock, 2012). Using language and pretend play (Fig. 8.2) are other characteristics of this substage (Santrock, 2012).

Although the ability to use symbols greatly increases the child's cognitive abilities, this substage is largely limited because of egocentrism and animism. *Egocentrism* is the inability to distinguish one's own perspective from another person's (Santrock, 2012). The child sees his or her view of the world only. For example, he or she expects that a parent who is away on a business trip still can see what he or she

TABLE 8.2 Piaget's Sensorimotor Substages

Age	Substage	Description and Examples
Birth to 1 month	Simple reflexes	Behaviors coordinate sensation and action; newborns suck reflexively when a nipple is placed in their mouths; focus is on infant's body
1–4 months	Primary circular reactions	Coordination of sensation and two types of schemes: reflexes and primary circular reactions (reproducing an event that initially happened by chance); main focus remains on infant's body; infant sucks on hand differently than on a nipple
4–8 months	Secondary circular reactions	Infant becomes more object oriented, moving beyond being preoccupied with the body; repeats actions that make interesting things happen, such as infant kicks and sees a mobile move and then kicks again to make the mobile move again
8–12 months	Coordination of secondary circular reactions	Infant is beginning to coordinate vision and touch as eye–hand coordination; coordination of schemes and intentionality, such as using one toy to reach another
12–18 months	Tertiary circular reactions	Infant experiments with new behavior; learning about the properties of objects and what they can do; toys can be dropped, pushed, pulled, and used to hit other toys
18–24 months	Internalization of schemes	Infants develop the ability to use simple symbols and form enduring mental representations; the infant sees another child have a tantrum and has one himself or herself the next day

From Santrock, J. (2012). *Life-span development* (14th ed.). New York, NY: McGraw-Hill.

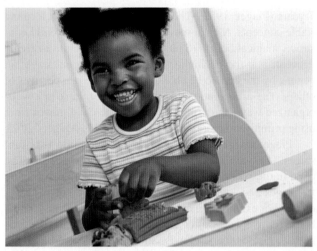

Figure 8.2 Children in the preoperational symbolic function substage rely on pretend play, with imagination and creative toys as part of their cognitive development.

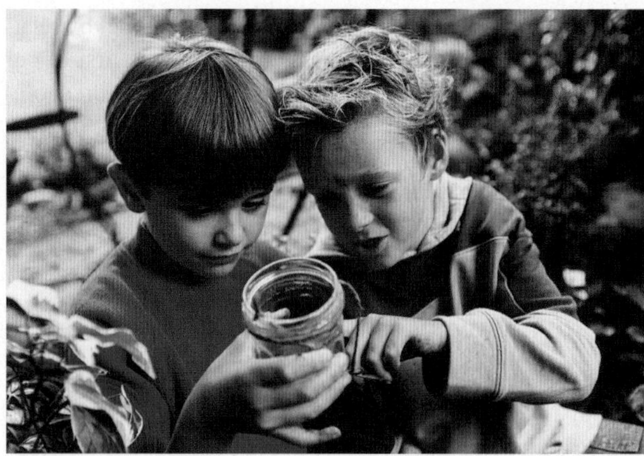

Figure 8.3 A characteristic of concrete operational cognition involves the ability to characterize and sort objects in complex ways. For example, children may have closely catalogued collections of action figures, science specimens, sports materials, or books and may spend a lot of time attending to and enhancing such collections.

sees and know what he or she knows; the child is very confused when the parent does not know what went on at home during the day. *Animism* is the belief that inanimate objects are capable of action and have lifelike qualities (Santrock, 2012). Dead leaves blowing down the street are still alive for the child; objects that cause the child to trip and fall have bad intentions. Imagination and invention are characteristic of children in this substage, and they are as comfortable in the world of make-believe as they are in the world of reality (Santrock, 2012).

The intuitive thought substage occurs from ages 4 to 7 years (Piaget, 1952). These children begin to use reasoning, although it is still very crude. They ask questions constantly and want to know the answers (Santrock, 2012). Piaget (1952) referred to this substage as intuitive because these children seem very sure about *what* they know but cannot tell *how* they know it. They have not used rational thinking to reach conclusions. An important characteristic of this stage is *centration*, which Piaget defined as the child centering attention on one aspect of a problem and failing to consider other dimensions. It is obvious to an adult that pouring water from a wide and short container to a long and narrow one has no effect on the volume of water. The child in the intuitive substage, however, can see only that the water level is higher in the new container. The child cannot reason that, if the adult poured the water back into the original container, it would be the same volume. This inability to conserve lasts until approximately age 7 or 8 years (Piaget, 1952).

School-Age Child: Concrete Operations

Piaget's next stage of cognitive development is the **concrete operational** stage, which lasts approximately from ages 7 to 11 years (Piaget, 1952). Piaget defined *operations* as internalized sets of actions that permit children to do mentally what they formerly did physically. Concrete operations are reversible mental actions; children now understand conservation and can tell the adult who pours water from one container to another that the volume remains the same and that to prove it, one could just pour the water back into the original container. These children recognize that the original container was short and wide, whereas the new container is tall and thin.

Concrete operational thinkers are also much better able to categorize objects (Fig. 8.3). For example, a school-age child may have a collection of baseball cards carefully organized by team and by each player's position on the team. The child understands that a player can be a pitcher and a team member at the same time. In addition, children at this stage can reason about relationships between classes, which Piaget called *seriation*. To continue the baseball card example, the child understands that one team has better players than another team and might organize the cards according to league standings. He or she might then rearrange the cards as teams win or lose during a season. Seriation also refers to the ability to arrange objects by quantitative dimensions.

Piaget's concept of *transitivity* refers to the child's ability to consider problems such as, if A is greater than B, and B is greater than C, then it must be true that A is greater than C. So the child understands that if John is taller than Jordan, and Jordan is taller than Justin, then John must also be taller than Justin as well.

Adolescent: Formal Operations

The last stage in Piaget's (1952) cognitive theory is the **formal operational** stage. The formal operator uses abstract reasoning far better than the concrete operator and can discuss theoretical concepts that escape younger children. Piaget contended that adolescence is the beginning of formal operations. The adolescent can now talk about "what if . . ." problems and can think logically about abstract solutions. Formal operations also include verbal problem-solving skills. The adolescent who uses formal operations can be presented verbally with "A = B, B = C, A ? C" and substitute the "=" for the question mark without having to see the written problem.

For the first time, those in the formal operations stage can use metacognition (Piaget, 1952), or the ability to "think about thinking." The adolescent also can now think idealistically and consider new possibilities. These abilities lead adolescents to wonder how they could become ideal and how they compare with role models and heroes. Such insights, however, may have drawbacks. The adolescent who can view world problems in a new light may wonder why those problems have not been solved. Additionally, the teen may find that he or she falls short of the qualities of role models and may then feel inadequate and hopeless about himself or herself.

Formal operations also encompass scientific thinking. The adolescent can now engage in what Piaget referred to as hypothetical–deductive reasoning. He or she can develop hypotheses about problems and deduce the best way to solve them. The concrete operational child uses much less efficient trial-and-error methods of problem solving. Hypothetical–deductive reasoning enables a person to reject some solutions as impractical or inefficient without having to test them and to use logic to arrive at the most likely and feasible solutions (Piaget, 1952).

Adolescent thinking, however, has fundamental shortcomings that result from physiological changes in the brain. Magnetic resonance imagery studies have shown two main changes before and after puberty. One is the development of myelin in the frontal cortex; the other is the development of additional synapses (Blakemore & Choudhury, 2006). Because the prefrontal cortex is involved in planning, setting priorities, suppressing impulses, and weighing behavioral consequences (Santrock, 2012), a natural outcome is that adolescents might struggle with these cognitive tasks as the brain undergoes changes in this region. In addition, the amygdala (that part of the brain involved in processing emotional information) matures sooner than the prefrontal cortex (Santrock, 2012). This finding may partially explain why teens frequently react emotionally before weighing the consequences of such behavior and why they may do things and not realize beforehand what the consequences might be.

Young Adult: Formal Operations

As the individual moves into young adulthood, Piaget (1952) contended that the person becomes more quantitatively advanced in formal operations. He also believed that the young adult increased knowledge in a specific area (e.g., skills regularly used in his or her career). Other developmental theorists have challenged this view.

It may be that the idealism that Piaget considered part of formal operational thinking decreases in early adulthood because the person moves into the professional world and must face the constraints of reality (Labouvie-Vief, 1986). It is not likely that adults go beyond the scientific thinking methods that accompany formal operational thinking but rather that adults surpass adolescents in their *use* of intellect (Schaie & Willis, 2000). Whereas adolescents are more concerned with acquiring knowledge (because they are usually engaged in educational settings or perhaps vocational training), adults move beyond acquisition to application. Pursuing long-term career goals and beginning to achieve professional success (e.g., as the person moves from an entry-level to a supervisory position) require much more application than acquisition of knowledge, although certainly the person never stops learning new things.

William Perry (1970, 1999) describes another perspective about changes in adult thinking. His view is that adolescents tend to look at the world in terms of polarities. Things are either right or wrong, people fall into the categories of "us and them," and decisions are either bad or good. Such thinking often proves less useful to adults who move into a broader environment and encounter diverse opinions, multiple perspectives, and cultural differences among the people they meet and situations they face. Over time, the reflective relativistic thinking of adulthood replaces the absolute dualistic thinking of adolescence. Perry's theory assumes that the individual encounters diverse opinions and values in his or her environment; however, it is possible that a person who isolates himself or herself from new people, situations, and value systems might not move from dualistic to relativistic thinking. The person may also simply choose not to accept others' viewpoints, rejecting their belief systems as simply untrue or misguided. The person may even find different ideas threatening instead of evaluating why another person from a certain group or belief system might value the things that are important to that group.

It may be that the changes in thinking that occur as the person moves into young adulthood are qualitatively different than Piaget's (1952) stage of formal operations. Such cognitive development has been termed *postformal thought*. Santrock (2012) explained postformal thought as

> . . . *understanding that the correct answer to a problem can require reflective thinking, that the correct answer can vary from one situation to another, and that the search for truth is often an ongoing, never-ending process. It also involves the belief that solutions to problems need to be realistic and that emotion and subjective factors can influence thinking.* (p. 452)

Clinical Significance

Young adults are more likely to use postformal thought than are adolescents. They deal directly with such realities as local and national politics, occupational issues, and relationships. They have had enough experience to understand that an approach to a work problem needs to differ from an approach to a romantic problem. Many young adults are skeptical about the notions of a single truth and one final answer (Santrock, 2012). Sometimes, thinking cannot simply be abstract but has to be realistic and practical. For example, a young adult may be more interested in whether she can afford to purchase a house and pay the mortgage than in debating how much closet space her dream home would have.

Middle Adult: Cognitive Expertise

Some people believe that cognitive abilities peak in adolescence or early adulthood and then begin to decline. Research with middle adults, however, shows that this pattern is not at all true. It is important to examine the types of intelligence that middle adults use to solve problems at work and in daily living to appreciate what happens with cognition.

There are two types of intellectual skills (Craig & Dunn, 2013). The first is *crystallized intelligence*, which is "accumulated knowledge and skills based on education and life experiences" (Craig & Dunn, 2013, p. 450). It can also be referred to as *cognitive pragmatics*. This intelligence is learned and influenced by the individual person's culture. The second type is *fluid intelligence*, which means "abilities involved in acquiring new knowledge and skills" (Craig & Dunn, 2013, p. 450). It can also be referred to as *cognitive mechanics*. This intelligence is a reflection of neurological functioning and more likely to be affected negatively by brain damage (Craig & Dunn, 2013). It appears that declines in memory actually do not appear until the last part of middle adulthood or into late adulthood (Santrock, 2012). What may look like memory declines may be attributable to using ineffective memory strategies. When middle adults use organization and imagery to remember things, they can improve their memories.

Another important aspect of intelligence is *expertise*, described by Santrock (2012) as "having an extensive, highly organized knowledge and understanding of a particular domain" (p. 515). Because expertise requires years of experience, learning, and work, middle adults are far more likely than young adults to have this type of intelligence. When resolving difficulties, expertise allows the person to rely on past experience, to use automatic processing of information and efficient analysis, to use better strategies and shortcuts, and to be more creative and flexible (Fig. 8.4). The novice must work much harder and less quickly than the expert because he or she is unfamiliar with the types of difficulties often encountered in a given area.

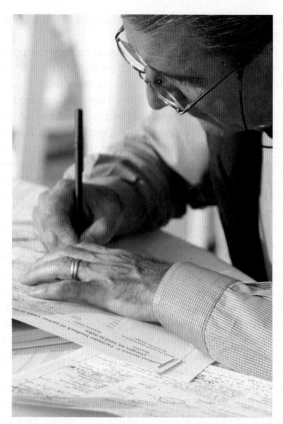

Figure 8.4 Expertise allows middle adults to automatically apply their experience to current situations, which facilitates efficiency and creativity.

Clinical Significance

Middle adults are usually more adept at solving practical difficulties than younger age groups because of their years of experience in doing so (Santrock, 2012). They have encountered everyday difficulties (e.g., cars that will not start and businesses that provide poor service) dozens of times. Although these difficulties remain irritating, a person in his or her 40s or 50s knows that they are solvable, what strategies to use to handle them, and how to survive them.

Older Adult: Wisdom

Cognition is multifaceted; aging affects some dimensions of intellectual functioning more than others (Craig & Dunn, 2013). Therefore, it is not true that all older adults are cognitively impaired.

Numerous studies have examined the speed of cognition in older adults, and the results have shown that older adults take about 50% longer than younger adults to do a simple comparison task (Craig & Dunn, 2013). With more complex tasks, older adults take even longer. These differences may partly result from neurological changes that occur with aging, but they may also be linked to the older adult's decreased use of different strategies to perform cognitive tasks (Craig & Dunn, 2013). Older adults may make fewer guesses and try harder to answer items correctly. If older adults are compared with college students, who are more accustomed to doing tests of recall, the older adults will appear less adept at such tests. Older adults may be able to learn new strategies to compensate for their lack of processing speed (Craig & Dunn, 2013).

Memory has been studied by numerous researchers. Table 8.3 shows different memory functions and the effects of aging on those functions.

Despite the small declines in memory in older adults, older adults are wiser comparatively (Craig & Dunn, 2013). *Wisdom* refers to an expert knowledge system composed of several characteristics:

- Wisdom appears to focus on important and difficult matters often associated with the meaning of life and the human condition.
- The level of knowledge, judgment, and advice reflected in wisdom is superior.
- The knowledge associated with wisdom has extraordinary scope, depth, and balance and is applicable to specific situations.
- Wisdom combines mind and virtue (character) and is employed for personal well-being as well as for the benefit of humankind.

TABLE 8.3 **Memory Functions**		
Type	**Description**	**Aging Effect**
Sensory memory	Retention of a sensory image for a very brief time	Slight or no decrease
Short-term memory	Memory for things the person is currently and actively thinking about	Slight or no decrease
Working memory	Active processing of information while it is held in short-term memory; active thinking	Decreases, but may use better strategies to limit decrease
Episodic long-term memory	Recollection of past events and personally relevant information	Decreases, but may be from slower processing speed
Semantic long-term memory	Retrieval of facts, vocabulary, and general knowledge	Decreases minimally

From Craig, G. J., & Dunn, W. L. (2013). *Understanding human development* (3rd ed). Upper Saddle River, NJ: Pearson Education.

- Although difficult to achieve, wisdom is easily recognized by most people, and it represents the capstone of human intelligence (Craig & Dunn, 2013, p. 511).

Although some older adults do not attain wisdom, it is only in older adulthood that the accumulation of life experience results in the acquisition of wisdom.

Cognitive Development for the Carr Family

- Emily Carr, 2 months old, is in the primary circular reactions substage of the sensorimotor stage.
- Jacob Carr is likely to be in the preoperational stage/symbolic function substage. At age 2 years, his thinking is still very primitive and he cannot see the perspectives of his parents or siblings.
- Madeline Carr, 5 years, is in the intuitive thought substage of the preoperational stage; her thinking is much more sophisticated than Jacob's. Although she may be very confident about the things she knows, she will not be able to tell her parents how her thought process worked to enable her to know things.
- The stage of postformal thought remains controversial among developmental theorists (Santrock, 2012), but considering some practical difficulties for the Carr family may demonstrate the challenges a young adult couple faces. Amber and Michael need to learn how to make decisions for their newly adopted children, and they need to consider that they make better decisions when they are not stressed, angry, or upset.
- Amber and Michael's parents, who are in the later years of middle adulthood, will have cognitive expertise. They should be able to expect that their numerical abilities and perceptual speed may have declined somewhat, but their superior abilities to solve practical difficulties may offset this decline. They may be able to offer wisdom to Amber and Michael and help them sort out which problems are major and which are not.

Language Development

All human societies use language as a means to communicate with one another. Language development consists of two parts. *Receptive language* is the understanding of spoken or written words and sentences and *productive language* is the individual's use of spoken or written words (Craig & Dunn, 2013). Receptive language leads productive language, and throughout the lifespan, receptive vocabulary tends to be larger than productive vocabulary (Craig & Dunn, 2013). A student who comes across an unfamiliar word while reading a book can relate to this phenomenon. One could stop reading to look up the meaning of the new word, figure out its meaning from the context of the sentence, or simply skip the new word and continue reading. Of course, the choice of options depends on whether the student really wants to understand the meaning of the word, incorporate the new word into productive vocabulary, or not bother to learn it at all. Using the new word in conversation is risky, however, if the student does not realize its cultural or social connotations before using it in conversation.

Table 8.4 shows the range of ages for the development of language skills in infants and young children.

Language Development for the Carr Family

- The Carr family can expect that Emily will make cooing sounds and listen to the language of the people around her.
- Jacob should have a vocabulary of some 50 words, although he may be frustrated when he cannot express all his emotions in words.
- Madeline should be easy for Amber and Michael to understand, and she may be able to translate some of Jacob's words because she knows Jacob better than his parents do early in the adoption process. Madeline needs to work on her skills with oral language to prepare her for school entry and the development of reading skills. Amber and Michael should make the time to read to all of the children each day to help them acquire language and use it appropriately.

TABLE 8.4 Language Development in Childhood

Age	Language Skill
Birth	Crying
1–2 months	Cooing
Middle of first year	Babbling
8–12 months	Gestures such as showing and pointing
10–15 months	Uses first word; has receptive vocabulary of 50 words
18 months	Has expressive vocabulary of 50 words
18–24 months	Uses two-word utterances (telegraphic speech) such as "more milk"
2 years	Expressive vocabulary of 200 words
3–6 years	Learns 5–8 new words a day; works on syntax and meaning
6 years	Expressive vocabulary of 8,000–14,000 words; learns 22 new words per day
7 years	Begins to categorize words by parts of speech; learns comparatives (bigger, longer, etc.) and subjective ("If you were the school principal . . . ")
6–12 years	Understands and uses more complex grammar; must be able to do this orally in order to read

From Santrock, J. (2012). *Life-span development* (14th ed.). New York, NY: McGraw-Hill.

Cultural Considerations

Culture profoundly affects individual development. Jean Piaget, Erik Erikson, and Uri Bronfenbrenner all came from Western European backgrounds; their theoretical frameworks clearly reflect the value their cultures placed on such characteristics as independence, self-motivation, and primacy of the individual. The Western viewpoint, however, is not universally supported. Some cultures value dependence and interdependence over independence. Through their choices about feeding, carrying, and dressing infants, and by sending messages about which temperamental qualities are desirable, parents, families, and communities convey to children which behaviors they consider positive and which they deem negative or unacceptable (Santrock, 2012). The toddler learns quickly whether independence is more valued than dependence on a caregiver for decision making and exploration. The preschooler may or may not receive formal early childhood education, depending on whether his or her parents place value on such preparation for school. Erikson's (1963) emphasis on the school-age child's acquisition of adult tools might mean, for some cultures, learning to read in a classroom, but for others, it might involve following older children to learn livestock herding skills, hunting strategies, how to care for younger siblings, or cooking, sewing, and other domestic skills. Adolescents may be required to stay in school until they are 14 years old, as in Brazil, or until they are 17 years old, as in Russia (Santrock, 2012). What a given culture views as a basic education to acquire the tools needed to enter adulthood clearly varies greatly; the curricula in secondary schools depend on what cultures value as important topics and the time it takes to teach those topics (Santrock, 2012). The value of educating both boys and girls (and whether they should attend school separately or together) is highly culturally driven, as is the chosen curriculum.

In addition, some cultures have rites of passage that mark the transition from childhood to adulthood. Santrock (2012) defines a rite of passage as "the avenue through which adolescents gain access to sacred adult practices, to knowledge, and to sexuality" (pp. 415–416). Examples include the Jewish ritual of bar mitzvah for boys and bat mitzvah for girls, Catholic confirmation, and the Hispanic girl's quinceanera (Fig. 8.5). In the United States, these rites do not necessarily give adolescents status as adults in the community outside their faith or ethnic communities. Graduation from high school may or may not lead to adulthood; the graduate may go on to a vocational school, college, or the world of work but may continue to live with or be economically dependent on parents for some years after (Santrock, 2012). The transition to adulthood is a long process for some cultures (particularly those with higher education opportunities) and a very short one in others.

Culture affects intimate relationships in adulthood as well. Desired characteristics in a long-term partner vary across cultures; for example, there are differences in how much people seek out attributes such as chastity, domesticity, spirituality, and a particular age (Santrock, 2012). The ideal age at which to marry is also culturally determined, as is whether it is acceptable to live with a potential spouse before marrying (Santrock, 2012).

By middle adulthood, culture still exerts a large influence on the developing person. Cultures that emphasize parenting as a key role in adulthood may leave the middle adult in an awkward position in a society where the expectation is that children will grow up and leave home; what is the adult's role when parenting is no longer central in his or her life (Santrock, 2012)? Grandparenting may vary greatly depending on cultural expectations for providing child care, advice, and support to children and grandchildren (Santrock, 2012).

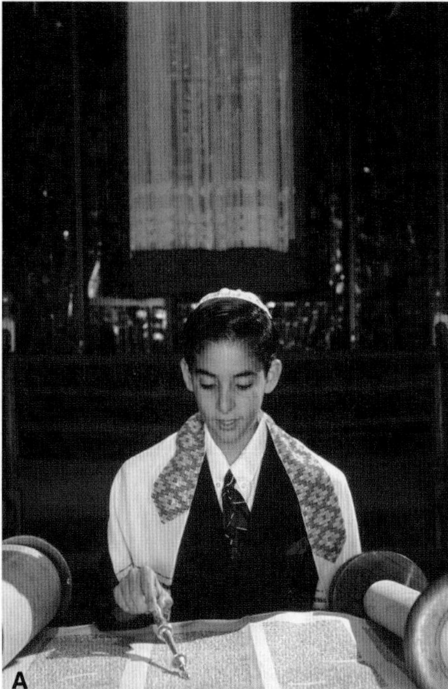

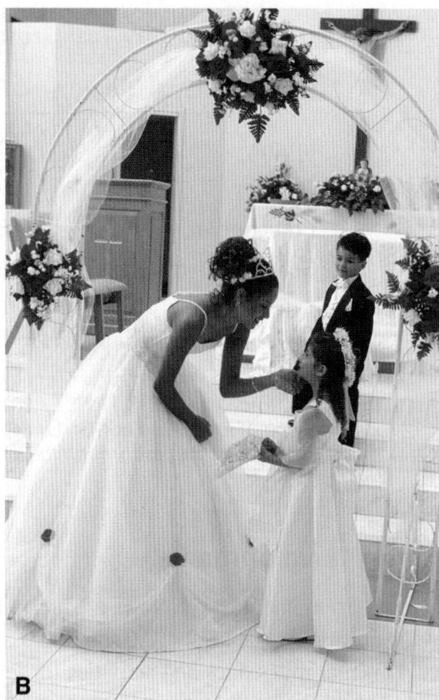

Figure 8.5 Culturally associated rites of passage in Western countries are often symbolic. Often, such occasions are accompanied by large parties with gatherings of family and friends to celebrate. **A.** The bar mitzvah marks that a boy has mastered the fundamental concepts of Judaism and is ready to worship with adults. **B.** The Hispanic *quinceanera* marks the occasion of a girl's 15th birthday.

Using technology to keep in touch with grandchildren across geographical distances may redefine what the family considers to be "close relationships" between grandchildren and grandparents.

For the older adult, cultural expectations are important in determining whether or not the individual engages in work and leisure activities. A society's acceptance of older adults may be limited by ageism and sexism (Santrock, 2012), so that the older adult finds no place in the social order even if he or she had wisdom and experience to share with younger generations. If a woman's role is limited to family maintenance and a man's role to financial productivity, they may be defined as no longer useful once their children are grown or they retire from work (Santrock, 2012). In addition, economic and health issues may determine when, or even whether, a person decides to retire from the world of paid work.

Objective Data

Physical **growth** refers to quantitative changes in a person over time. Increases in height and weight are examples (Leifer & Fleck, 2013). The ways in which nurses measure these changes involve universal tools and metrics (e.g., centimeters and kilograms). In addition, nurses can assess motor development more easily through physical examination and use of screening tools. Therefore, this chapter designates physical growth and motor development under the heading "Objective Data Collection."

Physical Growth

Physical growth takes place in an expected pattern but at a variable pace over time in childhood (Leifer & Fleck, 2013). Table 8.5 shows expected growth patterns in childhood and adolescence. It is important to assess children who are growing more slowly or more rapidly than usual for any potential underlying difficulties.

There are formulas for estimating potential adult height for children (Leifer & Fleck 2013). For boys, the formula is

$$\frac{\textit{Father's height} + \textit{mother's height in inches} + \textit{5 inches}}{2}$$

For girls, the formula is

$$\frac{\textit{Father's height} + \textit{mother's height in inches} - \textit{5 inches}}{2}$$

Expected Growth for the Carr Family

Amber and Michael will need to monitor the growth and nutrition patterns of their three newly adopted children. They need to monitor intake of all the children to ensure that each child consumes high-quality calories and sufficient protein, carbohydrates, and fats to sustain growth (Murray & Zentner, 2009).

- Two-month-old Emily should grow about 25 mm (1 in.) per month and gain 18 g (two-thirds oz) per day.
- Jacob, 2 years old, should have quadrupled his birth weight by now. His growth will slow in the next year; however, over the next 12 months, his height should increase by 64 mm (2.5 in.) to 90 mm (3.5 in.), and he should gain 1–2 kg (2–4 lb).
- Madeline, 5 years old, should grow 64 mm (2.5 in.) to 76 mm (3 in.) in the next year and gain slightly less than 2 kg (5 lb).

TABLE 8.5 Physical Growth in Childhood and Adolescence

Developmental Stage	Expected Growth
Infant	1½ times birth length and triple birth weight by age 1 year
Toddler	½ adult height and quadruple birth weight by age 2 years
Preschooler	6–8 cm (2½–3 in.) and 5–7 lb/year
School-age child	5 cm (2 in.) and 2.27–3.2 kg (5–7 lb)/year
Adolescent	Girls: Growth spurt of 6.4–12.7 cm (2.5–5 in.) and 3.6–4.5 kg (8–10 lb) Boys: Growth spurt of 7.6–15 cm (3–6 in.) and 5.45–6.36 kg (12–14 lb)

Data from Leifer, G., & Fleck, E. (2013). *Growth and development across the lifespan: A health promotion focus* (2nd ed). St. Louis, MO: Saunders; Murray, R. B., & Zentner, J. P. (2009). *Health promotion strategies through the life span* (8th ed.). Upper Saddle River, NJ: Prentice Hall.

Motor Development

Motor development also follows a pattern, but individuals develop at variable rates. Table 8.6 shows gross and fine motor developmental milestones and activities for infants, toddlers, and young children. It is important to recognize that there is a range of ages at which children acquire new skills. Parents concerned about a child's development may need education about the expected range of skill acquisition. Nevertheless, nurses should always take parental concerns about a child seriously so that health care providers can assess delays and intervene quickly, if needed.

TABLE 8.6 Gross and Fine Motor Development: Infancy to Early Childhood

Age	Gross Motor Skills	Fine Motor Skills
0–1 month	Lifts head up off of the bed when prone	Ruled by newborn reflexes
2–4 months	Lifts head and chest up off of the bed when prone, using arms for support	Begins to reach using shoulders and arms
2–4.5 months	Rolls over	Tracks moving objects well
3–6 months	Supports some weight with legs	Begins using hand–eye coordination to reach
5–8 months	Sits without support; some creeping/crawling	Uses visually guided reach; passes object hand to hand
5–10 months	Stands with support	Rolls a ball back and forth to an adult
6–10 months	Pulls self up to stand	Looks for a partially hidden object
7–13 months	Walks using furniture for support	Uses pincer grasp to pick up objects
10–14 months	Stands alone easily	Feeds self using spoon and cup, although not neatly
11–14 months	Walks alone easily	
13–18 months	May be able to climb stairs	Stacks 2–4 cubes or blocks, scribbles
19–24 months	Can pedal a tricycle, jumps on both feet, throws a ball	Pours water, molds clay, partially dresses self
2 years	Climbs, pushes, pulls, runs, hangs by both hands	Dresses self; stacks 6–8 cubes or blocks
3 years	Runs and moves smoothly	Builds high block towers, assembles large jigsaw puzzles but often forces pieces into place
4 years	Skips awkwardly, jumps; changes speed while running	Much more precise building and assembling skills
5 years	Skips smoothly, stands on one foot	Draws rectangle, circle, square, and triangle; ties own shoes

Data from Craig, G. J., & Dunn, W. L. (2013). *Understanding human development* (3rd ed). Upper Saddle River, NJ: Pearson Education; Santrock, J. (2012). *Life-span development* (14th ed.). New York, NY: McGraw-Hill.

Motor Development for the Carr Family

The Carr family should monitor the children's motor development as well as the physical growth.

- Baby Emily will soon be lifting her head off the mattress, although she will not yet be able to reach for objects.
- Toddler Jacob should be very active, learning to pedal a tricycle, jump with both feet, and throw a ball. He may be able to remove clothing and partially dress himself. However, Amber and Michael should not expect Jacob to completely dress himself without help. They will have to closely monitor Jacob because his ability to climb and run may get him into dangerous situations. Blocks and push or pull toys (e.g., wagon, toy lawnmower) are good toys for active and imitative play.
- Five-year-old Madeline should be able to dress herself independently and will run and jump much more easily than Jacob. She should be learning to tie shoes and will be able to draw figures beyond her brother's abilities. Toys could include those that encourage gross and fine motor development (e.g., riding toys, toys that she can assemble into different shapes).

Critical Thinking

When making decisions about how a patient is progressing along a developmental trajectory, the nurse needs to use evidence-based knowledge and critical thinking during assessment. Refer to Unit IV, Special Populations and Foci, for more information on pregnant women, infants, children, adolescents, and older adults.

Nurses are concerned with promoting health and wellness in individuals and families across the lifespan (Fig. 8.6). Healthy children are much more likely to grow into healthy adults; they need a great deal of support to make healthy and safe choices. Parents also need a great deal of support so that they can choose the healthiest possible lifestyles for themselves and their children. As adults move through the different stages of adulthood, they also need to make healthy and safe choices for themselves to lead productive, satisfying lives well into old age.

Diagnostic Reasoning

Nurses use the nursing process to assess, diagnose, plan, implement, and evaluate care. Some examples of nursing diagnoses commonly related to growth and development are included in Table 8.7.

Some outcomes that are related to growth and development difficulties include the following:

- The child will achieve developmental milestones without a delay of 25% or more in one or more areas of social or self-regulatory behavior or cognitive, language, or gross or fine motor skills (Moorhead, Johnson, Maas, & Swanson, 2013).
- The family members will report improvement in their communication, processes, and daily functioning.

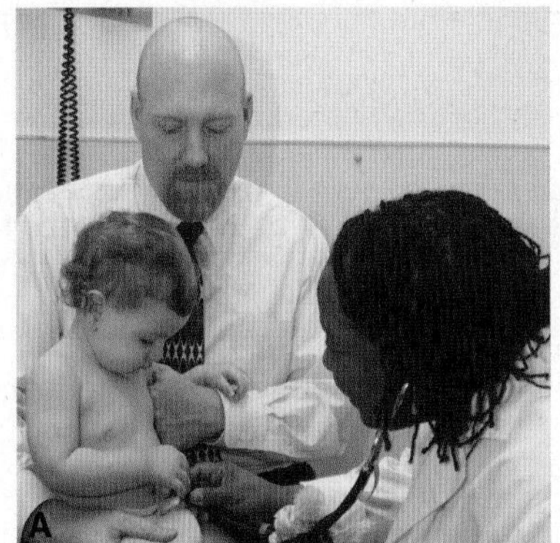

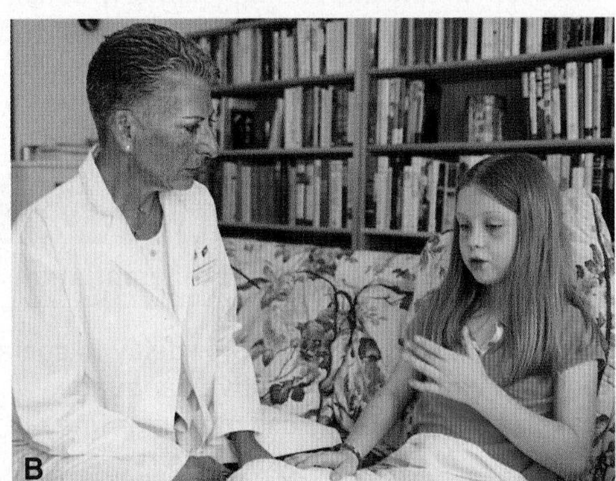

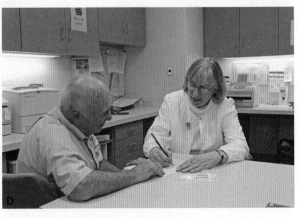

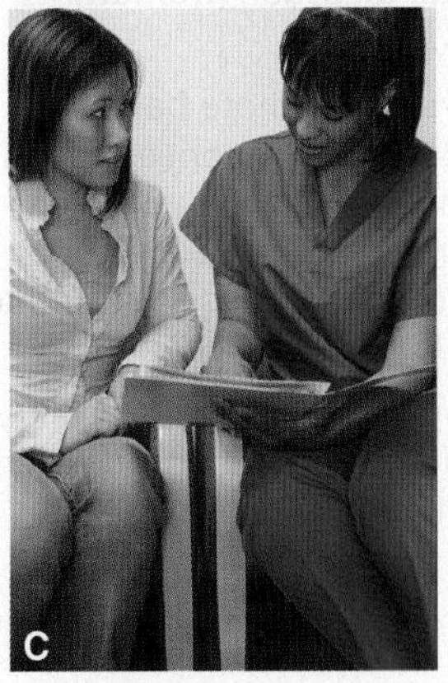

Figure 8.6 Nurses interact with patients at all stages of the lifespan. **A.** Infants and their caregivers. **B.** Older children. **C.** Young adults. **D.** Older adults.

Critical Thinking for the Carr Family

Amber and Michael require assistance to help them navigate the major life changes they are facing. They want information that can help them meet the needs of a preschooler, a toddler, and an infant. Specific concerns include caring for baby Emily, toilet training Jacob, and preparing Madeline for school.

In assessing and intervening with the Carr family, the nurse should rely on evidence-based information about childhood growth and development to advise the parents about the best ways to care for their children. It is also important to use accurate information to advise Amber and Michael about how they can make the healthiest choices for themselves. Doing so will help them maintain their relationship and personal wellness so that they are healthy and able to support their children effectively.

Amber and Michael's parents need careful, evidence-based information to guide them as they move through middle adulthood. Health promotion in middle adulthood is important because it sets the stage for health and wellness in older adulthood (Santrock, 2012).

Interventions for the Carr Family

A developmental assessment should be done for each of the Carr children to help identify any developmental delays quickly and begin intervention as early as possible.

The nurse can work to decrease the risk for developmental delay in the children by encouraging Amber and Michael to become attached to all of them (especially Emily), by managing the environment to ensure safety (e.g., installing gates at stairs in the home, using appropriate car seats for all children, designating safe play areas, supervising children in the bathroom and kitchen, ensuring lead-based paint is not a risk), and by teaching the parents about nutrition and social skills the boy should be acquiring.

The nurse should teach Amber and Michael that Emily needs environmental stimuli (auditory, visual, tactile, vestibular, and gustatory) each day, in short periods when she is awake, and that she must have a parent respond to her vocalizations. Emily needs a comfortable and safe environment to sleep well; Amber and Michael will want to consider factors such as noise, light, temperature, a firm mattress, and appropriate bedding (Wilkinson & Ahern, 2009). Jacob's bed needs to be safe and appropriate for him as well, and both he and Madeline may choose stuffed toys as comfort objects to help them sleep well. They should have regular bedtimes and sleep routines (putting on pajamas, which Jacob will need help with; brushing teeth; stories or songs; saying prayers if the parents wish; and quiet activities before bedtime) so that they are ready for sleep each night.

TABLE 8.7 Common Nursing Diagnoses Associated With Development

Diagnosis	Point of Differentiation	Assessment Characteristics	Nursing Interventions
Risk for delayed child development	At risk for delay in social, cognitive, language, gross motor, or fine motor skills	*Prenatal:* endocrine or genetic disorders, substance abuse *Individual:* adoption, brain damage, chronic illness, congenital disorder, prematurity	*Prenatal:* Avoid exposure to toxins, alcohol, and potentially dangerous substances. Teach caregivers appropriate developmental milestone interactions. *Child:* Provide adequate nutrition.
Readiness for enhanced family processes	Family patterns that support overall family unity and the well-being of its members	Activities promote balance between family cohesion and member autonomy. Boundaries are clear and respected. Communication is appropriate. Family adapts to change.	Assess the family stress level and coping abilities. Use family-centered care and role modeling. Identify resources. Provide parenting classes. Encourage family meals.
Risk for impaired attachment	Risk for disruption in the normal interactive process that fosters a nurturing relationship	If diagnosed, anxiety, inability to initiate contact or meet personal needs	Encourage mothers to breastfeed. Identify postpartum depression. Offer parents the opportunity to express their childhood experiences.

Pulling it All Together

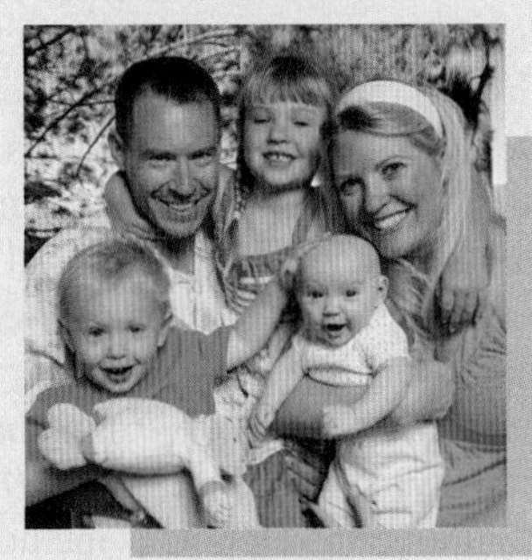

After completing evidence-based interventions, the nurse reevaluates the Carrs and documents findings in the chart to show progress toward outcomes. The nurse uses critical thinking and judgment to continue or revise the diagnosis, outcomes, or interventions. This is often in the form of a care plan or case note similar to the one below.

Nursing Diagnosis	Patient Outcomes	Nursing Interventions	Rationale	Evaluation
Risk for delayed child development related to recent adoption	Children will be within 25% of expected limits for growth, motor, and language development.	Teach that Emily needs environmental stimuli each day, in short periods when she is awake. Teach parents to respond to her vocalizations. Consider home health nurse visit to assess the environment for safety and comfort.	Interventions appropriate to developmental stages improve neurodevelopmental outcomes.	Performed screening on all children. Growth, motor, and language development are within expected limits. Continue regular well visits with the family. Allow time for the family members to ask questions as they adjust to the changes.

Applying Your Knowledge

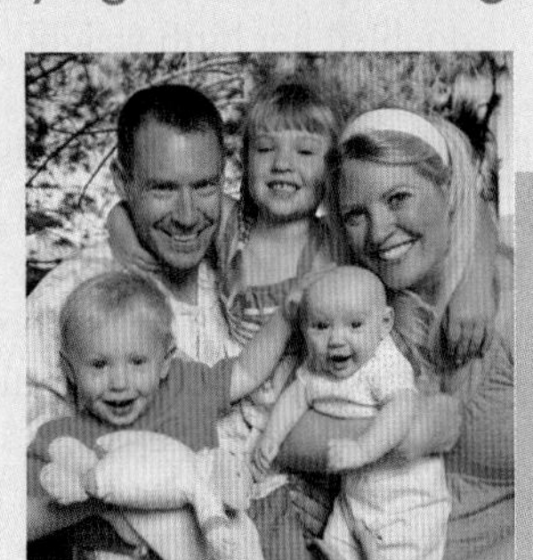

Understanding expected developmental processes is crucial for nurses so that they can recognize patients who are developing expectedly and also those who are deviating in some way from a expected developmental trajectory. Using the previous steps of nursing process and diagnostic reasoning, consider all the case study findings about the Carr family woven throughout this chapter. When answering the following questions, begin drawing conclusions and see how the pieces of assessment must work together to create an environment for personalized, appropriate, and accurate care.

- How much weight should 2-year-old Jacob have gained since birth?
- Why do Madeline and Jacob require supervision in the kitchen and bathroom?
- In what stage of psychosocial development is each member of the Carr family?
- In what stage of Piaget's cognitive thought is each member of the Carr family?
- What nursing diagnoses might be appropriate for members of the Carr family?
- How will the nurse individualize assessments of Emily, Jacob, and Madeline, considering their ages and that they are newly adopted?
- How will the nurse evaluate the success of health teaching with Amber and Michael about home hazards?

Key Points

- Each human experiences physical growth, psychosocial development, and cognitive development.
- Growth refers to changes in height and weight.
- Development refers to changes in motor, language, psychosocial, and cognitive developments.
- Erikson's stages of psychosocial development include (1) trust versus mistrust, (2) autonomy versus shame and doubt, (3) initiative versus guilt, (4) industry versus inferiority, (5) identity versus role confusion, (6) intimacy versus isolation, (7) generativity versus stagnation, and (8) ego integrity versus despair.
- Cognitive development includes sensorimotor, preoperational, concrete operational, and formal operational stages.
- Language development involves receptive and productive language.
- Physical growth takes place in an expected pattern but at a variable pace.
- Motor development follows a pattern, but individuals develop at variable rates.

Review Questions

1. Caitlyn was about 50 cm (20 in.) long at birth and weighed 3 kg (7 lb, 8 oz). At her 1-year well-child checkup, the nurse determines that Caitlyn is 66 cm (26 in.) and weighs 7 kg (16 lb). The nurse's reaction to these assessment findings is to be
   A. concerned; Caitlyn should have quadrupled her birth weight by now.
   B. unconcerned; Caitlyn is growing in height and weight at an expected pace.
   C. concerned because Caitlyn should have tripled her birth weight by now.
   D. unconcerned because Caitlyn has slightly more than doubled her birth weight.

2. The nurse's response to Emily's length, which is 66 cm (26 in.) now and was 51 cm (20 in.) at birth, is to be
   A. concerned because Emily should have grown 25 to 30 cm (10 to 12 in.) by now.
   B. unconcerned because Emily should have grown 15 cm (6 in.) by now.
   C. concerned because Emily should have doubled her birth length by now.
   D. unconcerned because Emily should have grown 7.6 to 10 cm (3 to 4 in.) by now.

3. Jasmyn, who has just had her second birthday, comes to the well-child clinic for an assessment. The nurse reviews her records and discovers that Jasmyn weighed 3.1 kg (7 lb) at birth. Today, the nurse expects that Jasmyn's weight should be
   A. 9.5 kg (21 lb).
   B. 12.7 kg (28 lb).
   C. 15.9 kg (35 lb).
   D. 19 kg (42 lb).

4. Tamika is often in a hurry with her toddler daughter Samantha and usually does things for her that Samantha could do herself if given more time. Erikson would say that Tamika's daughter
   A. will develop a healthy sense of autonomy because of her mother's help.
   B. will not develop shame and doubt because of these interactions with her mother.
   C. will develop a sense of autonomy no matter what her mother does.
   D. is at risk for developing a sense of shame and doubt because of her mother's behavior.

5. Oscar, 6 years old, has come to the well-child clinic for a visit. He is 1.16 m (46 in.) tall today. Assuming that he grows at an expected pace, how tall would the nurse expect Oscar to be at 10 years?
   A. 1.27 m (50 in.)
   B. 1.32 m (52 in.)
   C. 1.37 m (54 in.)
   D. 1.57 m (62 in.)

6. Mallory, 16 years old, is having difficulty in school and with her friends. She has not decided what she wants to do with the rest of her life after high school. Erik Erikson would say that Mallory is at risk for
   A. industry.
   B. inferiority.
   C. identity.
   D. role confusion.

7. At age 27 years, Steve is considering purchasing his first house. How might the nurse characterize Steve's cognitive processes now that he has entered into early adulthood?
   A. He will be very optimistic about the purchase regardless of the housing market.
   B. He will use only logical analysis to systematically consider all the pros and cons of the purchase.
   C. He will be less optimistic and more practical, considering the complexities of the situation.
   D. He will be more logical and more optimistic than he would have been a little earlier in development.

8. Nell, 50 years old, is worried about whether her intelligence will change as she continues to advance through middle age. What can the nurse tell Nell about what might happen to her cognitive skills in middle age?
   A. Nell can expect her vocabulary to gradually decrease over time.
   B. Nell can expect to be slightly slower as she does cognitive tasks.
   C. Nell will have great difficulty learning new skills.
   D. Nell will find that her life experience is unhelpful in problem solving.

9. Earl is healthy and vigorous at 68 years. Which of the following will NOT be true of his cognition as he ages?
   A. His long-term memory will definitely be impaired.
   B. His speed of processing information will slow down.
   C. His short-term memory should not be impaired.
   D. His sensory threshold will increase.

10. Amber and Michael Carr need to be taught that 2-month-old Emily
   A. needs stimuli each day in the short periods when she is awake.
   B. will benefit from as much attention as possible.
   C. needs to have stimuli limited to basic needs.
   D. will benefit from long periods of attention with rest.

The Jensen suite offers these additional resources to enhance learning and facilitate understanding of this chapter:

- thePoint online resource, http://thepoint.lww.com/Jensen2e
- *Laboratory Manual for Nursing Health Assessment: A Best Practice Approach*
- *Pocket Guide for Nursing Health Assessment: A Best Practice Approach*
- *Lippincott DocuCare,* an electronic health record simulation software, http://thepoint.lww.com/docucare
- *Adaptive Learning | Powered by PrepU*, http://thepoint.lww.com/prepu

References

Blakemore, S.-J., & Choudhury, S. (2006). Brain development during puberty: State of the science. *Developmental Science, 9*(1), 11–14.

Bronfenbrenner, U. (1977). Toward an experimental ecology of human development. *American Psychologist*, 32, 513–531.

Bronfenbrenner, U. (1979). *The ecology of human development.* Cambridge, MA: Harvard University Press.

Bronfenbrenner, U. (Ed.). (2005). *Making human beings human: Bioecological perspectives on human development.* Thousand Oaks, CA: Sage.

Craig, G. J., & Dunn, W. L. (2013). *Understanding human development* (3rd ed). Upper Saddle River, NJ: Pearson Education.

Erikson, E. H. (1963). *Childhood and society* (2nd ed.). New York, NY: W.W. Norton.

Labouvie-Vief, G. (1986, August). *Modes of knowing and life-span cognition.* Paper presented at the annual meeting of the American Psychological Association, Washington, DC.

Leifer, G., & Fleck, E. (2013). *Growth and development across the lifespan: A health promotion focus* (2nd ed.). St. Louis, MO: Saunders.

Moorhead, S., Johnson, M., Maas, M. L., & Swanson, E. (2013). *Nursing outcomes classification (NOC): Measurement of health outcomes* (5th ed.). St. Louis, MO: Elsevier.

Murray, R. B., & Zentner, J. P. (2009). *Health promotion strategies through the life span* (8th ed.). Upper Saddle River, NJ: Prentice Hall.

Perry, W. G. (1970). *Forms of intellectual and ethical development in the college years.* New York, NY: Holt, Rinehart and Winston.

Perry, W. G. (1999). *Forms of intellectual and ethical development in the college years: A scheme.* San Francisco, CA: Jossey Bass.

Piaget, J. (1952). *The origins of intelligence in children.* New York, NY: International Universities Press.

Santrock, J. (2012). *Life-span development* (14th ed.). New York, NY: McGraw-Hill.

Schaie, K. W., & Willis, S. (2000). A stage theory model of adult development revisited. In R. Rubinstein, M. Moss, & M. Kleban (Eds.), *The many dimensions of aging: Essays in honor of M. Powell Lawton.* New York, NY: Springer.

U.S. Department of Health and Human Services. (2013). *Healthy People 2020: Topics & Objectives – Objectives A-Z.* Retrieved from http://www.healthypeople.gov/2020/topicsobjectives2020/

9

Mental Health and Violence Assessment

Learning Objectives

1 Assess for risk factors for mental health conditions and identify appropriate health promotion measures.

2 Assess for alcohol or substance abuse.

3 Assess spirituality and sense of meaning.

4 Assess for suicidal ideations.

5 Analyze subjective and objective findings from assessment of patients victimized by violence to plan effective interventions.

6 Assess for depression.

7 Assess mental status including appearance, behavior, cognition, and thought processes.

8 Use the Mini-Mental State Examination (MMSE) to determine mental status.

Mr. Hart, a 75-year-old Caucasian male, arrives at the community health care walk-in clinic to have his blood pressure checked. He has been to the clinic several times in the last few weeks for the same purpose. His temperature is 37°C (98.6°F) orally, pulse 86 beats/min, respirations 16 breaths/min, and blood pressure 146/82 mmHg. Current medications include a multivitamin, an antihypertensive, and an antidepressant (citalopram).

You will gain more information about Mr. Hart as you progress through this chapter. As you study the content and features, consider Mr. Hart's case and its relationship to what you are learning. Begin thinking about the following points:

- What three techniques of mental health assessment the nurse could use to gain Mr. Hart's trust?
- How are the mental status assessment and mental health history integrated?
- How will the nurse assess for suicidal ideation, homicidal ideation, violence, and hallucinations?
- What developmental, behavioral, and life choices may contribute to Mr. Hart's symptoms?
- What recommendations for follow-up would the nurse suggest for Mr. Hart?
- How will the nurse evaluate whether he or she has gained the patient's trust and promoted respect?

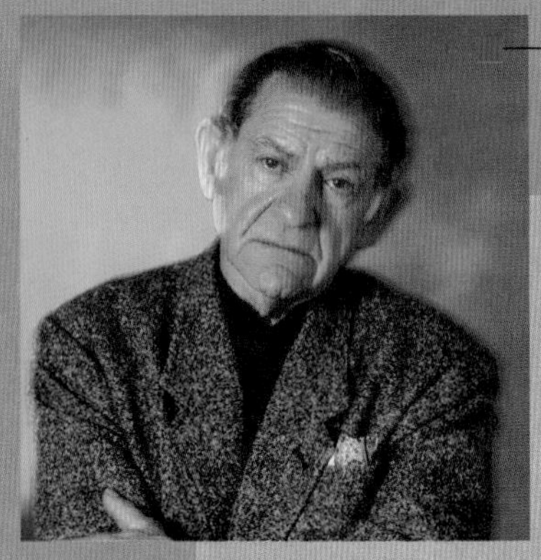

The World Health Organization (WHO) states the following regarding mental health:

> *There is no health without mental health . . . it [is a] state of well-being in which the individual realizes his or her own abilities, can cope with the normal stresses of life, can work productively and fruitfully, and is able to make a contribution to his or her community . . . mental health is the foundation for well-being and effective functioning for an individual and for a community. . . .* (WHO, 2013b).

Based on these definitions, mental health is an integral part of a patient's well-being; thus, the assessment of mental health status is essential. As a nurse, you are often the first health care practitioner a patient sees in any health care setting. The patient may be seeking care for a physical problem when a thorough nursing assessment uncovers an underlying mental health situation. It is not uncommon for a patient to have lived with a mental health condition for a long time, even since childhood, and not realize that he or she has a problem. The patient may be self-medicating with alcohol or other substances to feel better.

Common mental health disorders include depression, schizophrenia, and substance abuse. Nursing assessment of mental health consists of screening for preexisting, as well as current, mental health conditions for all age groups and also includes assessment for violence. Violence occurs in many forms, each with its unique risk factors and characteristics, and is often linked to mental health and coping skills. This chapter presents assessment techniques that nurses can use to identify risk factors, assess mental status and mental health, assess for violence, and guide patients in planning care.

Role of the Nurse in Mental Health and Violence Screening

You perform a mental health assessment while considering the patient within the context of his or her own culture. The mental health assessment is based on observation of the patient and the patient's responses to your questions. Mental health assessment questions are integral to any full medical or nursing examination, even in an examination of a patient without a history of mental illness. Assessment for violence is also included in the mental health assessment.

Assessment of mental health, unlike assessment of skin or lungs, must be inferred from answers to questions and behaviors because it cannot be observed directly. During the general nursing assessment, you determine whether there is a need to investigate an area in more depth; if indicated, you may add more assessment questions and observations.

Violence

About one third of women in the world are victims of violence. It is a common situation that often goes unreported (WHO, 2013a). There are many other forms of violence, including bullying, war violence, and elder abuse. The following paragraphs discuss various forms of violence in detail.

Family Violence

A crime is considered **family violence** if the victim is biologically related to the offender or is (or was) related to him or her through marriage, adoption, or legal guardianship. The term *family violence* is often used interchangeably with the terms *domestic violence*, *intimate partner violence*, and *male violence against women*. It is best to ask the patient for clarification and specifics if he or she uses any of these terms.

Types of family violence include child maltreatment, sibling violence, intimate partner violence, and elder abuse (Phillips, Phillips, Grupp, & Trigg, 2009). The nurse may encounter all these types during patient assessments. Some patients never disclose that they have been hurt or seek assistance from police, health care professionals, counselors, or lawyers.

Child Maltreatment

Child maltreatment covers a wide range of violent behaviors against children. Prevalence rates, however, have focused primarily on abuse of children by parents and are based mainly on reported cases of abuse investigated by child protective services (CPS). Violent practices rarely occur as isolated incidents; often, children have more than one victimization experience. Polyvictimization is highest in children who report rape and dating violence. Trauma symptoms such as anxiety, depression, anger, and aggression are "red flags" of polyvictimization.

Sibling Violence

Historically, violence between and among siblings has not been taken seriously. It often has been considered within the realm of normal sibling relationships and represented by such terms as sibling rivalry, roughhousing, and sibling competition (Phillips et al., 2009). Nevertheless, **sibling violence** is among the most common type of violence that children experience.

Intimate Partner Violence

Intimate partner violence (IPV) has been defined as behaviors between spouses or nonmarital partners involving threatened or actual physical or sexual violence, psychological/emotional abuse, and/or coercive tactics when prior physical or sexual violence took place. Nonmarital partners include those in adolescent and adult dating relationships and in long-term, committed, intimate heterosexual or homosexual relationships. No group is immune to IPV—it occurs in all cultures and populations and across all ages, ethnicities/races, education levels, and socioeconomic statuses. Perpetrators of IPV are most often male. Of women who report being raped, physically assaulted, or stalked since age 18 years, approximately two thirds are victimized by a current or former husband, cohabiting male partner, boyfriend, or date (Rape, Abuse & Incest National Network, 2008). Abusive and controlling behaviors and practices by perpetrators of IPV are described in Table 9.1.

TABLE 9.1 **Power and Control in Intimate Partner Violence**	
Intimate Partner Violence Behaviors and Practices by Perpetrators	**Descriptions**
Intimidation	Making victims afraid by using looks, actions, gestures; smashing things; destroying property; abusing pets; displaying weapons
Coercion and threats	Making and/or carrying out threats to do something to hurt victims; threatening to leave, commit suicide, report victims to welfare; making victims drop charges or do illegal things (i.e., take drugs)
Emotional abuse	Putting down victims or making them feel bad about themselves; calling victims names; making victims think they are crazy; playing mind games; humiliating or making victims feel guilty
Isolation	Controlling what victims do or read, whom they see or talk to, or where they go; limiting their involvement outside the home; using jealousy to justify actions
Minimizing, denying, and blaming	Making light of abuse and not taking concerns of victims seriously; saying abuse did not happen; shifting responsibility for abusive behavior; saying victims caused it
Using children	Making victims feel guilty about children; having children relay messages; using visitation to harass victims; threatening to take children away; using children as spies
Privilege	Treating victims like servants; making all big decisions; acting like the "master of the castle"; being the one who defines men's and women's roles
Economic abuse	Preventing victims from getting or keeping a job; making victims ask for money or giving them an allowance; taking money; not letting victims know about or have access to family income

Adapted from the Domestic Abuse Intervention Project, Duluth, MN 55306

Clinical Significance

Although rates of violence by female perpetrators are much lower than by male perpetrators, health care professionals who assume that women are not violent and, in particular, not sexually violent may mistakenly omit asking women in lesbian relationships or men in heterosexual relationships about female-perpetrated violence. Reexamining assumptions and stereotypes is integral to compassionate and respectful violence assessment.

Intimate Partner Violence Among Immigrants and Refugees. Female U.S. immigrants and refugees, particularly those who do not speak English or do not have U.S. legal documents, are especially vulnerable to IPV. Rates of IPV may be higher in female immigrants than in female U.S. citizens for several reasons. Some cultures more visibly accept violence against women than does the U.S. culture. In addition, U.S. immigrants who attempt to escape IPV face significant barriers. For example, they may not have access to bilingual safety shelters, financial assistance, food, or other support services. It is also unlikely that they have assistance from certified interpreters during court proceedings, when reporting complaints to police, or even when acquiring information about their rights and the legal system. Finally, perpetrators of IPV may use their partners' immigration status as a tool of control and force women to remain in the relationship, making it difficult for victims to escape the violence.

⚠ SAFETY ALERT

Murder or homicide is considered IPV when perpetrated by a current or former intimate partner. Most homicides in which the victim is a woman are preceded by a history of IPV before the woman's death. Just as males are perpetrators of most IPV, males also commit 90% of female homicides (U.S. Department of Justice, 2013).

Intimate Partner Violence in Pregnancy. IPV in pregnancy is a serious and widespread problem. Of women abused during pregnancy, more than half also experienced IPV before pregnancy. For nurses working with U.S. citizens, immigrants, and refugees, the high rates of abuse demonstrate that an assessment for violence in the prenatal, intrapartum, and postpartum periods is essential.

Elder Abuse

Maltreatment of adults can be in the form of **elder abuse**, neglect, financial exploitation, or abandonment. Abuse includes intentional actions, by a caregiver or other person who stands in a trust relationship to a vulnerable elder, that cause harm or create a serious risk to the elder (Fulmer, 2012). Examples include kicking, punching, slapping, or burning. Factors that put older adults at risk include dependency, cognitive decline, strained mental or physical health of caregivers, and financial issues. A commonly used tool to screen for maltreatment in older adults is the Elder Assessment Instrument (Fulmer, 2012).

Violence Against Adults With Disabilities

Violence against vulnerable adults, such as those with physical and mental disabilities, includes harmful acts of commission (abuse) or omission (neglect). Physical, sexual, psychological, and financial abuse and neglect may be intentional or unintentional. Adults with disabilities are more likely to experience severe and long-term abuse, be victims of multiple violent episodes, and be abused by many perpetrators. In addition, sexual assault is exceptionally high in women with developmental disabilities.

> *SAFETY ALERT*
> *Adults with disabilities are twice as likely to be victims of violence as those without disabilities (U.S. Department of Justice, 2013). Over the course of their lives, IPV occurs at disproportionate and elevated rates among men and women with disabilities (Hughes, Lund, Gabrielli, Powers, & Curry, 2011, p. 302).*

Youth and School Violence

Many young people witness, perpetrate, and are victimized by violence in and around their schools and neighborhoods. This includes daily nonfatal crimes, such as theft and simple assault, as well as serious violent crime. Violent practices include being slapped, hit, or punched at school; being beaten or mugged in neighborhoods; and being shot, shot at, or stabbed.

Punking and Bullying

Punking and bullying are common among middle and high school males, usually resulting in the victim's shame, humiliation, and anger. Similar to bullying and sometimes used interchangeably, **punking** is a practice of verbal and physical violence, humiliation, and shaming, usually done in public or with an audience (Phillips, 2007). **Bullying** in the form of verbal violence is common among middle and high school girls (Beaty & Alexeyev, 2008).

Sexual Violence

Sexual violence includes forced sex in dating and marital relationships, gang rape, sexual harassment, inappropriate touching, molestation, sex with a patient, forced prostitution, and forced exposure to sexually explicit behavior. Child sexual abuse and adult rape are two relatively common types of sexual violence. Marital rape is not a crime in all countries; in fact, it has been illegal in the United States only for 20 years. Strongly patriarchal societies, cultures, and religions are strictly organized around the supremacy of the father as head of the family or clan, with wives and children dependent (legally and otherwise) on him. Many women in some countries do not have the right or a voice to say "no" to sex in such relationships.

Hate Crimes

The U.S. Department of Justice (2013) defines a **hate crime** as one in which a perpetrator chooses a victim because of a characteristic such as race, ethnicity, gender, sexuality, or religion and provides evidence that hate motivated the crime. Psychological and emotional violence are the most common forms of hate crimes. Nurses and other health care professionals often meet people who have experienced hate crimes; however, such violence may never be disclosed by patients or asked about by professionals.

Human Trafficking

The United Nations Office on Drugs and Crime (2008) defines **human trafficking** as the recruitment, transportation, transfer, harboring, or receipt of people through threats, force, coercion, or deception. Misleading or false advertising (e.g., offers of good wages and "legitimate" work abroad) may entice men and women attempting to escape unemployment in their home countries. After responding to such advertising, these people may be abducted, bonded, or sold into indentured servitude. Reasons people are trafficked include sexual exploitation, forced marriage, and cheap labor for domestic or commercial purposes. Those who own and manage commercial "sex trade" businesses (i.e., forced prostitution, stripping, pornography, live sex shows) are the major perpetrators of human trafficking. Labor exploitation includes domestic servitude, sweatshop factories, and migrant agricultural work.

War-Related Violence

A relatively common form of violence is related to war. War-related fighting can involve witnessing killing, including of friends and fellow service people; intentionally killing and injuring other humans; and being intentionally injured or potentially killed. People who have experienced war violence may include veterans, families of veterans, and refugees who have witnessed war and its associated violence. Many refugees who have escaped war and who have spent time in a refugee camp before coming to the United States may have traumatic experiences that included actual or witnessed violence. Rates of IPV perpetration are higher in veterans with posttraumatic stress disorder (PTSD) related to combat exposure.

Interviewing Patients About Violence

Asking patients about personal experiences of violence is a key aspect of assessment. Of utmost importance is how such assessment is conducted. First and foremost in your mind should be the patient's physical and emotional safety. A universal rule is that patient interviews are done in private—including without significant others or anyone who may or could be the perpetrator (e.g., friend, mother-in-law). Do not make assumptions about who may or may not be a perpetrator or who may have power over the patient and thus prevent him or her from talking freely and safely.

Asking about violent experiences works best when it is a normal and natural part of nursing assessment. Your approach can be similar to asking about sleep or activity difficulties or dietary or sexual concerns. It is important to try to establish a connection with the patient first. In general, you should listen to patients more than you talk, using an 80% to 20% guideline (80% patient, 20% nurse). The possible exception is during patient education. Taking time to listen in a nonjudgmental, nondirective way and ensuring confidentiality helps create a safe, supportive atmosphere.

Basics to review when assessing for violence include the following:

- Perform assessment and screening only when the patient is alone in a safe private environment.
- Establish rapport and connection by showing interest in the patient and by listening.
- Be very patient as the patient talks.
- Move from general open-ended questions to specific questions.
- Demonstrate compassion, not judgment.
- Use interpreters if any question arises about understanding on the patient's or your part. Clarify and repeat back to the patient what he or she says and what you understand.
- Maintain comfortable and neutral body language.
- Remain close to and at eye level with the patient but not in his or her "personal" space.
- Use a relaxed and calm tone of voice at medium volume, with pacing appropriate to the patient's developmental level and level needed for clear understanding.
- Do not ask a patient if he or she wants to press charges against the perpetrator. This decision is up to a prosecutor and is not part of a violence assessment.
- Often, the best way to ask a patient about violence is simply and directly.

The above bullet points are generalizations. You should always ask a patient if he or she is comfortable with the approach taken and the interview space. Open-ended questions such as "What would you like to know?" "How can I help you understand?" or "What would you like me to know?" are especially helpful if a patient appears uncomfortable.

You can prepare patients for sensitive or difficult questions about violence by prefacing comments with statements such as, "Now is the point in the interview where I ask patients about relationships in their family. Who lives in your home with you? How do you feel in that relationship?" It is also common to ask, "Because violence is so common for so many people, I routinely ask all patients about violent experiences—in the past and currently. I wonder if you have experienced or are experiencing violence?" See Boxes 9.1 and 9.2 for other ways to phrase questions about violence to further assess potential victimization.

BOX 9.1 Abuse Assessment Screen

1. **Within the last year**, have you been hit, slapped, kicked, or otherwise physically hurt by someone? YES NO
   If YES, by whom? ____________
   Total number of times ________
2. **Since you've been pregnant**, have you been hit, slapped, kicked, or otherwise physically hurt by someone? YES NO
   If YES, by whom? ____________
   Total number of times ________
3. **Within the last year**, has anyone forced you to have sexual activities? YES NO
   If YES, by whom? ____________
   Total number of times ________

Score each of the following incidents according to the following scale. If any of the descriptions for the higher number apply, use the higher number.

1 = Threats of abuse including use of a weapon
2 = Slapping, pushing; no injuries and/or lasting pain
3 = Punching, kicking, bruises, cuts, and/or continuing pain
4 = Beating up, severe contusions, burns, broken bones
5 = Head injury, internal injury, permanent injury
6 = Use of weapon; wound from weapon

Developed by the Nursing Research Consortium on Violence and Abuse. Readers are encouraged to reproduce and use this assessment tool.

BOX 9.2 Assessment Questions: Violence Victimization and Perpetration

Assessing Violence Victimization Sample Questions

- "Because violence is so common in many people's lives, I ask all patients about it routinely."
- "Are you in a relationship with a person who physically or sexually hurts or threatens you?"
- "Did someone cause those injuries? Who?"
- "Injuries like yours could have been caused by someone hurting you. Did someone hurt you?"
- "Sometimes when people feel the way you do, it's because they have been hurt or abused at home. Is that happening to you?"
- "Many of the adults (children, teens) I work with have experienced violence in their past, and some are experiencing it in their current lives. I wonder if you have any experiences of violence."

Assessing Violence Perpetration

- "Some people think that under certain circumstances it's OK to hit a person you love. What are your thoughts about that?"
- "If you were faced with overwhelming stress (e.g., losing your job, spouse/partner leaving you), what behaviors might you display?"
- "Have you ever physically hurt someone in your family?" (Ask for specifics and think safety first.)
- "Have you ever physically hurt someone?"

Another way to begin assessment about controlling behaviors or emotional and psychological abuse is to assess daily routines. Examples of questions include, "Tell me what you did today from the time you got up until the time you got here.," or "Describe your last 3 days." Sometimes, asking patients about their daily lives and routines reveals detailed information about victimizing behaviors and isolation, even when abuse is by a sibling, peer, or parent (Phillips et al., 2009). In addition, this approach gives the patient a chance to share his or her story, connect with the nurse, and display strengths. It also provides opportunities for teaching, providing resources, affirming strengths, and giving support.

Include questions about adverse childhood and family events and about current living context; these questions may elicit information about adverse experiences. Psychosocial histories often include violence assessment, but they can be very sensitive areas for patients to discuss. Moving into this area of assessment toward the end of the patient history allows time to build rapport and to ask less sensitive questions first.

You should be calm and not pressure patients to disclose information, leave their partners, or otherwise make decisions that patients are not ready to make. This type of pressure can cause disconnection in your relationship with the patient and may result in the patient not returning for follow-up care, which could leave the patient in a less safe position and with fewer resources. The nurse's responsibility is to screen for and identify controlling and abusive behaviors, provide information about safety and resources, and report when mandatory reporting is required (see later discussion). Normally, patient information is confidential, which remains true when patients report violence, but some exceptions exist.

Urgent Assessment

Urgent mental health assessment includes questions about violence and harm to self or others. Acute situations include a risk for injury with psychotic states, depression, dementia, and delirium. Suspected violence and risk for harm is also a situation requiring urgent attention. It is important to ask the safety questions first and leave the presenting situation for last. This order of questioning prevents you from forgetting to ask about safety. It also allows you to have more time to focus on the presenting situation rather than rushing to ask the safety questions at the end of the interaction, when a patient may feel too rushed to speak frankly.

Subjective Data

Subjective data include what the patient says directly to you, what you overhear the patient telling someone else, and what family and friends report. The best way to obtain subjective data during an interview is to ask open-ended questions. Doing so encourages the patient to elaborate when answering. It also allows you to assess the patient's cognitive processes and understanding of the question. Common practice is to obtain information from family or friends to validate information that the patient provides in the interview. It is best to ask questions that family and friends can validate promptly, especially when assessing for level of memory, accuracy, or perception of the situation.

Assessing mental health and violence is an art as well as a science. The "art" lies in the nurse's ability to communicate and accurately assess the patient. You must listen not only for what is said but also for what remains unsaid. You must be comfortable asking questions about psychosis, suicide, history of abuse, and sexuality. If you are uncomfortable, the patient will sense it and be reluctant to respond. You may be tempted to avoid asking relevant questions because of emotions they evoke within you. It is important to practice asking these types of questions during the laboratory and clinical experiences to increase your skill and comfort level.

The "science" of mental health assessment lies in the knowledge base that you incorporate into the examination, including the accurate labeling of findings and the precise use of reliable and valid tools that screen for mental health issues.

When assessing a new patient, establish rapport first. If not much time is available to establish rapport, or if the patient is guarded or suspicious, you can say, "The questions I am about to ask you I ask all of my patients," and then proceed.

Patients may use diversionary tactics to avoid answering questions. Examples include laughing spontaneously, giving responses that do not follow a logical order, asking *you* personal questions, or being insulting. These tactics will likely disrupt the flow of communication and your thought processes. Assessing the reasons for such tactics is important. Patients may try to avoid answering questions because they are embarrassed, the topic is too emotionally overwhelming, or they cannot remember and do not want you to realize that. Patients might also fear being judged, or they may have difficulty concentrating. Focusing on what the patient is saying will help you identify when divergent tactics are being used as well as what is being left unsaid.

Assessment of Risk Factors

Assessment of risk factors involves assessment of violence and mental health conditions. Be aware that certain situations are considered risk factors for contributing to, or exacerbating, a mental health condition. Factors that cannot be changed include family history, age, and gender. Factors that can be changed are environmental factors; these include support systems, housing, health care accessibility, and literacy. Consider also metabolic issues and associated physiological processes such as Parkinson disease, cancer, HIV/AIDS, and other chronic conditions. Risk factors and causes for illness are often complex and interrelated. Nevertheless, identification of these risks helps identify topics for health promotion teaching.

History and Risk Factors	Rationale
Personal History What is your name? Age? Gender? Race?	This generic question opens a conversation about mental health concerns. *Age:* Children are at risk for abuse. Adolescence is a risk because of hormonal changes as well as growth and developmental stage. Older adults are at increased risk for depression. Diagnoses early in life may indicate more problems with developmental, cognitive, social, and coping skills. *Gender:* Females are more prone to depression, and males are more apt to commit suicide or violence. *Race:* Suicide rates among U.S. males are highest in Native Americans and Alaska Natives. Rates are lowest for African American women U.S. Department of Health & Human [USDHHS] Services, 2009a.
How are you feeling today? Do you have any medical difficulties, such as • Pain • Thyroid imbalance, diabetes mellitus • Hepatitis, renal disease • Cerebrovascular accidents, pulmonary diseases, asthma, chronic obstructive pulmonary disease (COPD) • Gastroinntestinal distress: irritable bowel syndrome, Crohn disease • Potentially terminal illnesses: HIV/AIDS, cancer • Surgery that has resulted or may result in disfiguring or incapacitating alteration of ability to function	Physiological changes with illness or emotional responses to illness can affect mental status. Also consider how the medical condition might affect any psychiatric medications, such as causing poor absorption or impaired elimination.
When did you first notice this mental health concern?	Response indicates how long the patient has had a difficulty. Patient responses also can be compared to family perceptions.
• Why do you think it started, when it did it start?	Identify any possible contributing factors.
• How often does it occur?	Response indicates how the patient's problem might be affecting functioning.
• What changes have you noticed?	Changes include frequency, intensity, or effects on functioning or well-being.
• Have you ever felt this way before?	This is to assess for any previous episodes, especially if untreated.
• What do you think is causing the problem?	Assess the patient's understanding of the situation and whether it is logical.
• How is this affecting your life now?	Assess implications of how this illness is affecting the patient's life. Assess feelings of self-worth from the patient's responses to the questions and statements the patient might make about himself or herself or the illness, such as, "I don't like feeling this way. I can't be a good mom when I'm feeling depressed."
Describe your typical day.	This helps to identify the ability to perform activities of daily living.
Have you experienced recent weight loss or gain?	Some medications cause weight gain and metabolic issues. Weight changes also may be related to anxiety, early-onset dementia, depression, or eating disorders. Physical difficulties can manifest with mental health issues.

(table continues on page 187)

History and Risk Factors	Rationale
Have you noticed any change in your sleeping habits?	Sleep disorders may be associated with anxiety, depression, bipolar disorder, or substance abuse.
Have you had any surgeries? If so, please list when and why.	Some patients with mental health conditions present with multiple surgeries and psychosomatic symptoms.
Have you ever been told that you have a mental health condition?	Assess for the patient's history of mental health conditions.
• Have you ever received treatment for a mental health condition before?	Treatment could be outpatient, inpatient, from a general practitioner, or from another health care practitioner.
• Have you ever been hospitalized for a mental health condition before?	Hospitalization indicates the severity of the condition. It is helpful to get the names of facilities and dates when admitted.
Have you ever been physically, sexually, or emotionally abused? If so, did this occur when you were a child?	Assess for situational stressors such as bullying at school, family violence, or war violence. Patients with a history of adverse childhood experiences, including abuse and violence, have been associated with increased risks of substance abuse, risky sexual behavior, psychological morbidity, and violence.
Psychosocial History	
Support Network. Do you have a support system? • Whom do you consider as part of your support system? • How well does your support system meet your needs?	Assess the patient's coping skills and resources. Assess patient's support system and its effectiveness. Some patients with chronic mental conditions have only their health care providers as a support system.
Do you have a significant other in your life, such as a spouse, partner, or close friend? • How do you get along? • How often do you get together with people with whom you do not live?	Assess the stability and effectiveness of the patient's relationships. Patients with high demands often move among relationships as family members, partners, or friends become fatigued.
Stressors. What are some stresses that you have been experiencing? • Have you experienced a loss recently, such as death of a family member or friend or loss of job or income?	Assess for the degree or amount of current stress.
• How do you cope with stress? • How is that working for you now?	Coping skills are used to deal with stress. Evaluate their effectiveness.
Are there any other factors in your life that may be contributing to your stress level? • What are your living arrangements? • How many hours a week do you work? • Is this problem affecting your work? • Is this problem affecting your level of functioning or thinking?	Factors that contribute to mental health situations include the following: • Isolation: lives alone or is withdrawn • Finances: lower socioeconomic status • Poor or diminished cognitive abilities • Housing: homeless or unsafe environment • Health care accessibility: have problems with cost, transportation, or ability to cognitively and safely use public transportation occurred? • Language: cannot speak or understand the predominant language • Literacy: cannot read or write
Do you have, or have you had, any legal problems? If so, please specify if you were sent to jail or prison for them and when.	Patients with problems of judgment, substance abuse, or anger management may become involved in the legal system.

(table continues on page 188)

History and Risk Factors	Rationale
Substance Use. Do you drink or use recreational substances? • What do you use (i.e., beer, wine, hard liquor, and/or recreational substances, such as marijuana, crack, or cocaine)? • How often do you use each substance? • How is the use of alcohol or recreational substances affecting your life? If you suspect that alcohol use might be a difficulty, the **CAGE** is a quick first-step questionnaire to use as an assessment tool. The acronym is easy to remember and use at any time. The tool is available online [Ewing, 1984].	Whenever a patient comes in for treatment of substance use, it is important to be aware of the possibility of an underlying mental health difficulty. Also, it is very important to know the effects that alcohol and other substances can have on mental health (Table 9.2). When screening for substance abuse, be aware that the patient will most likely deny a difficulty. The CAGE tool is valuable because it addresses this denial.
Spirituality. Do you have any religious beliefs regarding your illness? Should I be aware of any religious or cultural beliefs while caring for you? See **HOPE** tool (Box 9.3).	Asking how the patient views the mental health condition in the context of religion and beliefs allows the nurse to provide culturally sensitive nursing care.

(table continues on page 189)

TABLE 9.2 Substances That Can Affect Health

Substance Used	Effect on Health
Injectable drugs	Abscesses, sepsis, endocarditis, pulmonary fibrosis, renal disease
Narcotics	Dependence, addiction, drowsiness, respiratory arrest, overdose
Central nervous system stimulants	Possible dependence, weight loss, tooth decay
Club drugs (e.g., Ecstasy)	Possible loss of memory and subsequent sexual assault
Recreational drugs (specify)	Sherm—phencyclidine (PCP)-laced marijuana that causes irreversible brain damage
Herbals (specify)	Salvia—a psychedelic that, when misused, can cause errors in judgment, headaches, and vomiting
	Peyote/mescaline hallucinogenic herbs—used in Native American rituals under the guidance of a shaman; often misused by individuals; visual hallucinations may persist
Misused prescription medicines	
• Taking too much? (sleeping pills, diet pills, painkillers)	Sleeping pills and painkillers to ease emotional distress
• Using prescribed medicine for other purposes?	Patient experiences a "buzz" with no cognitive impairment
• Experimenting with other people's medications (common with adolescents)?	
• Intentionally taking other people's medications (e.g., parent taking a child's Ritalin)?	
• Taking benztropine (Cogentin)?	Reported in the news to be common in soldiers serving in Iraq
• Sniffing household chemicals, glue, or car exhaust fumes?	
• Misusing cold medicine or other over-the-counter drugs?	Contain chemical solvents that can cause fatal cardiac arrhythmias, rapid loss of consciousness, and respiratory arrest

History and Risk Factors	Rationale
Do you have a sense of hope for your future? • What provides you with your emotional support or sense of faith? • What is your religious affiliation? • What are your spiritual beliefs? • What spiritual practices are important to you?	No sense of hope for the future may be an indicator of risk for suicide. The last three questions meet The Joint Commission (2010) standards and recommendations for spiritual assessment. Refer to Box 9.3 for further assessment of spiritual beliefs using the HOPE assessment tool.
Medications What psychiatric medications are you taking? Are you taking them as prescribed? Do you use, or have you ever used, any alternative treatments, herbals, or other substances? If yes, list the specific treatments or substances.	Consider interactions between medications taken for psychiatric and medical conditions. For example, if the patient has a medical condition such as prolonged QT wave interval (a cardiac problem), the patient should not take or be prescribed some classes of antidepressants. Identify any psychiatric drugs taken, drug interactions, herbal–drug interactions, and alternative treatments that might cause psychiatric adverse effects. Patients may be taking substances to self-medicate. Keep in mind that some patients consider marijuana a natural herb or alternative medical treatment, not a recreational drug.
Family History Has anyone in your family been diagnosed with a mental health condition? • If so, which family member(s)? • What was the diagnosis and treatment plan for each family member diagnosed with a mental health condition? • Is the treatment plan working well for the particular family member?	A family history of mental health conditions is a risk factor for the patient. Answers may help direct the line of treatment or medication options for the patient.

BOX 9.3 HOPE Assessment of Spiritual Beliefs

H: Sources of Hope, Meaning, Comfort, Strength, Peace, Love, and Connection

- We have been discussing your support systems. I was wondering, what is there in your life that gives you internal support?
- What are your sources of hope, strength, comfort, and peace?
- What do you hold on to during difficult times?
- What sustains you and keeps you going?
- For some people, religious or spiritual beliefs act as a source of comfort and strength in dealing with life's ups and downs; is this true for you? (*If the answer is "Yes," go on to O and P questions. If the answer is "No," consider asking "Was it ever?" If the answer is "Yes," ask "What changed?"*)

O: Organized Religion

- Do you consider yourself part of an organized religion?
- How important is this to you?
- What aspects of your religion are helpful and not so helpful to you?
- Are you part of a religious or spiritual community? Does it help you? How?

P: Personal Spirituality/Practices

- Do you have personal spiritual beliefs that are independent of organized religion? What are they?
- Do you believe in God? What kind of relationship do you have with God?
- What aspects of your spirituality or spiritual practices do you find most helpful to you personally? (e.g., prayer, meditation, reading scripture, attending religious services, listening to music, hiking, communing with nature)

E: Effects on Medical Care and End-of-Life Issues

- Has being sick (or your current situation) affected your ability to do the things that usually help you spiritually? (Or affected your relationship with God?)
- Is there anything that I can do to help you access the resources that usually help you?
- Are you worried about any conflicts between your beliefs and your medical/mental situation/care/decisions?
- Would it be helpful for you to speak to a clinical chaplain/community spiritual leader?
- Are there any specific practices or restrictions I should know about in providing your care? (e.g., dietary restrictions, use of blood products)
- If the patient is dying: How do your beliefs affect the kind of medical care you would like me to provide over the next few days/weeks/months?

From Anandarajah, G., & Hight, E. (2001). Spirituality and medical practice: Using the HOPE questions as a practical tool for spiritual assessment. *American Family Physician, 63*, 81–89.

Risk Reduction and Health Promotion

Important patient education topics for health promotion and risk reduction include the following:

- Alterations in interest in life, motivation, energy, sleep, appetite, sexual behavior
- Current stressors and coping
- Physical or sexual abuse
- Violence
- Pervasive worry or anxiety
- Altered mood or affect
- Changes in behaviors, self-harm, or suicidal thoughts
- Alcohol or drug use
- Memory, concentration, and problem-solving abilities

Health goals for patients to maintain and promote health are the following:

- Reduce the suicide rate.
- Reduce the proportion of homeless adults who have serious mental illness (SMI).
- Reduce the proportion of adolescents and adults who experience major depressive episodes.
- Increase depression screening by providers.
- Increase the proportion of persons with substance abuse and mental disorders who receive treatment.
- Reduce maltreatment and maltreatment fatalities of children.
- Reduce the annual rate of rape or attempted rape and other sexual assaults.
- Reduce physical assaults.

(USDHHS, 2013)

Common Symptoms

Common Symptoms of Altered Mental Health

- Suicidal ideation
- Homicidal ideation and aggressive behavior
- Altered mood and affect
- Auditory hallucinations
- Visual hallucinations

Signs/Symptoms	Rationale/Abnormal Findings
Suicidal Ideation Do you have any thoughts of wanting to harm or kill yourself? *SAFETY ALERT* *Assess for safety. Some patients are not suicidal but perform self-mutilation, often to relieve emotional pain. The above question covers both suicidal and parasuicidal gestures. Identifying parasuicidal thoughts is important because patients can accidentally kill themselves while relieving emotional pain.*	Suicide is the 11th leading cause of death for U.S. citizens of all ages. It may accompany any psychiatric illness or occur without a psychiatric diagnosis. Suicide is one of the five leading causes of death in people 10–54 years of age (Centers for Disease Control and Prevention [CDC], National Center for Injury Prevention and Control, 2008). U.S. men older than 75 years of age have the highest suicide rate. Men are more than four times more likely to commit suicide than are women (CDC, 2012). Suicidal patients may present in any health care setting with various problems, not necessarily sad mood or suicidal thoughts. They may hint or joke about suicide or wanting to die to test the nurse's comfort with discussing the subject. In many cases, patients do not want to talk, but despondent behaviors indicate that they are suicidal. Failure to ask if these patients have had suicidal thoughts would be a lost opportunity to assist them. A patient is considered to have very "lethal" suicidal ideation if he or she has a history of suicide attempts, a specific plan, and access to the means (e.g., owns a gun, has medications).
Use the **SAD PERSONAS** mnemonic to assess for risk of suicide. See Box 9.4. This scale facilitates the systematic gathering of patient data and relevant psychosocial history.	**Clinical Significance** The strength of the SAD PERSONAS scale is not a precise risk predictor but is a way to alert the clinician that the patient may be at higher risk.

(table continues on page 191)

Signs/Symptoms	Rationale/Abnormal Findings
BOX 9.4 SAD PERSONAS Suicide Risk Assessment • **S**ex • **A**ge • **D**epression • **P**revious attempt • **E**thanol abuse • **R**ational thought loss • **S**ocial supports lacking • **O**rganized plan • **N**o spouse • **A**ccess to lethal means • **S**ickness The presence of each factor is given a point value of 1. Total scores range from 0 to 10. Higher scores indicate greater patient suicide risk. From Patterson, W. M., Dohn, H. H., Bird, J., & Patterson, G. A. (1983). Evaluation of suicidal patients: The SAD PERSON Scale. *Psychosomatics*, *24*(4), 343–349.	
Homicidal Ideation and Aggressive Behavior Do you have any thoughts of wanting to harm or kill anyone? **⚠ SAFETY ALERT** *Assess for safety of others. If the patient replies "yes" when asked about a desire to harm others, then ask if he or she wants to harm a specific person and if so, how. Notify the attending primary care provider who will determine whether there is a "duty to warn" the other person. The exact nature of the plan for harm and ability to carry it out are an important part of the assessment.*	Risk factors for aggressive behavior include male gender, history of violence, and substance abuse. Ethnicity, diagnosis, age, marital status, and education do not reliably identify this behavior (Moore & Pfaff, 2008). Patients with a history of violence are more likely to inflict serious injuries. Typically, the patient becomes angry, resists authority, and finally becomes confrontational. Violent behavior may occur without warning, however, especially when caused by medical problems or dementia. Trust your "gut feeling" about the potential for violence. Consider an obviously angry patient potentially violent. It is important to take actions to avoid injury. Signs of violence include the following: • Provocative behavior • Angry demeanor • Loud, aggressive speech • Tense posturing (e.g., gripping bed side rails tightly, clenching fists) • Frequently changing body position; pacing • Aggressive acts such as pounding walls, throwing objects, hitting self (Moore & Pfaff, 2008)
Altered Mood and Affect What has your mood been like? *Normal mood is pleasant.*	Mood is a sustained emotion. Assess the intensity, depth, and duration of altered mood.
On a scale of 0–10, with 10 being most intense, how depressed do you feel now?	Patients may describe mood as sad, tearful, depressed, angry, anxious, grandiose, or fearful. Mood inappropriate to the situation is abnormal.
Assess the patient's affect. Affect is an objective observation of how the patient expresses his or her feelings and mood. Assess whether affect matches what the patient says. *Normal affect is congruent with the situation.*	Affect may be temporary and changing compared with mood. Bland, apathetic, dramatic, bizarre, constricted, blunted, flat, labile, and euphoric are descriptors of altered affect. See Table 9.4 at the end of the chapter.

(table continues on page 192)

Signs/Symptoms	Rationale/Abnormal Findings
Auditory Hallucinations Do you hear voices that others do not hear? (Ask this question while closely observing the patient.)	A patient may answer "no" even though he or she is actually experiencing auditory hallucinations. The patient may not realize that others do not hear voices or not want to tell the nurse for fear of ramifications, such as continued hospitalization or starting medications. If the answer is "yes," alert the primary care provider; the patient may need more supervision if it seems that he or she cannot resist "command" hallucinations.
Assess the nature of auditory hallucinations. • Does the voice tell you what to do? • Must you listen or do what the voice says or does?	⚠ *SAFETY ALERT* *If the patient confirms auditory hallucinations, it is important to ask about their nature. Are they hostile or critical? Do they "command" or tell the patient to do things such as harm self or others?*
Visual Hallucinations Do you see things that other people do not see?	Common causes of visual hallucinations include adverse effects from medications, alcohol withdrawal, and Parkinson disease.
Other Hallucinations (If there is a history of hallucinations or if assessment indicates, continue to ask questions about other types of hallucinations such as olfactory and tactile.)	Some patients with psychotic disorders smell smoke or feel someone touching them.
Do you smell things that other people do not smell?	Brain tumors, toxins, and hallucinogens are common causes of olfactory hallucinations.
Do you have any unusual sensations on your skin such as bugs crawling on you?	Hallucinogen and methamphetamine use is associated with tactile hallucinations.

Documenting Normal Findings

Denies suicidal or homicidal thoughts. Mood pleasant, affect appropriate to situation. Denies visual, auditory, olfactory, or tactile hallucinations.

Lifespan Considerations: Older Adults

Additional Questions	Rationale/Abnormal Findings
Have you felt sad lately? Risk factors to assess include the following: • Female gender • African American or Hispanic background • Social isolation • Widowed, divorced, or separated marital status • Lower socioeconomic status • Comorbid medical conditions • Uncontrolled pain • Insomnia • Functional impairment • Cognitive impairment (Hirsch, Duberstein, & Unützer, 2009)	Females are at higher overall risk for depression. Older men and older African American and Hispanic adults are at higher risk for unrecognized depression. Assess for poor cognitive performance, sleep problems, and lack of initiative (Craven, Hirnle, & Jensen, 2012). Older adults may also have physical health changes or end-of-life issues. People who lose interest in work or hobbies, sleep too much, or live alone may be at risk for social isolation. Those experiencing financial pressure may have increased stress and potential depression.
Use the **Geriatric Depression Scale** to assess for the risk of depression in older adults. See Box 9.5.	The more "yes" answers the patient gives, the more depression is likely.
To family: Have you noticed any memory lapses or confusion?	Delirium, dementia, and depression are more common in older adults (Waszynski, 2007).

BOX 9.5 Geriatric Depression Scale: Short Form

Choose the best answer for how you have felt over the past week:

1. Are you basically satisfied with your life? YES/**NO**
2. Have you dropped many of your activities and interests? **YES**/NO
3. Do you feel that your life is empty? **YES**/NO
4. Do you often get bored? **YES**/NO
5. Are you in good spirits most of the time? YES/**NO**
6. Are you afraid that something bad is going to happen to you? **YES**/NO
7. Do you feel happy most of the time? YES/**NO**
8. Do you often feel helpless? **YES**/NO
9. Do you prefer to stay at home, rather than going out and doing new things? **YES**/NO
10. Do you feel you have more problems with memory than most? **YES**/NO
11. Do you think it is wonderful to be alive now? YES/**NO**
12. Do you feel pretty worthless the way you are now? **YES**/NO
13. Do you feel full of energy? YES/**NO**
14. Do you feel that your situation is hopeless? **YES**/NO
15. Do you think that most people are better off than you are? **YES**/NO

Answers in **bold** indicate depression. Score 1 point for each bold-faced answer.

A score higher than 5 points is suggestive of depression. A score higher than 10 points is almost always indicative of depression. A score higher than 5 points should warrant a follow-up comprehensive assessment.

From Yesavage, J. A., Brink, T. L., Rose, T. L., Lum, O., Huang, V., Adey, M., Leirer, V. O (1982). Development and validation of a geriatric depression screening scale: A preliminary report. *Journal of Psychiatric Research*, *17*, 37–49.

Cultural Considerations

Using an Interpreter for a Patient With a Mental Health Condition

When using an interpreter, it is not uncommon to ask the interpreter to sign a Health Insurance Portability and Accountability Act (HIPAA) statement or other confidentiality statement. The interpreter is not permitted to discuss any part of the communication with anyone other than the health care providers working with the patient. It is also unethical for an interpreter to meet with either party beforehand or to discuss the patient after the interview. If the interpreter has interpreted for other family members or friends in the community, he or she should not divulge that information to the patient. The interpreter may think such disclosure is a way of connecting and establishing rapport, when in reality it could cause the patient to feel uncomfortable or worry that the interpreter will share information with others.

Be aware of whether the interpreter appears not to be providing all the information the patient is stating. A professional interpreter only interprets what is said, as it is said, with no changes. After the interview, it is appropriate to ask the interpreter if the patient or family has any cultural beliefs of which health care providers should be aware. Be sure to include the interpreter's name in the nursing documentation of the interview.

Additional Questions	Rationale/Abnormal Findings
With what racial, cultural, or ethnic group do you identify?	Patients tend to selectively express or present symptoms in culturally acceptable ways. For example, Asian patients may be more likely to report physical symptoms (e.g., dizziness) than emotional symptoms (USDHHS, 2009a. Cultural attitudes and beliefs influence whether a patient considers an illness "real" or "imagined" and whether the illness is of the body or mind (or both). Cultural meanings of illness have real implications for whether people are motivated to seek treatment, how they cope with symptoms, how supportive families and communities are, and where patients seek help (mental health specialist, primary care provider, clergy, traditional healer).
Do you have an inherited family pattern of mental problems?	The prevalence of bipolar disorder and panic disorder is higher in parts of Asia, Europe, and North America (USDHHS, 2009a). Poverty, violence, and other stressful social environments increase risks for depression.
Are you concerned about seeking health care because of issues related to your living situation? Have you experienced traumatic situations in your life?	Traumatic experiences are common for combat veterans, inner city residents, and immigrants from countries at war, placing them at risk for PTSD.

Therapeutic Dialogue: Collecting Subjective Data

The nurse's role relative to subjective data collection is to gather information to improve the patient's health status and to help determine the cause of the patient's current symptoms. Remember Mr. Hart, introduced at the beginning of this chapter. This 75-year-old man has come to the health care walk-in clinic to have his blood pressure checked on several occasions. He is currently taking a prescription antidepressant.

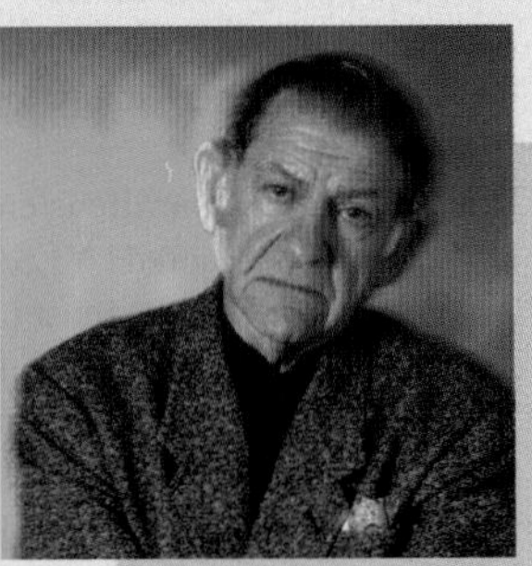

Nurse: Hi, Mr. Hart (pauses and smiles).

Mr. Hart: You're cute. Are you married?

Nurse: I'm sorry, but the hospital policy is not to disclose personal information. I would like to talk to you today.

Mr. Hart: Where do you live?

Nurse: I'm sorry, but I can't tell you that. How is that book that you're reading?

Mr. Hart: It's good. I like to read novels that have some mystery in them.

Nurse: (nods head and smiles) Reading is a good way to relax.

Mr. Hart: I don't have much time for relaxing. They keep us all busy with therapy and groups. I wish that I could rest more.

Nurse: You're here so that you can be safe. Do you have any thoughts of wanting to harm or kill yourself?

Mr. Hart: No. I did when I came here but not now.

Critical Thinking Challenge

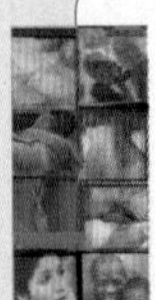

- Did any elements in the conversations make you feel uncomfortable?
- How can the nurse provide an environment so that Mr. Hart will feel comfortable and safe talking about feelings?
- What are some other ways that the nurse can ask either directly or indirectly about suicidal ideation?

Objective Data

Comprehensive Mental Health Assessment

For the **mental status examination**, you will collect objective data by observing the patient and the patient's behavior. This includes not only how the patient communicates and responds to questions but also physical presentation. A patient's physical presentation may be the first indication of toxicity, underlying medical problems, or psychosis.

Collecting objective data is an ongoing process throughout the time you spend with the patient. Data for the objective assessment are usually organized by **A** (appearance), **B** (behavior), **C** (cognitive function), and **T** (thought process) (**ABCT**), plus the MMSE.

Comprehensive Violence Assessment

Part of the mental health assessment is to observe and document any objective findings related to patients who have been victimized by violence. You assess nonverbal behaviors, such as the patient's eyes scanning the environment or the patient jumping or being startled when a door slams. You may notice that a child is very clingy to the person accompanying him or her, has a flat affect, or does not establish eye contact.

Technique and Normal Findings	Rationale/Abnormal Findings
A: Appearance	
Overall Appearance. Observe the overall physical appearance, including noticeable physical deformities, weight, and asymmetrical movements. *The patient appears stated age, is normal weight, and shows symmetrical movements without obvious deformity.*	Evidence of cutting or self-harm may be present. Physical problems such as stroke or dementia may exacerbate some mental health conditions. Cradle cap around the face of adults indicates long-term lack of care and is often seen in patients with schizophrenia.
Posture. Assess the posture. *Posture is erect but relaxed.*	Abnormal postures are rigid (indicates anxiety) or slouching (indicates withdrawal). A rigid posture might indicate that the patient is trying to hide, either from a real person or from his or her thoughts.
Movement. Assess baseline and additional movements. Observe their pace, range, and character. *Movements are voluntary, deliberate, coordinated, smooth, and even.*	Immobility (or tremor) might indicate Parkinson disease or schizophrenia. The patient may walk a lot to distract from "voices." He or she may feel the need to keep physically occupied to avoid having to deal with emotional thoughts. The patient might have a tic or tardive dyskinesia.
Assess the gait for steadiness and rhythm. *Gait is steady and even.*	Abnormal gaits include limping, fast or slow speed, pacing, shuffling, and stiffness. The gait is altered in some patients who take antipsychotic medications. Arm movements are lost with some gait abnormalities and in patients who have taken antipsychotic medications.
Observe the activity level. Is it under voluntary control? Do posture and motor activity change with topics under discussion or with activities or people around the patient? *Activity is moderately paced and relaxed.*	The activity level may be altered from hypomania or attention deficit hyperactivity disorder (ADHD), adverse effects of medications, or internal anxiety. Activity may be hypoactive, hyperactive, rigid, restless, agitated, gesturing, posturing, with inappropriate mannerisms, hostile or combative, or unusual. See Table 9.5 at the end of the chapter.
Hygiene and Grooming. Note hair, nails, teeth, skin, and, if present, beard. Observe hygiene and grooming, including body odor and condition of hair. If the patient is unwashed or unkempt, estimate for how long. Note a change in appearance in a previously well-groomed patient. Compare one side of the body with the other. *Patient is well groomed and has no unusual body odors.*	Poor hygiene may be from phobia of water, homelessness, severe depression, or incapacitation as a result of mental illness. Risk of lice increases with poor grooming. Excessive fastidiousness may accompany obsessive-compulsive disorder (OCD). One-sided neglect may result from stroke, brain trauma, or physical injury. An unkempt state might indicate depression or psychosis.
Observe for makeup and how it is worn. *Makeup is appropriate to weather, age, gender, culture, and social situation.*	Garish makeup applied in bold colors and outside the lines may indicate mania. Inappropriate makeup may also indicate a decline in mental status.
Observe the hands for coloration, cleanliness, tremors, pill rolling, or clubbing of the nail bed. Look for any signs of itching or scratching.	Hands may provide indicators of health problems, smoking status, drug withdrawal, low blood glucose level, or side effects of medications. Clubbing is seen in patients with emphysema or who use recreational drugs with talc in them; poor oxygenation affects cognition. Itching or scratching may be related to hallucinations, crystal methamphetamine use, or self-harm.
Dress. Observe how the patient is dressed. Is clothing clean, pressed, and fastened properly? How does it compare with clothing worn by people of comparable age and social group?	Clothing style and color may indicate an identified social group (e.g., gangs, Goth).

(table continues on page 196)

Technique and Normal Findings (continued)	Rationale/Abnormal Findings (continued)
Is clothing worn correctly such as right side out, not backward, shirt buttoned in alignment? How many layers is the patient wearing? *Clothing is clean and appropriate for culture and weather.*	Unfastened or incorrectly worn clothes might indicate physical difficulty, cognitive deficits, or altered mental status. Clothing may be slovenly, unkempt, overly meticulous, disheveled, inappropriate, provocative, unusual, inappropriate for weather, or with multiple layers. A patient wearing five shirts and three pairs of pants at once may be cold, homeless (and wearing so many clothes because there is nowhere to store them), or irrational.
B: Behavior ***Level of Consciousness.*** Is the patient awake and alert? To assess if the patient is arousable, gently shake the bed or chair that the patient is in; do not directly shake the patient.	Abnormal findings include drowsy, hyperalert, somnolent, intermittent alertness, or stupor. If the patient is not arousable, assess for breathing, stupor, or psychosis.
• Note if the patient is aware of surroundings and environmental situations. • Is the patient aware of self? • Does the patient respond appropriately to stimuli?	Abnormal findings are a lack of awareness of own physical needs and emotional responses. Refer to Chapter 22 for more information on neurological assessment and the Glasgow Coma Scale.
⚠ *SAFETY ALERT* *The patient's ability to correctly interpret the environmental cues and respond accordingly addresses safety.*	
Eye Contact and Facial Expressions. Assess eye contact. *The patient converses with eyes open and maintains eye contact.*	Abnormal findings are eyes closed, avoiding eye contact, staring, looking vacantly ahead, or twitching to side when discussing a traumatic event. A patient who looks away may be responding to voices or easily distracted by the environment. Poor eye contact may indicate low self-esteem, shame, embarrassment, depression, or a cultural trait.
Observe facial expressions at rest and when the patient is interacting with others. Watch for variations in facial expression with topics under discussion. Are they congruent? Is the face relatively immobile throughout? *The patient is calm, alert, and expressive. Facial expressions are congruent with subjects.*	Facial expressions indicate the emotional state. Abnormal expressions are perplexed, stressed, tense, dazed, grimacing, and lacking in expression. Facial expressions may give clues to depression, anxiety, hallucinations, physical injury, mania, side effects of medications, or possible extrapyramidal symptoms.
Speech. Assess speech for the following qualities: • Rate. *The rate is moderately paced.* • Rhythm. *The rhythm has normal fluctuations.* • Loudness. *Speech is audible with moderate loudness.* • Fluency. *Speech is fluent.* • Quantity. Does the patient respond only to direct questions? Assess for voluminous speech, poverty of speech, talkativeness, silence, or spontaneity. *There is usually a flow of conversation with pauses.* • Articulation. *Speech is articulate with words clear and distinct.*	Slow, fast, latent, pressured, monotone, or disturbed rates are abnormal. Determine if causes are anxiety, depression, or auditory hallucinations. Rhyming, slurring, mumbling, or unusual rhythm is abnormal. Determine if the cause is a hearing difficulty, anger or agitation, or mania. Note if barely audible or too loud. Determine if the cause is a hearing difficulty, auditory hallucination, or speech difficulty.

(table continues on page 197)

Technique and Normal Findings (continued)	Rationale/Abnormal Findings (continued)
	Note any lengthy pauses, hesitancy, or stuttering (specify the frequency). Determine if these are from difficulty speaking (aphasia) or hallucinations. Too much speech may be covering feelings of discomfort, embarrassment, not knowing answers, or avoiding questions. Too much or too little speech may indicate auditory hallucinations. Too little speech may indicate poverty of thought or developmental delay. Note any difficulty expressing self or finding words. See also Chapter 22.
• Content. *Content is organized and congruent with behavior or nonverbal communication.*	Disorganized, nonsensical, judgmental, religiously preoccupied, or sexually preoccupied speech may indicate impaired judgment and illogical thinking.
• Pattern. *There is a pattern of exchange in conversation.*	Note if the patient uses fragmented sentences, circuitous speech (talks in circles and cannot answer questions), confabulation (makes up answers to cover for loss of memory), or intellectualization (uses intellectual analysis to avoid dealing with emotions). Frequent or inappropriate laughter may indicate hallucinations or disordered perception. See also Table 9.6 at the end of the chapter.
C: Cognitive Function ***Orientation.*** Assess orientation through the following questions: • Tell me what day of the week, month, and year it is now. • Where are you right now? • What is your name (first and surname)? • Why are you here right now? *The patient is alert and oriented, which is commonly written as A&O × 3—alert and oriented times 3. It is also written as A&O × 4, indicating the additional information that the patient is aware of current situation (e.g., why hospitalized).*	Note any inconsistencies regarding orientation. Determine whether the patient is new to the area and might not know the place. If a woman provides her birth name instead of her married surname when questioned, determine whether she retained her birth surname or is confused. A confused patient will lose time first, then place, and finally, name. As confusion clears, the patient will regain knowledge in the reverse order (name, place, and time). If the patient is aware of person and time but not place (out of normal sequencing order), it is indicative of an organic process for the confusion. Refer to Chapter 22 for more information.
Attention Span. Can the patient follow the conversation? Is the patient easily distractible? *The patient can follow conversation and events.*	Attention span indicates the current level of cognitive functioning. Note if altered attention span is from restlessness, poor focus, ADHD, or hallucinations.
Memory. Assess memory using the MMSE or Mini-Cog (Box 9.6). • Does the patient have short-term memory? • Does the patient have long-term memory? *Short- and long-term memories are intact.*	Short- and long-term memories indicate the current level of cognitive functioning. Altered memory may be from dementia, Alzheimer disease, or other disorders. Refer to Chapter 22 for more information on the assessment of memory.

(table continues on page 198)

Technique and Normal Findings (continued)	Rationale/Abnormal Findings (continued)
Judgment. Assess judgment by noting the patient's responses to family situations, employment, interpersonal conflict, and use of money. Ask direct questions such as the following:	
• How will you get home if you have no money?	This question assesses the patient's ability to solve problems.
• What will you do if you feel the urge to use alcohol again (in patients with alcoholism)? (The patient might respond with answers such as seek help, call my AA sponsor, or talk myself out of it.)	This question assesses the patient's ability to choose among alternatives based on reality.
• What will happen if you hit someone you love, a neighbor, or someone else?	This question assesses the patient's ability to understand the consequences of behavior and take responsibility for actions.
• What is your part in this conflict? Or how might you have contributed to this situation?	Note whether the patient has poor insight, poor judgment, or poor impulse control and what these findings might indicate.
The patient makes good judgments and takes responsibility for own actions.	
T: Thought Processes and Perceptions Assess thought processes. *Patient's thoughts are easy to follow, logical, coherent, relevant, goal directed, consistent, and abstract.*	Illogical, incoherent, irrelevant, wandering, inconsistent, or concrete thought processes are indications that the patient is thinking less efficiently. Refer to Table 9.7 at the end of the chapter.
MMSE/Mini-Cog. Assess cognitive function by using the **MMSE** or Mini-Cog (Box 9.6). The self-explanatory MMSE has 11 questions about time and place orientation, serial 7s (subtract 7 from 100 and continue to subtract 7 from each subsequent remainder), naming objects (e.g., pencil), repeating phrases (e.g., "No ifs, ands, or buts"), following a 3-step direction, reading and responding, writing a sentence, and drawing intersecting pentagons (Folstein, Folstein, & McHugh, 1975). It takes 10–15 minutes to administer. The Mini-Cog takes about 3 minutes to administer and is perceived as less stressful. It includes recall and the clock drawing test. Registration is the ability to immediately state three words; recall is the ability to state them 3 minutes later. Recall is tested in both.	The MMSE and Mini-Cog are both scored tests. A score of 23 or lower on the MMSE indicates cognitive impairment (Folstein et al., 1975). For more information on this copyrighted tool, contact Psychological Assessment Resources, Inc., 16204 North Florida Avenue, Lutz, Florida 33549. Unsuccessful recall of three items or an abnormal clock drawing test indicates dementia on the Mini-Cog.

Documenting Normal Findings

Appears stated age and normal weight, no obvious deformity. Posture is erect and relaxed. Movements are symmetrical, voluntary, deliberate, coordinated, smooth, and even. Gait is steady and even. Activity is moderate and relaxed. Patient is well groomed with no unusual body odors. Makeup is appropriate to culture and social situation. Clothing is clean and appropriate for gender, age, culture, and weather. Patient is awake, alert, calm, and expressive, responding appropriately to voice cues. Patient converses with eyes open and good eye contact. Facial expressions are congruent with subjects. Speech is of moderate pace and volume, fluent with normal fluctuations, and articulate with clear and distinct words. Speech is organized and congruent with behavior and nonverbal communication. A&O $\times$ 3. Patient follows conversation and events; attention span is normal. Short- and long-term memory intact. MMSE completed with no deficits. Patient makes good judgments and takes responsibility for actions. Thought processes are easy to follow, logical, coherent, relevant, goal directed, consistent, and abstract.

BOX 9.6 The Mini-Cog

Administration

The test is administered as follows:

1. Instruct the patient to listen carefully to and remember three unrelated words and then to repeat the words.
2. Instruct the patient to draw the face of a clock, either on a blank sheet of paper or on a sheet with the clock circle already drawn on the page. After the patient puts the numbers on the clock face, ask him or her to draw the hands of the clock to read a specific time.
3. Ask the patient to repeat the three previously stated words.

Scoring

Give 1 point for each recalled word after the clock-drawing test (CDT) distractor.

Patients recalling none of the three words are classified as demented (Score = 0).

Patients recalling all three words are classified as non-demented (Score = 3).

Patients with intermediate word recall of 1-2 words are classified based on the CDT (Abnormal = demented; Normal = non-demented)

Note: The CDT is considered normal if all numbers are present in the correct sequence and position, and the hands readably display the requested time.

From Borson, S., Scanlan, J., Brush, M., Vitallano, P., & Dokmak, A. (2000). The Mini-Cog: A cognitive "vital signs" measure for dementia screening in multi-lingual elderly. *International Journal of Geriatric Psychiatry, 15*(11), 1021–1027.

The following signs are indicators of possible abuse or neglect:

- Injuries not consistent with the story of their cause
- Sexual activity in a child younger than age 14 years
- Inadequate supervision
- Serious injury
- Failure to seek timely medical care
- Multiple hospital or clinic visits for injuries
- Multiple previous fractures
- Bruises in multiple stages of healing

If any of the signs is evident, the nurse should perform a complete physical assessment to evaluate for other manifestations of violence.

Many additional indications, or "red flags," alert nurses to the possibility of past or current violence (Edwards, Anda, Gu, Dube, & Felitti, 2007) (Fig. 9.1). Common psychological red

Child Abuse Assessment Red Flags

- ✓ Mood changes, anger, isolating, sullenness
- ✓ Critical of self and/or others
- ✓ Risky behaviors
- ✓ Behavior changes
- ✓ Friend changes
- ✓ School troubles
- ✓ Short temper, difficulty getting along with others
- ✓ Verbal and physical violence with siblings, parents, peers
- ✓ Weight gain or loss
- ✓ Quitting teams and activities

IPV Assessment Red Flags

- ✓ Physical injury (facial fractures, dental, neurological, soft tissue, internal, "falls")
- ✓ Chronic pain (back, abdomen, chest, head)
- ✓ Fibromyalgia, chronic irritable bowel
- ✓ Hypertension, smoking
- ✓ Unintended pregnancy, adolescent pregnancy
- ✓ Abortion
- ✓ Anal and vaginal tearing, painful intercourse
- ✓ Depression

Sexual Abuse Assessment Red Flags

- ✓ Bruising or scratching around breasts, genitals
- ✓ Unexplained venereal or genital infections (children should not have STDs)
- ✓ Unexplained vaginal or anal bleeding
- ✓ Torn, stained, bloody underclothes
- ✓ Victim reports being sexually assaulted
- ✓ Victim withdrawn, personality changes, behavior changes

General Assessment Red Flags

- ✓ New-onset behaviors or change in behavior
- ✓ Withdrawal, depression
- ✓ Agitation, hyperarousal
- ✓ New displays of anger, noncompliance
- ✓ Sexualized behavior
- ✓ Bowel or bladder problems
- ✓ Sleep problems
- ✓ Unexplained and/or "curious" injuries

Elder/Vulnerable Adult Violence Assessment Red Flags

- ✓ Frailty, cognitive impairment
- ✓ Psychiatric disorder, depression, anxiety
- ✓ Alcohol abuse
- ✓ Decreased social network
- ✓ Shared living arrangements
- ✓ External stressors on family
- ✓ Vague excuses for missing activities, therapy
- ✓ Untrimmed, dirty nails
- ✓ Inadequate or absent assistive devices
- ✓ History of family violence
- ✓ Unexplained injuries
- ✓ Explanation not consistent with findings
- ✓ Recurrent UTIs or other infections
- ✓ Poor hygiene, poor oral hygiene, dirty clothes
- ✓ Weight loss/lack of interest in meals
- ✓ Recurrent or worsening pressure ulcers, dehydration

Abuse/Neglect Assessment Red Flags

- ✓ Bruises, welts, cuts, scratches, restraint marks
- ✓ Open wounds, punctures, untreated sores, maggots
- ✓ Sprains, dislocations, internal injuries
- ✓ Victim changes in behavior
- ✓ Caregiver refuses to allow visitors to see the victim
- ✓ Victim reports being hit and/or maltreated
- ✓ Soiled clothing or linens
- ✓ Overall bad hygiene, poor oral hygiene
- ✓ Dehydration, malnutrition, extreme weight loss

Violence in Pregnancy Assessment Red Flags

- ✓ Late or inconsistent prenatal care
- ✓ Preterm bleeding and/or labor
- ✓ Abruptio placentae–especially more than one time/with more than one pregnancy
- ✓ Low birth weight
- ✓ Unexplained fetal death
- ✓ Suicide attempts during pregnancy
- ✓ Postpartum depression
- ✓ Injuries during pregnancy
- ✓ Poor weight gain during pregnancy
- ✓ Partner unwilling to leave woman's side during prenatal visits, labor and delivery, and/or postpartum
- ✓ Partner speaks for woman and/or condescending to woman
- ✓ Partner makes negative comments about woman's appearance
- ✓ Woman speaks less or is very quiet especially when partner around, poor eye contact
- ✓ Partner oversolicitous with care providers

Figure 9.1 Assessing red flags for violence.

flags are mood and behavior changes from normal for the specific patient. Depression and anxiety can be manifest as a flat, quiet, and sullen affect (emotional dullness); withdrawal; or irritability and impulsive anger, which can further manifest as acting-out behaviors (e.g., impulsive aggression toward others, risky and dangerous behaviors). Some violence victims use substances such as alcohol, marijuana, methamphetamines, cocaine, and narcotics to feel better while simultaneously numbing feelings of anxiety, low self-worth, sadness, and fear. Nevertheless, a link between violence and mental health problems is usually hidden, and health care providers may overlook opportunities to plan effective interventions.

Mental health effects associated with violence that can be assessed during patient visits include depression, PTSD, panic disorders, dissociative symptoms, relationship and marital problems, acting out violently, and sexual and substance abuse. Symptoms common during assessment are easily triggered anxiety and panic episodes, isolation and social withdrawal, numbing or shutting down feelings, spacing out and forgetfulness, and difficulty focusing.

Among violence survivors, how each person experiences and is affected by violence depends on the type and severity and the lived experiences of a person in his or her family, community, and society. Age, ethnicity, socioeconomic status, education, sexual orientation, religion, urban or rural living, culture, and relationships can be highly influential. Thus, it is very important not to make assumptions but instead to use open-ended questions, such as, "How are you coping?" and "What has your experience been?"

Documentation

Documentation is an important aspect of violence assessment. Close listening and keen observation skills are necessary to capture key details. It is important to reassure adults that their patient records are available only with their consent and may be useful someday if needed for legal action. Nurses should document subjective data in direct quotes as much as possible (e.g., "pt states . . . ").

When documenting objective data, it is important to be detailed and descriptive and to note findings without bias.

Mandated Reporting

Nurses and other health care professionals are "mandated reporters" when child, elder, or vulnerable-adult abuse or neglect is disclosed, assessed, or suspected. Mandated reporters must call the protective services hotline when they suspect abuse or neglect. Provided the report is done in good faith and without malice, the nurse and other professionals mandated by the state to report are protected by the state.

> **Clinical Significance**
>
> Be aware of the mandatory reporting laws in the state where you practice. Also be aware of your institution or agency's policies and procedures regarding disclosure of violence perpetration and/or victimization and its appropriate documentation.

In addition to documenting findings from the patient assessment on forms approved by the health professional's institution, you should document the call to the protective services hotline in the patient's file, including the reason for the call, time of the call, full name of the person who took the call, and response of the worker. State laws on reporting domestic violence in adults or IPV vary from no mandatory reporting to requiring providers to report to a state agency (e.g., state health department, police).

Assessment of Dementia, Confusion, Delirium, and Depression

Dementia is more common in older adults. It is usually a gradual process over months to years. **Delirium** generally has an underlying medical cause that, after being treated, results in the delirium resolving.

Some cues that the patient may have dementia include the following:

- Seems disoriented
- Is a "poor historian"
- Defers to a family member to answer questions directed to the patient
- Repeatedly, and apparently unintentionally, fails to follow instructions
- Has difficulty finding the right words or uses inappropriate or incomprehensible words
- Has difficulty following conversations (Waszynski, 2007)

Delirium, dementia, and depression can also be acute conditions. Delirium usually has an acute onset; the disorganized thoughts can place the patient at risk for injury. The risk of suicide increases with depression. Refer to Table 9.8 at the end of the chapter for a comparison of findings.

Critical Thinking

Nursing Diagnoses, Outcomes, and Interventions

When formulating nursing diagnoses, it is important to use critical thinking to cluster data and identify patterns that fit together. Table 9.3 compares and contrasts nursing diagnoses, abnormal findings, and interventions commonly related to mental health assessment (Moorhead, Johnson, Maas, & Swanson, 2013). Note that altered thought processes and sensory perceptions are also related to the neurological system. Some coping behaviors are also relevant to other body systems and how patients cope with the effects of physical difficulties.

Nurses use assessment information to identify patient outcomes. Some outcomes related to mental health difficulties include the following:

- The patient does not harm self.
- The patient demonstrates appropriate social interactions.

TABLE 9.3 Nursing Diagnoses Associated With Mental Health			
Diagnosis	**Point of Differentiation**	**Assessment Characteristics**	**Nursing Interventions**
Risk for suicide	At risk for potentially fatal, purposefully self-inflicted injury	States desire to die, hopelessness, impulsiveness, loneliness	Establish a relationship. Assess for suicide risk. Refer for counseling. Remove lethal medications and weapons from the environment.
Risk for self-mutilation	At risk for deliberately injuring oneself to relieve stress and tension but not to end one's life	Cuts or scratches on body, picking at wounds, self-inflicted burns, insertion of objects into body orifices	Establish trust. Provide medical treatment for injuries.* Assess for depression, anxiety, impulsivity, and suicide. Secure a contract to notify staff when patient is experiencing a desire to mutilate self.
Altered thought processes	Alterations or disruption in cognition, thinking, and associated activities	Perceiving or interpreting one's surroundings incorrectly, non–reality-based thinking	Reorient as needed. Use concrete, nontechnical words and short phrases. Assess for hallucinations. Convey that you would like to understand what the patient is trying to say, but make sure that the patient does not follow through on harmful processes.
Sensory-perceptual alterations	Disturbances in and inappropriate responses to incoming stimuli	Poor concentration, auditory or visual hallucinations, irritability, agitation, change in behavior	Validate that the patient is the only person hearing or seeing the hallucination. Provide a safe environment. Encourage expression of responses to hallucinations. Encourage the use of alternate coping strategies, such as singing or wearing headphones.
Ineffective individual coping	Impairments in the way one appraises, responds to, or uses resources to deal with stressors	Substance abuse, ignoring problems, lack of concentration, sleep disturbances	Assess for causes. Build on the patient's strengths. Set realistic goals. Listen and avoid false reassurance.
Self-esteem disturbance	Negative self-evaluation; long-term view of self or self-capabilities that is focused on negative aspects	Does not believe or trust positive feedback from other people, exaggerates or fixates on negative feedback, displays shame or guilt	Listen to and respect the patient. Assess strengths and coping abilities. Reframe difficulties as learning opportunities.
Impaired social interaction	Engagement with others that is insufficient in frequency, lacking in quality, or both	Feeling ill-at-ease during social situations; interactions with peers, family, or others that are limited or result in negative consequences (e.g., arguments, poor communication)	Assess the social support system. List behaviors associated with being disconnected and alternative responses. Role-play social interactions and appropriate responses.
Rape-trauma syndrome	Long-term psychological, emotional, and physical consequences following one or more episodes of sexual abuse, sexual assault, or both	Use of drugs or alcohol, anger, aggression, anxiety, problems in relationships, confusion, embarrassment, fear, guilt, humiliation, loss of self-esteem	Stay with the patient. Explain the rationale for interventions. Warn before touching the patient in advance. Observe for signs of physical injury. Document according to forensic standards.

*Collaborative interventions.

Progress Notes: Analyzing Findings

Remember Mr. Hart, whose difficulties have been outlined throughout this chapter. Initial subjective and objective data collection is complete, and the nurse has spent time reviewing findings and other results. The following nursing note illustrates how subjective and objective data are collected and analyzed and nursing interventions are developed.

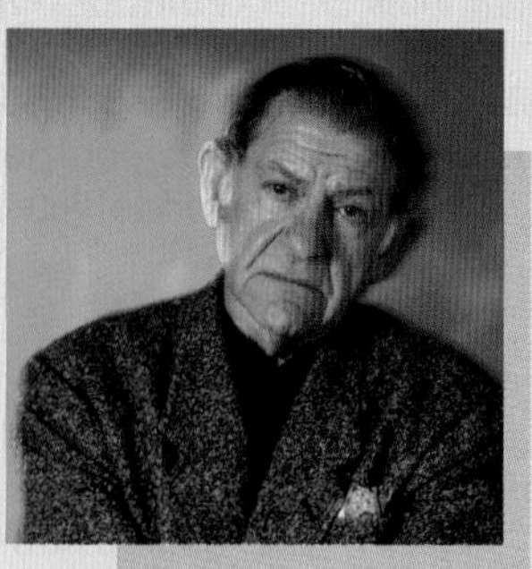

Subjective: "I'm scared when the voices tell me to run away. I know that I should stay here to stay safe."

Objective: A&O × 3. Some inappropriate comments, such as asking personal information. Denies thoughts of harming self or others. Hearing mumbling conversations with several people talking. He states that he can tell the difference between what the voices are saying and what is real. Talking to others usually makes the voices go away. Denies visual hallucinations. Somewhat distracted during initial conversation but attends more as conversation progresses.

Analysis: Altered auditory sensory perception. Risk for suicide.

Plan: Continue involuntary treatment hold. Monitor for effectiveness and side effects of medications. Encourage participation in both individual and group therapies. Assess for suicidal ideation and hallucinations every shift and whenever needed. Avoid asking questions about the past and focus on teaching skills to remain safe. Allow time to build a trusting relationship. Assist with problem solving. Avoid disclosing personal information.

Critical Thinking Challenge

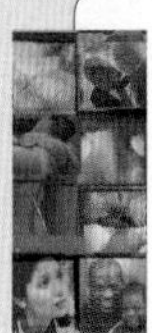

- What things will the nurse observe during the assessment of Mr. Hart?
- What other assessments might be indicated?
- What other nursing diagnoses might be considered?

- The patient identifies personal strengths (Bulechek, Butcher, Dochterman, & Wagner, 2013).

After outcomes have been established, the nurse implements care to improve the patient's status. The nurse uses critical thinking and evidence-based practice to develop interventions. Some examples of nursing interventions for mental health challenges are as follows:

- Assess for risk of harm to self or others.
- Provide a safe environment by removing items that might cause harm.
- Identify support systems and involve them in care (Bulechek et al., 2013).

Key Points

- During a mental health assessment, the nurse assesses the patient and family history, including gender, age, race, current health status, history of mental health concerns, functional status, weight gain or loss, sleeping difficulties, and medications.
- Risk factors for mental health conditions include abuse, family history, poor support network, exposure to violence, stressors, substance abuse, and loss of hope.
- Types of violence include family violence, child maltreatment, sibling violence, intimate partner violence, elder abuse, disabled, bullying and punking, sexual violence,

Applying Your Knowledge

Using the previous steps of the nursing process, consider all of the case study findings woven throughout this chapter. When answering the following questions, begin drawing conclusions and see how the pieces of assessment must work together to create an environment for personalized, appropriate, and accurate care.

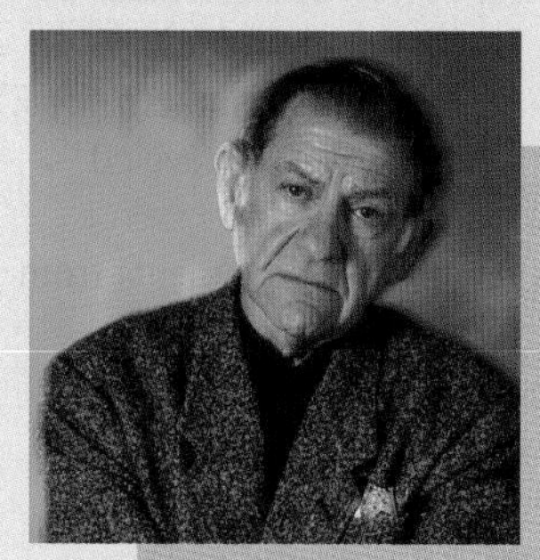

- What three techniques of mental health assessment the nurse could use to gain Mr. Hart's trust?
- How are the mental status assessment and mental health history integrated?
- How will the nurse assess for suicidal ideation, homicidal ideation, violence, and hallucinations?
- What developmental, behavioral and life choices may contribute to Mr. Hart's symptoms?
- What recommendations for follow-up would the nurse suggest for Mr. Hart?
- How will the nurse evaluate whether he or she has gained the patient's trust and promoted respect?

hate crimes, human trafficking, and war/ combat violence. The nurse assesses for alcohol or substance abuse using the CAGE tool.

- The nurse assesses spirituality and sense of meaning using the HOPE tool.
- Suicidal ideation is assessed by asking, "Do you have any thoughts of wanting to harm or kill yourself?"
- Homicidal ideation is assessed by asking, "Do you have any thoughts of wanting to harm or kill anyone?"
- Phrasing to normalize questions about the experience of violence is as follows: "Because violence is common in so many people's lives, I ask all patients about it routinely."
- Altered moods include sad, tearful, depressed, angry, anxious, grandiose, and fearful.
- Altered sensory perceptions include auditory, visual, tactile, and olfactory hallucinations.
- Depression may be assessed using the SAD PERSONAS.
- Assessment of mental status includes *A*ppearance (posture, movement, hygiene, and dress), *B*ehavior (level of consciousness, eye contact, facial expressions, speech), *C*ognitive function (orientation, attention span, memory, judgment), and *T*hought processes (ABCT).
- Assessment of mental status includes assessment of a patient's physical and emotional safety. Violence has psychological, mental, physical, emotional, and social consequences.
- The MMSE tool measures cognitive function and includes orientation, registration, attention and calculation, recall, and language to determine mental status.
- Common nursing diagnoses include risk for suicide, risk for self-mutilation, altered thought processes, sensory-perceptual alterations, ineffective individual coping, self-esteem disturbance, and impaired social interaction.

Review Questions

1. A nurse is working with a new patient, doing a standard assessment. To establish rapport, the nurse would use which of the following statements?
   A. "These are questions that I ask all my patients."
   B. "Don't worry because we are used to working with patients."
   C. "We're here because we want to help people with mental health issues."
   D. "These questions are silly, but I have to ask them."

2. The patient's family should not be present during the interview with the patient about violence because
   A. the patient may feel uncomfortable speaking openly with a relative present, especially if that person is contributing to the patient's stress.
   B. the patient may not answer questions related to the family member that could be perceived as insensitive or inappropriate.
   C. the family member may be ashamed or embarrassed by the patient's actions or statements and try to withhold or change the facts.
   D. the family member may be a perpetrator of abusive behavior, and thus the patient may be hesitant to honestly answer questions.

3. "Do you have any thoughts of wanting to kill or harm yourself?" is a common question to assess for suicidal ideation because it
   A. is blunt and patients cannot refuse to answer.
   B. will cover both suicidal and parasuicidal thoughts.
   C. is subtle, and patients will not know how to answer.
   D. will encourage patients who perform self-harm to stop cutting.

4. When charting general appearance and behavior, documentation may include which of the following?
   A. "Alert and oriented × 3."
   B. "Thought logical."
   C. "Judgment intact."
   D. "Clothes disheveled."

5. Abnormal movements from side effects of medications might be described as
   A. voluntary.
   B. deliberate.
   C. uncoordinated.
   D. smooth and even.

6. Normal speech is audible. This is a normal finding describing which quality of speech?
   A. Fluency
   B. Quality
   C. Loudness
   D. Articulation

7. A 90-year-old patient has a drooped body position, appears sad, and says that she has seasonal affective disorder. What tool would the nurse use to assess her?
   A. MMSE
   B. CAGE
   C. HOPE
   D. Geriatric Depression Scale

8. Which of the following represents the nurse's documentation of a patient with normal mood?
   A. Pleasant or appropriate to situation
   B. Grandiose or strongly confident
   C. Fearful but mildly humble and meek
   D. Sad and tearful during conversation

9. Patients may laugh spontaneously, provide inappropriate responses, ask the nurse personal questions, or insult the nurse. These are examples of
   A. perseveration.
   B. auditory hallucinations.
   C. divergent tactics.
   D. altered mood.

10. The MMSE is used to assess for severity of alterations in orientation, registration, attention and calculation, recall, and language. For which of the following patients would the MMSE be most appropriate?
    A. Women during the postpartum period
    B. Adolescents struggling with sexual orientation
    C. Various cultural groups not tested by other tools
    D. Adults, to assess for cognitive impairment

11. When questioning a patient about violence, it is best to
    A. ask to get the police involved to collect evidence.
    B. have the perpetrator present to assess his or her behaviors.
    C. move from general to specific questions.
    D. ask the patient what he or she did to provoke the violence.

12. Signs and symptoms that are "red flags" for violence include which of the following?
    A. Stating that everything is just fine.
    B. Displaying mood and behavior changes.
    C. Expressing sadness over loss.
    D. Wanting to have family involved.

The Jensen suite offers these additional resources to enhance learning and facilitate understanding of this chapter:

- thePoint online resource, http://thepoint.lww.com/Jensen2e
- *Laboratory Manual for Nursing Health Assessment: A Best Practice Approach*
- *Pocket Guide for Nursing Health Assessment: A Best Practice Approach*
- *Lippincott DocuCare,* an electronic health record simulation software, http://thepoint.lww.com/docucare
- *Adaptive Learning | Powered by PrepU,* http://thepoint.lww.com/prepu

References

Beaty, L. A., & Alexeyev, E. B. (2008). The problem of school bullies: What the research tells us. *Adolescence, 48*(169), 1–11.

Borson, S., Scanlan, J., Brush, M., Vitallano, P., & Dokmak, A. (2000). The Mini-Cog: A cognitive "vital signs" measure for dementia screening in multi-lingual elderly. *International Journal of Geriatric Psychiatry, 15*(11), 1021–1027.

Bulechek, G. M., Butcher, H. K., Dochterman, J. M., & Wagner, C. M. (2013). *Nursing interventions classification (NIC)* (6th ed). Philadelphia, PA: Elsevier.

Centers for Disease Control and Prevention. (2012). *Suicide facts at a glance.* Retrieved from http://www.cdc.gov/violenceprevention/pdf/Suicide-DataSheet-a.pdf

Centers for Disease Control and Prevention, National Center for Injury Prevention and Control. (2013). *WISQARS leading causes of death reports, 1999–2010.* Retrieved from http://webappa.cdc.gov/sasweb/ncipc/leadcaus10_us.html

Craven, R. C., Hirnle, C. J., & Jensen, S. (2012). *Fundamentals of nursing: Human health and function* (7th ed.). Philadelphia, PA: Wolters Kluwer Health/Lippincott Williams & Wilkins.

Edwards, V. J., Anda, R. F., Gu, D., Dube, S. R., & Felitti, V. J. (2007). Adverse childhood experiences and smoking persistence in adults with smoking-related symptoms and illness. *Permanente Journal, 11*, 5–7.

Ewing, J. A. (1984). Detecting alcoholism: The CAGE questionnaire. *Journal of the American Medical Association, 252*, 1905–1907.

Folstein, M. F., Folstein, S. E., & McHugh, P. R (1975). "Mini-mental state." A practical method for grading the cognitive state of patients for the clinician. *Journal of Psychiatric Research, 12(3)*, 189–198.

Fulmer, T. (2012). *Elder mistreatment assessment.* Retrieved from http://consultgerirn.org/uploads/File/trythis/try_this_15.pdf

Hirsch, J. K., Duberstein, P. R., & Unützer, J. (2009). Chronic medical problems and distressful thoughts of suicide in primary care patients: Mitigating role of happiness. *International Journal of Geriatric Psychiatry, 24*(7), 671–679.

Hughes, R. B., Lund, E. M., Gabrielli, J., Powers, L. E., & Curry, M. A. (2011). Prevalence of violence against community-living adults with disabilities: A literature review. *Rehabilitation Psychology*, *56*(4), 302–319. doi:10.1037/a0025620

Moore, G., & Pfaff, J. A. (2008). *Assessment and management of the acutely agitated or violent patient*. Retrieved from http://www.uptodateonline.com.proxy.seattleu.edu/online/content/topic.do?topicKey=ad_symp/6273&selectedTitle=2~6&source=search_result

Moorhead, S., Johnson, M., Maas, M. L., & Swanson, E. (2013). *Nursing outcomes classification (NOC): Measurement of health outcomes* (5th ed.). St. Louis, MO: Elsevier.

Phillips, D. A. (2007). Punking and bullying: Strategies in middle school, high school, and beyond. *Journal of Interpersonal Violence*, *22*(2), 158–178.

Phillips, D. A., Phillips, K. H., Grupp, K., & Trigg, L. J. (2009). Sibling violence silenced: Rivalry, competition, wrestling, playin', roughhousing, benign. *Advances in Nursing Science*, *32*(2), E1–E16.

Randall, T., Espinoza, R. T., and Unützer, J. (2008). *Diagnosis and management of late-life depression*. Retrieved February 1, 2009, from http://www.uptodateonline.com.proxy.seattleu.edu/online/content/topic.do?topicKey=psychiat/12560&selectedTitle=1~150&source=search_result

Rape, Abuse & Incest National Network. (2008). *Who are the victims?* Retrieved July 20, 2008, from http://www.rainn.com/get-information/statistics/sexual-assault-victims

The Joint Commission. (2010). *Advancing effective communication, cultural competence, and patient- and family-centered care: A roadmap for hospitals*. Oakbrook Terrace, IL: Author. Retrieved from http://www.jointcommission.org/assets/1/6/aroadmapforhospitalsfi nalversion727.pdf

United Nations Office on Drugs and Crime. (2008). *What is human trafficking?* Retrieved from https://www.unodc.org/unodc/en/human-trafficking/what-ishuman-trafficking.html?ref=menuside#What_is_Human_Trafficking

U.S. Department of Health & Human Services. (2009a). *Culture counts: The influence of culture and society on mental health, mental illness*. Retrieved from http://mentalhealth.samhsa.gov/cre/ch2_culture_of_the_patient.asp

U.S. Department of Health & Human Services. (2009b). *Mental health: A report of the surgeon general*. Rockville, MD: U.S. Department of Health & Human Services, Substance Abuse and Mental Health Services Administration, Center for Mental Health Services, National Institutes of Health, National Institute of Mental Health.

U.S. Department of Health & Human Services. (2013). *2020 Topics & Objectives - Objectives A-Z*. Retrieved from http://www.healthypeople.gov/2020/topicsobjectives2020/

U.S. Department of Justice. (2013). *NCVRW resource guide*. Retrieved from http://ovc.ncjrs.gov/ncvrw2014/

Waszynski, C. M. (2007). How to try this: Detecting delirium. *American Journal of Nursing*, *107*(12), 50–59.

World Health Organization. (2013a). *Global and regional estimates of violence against women*. Retrieved from http://apps.who.int/iris/bitstream/10665/85239/1/9789241564625_eng.pdf

World Health Organization. (2013b). *Mental health: A state of well-being*. Retrieved from http://www.who.int/features/factfiles/mental_health/en/

Tables of Abnormal Findings

TABLE 9.4 Abnormal Findings: Mood Disorders

Euphoria	Excessive sense of emotional and physical well-being inappropriate to the actual situation or environmental stimuli
Flat affect	No emotional tone or reaction
Blunted affect	Severe reduction in emotional expressiveness (often confused with flat affect)
Elation	High degree of confidence, boastfulness, uncritical optimism, and joy accompanied by increased motor activity
Exultation	Reaction extending beyond elation and accompanied by feelings of grandeur
Ecstasy	Overpowering feeling of joy and rapture
Anxiety	A feeling of apprehension or worry, especially about the future
Fear	An emotional reaction to an environmental threat
Ambivalence	Having two opposing feelings or emotions at the same time
Depersonalization	Feeling that oneself or one's environment is unreal
Irritability	Feeling of impatience, annoyance, and easy provocation to anger
Rage	Furious, uncontrolled anger
Lability	Quick change of expression of mood or feelings
Depression	Feeling characterized by sadness, dejection, helplessness, hopelessness, worthlessness, and gloom

Adapted from Department of Health. (2008). *Psychiatry*. Retrieved from http://www.doh.gov.ph/zcmc/index.php?option=com_content&task=view&id=101&Itemid=26

TABLE 9.5 Abnormal Findings: Motor Movements

Akathisia	Motor restlessness, inability to remain still; can also be a subjective feeling
Akinesia	No movement or difficulty with movement
Dystonia	Involuntary muscle contractions that cause slow repetitive movements or abnormal postures; can be painful or frightening
Parkinsonism	Slow, shuffling gait; masklike facial expression; tremors; pill-rolling movements of the hands; stooping posture; rigidity
Tardive dyskinesia	Involuntary and abnormal movements of the mouth, tongue, face, and jaw, may progress to the limbs; irreversible condition; may occur in months after antipsychotic medication use
Neuroleptic malignant syndrome	Develops as a potentially lethal adverse effect of antipsychotic medications, with muscle rigidity, tremors, altered consciousness, and incontinence; first warning signs are usually hyperthermia, hypertension, and tachycardia.
Choreiform movements	Irregular, involuntary actions of muscles of face and extremities
Waxy flexibility	Holding body posture that is imposed by another person for a long time
Hyperkinesias	Excessive movement; destructive or aggressive activity
Compulsive	Unwanted repetitive actions
Automatism	Not consciously controlled, automatic, undirected motor activity
Cataplexy	Temporary loss of muscle tone precipitated by strong emotions

(table continues on page 207)

TABLE 9.5 Abnormal Findings: Motor Movements *(continued)*

Catalepsy	Trancelike state with loss of voluntary motion
Stereotypy	Repetitive imitation of another person's movements
Psychomotor retardation	Decreased, slowed activity
Catatonic stupor	Extreme underactivity
Catatonic excitement	Extreme overactivity
Impulsiveness	Outbursts of unpredictable and sudden activity
Tics and spasms	Involuntary twitching and jerking of muscles, usually above the shoulders

Adapted from Department of Health. (2008). *Psychiatry*. Retrieved from http://www.doh.gov.ph/zcmc/index.php?option=com_content&task=view&id=101&Itemid=26

TABLE 9.6 Abnormal Findings: Speech Patterns

Verbigeration	Repetitive, meaningless expression of sentences, phrases, or words
Rhyming	Interjecting into conversation regular, recurring, corresponding sounds at the ends of phrases or sentences, as in poetry
Punning	Interjecting clever and humorous uses of a word or words
Mutism	No expression of words or lack of communication over a period of time
Selectively mute	Mostly mute with intermittent periods of verbal expression
Aphasia	Partial or total loss of the ability to express self through language or to understand the verbal communication of another person
Neologisms	Words created by the patient that are either not easily understood by others or unintelligible
Spontaneous	Communication initiated by a patient with others
Circumlocutions	Phrases or sentences substituted for a word that the person cannot think of (e.g., "what you write with" for a pen)
Paraphasias	Malformed, wrong, or invented words

Adapted from Department of Health. (2008). *Psychiatry*. Retrieved from http://www.doh.gov.ph/zcmc/index.php?option=com_content&task=view&id=101&Itemid=26

TABLE 9.7 Abnormal Findings: Thought Processes

Thought blocking	Sudden cessation of flow of thought and speech related to strong emotions
Flight of ideas	Rapid conversation with logically unconnected shifting of topics
Word salad	Disconnected and incoherent combination of phrases, words, and sentences
Perseveration phenomena	Repetitive behaviors such as lip licking, finger tapping, pacing, or echolalia
Circumstantiality	Interjection of great detail and incidental material with no primary significance to the central idea of the conversation
Tangential	Deviation from the central theme of conversation
Echolalia	Repetitive imitation of another person's speech
Delusion	False belief kept despite nonsupportive evidence
Phobia	Strong, persistent, abnormal fear of an object or situation
Obsession	Persistent, unwanted, recurring thoughts
Compulsions	Repetitive mental act or physical behavior that a patient feels driven to perform to reduce distress, prevent a dreaded event or situation, or respond to an obsession

(table continues on page 208)

TABLE 9.7 Abnormal Findings: Thought Processes *(continued)*

Hypochondriasis	Morbid concern for one's health and feeling ill without any actual medical basis
Psychosis	Disorderly mental state in which the patient has difficulty distinguishing reality from internal perceptions
Thought broadcasting	Delusion that others can hear one's thoughts
Thought control	Delusion that others can control a person's thoughts against one's will
Thought insertion	Delusion that others have the ability to put thoughts in a person's mind against one's will
Neologisms	Creating and using new words
Loose associations	Changes of conversation in an unrelated, fragmented manner
Incoherent	Not making any sense
Confabulation	Making up answers to cover for not knowing. Demonstrates the ability to think and reason with only short-term memory present. Symptom of Korsakoff syndrome
Ideas of reference	Perception that others or the media are talking to or about the patient
Ruminating	Getting "stuck" on, worrying, or thinking about an idea repetitively

Adapted from Department of Health. (2008). *Psychiatry.* Retrieved from http://www.doh.gov.ph/zcmc/index.php?option=com_content&task=view&id=101&Itemid=26

TABLE 9.8 Comparison of Delirium, Dementia, and Depression

	Delirium	**Dementia**	**Depression**
Onset	Acute over a few hours, lasting hours to weeks. Occurs in the context of medical illness, substance abuse, or withdrawal	Slow, lasting months to years	Slow
Description	Impaired recent and remote memory Fluctuating attention Thoughts disorganized Change in cognition Clouding of consciousness Perceptual disturbances—usually disorganized Does not usually present with mood components	Impaired remote memory Attention preserved Thoughts impoverished Global impairment of intellect Alert	Impaired memory Aware Attention intact Impaired concentration If psychosis is present, it is usually systematized and with normal emotional response Perceptual disturbances Sad affect or mood

Adapted from Sadock, B. J., Sadock, V. A., & Kaplan, H. I. (2014). *Kaplan & Sadock's comprehensive textbook of psychiatry* (11th ed.). Philadelphia, PA: Lippincott Williams & Wilkins; Edwards, N. (2003). Differentiating the three D's: Delirium, dementia, and depression. *MEDSURG Nursing, 12,* 347–358.

10

Assessment of Social, Cultural, and Spiritual Health

Learning Objectives

1. Identify "models of health" and how they relate to social, cultural, and spiritual assessment.
2. Identify the components of social assessment for individual patients, communities, and societies.
3. Describe the components of the core community assessment.
4. Identify the components of the Community as Partner Assessment Model.
5. Define the elements and use of cultural safety.
6. Demonstrate knowledge of the attributes and behaviors of a nurse practicing effective care within the nurse–patient cultural context.
7. Define spirituality and how it influences patient care in health care settings.
8. Discuss why it is important to be aware of the roles of religions and places of worship in sustaining patient development, national identity, and survival.
9. Discuss how spirituality often takes a central position during life transitions, such as loss of loved ones, accidents, or serious illnesses.
10. Identify nursing diagnoses related to social, cultural, and spiritual nursing assessments.

Mr. Farhan, a 54-year-old Somali Muslim immigrant, is being seen in an outpatient clinic for follow-up care related to his Type 2 diabetes mellitus. He works in maintenance at a local hospital during the day and also has a part-time job selling used goods at auction in the evening. He takes an oral hypoglycemic, metformin, for diabetes and is otherwise healthy. A focused assessment was documented during his last clinic visit 6 months ago.

You will gain more information about Mr. Farhan as you progress through this chapter. As you study the content and features, consider Mr. Farhan's case and its relationship to what you are learning. Begin thinking about the following points:

- What is the physiological effect of adjusting exercise, meal size, and timing of medication?
- How might Mr. Farhan's social network influence his healthy lifestyle?
- How will the nurse assess this patient's cultural needs?
- What effect might religion have on Mr. Farhan's diabetes management?
- Why did the nurse consider a combination of approaches to the patient's concern about Ramadan?
- How will the nurse assess this patient's understanding of the recommendations related to fasting during Ramadan?

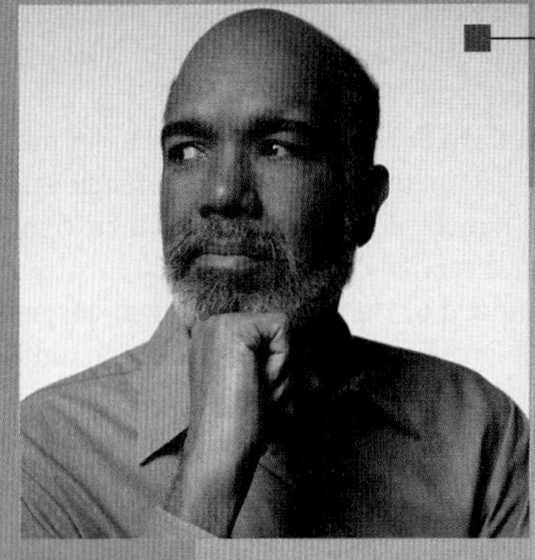

Most countries in the world have a multicultural population as well as a steady influx of new and diverse immigrants. Thus, an important aspect of health care consists of assessing patients' social and cultural backgrounds and spiritual beliefs and incorporating findings into the plan of care. The American Nurses Association, The Joint Commission, the American Psychological Association, and other accrediting agencies direct nurses to acknowledge and address the biopsychosocial and spiritual needs of patients. To facilitate this process, the Office of Minority Health of the U.S. Department of Health & Human Services published the *National Standards for Culturally and Linguistically Appropriate Services in Health Care* (Box 10.1). The accrediting agencies in health care mandated that the standards for culturally sensitive care must be upheld in every health care setting.

Many health care professionals already understand the importance of social, cultural, and spiritual assessments or are actively pursuing educational opportunities to enhance their knowledge. This chapter presents basic principles of conducting social, cultural, and spiritual assessments and ways to incorporate findings into plans of care for patients.

BOX 10.1 National Standards for Culturally and Linguistically Appropriate Services in Health Care (CLAS)

The CLAS standards are primarily directed at health care organizations; however, individual providers are also encouraged to use the standards to make their practices more culturally and linguistically accessible. The principles and activities of culturally and linguistically appropriate services should be integrated throughout an organization and undertaken in partnership with the communities being served.

The 14 standards are organized by themes: Culturally Competent Care (Standards 1–3), Language Access Services (Standards 4–7), and Organizational Supports for Cultural Competence (Standards 8–14). Within this framework, there are three types of standards of varying stringency: mandates, guidelines, and recommendations as follows:

CLAS mandates are current Federal requirements for all recipients of Federal funds (Standards 4–7).

CLAS guidelines are activities recommended by OMH for adoption as mandates by Federal, State, and national accrediting agencies (Standards 1–3, 8–13).

CLAS recommendations are suggested by OMH for voluntary adoption by health care organizations (Standard 14).

Standard 1: Health care organizations should ensure that patients/consumers receive from all staff members effective, understandable, and respectful care that is provided in a manner compatible with their cultural health beliefs and practices and preferred language.

Standard 2: Health care organizations should implement strategies to recruit, retain, and promote at all levels of the organization a diverse staff and leadership that are representative of the demographic characteristics of the service area.

Standard 3: Health care organizations should ensure that staff at all levels and across all disciplines receive ongoing education and training in culturally and linguistically appropriate service delivery.

Standard 4: Health care organizations must offer and provide language assistance services, including multilingual staff and interpreter services, at no cost to each patient/consumer with limited English proficiency at all points of contact, in a timely manner during all hours of operation.

Standard 5: Health care organizations must provide to patients/consumers in their preferred language both verbal offers and written notices informing them of their right to receive language assistance services.

Standard 6: Health care organizations must assure the competence of language assistance provided to limited English proficient patients/consumers by interpreters and bilingual staff. Family and friends should not be used to provide interpretation services (except on request by the patient/consumer).

Standard 7: Health care organizations must make available easily understood patient-related materials and post signage in the languages of the commonly encountered groups and/or groups represented in the service area.

Standard 8: Health care organizations should develop, implement, and promote a written strategic plan that outlines clear goals, policies, operational plans, and management accountability/oversight mechanisms to provide culturally and linguistically appropriate services.

Standard 9: Health care organizations should conduct initial and ongoing organizational self-assessments of CLAS-related activities and are encouraged to integrate cultural and linguistic competence-related measures into their internal audits, performance improvement programs, patient satisfaction assessments, and outcomes-based evaluations.

Standard 10: Health care organizations should ensure that data on the individual patient's/consumer's race, ethnicity, and spoken and written language are collected in health records, integrated into the organization's management information systems, and periodically updated.

Standard 11: Health care organizations should maintain a current demographic, cultural, and epidemiological profile of the community as well as needs assessment to accurately plan for and implement services that respond to the cultural and linguistic characteristics of the service area.

Standard 12: Health care organizations should develop participatory, collaborative partnerships with communities and utilize a variety of formal and informal mechanisms to facilitate community and patient/consumer involvement in designing and implementing CLAS-related activities.

Standard 13: Health care organizations should ensure that conflict and grievance resolution processes are culturally and linguistically sensitive and capable of identifying, preventing, and resolving cross-cultural conflicts or complaints by patients/consumers.

Standard 14: Health care organizations are encouraged to regularly make available to the public information about their progress and successful innovations in implementing the CLAS standards and to provide public notice in their communities about the availability of this information.

From U.S. Department of Health & Human Services, Office of Minority Health. (2013). *National standards for culturally and linguistically appropriate services in health care*. Retrieved from https://www.thinkculturalhealth.hhs.gov/Content/clas.asp

Models of Health

Across times and cultures, the concept of *health* has been defined from various perspectives (see Chapter 1). In the Western world, several models of health emerged in the 20th and 21st centuries.

The Biomedical Model

The most prominent, the **biomedical model**, views health as the absence of disease (Deacon, 2013). From the biomedical standpoint, health is restored by prompt diagnosis of illness, prevention of complications, and elimination of pathology. Social, cultural, and spiritual dimensions of health are not central to the biomedical perspective and generally considered private matters (Deacon, 2013).

The traditional biomedical model continues to serve as the philosophical basis for Western medical care. However, in recent decades, this approach has been openly criticized for its lack of attention to the broad determinants of health. Consequently, an appealing alternative to the traditional approach has emerged in the biomedical community—one that considers the social, cultural, and spiritual aspects of health when treatment decisions are made (Wade, 2009).

Complementary and Alternative Medicine

The **complementary and alternative medicine (CAM) model** of health, which emerged in the later 20th century, has been defined largely in relation to the biomedical perspective. CAM therapies used *instead of* conventional treatments to restore health are often termed **alternative**, whereas CAM therapies used *with* conventional medicine are often labeled **complementary** (Nissen & Manderson, 2013). The process of integrating the two perspectives evokes a new conceptual framework, which considers the complex interplay of mind, body, and spirit and offers opportunities to explore ways to facilitate healing.

Clinical interest in the use of alternative treatment modalities is driven in part by the medical community's interest in additional ways to treat people who have health problems that cannot be easily treated by conventional medicine (Karchmer, 2010). Patient dissatisfaction with biomedical health care has also resulted in a demand for more natural medical practices (Steel et al., 2014). The CAM model is said to view health in a considerably more holistic way than the biomedical model. Critics of the CAM approach, however, allege that research studies to date have not succeeded in demonstrating that alternative treatment methods are as effective as traditional Western medicine or pointed out the ineffectiveness of any alternative treatments (Offit, 2012). Research is needed to continue evaluating the effectiveness of numerous CAM therapies before skeptics will become more open to incorporating CAM treatments into plans of care (Offit, 2012).

The notion of wholeness is not a new concept to nursing. Florence Nightingale, the matriarch of modern nursing, described the nurse's duty as putting the patient in the best condition for nature (God) to act upon him or her (Nightingale, 1860/1992). She maintained that healing can occur only in an environment equipped with proper ventilation, adequate temperature control, pure air and water, efficient drainage, cleanliness, light, and diminished noise. These environmental features are as important to health and healing today as they were to Nightingale in the 19th century. Evidence is growing that care that embraces the patient's biopsychosocial and spiritual dimensions is important to health; this type of care puts the patient's life context and perceived needs first and offers healing for both body and spirit (Burkhardt, 2009). This holistic approach to care results in more favorable outcomes than conventional treatments alone (Bradwell, 2009; Burkhardt, 2009; Kerwin, 2009; Liu et al., 2008; McCaffrey, 2008; Morad, 2008; Palmer & Ward, 2007; Vance, Struzick, & Raper, 2008). Nursing must embrace the wholeness of individuals to properly manage the resources and constraints in their internal (biological, mental, and spiritual) and external (social and cultural) environments (Leininger & McFarland, 2005; Swanson, 1993; Swanson & Wojnar, 2004; Watson, 1999).

Roy's Adaptation Model

In addition to the biomedical and CAM models, several models of health emerged in nursing. **Roy's adaptation model** was one of the earliest conceptualizations (Roy & Andrews, 1999). Roy refers to health as the patient's ability to adapt, compensate, manage, and adjust to physiological–physical health-related setbacks (Hobfoll, 2001). The adaptation model holds that a person is a set of parts connected to function as a whole. The goal of nursing care is to assist the patient to attain an optimal level of

- *Physical health*: also described as physiological processes involved in the proper functioning of a living organism
- *Self-concept*: mental health
- *Role function*: ability to adequately perform in roles occupied in society
- *Interdependence*: satisfying interpersonal relationships (Roy & Andrews, 1999)

The healing environment is one that addresses symptoms of disease, supports bodily functioning, and sustains life by infection control, good oxygenation and nutrition, proper balance between activity and rest, and protection of the individual from harm (Roy & Andrews, 1999). The optimal level of adaptation is accomplished by educating the patient about the management of illness and health promotion activities (Swanson & Wojnar, 2004).

Gordon's Functional Health Patterns

Another widely used nursing model is **Gordon's functional health model** (Gordon, 2006). Gordon posits that people are considered healthy if they can fulfill their social roles by contributing to family and society in meaningful ways. She emphasizes the importance of personal role fulfillment. The primary focus of the functional health model is the use of the person's skills and talents to his or her full potential and avoidance of the risks associated with losing independence.

Gordon identified 11 categories of **functional health patterns**, which she refers to as behaviors that occur sequentially across time: (1) health perception–health management; (2) nutrition–metabolic; (3) elimination; (4) activity–exercise; (5) sleep–rest; (6) cognitive–perceptual; (7) self-perception–self-concept; (8) role–relationship; (9) sexuality–reproductive; (10) coping–stress tolerance; and (11) value–belief. Chapter 2 discusses these patterns in detail within the context of the patient's health history. From the functional health perspective, an optimal healing environment would sustain life to a level expected for and desired by the patient using various treatment modalities (Swanson & Wojnar, 2004).

The Eudaimonistic Model

The **eudaimonistic model of health** (Smith, 1981) emphasizes that wholeness of the individual is essential to maintaining good health. Basic dimensions of wholeness include biopsychosocial and spiritual well-being. In this model, biopsychosocial and spiritual health enables the person to achieve happiness and joy using aspirations as a measure of the value of each human act. This model opens the possibility of ongoing growth, learning, maturity, and positive transformation. The optimal healing environment is one in which providers of care respond to the patient's unique physical, psychosocial, and spiritual needs to promote the unity of mind, body, and spirit, which leads to restoration, maintenance, or promotion of good health (Swanson & Wojnar, 2004, p. 46).

Social Assessment

Social assessment refers to identifying the social context influencing the patterns of health and illness for individual patients, communities, and societies. Basic variables of social assessment include gender, age, ethnicity, race, marital status, occupational class, shelter, employment status, and education level. It is important to understand how these variables interact with the broader sociocultural environment. Knowledge obtained from social assessment helps nurses understand and address issues of equity and social justice related to health. It also helps health care providers to create new ways to improve patients' access to resources (Anderson et al., 1999; Anderson & McFarlane, 2011; Kaplan, 2006; Marmot & Wilkinson, 2006).

Social assessment is integral to quality nursing care at every level. It emphasizes the interconnectedness of physical, psychosocial, and spiritual dimensions of health for individual patients, communities, and populations studied. It helps health care providers and health care policy makers to refrain from compartmentalizing or making sweeping generalizations not grounded in data about individuals and communities. Although on the surface, social assessment might appear simple, it is a daunting task that requires knowledge, creativity, and skill to make the connections among the assessment variables and to interpret data accurately before incorporating them into plans of care.

There are three levels of social assessment: individual, community, and societal.

Social Assessment of the Individual

Social assessment of the individual is intended primarily to inform you about the patient's physical and mental health as related to the patient's existing resources, constraints, and demands. Resources might include education, income, housing, and support systems; constraints might be unemployment, single-parent family, minority status, unsafe neighborhood, and lack of social support; demands might involve struggling to live on a fixed income or caring for aging parents (Seid, 2008). Although information obtained from an individual's social assessment may not be necessary to diagnose illness or initiate treatment, it is essential for planning long-term management of illness as well as evidence-based health promotion activities for that patient (Melnyk & Fineout-Overholt, 2011).

Methods for individual social assessment predominantly entail personal interviews. Depending on assessment goals, interview questions vary from open-ended to specific, often guided by agency-designed assessment forms. A specific example of a comprehensive nursing assessment that attends to both social and cultural dimensions is the transcultural assessment shown in Figure 10.1. Because the list of suggested questions is extensive, it is recognized that you cannot conduct a complete assessment on admission to inpatient or outpatient care for every patient. Instead, you must determine which questions are most relevant based on the patient's symptoms and learning needs. You also must consider any potential effects of culturally based practices on health.

Social Assessment of the Community

At the community level, the scope of social assessment is broader and more complex than at the individual level. Community social assessment involves gathering data to identify community resources, constraints, and high-priority health concerns (Anderson & McFarlane, 2011).

Ideally, the process begins with the assessment of various social, economic, environmental, and quality-of-life health indicators and their relationship to the community's health concerns. Examples of findings from a community social assessment include the relationship between social determinants of health (family income, level of education, social support, and living conditions) and family violence (Bonomi, Anderson, Cannon, Slesnick, & Rodriguez, 2009; Romito et al., 2009), chronic illness (Lipstein, Perrin, & Kuhlthau, 2009; Seid, 2008), and teen pregnancy (Crittenden, Boris, Rice, Taylor, & Olds, 2009). This knowledge is invaluable for planning community-based health promotion campaigns, yet, one must keep in mind that every community is unique with different strengths, weaknesses, and

Cultural Nursing Assessment

Affiliations

- With what culture does the patient self-identify?
- To what degree does the patient identify with the cited cultural group?
- What is the patient's place of birth?
- Where has the patient lived? When? (If the patient is a recent U.S. immigrant, ask about or research prevalent diseases in the country of origin.)
- What is the patient's current residence?
- What is the patient's occupation?

Values

- How does the patient view birth and death?
- What is the patient's view of health versus illness?
- How does the patient regard health care providers?
- How does culture affect the patient's body image and any changes resulting from illness or treatment? For example, what emphasis does the patient's culture place on appearance, beauty, and strength?
- Is cultural stigma associated with any of the patient's illnesses or conditions?
- How does the patient view work?
- What is the patient's perspective on leisure?
- What are the patient's views on education?
- How does the patient feel about/perceive change?
- What effects on lifestyle do health, illness, treatments, and surgery pose for the patient?
- What is the patient's perspective on privacy? Courtesy? Touch? Age? Class? Gender?
- What perspective does the patient have regarding biomedical/scientific health care?
- How does the patient relate to those not from his or her culture?

Cultural Sanctions/Restrictions

- How do members of the patient's culture typically express emotion and feelings?
- How do they view dying, death, and grieving?
- How do men and women show modesty? Does the culture place expectations on male–female relationships? The nurse–patient relationship?
- Does the patient have restrictions related to sexuality, body exposure, or type of surgery?
- Are there restrictions about discussing the dead or fears related to the unknown?

Communication

- What is the patient's primary language? What other languages does the patient speak or read? In what language would the patient prefer to communicate with the nurse?
- What is the patient's level of fluency in English (written and spoken)?
- Does the patient need an interpreter?
- How does the patient prefer to be addressed?
- How does the patient's culture influence expectations about tempo of conversation, eye contact, topical taboos, confidentiality, and explanations?
- How does the patient's nonverbal communication compare with those from other cultural backgrounds? How does it affect the health care relationship?
- How does the patient view health care providers from different cultural backgrounds?
- Does the patient prefer to receive care from a nurse of the same cultural background, gender, or age group?
- What are overall cultural characteristics of the patient's language and communication?

Health-Related Beliefs/Practices

- To what cause(s) does the patient attribute illness and disease (e.g., punishment from God, imbalance in hot/cold or yin/yang)?
- What are the patient's beliefs about ideal body size and shape?
- What name does the patient give to his or her health-related conditions?
- What does the patient believe promotes health (e.g., certain foods, amulets)?
- What is patient's religious background (if any)?
- Does the patient rely on cultural healers (e.g., curandero, shaman, spiritualist, priest)?
- Who influences the patient's choice/type of healer and treatment?
- In what types of cultural healing practices does the patient engage (e.g., herbal remedies, potions, massage, talismans, healing rituals, incantations, prayers)?
- How does the patient perceive biomedical/scientific health care providers? Nurses? Nursing care?
- What comprises appropriate "sick " behavior? Who determines what constitutes symptoms? Who decides when the patient is no longer sick? Who cares for the patient?
- How does the patient's culture view mental disorders? Are there differences in acceptable behaviors for physical versus psychological illnesses?

Nutrition

- How does the culture influence the patient's nutritional factors?
- What is the meaning of food and eating for the patient?

Figure 10.1 Sample of a comprehensive cultural nursing assessment inventory.

(continued)

- With whom does the patient usually eat? What is the timing and sequencing of meals?
- What does the patient define as food? What is "healthy" versus "unhealthy" eating?
- Who shops for food? Where are groceries purchased? Who prepares the meals? How are foods prepared at home?
- Has the patient chosen a specific practice (e.g., vegetarianism, abstinence from alcohol)?
- Do religious beliefs/practices influence the patient's diet? Does the patient abstain from certain foods regularly, on specific dates determined by the religion, or at other times?
- If the patient's religion mandates or encourages fasting, what does "fast" mean (e.g., refraining from certain types or quantities of foods, eating only during certain times)? For how long does the patient fast?
- While fasting, does the patient refrain from liquid? Does the religion allow exemption from fasting during illness? Does the patient believe the exemption applies to him or her?

Socioeconomic Considerations
- Who comprises the patient's social network (family, friends, peers, and cultural healers)? How do they influence health or illness status?
- How do members of the patient's social support network define caring (e.g., being continuously present, doing things for the patient, providing material support, looking after family)?
- What is the role of various family members during health and illness?
- How does the patient's family participate in health promotion (e.g., dietary modifications, exercise) and nursing care (e.g., bathing, feeding, touching) of the patient?
- Does the cultural family structure influence the patient's response to health or illness? Does one key family member especially influence health-related decisions?
- Who is the principal wage earner in the family? What is the total annual income? (Note: This is a potentially sensitive question.) Is there more than one wage earner? Are there other sources of financial support?
- What insurance coverage does the patient have?
- What effects does economic status have on lifestyle, residence, living conditions, and ability to obtain health care? How does the home environment influence nursing care?

Organizations Providing Cultural Support
- What influences do ethnic/cultural organizations have on the patient?

Educational Background
- What is the patient's highest educational level obtained?
- Does the patient's educational background affect his or her knowledge of the health care delivery system, how to obtain needed care, teaching-learning, and any written material that he or she receives from health care providers?
- Can the patient read and write English, or is another language preferred? Are materials available in the other language?
- What learning style is most comfortable/familiar? Does the patient prefer to learn through written materials, oral explanation, or demonstration?

Religious Affiliation
- How does the patient's religious affiliation affect health and illness?
- What is the role of religious beliefs and practices during health and illness? Are there special rites or blessings for those with serious or terminal illnesses?
- Does the patient believe that any healing rituals or practices can promote well-being or hasten recovery from illness? If so, who performs these?
- What is the role of significant religious representatives during health and illness? Are there recognized religious healers?

Cultural Aspects of Disease
- Are there any specific genetic or acquired conditions more prevalent for the patient's cultural group (e.g., hypertension, sickle cell anemia, Tay Sachs)?
- Are socioenvironmental diseases more prevalent among a specific cultural group (e.g., lead poisoning, alcoholism, HIV/AIDS, ear infections)?

Biocultural Variations
- Does the patient have distinctive physical features characteristic of a particular ethnic or cultural group?
- Does the patient have any anatomical variations of a particular ethnic or cultural group (e.g., body structure, height, weight, facial shape and structure)?
- How do anatomic, racial, and ethnic variations affect the physical examination?

Developmental Considerations
- Do any developmental characteristics vary based on the patient's culture(s) (e.g., bone density)?
- What developmental factors are culturally influenced (e.g., expected growth, age for toilet training, feeding practices, gender expectations, methods of discipline)?
- What is the cultural perception of youthfulness?
- How does the culture view older adults?
- What are culturally acceptable roles for older adults?
- Are older adults isolated from culturally relevant supportive people?

Figure 10.1 *(continued)*

concerns. Hence, ongoing community assessments are essential to tailor interventions to each community's unique needs (Basara & Yuan, 2008).

Community-level social assessment techniques range from interviewing key informants through focus groups and mailed surveys to analyzing global housing situations, environmental concerns, and general access to health services. An example of a systematic community assessment framework is "**asset mapping**" (Kretzmann & McKnight, 1993). Core community assessment variables include the gender, age, ethnicity, race, marital status, housing, employment status, and education of members. Data generated from the assessment are grouped into three categories: **primary**, **secondary**, and **potential building blocks**. Formal institutions in the area, such as local businesses, schools, libraries, parks, police, and fire stations, constitute the primary building blocks. Secondary building blocks include agencies designed to serve the community that have outside overarching corporations that manage and operate these agencies. An example is a community's small primary care clinic that belongs to, and shares the values and mission of, a national corporate health care system. Potential building blocks are programs and services designed by an individual or agency outside the community to improve some aspect of community well-being. An example is a federally funded participatory action research study aimed at improving the cardiovascular health of a given community with an increased incidence of heart disease. Using the participatory action research approach, an investigator who is an "outsider" to the community strives to address and evaluate intervention outcomes by actively engaging with community members and facilitating change in a culturally sensitive way (McKnight & Kretzmann, 1977; Merzel & D'Afflitti, 2003).

A common community assessment framework is Anderson and McFarlane's (2011) **Community as Partner Assessment Model** (Fig. 10.2). It has been designed to help nurses thoroughly assess the demographics of a given community, including its values, beliefs, and history. It also assesses how resources (i.e., recreation, physical environment, education, safety and transportation, politics and government, health and social services, communications, and economics) affect and influence the community. This information is used to define community nursing diagnoses and to plan and implement interventions in collaboration with community members. Anderson and McFarlane's model mandates that every community assessment and intervention include systematic evaluation to identify the effects of interventions.

Social Assessment at the Societal Level

At the societal level, social assessment is intended to generate information about societal trends and relationships among the social variables and prevalent health concerns. Data collected through society-wide assessments are used to inform healthy public policy and broad health promotion initiatives. One specific example of societal-level social assessment is the population vulnerability analyses to identify areas of highest concern (Capistrano, Samper, Lee, & Raudsepp-Hearne, 2005; Cernea & McDowell, 2000). Not surprisingly, regions with high concentrations of low-income households, non–English-speaking immigrant families, and settlements of indigenous peoples emerged as areas of highest public health concern with respect to health vulnerabilities.

Collecting data and analyzing findings at the societal level is a very complex undertaking. Social assessments are conducted to identify human and material assets, social networks, and the norms and sanctions that govern character, which, in turn, influence health behavior and values. Societal-level social assessment can also be used to identify, for example, ecological risks, disaster preparedness, and posttraumatic stress. Social assessment at the society level can be conducted using diverse research methods ranging in complexity from mailed surveys, telephone assessments, Internet-based questionnaires, and opinion polls to focus groups in multiple locations. Data analyses include summary statistics from complex samples, population stratification, associations between variables, and predictions.

Cultural Assessment

Cultural health assessments and related care are known to promote health and healing. Hence, as a nurse, you have an ethical, moral, and professional responsibility to conduct cultural assessments and create safe, culturally congruent physical and emotional environments in which patients and their families feel cared for and well supported.

Characteristics of Culture

At the most basic level, **culture** can be defined as a shared, learned, and symbolic system of values, beliefs, and attitudes that shape and influence how people see and behave in the world (Hofstede, 1997). Major influences that shape world view, and the extent to which people identify with their culture of origin, are called **primary and secondary characteristics of culture** (Purnell & Paulanka, 2009). Primary characteristics include age, gender, nationality, and ethnicity. Secondary characteristics include cultural values, religious beliefs, morals, occupation, socioeconomic status, immigration status, reasons for migration, and beliefs about health held as important to life and healthy living. All people's cultural beliefs about health are important and they often powerfully influence health practices. Health care professionals, like their patients, add a unique dimension to the complexity of culturally based care (Purnell & Paulanka, 2009). The culturally based care model includes these domains: overview/heritage, communication, family roles and organization, workforce issues, biocultural ecology, high-risk health behaviors, nutrition, pregnancy and childbearing practices, death rituals, spirituality, and health care practices.

Aims of Cultural Assessment

From a holistic perspective, people of different cultures have the right to receive **cultural assessment** and have their health beliefs, values, and practices acknowledged and incorporated

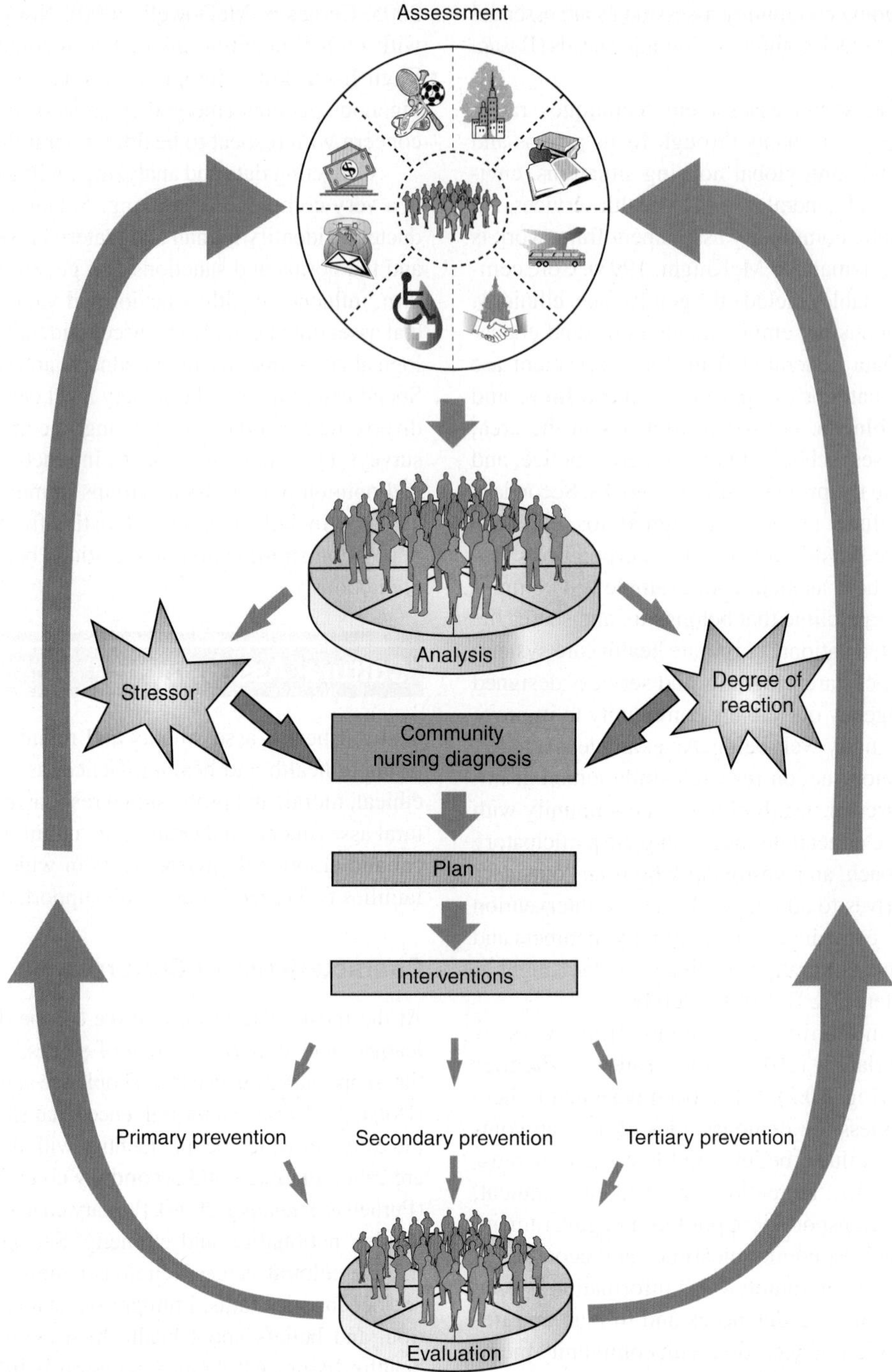

Figure 10.2 Community as Partner Assessment Model.

into plans of care, provided no safety concerns are present. Cultural assessment refers to systematic assessment of individuals, families, and communities regarding their health beliefs and values (Leininger & McFarland, 2005). The specific aim of cultural assessment is to provide an all-inclusive picture of the patient's culture-based health care needs by

1. Gaining knowledge about the patient's cultural beliefs and practices, including food and eating rituals, daily and nightly personal hygiene rituals, and sleeping habits
2. Comparing culture care needs of the specific person with the general themes of those of similar cultural background
3. Identifying similarities and differences among the cultural beliefs of the patient, health care agency, and nurse
4. Generating a holistic picture of the patient's care needs, on which a culturally congruent nursing care plan is developed and implemented (Leininger & McFarland, 2005)

The **Madeleine Leininger theory and the Sunrise Model** (Leininger & McFarland, 2005) proposes essential areas of assessment to better understand the relationship between one's culture and health. It identifies the relationships between cultural variables and health and highlights the nursing behaviors and skills necessary to carry out effective cultural assessment. (Cultural variables include cultural values and beliefs; religion, personal philosophy of life, and spiritual beliefs; educational and economic background; relationship with family and friends; views on and use of technology; politics; and the patient's legal status.)

Leininger suggests that the attributes and behaviors of a nurse practicing effective care within the patient's cultural context include the following:

- Genuine interest in a patient's culture and personal life experiences
- Active listening and awareness of meanings behind the patient's verbal communication (storytelling)
- Nonverbal communication (body language, eye contact, facial expressions, interpersonal space, and preferences regarding touch)
- Acknowledgement that the nurse's own beliefs and prejudices might create barriers to providing culturally sensitive care.

Consideration of patients' cultural backgrounds and incorporating their health beliefs and practices in care plans contribute to enhanced patient experiences with health care and improve health outcomes (Berry, 1999; Higgins, 2000; Lumberg, 2000; Sellers, Poduska, Propp, & White, 1999). Because of the comprehensive body of research showing the benefits of culturally based care, the mandate from accrediting professional organization, and the core values of nursing profession, you have an obligation to skillfully conduct cultural assessments and to incorporate findings into plans of care without bias, prejudice, or discrimination. See Figure 10.3.

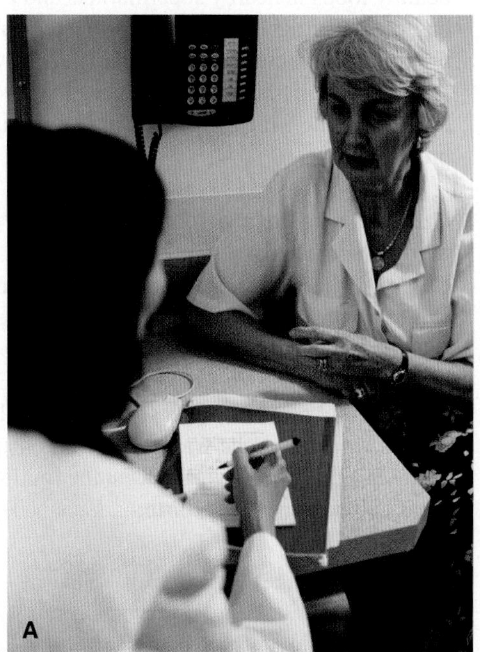

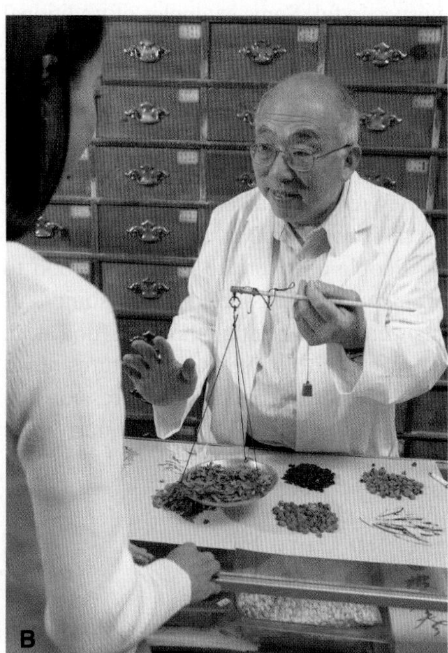

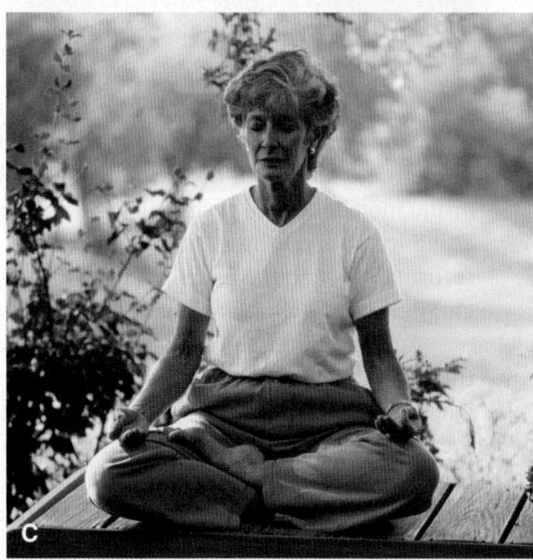

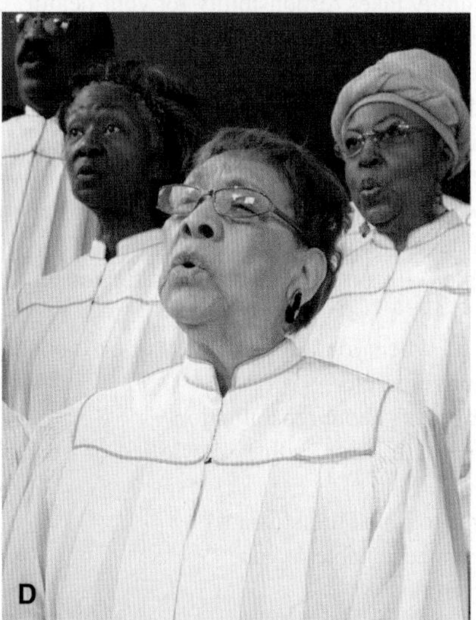

Figure 10.3 A. Patients benefit when nurses discuss cultural or spiritual practices that may influence their health. Examples include **(B)** Chinese traditional medicine, **(C)** meditation/relaxation, and **(D)** participation in religious services.

Cultural Health Beliefs and Practices

At the core of culturally based care is the assessment of the patient's beliefs and practices (Box 10.2) and, when no **cultural safety** concerns arise, incorporation of the patient's beliefs and practices into the plan of care. Seeking an understanding of patients' culturally based health care practices is essential to nursing because each culture has its own traditional values and beliefs about health and illness that may affect individuals' adherence to treatments. For example, for some individuals, health care services may not be affordable or culturally relevant, especially when dietary habits and preferences are not taken into consideration when treatments are ordered. Others, because of the unequal distribution and underrepresentation of ethnic minorities in health care, may reluctantly decide to seek conventional care from a health care provider who does not represent their own culture only after traditional healing remedies have proven unsuccessful. Some examples of traditional health and illness beliefs and practices of people from various minority groups are reviewed in Table 10.1.

Cultural Food and Nutrition Practices

Food and nutrition are an important part of cultural nursing assessment because they represent an expression of peoples' culture and, as such, their consumption may affect individuals' physical health. People all over the world use food to celebrate special events or religious holidays. In some cultures, food represents wealth and health; others use food as an offering to gods or a special gift to guests. All cultures relish ethnic dishes as symbols of identity or cultural expression that they often pass from generation to generation. As a nurse, you must be sensitive about the meaning of food to different people. You must be careful about not refusing food that accompanies special events such as childbirth or infant circumcision performed in hospitals for religious reasons because patients might perceive such refusal as personal rejection (Purnell & Paulanka, 2009).

In many cultures, ideal body weight is higher than medical experts recommend. Such cultures may not consider "dieting" healthy. People may prefer to consume foods high in fat, salt, and cholesterol and low in fruit and vegetables because they believe it is best for their health (Purnell & Paulanka, 2009). Others may have awareness that the ideal diet should be well balanced and rich in different nutrients, but they cannot afford it. Likewise, new immigrants may have difficulty finding ethnic food stores that carry healthy foods with which they are familiar and then unknowingly select unhealthy foods in nearby supermarkets and convenience stores based on affordability. It is therefore very important that you provide facts about the nutritional value of various foods and that you help patients make choices that promote health and are congruent with their cultural background and personal preferences.

BOX 10.2 Health Care Practices Assessment

1. In what prevention activities do you engage to maintain your health?
2. Who in your family takes responsibility for your health?
3. What over-the-counter medicines do you use?
4. What herbal teas and folk medicines do you use?
5. For what conditions do you use herbal medicines?
6. What do you usually do when you are in pain?
7. How do you express your pain?
8. How are people in your culture viewed or treated when they have mental illness?
9. How are people with physical disabilities treated in your culture?
10. What do you do when you are sick? Stay in bed, continue your normal activities, etc.?
11. What are your beliefs about rehabilitation?
12. How are people with chronic illnesses viewed or treated in your culture?
13. Are you adverse to blood transfusions?
14. Is organ donation acceptable to you?
15. Are you an organ donor?
16. Would you consider having an organ transplant if needed?

Adapted from Purnell, L. D., & Paulanka, B. J. (2009). *Guide to culturally competent health care* (2nd ed) . Philadelphia, PA: F. A. Davis.

Cultural Beliefs and Practices of Pregnancy and Childbirth

Cultural beliefs and practices surrounding pregnancy care and childbirth are powerful and cannot be ignored. Many culture-specific taboos are believed to promote well-being and prevent bad outcomes for mother and child (Enang, Wojnar, & Harper, 2002). For example, some women claim that the fetus signals what he or she wants them to consume via cravings, and that if the mother does not eat the food she is craving, the child will be born with a birthmark shaped like the food.

SAFETY ALERT

Certain cravings in women who are pregnant may be unhealthy. You need to provide evidence-based information about the benefits of a well-balanced diet and avoiding substances that might harm mother and fetus.

Women in many cultures believe that buying infant clothing before birth is bad luck and may contribute to a stillbirth. Therefore, you should not assume that the baby is unwanted or the mother "doesn't care" if she arrives at the hospital for childbirth without infant clothing. Instead, you should seek information about her beliefs regarding pregnancy and childbirth (Purnell & Paulanka, 2009).

Across cultures, childbirth is a time of celebration. Relatives and friends might congregate in a hospital or house where childbirth is occurring. Although some cultures permit the presence of relatives in birthing rooms, others might forbid even the father to visit the mother until after the baby is born. Understanding and accepting cultural differences and preferences surrounding childbirth help to alleviate interpersonal barriers between nurses and clients, make families feel more at ease to discuss their beliefs and needs, and help to enhance the experience (Enang et al., 2002).

TABLE 10.1 **Health Characteristics of Minority Populations**

Characteristic	African Americans	American Indians/ Alaska Natives	Asian Americans/Pacific Islanders	Hispanics/Latinos
Demographics	14% of U.S. population (second largest minority). Many live in the South.	2% of U.S. population. 60% live in metropolitan areas.	Consists of people of Far Eastern, Southeast Asian, or Indian subcontinent descent. 5.8% of U.S. population.	Largest U.S. minority group with 17%. Consists of people of Cuban, Mexican, Puerto Rican, South or Central American, or other Spanish culture or origin
Educational Attainment	Fewer Blacks earn a high school diploma than Whites. More Black women than Black men earn a bachelor's degree.	76% have a high school diploma. 14% have a bachelor's degree.	62% of Vietnamese, 50% of Chinese, 24% of Filipinos, and 23% of Asian Indians are not fluent in English. 86% have a high school diploma. 50% of Asian Americans compared with 28% of total U.S. population have a bachelor's degree. 45% are professional compared to 34% of total.	Language fluency varies among subgroups; nationally, 12% of Mexicans speak Spanish at home. 81% have a high school diploma. 13% have a bachelor's degree.
Economics	Average family income is $34,000 compared with $55,000 for White families. 25% of families live at poverty level. Rate of unemployment is twice that of Whites.	Median family income is about $34,000. 26% work in professional occupations. 25% live at poverty level.	Median family income is $55,600, higher than the national average.	25% work in service occupations, compared with 14% of Whites. 17% work in professional occupations, compared with 40% of Whites.
Health Insurance Coverage	About 50% of African Americans have health insurance, compared with 66% of Whites. Twice as many African Americans are uninsured, compared with Whites.	36% have insurance; 33% have no health insurance	Public insurance rates vary according to subgroup, from 76% to 84%. Overall insurance coverage is 84% compared with 90% of Whites.	Hispanics have the highest uninsured rates of any U.S. racial or ethnic group. Uninsured rate ranges from 23% to 38%.
Cancer	African American men are more likely to have lung, prostate, and stomach cancer. African American women are less likely to be diagnosed with stomach and breast cancer but 34% more likely to die from breast cancer and 2.4 times more likely to die from stomach cancer.	Men are twice as likely to have liver and bowel cancer. Native Americans have higher rates of stomach, liver, kidney, and pelvic cancers.	Asian men are 40% less likely to have prostate cancer. Women are 30% less likely to have breast cancer. Asian Americans have three times the incidence of liver, bowel, and stomach cancers as Whites.	Hispanic men are 16% less likely to have prostate cancer. Women are 33% less likely to have breast cancer. They have higher rates of stomach, liver, and cervical cancer than Whites.
Diabetes	African Americans are twice as likely to be diagnosed with diabetes. They are about twice as likely to die from complications of diabetes.	American Indians are 2.3 times more likely to be diagnosed with diabetes and twice as likely to die from it. They are more likely to be obese and have hypertension.	Native Hawaiians have twice the rate of diabetes and are six times more likely to die from it.	They are twice as likely to have diabetes. Hispanics are more likely to have treatment for end-stage renal disease and die from diabetes.

(table continues on page 220)

TABLE 10.1 **Health Characteristics of Minority Populations** *(continued)*

Characteristic	African Americans	American Indians/ Alaska Natives	Asian Americans/Pacific Islanders	Hispanics/Latinos
Heart Disease	African American men are 30% more likely to die from heart disease. African Americans are 1.5 times as likely to have high blood pressure. Women are 1.7 times more likely to be obese.	They are more likely to have heart disease, smoke cigarettes, be obese, and have high blood pressure.	Asian adults are less likely to have heart disease and die from it than Whites.	Hispanics are 10% less likely to have heart disease and 30% less likely to die from it.
HIV/AIDS	Although African Americans make up only 14% of the population, they represent almost 50% of cases of HIV/AIDS.	American Indians are more likely to have AIDS. Women have twice the AIDS rate of White women.	They have lower AIDS rates than Whites and are less likely to die from it.	Hispanic men have almost three times the AIDS rate as Whites. Women have almost five times the rate as Whites. Hispanics are 2.5–3 times more likely than Whites to die from AIDS.
Immunization	Older adults are 30% less likely to receive a flu shot and 40% less likely to receive a pneumonia shot.	Children were immunized at the same rate as White children. They are more likely to die from sudden infant death syndrome (SIDS), low birth weight, and congenital malformations.	Older adults are 40% less likely to receive a pneumonia shot. Children reached the Healthy People goal for immunizations.	Older adults are 10% less likely to receive the flu shot and 50% less likely to receive a pneumonia shot. Children have comparable rates of immunization.
Infant Mortality	African Americans have 2.3 times the infant mortality rate of Whites. They have higher rates of SIDS, low-birth-weight babies, and failure to receive prenatal care.	American Indians have 1.4 times the mortality as Whites. They are 3.7 times as likely to begin prenatal care in the third trimester.	SIDS is the fourth leading cause of mortality. It is higher for babies born to mothers younger than 20 years of age.	Infant mortality varies among subgroups from 4.4 to 8.3 compared with 5.8 for Whites. Puerto Ricans have 1.4 times the infant mortality rate of Whites.
Stroke	African Americans are 1.6 times more likely to have a stroke and 60% more likely to die from it.	American Indian adults are 60% more likely to have a stroke. Women have twice the rate of stroke.	Adults are less likely to die from stroke, be overweight or obese, have hypertension, or smoke.	Hispanic men and women are 15%–25% less likely to die from stroke than Whites.

From U.S. Department of Health, Office of Minority Health. (n.d.). *Home page*. Retrieved from http://minorityhealth.hhs.gov/templates/browse.aspx?lvl=2&lvlID=9

Culturally based postpartum practices are also diverse. Generally, most cultures recognize that, after childbirth, women must rest, take care of the baby, and "eat for two" when breastfeeding. In some cultures, people may believe that a fat baby is a healthy baby, and new parents might be advised to offer their baby a bottle after breastfeeding to ensure that the infant is "not starving" and "puts some meat on the bones fast." In these situations, you must provide facts about infants' nutritional needs and weight gain patterns as well as health risks associated with infant formula consumption and overfeeding (Riordan & Auerbach, 2005).

In some situations, adhering to culture-based postpartum practices is difficult. For example, women who are practicing Muslims are expected to rest, eat well, take care of the baby, and stay at home for 40 days. Traditionally, they are cared for by other women in the community and not expected to have demands put on them during this time. This may be difficult, if not impossible, when they arrive in the United States as new immigrants and give birth before they make new friends or have a community network. In such cases, you might help by making arrangements for visitations of volunteer women in the community (Purnell & Paulanka, 2009).

Cultural Beliefs and Expressions of Illness and Pain

In some cultures, the roles of men and women and of young and old can vary greatly. Also, it is important to consider differences in culture and religion—for example, a U.S.-born Muslim may have a different kind of cultural orientation than a Muslim who has immigrated to the United States Although many U.S. immigrants transition to Western medicine, some continue to maintain their roots in traditional healing practices, and others mix traditional and Western therapies to restore health. When you conduct cultural health assessment, you might find that an African American patient, especially an older person, mentions already consulting the *Farmer's Almanac* for information on natural cures. Patients of Hispanic background may mention that they have already turned for help to a "curandero(a)," spiritualist, herbalist, or traditional healer. Asian patients may report that they received care from an herbalist, acupuncturist, or bonesetter (Andrews & Boyle, 2011; Purnell & Paulanka, 2009).

> ⚠ *SAFETY ALERT*
> *It is imperative that you ask patients whether they are currently using any traditional remedies to better understand their perspectives on health and illness and to impress upon them the potential for antagonistic or adverse reactions when some traditional and conventional therapies are used at the same time.*

Pain assessment is an integral feature of culturally based health assessment. For example, many people perceive pain as a sign of disease. In the absence of pain, they may decide to not take prescribed medications or take them only when they feel discomfort, which could have grave consequences. Others believe that pain is an inevitable part of being human and endure pain in silence. This belief might contribute to a high pain tolerance or complete refusal of pain medication. Therefore, you must rely both on patients' verbal and nonverbal manifestations when assessing and treating pain (Purnell & Paulanka, 2009).

Some cultures believe that praying and laying on of hands or using holy water and religious symbols will free the person of all pain and suffering. Hence, in some circumstances, sick patients who still report pain may be considered to have little faith. In contrast, other cultures encourage sick patients to be pampered and to express pain freely. Whatever the situation, you must display a nonjudgmental attitude, provide facts, and use a culturally specific approach when administering prescribed treatments. You must never interpret patients' inactivity and dependence as apathy, depression, or "being difficult" without first conducting a cultural assessment and gaining insight into the patient's medical diagnosis and behavior.

Spiritual Assessment

Spirituality, in the most fundamental sense, pertains to matters of the human soul, be it a state of mind, a state of being in the world, a journey of self-discovery, or a place outside the five senses (Holt, Lewellyn, & Rathweg, 2005). In general, spirituality emphasizes a notion of a path to achieve better understanding and connectedness with nature, inner harmony, other people, or an improved relationship with the Divine (Fig. 10.4). Spirituality is also considered an integral part of one's religion or self-directed path modeled after several different religions. In all cases, spirituality is concerned with matters of the soul rather than the world of senses and material things (Borysenko, 2005). Similar to social and cultural assessments, spiritual assessment involves understanding the relationship between spirituality and health.

To be meaningful, spiritual care within the health care context must be congruent with the patient's spiritual beliefs. Just as with social and cultural assessment, making

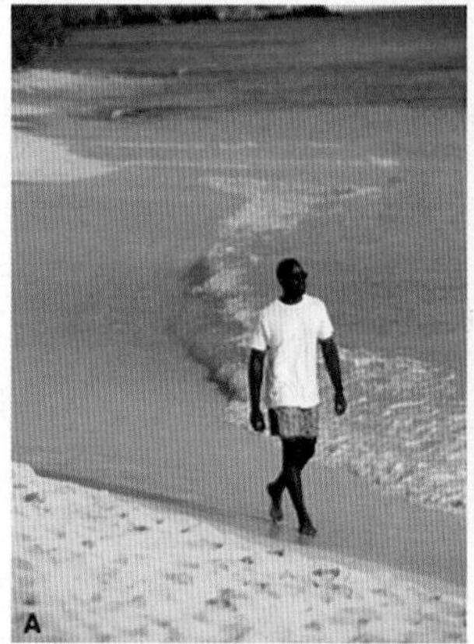

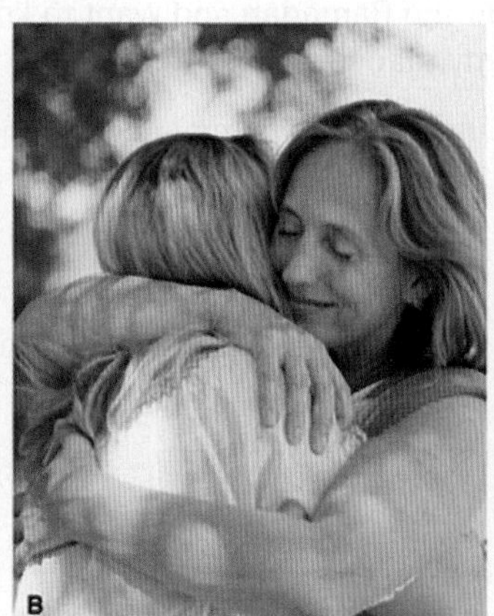

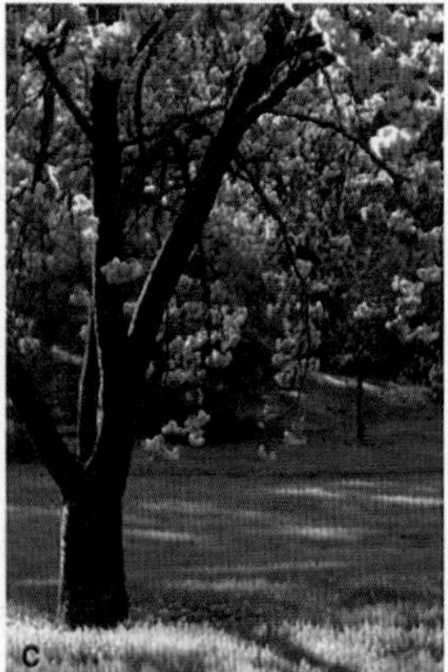

Figure 10.4 A sense of spirituality can be manifested through a relationship with **(A)** oneself, **(B)** other people, or **(C)** transcendent forces, such as God or nature.

BOX 10.3 Spiritual Assessment

1. What is your religion?
2. Do you consider yourself deeply religious?
3. How many times a day do you pray?
4. What do you need in order to say your prayers?
5. Do you meditate?
6. What gives strength and meaning to your life?
7. In what spiritual practices do you engage for your physical and emotional pain?

Adapted from Clancy, C. (2006). Care transitions: A threat and opportunity for patient safety. *American Journal of Medical Quality, 21*(6), 414–417.

assumptions or generalizations about a patient's spiritual needs based on ethnic or religious affiliation is almost certain to be an oversimplification. Nevertheless, it is important to be aware that for people of many cultures, church and religion play important roles in sustaining their development, national identity, and survival and must be treated as such. For example, patients of Polish descent may identify the Roman Catholic Church as a symbol of their national identity and sustainability because it helped the nation to survive and maintain native language and culture for more than 150 years of foreign occupation. Similarly, African American churches played a major role in the development and survival of African American culture. Hence, many African Americans make no distinction between the African American church and the African American community. These specific examples are not isolated. Having faith in God and participating in organized religious life are important to people of diverse cultures and ethnicities and are often seen as a source of inner strength and spirituality. It is therefore important to assess the meaning of the church and organized religion in the patient's life and how it might best be incorporated in the plan of care to promote health and healing. An example of spiritual assessment is presented in Box 10.3 and in Chapter 9 (HOPE tool).

Therapeutic Dialogue: Collecting Subjective Data

Consider the cultural background of Mr. Farhan, who is mentioned at the beginning of this chapter. How would the nurse address his concerns related to diabetes care during the Muslim religious holiday of Ramadan? Through therapeutic dialogue, nursing assessment seeks to incorporate the patient's social, cultural, and spiritual dimensions of health. It is important that the nonverbal behaviors are congruent with the verbal communication.

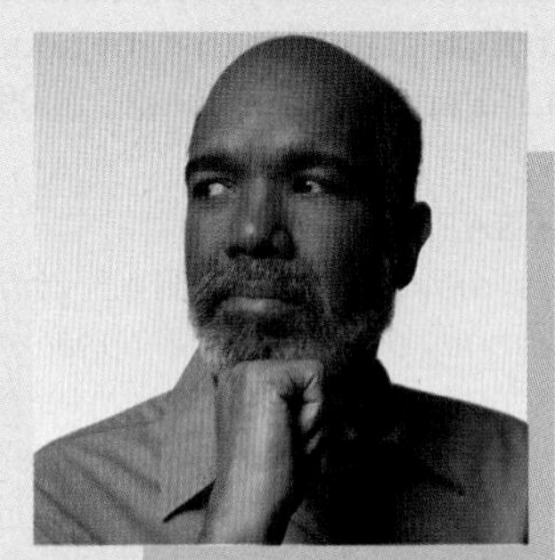

Nurse: Hello, Mr. Farhan. How are you doing today? (smiles)

Mr. Farhan: Very well, thank you.

Nurse: How are you doing with managing your diabetes?

Mr. Farhan: I think, well. I am going to fast during Ramadan and want to know if I should do anything special with managing my diabetes.

Nurse: I am glad that you came in to talk to us about it. We may need to make some changes in your medication and diet regimen. (smiles)

Mr. Farhan: Allah will take care of me.

Nurse: When do you usually take your metformin? We may need to adjust the timing.

Mr. Farhan: In the morning.

Nurse: How do you usually break your daily fast?

Mr. Farhan: We have a big meal together after sunset.

(case study continues on page 223)

Nurse: You might want to have a few small meals after sunset instead. And what is your typical daily exercise?

Mr. Farhan: I go for a 30-minute brisk walk after work on most days.

Nurse: During Ramadan, you may want to exercise a few hours after eating so that you don't get hypoglycemia. We can talk with your doctor about making adjustments so that your diet, exercise, and medication management all fit together during Ramadan.

Mr. Farhan: Thank you so much.

Critical Thinking Challenge

- What might be the social, cultural, or spiritual influences on Mr. Farhan's decision to fast?
- What communication skills did the nurse use with Mr. Farhan?
- What is the role of a nurse when counseling a patient making this decision?

During **spiritual assessment**, you might learn that a practicing Muslim wishes to combine conventional biomedical treatments with spiritual nourishment consisting of daily prayers and reading or listening to the Qur'an. The patient may request that the hospital bed be turned to face Mecca and may ask to have a hospital gown changed and a basin of water placed near the bed for ritualistic washing of hands before praying. By making simple accommodations, you can create an environment in which a Muslim patient may not only have his or her spiritual needs met but also experience a general sense of respect and understanding (Purnell & Paulanka, 2009).

For practicing Jews, observance of Jewish holidays and participating in religious rituals are also important to health and healing. Some Jews may want to pray three times a day and bring their prayer items such as yarmulke or *kippah*, *tallit*, tzitzit, and tefillin to the hospital. They may refuse medical or surgical procedures on the Jewish Sabbath or other religious holidays unless the situation is life threatening. You may also find many visitors in the patient's room because, among other reasons, visiting the sick is a social obligation for Jews. It is important that you and others be accommodating and respectful of the patient's wishes and that you create an environment in which the physical and spiritual healing of the patient occurs concurrently (Robinson, 2000).

For many practicing Hindus, spirituality and religion are also closely related. Those who live far away from temples often pray, sing, recite scriptures, and repeat the names of deities at home or in other places. Shrines that represent symbols of one or more deities may therefore be set at the back of the house or even by the sick person's bedside in the hospital. It is important that you assess the extent to which the patient who states Hinduism as his or her religion practices it and how beliefs relate to health and illness and to daily religious prayer. Assessing the spiritual needs of these patients may assist you in accommodating their need for prayer in privacy (Jambunathan, 2009).

Even when daily prayers or other religious practices are not a routine part of a patient's life, they often take a central position during life transitions, such as loss of a loved one, accident, or serious illness (Hudson & Rumbold, 2003; Rumbold, 2003). Assessment of spiritual needs might reveal that the use of blood products or modern technologies to sustain life may not be congruent with their beliefs. On the other hand, another patient's spirituality allows aggressive medical treatments until the end of life. In each instance, if the health care provider imposes his or her own values on the patient, this may be stress provoking and counterproductive (Holt et al., 2005). Thus, individual patient assessment and incorporation of spiritual assessment findings into plans of care are essential to promote acceptance and spiritual well-being of individuals across the lifespan.

Critical Thinking

Nursing Diagnoses, Outcomes, and Interventions

Table 10.2 compares and contrasts nursing diagnoses, abnormal findings, and interventions commonly related to social, cultural, or spiritual assessment (NANDA International, 2012).

TABLE 10.2 Common Nursing Diagnoses Associated With Social and Spiritual Domains

Diagnosis	Point of Differentiation	Assessment Characteristics	Nursing Interventions
Social interaction, impaired	Engagement with others that is insufficient in frequency, lacking in quality, or both	Failure to maintain eye contact (as culturally appropriate); minimal verbal communication; decreased interaction with friends, neighbors, family, work, and groups	Assess cause of discomfort. Use listening skills. Encourage feelings. Role-play situations. Use humor as appropriate.
Social isolation	Loneliness experienced as a negative condition	Hostility, withdrawal, lack of communication, inappropriate activities for age, rejection of others, expressions of loneliness	Discuss causes of isolation. Recommend support groups. Identify support system. Offer choices of activities. Provide physical activities.
Spiritual distress	Disruption in larger life concepts that integrate the meaning of life	Expresses concern with meaning of life or death, questions the meaning of suffering, questions the meaning of own existence, and expresses anger toward higher power	Assess sources of support and make appropriate referrals. Ask how to be most helpful. Listen to feelings. Assist with providing appropriate religious materials. Provide privacy for praying.
Readiness for enhanced spiritual well-being	Developing of inner strengths to understand life's purpose and harmony with all	Expresses feelings of hope; recognizes inner strength; states purpose of life; feels at peace with self, others, and higher power	Assess spiritual or religious preferences. Make referrals when indicated. Promote support from friends and family. Allow time for praying, talking, or journaling. Provide music.

Note the differences between the two diagnoses for social interaction and spirituality.

As a nurse you use assessment information to identify patient outcomes. Some outcomes related to social, cultural, and spiritual issues include the following:

- The patient will express a sense of connectedness with self, others, arts, music, or power greater than oneself.
- The patient will express meaning and purpose in life.
- The patient will initiate interactions with others (Moorhead, Johnson, Maas, & Swanson, 2013).

After the outcomes have been established, you implement nursing care to improve the patient's status. You use critical thinking and evidence-based practice to develop the interventions. Some examples of nursing interventions for the social, cultural, and spiritual domains are as follows:

- Monitor and promote supportive social contact.
- Integrate family into spiritual practices as appropriate.
- Offer visits with spiritual or religious advisors (Bulechek, Butcher, Dochterman, & Wagner, 2013).

You then evaluate care according to the patient outcomes that you developed by reassessing the patient and continuing or modifying the interventions as appropriate. An accurate and complete nursing assessment is an essential foundation for holistic nursing care. Even as a beginner, you can use the patient assessment to implement new interventions, evaluate their effectiveness, and make a difference in the quality of patient care.

Progress Note: Analyzing Findings

Remember Mr. Farhan, the patient with diabetes who was planning on fasting for Ramadan. Initial subjective and objective data collection is complete, and the nurse has spent time reviewing findings with the primary care provider. The following nursing note illustrates how subjective and objective data are collected and analyzed and nursing interventions are developed.

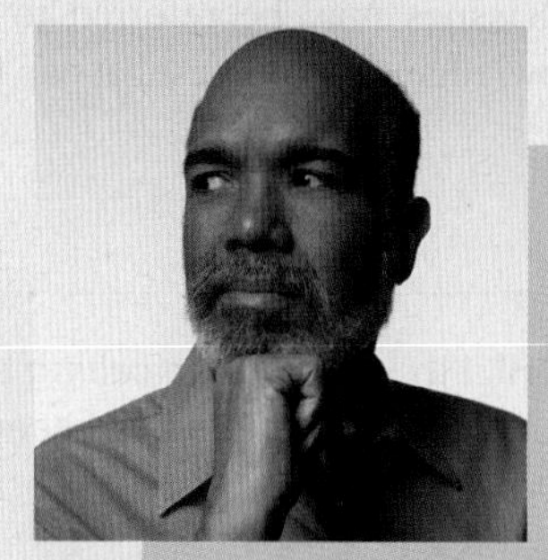

Subjective: Mr. Farhan, a 54-year-old Somali immigrant seen in the clinic for 6-month follow-up appointment related to Type 2 diabetes mellitus. Plans on fasting for Ramadan next month. Asks for advice on how to best manage diabetes during this time. Usually takes metformin in the morning and takes a walk after work in the evening. States that he has a large family with seven children and that some of his children live away from home. During Ramadan, his entire family gathers together at his home to break the fast each night. Prays to Allah five times daily and attends mosque weekly and on holidays. Allah is a source of strength for him and he reads the Qur'an daily. He is involved in a community of Somali immigrants in the Somali Community Services agency. He is also very much involved in a Sunni mosque in the central district of town. He feels well supported and connected to others.

Objective: Wearing Western clothing, well groomed with good personal hygiene. Conversing appropriately, maintaining distance because of gender roles. Affect appropriate, interested, and animated. T 36.8°C tympanic, P 78 beats/min, R 16 breaths/min, BP 112/68 mmHg. Height 1.57 m, weight 66 kg, BMI 26.8. Skin with pink undertones, erect posture, and breathing easily.

Analysis: Health-seeking behaviors related to anticipated fast for Ramadan.

Plan: Consult with physician to establish risk for fasting and modifications to usual routine. May need adjustments in medication, diet, and activity to prevent hypoglycemic complications and dehydration. Further assess types of food eaten and nutritional content to promote a healthy diabetic diet. Assess knowledge of symptoms of hypoglycemia and hyperglycemia and the actions that should be taken.

Critical Thinking Challenge

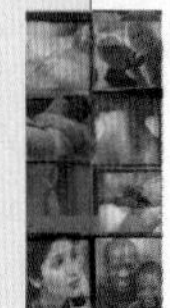

- What are your beliefs about a diabetic patient fasting? How might such beliefs influence care provided?
- What information on the social, cultural, and spiritual practices of Mr. Farhan is needed to provide culturally competent care?
- How will Mr. Farhan recognize whether his fasting has been successful?

In many health care facilities, nurses initiate referrals to social or spiritual care based on assessment findings. Results that might trigger a consult include patients and families expressing social concerns, cultural concerns, or spiritual concerns; death; receiving a terminal diagnosis; comfort care; family conferences; and families in crisis. It is important to assess whether the patient or family is interested in receiving social or spiritual care. Because of the personal nature of religion and the meaning of spirituality, an open-ended question such as, "How would you feel about talking to someone about your spiritual needs?" or "Tell me about whether you want someone to talk or pray with you?" can offer support. Follow-up questions, such as "Do you have a religious preference?" or "Would you like to have someone important from your church to visit with you?" can help identify the most appropriate person to contact. Many patients appreciate spiritual guidance, especially during challenging times. Social issues may be referred to social workers who have knowledge of resources that can be gathered during times of need. Cultural understandings can be learned through Web sites such as Ethnomed or through the Office of Minority Health. It is especially important to interpret these issues within the context of the individual patient, family, and community.

Collaborating With the Interprofessional Team

S: "Hi, I'm Lisa and I'm calling to ask if you could see Mr. Farhan, a 54-year-old Somali immigrant we have seen in clinic for 6-month follow-up appointment related to Type 2 diabetes."

B: "He plans on fasting for Ramadan next month and asking for advice on how to best manage diabetes during this time."

A: "He has a large family with seven children, and some of his children live away from home. During Ramadan, his entire family gathers together at his home to break the fast each night."

R: "I am wondering if he may be able to get permission from you not to fast for medical reasons. This is something that we can work together on because he is a very religious person. After talking with him and deciding about fasting, can you call and let me know and we can adjust his plan accordingly. Thanks very much."

Applying Your Knowledge

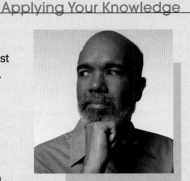

Using the previous steps of diagnostic reasoning, organizing, and prioritizing, consider all the case study findings woven throughout this chapter. When answering the following questions, begin drawing conclusions and see how the pieces of assessment must work together to create an environment for personalized, appropriate, and accurate care.

- What is the physiological effect of adjusting exercise, meal size, and timing of medication?
- How might Mr. Farhan's social network influence his healthy lifestyle?
- How will the nurse assess this patient's cultural needs?
- What effect might religion have on Mr. Farhan's diabetes management?
- Why did the nurse consider a combination of approaches to the patient's concern about Ramadan?
- How will the nurse assess this patient's understanding of the recommendations related to fasting during Ramadan?

Key Points

- The *National Standards for Culturally and Linguistically Appropriate Services in Health Care* mandate the standards to be upheld in every health care setting.
- CAM therapies used *instead of* conventional treatments to restore health are often termed alternative, whereas CAM therapies used *with* conventional medicine are often labeled complementary.
- Social assessment refers to identifying the social context influencing the patterns of health and illness for individuals, communities, and societies.
- With the transcultural assessment, the nurse must determine which questions to ask based on the patient's symptoms, learning needs, and potential effects of the patient's culturally based practices on health.
- Core community assessment variables include gender, age, ethnicity, race, marital status, housing, employment status, and education of community members.
- The Community as Partner Assessment Model has been designed to help nurses thoroughly assess the demographics of a given community and its values, beliefs, and history and to determine how the community is affected and influences resources (e.g., recreation, physical environment, education,

safety and transportation, politics and government, health and social services, communications, economics).

- Culture can be defined as a shared, learned, and symbolic system of values, beliefs, and attitudes that shapes and influences the way people see and behave in the world.
- The goal of cultural assessment is to provide a picture of the patient's culture-based health care needs by (1) gaining knowledge about the patient's cultural beliefs and practices including food and eating rituals, daily and nightly personal hygiene rituals, and sleeping habits; (2) comparing cultural care needs of the specific individual with the general themes of people from similar cultural backgrounds; (3) identifying similarities and differences between the cultural beliefs of the patient, health care agency, and the nurse; and (4) generating a holistic picture of the patient's care needs, on which culture-congruent nursing care plan is developed and implemented.
- The attributes and behaviors of a nurse practicing effective care within the patient's cultural context include genuine interest in culture and personal life experiences, active listening, and effective nonverbal communication.
- Seeking understanding of one's culturally based health care practices is essential to nursing because each culture has its own traditional values and beliefs about health and illness that may affect patients' adherence to treatments.
- Spirituality pertains to the matters of human soul—be it a state of mind, state of being in the world, journey of self-discovery, or place outside of our five senses.
- For people of many cultures, church and religion play important roles in sustaining their development, national identity, and survival.
- Even when daily prayer or other religious practices are not part of a patient's life routine, they often take a central position during life transitions, such as loss of a loved one, accident, or serious illness.
- Common nursing diagnoses related to social, cultural, and spiritual assessments include impaired social interaction, social isolation, spiritual distress, and readiness for enhanced spiritual well-being.

Review Questions

1. The *National Standards for Culturally and Linguistically Appropriate Services in Health Care* mandate that the standards
   A. should be applied in private offices.
   B. may be used in public settings.
   C. should be used in hospitals.
   D. be upheld in every health care setting.

2. CAM therapies used *instead of* conventional treatments to restore health are often termed
   A. alternative.
   B. advantaged.
   C. complementary.
   D. conventional.

3. The social context influences the patterns of health and illness for individuals, communities, and societies. An example is assessment of
   A. the patient's health beliefs and practices.
   B. focus groups in multiple locations.
   C. culturally based postpartum practices.
   D. the religious practices of the patient.

4. The purpose of comparing culture care needs of the specific individual to the general themes of people from similar cultural background is to
   A. identify the dietary needs of a specific religious preference.
   B. determine if the patient needs a spiritual consultation.
   C. provide a picture of the individual's culture-based health care needs.
   D. consider how closely the patient follows his or her religion.

5. With transcultural assessment, the nurse must
   A. ask all the questions for completeness.
   B. determine which questions to ask.
   C. include all the questions as part of an admitting assessment.
   D. wait until the relationship is established to ask questions.

6. A shared, learned, and symbolic system of values, beliefs, and attitudes that shapes and influences the way people see and behave in the world is defined as
   A. society.
   B. community.
   C. culture.
   D. spirituality.

7. Even when daily prayers or other religious practices are not a part of a patient's life routine, they often take a central position during life transitions, such as loss of a loved one, accident, or serious illness. A related nursing diagnosis might be
   A. spiritual distress.
   B. impaired social interaction.
   C. readiness for enhanced spiritual well-being.
   D. social isolation.

8. It is important to identify similarities and differences among the cultural beliefs of the patient, health care agency, and the nurse to
   A. get the proper diet.
   B. perform a spiritual consult.
   C. communicate with family.
   D. avoid making assumptions.

9. Seeking understanding of patients' culturally based health care practices is essential to nursing because each culture has its own traditional values and beliefs about health and illness that
   A. has things that need to be avoided.
   B. affect the body image and habits that may lead to becoming overweight.
   C. may affect patients' adherence to treatments.
   D. use various health methods that might be harmful.

10. What is the nurse's best response when a Muslim patient has a basin of water on his bedside stand that he does not want emptied?
   A. Tell him that the water is a health hazard.
   B. Empty it because it could spill and get the bed wet.
   C. Talk with him about why he should not have it there.
   D. Support and accommodate his preference.

The Jensen suite offers these additional resources to enhance learning and facilitate understanding of this chapter:

- thePoint online resource, http://thepoint.lww.com/Jensen2e
- *Laboratory Manual for Nursing Health Assessment: A Best Practice Approach*
- *Pocket Guide for Nursing Health Assessment: A Best Practice Approach*
- *Lippincott DocuCare,* an electronic health record simulation software, http://thepoint.lww.com/docucare
- *Adaptive Learning | Powered by PrepU*, http://thepoint.lww.com/prepu

References

Anderson, L. M., Fullilove, M., Scrimshaw, S., Fielding, J., Normand, J., Zaza, S., . . . Higgins, D. A. (1999). A framework for evidence-based reviews of interventions for supportive social environments. In N. E. Adler, M. Marmot, B. S. McEwen, & J. Steward (Eds.), *Socioeconomic status and health in industrial nations: Social, psychological and biological pathways*. New York, NY: New York Academy of Sciences.

Anderson, E. T., & McFarlane, J. (2011). *Community as partner. Theory and practice in nursing* (6th ed.). Philadelphia, PA: Lippincott Williams & Wilkins.

Andrews, M. M., & Boyle, J. S. (2011). *Transcultural concepts in nursing care* (4th ed.). Philadelphia, PA: Lippincott Williams & Wilkins.

Basara, H. G., & Yuan, M. (2008). Community self assessment using self organizing maps and geographic information systems. *International Journal of Health Geography*, *7*(1), 67.

Berry, A. (1999). Mexican American women's expressions of the meaning of culturally congruent prenatal care. *Journal of Transcultural Nursing*, *10*(3), 229–236.

Bonomi, A. E., Anderson, M. L. Cannon, E. A., Slesnick, N., & Rodriguez, M. A. (2009). Intimate partner violence in Latina and non-Latina women. *American Journal of Preventive Medicine*, *36*(1), 43–48.

Borysenko, J. (2005). *Healing and spirituality: The sacred quest for transformation of body and soul*. Carlsbad, CA: Hay House Audio.

Bradwell, M. (2009). Survivors of childhood cancer. *Pediatric Nursing*, *21*(4), 21–24.

Bulechek, G. M., Butcher, H. K., Dochterman, J. M., & Wagner, C. M. (2013). *Nursing interventions classification (NIC)* (6th ed). Philadelphia, PA: Elsevier.

Burkhardt, M. A. (2009). Commentary on "Existential and spiritual needs in mental health care: An ethical issue." *Journal of Holistic Nursing*, *27*, 43–44.

Capistrano, D., Samper, C., Lee, M., & Raudsepp-Hearne, C. (2005). *Ecosystems and human well being: Multi-scale assessments*. Washington, DC: Island Press.

Cernea, M. M., & McDowell, C. (2000). *Risks and reconstruction: Experiences of resettlers and refugees*. Washington, DC: The World Bank.

Crittenden, C. P., Boris, N. W., Rice, J. C., Taylor, C. A., & Olds, D. L. (2009). The role of mental health factors, behavioral factors, and past experiences in the prediction of rapid repeat pregnancy in adolescence. *Journal of Adolescent Health*, *44*(1), 25–32.

Deacon, B. J. (2013). The biomedical model of mental disorder: A critical analysis of its validity, utility, and effects on psychotherapy research. *Clinical Psychology Review*, *33*(7), 846–861.

Enang, J., Wojnar, D., & Harper, F. (2002). Childbearing among diverse populations. How one hospital is providing multicultural care. *Lifelines*, *6*(2), 153–158.

Gordon, M. (2006). *Manual of nursing diagnosis* (11th ed.). Boston, MA: Jones & Bartlett.

Higgins, B. (2000). Puerto Rican cultural beliefs: Influence on infant feeding practices in western New York. *Journal of Transcultural Nursing*, *11*(1), 19–30.

Hobfoll, S. E. (2001). Social and psychological resources and adaptation. *Review of General Psychology*, *6*, 307–324.

Hofstede, G. (1997). *Cultures and organizations: Software of the mind*. New York, NY: McGraw-Hill.

Holt, C. L., Lewellyn, L. A., & Rathweg., M. J. (2005). Exploring religion-health mediators among African American parishioners. *Journal of Health Psychology*, *10*(4), 511–527.

Hudson, R., & Rumbold, B. (2003). Spiritual care. In M. O'Connor & S. Aranda (Eds.), *Palliative care nursing* (2nd ed.). Melbourne, Australia: Ausmed.

Jambunathan, J. (2009). People of Hindu heritage. In L. Purnell & B. Paulanka (Eds.), *Transcultural care: A culturally competent approach* (2nd ed.). Philadelphia, PA: F. A. Davis.

Kaplan, G. (2006). Book review: *Social determinants of health* (2nd ed.). In M. Marmot and R. Wilkinson (Eds.). Oxford. *International Journal of Epidemiology*, *35*(4), 1111–1112.

Karchmer, E. (2010). Chinese medicine in action: On the postcoloniality of medical practice in China. *Medical Anthropology*, *29*(3), 226–252.

Kerwin, R. (2009). Connecting patient needs with treatment management. *Acta Psychiatrica Scandinavica*, *438*, 33–39.

Kretzmann, J. P., & McKnight, J. L. (1993). *Building communities from the inside out: A path toward finding and mobilizing a community's assets*. Evanston, IL: Institute for Policy Research.

Leininger, M. M., & McFarland, M. (2005). *Culture care diversity and universality: A worldwide nursing theory* (2nd ed.). Boston, MA: Jones & Bartlett.

Lipstein, E. A., Perrin, J. M., & Kuhlthau, K. A. (2009). School absenteeism, health status, and health care utilization among children with asthma: Associations with parental chronic disease. *Pediatrics*, *123*(1), e60–e66.

Liu, C. J., Hsiung, P. C., Chang, K. J., Liu, Y. F., Wang, K. C., Hsiao, F. H., . . . Chan, C. L. (2008). A study on the efficacy of body-mind-spirit group therapy for patients with breast cancer. *Journal of Clinical Nursing*, *17*(19), 2539–2549.

Lumberg, P. (2000). Culture care of Thai immigrants in Uppsala: A study of the effects of transcultural nursing in Sweden. *Journal of Transcultural Nursing*, *11*(4), 274–280.

Marmot, M. G., & Wilkinson R. G. (2006). *Social determinants of health* (2nd ed.). Oxford, United Kingdom: Oxford University Press.

McCaffrey, R. (2008). Music listening: Its effects in creating a healing environment. *Journal of Psychosocial Nursing and Mental Health Services*, *46*(10), 39–44.

McKnight, J. L., & Kretzmann, J. P. (1977). Mapping community capacity. In M. Minkler (Ed.), *Community organizing and community building for health*. New Brunswick, NJ: Rutgers University Press.

Melnyk, B., & Fineout-Overholt, E. (2011). *Evidence-based practice in nursing and healthcare. A guide to best practice* (2nd ed.). New York, NY: Lippincott Williams & Wilkins.

Merzel, C., & D'Afflitti, J. (2003). Reconsidering community-based health promotion: Promise, performance, and potential. *American Journal of Public Health*, *93*(4), 557–574.

Moorhead, S., Johnson, M., Maas, M. L., & Swanson, E. (2013). *Nursing outcomes classification (NOC): Measurement of health outcomes* (5th ed.). St. Louis, MO: Elsevier.

Morad, M. (2008). Focus on holistic care for children and adolescents with diabetes. *International Journal of Adolescent Med Health*, *20*(4), 387–388.

NANDA International. (2012). *Nursing diagnoses: Definitions and classification 2012–2014* (9th ed). Oxford, United Kingdom: Wiley-Blackwell.

Nightingale, F. (1992). *Notes on nursing: What nursing is, what nursing is not*. New York, NY: Lippincott Williams & Wilkins. (Original work published 1860)

Nissen, N., & Manderson, L. (2013). Researching alternative and complementary therapies: Mapping the field. *Medical Anthropology, 32*(1), 1–7.

Offit, P. A. (2012). Studying complementary and alternative therapies. *Journal of the American Medical Association, 307*(17), 1803–1804.

Palmer, D., & Ward, K. (2007). "Lost": Listening to the voices and mental health needs of forced migrants in London. *Medicine, Conflict, and Survival, 23*(3), 198–212.

Purnell, L. D., & Paulanka, B. J. (2009). *Guide to culturally competent health care* (2nd ed.). Philadelphia, PA: F. A. Davis.

Riordan, J., & Auerbach, K. (2005). *Breastfeeding and human lactation*. Boston, MA: Jones & Bartlett.

Robinson, G. (2000). *Essential Judaism: A complete guide to beliefs, customs, and rituals*. New York, NY: Pocket Books.

Romito, P., Turan, J. M., Neilands, T., Lucchetta, C., Pomicino, L., & Scrimin, F. (2009). Violence and women's psychological distress after birth: An exploratory study in Italy. *Health Care for Women International, 30*(1–2), 160–180.

Roy, C., & Andrews, H. (1999). *The Roy adaptation model* (2nd ed.). Stamford, CT: Appleton & Lange.

Rumbold, B. (2003). Caring for the spirit: Lessons from working with the dying. *Australian Medical Journal, 179*(6 Suppl), S11–S13.

Seid, M. (2008). Barriers to care and primary care for vulnerable children with asthma. *Pediatrics, 122*(5), 994–1002.

Sellers, S. C., Poduska, M. D., Propp, L. H., & White, S. I. (1999). The health care meanings, values and practices of Anglo American males in the rural Midwest. *Journal of Transcultural Nursing, 10*(4), 320–330.

Smith, J. A. (1981). The idea of health. A philosophic inquiry. *Advances in Nursing Science, 3*, 43–50.

Steel, A., Adams, J., Sibbritt, D., Broom, A., Gallois, C., & Frawley, J. (2014). Determinants of women consulting with a complementary and alternative medicine practitioner for pregnancy related health conditions. *Women & Health.* Advance online publication.

Swanson, K. M. (1993). Nursing as informed caring for the well-being of others. *Image, 25*(4), 352–357.

Swanson, K. M., & Wojnar, D. M. (2004). Optimal healing environments in nursing. *Journal of Alternative and Complementary Medicine, 10*(1), 43–48.

Vance, D. E., Struzick, T. C., & Raper, J. (2008). Biopsychosocial benefits of spirituality in adults aging with HIV: Implications for nursing practice and research. *Journal of Holistic Nursing, 26*(2), 119–125.

Wade, D. T. (2009). Goal setting in rehabilitation: An overview of what, why and how. *Clinical Rehabilitation, 23*, 291–295.

Watson, J. (1999). *Postmodern nursing and beyond*. New York, NY: Churchill Livingstone.

UNIT

3

Regional Examinations

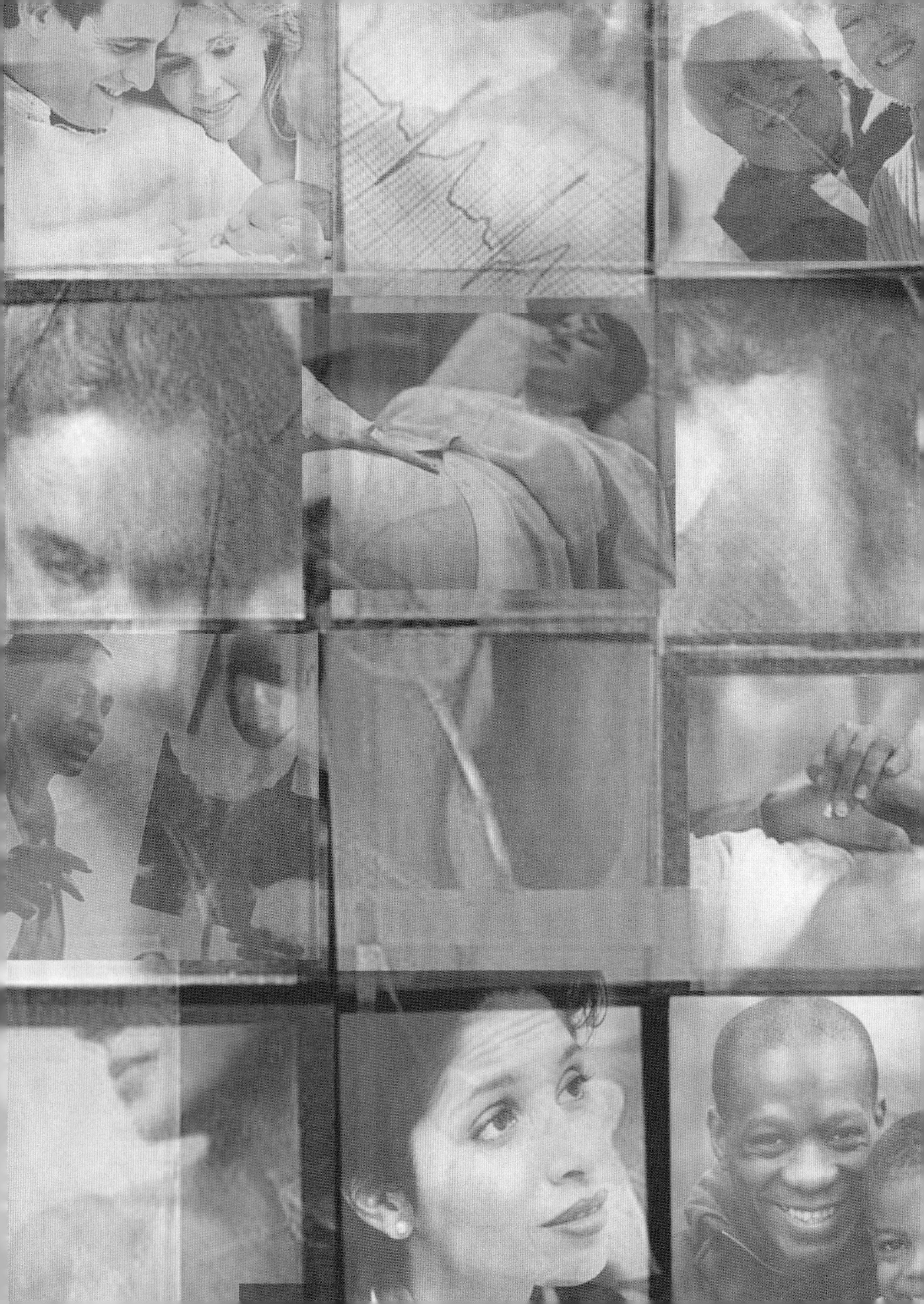

11

Skin, Hair, and Nails Assessment

Learning Objectives

1. Demonstrate knowledge of anatomy and physiology of the integumentary system.
2. Identify important topics for health promotion and risk reduction related to the integumentary system.
3. Collect subjective data relating to various skin lesions and risk factors for altered skin integrity (e.g., cancer, pressure ulcer).
4. Collect objective data on the skin, including turgor, temperature, color, and moisture.
5. Identify normal and unexpected findings related to the integumentary system.
6. Analyze subjective and objective data from assessment of the integumentary system and consider initial interventions
7. Document and communicate data from the integumentary assessment using appropriate medical terminology and principles of recording.
8. Consider condition, age, gender, and culture of the patient to individualize the integumentary assessment.
9. Use integumentary assessment data to identify diagnoses and initiate a plan of care.

Mr. Sholokhov, a 65-year-old Russian immigrant, has been in an acute care unit since yesterday for a venous ulcer. He is scheduled to have a wound vacuum applied later today. Current medications include a thiazide diuretic for high blood pressure, platelet inhibitor for peripheral vascular disease (PVD), and insulin for Type 2 diabetes mellitus. The nurse documented assessment findings last shift. Mr. Sholokhov's temperature was 37.4°C (99.3°F) orally, pulse 92 beats/min, respirations 16 breaths/min, and blood pressure 142/78 mm Hg.

You will gain more information about Mr. Sholokhov as you progress through this chapter. As you study the content and features, consider Mr. Sholokhov's case and its relationship to what you are learning. Begin thinking about the following points:

- What are the major functions of the skin?
- What other assessments are indicated given Mr. Sholokhov's history?
- What information will you teach Mr. Sholokhov about managing his wound care at home?
- What factors in Mr. Sholokhov's home might aggravate his wound?
- What precautions at home and during leisure will benefit Mr. Sholokhov?
- How will you evaluate Mr. Sholokhov's understanding of the teaching you have done?

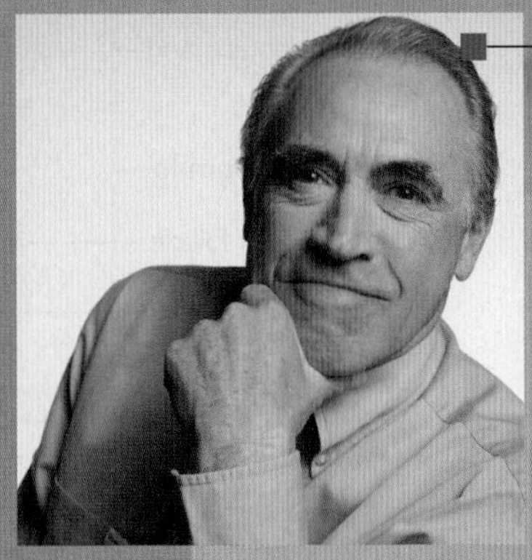

The integumentary system—skin, hair, nails, and sweat glands—provides vital information about a patient's health status. It can indicate whether functioning of the thermoregulatory, endocrine, respiratory, cardiovascular, gastrointestinal, neurological, urinary, and immune systems is adequate. Integumentary findings also reflect the patient's hydration, nutrition, and emotional status and help point you in the direction of other systems or organs that may be compromised. For example, cyanosis in a patient's lips may prompt you to further evaluate the respiratory and circulatory systems. Skin assessment is ongoing; as a nurse, you will integrate integumentary assessment into the examination of other body areas.

This chapter reviews normal anatomy and physiology of the skin, hair, and nails. It presents common variations of normal integumentary findings as well as findings that relate to systemic disorders. It outlines data collection strategies related to common skin lesions, alterations in skin integrity, risk factors for skin cancer (e.g., excessive sun exposure, inadequate skin protection), current health promotion practices, and wound assessment. It presents a systematic method for skin assessment and strategies for interweaving such assessment with examination of other systems. This chapter discusses approaches for accurately documenting subjective and objective integumentary findings and presents information relating to health promotion and disease prevention, such as skin self-assessment, dry skin care, pressure ulcer prevention, and skin protection.

Structure and Function

Skin

The skin is composed of three layers with distinct and separate functions: the epidermis, dermis, and subcutaneous layer (Fig. 11.1).

Epidermis

As the outermost skin layer, the epidermis serves as the body's first line of defense against pathogens, chemical irritants, and moisture loss. The five layers of the epidermis are (1) stratum corneum, (2) stratum lucidum, (3) stratum granulosum, (4) stratum spinosum, and (5) stratum germinativum.

The stratum germinativum contains keratinocytes and melanocytes. Keratinocytes are composed chiefly of keratin, a tough protein providing resistance against friction and trauma. Keratinocytes differentiate over time; they move through the more superficial strata, become anuclear, and eventually are shed from the stratum corneum. Melanocytes produce two types of melanin—eumelanin and pheomelanin—which contribute to integumentary variations based on their amounts and proportions in each person. Larger amounts of eumelanin produce darker skin and hair, whereas larger amounts of pheomelanin are responsible for lighter skin and hair. The absolute number of melanocytes, however, is consistent in all people (Barsh, 2003).

The epidermis contains specialized cells responsible for perception of pain, light touch, vibration, and temperature as well as detection of foreign antigens. In other words, the epidermis is the first part of the body to initiate the immune response. Thickness of the epidermis remains constant throughout the lifespan and across genders.

Dermis

The second layer, the dermis, supports the epidermis. The dermis contains blood vessels, nerves, sebaceous glands, lymphatic vessels, hair follicles, and sweat glands, which support the nutritional needs and protective function of the epidermis. The two layers of the dermis are the papillary and the reticular layers. The papillary dermis, composed primarily of loose connective tissue and elastin, contains capillaries, smaller blood vessels, and nerve endings. It connects directly to the epidermis, facilitating exchange of oxygen, nutrients, and

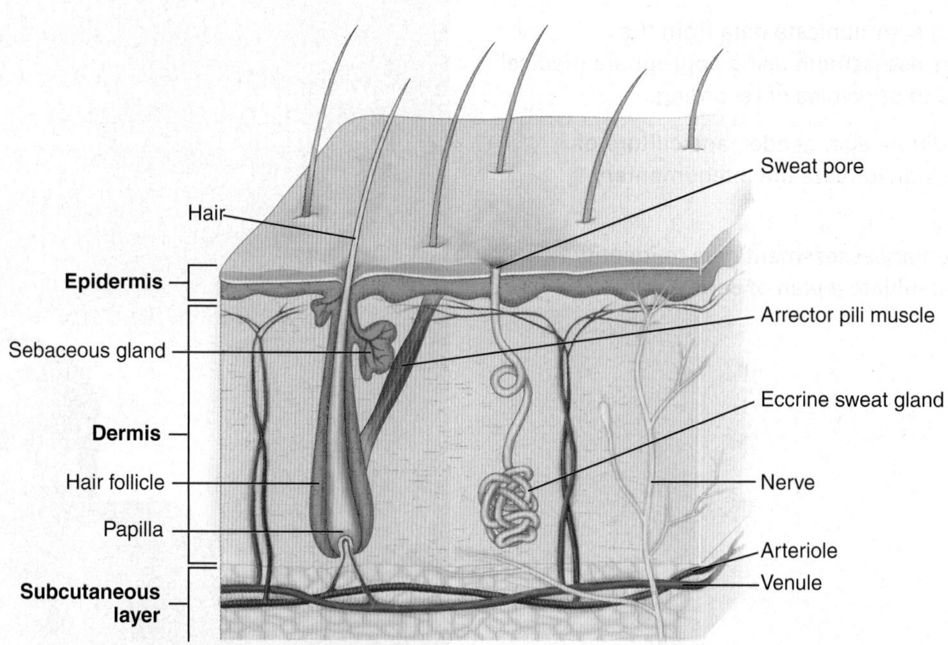

Figure 11.1 Anatomy of the skin.

waste products. The deeper reticular dermis, composed of collagen and elastin, provides the resilience, distensibility, elasticity, and turgor of the skin.

Variations in skin thickness result from changes in dermal thickness, with the thinnest example being the eyelids and the thickest being the palms and soles. Dermal thickness varies across the lifespan and with gender. Skin is thinnest at birth but gradually increases in thickness until the fourth or fifth decade of life, when thickness begins to decline. Men have consistently thicker skin than women as a result of men's greater amount of androgens (Zouboulis, Chen, Thornton, Qin, & Rosenfield, 2007).

Subcutaneous Layer

The subcutaneous layer provides insulation, storage of caloric reserves, and cushioning against external forces. Composed mainly of fat and loose connective tissue, it also contributes to the skin's mobility.

> **Clinical Significance**
>
> The integumentary system is a window to other body systems. Changes in skin, hair, or nails may be the first clue to other health problems.

Hair

Hair is an appendage of skin. It protects various body areas from debris and invasion, provides insulation, enables the conduit of sensory stimulation to the nervous system, and contributes to gender identification. Vellus hair is fine, short, hypopigmented, and located all over the body. Terminal hair is darker and coarser than vellus hair. It varies in length and is generally found on the scalp, brows, and eyelids. In postpubertal males and females, terminal hair also is found on the axillae, perineum, and legs; on postpubertal males, it also appears on the chest and abdomen.

Hair, composed of keratin, is produced by hair follicles located deep in the dermis. Hair follicles are present in all body areas except the palms and soles. The shape of the hair shaft determines the curliness of hair, with an oval shape producing curlier hair than a rounded shape. The amount and proportion of eumelanin and pheomelanin produced by melanocytes in the hair bulb influence hair color.

Arrector pili muscles attached to each hair follicle contract in response to environmental and nervous stimuli, causing erection of the hair and follicle. Sebaceous glands supporting each follicle secrete sebum, maintaining hair moisture and condition. Sebum production declines with increasing age (Fig. 11.2).

Nails

The nails are epidermal appendages that arise from a nail matrix in the epidermal layer, near the distal portions of each finger and toe. The nail plate, composed of hardened keratin, grows at varying rates, with fingernails growing faster than toenails. The highly vascular nail bed appears pink through the transparent

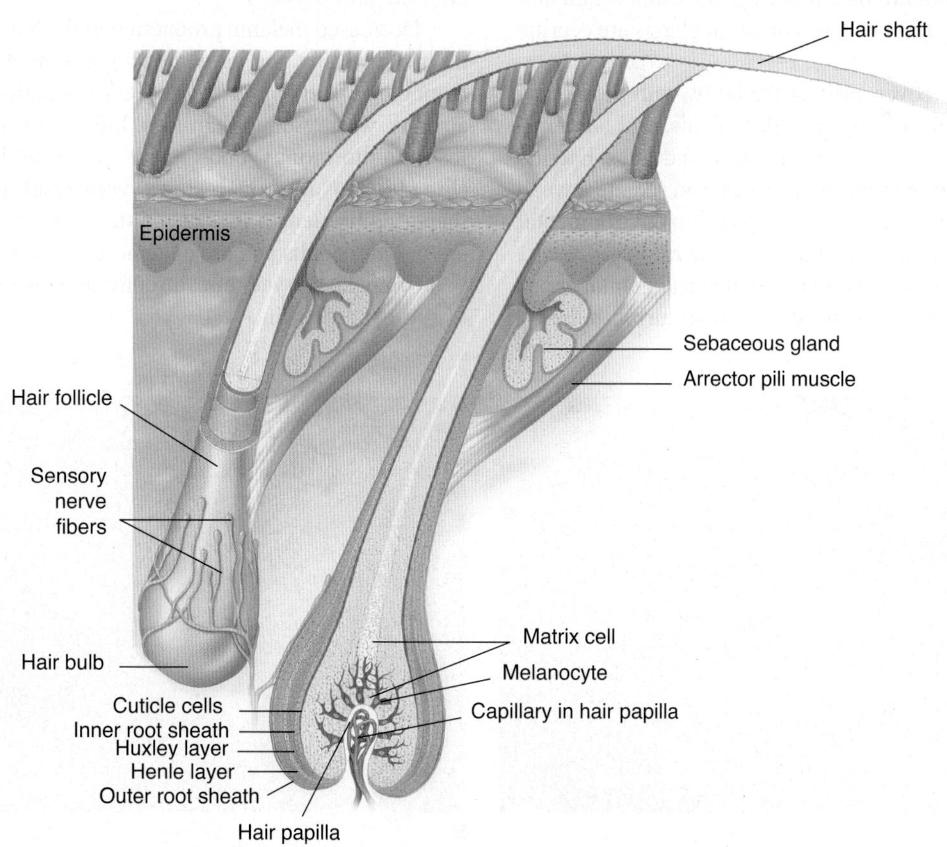

Figure 11.2 Anatomy of hair.

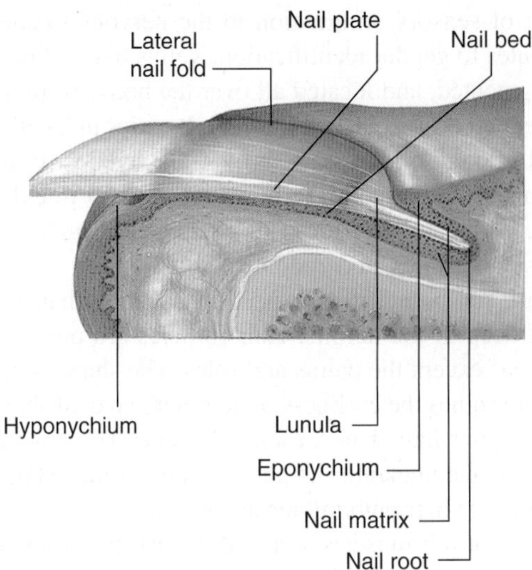

Figure 11.3 Anatomy of nails.

nail plate. Lateral folds of skin on each side and a proximal fold of skin at the base border each nail plate (Fig. 11.3).

Some systemic diseases and infectious processes affect the growth rate and thickness of nails. Changes caused by disease or infection generally are not visible for some time after the incident.

Glands

Sweat-producing (sudoriferous) glands function to maintain normal body temperature by controlling the evaporation and resorption of water. The two types of sweat glands are eccrine and apocrine.

Eccrine glands cover most of the body, with the exception of the nail beds, lip margins, glans penis, and labia minora. They are most numerous on the palms and soles. Eccrine glands open directly onto the skin surface and secrete a weak saline solution known as sweat in response to environmental or psychological stimuli. Sweat assists in thermoregulation.

Apocrine glands, located in the axillae and genital areas, open into hair follicles and become active during puberty. Apocrine glands secrete a thicker, milky sweat into the hair follicle that, after being mixed with bacterial flora on the skin, produces a characteristic musky odor. Functioning of the apocrine glands decreases with aging.

Sebaceous glands are located throughout the body, except the palms and soles, and open into hair follicles. These glands secrete sebum, an oil-like substance that assists the skin with moisture retention and friction protection. Inflammation of the sebaceous glands may result in acne (Fig. 11.4).

Lifespan Considerations: Older Adults

As skin ages, it gradually loses elastin, collagen, and subcutaneous fat, resulting in overall thinner skin (Merck Manual of Geriatrics, 2013). Effects of these changes include decreased resilience, sagging and wrinkling of skin structures, and increased visibility and fragility of superficial vascular structures. Elders are prone to increased bruising and shearing injury.

Turgor, a measure of skin elasticity, decreases as a result of thinning of the dermis and reduced elastin production. The patient's hydration status also can affect skin turgor (Fig. 11.5). The rate of replacement of the epidermal layer decreases with aging, resulting in rougher skin texture and prolonged time for wound healing. These changes affect thermoregulation, resulting in increased hypothermia and increased risk for heat stroke. Function of the eccrine and apocrine glands is reduced, causing increased skin dryness.

Decreased melanin production in the hair matrix and epidermis results in gray or white hair and increased risk for the damaging effects of ultraviolet (UV) radiation. Hair follicles atrophy, with resultant hair loss. Influences from both genetics and hormones may result in androgenic hair loss (Fig. 11.6). Nail growth slows, with resulting thinning and increased brittleness. Effects of sun damage are more apparent in older adults and are evidenced by increased wrinkling, yellowing, leathery texture, atrophy, and uneven pigmentation of sun-exposed skin.

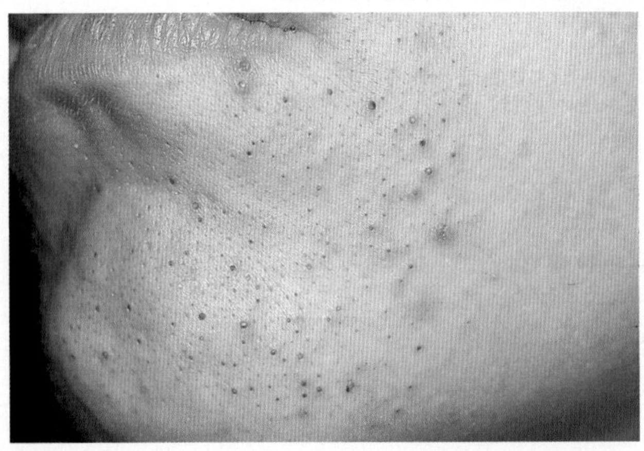
A

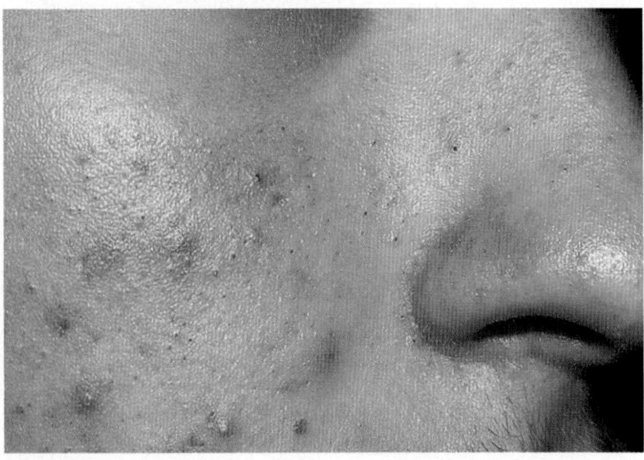
B

Figure 11.4 Acne. **A.** Comedones. **B.** Papular and pustular acne.

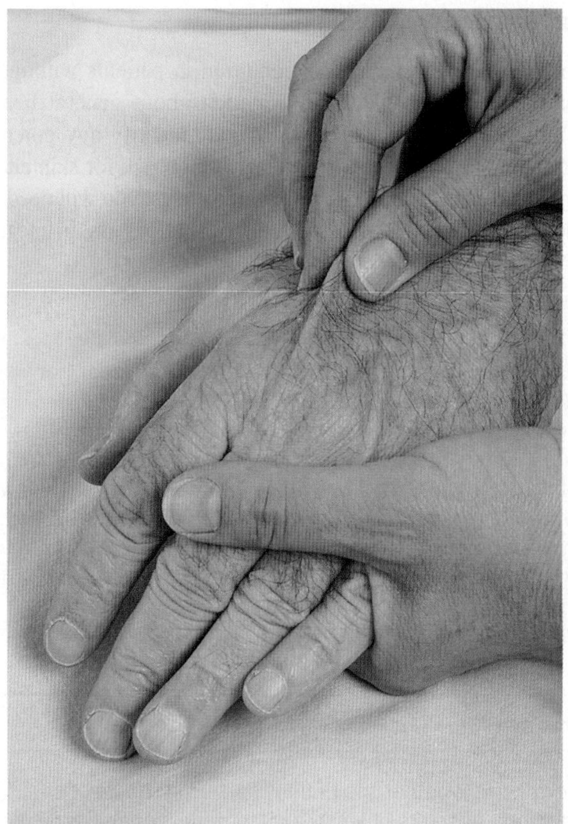

Figure 11.5 Assessing skin turgor. Note thinning of the dermis.

Cultural Considerations

Culturally sensitive assessment includes consideration of the patient's cultural beliefs and practices. Cultural variations can include a patient's refusal to remove a head covering and a requirement for the presence of a chaperone during skin examination, particularly if the health care provider is of a different sex than the patient. Some cultures prohibit directly touching a patient, requiring a nurse to wear gloves to avoid skin-to-skin contact. Becoming familiar with such cultural practices facilitates communication, accurate assessment, and necessary patient education. When you are working with a patient from an unfamiliar culture, inquire about cultural practices and norms before beginning the examination.

Common integumentary findings in African Americans include keloid formation, traction alopecia, and pseudofolliculitis barbae (Juckett, 2005). African American women have increased incidence of melasma in pregnancy; Mongolian spots are fairly common in African American newborns. Curly hair in these patients tends to be coarser than in Caucasians because of a lesser ability of secreted sebum to travel along the hair shaft from the skin. Skin is commonly dry, resulting in ashy dermatitis. Pityriasis rosea, which presents as a macular hyperpigmented viral dermatitis in Caucasians, commonly presents with papular, maroon, or purple lesions in African Americans. Skin cancers are more common on the palms, soles, and nail beds in African Americans than in other groups (Hemenway, 2006).

Southeast Asian men have less body and facial hair than patients of other genetic heritages. Tattoos, body piercings, and other skin adornments are common in various Asian cultures (Ethnomed, 2013). Skin discolorations from cupping or coining may be found. Pigmentary disorders such as vitiligo or melasma in darker skinned Asian populations carry a higher degree of psychosocial and emotional distress than in Caucasian patients (Parsad & Kumarasinge, 2006). Other lesions rarely found outside Asian populations include Hori nevus and nevus of Ota. Other common lesions include solar lentigo, dark eye circles, postinflammatory hyper-/hypopigmentation, ashy dermatoses, and melanocytic nevi. Many Asian men request removal of nevi from body parts for cultural rather than cosmetic reasons (Ethnomed, 2013). Henna tattoos are common in Arabic and Indian females. Newborns of Arabic descent commonly have Mongolian spots, café au lait spots, and congenital nevi (Kahana, Feldman, Abudi, & Yurman, 1995).

Urgent Assessment

Skin findings indicating dehydration, cyanosis, or impaired skin integrity (acute lacerations) require prompt evaluation and intervention with fluids, oxygen administration, skin repair, or a combination. Most skin findings are nonemergent, but you must report them to other health care providers for further evaluation and management.

If a patient has a suspicious lesion, the primary care provider needs to assess and biopsy the site. Concern about cancer can be anxiety provoking; to minimize stress for the patient, you should facilitate these actions in a timely manner.

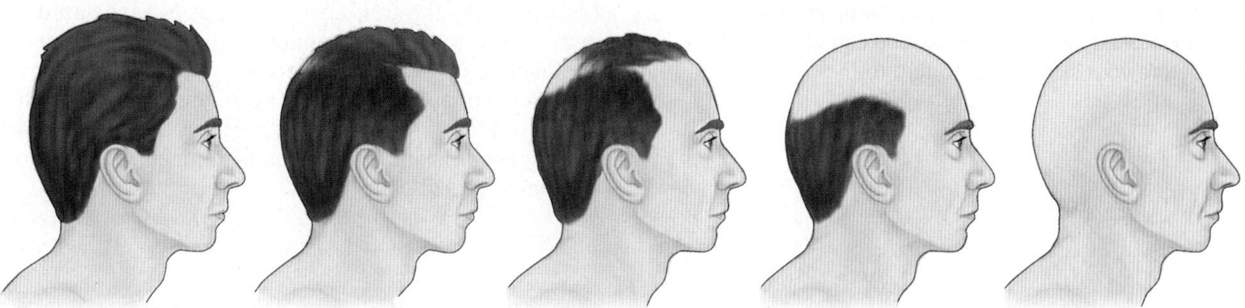

Figure 11.6 Common hair loss patterns in men beginning at age 40 years.

A patient may present with infections or infestations that necessitate use of gloves or, in the case of measles, isolation. Rash and fever in a patient should raise suspicion of an infectious process. The patient should avoid contact with others to avoid infecting them.

Acute trauma and burns may require immediate attention, depending on severity. With large lacerations, you must control bleeding and then work with colleagues to manage the wound. Patients with burns can lose large amounts of fluid through their wounds, so rapid fluid replacement is a necessity. Both large wounds and burns are urgent and potentially life-threatening situations that require advanced interventions.

Subjective Data

During subjective data collection, you have the opportunity to integrate health teaching with history taking. For the integumentary system, a major focus of such teaching relates to prevention of skin cancers, including melanoma.

Assessment of Risk Factors

When assessing general skin condition in patients without an identified concern, gather information about general health, including nutritional status, which may identify any potential causes for skin disorders. In patients at high risk for skin alterations, such as immobile or bed-bound patients, you will need additional information related to potential alterations in skin integrity.

Clinical Significance

If a patient has a specific concern about his or her skin, inspect the area or lesion before asking questions. Often, once you have identified the type of lesion (inflammatory, infectious, tumor, or altered integrity), you can focus questions to address the specific type of lesion. For instance, if a patient is scratching a deep, pink, scaly lesion on his elbow, you may want to inquire about atopic illness or contact irritants instead of about melanoma.

History and Risk Factors	Rationale
Personal History Do you examine your skin for new lesions or changes in current lesions monthly? When was your last clinical skin examination?	Determining whether the patient performs regular skin screenings or seeks at least annual professional examinations will help you provide appropriate education and reinforcement. Give the patient information related to identifying potentially serious skin lesions by teaching what changes warrant further evaluation. A simple method is to use the **ABCDEs** of melanoma detection (Table 11.1): • **A**symmetry • **B**order irregularity • **C**olor • **D**iameter of more than 6 mm • **E**volution of lesion over time
Do you have any pigmented skin lesions? • How many lesions? • Where are they located? • Are any larger than a pencil eraser? • Have any lesions changed (itching, bleeding, nonhealing, color change, size change, change in borders)?	Any **dysplastic nevi** (Fig. 11.7) or more than 50 normal moles increases risk for melanoma. These moles can be in sun-exposed or sun-protected skin areas. Melanomas are most common on the face, shoulder, and upper arms for both genders; back for men; and legs for women, most likely related to sun exposure (Bulliard, De Weck, Fisch, Bordoni, & Levi, 2007). Evolving changes in moles that warrant further evaluation are alterations in size, color, texture, or shape; onset of itching or bleeding; and nonhealing wounds.
Did you ever have severe sunburn, particularly during childhood or adolescence? How long can you be in the sun before your skin begins to turn red?	Melanoma on the trunk, arms, or legs is associated with severe (blistering) sunburn during childhood or adolescence. Fair-skinned people who turn red after minimal exposure to sunlight have less melanin, with less protection from the sun's harmful UV rays, and are at increased risk for melanoma (American Academy of Dermatology, 2013b).

(table continues on page 10)

TABLE 11.1 ABCDEs for Assessment of Melanoma

A: *A*symmetry

Does one half look like the other half?

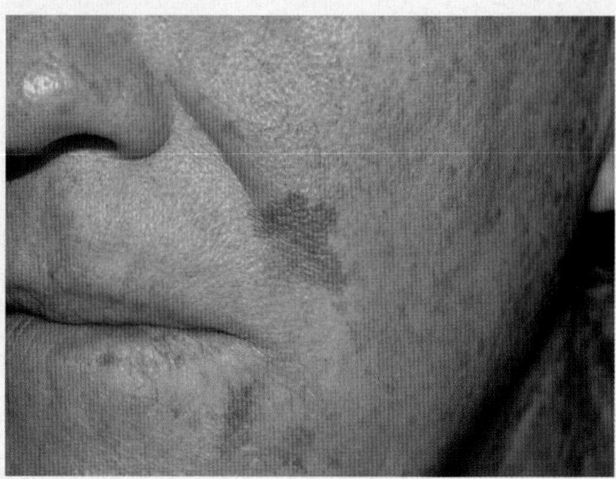

B: *B*order irregularity

Is the border ragged or notched?

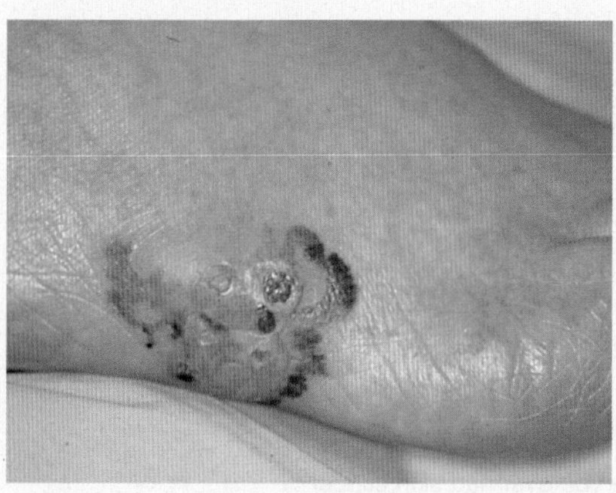

C: *C*olor

Does the mole have a variety of shades or different colors?

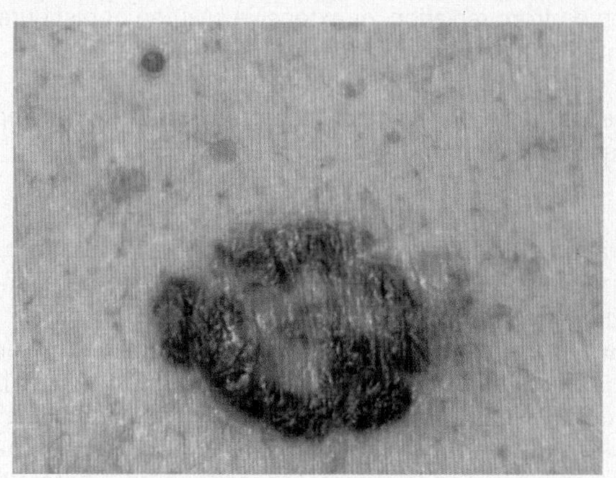

D: *D*iameter

Is the diameter greater than 6 mm (about the size of a pencil eraser)?

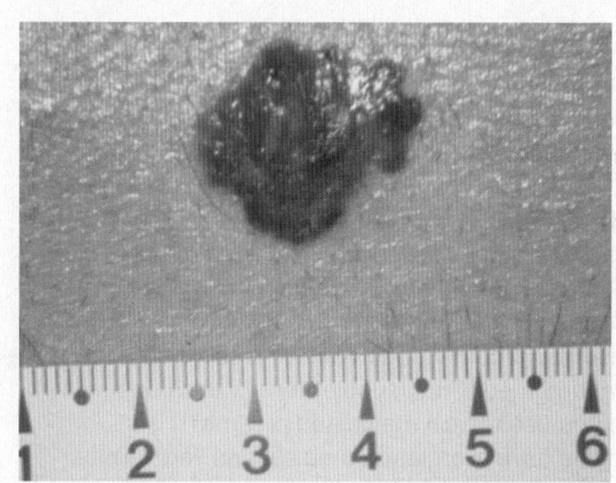

E: *E*volution

Has the lesion evolved or changed over time?

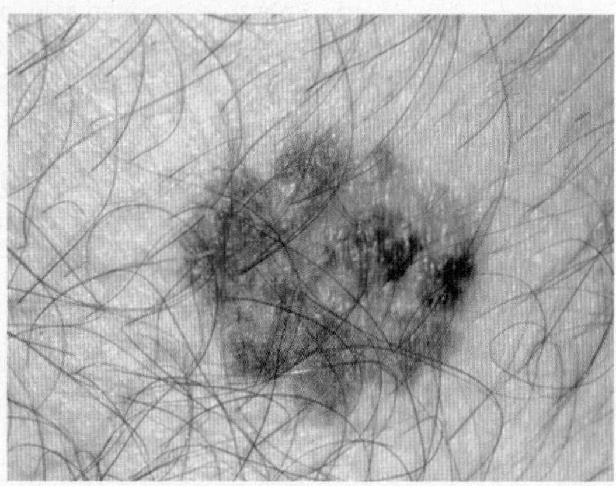

History and Risk Factors	Rationale
	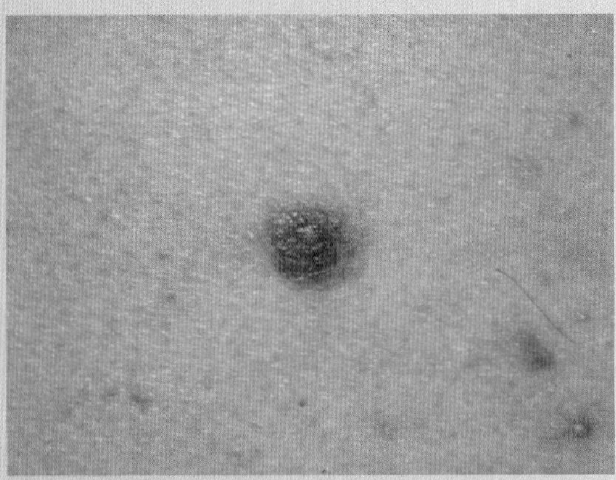 **Figure 11.7** Dysplastic nevus.
Have you ever had skin cancer? • When did you have skin cancer? • Where was it located? • How deep was it? • How was it treated?	Previous history of any skin cancer (squamous cell, basal cell, or melanoma) significantly increases the risk of developing additional cancerous skin lesions (National Cancer Institute, 2011). Deeper melanomatous lesions indicate advanced staging and increased risk for metastases. Previous treatment may have caused additional skin problems, such as burns from radiation, or extensive scarring or disfigurement from surgical excision.
Do you have a history of organ transplant, HIV/AIDS, chemotherapy, or radiation therapy?	A weakened immune system increases the risk for developing melanoma (American Cancer Society [ACS], 2013).
Medications Are you taking any medications, including herbal or nutritional supplements, vitamins, or over-the-counter medications? • Have you recently begun a new prescription or nonprescription medication/supplement? Which one(s)? • Do you use topical medicated creams? • Do you have allergies to medications, latex, nuts, bees, or other items? • What was your reaction to the allergy? • Have you ever had a reaction to sunscreen?	Certain medications (Box 11.1), sunscreens, perfumes, cosmetics, and topical skin creams can cause photosensitivity reactions (Skin Cancer Foundation, 2013), which usually present with rash following sun exposure. Other medications stimulate phototoxicity, a reaction caused by a drug's molecules absorbing energy from a particular UV wavelength and then damaging surrounding tissues. The result is marked and severely tender sunburn. Phototoxicity usually develops immediately (within 24 hours of initial ingestion of the photoreactive medication) and resolves readily upon removal of the offending substance, UV exposure, or both. Photoallergy manifests with blisters and redness on exposed skin, occurs only after repeated exposure to an offending substance, and persists for some time after removal of the offending substance, UV exposure, or both.

BOX 11.1 Medications That Cause Photoreactions

Antimicrobials	Disease-modifying agents
Psychotropics and other psychiatric agents	Chemotherapeutic agents
Cardiovascular agents	Hypoglycemics
Herbals and topicals	Topical agents
Antihistamines	Nonsteroidal antiinflammatory drugs

(table continues on page 241)

History and Risk Factors	Rationale
Risk Factors • What is your occupation? Hobbies? • Are you exposed to excessive sunlight or other sources of radiation? • What do you do to protect yourself from excessive sun exposure?	Work or hobbies involving excessive exposure to sunlight, especially during intense midday hours, increase risk for melanoma. Determining what protection the patient uses (e.g., gloves, hats, long-sleeved shirts, pants, shoes, socks, sunscreens, sunblocks) helps you ascertain the patient's risk level for melanoma.
• How often do you shower or bathe? • What is the water temperature? • Do you apply moisturizer after you bathe?	Excessively dry skin may result from frequent bathing and inadequate moisturizing. Showering or bathing more than once daily in the normal adult causes excessive loss of skin oils. Elderly patients need to bathe less often, usually every 2–3 days. Using hot water to bathe increases loss of skin oils; bathing should be with warm water only and for the shortest time necessary to cleanse all body areas. Use of moisturizing creams (not lotions) immediately after toweling dry decreases the effect of loss of skin oils from bathing.
Determine risk for skin breakdown. • Are you confined to bed? • Do you have a cast, brace, or other immobilizing device on any body part? • Can you change your body position or position of the immobilized body part? • How often are you changing position or shifting weight from one part of your body to another? • Do you have any difficulty with loss of sensation or position sense of any part of your body? • Do you have diabetes mellitus, PVD, or any known sensory loss? • How is your nutritional intake? • What is your age? • What is your weight?	Immobility of the body or a body part increases risk for pressure ulcers. The National Pressure Ulcer Advisory Panel (2012) defines a **pressure ulcer** as a "localized injury to the skin and/or underlying tissue usually over a bony prominence, as a result of pressure or pressure in combination with shear and/or friction." Casts, splints, or other immobilizing devices may exert pressure on bony prominences of an immobilized extremity or part and increase risk for pressure ulcer. This risk is amplified in patients with decreased sensory perception of the immobilized extremity or body part (e.g., in diabetic neuropathy, venous insufficiency, other sensory deficits) because they cannot sense discomfort associated with decreased circulation to an area caused by prolonged pressure. Elderly patients are at increased risk for pressure ulcers from age-related loss of subcutaneous fat and decreased cushioning. Thin patients have less subcutaneous fat to cushion the skin against pressures exerted on it.

Risk Assessment and Health Promotion

Risk assessment identifies areas of concern and provides direction for patient education. Excessive UV radiation is the most important focus area for the integumentary system because exposure to it has been shown to cause skin cancers, particularly melanoma. *Healthy People 2020* goals for integumentary health are as follows:

- Reduce the rate of melanoma cancer deaths.
- Increase the proportion of persons who use at least one of the following protective measures that may reduce the risk of skin cancer: avoid the sun between 10 AM and 4 PM, wear sun-protective clothing when exposed to sunlight, use sunscreen with a sun protection factor (SPF) of 15 or higher, and avoid artificial sources of UV light. (U.S. Department of Health & Human Services, 2013)

Self skin-examination (SSE) helps patients identify potentially problematic lesions through the detection of moles (Fig. 11.8). Educate the patient that a normal mole has the following features (American Academy of Dermatology, 2013a):

- A solid tan, brown, black, or skin-toned color
- Size smaller than 6 mm in diameter (approximately the size of a pencil eraser)
- Well-defined edges
- Usually round or oval shape with a flat or dome-like surface
- Emergence before 30 years of age

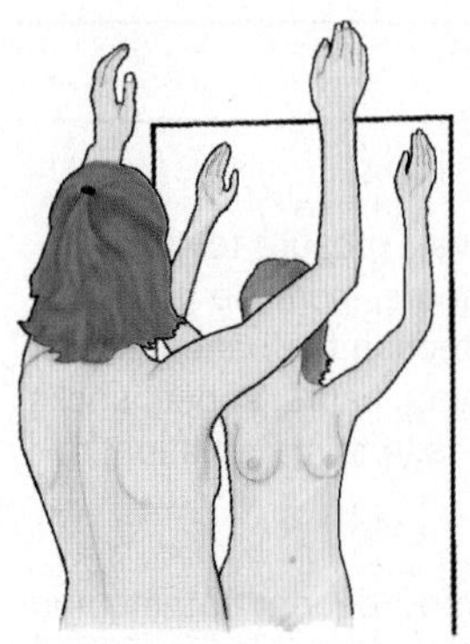

1. Examine the body front and back in the mirror, then the right and left sides, with the arms raised.

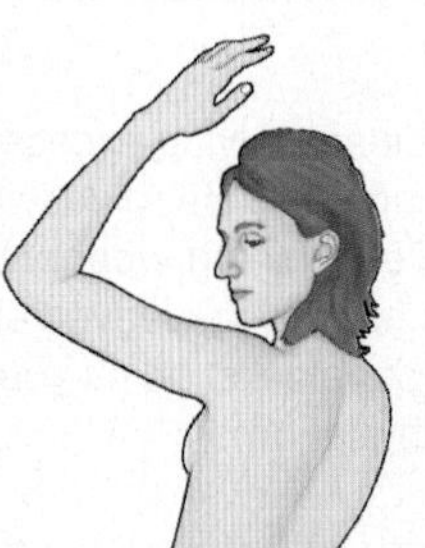

2. Bend the elbows, looking carefully at the forearms, back of the upper arms, and palms

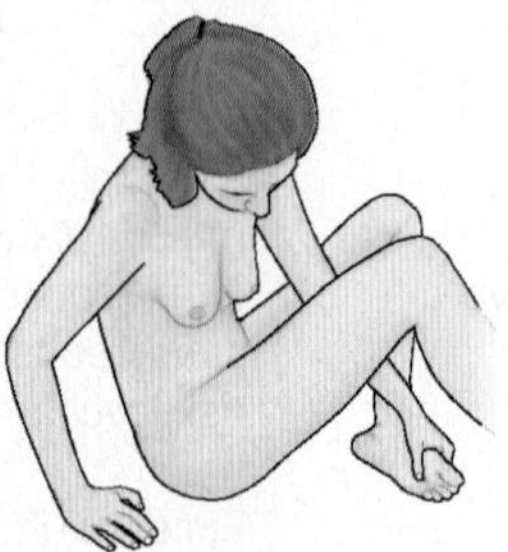

3. Next, look at the back of the legs and feet, the spaces between the toes, and the soles of the feet.

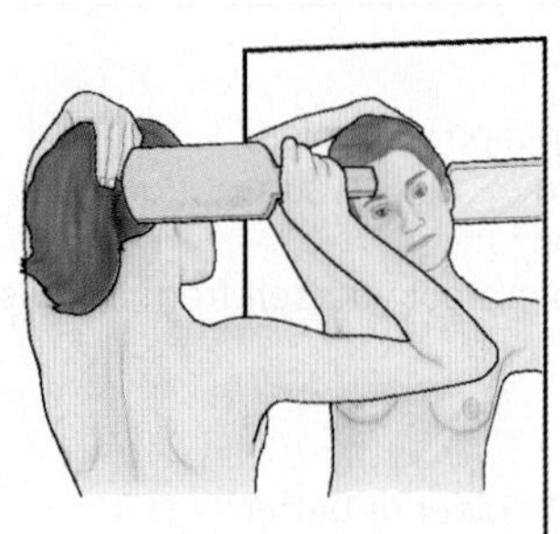

4. Examine the back of the neck and the scalp with a handheld mirror. Part the hair to lift.

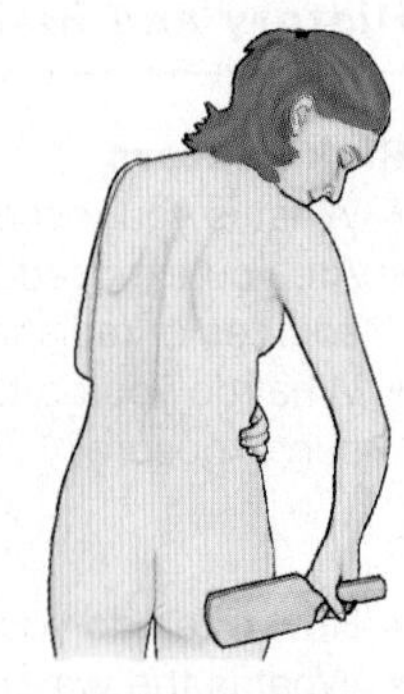

5. Finally, check the back and buttocks with a hand mirror.

Figure 11.8 Skin self-examination.

The nurse emphasizes to the patient the following steps of the SSE:

1. Get fully undressed and stand in front of a full-length mirror.
2. Carefully scan the entire body, using a handheld mirror to look at areas difficult to see (e.g., soles of feet).
3. When examining the scalp, use a comb or blow dryer to part the hair and examine the scalp section by section.
4. Report any suspicious lesion to the health care provider.

Both natural and artificial forms of UV light are carcinogenic; exposure to UV light directly increases the risk of skin cancer (American Academy of Dermatology, 2013b). Ultraviolet B (UVB) waves, which are shorter than ultraviolet A (UVA) waves, are more likely to cause sunburn. UVB waves are directly linked with skin cancers, especially basal cell and squamous cell cancers. UVA waves are longer and have deeper skin penetration than UVB waves (U.S. Environmental Protection Agency 2013b). UVA waves are responsible for some melanomas but are chiefly responsible for the effects of photoaging, specifically wrinkling and leathering of the skin. Intensity of UV waves is greatest during midday; exposure between 10 AM and 4 PM increases potentially damaging effects. Reflection of UV waves off sand, concrete, snow, and water doubles UV exposure and its damaging effects.

You can help patients remember to limit UV light exposure by teaching the phrase "Slip! Slop! Slap! . . . and Wrap!" Coined by the ACS (2013), it reminds people to slip on a shirt, slop on sunscreen, slap on a hat, and wrap on sunglasses to increase protection against UV exposure. Sunburn protection from clothing depends on how much skin is covered, fabric color, and fabric weave. Dark colors reflect UV rays better than light colors; tightly woven fabrics afford less penetration by harmful UV rays. Some fabrics provide less protection than sunscreen with an SPF of 15 or higher. Wearing a hat with a wide all-around brim protects the face, neck, and ears, which are common sites for skin cancer (American Academy of Dermatology, 2013b).

The SPF is defined as the amount of time a product protects the skin from reddening, as compared to the amount of time for unprotected skin to redden (U.S. Food and Drug Administration, 2013). For example, if it normally takes 10 minutes for unprotected skin to redden, use of a product with SPF 15 would protect the skin from reddening for 15 × 10 minutes, or 150 minutes. Applying sunscreen 15 to 30 minutes before exposure enhances absorption of the sunscreen into the skin and increases protection. Sunscreen must be applied every 2 hours for maximum benefit. Sunscreens absorb harmful UV rays; sunblocks deflect rays, preventing absorption. People also should apply lip balm with SPF repeatedly during sun exposure to protect the lips. Sunglasses with at least 99% UVA and UVB protection should be worn when extended sun exposure is anticipated.

Another helpful reminder to limit excessive UV exposure is "short shadow, seek shade" (U.S. Environmental Protection Agency, 2013a). Sun that is overhead casts a shadow shorter than the actual person and should serve as an alert to seek more shade for protection. As a shadow lengthens, it signifies decreased UV intensity and thus a lessening need for protection. Changes in the weather, seasons, and ozone layer affect the intensity of UV rays (World Health Organization, 2013). The UV Index, published daily, uses a scale from 0 to 11 or higher to indicate the degree of predicted UV radiation based on weather, season, and ozone layer changes (Table 11.2). The higher the number, the greater the risk, and the greater degree of protection that is required.

Common Symptoms

Common Integumentary Symptoms

- Pruritus
- Rash (multiple lesions)
- Single lesion or wound

TABLE 11.2 Ultraviolet Light Index and Skin Protection Recommendations

UV Index	Level	Minutes to Reddened Skin: *Fair Skin*	*Medium Skin*	*Dark Skin*	Recommended Skin Protection
0–2	Low	44–120+	74–120+	120+	Wear sunglasses when it is bright outside. Wear sunscreen, especially fair-skinned patients and others who burn easily.
3–5	Moderate	26–43	44–71	77–120	Wear sun-protective clothing. Follow "short shadow, seek shade."
6–7	High	18–26	31–43	55–76	Unprotected skin can burn quickly. Wear SPF ≥ 15 sunscreen or sunblock, protective clothing, sunglasses, shade, or hat. Reduce exposure between 10 AM and 4 PM.
8–10	Very high	13–18	22–31	38–54	Risk of harm from unprotected sun exposure is high. Wear SPF ≥15 sunscreen or sunblock, protective clothing, sunglasses, shade, and hat. Reduce exposure between 10 AM and 4 PM.
11+	Extreme	9–13	14–21	25–38	Avoid UV light exposure if possible. Use liberal application of SPF ≥15 sunscreen or sunblock. Wear protective clothing, sunglasses, shade, and hat. Reduce exposure between 10 AM and 4 PM.

From U.S. Environmental Protection Agency. (2008). *UV index.* Retrieved from http://epa.gov/sunwise/uvindex.html

Signs/Symptoms	Rationale/Abnormal Findings
Pruritus (Itching) Do you experience discomfort with itching? • How long have you had the discomfort? • Where do you itch? • *If there are signs of a rash*: Did you first have itching followed by rash, or did the rash come first? • What makes the itching worse? What makes it better? • Does itching disrupt rest and sleep? • Have you tried any remedies for the itching? What was the result? • What do you think the discomfort is?	Skin lesions or conditions are pruritic, occasionally pruritic, or never pruritic. **Pruritus** frequently precedes atopic lesions but follows inflammatory lesions. Recent pruritus may indicate toxic exposure, insect bites, parasite infestations, or viral exanthems such as varicella. Localized pruritus may indicate infestation, insect bite, allergic reaction, or toxic exposure. Generalized pruritus is common in medication or food allergies. Severe pruritus interfering with sleep is frequently from scabies. Psoriasis is occasionally pruritic. Moles usually do not itch. Noting what, if any, remedies the patient tried and their effectiveness may help identify cause.
Rash Where is/are the lesion(s) located? • Do you have a single lesion or are there several lesions? • Is the rash all over or just in one area? • Does the rash appear to have a pattern? (See Table 11.12.)	Lesions from contact or allergic dermatitis are usually on the body part exposed to an irritant or allergen. Lesions over the entire body, including palms and soles, may be linked to syphilis. Seborrheic dermatitis is often found on the face, head, and hair-covered body areas. Herpes zoster follows a dermatome and is often found on the chest, back, abdomen, and face and rarely on the extremities. Genital lesions are commonly from sexually transmitted infections. Single lesions could be cancer; multiple lesions could indicate an infection.

(table continues on page 244)

Signs/Symptoms	Rationale/Abnormal Findings
Has the rash changed since you first noticed it?	Varicella begins with macular lesions, progresses to papular, then vesicular, and ultimately superficial ulcers. Lesions changing in size, color, or other characteristics may indicate cancer. Pityriasis rosea begins as a single large macular lesion on the trunk and progresses to multiple macular lesions of similar shape but smaller size distributed predominantly over the chest and back. Contact dermatitis spreads from initial point of contact; in severe cases, lesions appear in unexposed areas.
Have you been exposed to anything that would cause itching or the rash? • Have you been exposed to any chemicals, either at work or play? • Do you have pets or frequent contact with animals? • Have you worked in the yard recently? • Have you had any close contacts with people with a similar skin problem? • Have you started any new medications, vitamins, or herbal/nutritional supplements recently? • Have you eaten unusual foods recently? • Have you recently traveled, especially foreign travel? • Have you shared clothing, hats, bed linens, or sleeping bags, or slept in someone's house on sofa/upholstered furniture recently? • Do you live in a community dwelling?	Skin exposure to an allergen releases histamine from mast cells, resulting in pruritus. Scratching causes additional histamine release, stimulating further pruritus; this prompts further scratching, and develops into a persistent cycle of itching and scratching. Determining recent occupational and leisure activities, animal or plant contacts, and outdoor activities may identify exposures to poison ivy, insects, microbials such as dermatophytes or bacteria, chemicals, and pesticides. Medications, vitamin or herbal supplements, and foods new to the patient may be causes of allergic dermatitis. Insect bites or contact with foods or other products not found in the patient's home country may cause lesions that present during or shortly after travel. Wearing another person's clothes, sleeping in someone else's bed, or living in communal dwellings may expose the patient to scabies or lice.
How would you describe your rash? • Flat? • Raised? • Blister-like? • Pus-filled? • Looks like thickened skin?	**Macular** lesions could be **ecchymosis**, pressure point, or tinea versicolor. **Papular** lesions may indicate acne, warts, nevi, insect bites, or early varicella. **Pustular** lesions include acne, furuncles, and carbuncles. **Vesicular** lesions may be herpes simplex, varicella, or impetigo. **Plaque** lesions are commonly psoriasis or lichen simplex.
Do you have any other symptoms related to this rash or skin lesion? • Have you had a recent illness? • Any fever, chills, or headache?	Fevers and chills often accompany infectious skin disorders, such as measles, rubella, and varicella. Headache often accompanies mumps and meningitis.
Single Lesion or Wound • Is this wound acute or chronic? • Is it related to medical, surgical, or traumatic causes? • Would any factors delay healing, such as malnutrition, impaired circulation, immune suppression, obesity, smoking, diabetes mellitus, or infection?	Obtain additional information about the wound, when it first appeared, if it has increased or decreased, and associated symptoms. If the wound is related to an injury, evaluate the nature of the events leading to the trauma. If the patient provides vague or suspicious explanations, be alert to the possibility of abuse and make appropriate referrals. Also ask about any treatments including natural and over-the-counter remedies.

Documenting Expected Findings

Patient denies pruritus, skin lesions, excessive dryness of skin. Denies changes to existing moles.

Lifespan Considerations: Older Adults

Additional Questions	Rationales/Abnormal Findings
Do you have easy or excessive bruising? Does your skin tear or split easily?	Multiple ecchymoses may be from repeated trauma (falls), clotting disorder, or physical abuse. Aging causes the junction between the dermis and epidermis to flatten, increasing the tendency of the skin to tear. Decreased eccrine gland function results in a decreased sweat response. Nerve endings in skin decrease with age, causing decreased sensation to 2-point discrimination, touch, and vibration.
Are your nails brittle or splitting?	Nail growth decreases with aging, leading to the formation of concave, flat, or dry and brittle nails. Pigmented nail bands present earlier in life are more pronounced in aging patients.

Cultural Considerations

Additional Questions	Rationales/Abnormal Findings
• What are some treatments you use at home for this skin situation? • What would your parents do for you if you had this skin situation? • Do health care practitioners in your culture apply any health or beauty aids directly to the skin? • Why do you think this skin situation began when it did? • What do you think caused this situation? • What kind of treatment do you think you need to correct the skin situation? • What do you fear the most about this skin situation?	A common practice among Southeast Asians is **coining**, in which they rub a coin or other object across the skin in a specific manner to treat various health concerns (Fig. 11.9). Coining frequently results in bruising and abrasions and is often mistaken as a sign of physical abuse. **Cupping** involves placement of a cup on the skin surface, and then applying heat to form a vacuum. This practice often leaves circular bruises on the skin. The patient's perception of the cause, reason for onset, type of treatment needed, and fears related to any illness will affect the approach and effectiveness in treating the patient's skin condition. 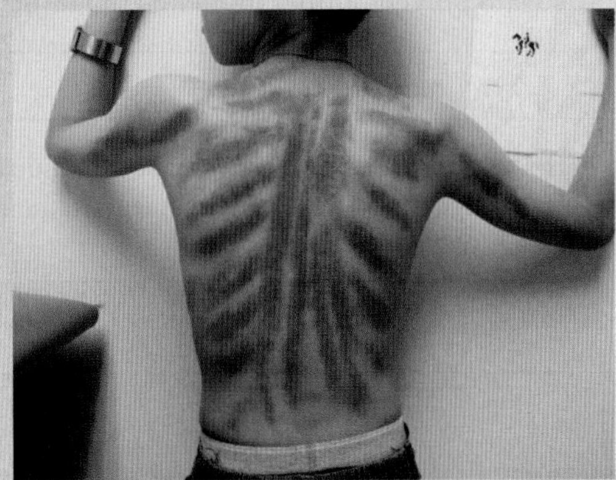 **Figure 11.9** Effects of coining. Another common cultural practice is the application of henna tattoos in an array of patterns and at specific locations to represent a particular occasion in the patient's life and culture (Ethnomed, 2013).

Therapeutic Dialogue: Collecting Subjective Data

Remember Mr. Sholokhov, the patient described at the beginning of this chapter, who was admitted to the hospital with a venous ulcer. The nurse uses professional communication techniques to gather subjective data from Mr. Sholokhov.

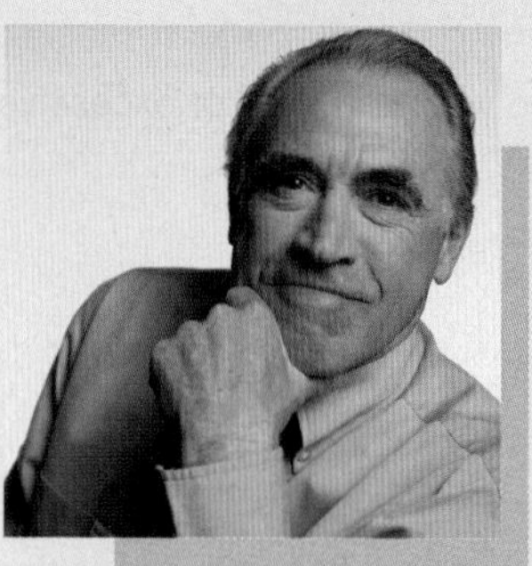

Nurse: Hello, Mr. Sholokhov. I'm going to be your nurse today. My name is Lin. (smiles, pauses) How are you feeling?

Mr. Sholokhov: Fine.

Nurse: Your chart says that you came to the hospital because of your foot. Is that right?

Mr. Sholokhov: Yeah, I have kept it up at home, you know, but the doctor wanted me to come here.

Nurse: What other things did you do to get it better?

Mr. Sholokhov: My wife, she told me to stay home. I didn't do that.

Nurse: It sounds like you really like to be active.

Mr. Sholokhov: I don't like being here. I can take care of my foot myself, you know.

Nurse: It sounds like you like being independent. It must be hard for you to be in the hospital.

Mr. Sholokhov: (silent)

Nurse: Can I look at your foot? Maybe we can talk about how it has changed. I know that it's difficult to have us help you, but we really want to help you to get better (smiles). Perhaps we can talk about other things you can do at home to help your foot improve and prevent further problems requiring hospitalization.

Critical Thinking Challenge

- How might the nurse's nonverbal communication promote a therapeutic relationship?
- How might the patient's Russian cultural heritage influence his perceptions, values, and beliefs about his diagnosis and healing?
- What is the role of the nurse in giving advice versus listening to the patient's perspective?

Objective Data

Common and Specialty or Advanced Techniques

Objective assessment of the skin is performed in a head-to-toe format if the patient is seeking a complete skin assessment, usually in a dermatology clinic for cancer screening. More commonly, you assesses skin with inspection of each body area, such as abdominal skin when inspecting the abdomen. General skin assessment includes color, texture, moisture, turgor, and temperature. Additionally, you might assess a specific problem, such as a rash on the thorax. You assess and describe wounds, lesions, rashes, and hematomas separately during the focused assessment. The table summarizes comprehensive assessment techniques. Additional examinations may be added if indicated by the clinical situation.

Basic Versus Focused/Specialty or Advanced Techniques Related to Skin, Hair, and Nails Assessment			
Comprehensive Assessment Technique	**Purpose**	**Screening or Registered Nurse Assessment**	**Focused or Advanced Practice Examination**
Inspect skin of each body area	To collect data on rashes, lesions, wounds	X	
Inspect fingernails and toenails	To assess hygiene, circulation	X	
Inspect wounds	To evaluate wound and wound healing	X	
Palpate skin	To assess temperature, turgor, vascularity	X	
Inspect hair	To look for lesions, nits	X	
Inspect entire body thoroughly	To screen for cancer or other conditions		X Skin cancer screen

Equipment

- Examination gown
- Tape measure
- Adequate light source
- Magnifying glass

Preparation

Ensure a comfortable room temperature. Wash your hands thoroughly. Apply clean gloves if you anticipate contact with a skin lesion and during inspection of the scalp. Examination of the skin involves inspection and palpation. Expose only areas being directly examined to facilitate privacy, decrease the patient's anxiety, and show consideration for possible cultural concerns.

Comprehensive Skin Assessment

First, assess the overall skin appearance, and inspect the face and exposed skin surfaces for color and pigmentation. Move the bedbound patients to visualize all body surfaces. If a patient cannot help with the movement, additional help may be necessary to position the patient safely.

Bedridden patients require frequent detailed inspection of dependent areas, especially bony prominences, to detect early evidence of skin breakdown. Additionally, it is important to evaluate skin folds for infection or irritation, especially under the breasts, in the groin, and in the abdominal pannus.

Individual lesions may be generally categorized as primary or secondary. **Primary lesions** arise from previously normal skin and include **maculae**, **papules**, **nodules**, **tumors**, **polyps**, **wheals**, **blisters**, **cysts**, **pustules**, **vesicles**, **and abscesses**. Primary lesions may be further described as nonelevated, elevated-solid, or fluid-filled. **Secondary lesions** follow primary lesions (e.g., scar tissue, crusts from dried burns). Review the Tables of Unexpected Findings at the end of this chapter for more details.

The language of the integumentary system can be very complex and intimidating. Remember, it is best to describe lesions if you are unsure about how to label them. A complete and accurate description can be used to identify if the patient is healing.

Technique and Normal Findings	Abnormal Findings
Inspection If performing a complete skin assessment, inspect all body areas, beginning at the crown of the head, parting the hair to visualize the scalp, and progressing caudally to the feet. Make sure to assess the undersides of the feet and to separate the toes. Note general skin color. Pigmentation is consistent throughout the body. Patients with dark skin may have hypopigmented skin on the palms and soles.	Note changes in pigmentation in any areas. **Vitiligo** is characterized by areas of no pigmentation. Other unexpected color changes include **flushing**, **erythema** (redness), **cyanosis** (bluish discoloration), **pallor** (paleness), **rubor** (dependent redness), **brawny** (dark leathery appearance), and **jaundice** (yellow discoloration of skin and sclerae). The tongue, lips, nail beds, and buccal mucosa are less pigmented areas and may be the best indicators of pallor or cyanosis. **Uremic frost** is a whitish coating noted with severe kidney failure.

(table continues on page 248)

Technique and Normal Findings (continued)	Abnormal Findings (continued)
Inspect for any lesions. If observed, identify the configuration pattern, morphology, size, distribution, and exact body location. Common benign lesions include freckles, birth marks, skin tags, moles, and cherry angiomas.	Configurations may be anular, arciform, iris, linear, polymorphous, punctuate, serpiginous, nummular/discoid, umbilicated, filiform, or verruciform (see Table 11.11 at the end of the chapter). Patterns include asymmetrical, confluent, diffuse, discrete, generalized, grouped, localized, satellite, symmetrical, or zosteriform (see Table 11.12). Lesion morphology is a key determinant in identifying a skin disorder. Primary morphology is the type. Secondary morphology includes shape, size, arrangement, and distribution, which further defines the underlying problem (or normal variant). Vitiligo, a miscellaneous lesion, causes skin depigmentation. See Tables 11.9 and 11.10 at the end of this chapter.
Identify any infections. Be sure to use infection control principles if infection is suspected.	Infections include acne, cellulitis, impetigo, German measles (rubella), herpes simplex (cold sores), measles (rubeola), pityriasis rosea, roseola, warts, candida, tinea corporis, and tinea versicolor. See also Table 11.13 at the end of the chapter.
Note any inflammatory lesions.	These include psoriasis, eczema, urticaria, contact dermatitis, allergic drug reaction, insect bites, or seborrhea. See Table 11.14 at the end of the chapter.
Assess for any infestations.	Lice (pediculosis), scabies, or ticks may infest the skin and produce lesions. See Table 11.15 at the end of the chapter.
Observe for growths, tumors, or vascular or other miscellaneous lesions.	Growths and tumors include moles or nevi, skin tags, lipoma, lentigo, actinic keratosis, basal or squamous cell carcinoma, malignant melanoma, and Kaposi sarcoma (see Table 11.16 at the end of the chapter). Vascular lesions include hemangiomas, nevus flammeus (port-wine stain), spider or star angiomas, and venous lakes. See also Table 11.17 at the end of the chapter.
Inspect any wounds or incisions. If observed, note the shape and measure the length, width, and depth with a ruler. If a wound is deep or tunneled, insert a cotton applicator to measure depth. Wounds can be intentional (surgical) or unintentional (trauma); open or closed; acute or chronic; superficial or deep; and clean, contaminated, or infected (Table 11.3). Wound assessment involves some knowledge of the healing process, which is divided into inflammatory, proliferative, and remodeling phases.	Partial-thickness wounds involve the epidermis; full-thickness wounds involve the dermis and subcutaneous tissue. Healthy-healing tissue appears pink to red; necrotic tissue may be yellow, white, brown, or black (eschar). Pale tissue may indicate poor circulation and may be slow to heal. The surrounding area may be inflamed and red or pale with poor circulation. See Table 11.19 at the end of this chapter.
Describe any wounds related to trauma. Assess status of the blood supply to the skin, making note of any bleeding or ecchymosis (bruising).	Lesions from trauma may be **petechiae, purpura, ecchymoses, hematomas, lacerations, abrasions, puncture wounds, or avulsions**. See also Table 11.18.

(table continues on page 249)

TABLE 11.3 Wound Classification

Wound Healing Phase	Description
Inflammatory phase: Begins within 30 minutes of injury; lasts 2–3 days	Upon injury, vasoconstriction, platelet aggregation, and release of thromboplastin promote hemostasis. An inflammatory reaction follows, initially through polymorphonuclear cells to cleanse the wound of debris and kill bacteria. Mononuclear cells follow and become macrophages to further cleanse the wound of debris, dead bacteria, and spent neutrophils.
Proliferative phase: Begins at end of inflammatory phase; may last up to 4 weeks	Fibroblasts migrate into the wound bed to deposit collagen and secrete growth factors. Macrophages now produce enzymes to stimulate tissue growth and generate blood vessels. The wound bed has the appearance of granulation. As the wound bed continues to regenerate, the wound edges begin to contract and move centrally to close the defect. Finally, epithelial regrowth closes the defect.
Remodeling phase: Begins at end of proliferative phase; may last as long as 2 years	Once deposition of new collagen is maximized (at approximately 3 weeks), macrophages stimulate a gradual replacement of the new, rapidly replaced collagen with mature collagen, which greatly increases the tensile strength of the wound.
Wound Classification	**Description**
Clean	Made under sterile conditions and not at risk for infection. Usually skin or vascular incisions
Clean-contaminated	Made under sterile conditions but involving the respiratory, gastrointestinal, genital, or urinary tracts without unusual contamination. Includes appendectomies, hysterectomies, cholecystectomies, and oropharyngeal surgeries
Contaminated	Exposed to contents of the gastrointestinal tract or infected fluids from the genitourinary systems. Also includes open, traumatic wounds such as lacerations, puncture wounds, and open fractures
Infected	Exposed to contaminants or exhibiting evidence of infection prior to surgery. Includes any traumatic wound because of the high risk for foreign body, bacteria, and chemical or other organic contaminant

Technique and Normal Findings (continued)	Abnormal Findings (continued)
Identify risk for skin breakdown, which is especially important in hospitalized or inactive patients. Many health care facilities use the Braden Scale (Table 11.4) to assess risk in patients, with interventions based on the total score (Bergstrom, Braden, Laguzza, A., & Holman, 1987). Alternatively, the similar Norton Scale includes incontinence and other variables (Norton, 1989).	The Braden Scale scores patients from 1 to 4 in each of six subscales: sensory perception, moisture, activity, mobility, nutrition, and friction (Braden & Bergstrom, 1989). The Norton Scale rates patients from 1 to 4 in each of 5 subscales: physical condition, mental condition, activity, mobility, and incontinence. A score of 14–18 on the Braden Scale or less than 14 on the Norton Scale indicates a high risk of pressure ulcer development.
Classify the wound as partial or full thickness; if a pressure ulcer is present, identify the stage. When assessing any ulcer, it is important to observe and document the size in depth and diameter, margins, condition of surrounding tissues, any varicosities or telangiectasias, status of granulation tissue and epithelial growth, and any drainage, odor, or necrotic tissue. Describe the color and texture of the tissue. Identify the amount, color, consistency, and odor of exudate (drainage). Describe the location using appropriate landmarks. Use an objective tool to measure associated pain (see Chapter 6).	Pressure ulcers may be Stage I, Stage II, Stage III, Stage IV, or unstageable (Black et al., 2007). Stages I and II are partial thickness into the dermis. Stages III and IV are full thickness. **Wound drainage** is classified as serous (clear), sanguinous (bloody), serosanguineous (mixed), fibrinous (sticky yellow), or purulent (pus). Note any signs or symptoms of infection.

(table continues on page 252)

TABLE 11.4 **The Braden Scale for Predicting Pressure Sore Risk**

Sensory Perception	**1. Completely Limited**	**2. Very Limited**	**3. Slightly Limited**	**4. No Impairment**	**Indicate Appropriate Numbers Below**
Ability to respond meaningfully to pressure-related discomfort	Unresponsive (does not moan, flinch, or grasp) to painful stimuli, due to diminished level of consciousness or sedation. *Or* limited ability to feel pain over most of body surface.	Responds only to painful stimuli. Cannot communicate discomfort except by moaning or restlessness. *Or* has a sensory impairment which limits the ability to feel pain or discomfort over one half of body.	Responds to verbal commands but cannot always communicate discomfort or need to be turned. *Or* has some sensory impairment which limits ability to feel pain or discomfort in one or two extremities.	Responds to verbal commands. Has no sensory deficit which would limit ability to feel or voice pain or discomfort.	
Moisture	**1. Constantly Moist**	**2. Very Moist**	**3. Occasionally Moist**	**4. Rarely Moist**	
Degree to which skin is exposed to moisture	Skin is kept moist almost constantly by perspiration, urine, or other moisture source. Dampness is detected every time patient is moved or turned.	Skin is often, but not always, moist. Linen must be changed at least once a shift.	Skin is occasionally moist, requiring an extra linen change approximately once a day.	Skin is usually dry. Linen only requires changing at routine intervals.	
Activity	**1. Bedfast**	**2. Chairfast**	**3. Walks Occasionally**	**4. Walks Frequently**	
Degree of physical activity	Confined to bed.	Ability to walk severely limited or nonexistent. Cannot bear own weight and/or must be assisted into chair or wheelchair.	Walks occasionally during day but for very short distances, with or without assistance. Spends majority of each shift in bed or chair	Walks outside the room at least twice a day and inside room at least once every 2 hours during waking hours.	
Mobility	**1. Completely Immobile**	**2. Very Limited**	**3. Slightly Limited**	**4. No Limitations**	
Ability to change and control body position	Does not make even slight changes in body or extremity position without assistance.	Makes occasional slight changes in body or extremity position but unable to make frequent or significant changes independently.	Makes frequent though slight changes in body or extremity position independently.	Makes major and frequent changes in position without assistance.	

Nutrition	1. Very Poor	2. Probably Inadequate	3. Adequate	4. Excellent
Usual food intake pattern	Never eats a complete meal. Rarely eats more than one third of any food offered. Eats two servings or less of protein (meat or dairy products) per day. Takes fluids poorly. Does not take a liquid dietary supplement. *Or* is under orders to take nothing by mouth (NPO) and/or maintained on clear liquids or IVs for more than 5 days.	Rarely eats a complete meal and generally eats only about one half of any food offered. Protein intake includes only three servings of meat or dairy products per day. Occasionally will take a dietary supplement. *Or* receives less than optimal amount of liquid diet or tube feeding.	Eats over half of most meals. Eats a total of four servings of protein (meat, dairy products) each day. Occasionally will refuse a meal but will usually take a supplement if offered. *Or* is on a tube feeding or total parenteral nutrition regimen that probably meets most of nutritional needs.	Eats most of every meal. Never refuses a meal. Usually eats a total of four or more servings of meat and dairy products. Occasionally eats between meals. Does not require supplementation.
Friction and Shear	**1. Problem**	**2. Potential Problem**	**3. No Apparent Problem**	
	Requires moderate-to-maximum assistance in moving. Complete lifting without sliding against sheets is impossible. Frequently slides down in bed or chair, requiring frequent repositioning with maximum assistance. Spasticity, contractures or agitation lead to almost constant friction.	Moves feebly or requires minimal assistance. During a move, skin probably slides to some extent against sheets, chair restraints, or other devices. Maintains relatively good position in chair or bed most of the time but occasionally slides down.	Moves in bed and in chair independently and has sufficient muscle strength to lift up completely during move. Maintains good position in bed or chair at all times.	

NOTE: Bed- and chair-bound patients or those with impaired ability to reposition themselves should be assessed upon admission for their risk of developing pressure ulcers. Patients with established pressure ulcers should be reassessed periodically. Patients with a total score of 16 or less are considered to be at risk of developing pressure ulcers (15 or 16 = low risk; 13 or 14 = moderate risk; 12 or less = high risk).

Total Score:

Technique and Normal Findings (continued)	Abnormal Findings (continued)
Assess for nonpressure ulcers; note the characteristics of the wound.	Examples include neuropathic, venous (vascular), and arterial (vascular) ulcers (Table 11.5). See also Table 11.20 at the end of this chapter.

TABLE 11.5 Wagner Classification of Ulcers

Grade	Classification
0	Preulcerative lesion, healed ulcers, presence of bony deformity
1	Superficial ulcer without subcutaneous tissue involvement
2	Penetration through the subcutaneous tissue (may expose bone, tendon, ligament, or joint capsule)
3	Osteitis, abscess, or osteomyelitis
4	Gangrene of the forefoot
5	Gangrene of the entire foot

Technique and Normal Findings (continued)	Abnormal Findings (continued)
Burns are classified based on depth of tissue destruction and percentage of total body surface area (TBSA) affected. Depth involves assessing vascular and sensory status and appearance and blanching of the burn. Assess blanching by applying pressure with a sterile cotton-tipped applicator and observing capillary refill time. Calculate the percentage of TBSA affected using the Wallace Rule of Nines (Fig. 11.10) (the Lund and Browder chart is used for pediatric patients; see Chapter 27).	Superficial burns involve the epidermal layers, superficial dermal burns involve the epidermis and part of the dermis, deep dermal burns involve the epidermis and all of the dermis, and total thickness burns involve all layers of the skin and may extend into the supportive fascia below (Nam et al., 2014). See also Table 11.6.
Inspect each fingernail and toenail. Assess for color, thickness, and consistency. Nails are smooth, translucent, and consistent in color and thickness. Longitudinal ridging is common in aging patients. Longitudinal pigmentation in dark-skinned patients is a normal variant.	Dietary deficiencies lead to splitting of nail tips (Fawcett, Linford, & Stulberg, 2005). Thickened nails may be from fungal infection. Discoloration of the nail bed may indicate trauma, fungal infection, or melanoma.
Have the patient place the fingernails of both index fingers together to assess the nail angle. A diamond-shaped opening is visible between the two fingernails, indicating a nail angle of at least 160 degrees.	**Clubbing** of the nails indicates chronic hypoxia. Clubbing is identified when the angle of the nail to the finger is more than 160 degrees. Also see Table 11.21 at the end of the chapter for common nail abnormalities.
Inspect the hair, noting color, consistency, distribution, areas of hair loss, and condition of the hair shaft. Hair is equally and symmetrically distributed across the scalp. Hair shafts are smooth, shiny, of even consistency, and without evidence of breakage.	In female patients, ovarian dysfunction may be characterized by hair on the beard area, abdomen, upper back, shoulders, sternum, and inner upper thighs.

(table continues on page 253)

TABLE 11.6 **Burn Classification**

Depth of Burn	Bleeding	Sensation	Appearance	Blanching
Superficial	Brisk	Pain	Rapid capillary refill	Moist, red
Superficial-dermal	Brisk	Pain	Slowed capillary refill	Dry, pale pink
Dermal	Delayed	No pain	No capillary refill	Mottled cherry red color
Full thickness	None	No pain	No blanching	Dry, leathery, or waxy hard wound surface

Technique and Normal Findings (continued)	Abnormal Findings (continued)
9% · Anterior 18% · 9% · Posterior 18% · 9% · 1% · 18% · 18% **Figure 11.10** Wallace Rule of Nines to estimate percentage of total body surface area burned in adults. Different areas are sectioned into numerical values related to the figure nine (9). Note that the anterior and posterior head equate to 9% each.	
Note areas of decreased or absent hair. Parting the hair enables visualization of the scalp skin. Note any lesions or color changes there. ■ Scalp skin is of consistent color with the rest of the body.	Brittle or broken hair shafts may indicate endocrine or metabolic dysfunction. Lice or their nits (eggs) may be on the hair shaft. The closer to the scalp the nit is located, the more recent the infestation. Excessive dryness and scaling of the scalp is often present in seborrheic dermatitis. See Table 11.22 at the end of this chapter.
Observe hair shafts near the root for lice or nits.	
Palpation Using the dorsal surface of the hands, assess skin temperature. ■ Skin temperature is consistently warm or cool and appropriate, considering the environmental temperature.	Further assess any areas of increased temperature for lesions, swelling, and color changes.

(table continues on page 254)

Technique and Normal Findings (continued)	Abnormal Findings (continued)
Using the palmar surface of the fingers and hands, assess for skin moisture and texture. ▪ Moisture is consistent throughout, with evenly smooth skin texture.	Excessive dryness may be from too frequent bathing or hyperthyroidism. Excessive moisture may signify a problem with temperature regulation. Cracked or fissured skin may indicate hydration disorders, infections, or chemical injuries.
Assess skin turgor. Gently grasp a fold of the patient's skin between your fingers and pull up, then release. This is most easily performed on the dorsal surface of the patient's hand or lower arm, but the most accurate reflection of turgor in the adult is on the anterior chest, just below the midclavicular area (Dains, Baumann, & Scheibel, 2012). ▪ The skin promptly recoils to its normal position.	A persistent pinch, or **tenting**, indicates dehydration.
Assess for vascularity by applying direct pressure to the skin surface with the pads of your fingers. This will cause the patient's skin to blanch, or pale, in comparison with surrounding skin. ▪ On releasing pressure, color promptly returns to normal.	Decreased vascular supply is often initially found in the extremities, particularly the hands and feet. Delayed return of skin color to normal after direct pressure indicates decreased circulation. Altered circulation can result in pallor or rubor of an extremity.
Palpate lesions for tenderness, mobility, and consistency. Apply gentle pressure and attempt to move the skin under your finger. ▪ Skin shifts slightly without adherence.	Tenderness of a lesion or dermatitis may indicate infection. Lesions seemingly fixed in place may be cancerous. Consistency of skin lesions will assist in diagnosis of the problem.
Palpate each fingernail and toenail. ▪ Nails are smooth, nontender, and firmly adherent to the nail bed. Lateral and proximal folds are not tender or swollen.	Swelling, redness, or tenderness in the lateral or proximal folds may indicate paronychia (bacterial or fungal infection). Sponginess of the nail bed may indicate clubbing.
Palpate the hair. ▪ Hair is smooth. Grasp 10–12 hairs and gently pull. ▪ Just a few hairs come off in your hand.	Note excessive hair loss (more than six hairs) and then assess for presence or absence of the hair bulb. Absent hair bulb may indicate chemical damage to the hair shaft (excessive dyeing or bleaching). Presence of the hair bulb may indicate endocrine dysfunction.

Documenting Normal Findings

Skin evenly colored, smooth, soft, consistently warm, with intact turgor. No suspicious lesions. Nails smooth and translucent, lateral and proximal folds without swelling or erythema. Hair smooth texture, symmetrically distributed on the scalp, consistent coloration and hydration, without evidence of excessive breakage or loss. Scalp with consistent pigmentation, no lesions noted.

Lifespan Considerations: Older Adults

As discussed earlier, common skin assessment findings for older adults include decreased elasticity, thinness, excessive dryness, and lesions associated with aging such as seborrheic keratosis, actinic keratosis, and lentigines (Merck Manual of Geriatrics, 2013). In addition, older adults are at increased risk for skin cancer, abnormal ecchymoses or purpuric lesions, and trauma.

Cultural Considerations

More than half of all patients are likely to self-treat a skin lesion or dermatitis with what is culturally familiar to them before seeking assistance from a health care professional. Inquiring about cultural practices and home remedies provides insight into the patient's specific culture and assists in designing appropriately sensitive therapeutic interventions.

Documenting Case Study Findings

The nurse has just finished a physical examination of Mr. Sholokhov, the 65-year-old patient with a venous ulcer secondary to peripheral vascular disease. Unlike the samples of normal documentation previously charted, Mr. Sholokhov has abnormal findings. Review the following important findings revealed in each step of objective data collection for Mr. Sholokhov. Consider how these results compare with expected findings. Note that inspection is the major technique used in wound assessment.

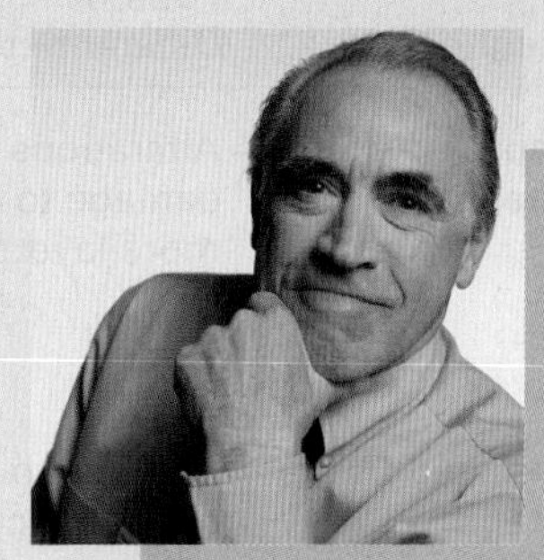

Inspection: A 6 × 8 cm wound on left lateral ankle above the medial malleolus. Irregular wound margins with some pallor at the edges. Wound is partial thickness with 80% beefy red and 20% yellow. Large fibrinous exudate on dressing. Left leg skin hyperpigmented and ruddy. Some flaking is present, no hair on leg. 3+ edema, capillary refill 4 seconds. Full range of motion present, strength 2+ and slightly decreased.

Palpation: Leg is cool, sensation decreased.

Critical Thinking

Integumentary findings often reflect the status of other systems (see Table 11.8). You must constantly observe the skin while assessing other systems and interpret skin findings in conjunction with other systemic findings to determine underlying function. Interpreting these findings assists in planning appropriate interventions and making necessary referrals.

Laboratory and Diagnostic Testing

After a dermatologic problem has been identified, inspected, and palpated, one of several laboratory tests may be indicated to determine the most effective treatment. A superficial scraping of disordered skin for microscopic examination may help to identify the type of lesion. If exudate or signs of infection are present, a culture and sensitivity test for bacteria may reveal specific organisms. Methicillin-resistant *Staphylococcus aureus* (MRSA) is an organism that may be found in wounds. For suspected fungal infections, a culture using a preparation of potassium hydroxide (KOH) may confirm diagnosis. The Wood light test may diagnose scalp infections caused by a particular group of spore-producing microorganisms. The spores, located on hair strands, fluoresce apple green under the Wood light. Special skin tests (e.g., patch tests) may detect sensitivity to allergens.

Biopsy of skin tissue is indicated for those disorders that manifest changes in color, size, or shape. Nonhealing lesions, abnormal growths, or tumors are also biopsied. Nursing responsibilities include preprocedure discussion with the patient regarding the reason for the biopsy, procedure involved, and time required for results. Also ensure that the patient signs consent forms. Assist with procedures, ensure samples are appropriately labeled, apply necessary dressings, and gives postoperative instructions to the patient.

Diagnostic Reasoning

Nursing Diagnosis, Outcomes, and Interventions

When formulating a nursing diagnosis, it is important to use critical thinking to cluster data and identify patterns that fit together. Compare these data clusters with defining characteristics for the diagnosis to ensure the most accurate labeling and appropriate interventions. See Table 11.7 (NANDA International, 2012).

Use assessment information to identify patient outcomes. Some outcomes related to integumentary problems include the following:

- Skin and mucous membranes are intact.
- Patient reports no altered sensation or pain at site.
- Patient demonstrates measures to protect and heal the skin (Moorhead, Johnson, Maas, & Swanson, 2013).

After outcomes are established, interventions are enacted to improve the patient's status. Use critical thinking and evidence-based practice to develop interventions. Some examples for integumentary care are as follows:

- Assess skin and risk for skin breakdown.
- Change dressing as ordered with topical agent that promotes a moist healing environment.
- Evaluate for specialty mattress (Bulechek, Butcher, Dochterman, & Wagner, 2013).

TABLE 11.7 Common Nursing Diagnoses Associated With the Integumentary System

Diagnosis	Point of Differentiation	Assessment Characteristics	Nursing Interventions
Impaired skin integrity	Alterations in or damage to one or more layers of the skin	Wound, surgical incision, break in skin integrity	Classify wound as partial or full thickness (Stage I or II). Document wound assessment. Assess for risk of skin breakdown. Apply appropriate dressing. Evaluate for use of specialty mattress. Avoid positioning over bony prominences.
Impaired tissue integrity	Damage to tissues of the subcutaneous layer of the skin, mucous membrane, cornea, or all of these	Damaged or destroyed subcutaneous, muscle, bone, mucous membrane, or corneal tissues	Determine size and depth of wound (Stage III or IV), skin around wound, continence status, tube/incision placement. Apply appropriate dressing. Collaborate with physician on necessary débridement and surgical intervention.*
Pain	An unpleasant sensory and emotional experience directly related to skin or tissue damage	Self-report of pain is subjective. Expressions are variable and include facial grimace, guarding, muscle tension, tachycardia, tachypnea, and nausea (see Chapter 6).	Use pain scale to identify current pain intensity and effectiveness of medication. Develop pain goal with patient. Provide pain medications as ordered.* Provide alternatives such as distraction, breathing, and relaxation.
Risk for infection	At risk for pathogenic organisms from break in the skin or tissue, the body's primary defense	Break in skin integrity, tubes and procedures, exposure to pathogens, malnutrition, inadequate immunity, chronic disease	Practice frequent handwashing and universal precautions. Protect wound with dressing. Monitor for fever, elevated white blood cell count, wound drainage, or erythema. Discontinue tubes as soon as possible. Encourage adequate nutrition.

*Collaborative interventions.

Progress Note: Analyzing Findings

Mr. Sholokhov's problems have been outlined throughout this chapter. Initial subjective and objective data collection is complete; the nurse has spent time reviewing findings and results. The following note illustrates how the nurse collects and analyzes subjective and objective data and develops interventions.

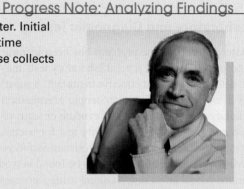

Subjective: States throbbing 4/10 pain that increases when legs are dependent and with ambulation, decreases when lying in bed. Refuses medication for pain. States "Those pills make me sleepy, and I don't like that."

Objective: Grimacing with movement. Ambulates in room to bathroom, sits in chair for meals with legs elevated. A 6 × 8 cm wound on left lateral ankle above the medial malleolus. Irregular wound margins with some pallor at the edges. Tissue

(case study continues on page 257)

80% beefy red and 20% yellow. Large fibrinous exudate on dressing. Left leg skin hyperpigmented and ruddy. Some flaking is present, no hair growth. 3+ edema, capillary refill 4 seconds. Leg is cool, sensation decreased. Full range of motion, strength 2+ and slightly decreased.

Analysis: Impaired skin integrity related to venous impairment as evidenced by ulcer on left lateral ankle. Pain related to ulcer.

Plan: Hydrocolloid dressing changed. Consult with wound care nurse about placement of wound vacuum. Elevate legs when awake. Monitor temperature every 4 hours. Monitor wound for signs of infection, drainage, increased pain, and erythema. Encourage 1 L of fluid a day and 50% of meals.

Critical Thinking Challenge

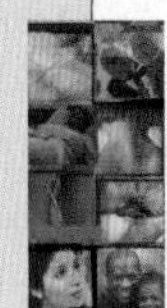

- What type of ongoing assessment would you predict?
- How should the nurse address the issue of pain assessment and management?
- What teaching should the nurse provide related to venous stasis, ulcer, and treatment?

Collaborating With the Interprofessional Team

In many facilities, nurses initiate referrals based on assessment data. Findings that might increase urgency of a referral to the skin care team include decreased vascularity, new infection, and increased pressure/shearing forces. Wound and ostomy nurses are available for consultation on complex wounds, ostomy management, and monitoring for pressure ulcers.

A wound care consult is indicated for placement of the wound vacuum. The following conversation illustrates how the nurse might organize data and make recommendations about Mr. Sholokhov when the wound care nurse arrives.

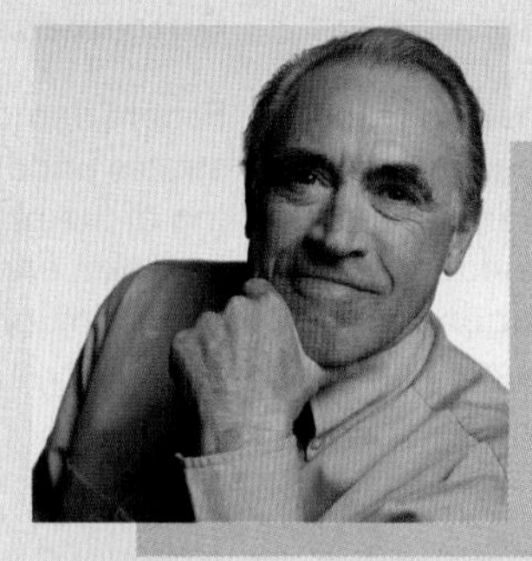

Situation: "Hello. I'm taking care of Mr. Sholokhov. He's 65 years old and was admitted yesterday for placement of a wound vacuum because his left leg ulcer isn't healing."

Background: "He has a history of PVD, high blood pressure, and diabetes. Blood pressure and diabetes have been under fairly good control. He's had the ulcer for about 3 months, and the physician would like a wound vacuum applied. Mr. Sholokhov can potentially go home with it tomorrow."

Assessment: "The wound doesn't look infected. It's fairly clean and about 6 × 8 cm just above his left medial malleolus. He's fairly independent and eager to get home. He also doesn't like taking pain medications because they make him drowsy."

Recommendations: "When you place his wound vac, I think that you might discuss how he can manage with it at home. His wife should be there, so that will be a good teaching opportunity. He's really anxious to get back home, so if you can work with him to get prepared, he'll appreciate it. He prefers to be as independent as possible."

(case study continues on page 258)

Critical Thinking Challenge

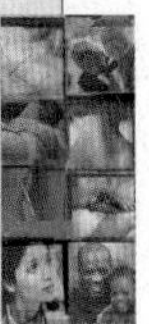

- Why is the information on the wound assessment summarized in this verbal communication versus the level of detail in the documentation?
- What other assessments might be performed related to the patient's history?
- What further assessment information might need collection before discharge?

Pulling It All Together

The nurse uses assessment data to formulate a nursing care plan with patient outcomes and interventions for Mr. Sholokhov. After interventions are completed, the nurse reevaluates Mr. Sholokhov and documents findings in the chart to show progress. The nurse uses critical thinking and judgment to continue or revise diagnoses, outcomes, or interventions. This is often in a form similar to the one below.

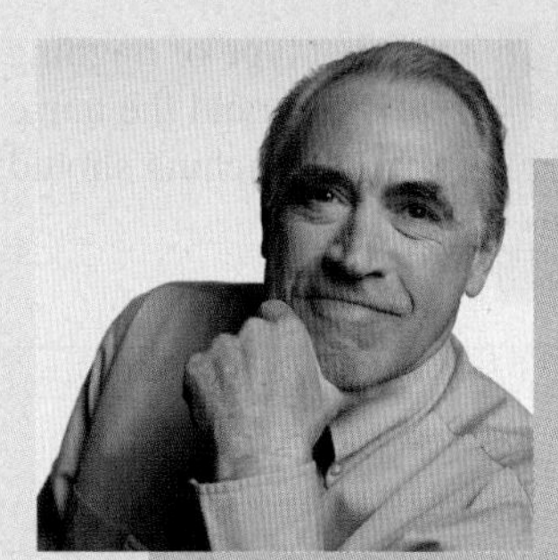

Nursing Diagnosis	Patient Outcomes	Nursing Interventions	Rationale	Evaluation
Impaired skin integrity related to venous stasis as evidenced by ulcer on left lateral malleolus	Patient demonstrates understanding of the plan to heal skin and prevent reinjury.	Teach care for wound vacuum. Initiate home care consultation. Teach patient signs of healing, infection, and complications. Involve wife in care.	Knowledge of the function and purpose of the wound vacuum promotes patient autonomy. He should know when to call the physician if the wound is worsening.	Patient and wife asked multiple questions about wound vacuum at home; especially related to mobility. Wife appreciates home health visit and looks forward to patient returning home.

Applying Your Knowledge

Using the previous steps of diagnostic reasoning, organizing, and prioritizing, consider all the case findings woven through this chapter. When answering the following questions, begin drawing conclusions and see how pieces of assessment work together to create an environment for personalized, appropriate, and accurate care.

- What are the major functions of the skin?
- What other assessments are indicated given Mr. Sholokhov's history?
- What information will you teach Mr. Sholokhov about managing his wound care at home?
- What factors in Mr. Sholokhov's home might aggravate his wound?
- What precautions at home and during leisure will benefit Mr. Sholokhov?
- How will you evaluate Mr. Sholokhov's understanding of the teaching you have done?

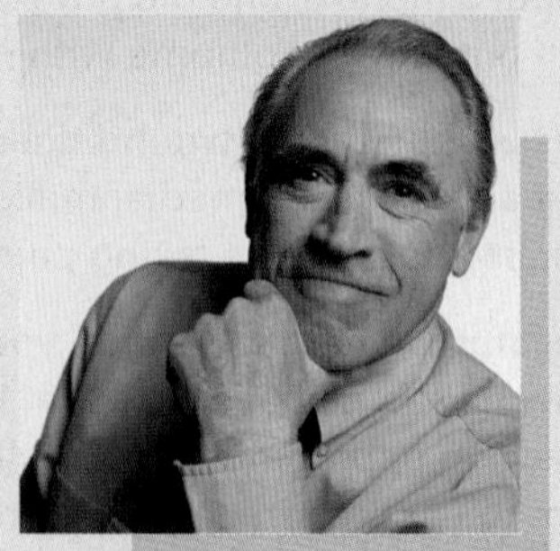

Key Points

- Skin assessment findings reflect overall health, hydration, and nutritional status.
- Skin color variations largely result from the amounts and proportions of pheomelanin and eumelanin produced by the melanocytes.
- Skin changes during pregnancy include melasma, linea nigra, increased sebaceous and cutaneous gland function, and hair loss following pregnancy.
- Loss of elastin, collagen, and subcutaneous fat result in decreased resilience, sagging, wrinkling, and increased fragility of the skin in the older adult.
- The ABCDEs of melanoma detection include *A*symmetry, *B*order irregularity, *C*olor, *D*iameter of more than 6 mm, and *E*volution of the lesion over time.
- Skin self-examination helps patients identify problematic lesions.
- Common integumentary symptoms include pruritus, rash, lesions, or wounds.
- Coining and cupping are self-treatments performed as cultural home remedies.
- Skin assessment involves inspection of general color, texture, moisture, turgor, and temperature, and focused inspection and palpation of rashes, lesions, and wounds.
- When assessing a lesion, identify configuration, pattern, morphology, size, distribution, and exact body location.
- Assess a wound for location, size, color, texture, drainage, margins, surrounding skin, and healing status.
- Depth of a burn can be superficial, superficial-dermal, dermal, or full thickness.
- Assessment of the nails and hair is performed as a part of the skin assessment.
- Unexpected skin findings include infection, inflammation, infestation, growths and tumors, trauma, and ulcers.
- Common nursing diagnoses related to the integumentary system include impaired skin integrity, impaired tissue integrity, pain, and risk for infection.

Review Questions

1. The nurse is admitting a 75-year-old man with a 50-year history of smoking one pack of cigarettes per day. Among the patient's concerns is his chronic shortness of breath. One nail finding that demonstrates chronic hypoxia is
   A. pitting.
   B. thickening and discoloration of the nail bed.
   C. clubbing.
   D. brittleness and cracking of the nails.

2. All of the following skin lesions are papular *except*
   A. warts.
   B. acne.
   C. moles.
   D. herpes zoster.

3. The ABCDs of melanoma identification include (select all that apply)
   A. *A*symmetry: one half does not match the other half.
   B. *B*irthmark: recently changed in appearance.
   C. *C*olor: pigmentation is not uniform; there may be shades of tan, brown, and black as well as red, white, and blue.
   D. *D*iameter: greater than 6 mm.

4. A nurse observes a skin lesion with well-defined borders on the upper left thigh. It is 1.5 cm in diameter, flat, hypopigmented, and nonpalpable. What is the correct terminology for this lesion?
   A. Patch
   B. Plaque
   C. Papule
   D. Macule

5. When assessing hydration, the nurse will
   A. pinch a fold of skin on the medial aspect of the forearm and observe for recoil to normal.
   B. pinch a fold of skin on the abdomen and observe for recoil to normal.
   C. pinch a fold of skin just below the midpoint of one of the clavicles and allow the skin to recoil to normal.
   D. pinch a fold of skin on the head and allow for skin to recoil in children.

6. A fair-skinned, blonde, 18-year-old woman is at the clinic for a skin examination. She reports that she always turns red within 10 minutes of going outside. She is planning a trip to Mexico and wants to avoid getting sunburned. Which of the following would be included in the teaching?
   A. Excessive exposure to UVA and UVB rays increases risk of sunburn and skin cancer.
   B. Apply a sunscreen or sunblock at least 15 to 30 minutes before sun exposure.
   C. Avoid sun exposure between 10 AM and 4 PM to reduce UVA and UVB exposure.
   D. A mild sunburn is acceptable in a fair-skinned blonde person.

7. A patient presents to the clinic with erythematous vesicles on the face and chest. Some vesicles have broken open, revealing a moist, shallow, ulcerated surface; some have scabbed over. The nurse suspects which of the following infectious illnesses?
   A. Varicella
   B. Measles
   C. Roseola
   D. Herpes simplex

8. A 24-year-old patient reports an itchy red rash under her breasts. Examination reveals large, reddened, moist patches under both breasts in the skin folds. Several smaller, raised, red lesions surround the edges of the larger patch. What is the correct terminology for the distribution pattern of these smaller lesions?
   A. Satellite
   B. Discrete
   C. Confluent
   D. Zosteriform

9. A 22-year-old patient presents to the clinic with a large firm mass on her left earlobe. She had her ears pierced approximately 3 weeks ago. The mass began as a small bump and progressively enlarged to its current size of approximately 2.5 cm (1 in.) in diameter. It is not tender, reddened, or seeping any drainage. What is the term used to describe this secondary skin lesion?
   A. Crust
   B. Lichenification
   C. Keloid
   D. Scale

10. An 83-year-old woman is undergoing a routine physical examination. Which of the following assessment findings would the nurse consider an expected age-related variation?
   A. Thinning of the skin
   B. Increased skin turgor
   C. Hypopigmented flat macules and patches over sun-exposed areas
   D. Multiple purplish bruises on the arms and legs

11. A patient has several red, inflamed, superficial, palpable lesions containing a thickened yellowish substance. How would the nurse document this lesion?
   A. Papule
   B. Pustule
   C. Cyst
   D. Vesicle

The Jensen suite offers these additional resources to enhance learning and facilitate understanding of this chapter:

- thePoint online resource, http//thepoint.lww.com/Jensen2e
- *Laboratory Manual for Nursing Health Assessment: A Best Practice Approach*
- *Pocket Guide for Nursing Health Assessment: A Best Practice Approach*
- *Lippincott DocuCare,* an electronic health record simulation software, http://thepoint.lww.com/docucare
- *Adaptive Learning | Powered by PrepU*, http://thepoint.lww.com/prepu

References

American Academy of Dermatology. (2013a). *How do I check my moles?* Retrieved from http://www.aad.org/spot-skin-cancer/understanding-skin-cancer/how-do-i-check-my-skin

American Academy of Dermatology. (2013b). *How do I prevent skin cancer?* Retrieved from http://www.aad.org /spot-skin-cancer/understanding-skin-cancer/how-do-i-prevent-skin-cancer

American Academy of Dermatology. (2013c). *Skin cancer: A fact of life in skin of color*. Retrieved, from http://www.skincarephysicians.com/SkinCancerNet/skin_of_color.html

American Academy of Dermatology. (2013d). *Tattoos and body piercings*. Retrieved from http://www.aad.org/media-resources/stats-and-facts/prevention-and-care/tattoos-and-body-piercings

American Cancer Society. (2008). *Detailed guide: Skin cancer—melanoma*. Retrieved from http://www.cancer.org/cancer/skincancer-melanoma/detailedguide

American Cancer Society. (2013). *Skin cancer prevention activities*. Retrieved from http://www.cancer.org/healthy/morewaysacshelpsyoustaywell/acs-skin-cancer-prevention-activities

Barsh, G. (2003). What controls variation in human skin color? *PLoS Biology, 1*(1), *e27. Retrieved* from http://biology.plosjournals.org/perlserv/?request=get-document&doi=10.1371/journal.pbio.0000027

Bergstrom, N., Braden, B. J., Laguzza, A., & Holman, V. (1987). The Braden Scale for predicting pressure sore risk. *Nursing Research, 36*, 205.

Black, J., Baharestani, M., Cuddigan, Dorner, B., Edsberg, L., Langemo, D., . . . Ratliff, C (2007). National Pressure Ulcer Advisory Panel's updated pressure ulcer staging system. *Dermatological Nursing, 19*(4), 343–349.

Braden, B., & Bergstrom, N. (1989). Clinical utility of the Braden scale for predicting pressure sore risk. *Decubitus, 2*(3), 44–51.

Bulechek, G. M., Butcher, H. K., Dochterman, J. M. & Wagner, C. M (2013). *Nursing interventions classification (NIC)* (6th ed.). St. Louis, MO: Mosby

Bulliard, J.-L., De Weck, D., Fisch, T., Bordoni, A., & Levi, F. (2007). Detailed site distribution of melanoma and sunlight exposure: Aetiological patterns from a Swiss series. *Annals of Oncology, 18*(4), 789–794.

Dains, J., Baumann, L., & Scheibel, P. (2012). *Advanced health assessment and clinical diagnosis in primary care* (4th ed.). St. Louis, MO: Mosby.

Ethnomed. (2013). *Self-teaching module for the influence of culture on skin conditions in children*. Retrieved from http://ethnomed.org/ethnomed/clin_topics/dermatology/pigmented_main.html

Fawcett, R., Linford, S., & Stulberg, D. (2005). Nail abnormalities: Clues to systemic disease. *American Family Physician, 69*(6), 1417–1424.

Hemenway, M. (2006). Skin cancer: Skin color doesn't matter. *EastWest Magazine*. Retrieved from http://www.eastwestmagazine.com/content/view/39/40

Juckett, G. (2005). Cross-cultural medicine. *American Family Physician, 72*(11), 2267–2274.

Kahana, M., Feldman, M., Abudi, Z., & Yurman, S. (1995). The incidence of birthmarks in Israeli neonates. *International Journal of Dermatology, 34*(10), 704–706.

Merck Manual of Geriatrics. (2013). *Evaluation of the elderly patient*. Retrieved from http://www.merckmanuals.com/professional/geriatrics/approach_to_the_geriatric_patient/evaluation_of_the_elderly_patient.html

Moorhead, S., Johnson, M., Maas, M. L., & Swanson, E. (2013). *Nursing outcomes classification (NOC): Measurement of health outcomes* (5th ed.). St. Louis, MO: Mosby.

Nam, J. J., Chung, K. K., King, B. T., Jones, J. A., Cancio, L. C., Baer, D. G., . . . Orman, J. A. (2014). Citation classics in the burn literature during the past 55 years. Journal of Burn Care & Research, 35, 176 -185. Retrieved from http://journals.lww.com/burncareresearch/Abstract/publishahead/Citation_Classics_in_the_Burn_Literature_During.99033.aspx

NANDA International. (2012). *Nursing diagnoses: Definitions and classification 2012-2014* (9th ed). Oxford, United Kingdom: Wiley-Blackwell

National Cancer Institute. (2011). *What you need to know about melanoma and other skin cancers*. Retrieved from http://www.cancer.gov/cancertopics/wyntk/melanoma/page7

National Pressure Ulcer Advisory Panel. (2012). *Updated staging system*. Retrieved from http://www.npuap.org/?s=staging+system

Norton, D. (1989). Calculating the risk: Reflections on the Norton scale. *Decubitus, 2*, 24.

Parsad, D., & Kumarasinge, S. (2006). *Psycho-social implications of pigmentary disorders in Asia*. Retrieved, from http://paspcr.med.umn.edu/Commentary/Parsad_Kumarasingecommentary.pdf

Skin Cancer Foundation. (2013). *The photosensitivity report*. Retrieved on from http://www.skincancer.org/publications/photosensitivity-report

U.S. Department of Health & Human Services. (2013). *2020 Topics & objectives - Objectives A-Z.* Retrieved from http://www.healthypeople.gov/2020/topicsobjectives2020/

U.S. Environmental Protection Agency. (2013a). *SunWise program.* Retrieved from http://www.epa.gov/sunwise

U.S. Environmental Protection Agency. (2013b). *UV index*. Retrieved from http://epa.gov/sunwise/uvindex.html

U.S. Food and Drug Administration. (2013). *Tanning*. Retrieved, from http://www.fda.gov/Radiation-EmittingProducts/RadiationEmittingProductsandProcedures/Tanning/default.htm

World Health Organization. (2013.). *Ultraviolet radiation and the INTERSUN Programme*. Retrieved from http://www.who.int/uv/intersunprogramme

Zouboulis, C. C., Chen, W. C., Thornton, M. J., Qin, K., & Rosenfield, R. (2007). Sexual hormones in human skin. *Hormone and Metabolic Research*, *39*(2), 85–95.

Tables of Abnormal Findings

TABLE 11.8 Manifestations in Integument of Systemic Disorders

Integument Finding	Associated Disorder	Other Considerations/Depictions
	Cardiovascular	
Flushing	Increased permeability of the peripheral capillaries, as with fever	May be normal with exercise 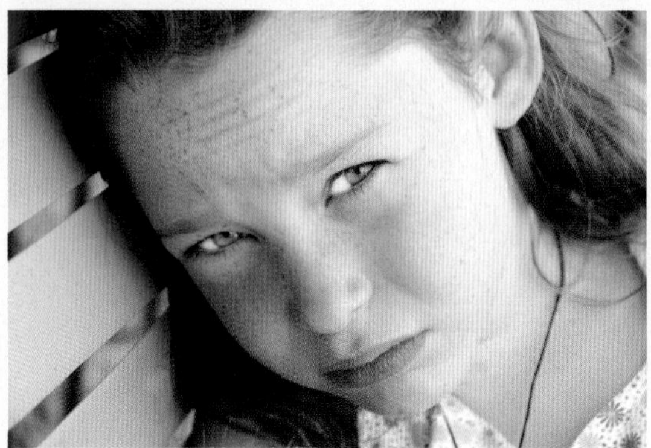
Pallor	Decreased arterial blood flow of arterial insufficiency	
Rubor and brawny skin	Decreased venous return in venous insufficiency	Skin is cool or cold over areas of decreased circulation.
Cyanosis	Circumoral cyanosis in association with congestive heart failure or chronic obstructive pulmonary disease	Bluish skin discoloration occurs in areas of decreased blood flow or poor blood oxygenation. Cyanosis in dark-skinned patients is not readily observed on the skin but can be assessed in buccal mucosa or conjunctivae.
	Peripheral cyanosis in areas of impaired circulation with oxygenated blood	Cyanosis appears along with fingernail clubbing in the photo below.
Fingernail clubbing	Disease states with prolonged hypoxia (e.g., emphysema)	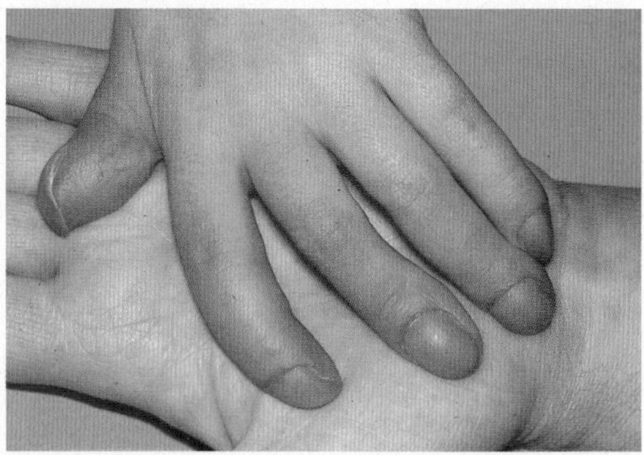
	Gastrointestinal	
Thinning of the skin, hair, and nail and hair loss	Nutritional deficiencies, inadequate absorption of vitamins A, B_6 (riboflavin), and C	

(table continues on page 263)

TABLE 11.8 Manifestations in Integument of Systemic Disorders *(continued)*

Integument Finding	Associated Disorder	Other Considerations/Depictions
Jaundice (yellow discoloration of the skin, sclera, or buccal mucosa; shown)	Liver disease	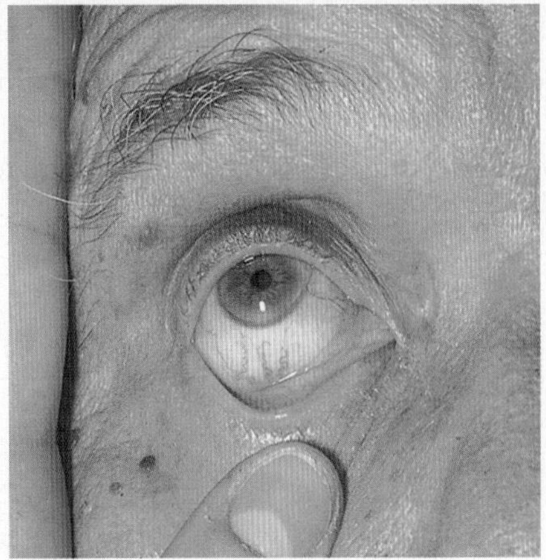
Pigmented macules	Peutz-Jeghers disease	Pigmented areas may be on hands, lips, or buccal mucosa. 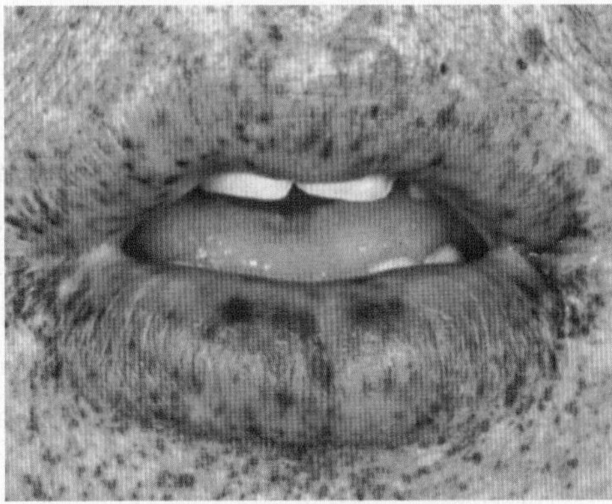
	Genitourinary	
Uremic frost	Marked renal failure	Results from precipitation of renal urea and nitrogen waste products through sweat onto skin
Hirsutism (shown)	Polycystic ovarian syndrome	Affected women show male-pattern hair distribution, usually on face, chest, abdomen, or genital area. 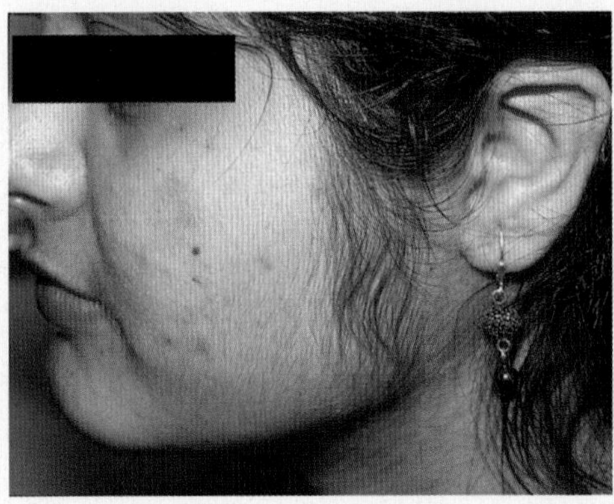

(table continues on page 264)

TABLE 11.8 Manifestations in Integument of Systemic Disorders *(continued)*

Integument Finding	Associated Disorder	Other Considerations/Depictions
	Endocrine	
Thick coarse hair, dry skin, and cool skin temperature	Hypothyroidism	
Smooth skin, thin, silky hair, and brittle nails	Hyperthyroidism	Cushing disease 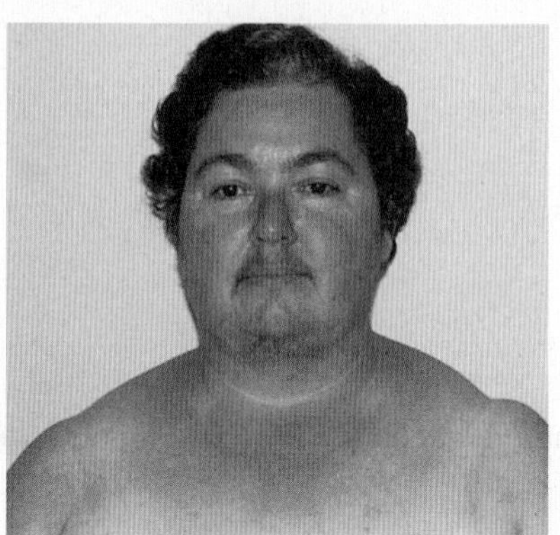
Excessive hair growth or thinning; development of or worsening of acne	Androgen disorders	
Striae	Cushing syndrome	
Hyperpigmentation of skin and mucous membranes; nevi	Addison disease	
Flushing	Pheochromocytoma	
Thickened skin	Pituitary tumor	
Decreased sweating (hypohidrosis), frequent cutaneous yeast infections, and hair loss on distal extremities	Diabetes mellitus	
Acanthosis nigricans (hyperpigmentation)	Diabetes mellitus and many other endocrine disorders	
	Neurological	
Neuropathic ulcers on distal extremities	Peripheral neuropathy in diabetes	Decreased sensation of any body area increases risk for injury, including burns and pressure ulcers. 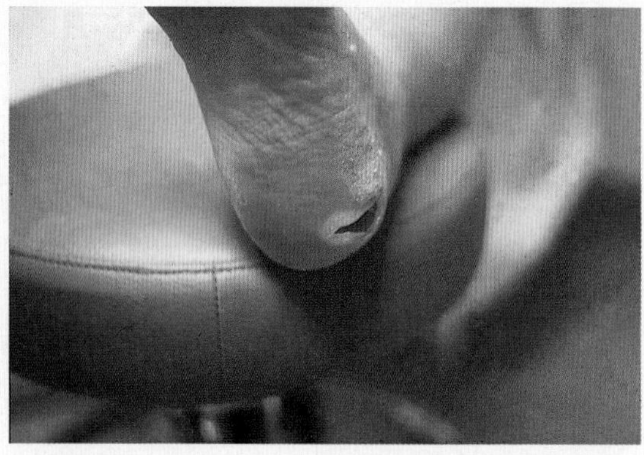

(table continues on page 265)

TABLE 11.8 **Manifestations in Integument of Systemic Disorders** *(continued)*

Integument Finding	Associated Disorder	Other Considerations/Depictions
Café au lait macules (shown)	Neurofibromatosis	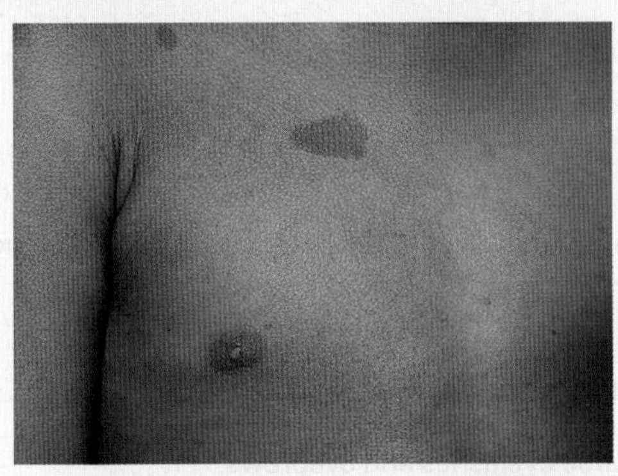
	Musculoskeletal	
Photosensitivity, malar rash (red macular lesions distributed over forehead, cheeks, and chin, resembling a butterfly, as shown), coin-shaped lesions on trunk and extremities, and aphthous ulcers on buccal mucosa	Systemic lupus erythematosus	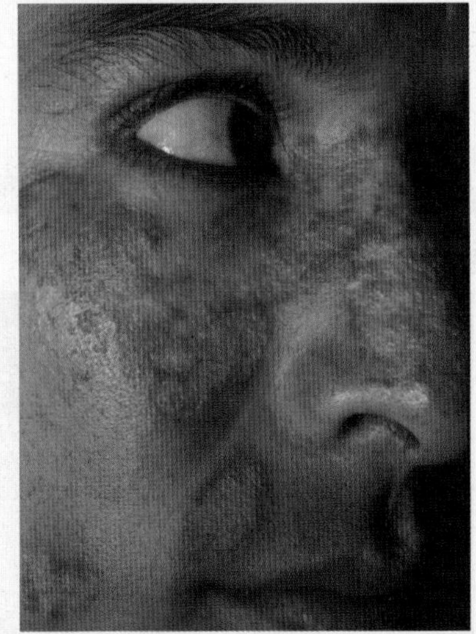
Anular erythema	Sjögren syndrome	
Pallor of fingers and toes in response to cold (shown)	Raynaud phenomenon	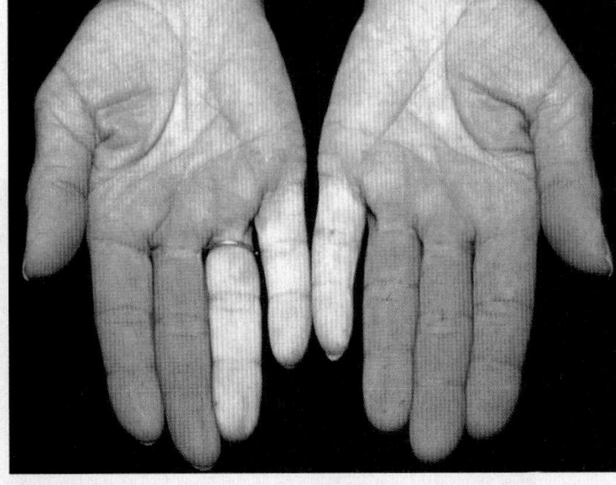
Erythema and increased temperature over a joint	Sepsis or acute inflammation of the joint	

(table continues on page 266)

TABLE 11.8 Manifestations in Integument of Systemic Disorders *(continued)*

Integument Finding	Associated Disorder	Other Considerations/Depictions
	Hematology/Lymph	
Generalized pallor	Anemia	
Pruritus	Polycythemia, mastocytosis, lymphoma, or leukemia	
Spooning of nails	Iron deficiency states	
	Psychiatric	
Patchy alopecia on the scalp or body as well as missing or sparse eyelashes and eyebrows	Trichotillomania (compulsive hair pulling)	
Small linear cuts on patient's arms, legs, or anterior torso	"Cutting"	This self-injury coping method occurs in patients with borderline personality disorder, depression, and other psychiatric states.

TABLE 11.9 Primary Skin Lesions

Macule

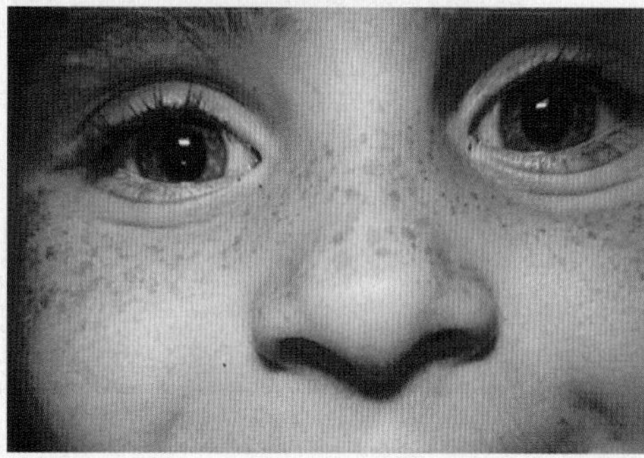

Flat, circumscribed, discolored, less than 1 cm diameter

Examples: Freckles (shown), tattoo, stork bite (birthmark type seen in newborns)

Patch

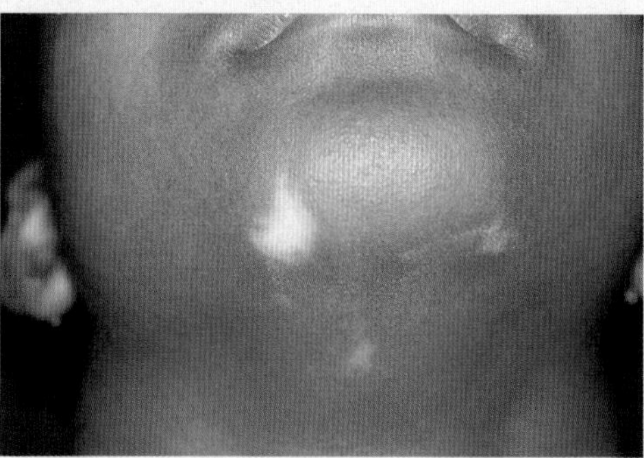

Flat, circumscribed, discolored, greater than 1 cm diameter

Examples: Vitiligo (shown), melasma, tinea versicolor

Papule

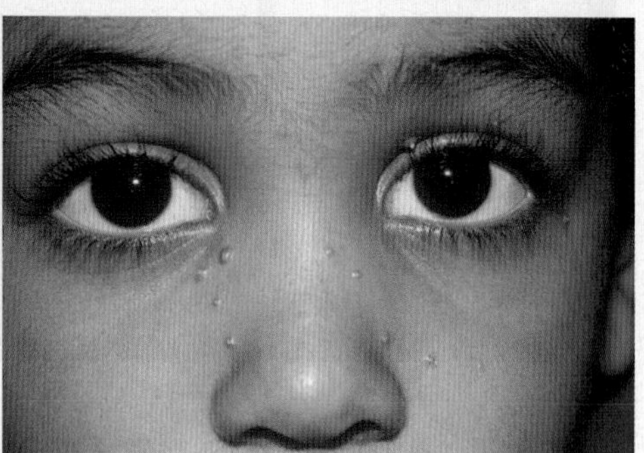

Raised, defined, any color, less than 1 cm diameter

Examples: Wart, insect bite, molluscum contagiosum (shown)

Plaque

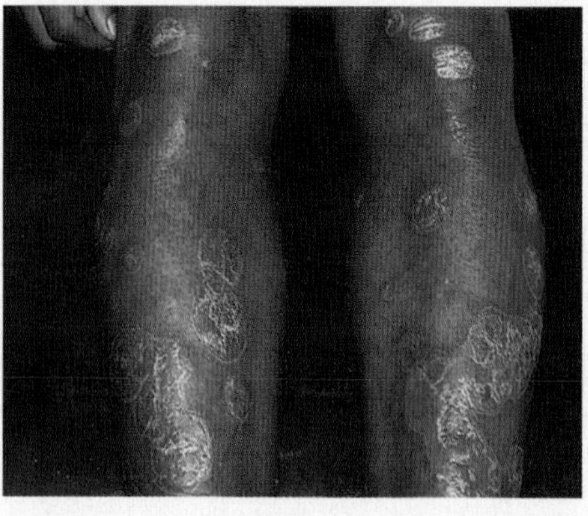

Raised, defined, any color, less than 1 cm diameter

Examples: Psoriasis (shown), lichen sclerosus

(table continues on page 267)

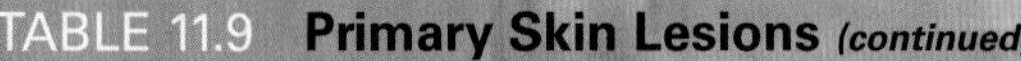

TABLE 11.9 Primary Skin Lesions *(continued)*

Wheal

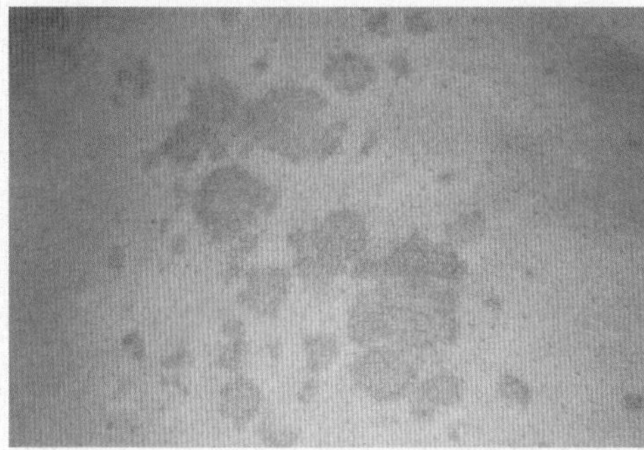

Raised, flesh-colored, or red edematous papules or plaques; vary in size and shape

Example: Urticaria (shown)

Nodule

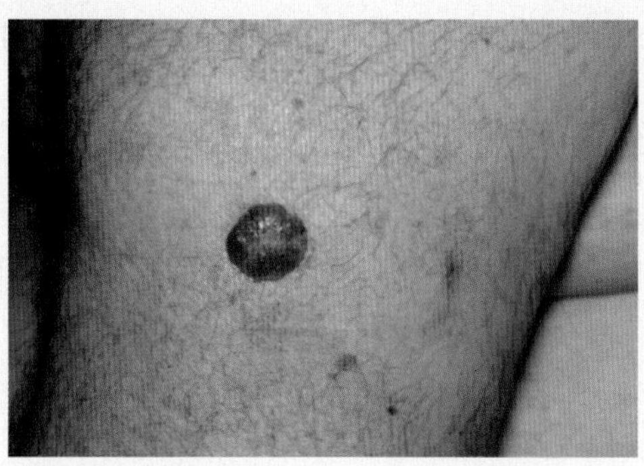

Solid, palpable, less than 1 cm diameter, often with some depth

Example: Basal cell carcinoma (shown)

Tumor

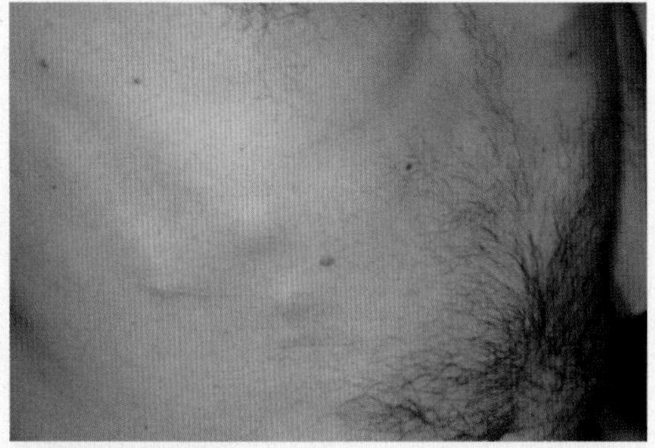

Large nodule

Examples: Large nevus, basal cell carcinoma, lipoma (shown)

Vesicle

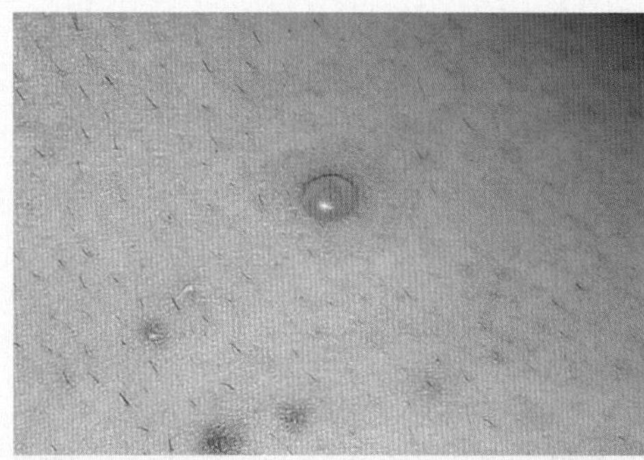

Fluid-filled, less than 1 cm diameter

Examples: Herpes simplex, chicken pox (shown)

Bulla

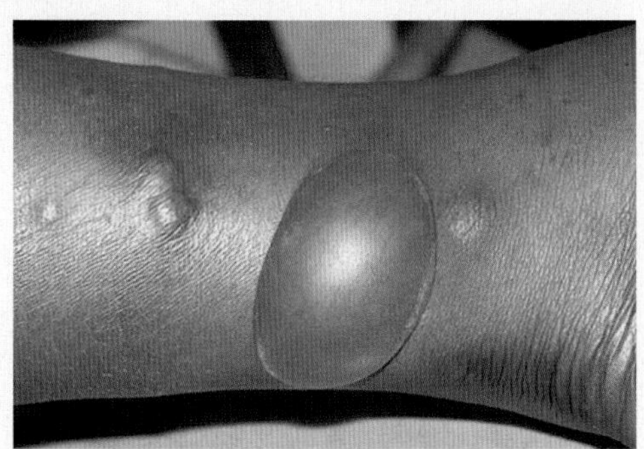

Fluid-filled, less than 1 cm diameter

Examples: Partial-thickness burns, bullous impetigo (shown)

Pustule

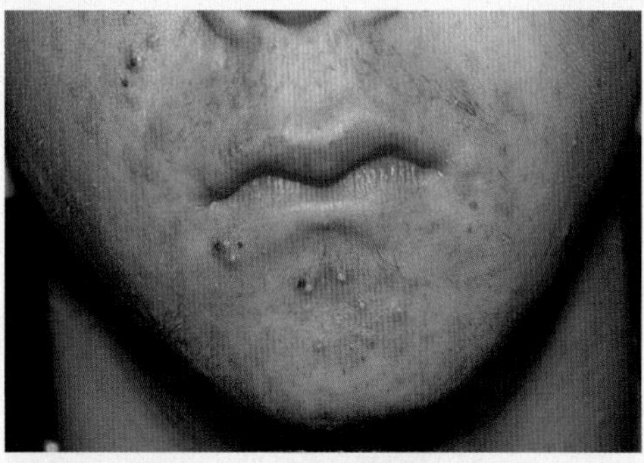

Purulent, fluid-filled, raised of any size

Examples: Pustular acne (shown), folliculitis

(table continues on page 268)

TABLE 11.9 Primary Skin Lesions *(continued)*

Cyst

Distinct and walled-off, containing fluid or semisolid material, varies in size

Examples: Epidermal cyst (shown), cystic acne

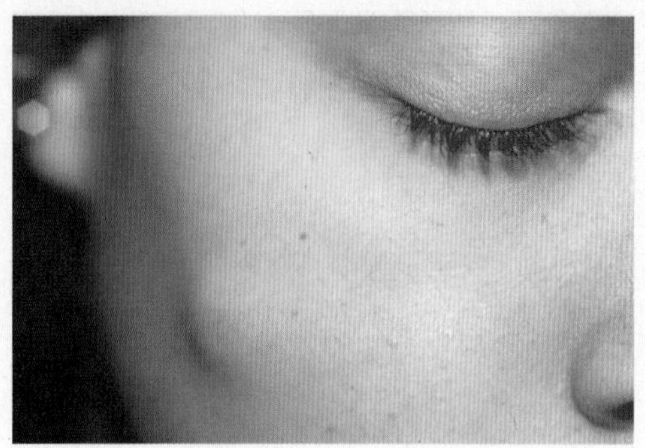

TABLE 11.10 Secondary Skin Lesions

Atrophy

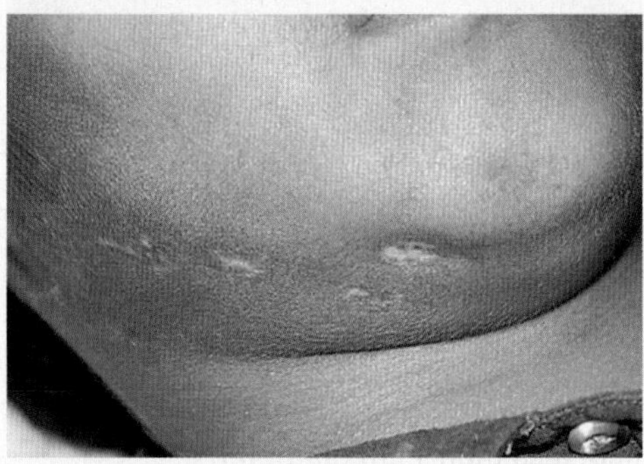

Thinning of skin from loss of skin structures

Examples: Steroid-induced atrophy, scleroderma (shown)

Scar

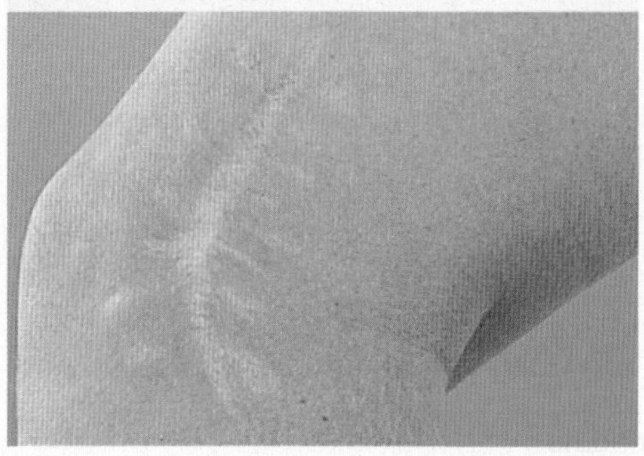

Fibrous replacement of lost skin structure

Example: Surgical scar (shown)

Keloid

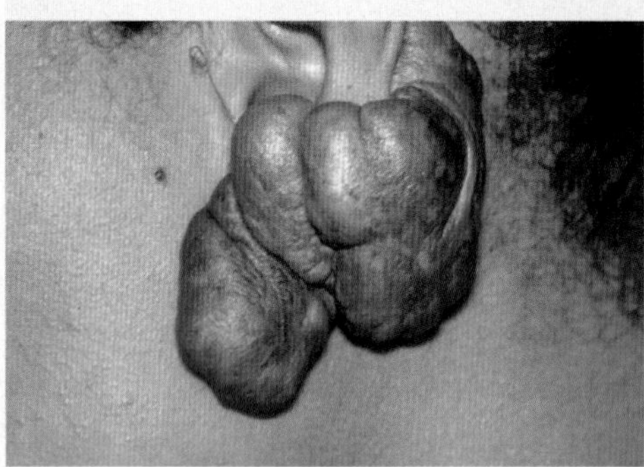

Excessive fibrous tissue replacement resulting in enlarged scar and deformity

Crust

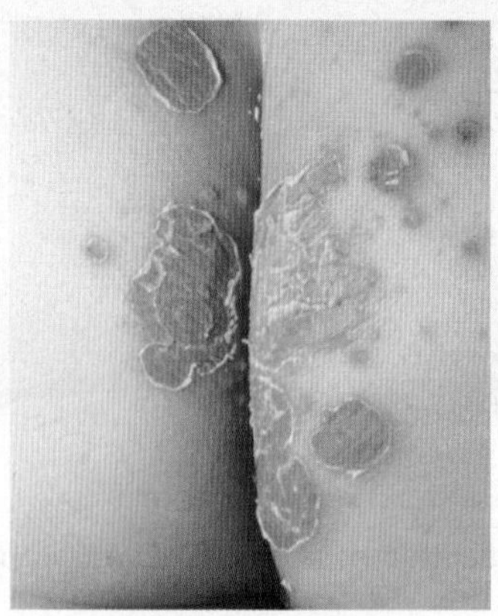

Dried secretions from primary lesion

Example: Impetigo (shown)

(table continues on page 269)

TABLE 11.10 Secondary Skin Lesions *(continued)*

Scale

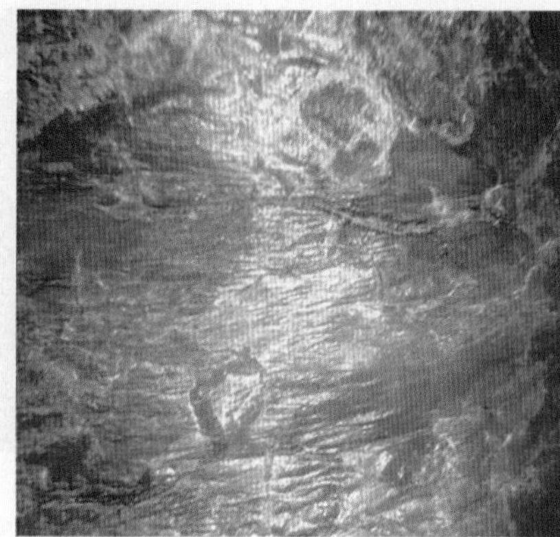

Rapid turnover of epidermal layer resulting in accumulation of and delayed shedding of outermost epidermis

Examples: Psoriasis (shown), tinea corporis

Lichenification

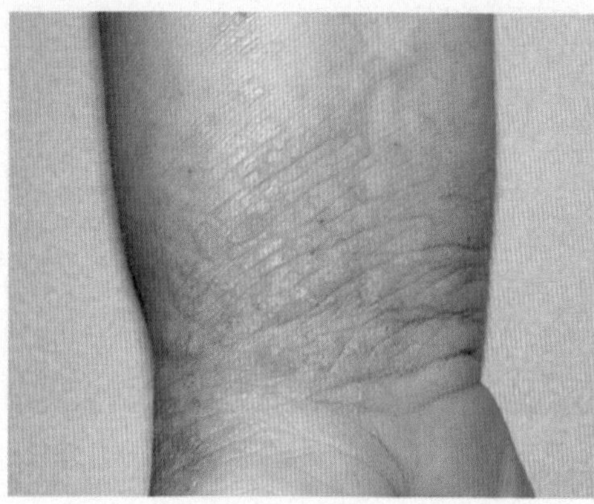

Accentuation of normal skin lines resembling tree bark, commonly caused by excessive scratching

Examples: Lichen simplex chronicus (shown), psoriasis, chronic contact dermatitis

Excoriation

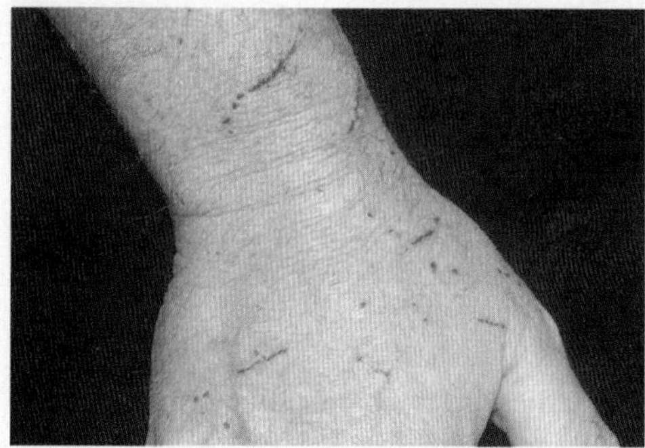

Lesion resulting from scratching or excessive rubbing of skin

Example: Cat scratches (shown)

Erosion

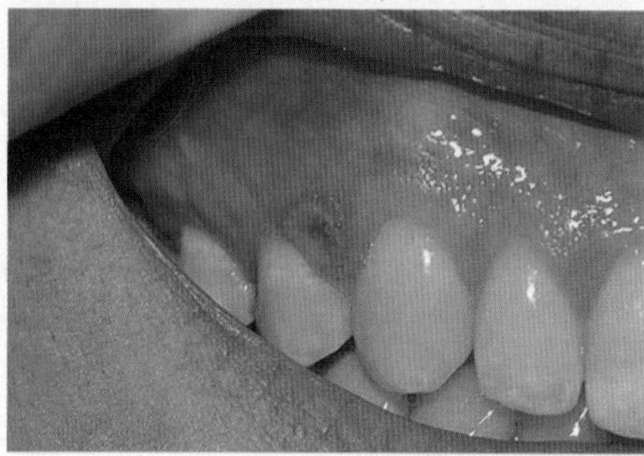

Loss of epidermal layer, usually not extending into dermis or subcutaneous layer

Examples: Aphthous stomatitis (shown), varicella

Fissure

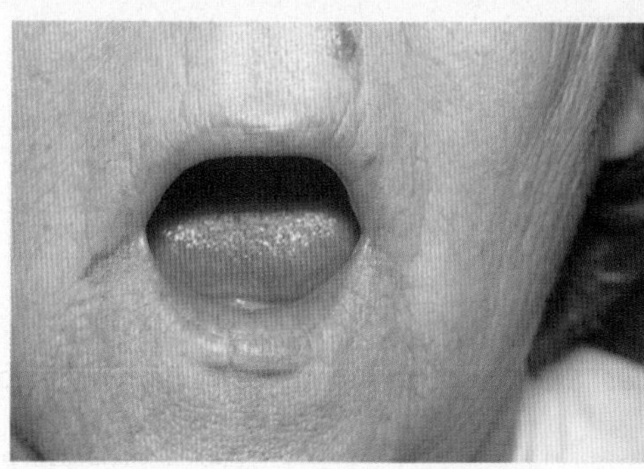

Linear break in skin surface, not related to trauma

Examples: Cheilitis, angular stomatitis (shown)

Ulcer

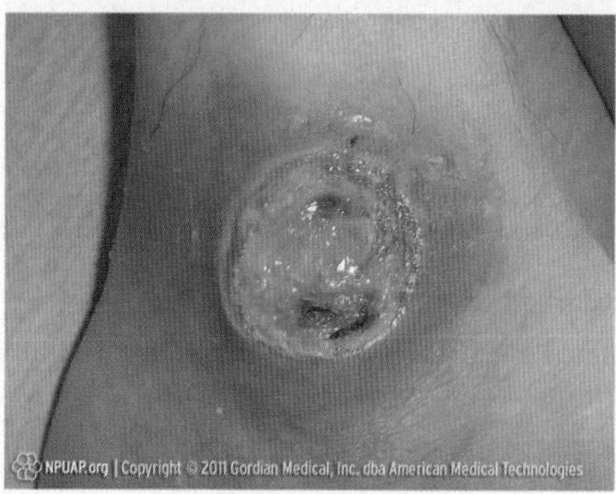

Loss of skin surface, extending into dermis, subcutaneous, fascia, muscle, bone, or all

Examples: Pressure ulcers, vascular ulcers, neuropathic ulcers (shown)

(table continues on page 270)

TABLE 11.11 Configurations of Lesions

Annular

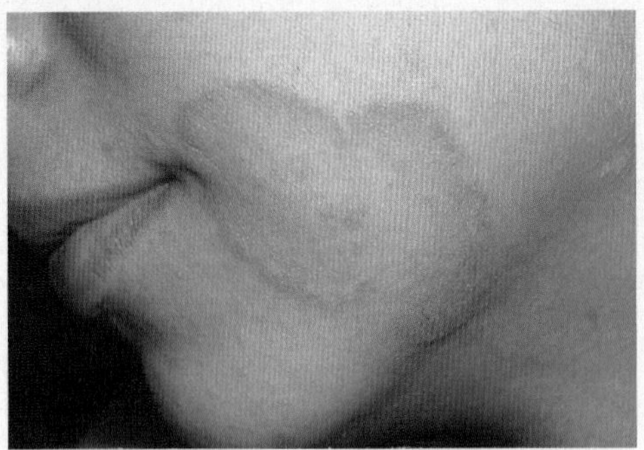

Ringlike, circular

Example: Tinea corporis (shown)

Iris

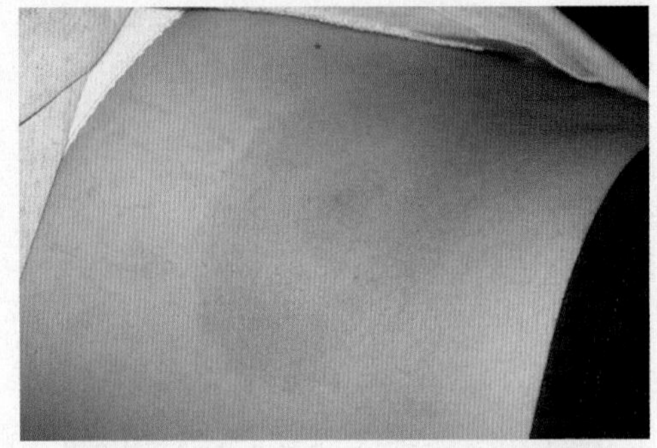

Bull's eye

Examples: Lyme disease (shown), erythema nodosum

Linear

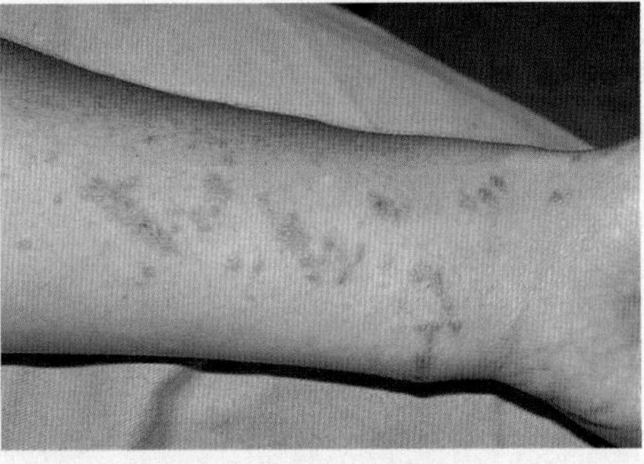

Line shape

Example: Contact dermatitis (shown)

Polymorphous

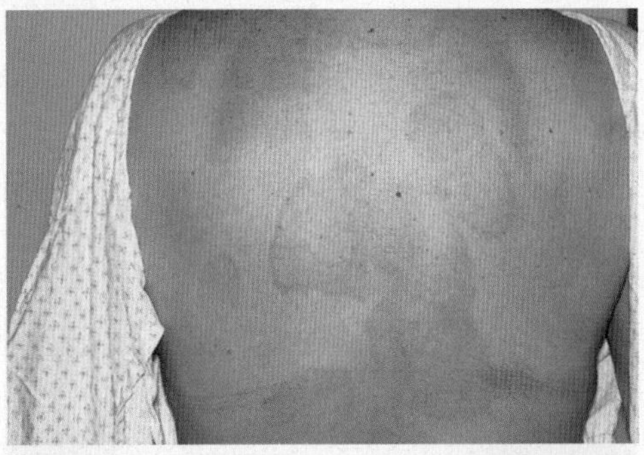

Several different shapes

Examples: Urticaria, tinea corporis (shown)

Punctuate

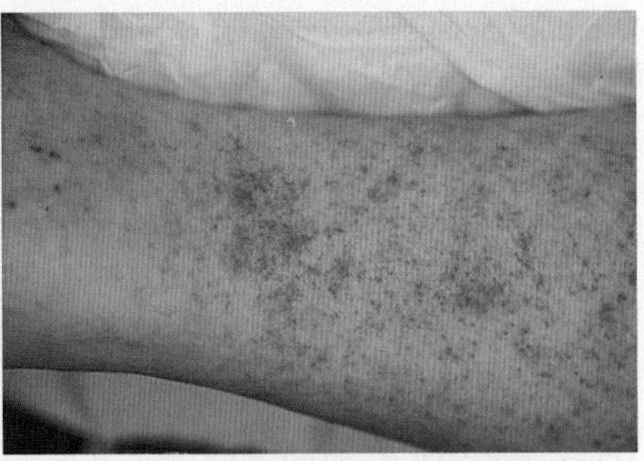

Small, marked with points or dots

Examples: Petechiae, Rocky Mountain spotted fever (shown), meningococcemia, vasculitis

Serpiginous

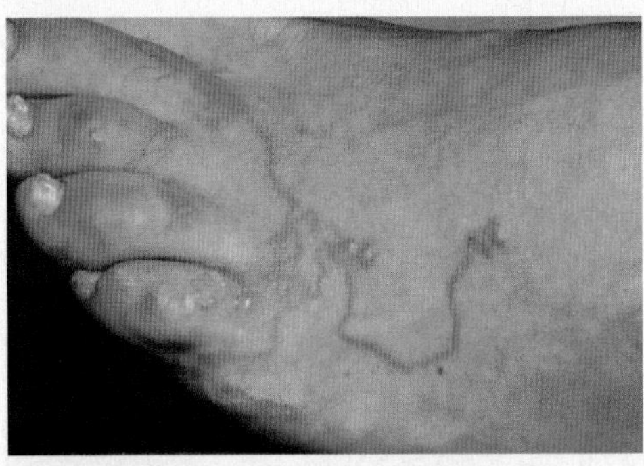

Curving, snakelike

Examples: Cutaneous larva migrans (shown), scabies

(table continues on page 271)

TABLE 11.11 Configurations of Lesions *(continued)*

Nummular/Discoid

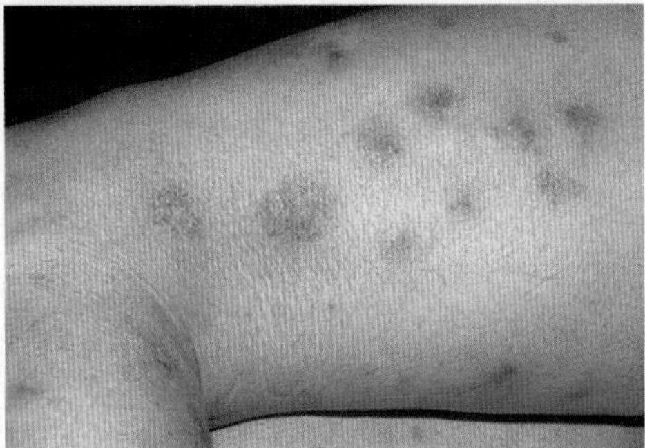

Coin-shaped

Examples: Nummular psoriasis, nummular eczema (shown)

Umbilicated

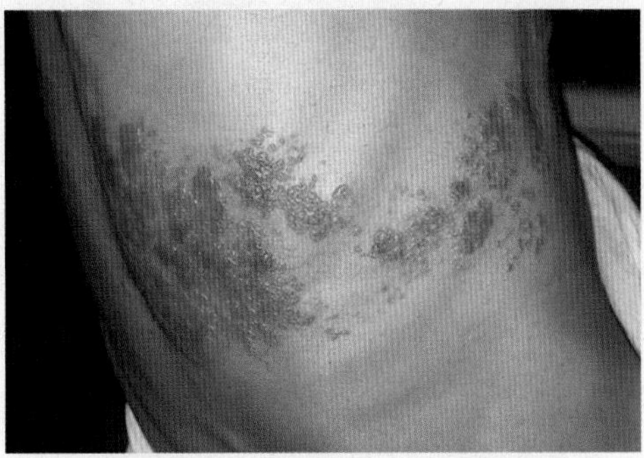

Central depression

Examples: Herpes zoster (shown), basal cell carcinoma

Filiform

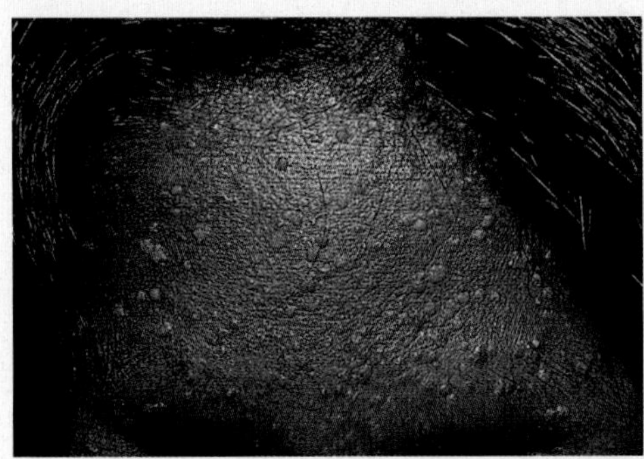

Papilla-like or fingerlike projections (similar to tongue papillae)

Example: Warts (shown)

Verruciform

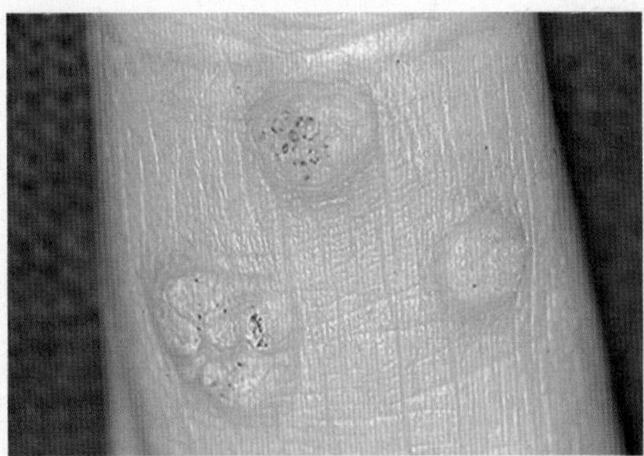

Circumscribed, papular with rough surface

Example: Warts (shown)

TABLE 11.12 Distribution Patterns of Lesions

Assymetrical

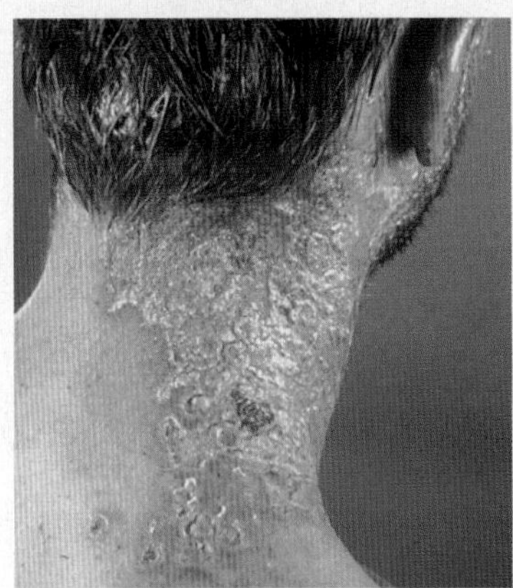

Distributed solely on one side of body

Examples: Contact dermatitis (shown), herpes zoster

Confluent

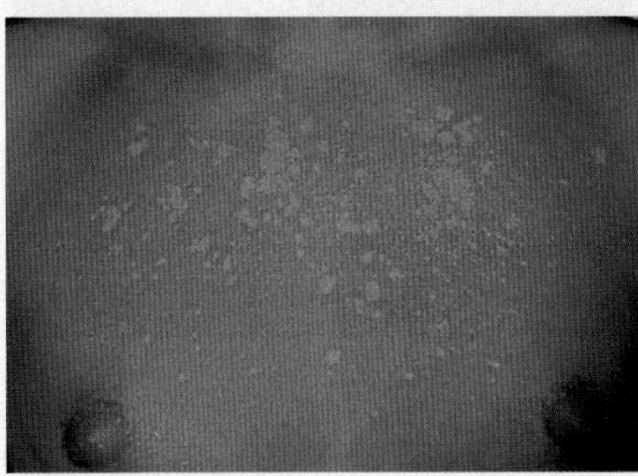

With enlargement or multiplication, begins to coalesce to form larger lesion

Examples: Urticaria, tinea versicolor (shown)

(table continues on page 272)

TABLE 11.12 Distribution Patterns of Lesions *(continued)*

Diffuse

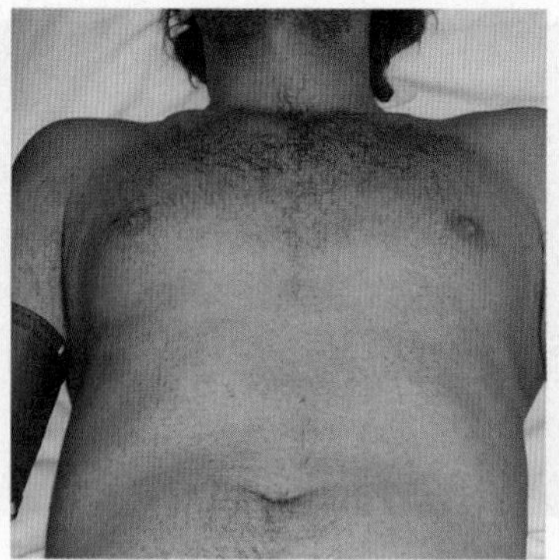

Distributed widely across affected area without any pattern

Examples: Drug reaction (shown), rubella, rubeola

Discrete

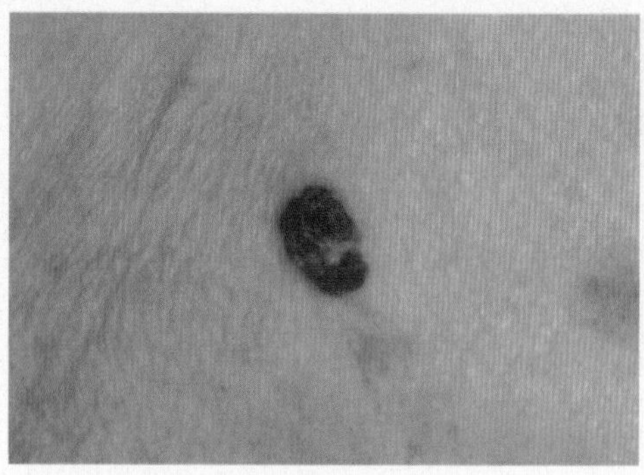

Single, separated, well-defined borders

Examples: Melanoma (shown), wart

Generalized

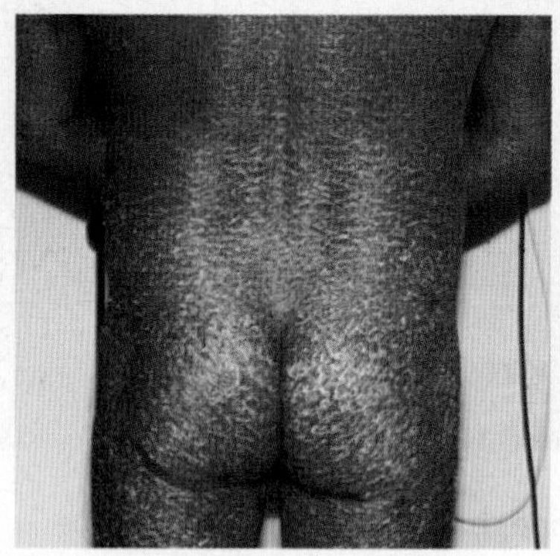

Distributed over large body area

Examples: Psoriasis (shown), acne vulgaris, exfoliative dermatitis

Grouped

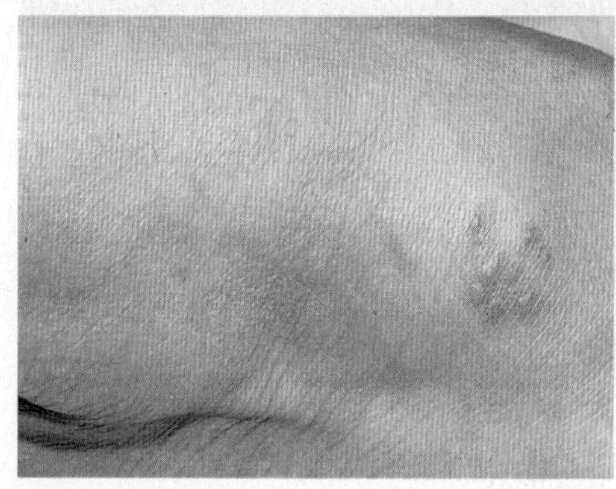

Clustered

Examples: Herpes simplex (shown)

Localized

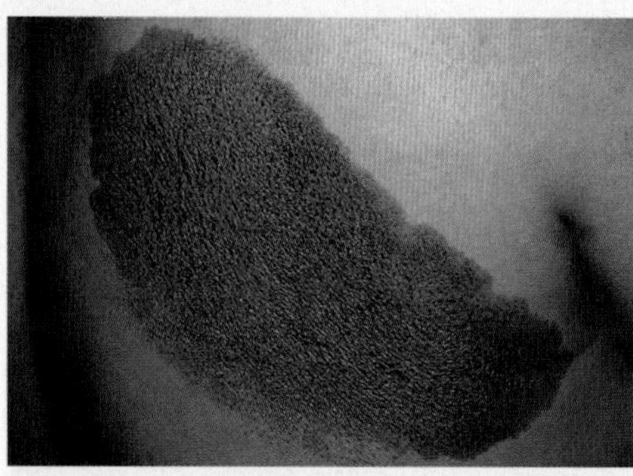

Located at distinct area

Examples: Giant nevus (shown), contact dermatitis, vitiligo

Satellite

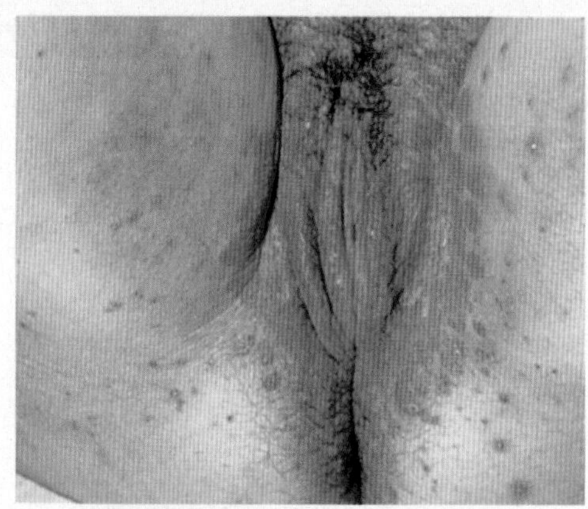

Single lesion(s) in close proximity to larger lesion, as if "orbiting"

Example: Cutaneous candidiasis (shown)

(table continues on page 273)

TABLE 11.12 Distribution Patterns of Lesions *(continued)*

Symmetrical

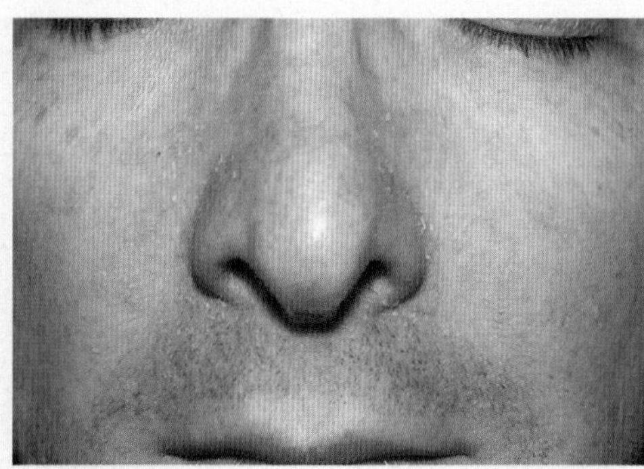

Distributed equally on both sides of body

Examples: Pityriasis rosea, freckles, seborrheic dermatitis (shown)

Zosteriform

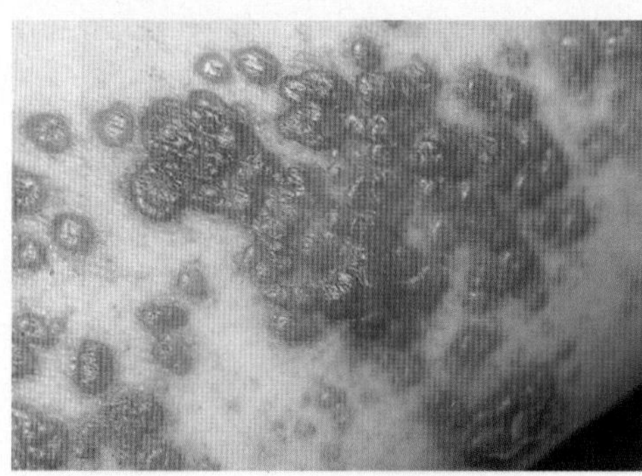

Distributed along dermatome

Example: Herpes zoster (shown)

TABLE 11.13 Common Skin Infections

Acne

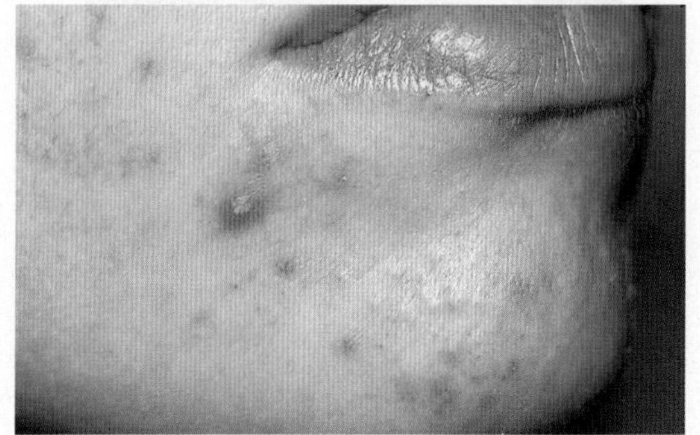

Pustular acne

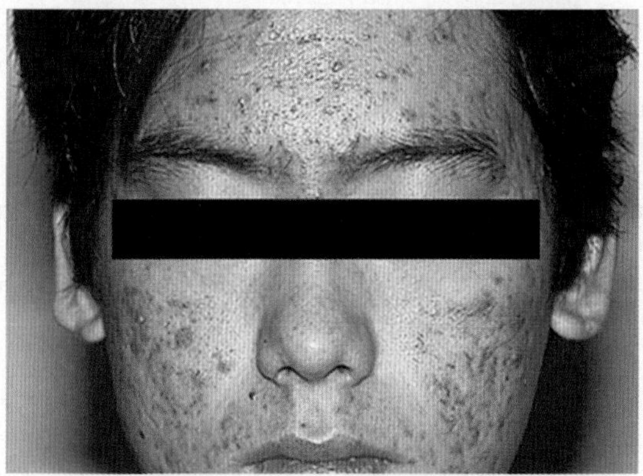

Cystic acne

Acne presents as an inflammatory and noninflammatory skin disorder characterized by one or a combination of the following lesions: comedo, papule, pustule, or cyst. Distribution of acne is frequently on the face, neck, torso, upper arms, and legs, although lesions may occur in other areas.

Warts

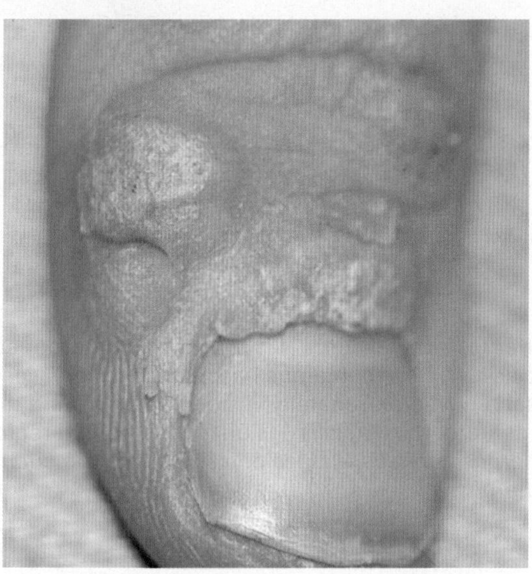

Warts are flesh-colored papules commonly caused by viruses. Their surface is usually rough and textured without scale.

(table continues on page 274)

TABLE 11.13 Common Skin Infections *(continued)*

Cellulitis

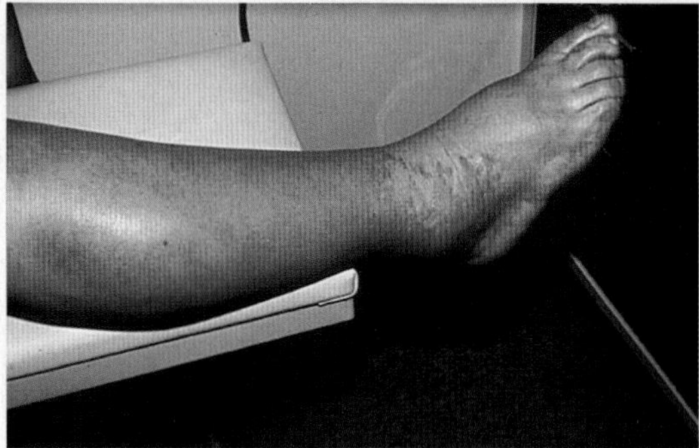

Cellulitis is a bacterial infection of deep skin tissues, often preceded by a minor wound to the area allowing bacteria to invade the tissue. Cellulitis can occur anywhere and is characterized by swelling, redness, warmth, and tenderness or pain.

Impetigo

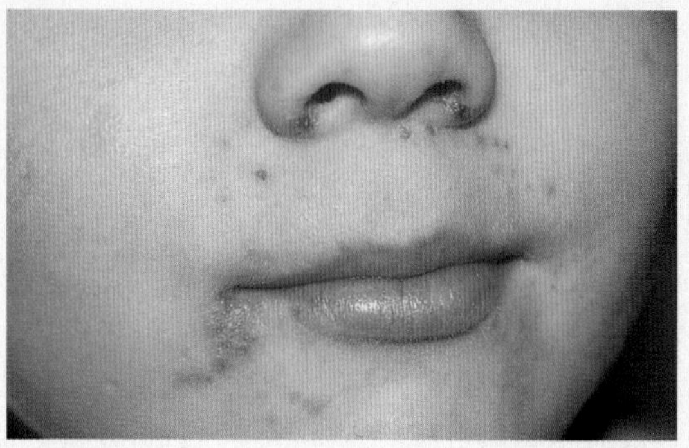

This highly contagious superficial skin infection commonly results from *Staphylococcus aureus* or group A beta-hemolytic streptococci. It is characterized by vesicles or bullae that eventually rupture and ooze serous fluid that forms the classic honey-colored crust.

Herpes Simplex (Cold Sores)

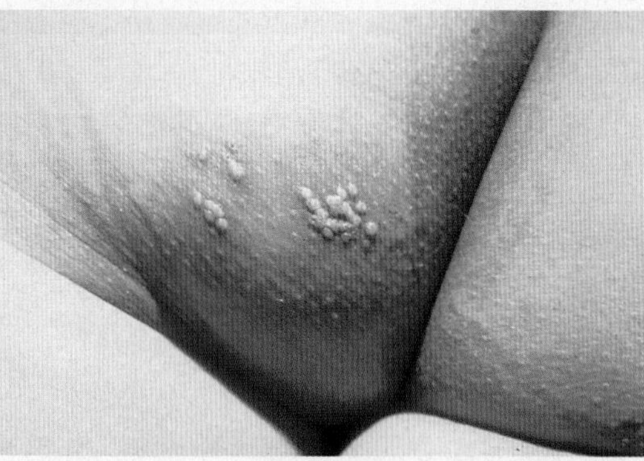

The herpes simplex virus is characterized by grouped vesicles on an erythematous base. These lesions can appear anywhere. Generally, lesions on or around the mouth are *herpes labialis*, lesions in the genital regions are *herpes genitalis*, and lesions elsewhere are *cutaneous herpes*.

Measles (Rubeola)

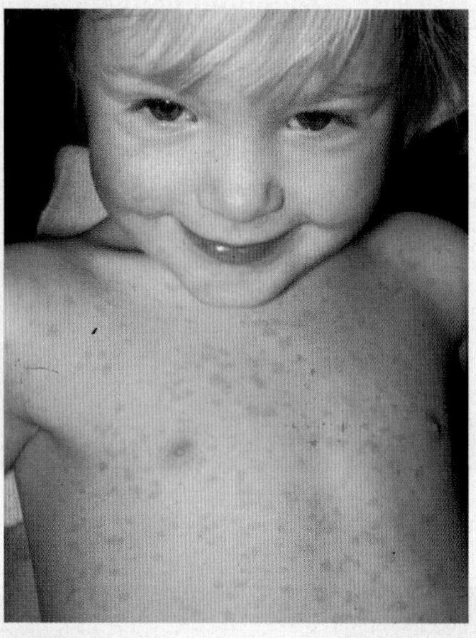

Commonly called hard measles, rubeola is a virus characterized by pinkish, erythematous macules and papules initially on the face, with progressive caudal spread. In 3–4 days, the rash becomes brownish with a fine desquamation.

(table continues on page 275)

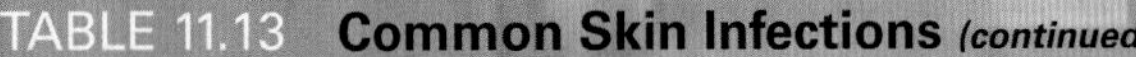

TABLE 11.13 Common Skin Infections *(continued)*

Pityriasis Rosea

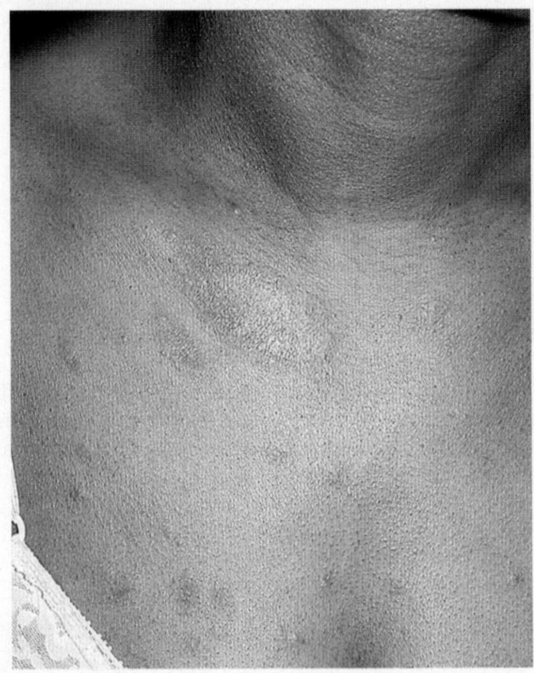

This viral infection is initially characterized by a "herald patch"—a large oval hyperpigmented lesion with a fine scale, usually on the chest or back. Over subsequent days, additional similar but smaller lesions develop and are distributed generally over the torso and extremities, with the face usually spared.

German Measles (Rubella)

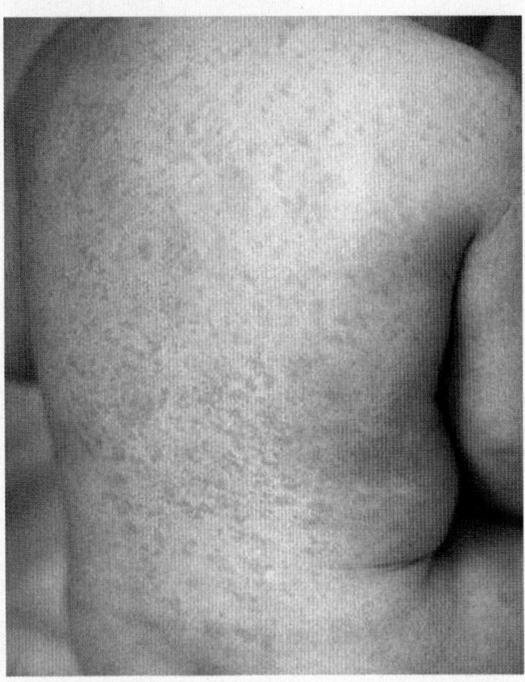

Commonly called the 3-day measles and largely vaccine preventable, this viral illness presents as a pinkish discrete macular and papular rash covering the entire body. It usually resolves in 3 days.

Roseola

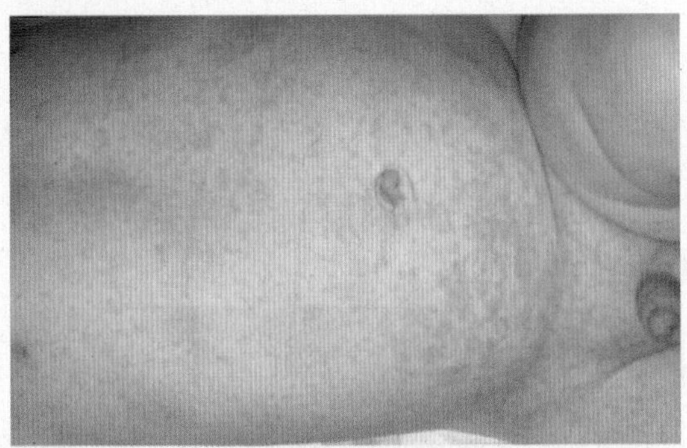

Roseola is a viral illness whose rash appears as the fever resolves. The rash of roseola is described as discrete macules and papules, usually no more than 1–5 mm diameter, with an area of pallor surrounding each lesion.

Candida

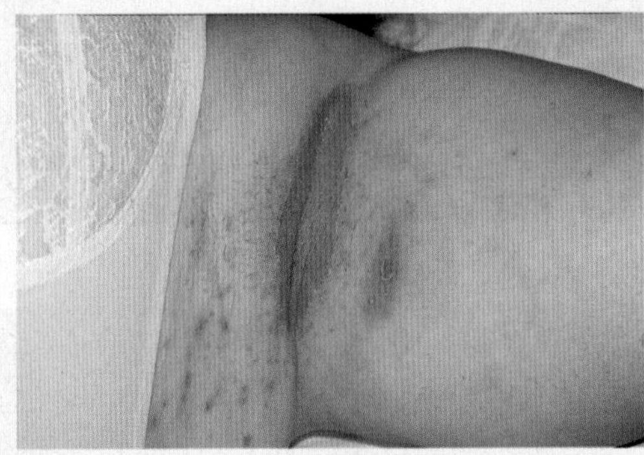

Candida is a fungus commonly found in skinfolds or generally warm and moist areas. Commonly affected sites are the axillae, inframammary areas, and groin. Satellite pustules commonly surround the erythematous macules.

(table continues on page 276)

TABLE 11.13 Common Skin Infections *(continued)*

Tinea Corporis

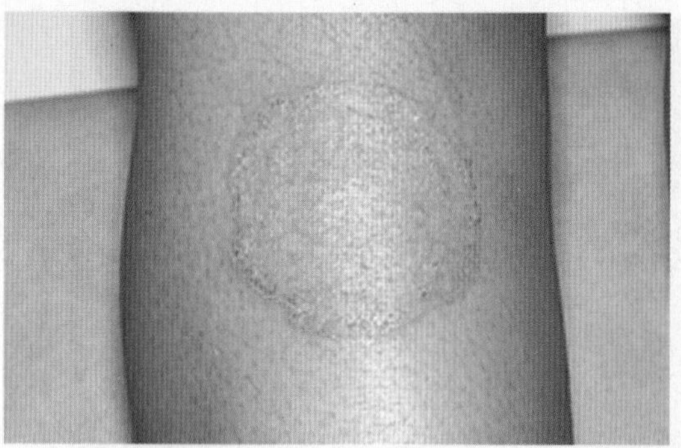

Commonly called *ringworm*, this dermatophytic skin infection results in an erythematous, commonly pruritic, anular lesion with a raised border and central clearing.

Tinea Versicolor

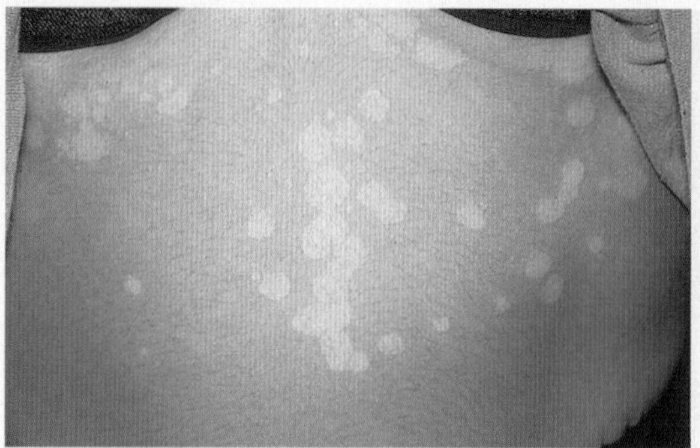

This dermatophyte infection caused by normal skin flora results in hypopigmented patchy lesions generally distributed on the upper chest, upper back, and proximal extremities. It rarely occurs on the face and legs.

TABLE 11.14 Inflammatory Skin Lesions

Psoriasis

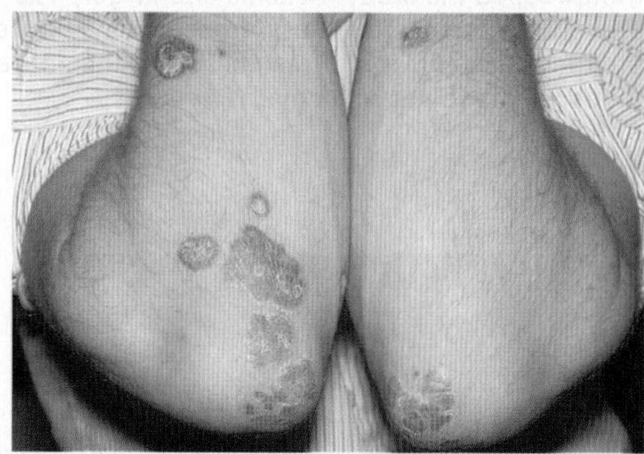

This chronic skin disorder is commonly characterized by reddish-pink lesions covered with silvery scales. It commonly occurs on extensor surfaces (e.g., elbows and knees) but can appear anywhere on the body.

Eczema

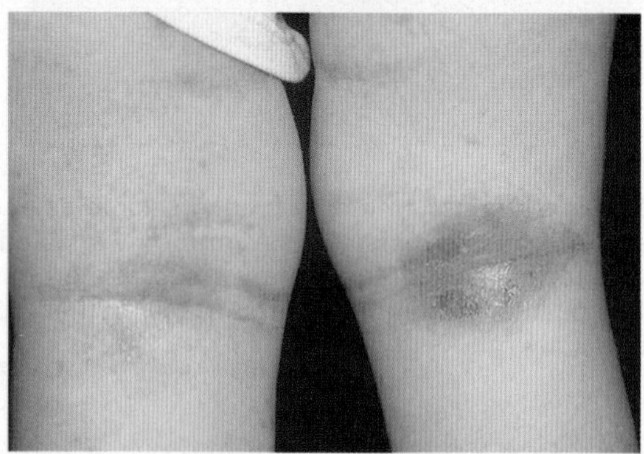

Also known as *atopic dermatitis*, eczema is characterized by itchy pink macules or papules, commonly on flexural areas (e.g., inner elbows and posterior knees). Eczema can occur anywhere on the body.

Contact Dermatitis

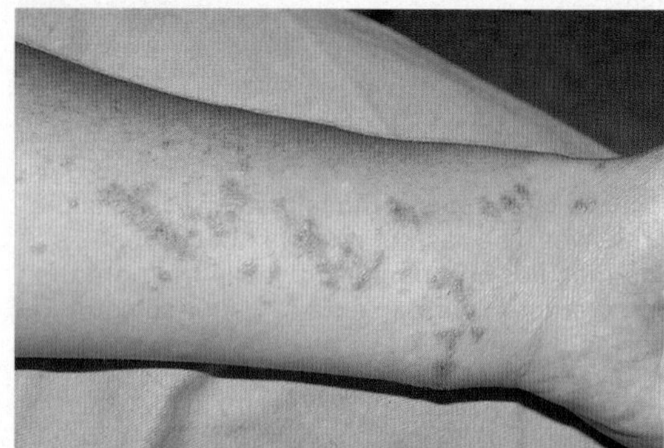

This inflammatory response to an antigen that has contact with exposed skin initially causes stimulation of the histamine receptors, which results in the classic erythematous and pruritic lesions.

(table continues on page 277)

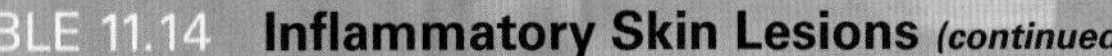

TABLE 11.14 Inflammatory Skin Lesions *(continued)*

Urticaria

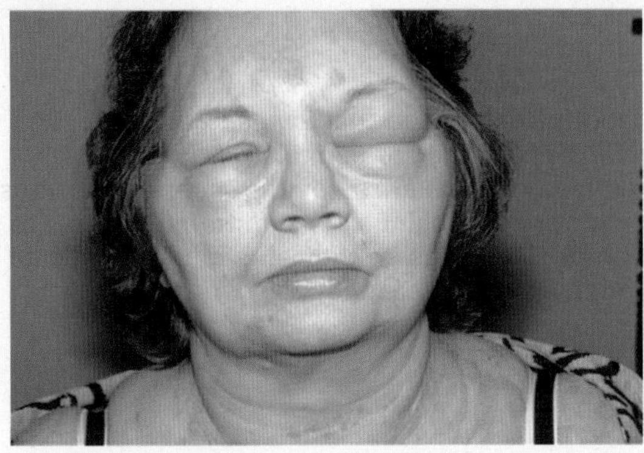

Commonly called *hives*, urticaria is the accumulation of fluid in the dermal layer of the skin as a direct result of histamine release.

Allergic Drug Reaction

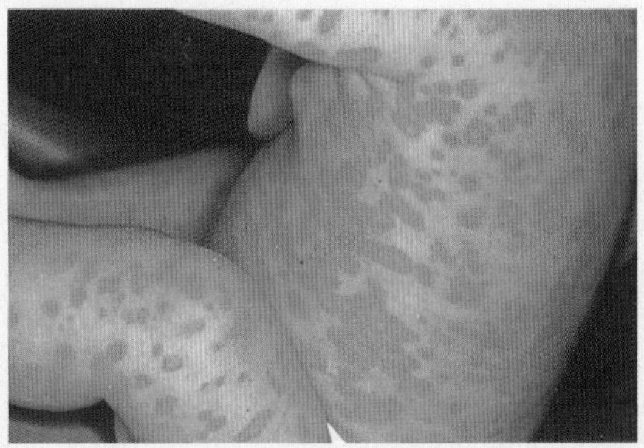

Drug allergies can occur immediately or have a delayed response after exposure to the offending agent.

Insect Bites

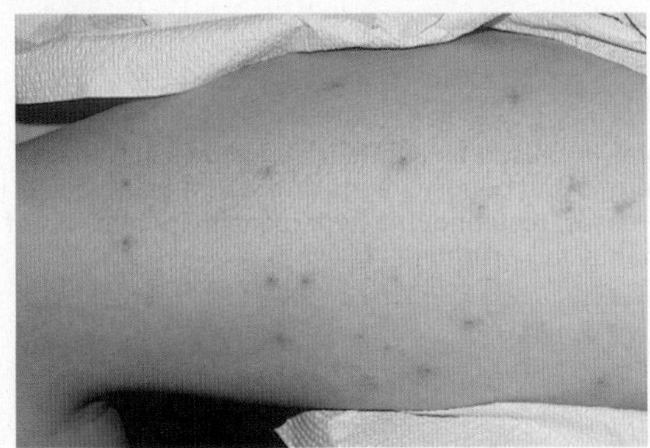

Insect bites usually cause an inflammatory and pruritic response at the site. Lesions are usually erythematous and papular with a visible punctum at the central part.

Seborrhea

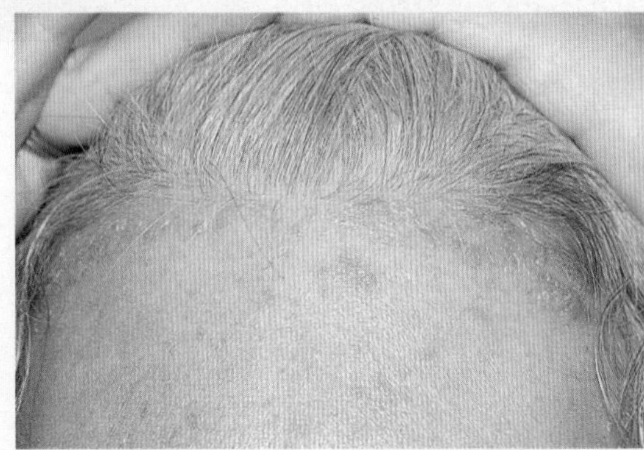

Seborrhea (seborrheic dermatitis) is an inflammatory skin disorder characterized by macular pink, red, or orange-yellow lesions that may or may not have a fine scale. Distribution is usually on the face, scalp, and ears.

TABLE 11.15 **Skin Lesions From Infestations**

Lesion	Description
Lice (Pediculosis)	
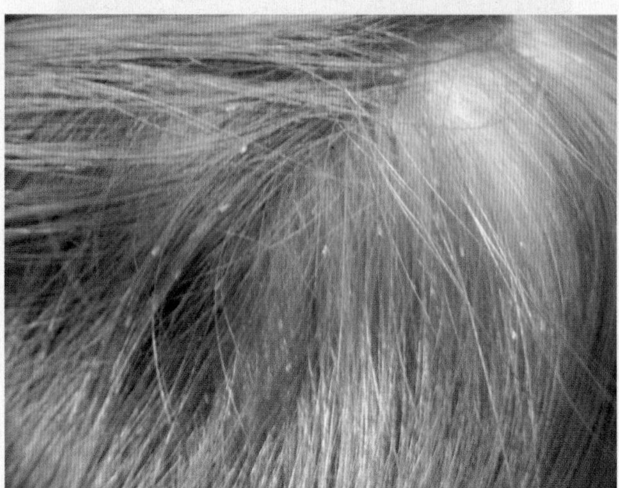	Infestations on the head (*pediculosis capitis*), body (*pediculosis corporis*), or genitals (*Phthirus pubis*) are frequently characterized by the secondary lesions resulting from scratching. It is common to be able to see one or more lice; eggs on the hair shaft also indicate infestation even if lice cannot be seen.
Scabies	
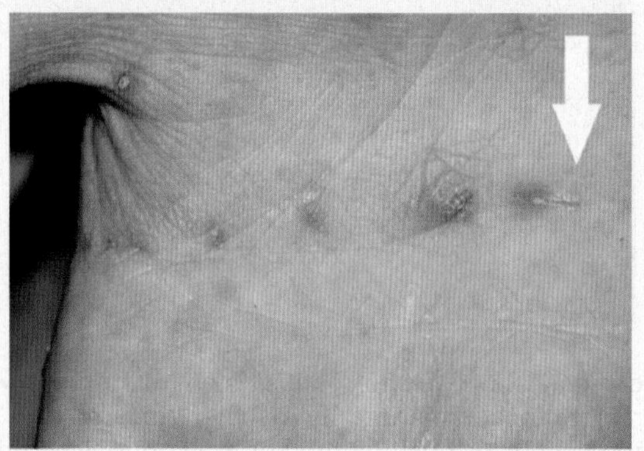	Scabies is caused by a mite that burrows into the epidermis and deposits eggs and waste materials as it progresses, resulting in a hypersensitivity reaction of erythema and pruritus.
Ticks	
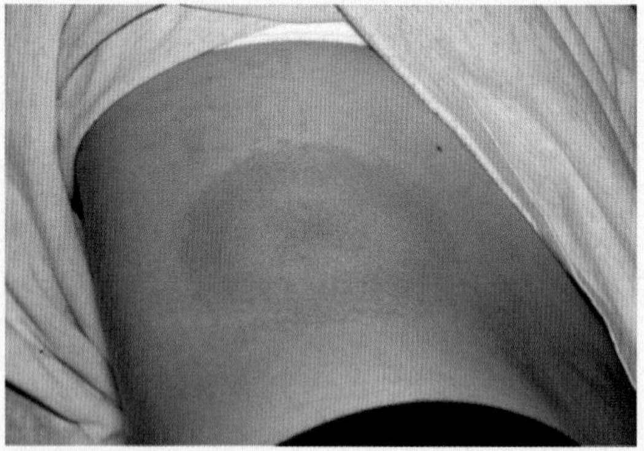	Tick bites frequently resemble simple insect bites. Nevertheless, certain ticks cause systemic illness, with a characteristic erythematous target lesion that appears at the site of the bite, which requires prompt medical evaluation.

TABLE 11.16 Skin Tumors and Growths

Moles or Nevi

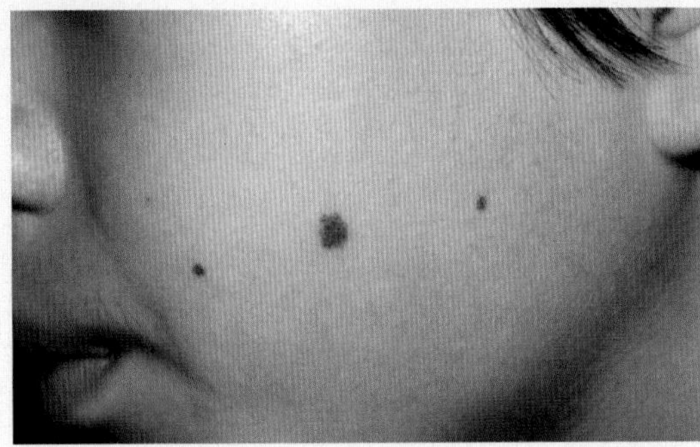

Nevi (moles) are normal variants. They can be macular or papular and distributed anywhere. They are congenital or acquired. *Congenital nevi* exist from birth and are commonly referred to as "birth marks." *Acquired nevi* occur most commonly in childhood and adolescence.

Skin Tags

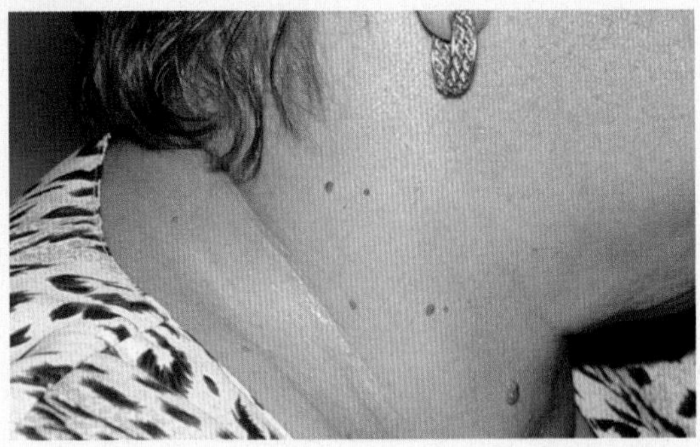

These normal papules are generally less than 1 cm and commonly distributed on the neck, axillae, inframammary area, and groin. Skin tags are common in pregnancy and in aging skin.

Lipoma

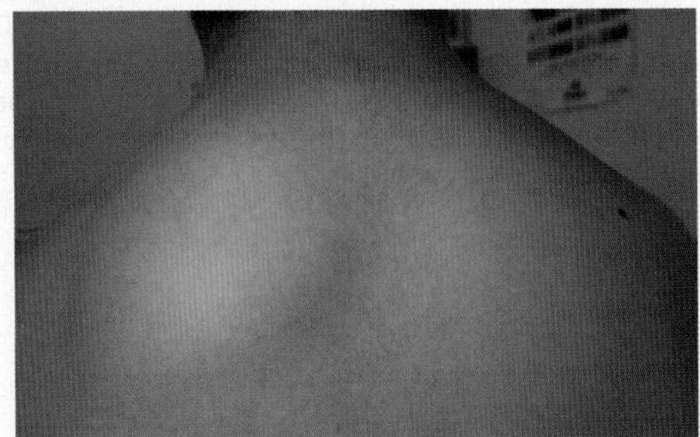

Lipomas are tumors composed of fat cells that are commonly located on the back of the neck, torso, arms, and legs. Although benign, some varieties are painful. Lipomas occur singly and multiply, and range in size.

Lentigo

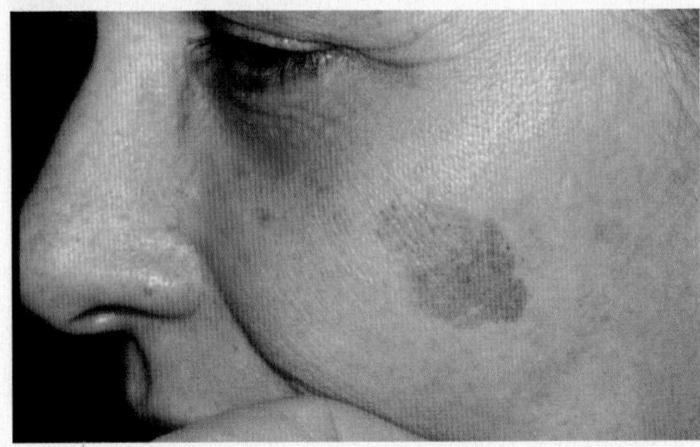

Lentigines are benign, acquired, circumscribed, pigmented macules found generally on sun-exposed skin.

Actinic Keratosis

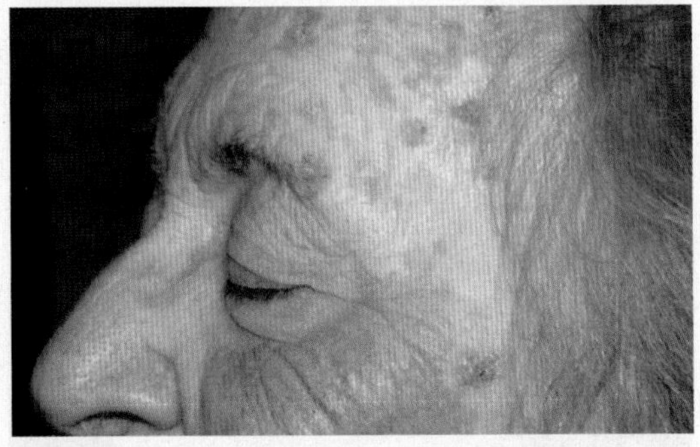

Also commonly called solar keratosis, they usually are found on sun-exposed skin and are thought to result from UV damage. These macular or papular lesions are discrete, with a rough or scaly surface.

Basal Cell Carcinoma

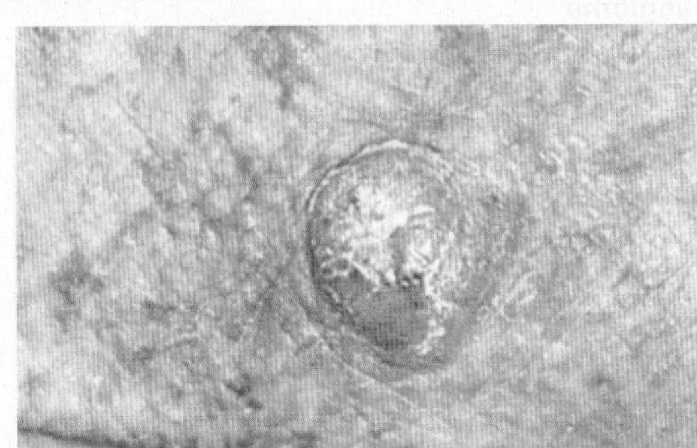

This nodular or popular lesion appears shiny with a rolled pearly border; it typically has telangiectases (small spider veins) on its surface. This skin cancer grows slowly and rarely metastasizes.

(table continues on page 280)

TABLE 11.16 Skin Tumors and Growths *(continued)*

Squamous Cell Carcinoma

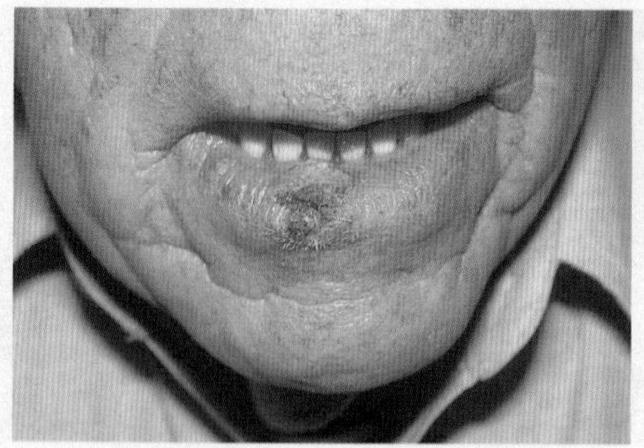

The second most frequently found skin cancer is related to actinic keratosis and sun exposure. Lesions are typically papular, nodular, or plaques located on sun-exposed skin surfaces.

Kaposi Sarcoma

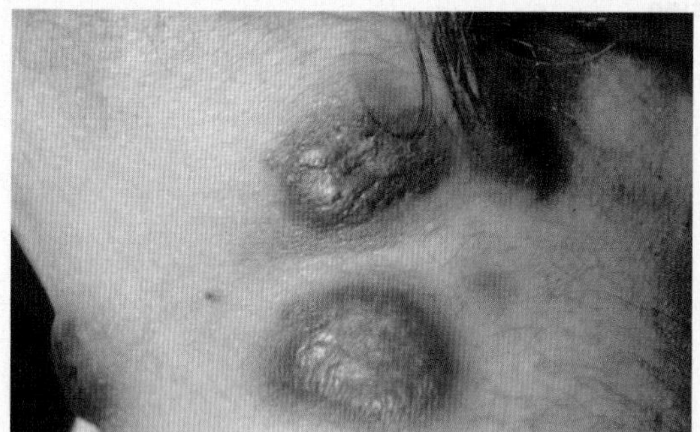

This opportunistic skin infection is a consequence of impaired immune status, such as associated with AIDS. Lesions generally occur on the nose, penis, and extremities, although with advanced HIV, distribution may be more generalized. Improved immune status may cause resolution.

Melanoma

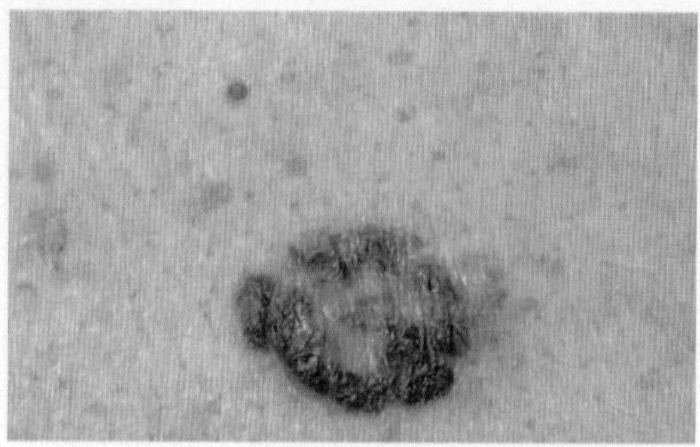

Malignant melanoma is identified by the ABCDEs of skin cancer detection

TABLE 11.17 Common Vascular Lesions

Hemangioma

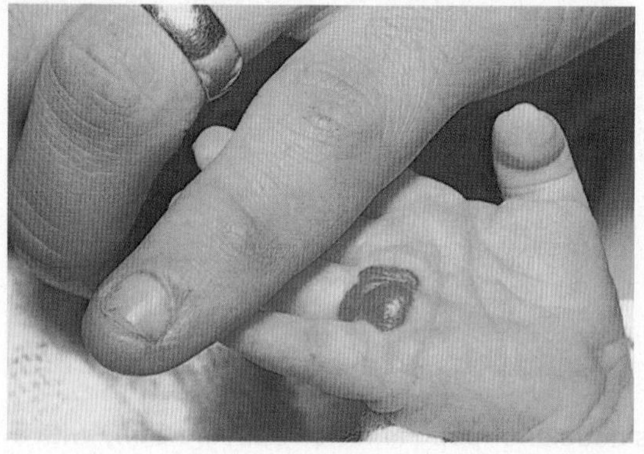

These vascular lesions, present at birth, rapidly develop and grow but spontaneously resolve by age 9 years. Made up of endothelial cells that form caverns and fill with blood, they blanch with applied pressure.

Nevus Flammeus (Port Wine Stain)

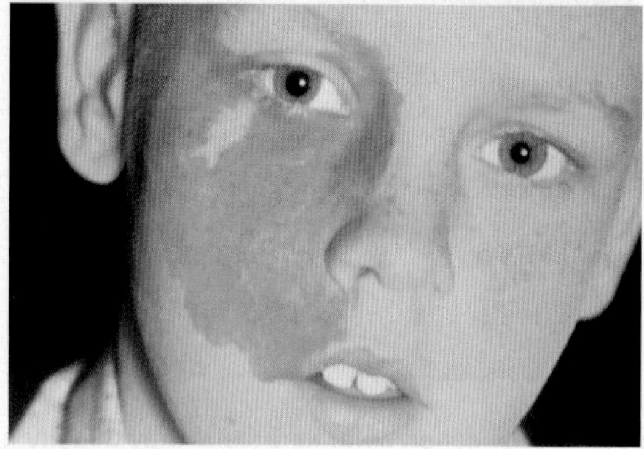

Malformation of superficial dermal blood vessels is present at birth. The lesion grows with the child and never resolves on its own.

(table continues on page 281)

TABLE 11-17 Common Vascular Lesions *(continued)*

Spider or Star Angioma

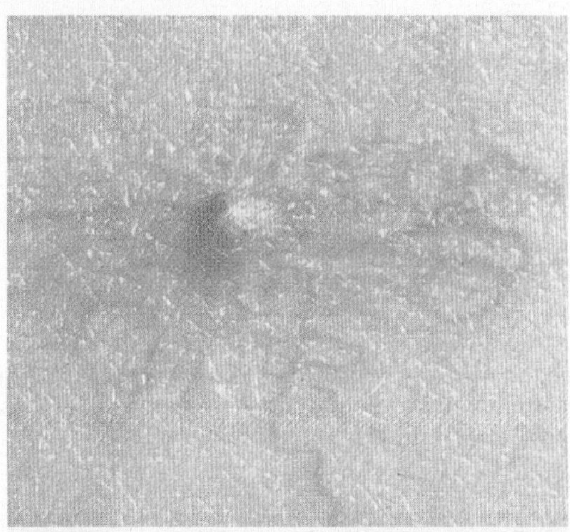

This vascular lesion arises from a central dermal arteriole with multiple extensions forming the appearance of spider legs. Distribution can be anywhere but is commonly found on the face, arms, and torso.

Venous Lake

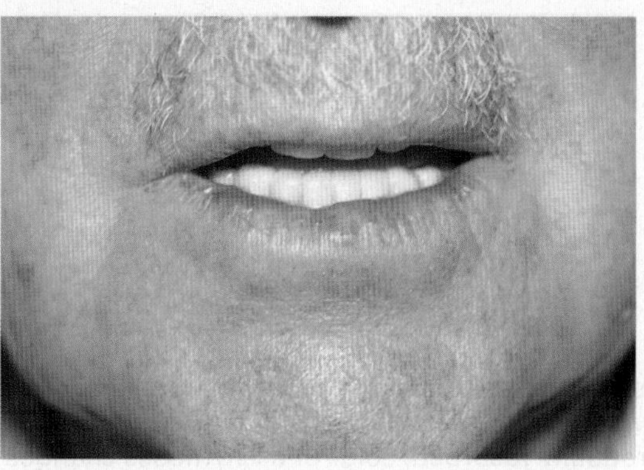

This papular bluish-to-purple lesion blanches on pressure and is generally found on the face, especially on the lips or ears. It is benign and often associated with sun exposure.

TABLE 11.18 Acute Wounds and Lesions From Trauma

Petechiae

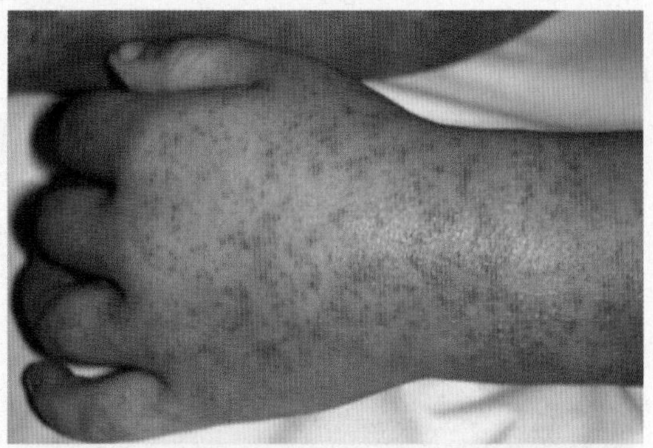

These small reddish to purple macules or papules can develop anywhere on the body in response to physical trauma.

Purpura

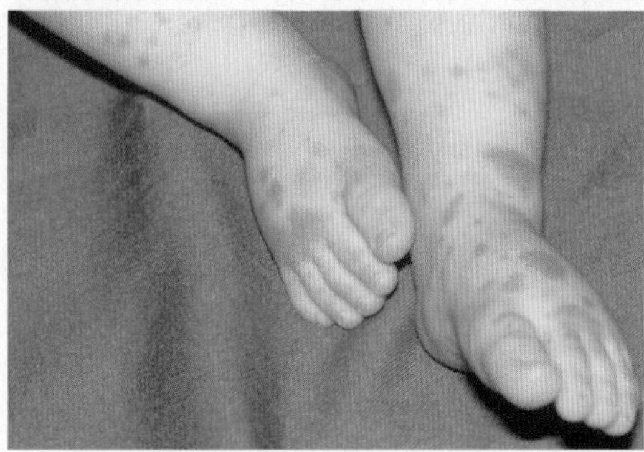

Purplish macules or papules result from bleeding under the skin secondary to inadequate clotting mechanisms.

(table continues on page 282)

TABLE 11.18 Acute Wounds and Lesions From Trauma *(continued)*

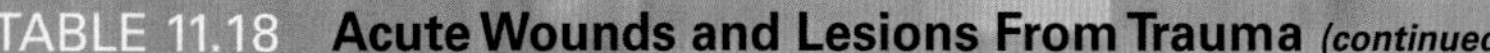

Ecchymosis

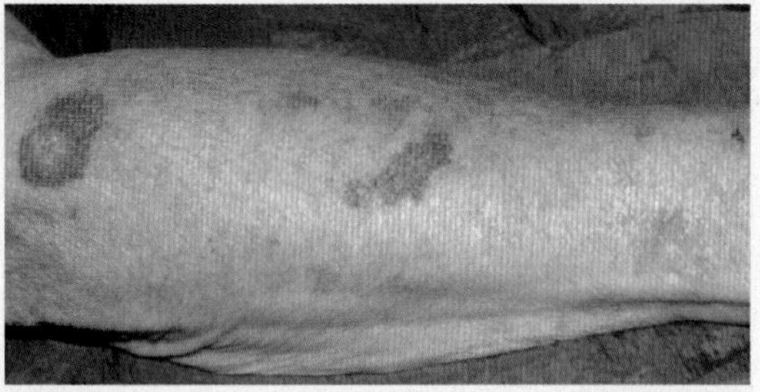

Physical trauma to the skin damages capillaries and allows blood to seep into surrounding tissues. As blood is gradually resorbed, color of ecchymoses changes and may be purple, blue, green, yellow, or brown.

Hematoma

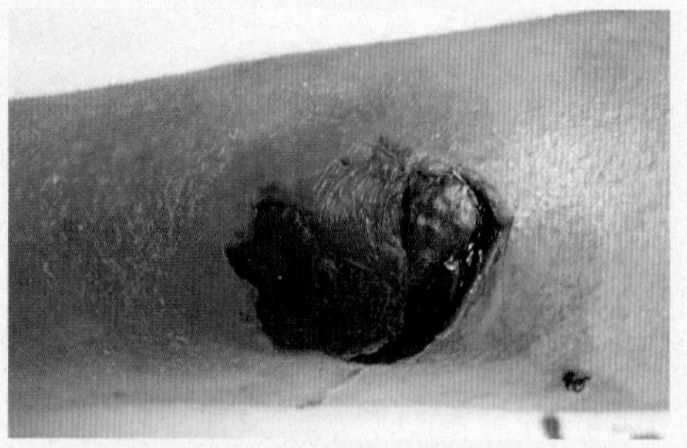

Collection of blood under the skin usually results from blunt-force trauma. Hematomas are palpable lesions, and coloration mimics that of ecchymoses.

Laceration

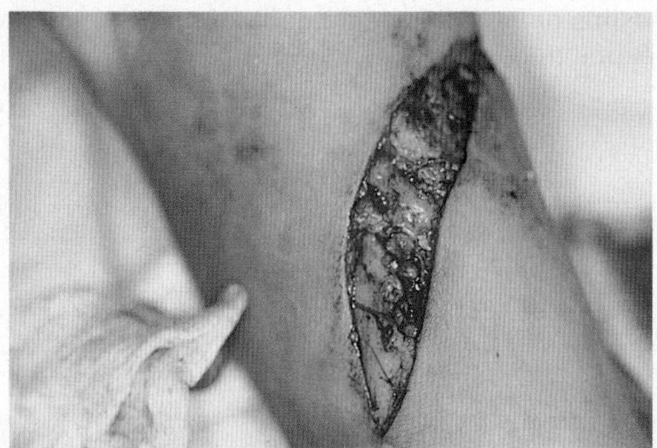

Tears in the skin can be superficial or deep, short or long, and frequently require suturing to heal correctly.

Abrasions

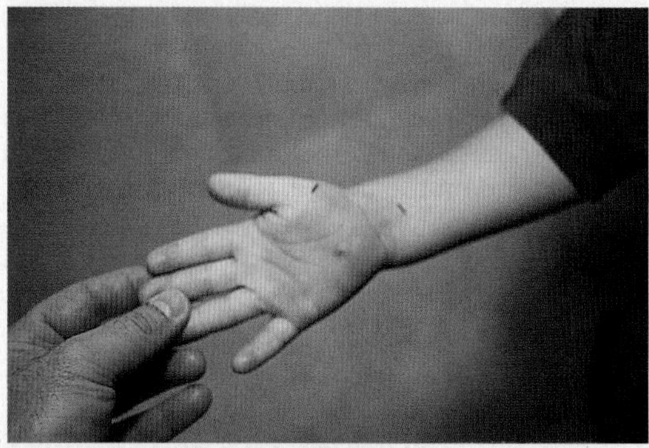

Abrasions are caused by shear force or friction against the skin, removing several layers and exposing the dermis.

Puncture Wound

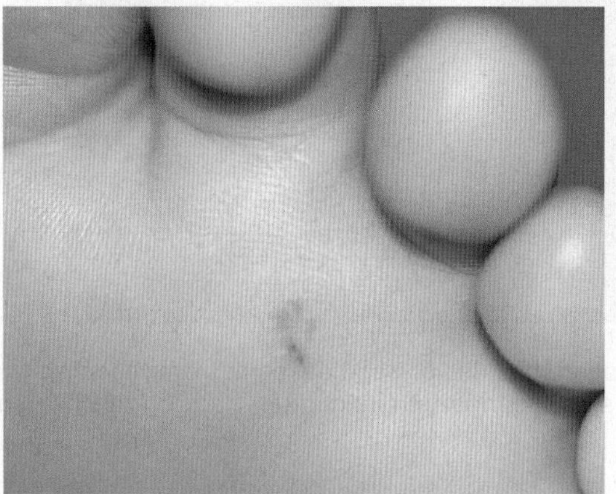

A sharp object pierces the skin, causing a wound with greater depth than width.

Avulsion

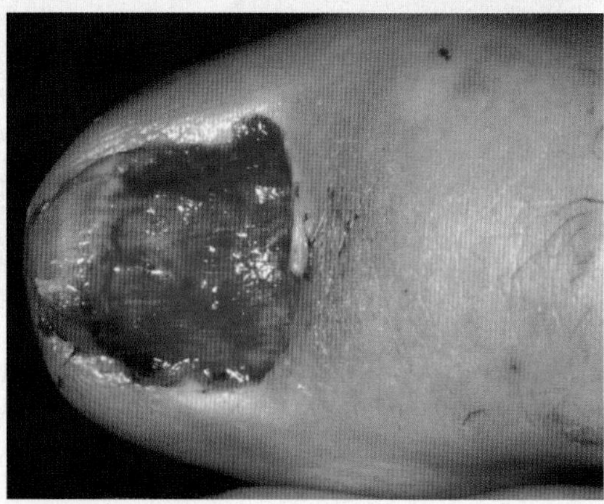

Trauma forces the skin to separate from underlying structures, leaving an open ragged wound.

TABLE 11.19 Pressure Ulcers

Stage I

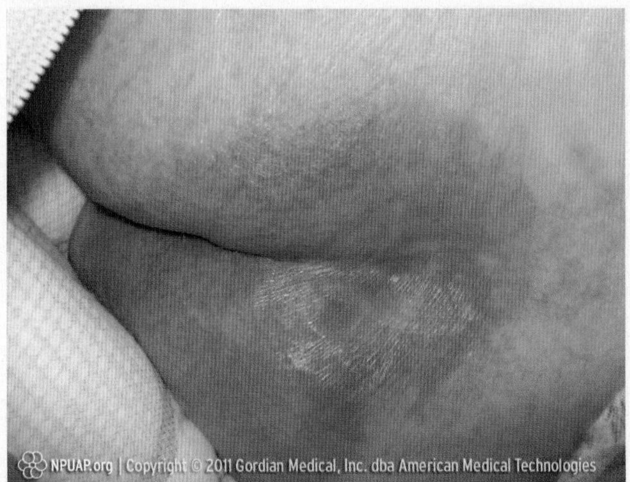

Intact skin with nonblanchable redness of a localized area, usually over a bony prominence. Darkly pigmented skin may not have visible blanching; its color may differ from the surrounding area. The area may be painful, firm, soft, warmer, or cooler as compared with adjacent tissue. Stage I may be difficult to detect in people with dark skin. May indicate "at risk" people (a heralding sign of risk).

Stage II

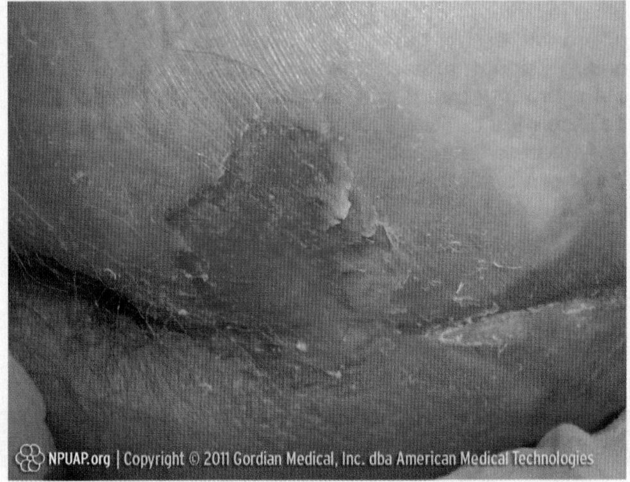

Partial-thickness loss of dermis presenting as a shallow open ulcer with a reddish pink wound bed, without slough. May also present as an intact or open/ruptured serum-filled blister. Presents as a shiny or dry shallow ulcer without slough or bruising (indicates suspected deep tissue injury). This stage should not be used to describe skin tears, tape burns, perineal dermatitis, maceration, or excoriation.

Stage III

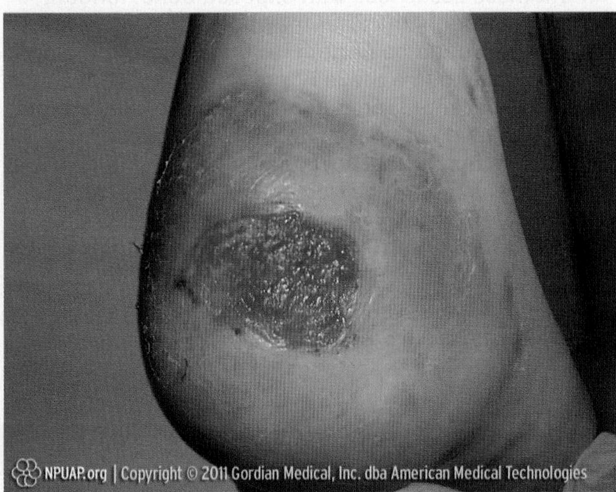

Full-thickness tissue loss. Subcutaneous fat may be visible, but bone, tendon, or muscle is not exposed. Slough may be present but does not obscure the depth of tissue loss. May include undermining and tunneling. The depth of a stage III pressure ulcer varies by anatomical location. The bridge of the nose, ear, occiput, and malleolus do not have subcutaneous tissue; stage III ulcers can be shallow. In contrast, areas of significant adiposity can develop extremely deep Stage III pressure ulcers. Bone/tendon is not visible or directly palpable.

(table continues on page 284)

TABLE 11.19 Pressure Ulcers *(continued)*

Stage IV

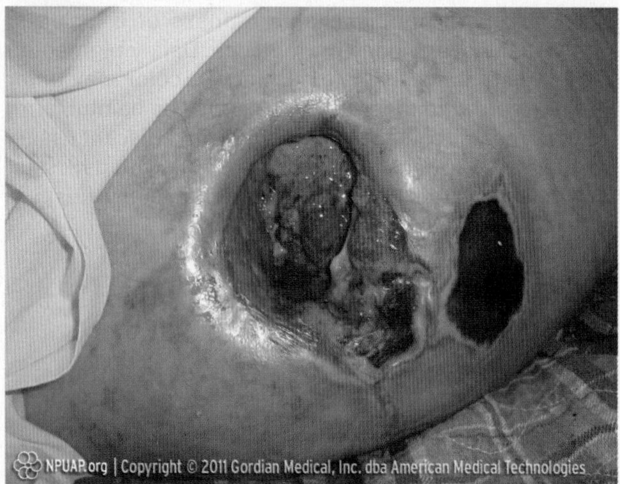

Full-thickness tissue loss with exposed bone, tendon, or muscle. Slough or eschar may be present on some parts of the wound bed. Often include undermining and tunneling. Depth of a Stage IV pressure ulcer varies by anatomical location. The bridge of the nose, ear, occiput, and malleolus do not have subcutaneous tissue so these ulcers may be shallow. Stage IV ulcers can extend into muscle, supporting structures (e.g., fascia, tendon, joint capsule), or both, making osteomyelitis possible. Exposed bone/tendon is visible or directly palpable.

Unstageable

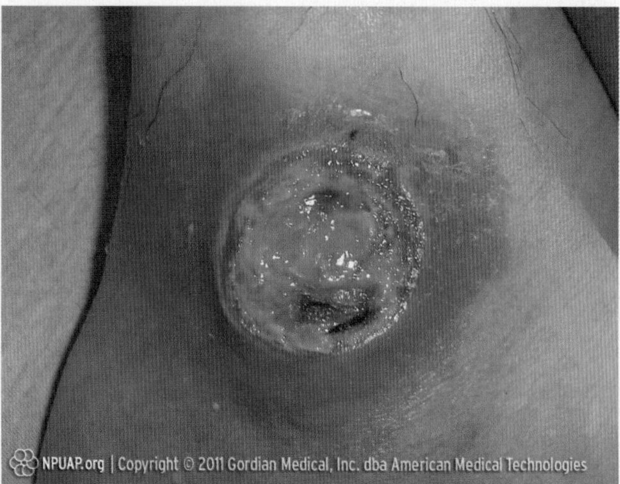

Full-thickness tissue loss in which the base of the ulcer is covered by slough (yellow, tan, gray, green, or brown), eschar (tan, brown, or black), or both. Until enough slough or eschar is removed to expose the base of the wound, true depth, and therefore stage, cannot be determined. Stable (dry, adherent, intact without erythema or fluctuance) eschar on the heels serves as "the body's natural (biological) cover" and should not be removed.

From National Pressure Ulcer Advisory Panel. (2007). *Updated staging system.* Retrieved, from http://www.npuap.org/pr2.htm

TABLE 11.20 Nonpressure Ulcers

Neuropathic Ulcer

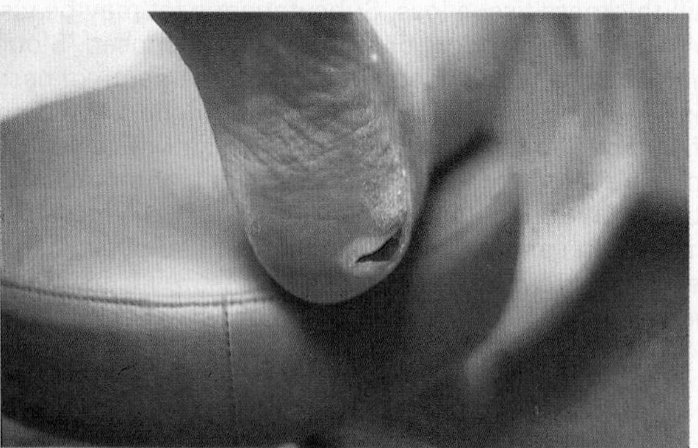

Loss of sensation in an extremity impairs the patient's ability to detect pressure on the feet. Sustained pressure or friction results in lost skin surface, which often remains unnoticed because the patient is not detecting pain. Diabetes mellitus is a common cause of this type of ulcer. Use the Wagner classification to determine grade (severity).

Venous Ulcers (Vascular)

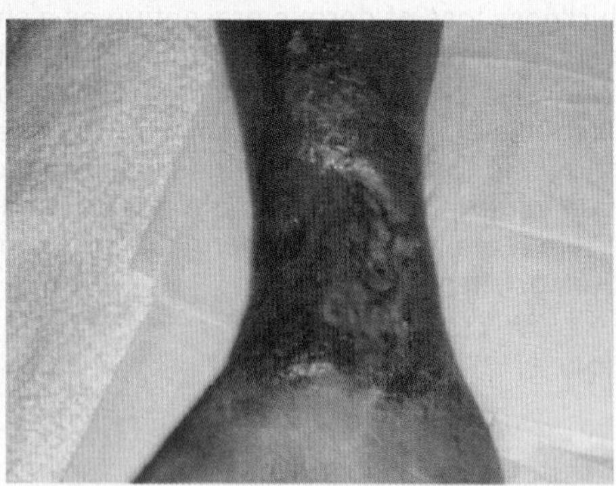

Venous ulcers develop from chronic pooling of blood in the extremity. See Chapter 18. Venous ulcers usually occur between ankle and knee in a "gaiter" distribution. Wound edges are ragged and irregular; the base is beefy red with evident granulation tissue with profuse exudation. Some ulcers can be deep. These ulcers are generally painless. The surrounding tissue commonly is hyperpigmented.

(table continues on page 285)

TABLE 11.20 Nonpressure Ulcers *(continued)*

Arterial Ulcer (Vascular)

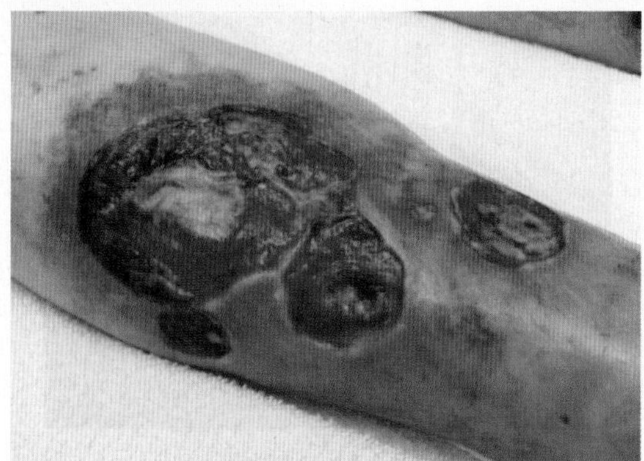

Arterial ulcers result from chronic ischemia as a consequence of impaired arterial circulation to an extremity. See Chapter 18. Arterial ulcers are usually located distally, such as at the ends of the toes or fingers. Wound edges are sharply defined; the base is pale when elevated and appears ruddy when dependent. These ulcers may be deep, frequently infected, and painful; they exhibit minimal granulation tissue.

TABLE 11.21 Nail Findings

Longitudinal Ridging

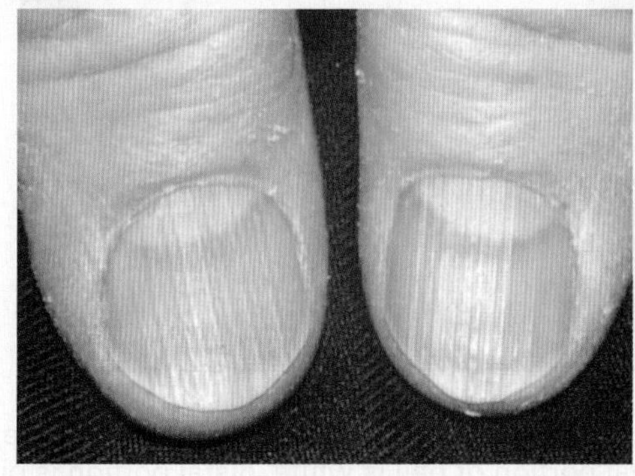

Normal variation, especially in elderly. Common cause is normal aging.

Onycholysis

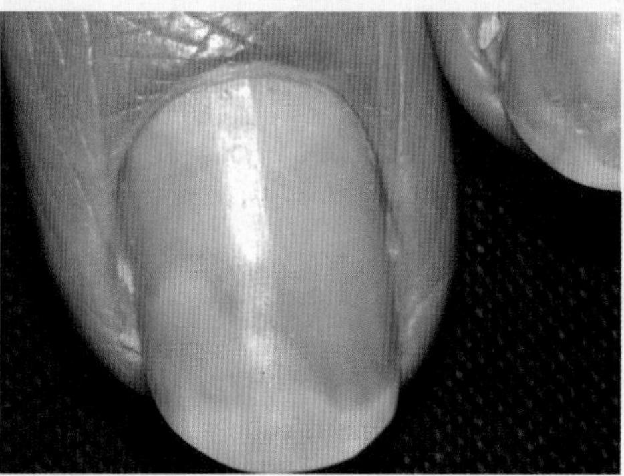

Separation of a portion of the nail plate from the nail bed; results in opacity to the affected part of the nail, appearing white to yellow to green. Common causes include trauma, fungal infections, topical irritants, psoriasis, and subungual neoplasms or warts.

Koilonychia (Spoon Nails)

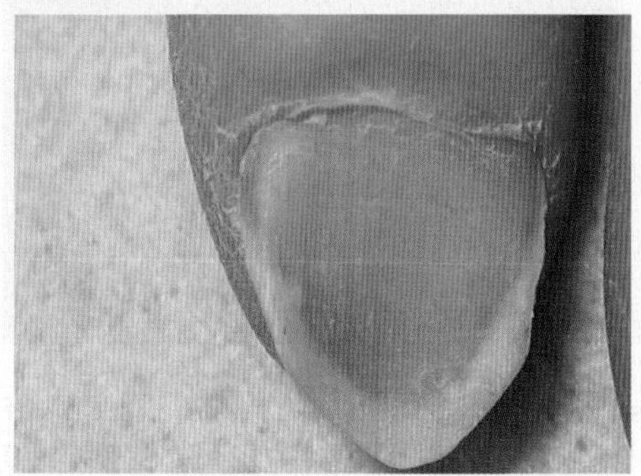

Transverse and longitudinal concavity of the nail, giving the appearance of a spoon. May be normal in infants (usually resolves in few months). Other causes include trauma, iron-deficiency anemia, and hemochromatosis.

Pitted Nails

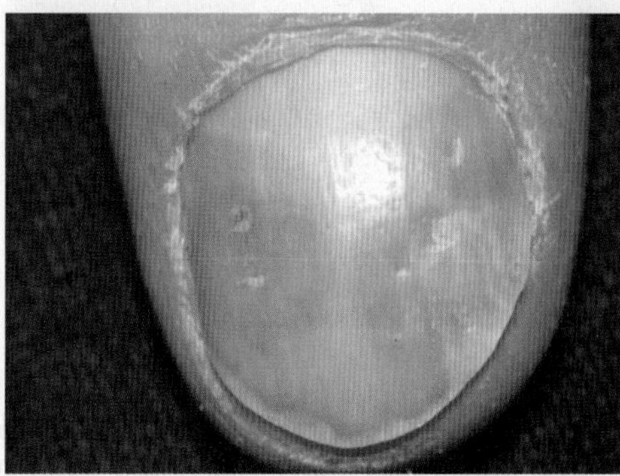

Lesions from psoriasis; arise from nail matrix that causes pitting on the nail plate as it grows

(table continues on page 286)

Beau Lines

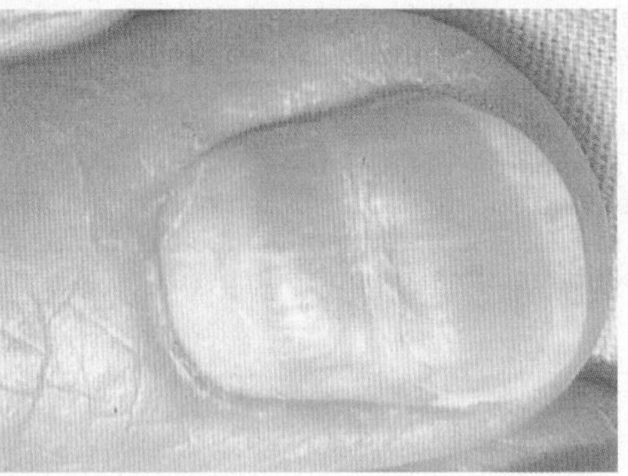

Results from slowed or halted nail growth in response to illness, physical trauma, or poisoning.

Clubbing

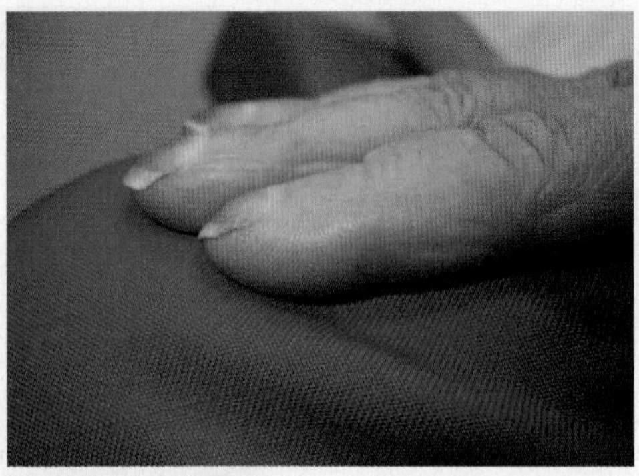

Results from chronic hypoxia to distal fingers, such as in emphysema or congestive heart failure.

Yellow Nails

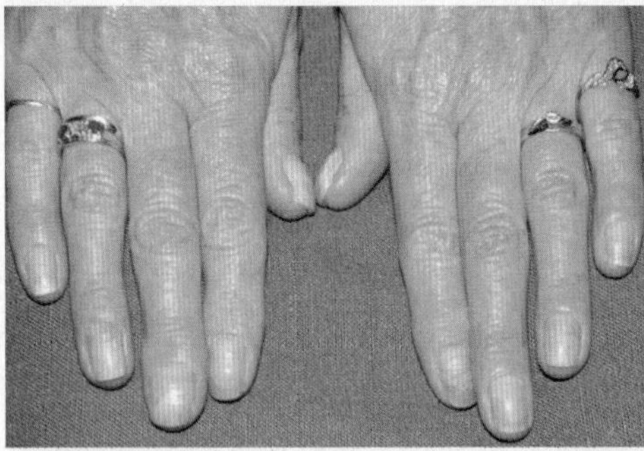

Slowly growing nail, without cuticle, and onycholysis resulting in thickening of nail and yellowish appearance. Causes include lung disorders and lymphedema.

Half-and-half Nails

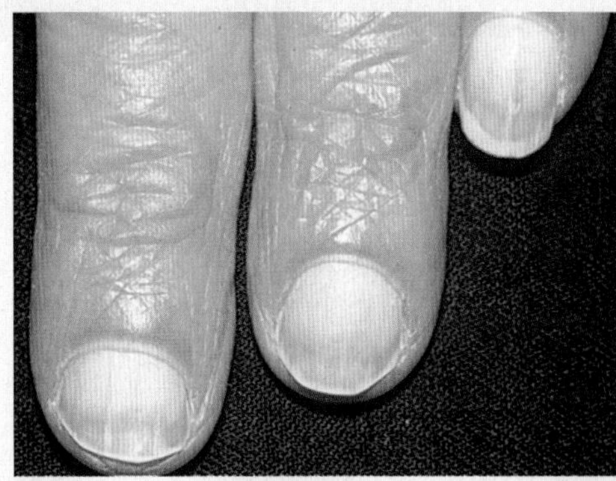

Color changes associated with chronic renal failure; proximal portion of nail is white, distal portion is pink or brown

Dark Longitudinal Streaks

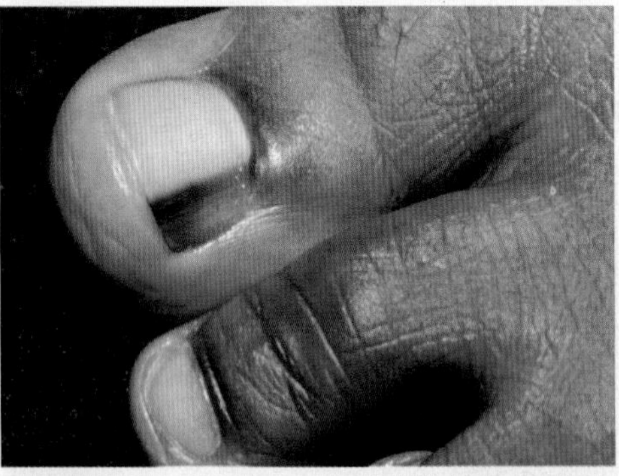

Often a normal variant in dark-skinned patients from junctional nevus of nail matrix. Suspicious for malignancy if the streaks blur, spread, or are not solid the full length of the nail.

Splinter Hemorrhages

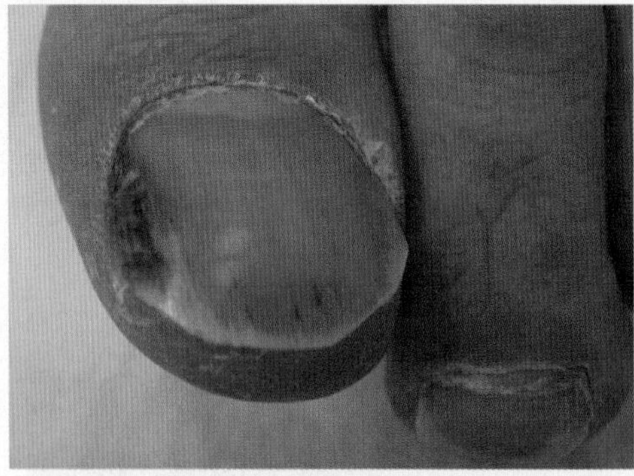

Brownish red longitudinal lines in the direction of nail growth that result from damage to capillaries (e.g., endocarditis, vasculitis, antiphospholipid syndrome) supplying the nail matrix caused by microemboli.

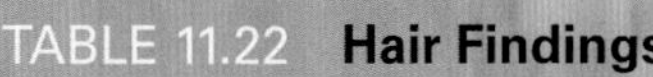

TABLE 11.22 Hair Findings

Alopecia Areata

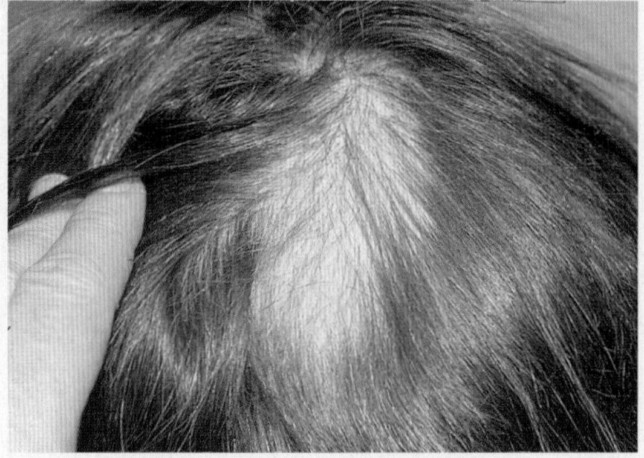

This autoimmune disorder results in noninflammatory loss of hair in a circumscribed distribution.

Hirsutism

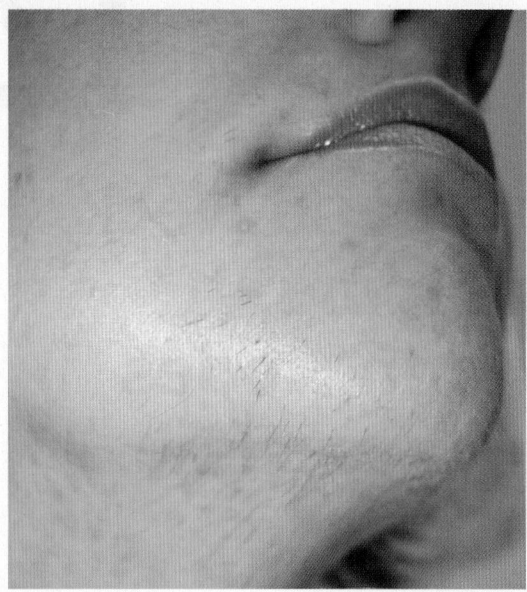

Excessive androgenic hormones in a female patient can cause masculinization changes including hair in male distribution patterns (i. e., beard, chest, back, upper thighs).

Traction Alopecia

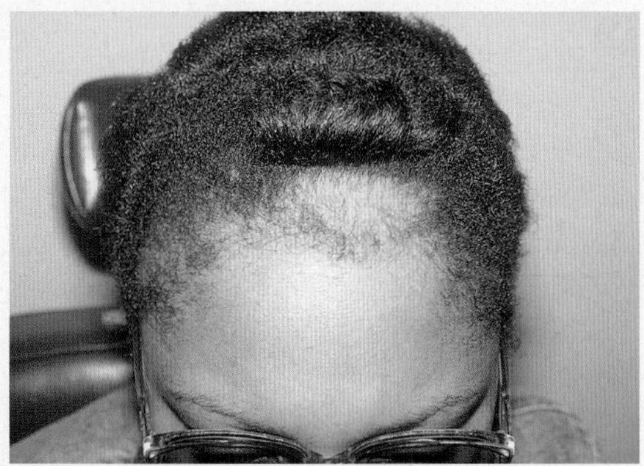

Tight hair braiding practices exert traction force on the hair bulb with subsequent hair loss.

Trichotillomania

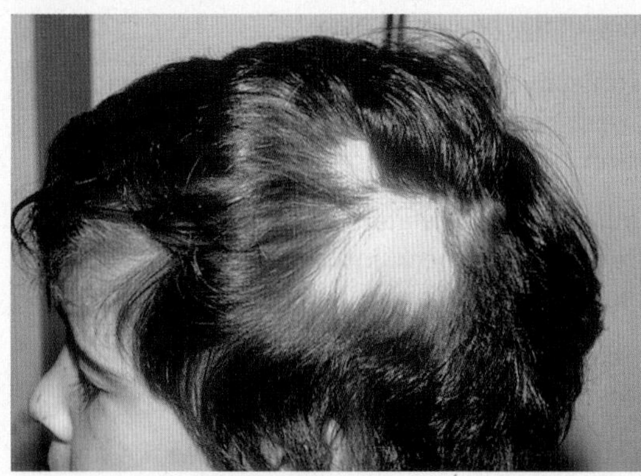

Compulsive hair pulling causes breakage of hair and thinned or balding areas on scalp, although some hair remains present and visible in the affected area.

12

Head and Neck, Including Lymph Nodes and Vessels

Learning Objectives

1 Demonstrate knowledge of anatomy and physiology of the head, neck, and associated lymphatics.

2 Identify important topics for health promotion and risk reduction related to the cranium, thyroid, and lymphatics of the head and neck.

3 Collect subjective data related to headache, head trauma, neck pain, neck masses, and thyroid dysfunction.

4 Collect objective data related to the scalp, cranium, facial structures, and neck, including lymphatics and thyroid, using physical examination techniques.

5 Identify expected and unexpected findings from inspection and palpation of the head and neck.

6 Analyze subjective and objective data from the head and neck assessment using appropriate medical terminology and principles of recording.

7 Document findings from head and neck examinations using appropriate terminology.

8 Consider age, gender, genetic background, and culture of the patient to individualize the head and neck assessment.

9 Identify nursing diagnoses and initiate a plan of care based on findings from the head and neck assessment.

Faye Davis-Pierce, 21 years old, is visiting her college clinic for the first time. She reports fatigue and a weight gain of about 9 kg (20 lb) over the past 3 months. She is also concerned because her hair has been falling out. Her temperature is 36.8°C (98°F) orally, pulse 64 beats/min, respirations 12 breaths/min, and blood pressure 98/66 mmHg. Her height is 1.72 m (5 ft 8 in.), her weight is 94 kg (208 lb), and her body mass index is 31.6 (which indicates that she is obese). Faye's current medications include an oral contraceptive and a multivitamin.

You will gain more information about Faye as you progress through this chapter. As you study the content and features, consider Faye's case and its relationship to what you are learning. Begin thinking about the following points:

- What are the signs and symptoms of hypothyroidism?
- How do the symptoms and signs of hypothyroidism and hyperthyroidism differ?
- What other physical findings might be present, and what other body systems might be involved?
- How might Faye's physical issues relate to her psychosocial health, including potential issues related to her age and status as a college student?
- What type of follow-up care and reassessment might the patient need at subsequent visits?
- How will you evaluate Faye's understanding of her diagnosis and determine any additional needed teaching?

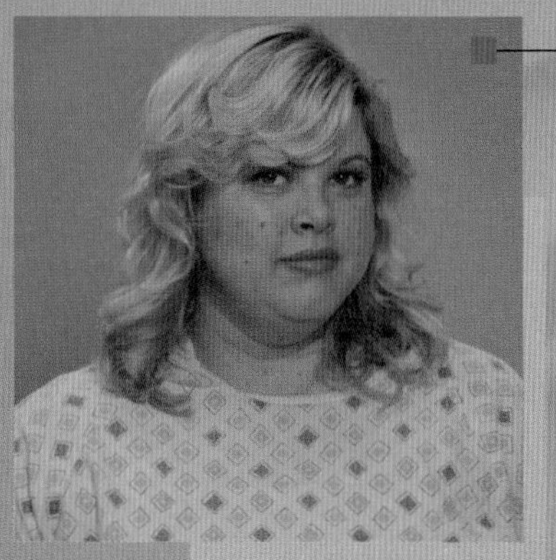

This chapter describes assessment of the head and neck regions, which include the scalp, cranium, lymphatic system, parathyroid glands, and thyroid gland. It explores pertinent anatomy and physiology as well as variations based on age, gender, and culture. Methods for collecting subjective and objective data related to cranium or scalp injury, lymphatic function, and thyroid function are included. Other key components of the chapter include the signs and symptoms of headache, lymphadenopathy, and parathyroid and thyroid imbalances; correct techniques for inspection and palpation of the structures of the head and neck; and descriptions of common normal and unexpected findings.

Structure and Function

Structures of the head and neck interact with multiple body systems—integumentary, neurological, musculoskeletal, respiratory, vascular, gastrointestinal, lymphatic, and endocrine.

The Head

Skeletal Structure

The head includes the cranium and facial skeleton, which together encompass 22 bones that support and contain soft tissue organs, including the eyes (see Chapter 13), ears (see Chapter 14), and brain (see Chapter 22).

The bones of the **cranium** are the frontal, parietal, occipital, and temporal (Fig. 12.1). **Sutures** join these bones together. The major sutures are the coronal, which crosses the top of the scalp from ear to ear; the sagittal, which crosses the cranium from anterior to posterior; and the lambdoidal, which separates the parietal and occipital bones. In the fetus, these sutures are not tightly joined; this allows the cranium to mold and pass through the maternal birth canal more easily. The sutures remain somewhat loose during infancy to facilitate growth of the head and brain; they knit together by approximately 12 to 18 months. See Table 12.3 at the end of the chapter for abnormal conditions common in children.

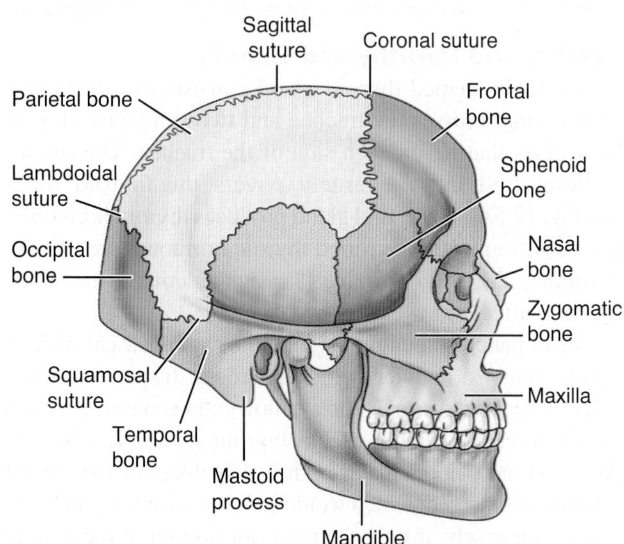

Figure 12.1 Bones and sutures of the cranium.

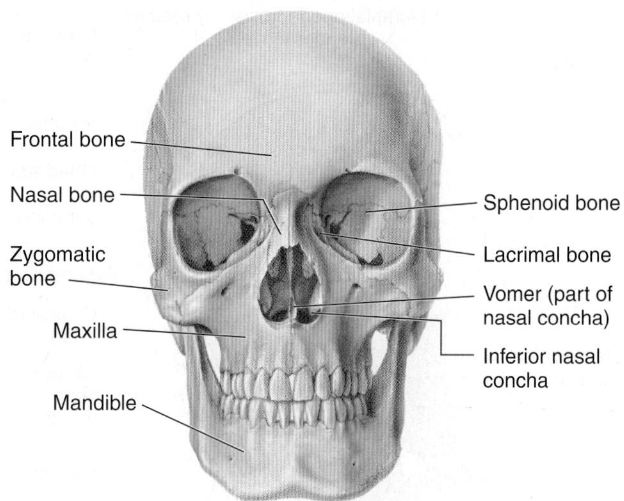

Figure 12.2 The facial bones.

When documenting the physical assessment, the nurse must take care to describe the location of scalp or cranium findings according to the bones and sutures (Ellis, 2010). The largest facial bones are the **maxilla**, **mandible**, nasal, lacrimal, and vomer (Fig. 12.2). The mastoid process—part of the temporal bone—has particular relevance during assessment of the ear.

Muscles

The major facial muscles are the frontalis, temporalis, zygomaticus, masseter, buccinators, orbicularis oculi, and orbicularis oris.

> **Clinical Significance**
>
> The major facial muscles and other smaller muscles enable chewing, speaking, smiling, and frowning (Fig. 12.3).

Blood Supply

Blood is supplied to the head through the carotid arteries, which split into the internal and external branches. The temporal artery is a branch of the external carotid artery that supplies the face. The veins are the external and internal jugular. See Chapter 17 for further information.

Nerve Supply

Cranial nerve (CN) V—the trigeminal nerve—supplies both motor and sensory innervations to the forehead, cheeks, and chin. See Chapter 22 for further information.

Salivary Glands

There are three pairs of **salivary glands**. The parotid glands are in the cheek anterior to the bottom half of the ear. The submandibular glands are at the angle of the jaw below the mandible. The sublingual glands are in the mouth and under the tongue. See Chapter 15 for further information.

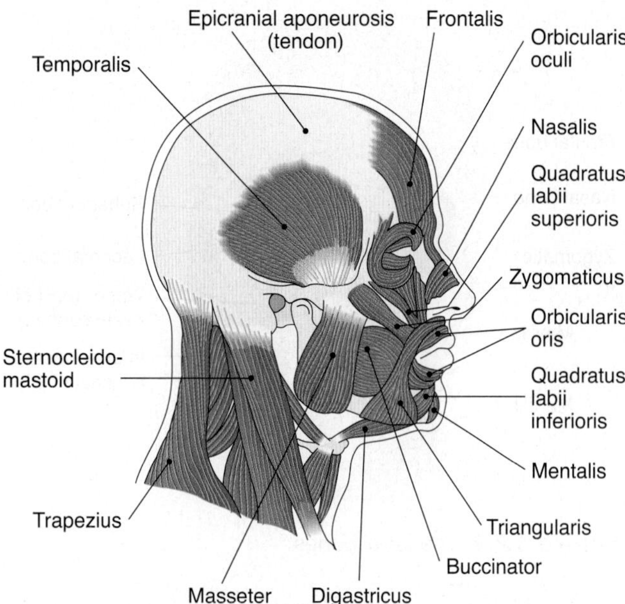

Figure 12.3 The facial muscles. The **anterior triangle** is between the sternocleidomastoid and midline of the neck. The **posterior triangle** is between the sternocleidomastoid and the trapezius.

The Neck

The neck is supported by the cervical vertebrae, C1–C7. A useful neck landmark is the vertebral prominence, which is the spinous process of C7, the longest cervical vertebrae (Ellis, 2010). Of the vertebrae of the neck, C7 and T1 are usually the most easily palpable; C7 protrudes the farthest (Fig. 12.4). Locating C7 during assessment of the head, neck, and posterior thorax facilitates a more accurate description of findings.

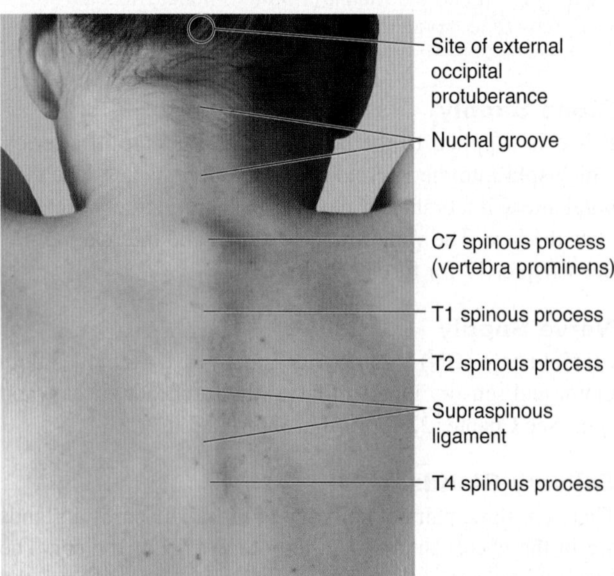

Figure 12.4 Posterior surface anatomy of the neck. Note the location of C7.

> **SAFETY ALERT**
> *Falls or sudden jerking of the head and neck (whiplash) are particularly likely to result in dislocation of the cervical vertebrae. Fractures also may occur with head-first falls. Any history of falls or sudden jerks of the neck requires careful investigation.*

The major neck muscles are the sternocleidomastoid and the trapezius. The **sternocleidomastoid muscle** arises from the sternum and medial clavicle and extends to behind the ear. The **trapezius muscle** arises from the occipital bone and vertebra and fans out to the clavicle and scapula.

> **Clinical Significance**
> The major neck muscles may be used as accessory muscles of respiration when the patient has difficulty breathing.

Trachea

The trachea passes down the midline of the neck and is part of the upper respiratory system (see Chapter 16). Important landmarks for the head and neck region are in the tracheal area (Fig. 12.5). The usually palpable U-shaped hyoid bone is located midline just beneath the mandible. The large thyroid cartilage consists of two flat, platelike structures joined together at an angle and with a small, sometimes palpable notch at the superior edge. Usually more prominent in males, the thyroid cartilage is also called the "Adam's apple." The palpable cricoid cartilage is a ringed structure just inferior to the thyroid cartilage. The thyroid isthmus crosses the trachea just below the cricoid cartilage.

> **Clinical Significance**
> Palpation of the thyroid gland reveals important landmarks of the trachea. Such landmarks are noted when assessing for tracheal deviation, which accompanies a potentially life-threatening condition called *tension pneumothorax* (see Chapter 16).

Thyroid and Parathyroid Glands

The butterfly-shaped thyroid gland consists of a band (the isthmus) that crosses the trachea and two symmetrical 3- to 4-cm lobes that lie on each side of the trachea. The sternocleidomastoid muscle largely covers the thyroid lobes (see Fig. 12.5). The thyroid gland produces thyroid hormones. The most frequently measured thyroid hormones are triiodothyronine (T_3), and thyroxine (T_4), which control metabolic rates and affect almost every body system.

In all patients, the thyroid should be symmetrical without discrete masses, nodularity, or tenderness. Inspection of the patient's neck while he or she swallows can sometimes reveal up-and-down movement of the thyroid gland. The thyroid gland is usually not palpable; if it *is* palpable, this means that the gland is enlarged, which would indicate a pathological condition. Conversely, if only the posterior portion of the thyroid gland is enlarged, it may not be palpable. Nurses must take care

Internal carotid artery
Thyroid cartilage
Sternocleidomastoid (SCM)
Cricoid cartilage
Trapezius
External jugular vein (EJV)
Trachea
Mandible
Hyoid bone
Thyroid gland
External jugular vein
Common carotid artery
Left vagus nerve
Internal jugular vein (IJV)
Deep cervical lymph node
Thoracic duct
Subclavian vein
Thyroid gland

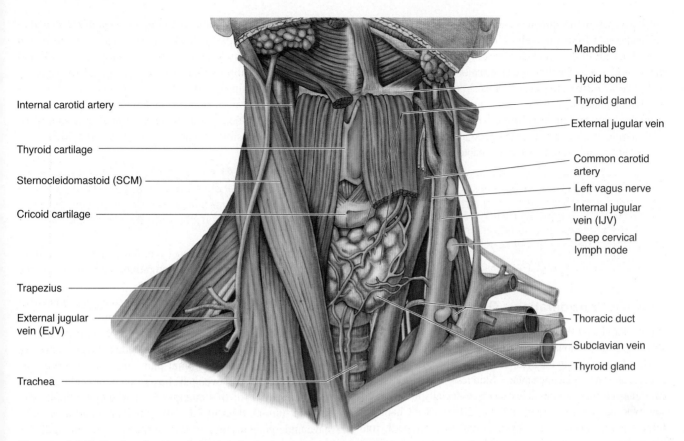

Figure 12.5 Key head and neck landmarks in the region of the trachea.

to gather thorough data in history taking that may identify symptoms of hypothyroid or hyperthyroid function, even in the absence of an enlarged thyroid gland (McDermott, 2012).

Two pairs of parathyroid glands are embedded in the thyroid lobes and produce the hormone calcitonin, which helps move calcium into bones. The parathyroid glands are usually not palpable.

Lymphatics

The major chains of **lymph nodes** in the neck are the preauricular, posterior auricular, occipital, superficial cervical (extending from the tonsillar to supraclavicular nodes), deep cervical, posterior cervical, submental, and submandibular (Fig. 12.6A). Approximately 80 lymph nodes are in the head and neck region,

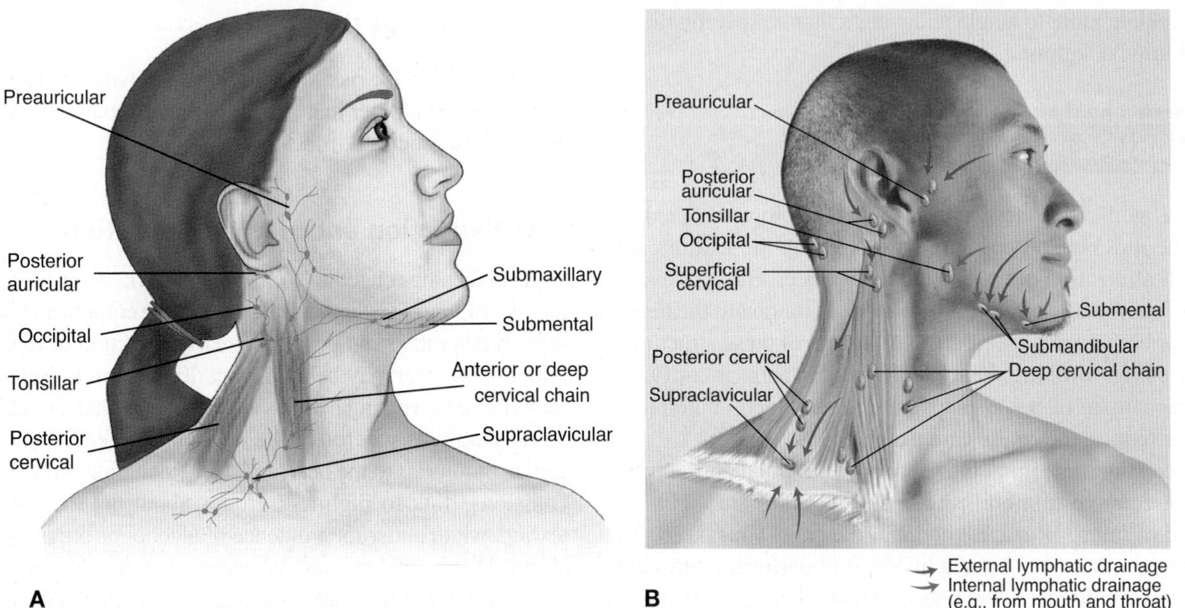

Figure 12.6 Lymphatic system of the head and neck. **A.** Major chains of lymph nodes in the neck. **B.** Direction of lymphatic flow and drainage.

serving as part of the immune system. These vessels filter potential pathogens from the body. They also drain fluid that has moved outside of the circulation back into the vessels. There are many more nodes than those of the major chains listed earlier, and some are difficult to palpate (Drake, Vogl, & Mitchell, 2010). The lymph nodes are named for their anatomical locations. They drain fluid along a path in a chain and have a particular direction of flow (Fig. 12.6B). An enlarged node indicates inflammation that is "upstream" from it. See also Chapters 17 and 18.

Clinical Significance

It is important to understand the drainage patterns of the lymphatics because enlargement of a node may be a sign of pathology that is not directly adjacent to that node.

Lifespan Considerations: Older Adults

With aging, facial subcutaneous fat decreases, making the bony structure more pronounced. Skin may sag and wrinkle across the forehead, surrounding the eyes, at the tip of the nose, and on the cheeks, altering facial appearance. Skin lesions are more likely; careful assessment for possible cancers, especially in commonly sun-exposed areas, is important (Ellis, 2010). (See Chapter 11 for further information.) Both hypothyroidism and hyperthyroidism occur more frequently in the elderly, with hypothyroidism the more common condition, affecting 10% to 16% of adults ages 65 to 74 years (Papaleontiou & Haymart, 2012). Thus, elderly patients should be evaluated for thyroid dysfunction.

Cultural Considerations

The most noticeable difference among racial groups is skin color. Shape of the eyes, nose, and lips also varies based on background and genetics. Variations in cranium or neck shape or size relate more to height and weight than to specific racial or cultural background.

Urgent Assessment

Patients with acute head injuries and neurological changes must be quickly and accurately assessed by the health care team. Stabilization of the head and neck is essential to avoid further neurological injury. Any history of trauma to the head, neck, or both warrants a careful assessment of these structures for bleeding, swelling, loss of mobility, or pain. Identifying the mechanism of injury helps determine which anatomical regions require the health care team's focus.

Keep the spine immobilized to prevent spinal cord injury. Do not remove immobilization devices until the spine is cleared of injury (Raza, Elkhodair, Zaheer, & Yousaf, 2013). It is critical that you obtain a history and perform a physical examination focused on neurological changes (Abrams, 2013). Note that the patient with a severe headache may be unable to provide a complete history.

Neck pain, a common symptom, is most often related to muscle tension or spasm. Neck pain associated with fever and headache may signify serious illness such as meningitis and should be carefully evaluated (see Chapter 22 for signs of conditions affecting the meninges). Patients experiencing a myocardial infarction may present with neck pain, so any patient with sudden onset of neck or jaw pain should be evaluated for possible cardiac etiologies (Swartz, 2010).

⚠ SAFETY ALERT

Patients may experience referred neck pain from myocardial infarction. If cardiac origin is suspected, focus assessments and interventions on the heart (see Chapter 17).

Lymph nodes larger than 1 cm, fixed, irregular, hard, or rubbery require emergency investigation. Such signs raise the possibility of cancer.

Hyperthyroidism may present as an emergency known as "thyroid storm" or "thyroid crisis," with symptoms of hypermetabolism in all systems. The most common sign is tachycardia, but other possibilities include tachypnea, nausea, vomiting, diarrhea, abdominal pain, anxiety, hyperkinesis, fever, weakness, and even psychosis, coma, or death. Patients at greatest risk for this emergency state include those with thyroid tumors, thyroid infection, or trauma and those who have undergone thyroid or other surgery (McDermott, 2012).

Acute bacterial thyroiditis is another emergency condition. Patients presenting with anterior neck swelling, pain, and fever must be evaluated carefully to determine whether the thyroid gland is acutely infected. Emergency referral is essential because the patient is at high risk for airway compromise as well as thyroid dysfunction (Paes et al., 2010).

Subjective Data

Assessment of Risk Factors

When assessing for risk factors associated with head and neck pathology, remember that multiple systems may influence the structure or function of these regions.

Risk Reduction and Health Promotion

Patient teaching related to the head and neck involves reducing the risk of injury to these areas, preventing complications from thyroid disorders, and promoting early detection of masses or lymph nodes that may be malignant. Emphasize to patients the importance of wearing helmets and the use of seatbelts and child safety restraints to protect the head and neck. Review other causes of injuries to the head and neck, including motor vehicle collisions. Talk to high-risk groups about not driving while texting, while under the influence of alcohol or drugs, or when sleepy. Discuss fall prevention, especially with older adults.

For women who are pregnant, review the need for regular examinations that include thyroid assessment. Such prenatal care helps to ensure that thyroid levels remain within

History and Risk Factors	Rationale
Personal History	
Have you ever had an accident that resulted in a head injury or loss of consciousness? Do you wear a seat belt? Do you wear a bicycle or motorcycle helmet? (Refer to Chapter 22 for more information.)	Head injuries are a major cause of disability, which can be permanent. They may be preventable with appropriate use of protective gear, such as a helmet. Nurses can promote use of appropriate safety equipment for patients across the lifespan.
Were you ever treated with radiation to the neck, chest, or back?	Before the 1950s, acne on the neck and upper thorax was sometimes treated with radiation therapy. Patients who received such treatment are at significantly increased risk for thyroid, parathyroid, and salivary gland malignancies (Swartz, 2010).
Have you had any surgeries involving your head or neck?	Because the head and neck have multiple structures, surgeries there may result in dysfunction of nerves, muscles, or vascular flow or in endocrine changes. Nurses should understand the specific procedure and assess for any functional changes that could occur.
Medications	
Do you take any regular medications? How much alcohol do you drink? Do you take any herbal products?	Many medications (e.g., bronchodilators, oral contraceptives) and alcohol can precipitate headaches. Some randomized studies have found acupuncture to be an effective treatment for migraine headaches, but other alternative and complementary therapies have not been adequately studied. Both butterbur and vitamin B_2 have been found to be effective in some randomized clinical trials (Nicholson, Buse, Andrasik, & Lipton, 2011). Patients may use alternative or herbal products for relief of symptoms such as headaches, but these potentially potent chemicals could actually cause headache and other neurological adverse effects. Patients should be encouraged to always tell their health care provider about any alternative, herbal, or natural therapies they are using for any and all conditions.
Family History	
Do you have a family history of thyroid difficulties? • Who had the illness? • Was it hypothyroidism or hyperthyroidism? • When did the person have it? • How was it treated? • What were the outcomes?	Graves disease, the most common type of hyperthyroidism, is an autoimmune disease that may also have genetic causes. Some evidence supports a genetic link for medullary thyroid cancer as well (McDermott, 2012).

normal limits, protecting both mother and fetus (Alamdari et al., 2013).

Risk factors for cancers of the neck include male gender, age over 50 years, tobacco use, and alcohol consumption (National Cancer Institute, 2013). For patients with such risk factors, emphasize teaching related to smoking prevention or cessation.

Health goals for the nation are wide and vary depending on the age and gender of the patient. The goals that are significant to the developed countries include the following:

- Reduce the occurrence of developmental disabilities.
- Reduce fatalities and hospitalizations from traumatic brain injuries and spinal cord injuries.
- Increase the proportion of bicyclists and motorcyclists using helmets.
- Reduce deaths caused by motor vehicle crashes (U.S. Department of Health & Human Services, 2013).

Common Symptoms

Common Head and Neck Symptoms

- Headache
- Neck pain
- Limited neck movement
- Facial pain
- Lumps or masses
- Hypothyroidism
- Hyperthyroidism
- Sleepiness

Signs/Symptoms	Rationale/Abnormal Findings
Headache Have you had any unusually frequent or severe headaches? • Where is the headache? Does it radiate? Is it on one or both sides? • Describe the headache. What does it feel like? • How bad is it on a scale from 1 to 10, with 10 being the worst? • When did it start? How long has it lasted? How often do you get headaches? Do you ever have milder headaches? Is a pattern evident? • What makes it worse? What makes it better? What brings it on? Is there a relationship with food or alcohol? With activity? With menstrual cycle? • Do any other symptoms accompany the pain, such as nausea, visual changes, or an aura? • Have you tried any treatments? How often do you take headache relievers or pain pills? Is it difficult to function without treatment? • Has there been any recent change in your headaches?	When taking history, pay attention to characteristics such as pain worse in the morning on awakening, precipitated or made worse by straining or sneezing (potentially elevated intracranial pressure), or worsening as the day progresses (more likely tension). A throbbing, severe, unilateral headache that lasts 6–24 hours and is associated with photophobia, nausea, and vomiting suggests migraine, whereas a constant, unremitting, general headache that is described as a feeling of a tight band around the head and lasts for days, weeks, or even months is usually characteristic of a tension muscle contraction headache. Headaches may be categorized as primary or secondary. Primary headaches are benign, often recurring, and not associated with underlying pathology. Secondary headaches are associated with underlying pathology that ranges from mild (e.g., common cold) to severe (e.g., subarachnoid hemorrhage, brain tumor, meningitis).
Neck Pain • Where exactly is the pain? • How long have you had it? • On a scale of 1–10, how bad is it? • Describe the pain. • What makes it better? Worse? • What is your pain goal?	Neck pain can be from musculoskeletal injury, tension, or pathological changes. Common causes include trauma at any age, muscle tension in adolescents or adults, and arthritis in older patients.
Limited Neck Movement Are you having any difficulty turning or flexing/extending your neck?	Limitation of neck mobility may be from muscle tension/strain or cervical vertebral joint dysfunction.
Facial Pain • Where exactly is the pain? • How long have you had it? • On a scale of 1–10, how bad is it? • Describe the pain. • What makes it better? Worse?	Trauma, infection, and neurological disorders may result in facial pain, which also can be referred from another organ or system. Common causes of facial pain include the following: • Muscle overuse • Mouth/tooth infections • Sinusitis • Herpes zoster • Trauma • Migraine or cluster headaches **⚠ SAFETY ALERT** *Jaw pain, especially if associated with shoulder or arm pain, could indicate cardiac involvement. This is a medical emergency that requires immediate evaluation and treatment.* • Cranial pain, which may be related to tension headaches or tension of the neck muscles. Other possible causes include skin lesions, trauma, and infection.
Lumps or Masses Have you noted any lumps or masses in your head or neck? • How long have you had this? • How many are there? • How large are they, if any? • Are they changing? • Are they tender or painful?	You must differentiate the many structures in the neck by careful questioning of the characteristics of any neck lump, followed by careful physical examination grounded in knowledge of the anatomy of this region.

(table continues on page 295)

Signs/Symptoms	Rationale/Abnormal Findings
Hypothyroidism Do you have any of these symptoms: fatigue; anorexia; cold intolerance; dry skin; brittle, coarse hair; menstrual irregularities; weight gain or difficulty losing weight; decreased libido?	Signs and symptoms of thyroid dysfunction are often nonspecific (Swartz, 2010). Consider that the patient has a thyroid difficulty when several symptoms are "clustered together." Metabolism is slow.
Hyperthyroidism Do you have any of these symptoms: fatigue; weight loss; anxiety; palpitations; rapid pulse; heat intolerance; fine, limp hair; diaphoresis; muscle weakness?	Hyperthyroidism usually presents with several of these signs or symptoms (Swartz, 2010). An overactive thyroid gland increases the metabolic rate.

Documenting Normal Findings

Patient reports no unusual, severe, or frequent headaches. Denies loss of neck mobility or neck pain. Denies any lumps or masses in the neck. Reports no difficulties with fatigue, weight change, temperature discomfort, skin changes, sweating, or other unusual findings.

Older Adults

Additional Questions	Rationale/Abnormal Findings
• Have you noticed any lumps/masses in your neck? • Do you have a new type of headache? • Do you have any pain in your neck? • Any weakness, numbness, or tingling in your arms?	Cervical lymph nodes are usually not palpable, but submandibular glands may be more prominent because of less subcutaneous fat. New headache in a patient older than 50 years of age requires thorough investigation to determine etiology. Arthritic changes in the cervical spine may present as neck pain or loss of sensation or strength in the upper extremities.
Cultural Considerations	
Do you feel that you have a neck injury that has not been treated?	Diagnosis of a cervical spine injury is challenging and in many cases goes undiagnosed, especially in those lacking adequate health insurance (Rubenstein & van Tulder, 2008). Patients at risk include those who have experienced a fall or collision and patients with osteoporosis, advanced arthritis, cancer, or degenerative bone disease (Harris, Blackmore, Mirza, & Jurkovich, 2008).

Objective Data

Equipment

- Ambient lighting
- Penlight or flashlight for tangential lighting
- Gloves, if any lesions of the scalp or skin of head and neck are suspected
- Small cup of water

Preparation

If the patient is wearing a wig or hairpiece, ask him or her to remove it. Wash your hands. The patient is usually seated, facing the examiner. Instruct the patient that the head and neck will be inspected, palpated, and manipulated but that the procedures should not be painful. Instruct the patient to tell you if any part of the head and neck examination causes discomfort.

Common and Specialty or Advanced Techniques

The routine head-to-toe assessment includes the most important and common assessment techniques. You may add specialty or advanced steps if you are concerned about a specific finding.

The most common basic and advanced techniques used in the comprehensive assessment of the head and neck are summarized in the table. These techniques are essential for clinical practice. Additional techniques may be added if the clinical situation warrants them.

Basic Versus Focused/Specialty or Advanced Techniques Related to Head and Neck Assessment			
Technique	**Purpose**	**Screening or Registered Nurse Assessment**	**Focused or Advanced Practice Examination**
Inspection of the head	Observe for symmetry, deformities	X	
Inspection of the hair	Observe for texture, color	X	
Inspection of the neck	Observe for lesions, limitations of movement	X	
Palpation of the scalp	Assess masses or lesions	X	
Palpation of the thyroid	Assess for enlargement		X Assess risk for thyroid disorders
Palpation of lymph nodes	Assess for enlargement or tenderness		X Assess for cancer risk
Auscultation of the thyroid	Listen for bruit		X Assess increased blood flow

Therapeutic Dialogue: Collecting Subjective Data

Remember Faye Davis-Pierce, introduced at the beginning of this chapter. This 21-year-old college student has presented to the campus clinic with fatigue and weight gain. The nurse uses professional communication techniques to gather subjective data from the patient.

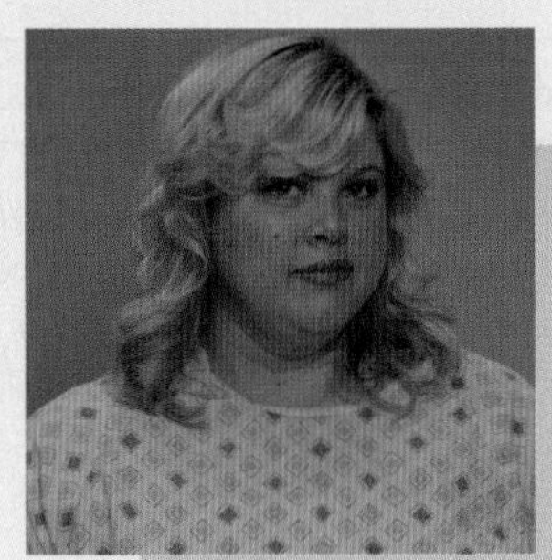

Nurse: Hi, I'm Brenda. What name do you prefer to be called?

Faye: Faye is fine. Thanks for asking.

Nurse: Sure. So, how are you doing today?

Faye: I've just been feeling really tired.

Nurse: Tell me a little about that.

Faye: Well, I've been really stressed out and having trouble sleeping. It's hard to get out of bed sometimes in the morning.

Nurse: College can be stressful.

Faye: Yes, it really can be.

Nurse: Have you noticed any other symptoms with your fatigue?

Faye: Yeah, I've gained 20 lb. I think that it's the dorm food.

Nurse: We can talk about some strategies for your nutrition later if you would like.

Faye: Yes, I would.

Nurse: Have you noticed anything else, such as loss of appetite, dry skin, or hair?

Faye: Well, yes, my skin and hair have been dry. You know, my mother has been saying that she had a low thyroid when she was around my age. Could it be related?

Nurse: It's possible. I'll make sure to report this information to the nurse practitioner when she sees you.

(case study continues on page 297)

Critical Thinking Challenge

- What did the nurse do to establish a therapeutic relationship?
- How did the nurse use interview skills to collect pertinent data?
- How will the nurse prioritize Faye's difficulties?

Comprehensive Physical Examination

Technique and Normal Findings	Abnormal Findings
Inspection Inspect the head (Fig. 12.7). The head is centered, proportional to the body (1/7), erect, and without tremors, tics, or unusual movements. The cranium is round without obvious deformities. The neck muscles are symmetrical. 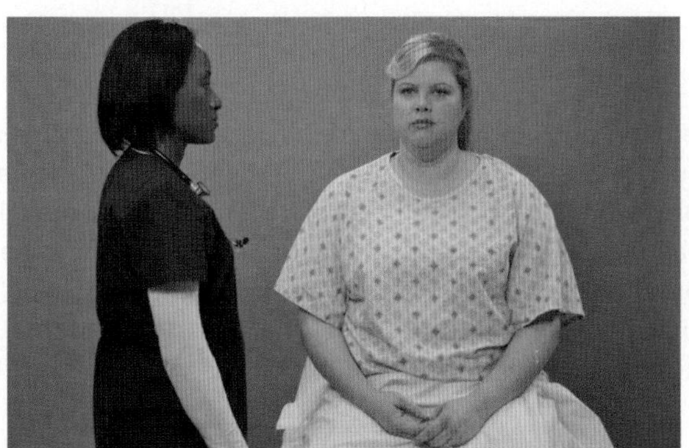 **Figure 12.7** Inspecting the head.	Facial asymmetry may indicate inflammation of CN VII with Bell palsy or a serious condition such as a stroke (see Chapter 22). Enlarged bones or tissues are associated with acromegaly. A puffy "moon" face may be associated with Cushing syndrome. Increased facial hair in females may be a sign of Cushing syndrome or endocrinopathy. Periorbital edema is seen with congestive heart failure and hypothyroidism (myxedema). See Tables 12.4 and 12.5 at the end of this chapter for visual examples.
Inspect facial features for symmetry and size. **Nasolabial** folds are symmetrical.	If asymmetrical, look for signs of trauma. Carefully assess any lesions for infection.
Inspect the hair (Fig. 12.8) for the following: • Distribution and quantity • Texture • Cleanliness 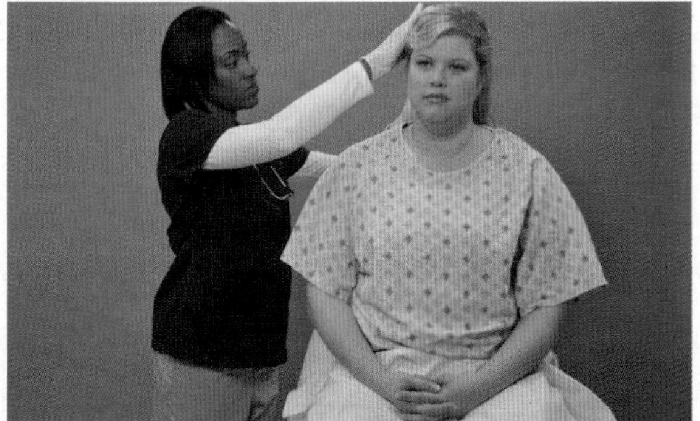 **Figure 12.8** Examining the hair and scalp. The nurse wears gloves if there is any possibility of contact with an open sore or lesion.	Testosterone stimulates hair growth on the face, pubic area, axillae, and chest but diminishes scalp hair growth. Male pattern baldness occurs when there is both a genetic predisposition and increased testosterone or other male hormones. Adult men may present with male pattern baldness in either an "M" pattern on the scalp or, as hair loss continues, a "U" pattern with hair growth around the cranium at the level of the temples. These are considered to be normal variants. Such hair loss can occur any time after puberty but is usually more noticeable in middle-aged and older adults (Hall, 2011). Unusual distribution or patterns of hair growth on the face or cranium are often associated with endocrine abnormalities.
Hair is evenly distributed across the scalp, extending from the superior aspect of the forehead to the base of the cranium and to the top of the ears bilaterally.	Any nits (white to brown, small, 1-mm specks) attached to hair shafts may be signs of pediculosis (head lice); intense itching usually accompanies infestation. Traction alopecia may occur with tight braiding (see Chapter 11).

(table continues on page 298)

Technique and Normal Findings (continued)	Abnormal Findings (continued)
Inspect the neck (Fig. 12.9). Look at the neck muscles, the sternocleidomastoid muscle, the thyroid gland, and the aortic isthmus (may be visualized with tangential light and by asking the patient to swallow a sip of water). Trachea is midline. A slight symmetrical elevation may be observed in the mid-neck. 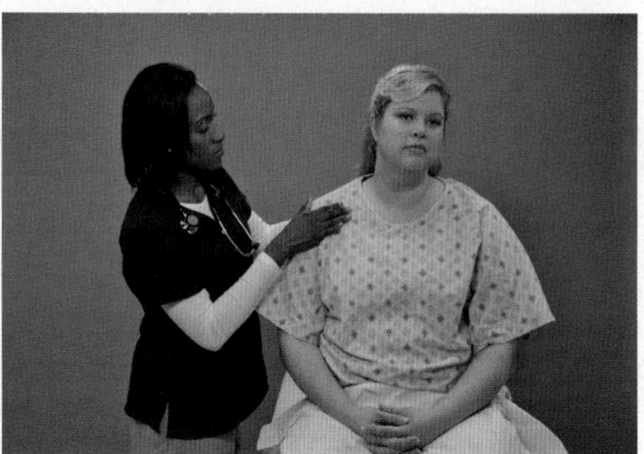 **Figure 12.9** Inspecting the neck.	Thyroid asymmetry, enlargement, or masses can be seen more easily when the patient swallows and while illuminating the neck with a tangential light.
With the patient standing, inspect the cervical spine from all sides. It should position the head above the trunk. Observing from the side, check for the concave curve of the cervical spine. As viewed from behind, the patient holds the head erect, and the cervical spine is in straight alignment. From the side, the neck has a concave curve.	Degenerative joint disease of the cervical vertebrae may cause lateral tilting of the head and neck. Lateral deviation of the neck (torticollis) may be due to acute muscle spasms, congenital difficulties, or an adjustment in head posture to correct vision problems. Weight lifting will cause hypertrophy of the neck muscles, resulting in a thickened appearance of the neck.
Palpation Palpate the temporal artery in the space above the cheekbone near the scalp line. The temporal artery pulse is 2–3 on a 4-point scale. Palpate the scalp. (Refer to Chapter 11.)	Temporal arteritis is a painful inflammation of the temporal artery. Patients report severe unilateral headache sometimes accompanied by visual disturbances. This condition needs immediate care. A biopsy may be necessary for diagnosis.
The scalp is symmetrical without tenderness, masses, lesions, or differences in firmness.	Bulging or depression of the bony structure of the scalp may result from trauma or tumor growth. Bulging fontanelles in an infant may be a clinical sign of hydrocephalus or simply the result of vigorous crying (see Table 12.3 at the end of the chapter). Depressed fontanelles are most often associated with dehydration.
Palpate the thyroid, either from the anterior or posterior approach. • For the *anterior approach*, have the patient tilt the head slightly back. Locate the thyroid and cricoid cartilages. The thyroid cartilage is larger, shield shaped, and in the mid-neck; it is sometimes referred to as the *Adam's apple* in males. Below is the ringed cricoid cartilage. Just below the cricoid cartilage, the isthmus of the thyroid should be palpable as a smooth, rubbery band that rises and falls with swallowing. With the pads of	Unilateral bulging may indicate a thyroid goiter, cyst, or tumor. Neck masses may also originate from a lymph node or cyst. **SAFETY ALERT** *Any new neck mass in a patient older than 35 years of age should be carefully evaluated to rule out cancer. It could be a lymph node enlarged by metastatic cancer, a primary lymphoma, or a tumor of structures of the neck.*

(table continues on page 299)

Technique and Normal Findings (continued)	Abnormal Findings (continued)
the fingers of one hand, gently palpate the thyroid isthmus. Ask the patient to lower the head slightly and turn it slightly to one side. The sternocleidomastoid muscle will relax on the side to which the patient turns. Palpate behind the sternocleidomastoid muscle (Fig. 12.10).	Unusual hardness is a dangerous finding, possibly associated with cancer (Swartz, 2010). Toxic goiter may feel softer than normal thyroid tissue during palpation. Tenderness is common with subacute infections, traumatic injury, and radiation thyroiditis The parathyroid gland is not normally palpable, but it may be when enlarged or inflamed. Parathyroid carcinoma is a rare form of cancer; the associated tumors usually secrete parathyroid hormone, producing hyperparathyroidism and increased calcium levels. Parathyroid carcinoma may be suspected if the symptoms mentioned earlier are present, but it usually can only be confirmed surgically.
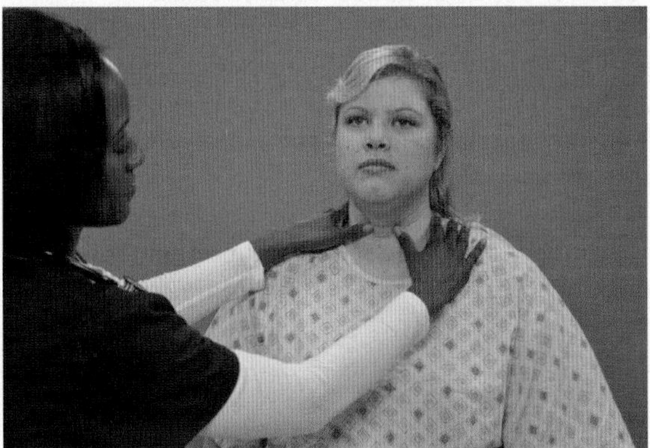 **Figure 12.10** Palpating behind the sternocleidomastoid muscle for the anterior thyroid.	
• For the *posterior approach*, locate the thyroid and cricoid cartilages and the thyroid isthmus by palpation while standing behind the patient. Have the patient bend the head slightly forward and toward one side. Use your index finger to slightly retract the sternocleidomastoid muscle on the side toward which the patient has tilted the head. Use the middle two or three fingers to locate the lobe of the thyroid. Use the fingers of the other hand to gently displace the trachea and thyroid cartilage on the opposite side, which helps to move the thyroid gland slightly forward, making it more prominent and allowing for easier palpation. It is, however, not unusual for the thyroid lobes to also be nonpalpable with this approach (Fig. 12.11).	
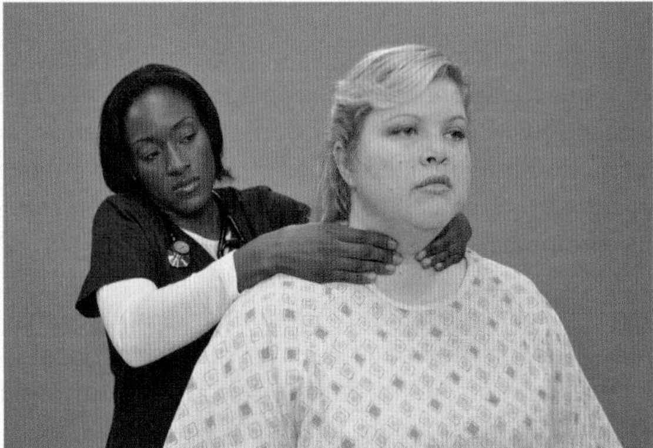 **Figure 12.11** Palpating the thyroid from the posterior approach.	
If palpable, the thyroid is smooth, rubbery, nontender, symmetrical, and barely palpable beneath the sternocleidomastoid.	(table continues on page 300)

Technique and Normal Findings (continued)	Abnormal Findings (continued)
Following a systematical pattern, palpate for discernible lymph nodes in the head and neck (Fig. 12.12). The order of examination is usually preauricular, posterior auricular, occipital, submental, submandibular, tonsillar, anterior cervical chain, posterior cervical chain, and supraclavicular. Using the pads of the second, third, and fourth fingers, gently palpate in small circles, varying the amount of pressure over each lymphatic region. *Usually, no lymph nodes are palpable in the adult.* If a node is palpable, it is important to describe the following characteristics: • Location—which lymphatic chain and where along that chain is the node • Size—in millimeters or centimeters • Consistency—how hard or soft is the node? It should be smooth and slightly soft. • Tenderness—with an acute infection or inflammation, a node may be tender. With malignancy, nodes are usually nontender. • Mobility—It should be freely movable. • Delimitation—There should not be any matting together of lymph nodes. 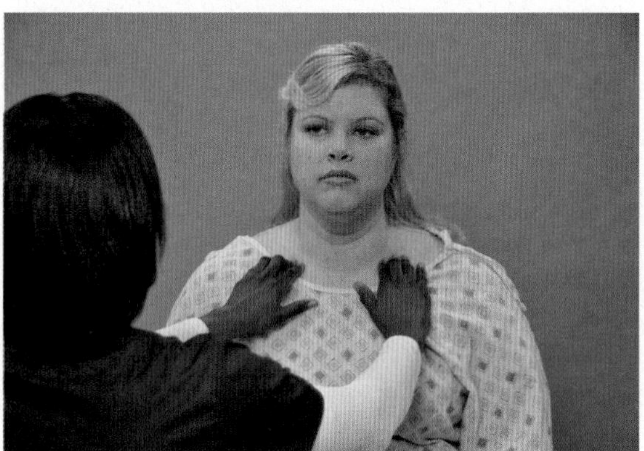 **Figure 12.12** Palpating for any discernible lymph nodes.	Palpable, tender, and warm lymph nodes usually indicate an infection in the area from which the lymph vessels drain to that node (Ellis, 2010): • Anterior cervical nodes: pharyngitis • Posterior cervical nodes: mononucleosis • Posterior auricular nodes: otitis media • Supraclavicular nodes: these must be carefully evaluated as a possible sign of metastatic cancer. The Virchow node (also called the signal node, found on the left supraclavicular) is associated with lung and abdominal cancers. Hard, rubbery, irregular, fixed, and nontender lymph nodes are a possible sign of lymphoma.
Palpation Stand behind the patient to palpate the cervical spine and neck. C7 and T1 spinous processes should be prominent. The paravertebral, sternocleidomastoid, and trapezius muscles should be fully developed, symmetrical, and nontender.	Osteoarthritis, neck injury, disk degeneration because of aging or occupational stress, and spondylosis can cause decreased ROM, pain, and tenderness on palpation. Pain on palpation may indicate inflammation of the muscles (myositis). Neck spasm may indicate nerve compression or psychological stress.
Palpate the neck. Ask the patient to touch the chin to the chest (flexion), look up toward the ceiling (hyperextension), attempt to touch each ear to the shoulder without elevating the shoulder (lateral flexion or bending), and turn the chin to the shoulder as far as possible (rotation). Neck range of motion (ROM) is normal: flexion 45 degrees, hyperextension 55 degrees, lateral flexion 40 degrees, and rotation 70 degrees to each side.	Pain or muscle spasms may impair ROM. Hyperextension and flexion may be limited because of cervical disk degeneration, spinal cord tumor, or osteoarthritic changes. Pain may radiate to the back, shoulder, or arms. Pain, numbness, or tingling may indicate compression of spinal root nerves.

(table continues on page 301)

Technique and Normal Findings (continued)	Abnormal Findings (continued)
Muscle strength: Ask the patient to rotate the neck to the right and left, against the resistance of your hand. This tests CN XI. Muscle strength should be sufficient to overcome resistance.	Weakness or loss of sensation in arms may result from cervical cord compression.
Clinical Significance Following any trauma, do not move patients with neck pain until the neck has been stabilized. Moving the patient could cause subluxation or dislocation of the cervical vertebrae and permanent injury to the spinal cord.	
Auscultation If the thyroid is enlarged, either unilaterally or bilaterally, auscultate over each lobe for a bruit using the bell of the stethoscope (Fig. 12.13). No bruit or vascular sounds are audible.	Bruits are most often associated with a toxic goiter, hyperthyroidism, or thyrotoxicosis.
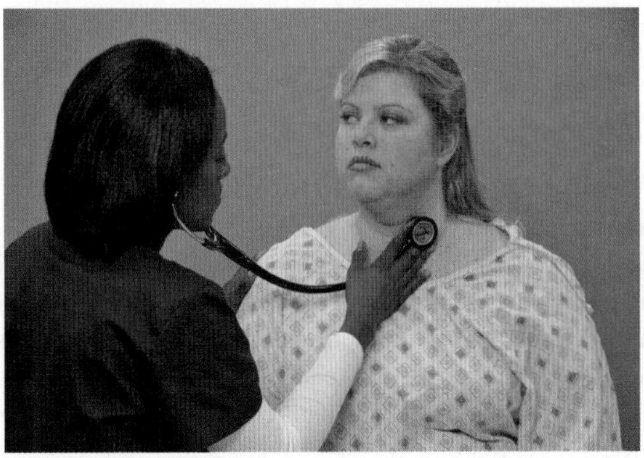 **Figure 12.13** Auscultating the thyroid.	

Documenting Normal Findings

Hair evenly distributed, clean, brown. Scalp with even coloration, skin intact. Cranium size proportional to body, symmetrical. Face with symmetrical movement of facial muscles. Skin smooth, consistent color, intact. Neck with full range of motion, symmetrical. Lymph nodes and salivary glands nonpalpable, nontender. Thyroid gland palpable midline, symmetrical, smooth, rubbery, and nontender. Thyroid isthmus midline. No bruit.

Lifespan Considerations: Older Adults

The facial skin may appear more wrinkled and less elastic in the older adult. Thinning of the hair is also an expected process of aging. The neck may have reduced range of motion if the patient has a chronic condition such as arthritis. Additionally, the spine may have an exaggerated concave curve.

The older adult with hypothyroidism often lacks the classic symptoms seen in younger patients (Papaleontiou & Haymart, 2012). This is because hypothyroidism has a more subtle onset in the older adult and also because the typical signs and symptoms (fatigue, cold intolerance, constipation, and depression) may be attributed to aging or chronic diseases. The older adult is more prone to hyperthyroidism than a younger person (McDermott, 2012). Unexplained weight loss, diarrhea or constipation, nausea, and vomiting may be presenting symptoms. Depression and mania can also be presenting symptoms of hyperthyroidism in the elderly.

Cultural Considerations

The prevalence of goiter decreases with age; the greatest prevalence is in premenopausal women. Women are four times more likely to have goiter than men.

Hypothyroidism is more common in older women and 10 times more common in women than in men. African Americans have a lower prevalence of hypothyroidism compared with Caucasians (Vanderpump, 2011).

The prevalence of hyperthyroidism in women is 10 times more common than in men. There is 10-fold lower incidence

Documenting Case Study Findings

The registered nurse (RN) reports her findings and history to the advanced practice registered nurse (APRN), who finishes conducting a physical examination of Faye Davis-Pierce, the 21-year-old college student presenting with fatigue and weight gain. Review the following important findings revealed in each of the steps of objective data collection. Consider how the RN and APRN will collaborate related to these findings.

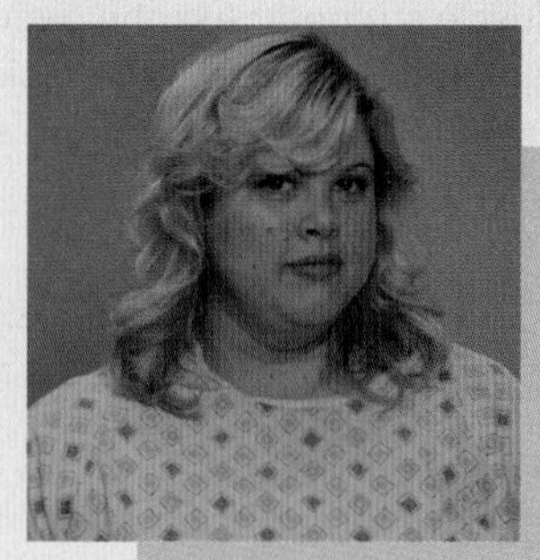

Inspection: Cranium is normocephalic, atraumatic. Hair blondish and slightly dry. Skin dry and intact. Trachea midline. Skin color slightly pale, appears puffy.

Palpation: Thyroid gland palpable and enlarged, symmetrical, smooth, rubbery, and nontender. No lumps or masses.

Auscultation: No bruit over thyroid.

of hyperthyroidism in African American populations than in Caucasians (Vanderpump, 2011).

Critical Thinking

Laboratory and Diagnostic Testing

Evaluation of headaches may indicate the need for several diagnostic tests, which would be determined by an advanced health care professional. Examples of such tests include computed tomography (CT), magnetic resonance imaging (MRI), and lumbar puncture.

Musculoskeletal injury or disease can be confirmed with a radiograph, CT scan, or MRI (see Chapter 21). If test results are negative, assess for complete range of motion of the neck, looking for any muscle tension, loss of mobility, or pain. Recall that cardiac disease may present with referred pain to the neck or jaw, making it important to assess for signs of cardiovascular disease.

Tests of thyroid function are commonly performed for patients at any age presenting with signs or symptoms of hyperthyroidism or hypothyroidism. Usually thyroid-stimulating hormone (TSH), T_3, and T_4 are measured. Table 12.1 shows expected and abnormal values.

Diagnostic Reasoning

Nursing Diagnosis, Outcomes, and Interventions

Table 12.2 compares nursing diagnoses, abnormal findings, and interventions commonly related to assessment of the head and neck (NANDA International, 2012). Nurses use assessment information to identify patient outcomes. Some outcomes related to head and neck difficulties include the following:

- Patient participates in physical activity with appropriate changes in vital signs.
- Patient verbalizes increased energy and well-being.
- Pain goals are met (Moorhead, Johnson, Maas, & Swanson 2013).

After the outcomes area has been established, implement nursing care to improve the status of the patient. Use critical thinking and evidence-based practice to develop the interventions. Some examples of nursing interventions for the head and neck are as follows:

- Allow for periods of rest before planned activities.
- Set small, achievable, short-term goals for activity; this can help motivate the patient.
- Treat pain before it becomes severe (Bulechek, Butcher, Dochterman, & Wagner, 2013).

TABLE 12.1 **Thyroid Hormone Levels**

Test	TSH	Free T_4	Total T_3	Total T_4
Normal values	0.3–5.0 mU/L	0.8–2.3 ng/dl	80–200 ng/dl	5–12 mcmg/dl
Hypothyroidism	High	Low	Low	Low
Hyperthyroidism	Low	High	High	High

TABLE 12.2 Common Nursing Diagnoses Associated With the Head and Neck

Diagnosis	Point of Differentiation	Assessment Characteristics	Nursing Interventions
Activity intolerance	Inability to complete or continue daily activities as a result of a lack of physical or mental energy, which is symptomatic of the thyroid problem	Verbal report of weakness, abnormal pulse or BP during activity, dyspnea, electrocardiographic changes	Determine cause.* If appropriate, gradually increase activity. Monitor response to activity. Refer patient to physical therapy.
Fatigue	A continual and overwhelming feeling of exhaustion or tiredness despite sleep that is normally sufficient for age, health, and lifestyle	Lack of energy, increased rest and sleep requirements, lethargy or listlessness, drowsiness	Assess severity. Evaluate sleep and nutritional status. Gather data to help determine if cause is physiological or psychological.
Chronic pain	Pain lasting more than 6 months. Use pain scale to describe.	Report of pain; facial grimace; muscle tension; increased pulse, respiratory rate, or BP; shifting or guarding	Assess characteristics. Work with pain team to determine appropriate medical treatment. Use nonpharmacological interventions.

BP, blood pressure.
*Collaborative interventions.

Progress Notes: Analyzing Findings

Remember Faye Davis-Pierce, whose difficulties have been outlined throughout this chapter. Initial subjective and objective data collection is complete. Tests of Faye's thyroid levels reveal an elevated TSH and low T_3 and T_4, indicating hypothyroidism. The following nursing note illustrates how the assessment data are analyzed and nursing interventions are developed.

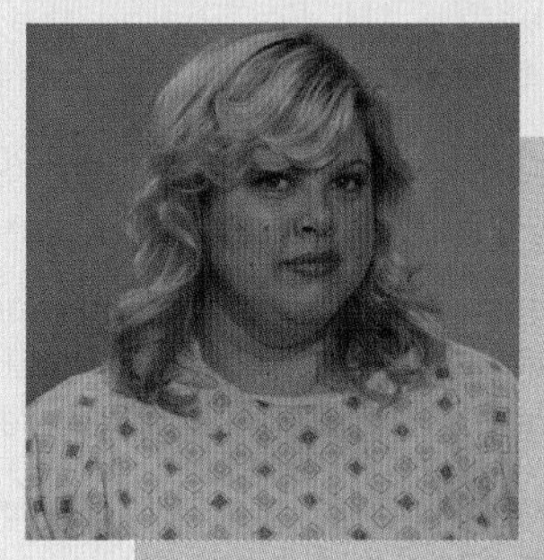

Subjective: "I've just been feeling really tired. I've had some weight gain and I've been really cold."

Objective: Hair blondish, slightly dry. Skin dry and intact. Skin color slightly pale, appears puffy and tired. TSH high and T_3 and T_4 are low. Cranium is normocephalic, atraumatic. Trachea midline. Thyroid gland palpable and enlarged, symmetrical, smooth, rubbery, and nontender. No discrete lumps or masses. No bruit over thyroid.

Analysis: Symptoms are related to low thyroid. Need for teaching about new prescription for thyroid replacement medication.

Plan: Provide teaching about new thyroid replacement medication. Provide materials on nutrition for healthy food choices. Suggest calorie limitation of 1,500 per day, including foods that she likes and can eat. Consult with dietary on written materials. Also stated exercise plan of yoga and walking daily. Continue on oral contraceptive and multivitamin daily. See back in clinic in 1 month. Give numbers and contact information. Assess college stressors at next visit.

(case study continues on page 304)

Critical Thinking Challenge

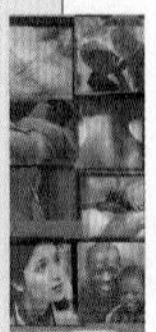

- What role and responsibility does the RN have for assessment of the laboratory values?
- How will the nurse approach teaching about diet and exercise, given sensitivity in many patients about weight gain?
- Why did the RN decide to defer assessment of college stressors until the next visit?

Collaborating With the Interprofessional Team

Faye will benefit by involvement of other members of the health care team participating in her care. The dietician can help her with planning a healthy weight loss diet. The pharmacist will help her understand the importance of taking her thyroid replacement therapy daily at the same time. Faye will obtain her prescription thyroid medication from the same pharmacy each time, making certain that it comes from the same manufacturer each time to ensure consistent dosing. The health care team will work together to evaluate Faye's response to treatment.

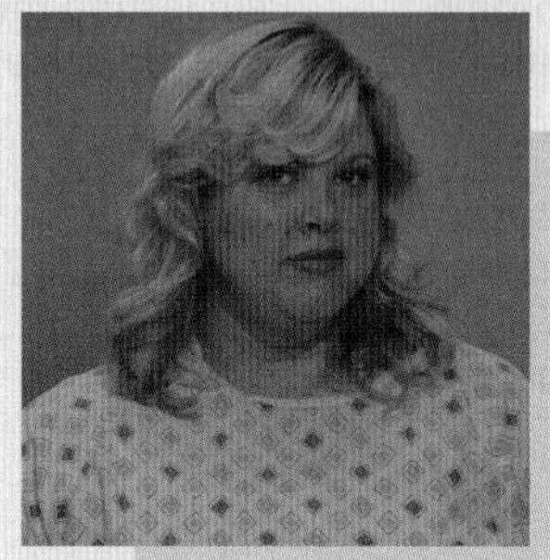

Situation: "Hi, I'm Sharon, the nurse who has been working with Faye Davis-Pierce, a 21-year-old woman who has just been diagnosed with hypothyroidism."

Background: She has gained 20 lb over the past 3 months and is concerned about her weight gain."

Assessement: She is being placed on a thyroid replacement medication Synthroid (levothyroxine) and additionally would like some information about diet, weight control, and exercise to reduce weight."

Recommendations: "Would you be able to come and see her to assess her current nutritional status and make recommendations on a plan for after she leaves? It would be great if you could provide her with written recommendations on diet plan."

Pulling It All Together

The nurse uses assessment data to formulate a nursing care plan with patient outcomes and interventions for Faye Davis-Pierce. After completion of interventions, the nurse reevaluates Ms. Davis-Pierce and documents findings in the chart to show progress toward goals. The nurse uses critical thinking and judgment to continue or revise the diagnosis, outcomes, or interventions. This is often in the form of a care plan or case note similar to the one below.

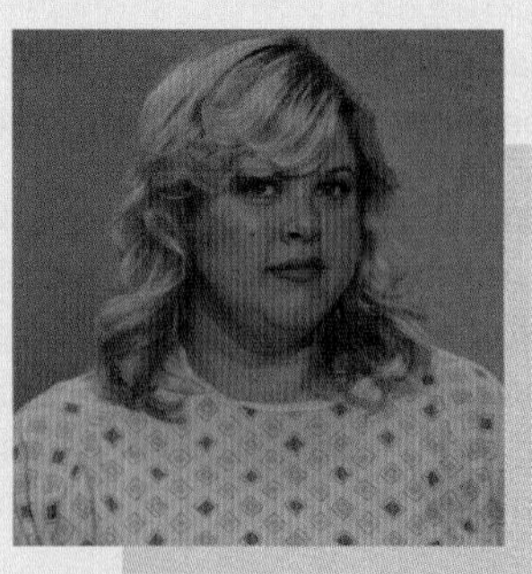

(case study continues on page 305)

Nursing Diagnosis	Patient Outcomes	Nursing Interventions	Rationale	Evaluation
Knowledge deficit related to new diagnosis of hypothyroidism as evidenced by no knowledge of new medication	Patient will state intended effect and adverse effects of medication.	Teach patient not to take medication with food. Review effects and adverse effects of medication, making sure the patient is aware that it may take several weeks to notice a change. Provide written information. Give a phone number in case the patient has questions or experiences adverse effects.	Written instructions are a resource that the patient can use after leaving the clinic. Questions may not arise until the patient is at home.	The patient stated the intended effect of resolution of her symptoms. She also stated the adverse effects of too high a level of medication, including weight loss; anxiety; palpitations; rapid pulse; heat intolerance; fine, limp hair; and diaphoresis. The patient scheduled a follow-up appointment in 3 weeks.

Applying Your Knowledge

Using the previous steps of diagnostic reasoning, organizing, and prioritizing, consider all the case study findings woven throughout this chapter. When answering the following questions, begin drawing conclusions and notice how the pieces of assessment must work together to create an environment for personalized, appropriate, and accurate care.

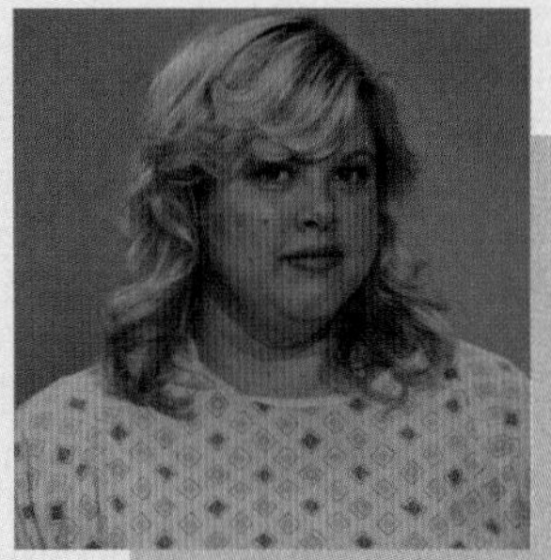

- What are the signs and symptoms of hypothyroidism?
- How do the symptoms and signs of hypothyroidism and hyperthyroidism differ?
- What other physical findings might be present, and what other body systems might be involved?
- How might Faye's physical issues relate to her psychosocial health, including potential issues related to her age and status as a college student?
- What type of follow-up care and reassessment might the patient need at subsequent visits?
- How will you evaluate Faye's understanding of her diagnosis and determine any additional needed teaching?

Key Points

- Structures of the head and neck also include the trachea, thyroid, and lymphatics.
- Urgent situations that need emergency assessment and intervention include head or neck injuries, neck pain (may be cardiac), enlarged hard nodes (which may indicate cancer), and thyrotoxicosis.
- Common symptoms of the head and neck include pain, limited neck movement, lumps or masses, hypothyroidism, and hyperthyroidism.
- The neck muscles, sternocleidomastoid muscle, thyroid gland, and aortic isthmus are inspected in the neck.
- The thyroid is normally smooth, rubbery, and moveable. It is also common for the thyroid to be nonpalpable.
- A bruit may be present with hyperthyroidism or thyrotoxicosis.
- Common nursing diagnoses for the head and neck include activity intolerance, fatigue, chronic pain, and knowledge deficit.

Review Questions

1. While examining the patient's neck, the nurse finds the trachea midline but has difficulty palpating the thyroid. What action would the nurse take next?
   A. Document this finding as normal.
   B. Tell the patient that this finding is unexpected.
   C. Report to the physician a suspicion of a slow growing goiter.
   D. Look for signs of hypothyroidism.
2. The lymph nodes that lie in front of the mastoid bone are the:
   A. Preauricular nodes
   B. Occipital nodes
   C. Superficial cervical nodes
   D. Supraclavicular nodes
3. Which of the following descriptions is most consistent with a patient who has hypothyroidism?
   A. Slightly obese, perspiring female, who complains of feeling cold all the time and having diarrhea

B. Slightly obese female with periorbital edema and a flat facial expression, who complains of constipation, deceased appetite, and fatigue
C. Thin, anxious-appearing female with exophthalmos and a rapid pulse, and who complains of diarrhea
D. Thin, perspiring male with a deep hoarse voice, facial edema, a thick tongue, and reports of diarrhea

4. Physical examination of a patient reveals an enlarged tonsillar node. Acutely infected nodes would be
A. Hard and nontender
B. Fixed and soft
C. Firm but movable and tender
D. Irregular and hard

5. While assessing the skin of a 24-year-old patient, the nurse notes decreased skin turgor. The nurse should further assess for signs and symptoms of
A. hyperthyroidism
B. hypothyroidism
C. malnutrition
D. dehydration

6. The nurse can best evaluate the strength of the sternocleidomastoid muscle by having the patient
A. clench his or her teeth during muscle palpation
B. bring his or her head to the chest
C. turn his or her head against resistance
D. extend his or her arms against resistance

7. Which of the following best describes the instructions the nurse should give a patient when assessing the thyroid from the posterior approach?
A. Please tilt your head back as far as possible.
B. Please turn your head as far to the right as you can.
C. Please bring your chin down toward your neck.
D. Please tilt your head slightly down and to one side.

8. While assessing a patient, the nurse finds a palpable lymph node in the left supraclavicular region. Which of the following should be the next action?
A. Recognize that it is not common to palpate lymph nodes in this region and they must be carefully evaluated.
B. Recognize that a palpable node in this region is a dangerous indication of metastatic cancer that requires further evaluation.
C. Recognize that this is a common area for lymph nodes to be enlarged with minor infections.
D. Recognize that a palpable lymph node in this region is always indicative of malignancy.

9. While reviewing laboratory values for thyroid function on an adult patient, the nurse sees that the TSH is elevated, and the T3 and T4 are decreased. The nurse recognizes that these findings are indicative of
A. normal thyroid function
B. hypothyroidism
C. hyperthyroidism
D. thyroid cancer

10. A patient presents with a complaint of drooping of his eyes, cheeks, and mouth on one side. This finding is most likely associated with pathology of which cranial nerve?
A. Cranial nerve III
B. Cranial nerve V
C. Cranial nerve VII
D. Cranial nerve IX

The Jensen suite offers these additional resources to enhance learning and facilitate understanding of this chapter:

- *thePoint online resource, http://thepoint.lww.com/Jensen2e*
- *Laboratory Manual for Nursing Health Assessment: A Best Practice Approach*
- *Pocket Guide for Nursing Health Assessment: A Best Practice Approach*
- *Lippincott DocuCare, an electronic health record simulation software, http://thepoint.lww.com/docucare*
- *Adaptive Learning | Powered by PrepU, http://thepoint.lww.com/prepu*

References

Abrams, B. M. (2013). Factors that cause concern. *Medical Clinics of North America, 97*(2), 225–242.

Alamdari, S., Azizi, F., Delshad, H., Sarvghadi, F., Amouzegar, A., & Mehran, L. (2013). Management of hyperthyroidism in pregnancy: Comparison of recommendations of American Thyroid Association and Endocrine Society. *Journal of Thyroid Research, 2013*, 878467. doi:10.1155/2013/878467

Bulechek, G. M., Butcher, H. K., Dochterman, J. M., & Wagner, C. M. (2013). *Nursing interventions classification (NIC)* (6th ed.) St. Louis, MO: Mosby.

Drake, R. L., Vogl, W., & Mitchell, A. W. M. (2010). *Gray's anatomy for students* (2nd ed.). Philadelphia, PA: Churchill Livingstone

Ellis, H., & Mahadevan, V. (2010). *Clinical anatomy: Applied anatomy for clinical students* (12th ed.). West Sussex, United Kingdom: Wiley-Blackwell.

Hall, J. E. (2011). *Guyton and Hall textbook of medical physiology* (12th ed.). Philadelphia, PA: Elsevier Saunders.

Harris, B. A., Blackmore, C. C., Mirza, S., & Jurkovich, J. (2008). Clearing the cervical spine in obtunded patients. *Spine, 33*(14), 1547–1553.

McDermott, M. T. (2012). Hyperthyroidism. *Annals of Internal Medicine, 157*(1), ITC1–ITC16. doi:10.7326/0003-4819-157-1-20120703-01001.

Moorhead, S., Johnson, M., Maas, M. L., & Swanson, E. (2013). *Nursing outcomes classification (NOC): Measurement of health outcomes* (5th ed.). St. Louis, MO: Elsevier

National Cancer Institute. (2013). *Head and neck cancers.* Retrieved from http://www.cancer.gov/cancertopics/factsheet/Sites-Types/head-and-neck

Nicholson, R. A., Buse, D. C., Andrasik, F., & Lipton, R. B. (2011). Non-pharmacologic treatments for migraine and tension-type headache: How to choose and when to use. *Current Treatment Options in Neurology, 13*(1), 28–40. doi:10.1007/s11940-010-0102-9

NANDA International. (2012). *Nursing diagnoses: Definitions and classification 2012-2014* (9th ed). Oxford, United Kingdom: Wiley-Blackwell.

Paes, J. E., Burman, K. D., Cohen, J., Franklyn, J., McHenry, C. R., Shoham, S., & Kloos, R. T. (2010). Acute bacterial suppurative thyroiditis: A clinical review and expert opinion. *Thyroid, 20*(3), 247–255. doi:10.1089/thy.2008.0146

Papaleontiou, M., & Haymart, M. R. (2012). Approach to and treatment of thyroid disorders in the elderly. *Medical Clinics of North America, 96*(2), 297–310.

Raza, M., Elkhodair, S., Zaheer, A., & Yousaf, S. (2013). Safe cervical spine clearance in adult obtunded blunt trauma patients on the basis of a normal multidetector CT scan-a meta-analysis and cohort study. *Injury, 44*(11), 1589–1595.

Rubenstein, S. M., & van Tulder, M. (2008). A best-evidence review of diagnostic procedures for neck and low-back pain. *Best Practice and Research: Clinical Rheumatology, 22*(3), 471–482.

Swartz, M. H. (2010). *Textbook of physical diagnosis: History and examination* (6th ed.). Philadelphia, PA: Elsevier Saunders.

U.S. Department of Health & Human Services. (2013). 2020 *Topics & objectives: injury and violence prevention.* Retrieved from http://www.healthypeople.gov/2020/topicsobjectives2020/objectiveslist.aspx?topicId=24

Vanderpump, M. P. J. (2011). The epidemiology of thyroid disease. *British Medical Bulletin, 99*(1), 39–51. doi:10.1093/bmb/ldr030

Tables of Abnormal Findings

TABLE 12.3 Head and Neck Problems More Common in Childhood

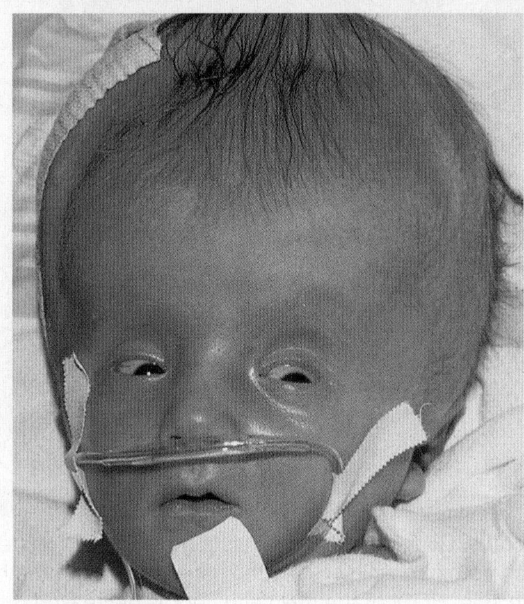

Hydrocephalus. An abnormal collection of cerebrospinal fluid in the ventricles of the brain causes enlargement of the cranium. Infants with hydrocephalus may have separation of the cranial sutures, bulging fontanelles, and dilated veins across the scalp.

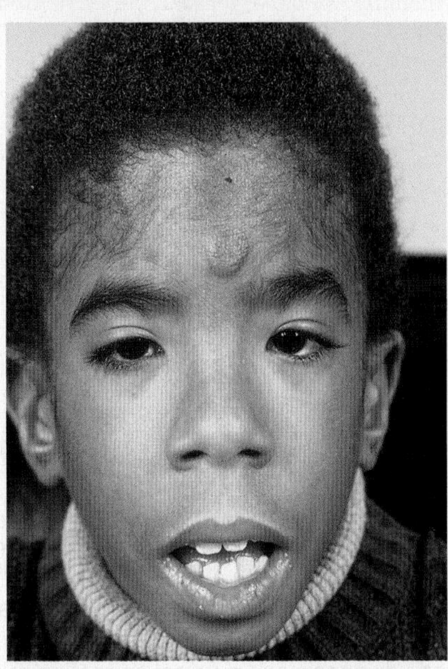

Fetal Alcohol Syndrome (FAS). Developmental delays and congenital abnormalities are associated with maternal intake of alcohol during pregnancy. Physical manifestations include microcephaly, flattened cheekbones, small eyes, and a flattened upper lip. Children with FAS have multiple developmental and learning disabilities.

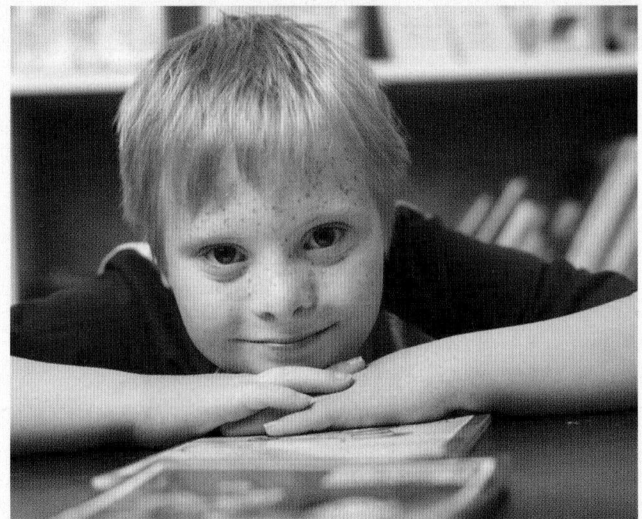

Down Syndrome (Trisomy 21). This congenital condition results from either an extra chromosome 21 or translocation of chromosome 14 or 15 with 21 or 22. Manifestations in the head and neck region include microcephaly, a flattened occipital bone, slanted small eyes, a depressed nasal bridge, low-set ears, and a protruding tongue.

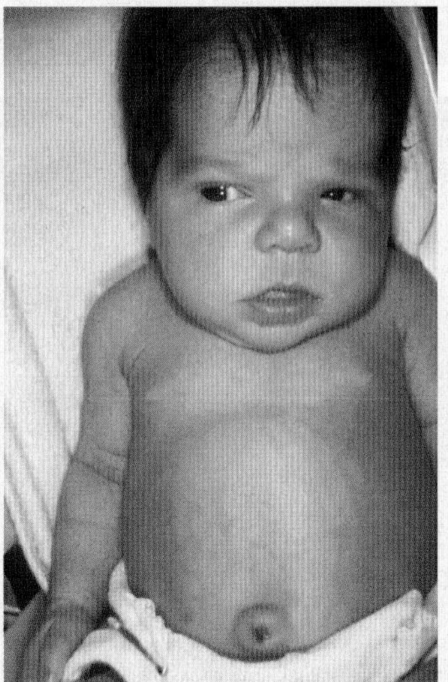

Congenital Hypothyroidism. Affected infants have puffy facial features and often a larger-than-normal tongue. This syndrome is more common in parts of the world where diets are deficient in iodine.

(table continues on page 308)

TABLE 12.3 Head and Neck Problems More Common in Childhood *(continued)*

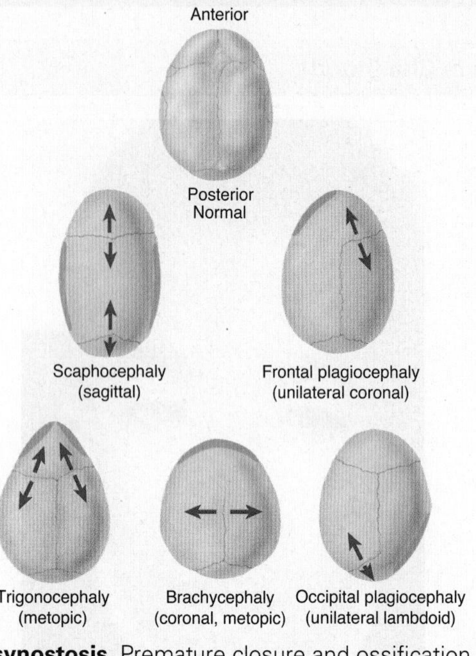

Craniosynostosis. Premature closure and ossification of the fontanelles results in cranial deformities and microcephaly. Early diagnosis and surgical correction minimize malformations.

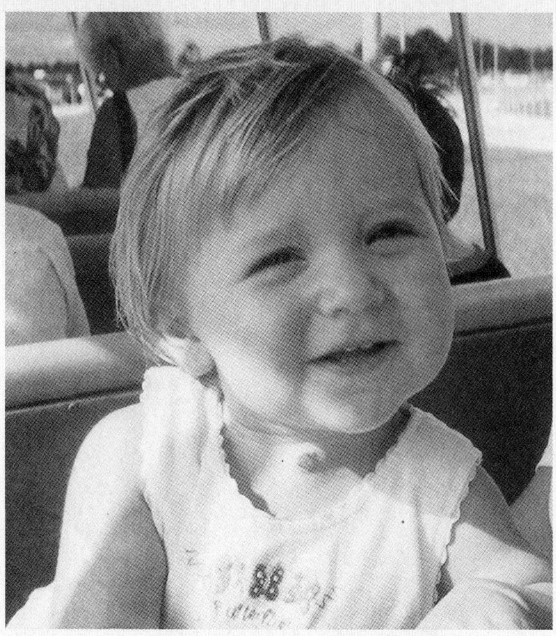

Torticollis. Congenital or acquired contraction of the sternocleidomastoid muscle causes the patient to incline the head to one side. ROM of the head and neck is decreased.

TABLE 12.4 Head and Neck Problems Common in Adults

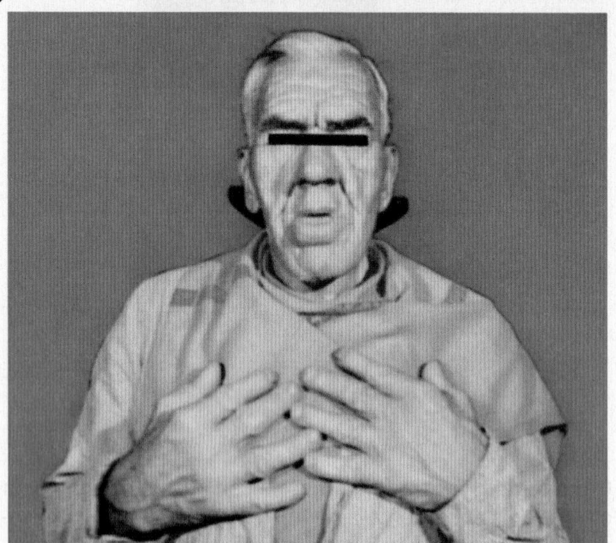

Acromegaly. Overproduction of growth hormone in adults results in thickening of the skin, subcutaneous tissue, and facial bones, and coarsening of facial features (see also Chapter 5).

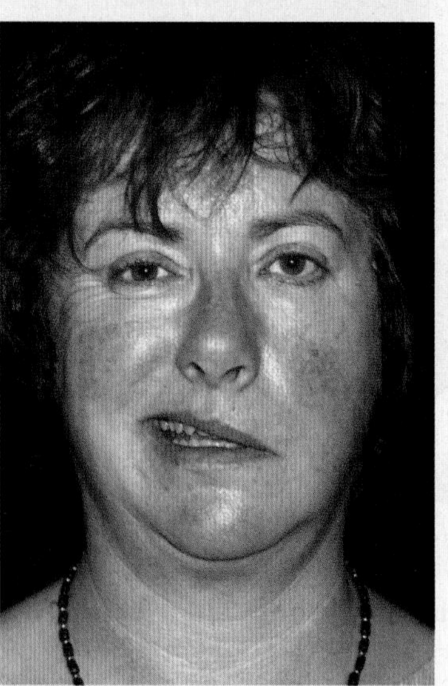

Bell Palsy. Paralysis, usually unilateral, of the facial nerve (CN VII) can be transient or permanent. Causes include trauma, compression, and infection.

(table continues on page 309)

TABLE 12.4 Head and Neck Problems Common in Adults *(continued)*

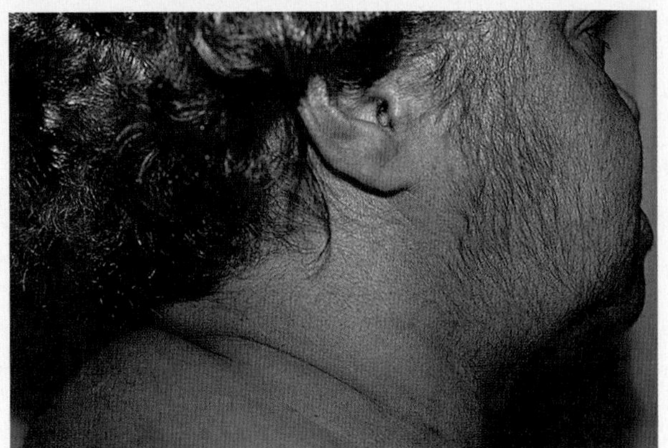

Cushing Syndrome. Excessive production of exogenous adrenocorticotropic hormone results in a round "moon" facies, fat deposits at the nape of the neck, "buffalo hump," and sometimes a velvety discoloration around the neck (acanthosis nigricans).

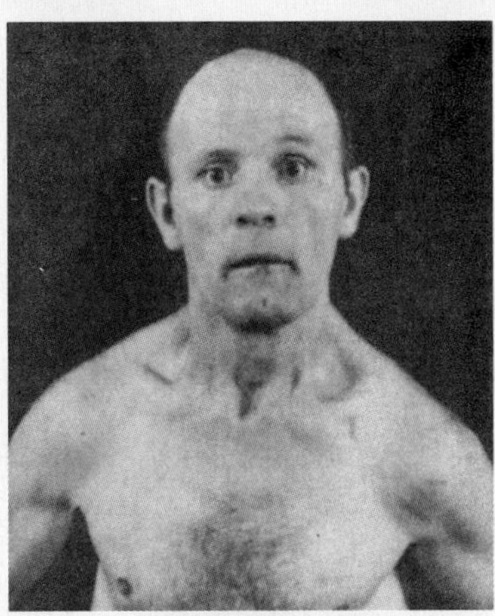

Parkinson Disease. With this degenerative neurological disease, patients present with a masklike facial appearance, rigid muscles, diminished reflexes, and a shuffling gait.

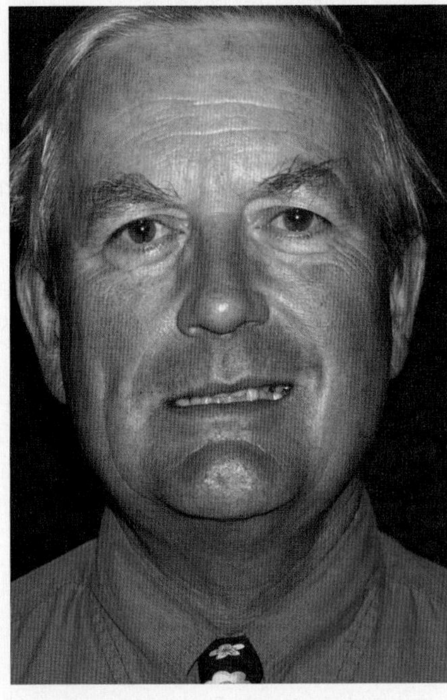

Cerebrovascular Accident (CVA/Stroke). Also known as a "brain attack." Embolism, hemorrhage, or vasospasm in the brain results in ischemia of surrounding tissue and neurological damage. Symptoms depend on the part of the brain affected.

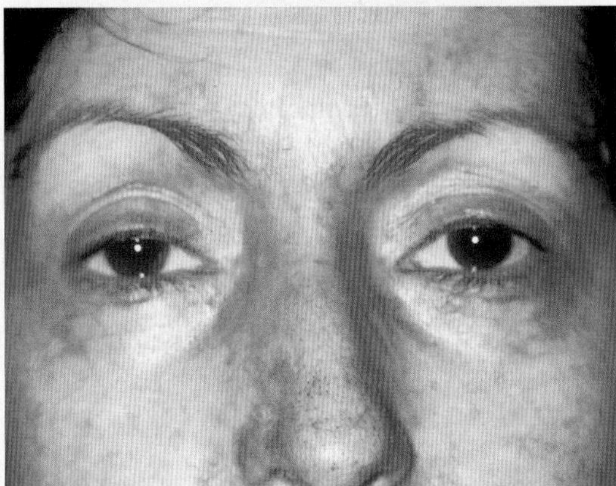

Scleroderma. Hardening of the skin usually is noted first in the hands and face. Skin becomes firm and loses mobility, seemingly fixed to underlying tissues. Facial scleroderma presents with shiny, taut, immobile skin, which may make it difficult for patients to speak, chew, or even swallow. It can affect other organs and tissues.

(table continues on page 310)

TABLE 12.4 **Head and Neck Problems Common in Adults** *(continued)*

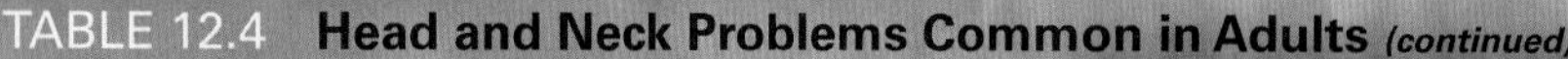

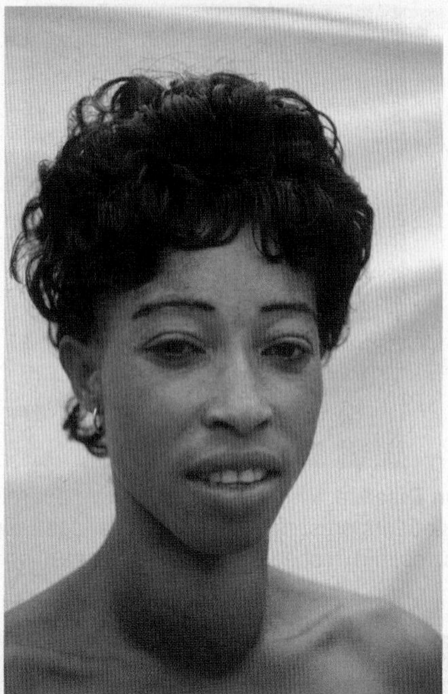

Goiter. Enlarged thyroid gland can be associated with hyperthyroidism, hypothyroidism, or normal thyroid function. Enlargement can compress other structures in the neck, making surgical removal of the thyroid necessary. After thyroidectomy, patients must be treated with exogenous thyroid hormone for the rest of their lives.

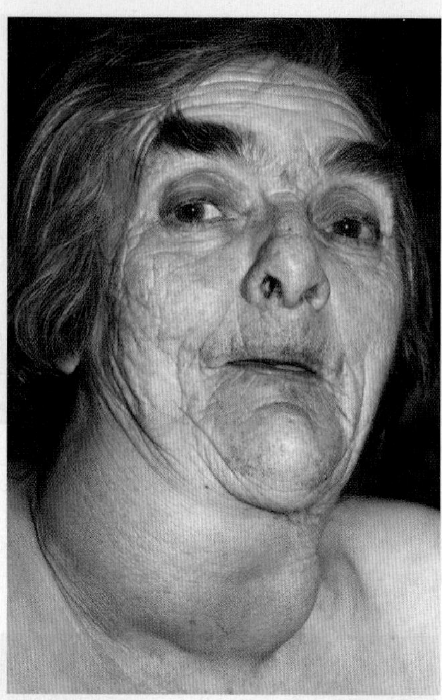

Myxedema. With severe hypothyroidism, patients present with periorbital swelling and edema of the face, hands, and feet. These patients must be identified and treated quickly and over the long term with exogenous thyroid hormone.

13

Eyes Assessment

Learning Objectives

1 Identify common landmarks of the eye. Relate periorbital landmarks to eye structures.

2 Demonstrate knowledge of the anatomy and physiology of the eye.

3 Identify important topics for health promotion and risk reduction related to the eye and vision.

4 Collect subjective data related to the eye.

5 Collect objective data related to the eye using physical examination techniques.

6 Identify normal and abnormal findings related to the eye.

7 Analyze subjective and objective data from assessment of the eye and consider initial interventions.

8 Document and communicate data from the eye assessment using appropriate terminology and principles of recording.

9 Consider the condition, age, gender, and culture of the patient to individualize eye assessment.

10 Identify nursing diagnoses and initiate a plan of care based on findings from the eye assessment.

Mr. Harris, a 61-year-old African American man, is in the adult medicine clinic for a routine physical examination. His temperature is 37°C (98.6°F), pulse 86 beats/min, respirations 16 breaths/min, and blood pressure 118/68 mm Hg. Upon reviewing documentation from his last annual assessment, the nurse notes that Mr. Harris takes a blood pressure medication and a cholesterol-lowering agent. The patient previously worked as a janitor for the school system and now is a school bus driver. He has a 5-year history of glaucoma, for which he uses eye drops. Today, he states that his vision seems worse than usual.

You will gain more information about Mr. Harris as you progress through this chapter. As you study the content and features, consider Mr. Harris's case and its relationship to what you are learning. Begin thinking about the following points:

- What are the signs and symptoms of glaucoma?
- How can examination findings distinguish glaucoma from other eye conditions such as macular degeneration?
- How will you teach Mr. Harris about preventing falls associated with vision loss?
- What factors may have contributed to Mr. Harris's glaucoma?
- What recommendation for additional screening and follow-up would you recommend for Mr. Harris?
- How can you evaluate Mr. Harris's understanding of what you taught him about preventing vision loss related to falls at home?

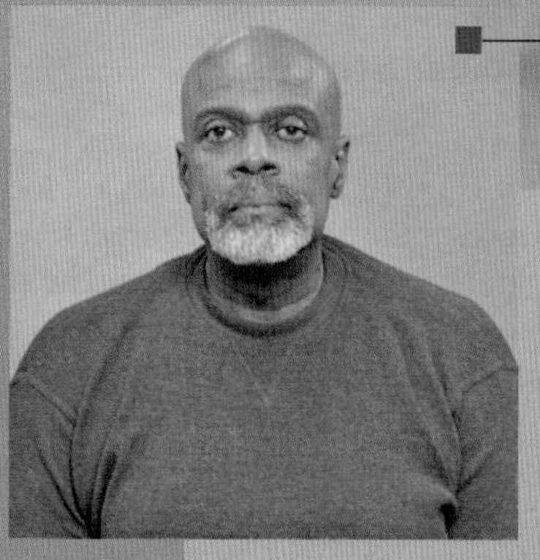

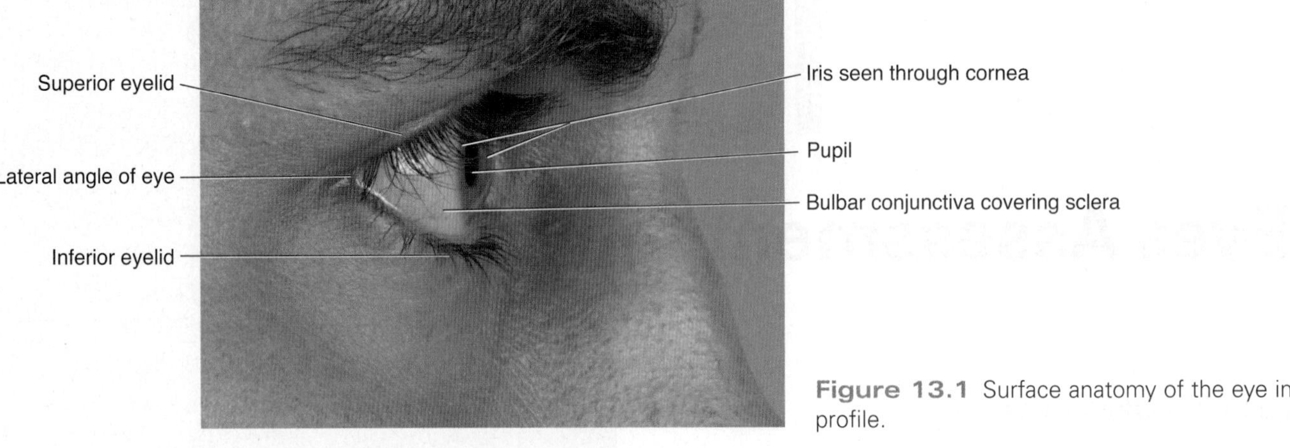

Figure 13.1 Surface anatomy of the eye in profile.

This chapter reviews anatomy and physiology pertinent to ocular and visual function, along with key variations in eye assessment related to lifespan and culture. It explores subjective data collection for eye health, including assessment of risk factors and focused history related to common symptoms. Content on objective data collection includes correct techniques for assessing vision, ocular movements, the external eye, and exterior and interior ocular structures; expected and unexpected visual and ocular findings; and appropriate documentation. Tests of visual acuity are part of the screening process during the complete physical examination and ongoing assessments for patients with identified ocular and visual problems or diseases. Although challenging, ocular and retinal assessments provide information that can assist with accurate diagnosis and related early interventions.

Structure and Function

The eye (commonly referred to as the eyeball) is the sensory organ of sight. The orbital socket of the cranium protects the complex internal structures of the eye; only the anterior portion of the eyeball is visible.

The eye is small, with an approximate diameter of 2.5 cm (1 in.). It takes in information in the form of light, which internal structures then analyze and interpret to produce shapes, colors, and objects.

Extraocular Structures

The external (extraocular) structures of the eye support and protect it (Fig. 13.1). The eyelids are loose mobile folds of skin that cover the eye, protect it from foreign bodies, regulate light entrance, and distribute tears. The **palpebral fissure** is the almond-shaped open space between the eyelids. The lid margins normally approximate completely when the palpebral fissure is closed. The upper eyelid normally covers the upper portion of the iris. The lower eyelid's margin is at the **limbus**, which is the border between the cornea and sclera.

The conjunctiva is a thin mucous membrane that lines the inner eyelid (palpebral conjunctiva) and also covers the sclera (bulbar conjunctiva). The lacrimal apparatus (which consists of the lacrimal gland, punctum, lacrimal sac, and nasolacrimal duct) protects and lubricates the cornea and conjunctiva by producing and draining tears (Fig. 13.2).

Extraocular Muscle Function

The six extraocular muscles control eye movement and hold the eye in place in the socket. These muscles coordinate their actions to produce vision within both eyes (Fig. 13.3). Proper functioning of these muscles determines normal alignment or position of the eye. The muscles and their functions are as follows:

- *Superior rectus*: elevates the eye upward and adducts (toward the nose) and rotates the eye medially (inward)
- *Inferior rectus*: rotates the eye downward and adducts and rotates the eye medially
- *Lateral rectus*: moves the eye laterally (toward the temple)

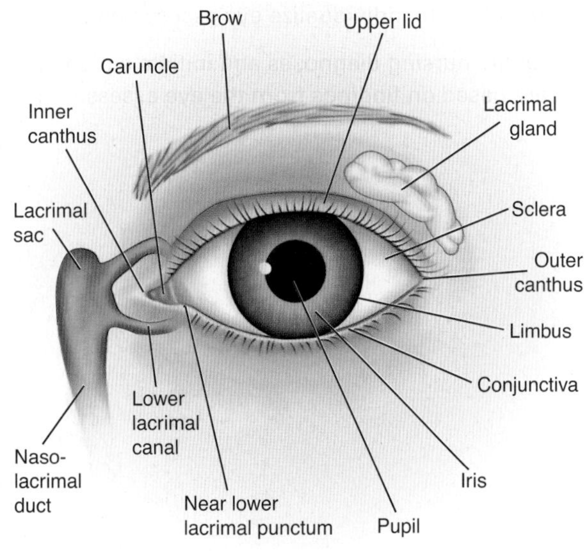

Figure 13.2 Structures of the eye and lacrimal apparatus.

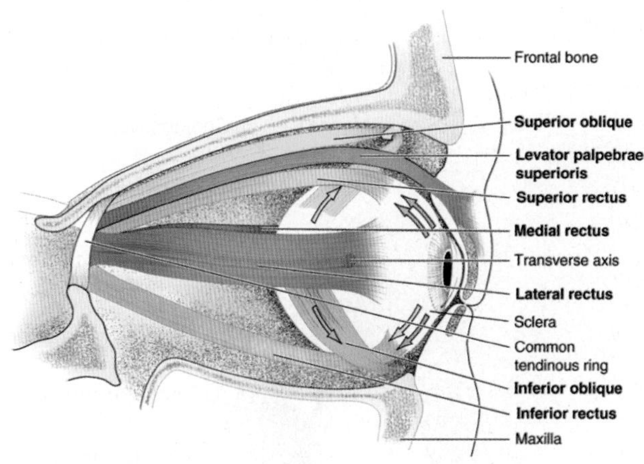

Figure 13.3 The extraocular muscles.

- *Medial rectus*: moves the eye medially
- *Superior oblique*: turns the eye downward and abducts (toward the temple) and rotates the eye laterally
- *Inferior oblique*: turns the eye upward and abducts and turns the eye laterally

The oculomotor (CN III), trochlear (CN IV), and abducens (CN VI) nerves innervate and control the motor nerve activities of the eye (Table 13.1).

The extraocular muscles oppose one another, much like the muscles surrounding joints of the skeleton. One muscle's contraction causes a relaxation of the corresponding muscle.

Intraocular Structures

The internal (intraocular) structures are involved in vision directly. The eye itself contains three layers of tissue:

1. An outer fibrous layer contains the sclera and cornea.
2. A vascular middle layer is composed of the iris, ciliary body, and choroids.
3. An inner neural layer is the retina.

The white sclera helps to maintain the size and shape of the eye. The transparent and avascular cornea allows light rays to enter the eye. It is highly sensitive to touch. The iris regulates the amount of light that enters the pupil. The color of the eye depends on the type and amount of pigment in the smooth muscles of the iris. The pupil opens and closes to permit light to enter the eye. Pupil size can range from 3 to 5 mm. The lens, which sits directly behind the pupil, refracts and focuses light on to the retina. The ciliary body produces aqueous humor and contains the muscle that controls the shape of the lens. The choroids, which cover the recessed portion of the eye, are a network of blood vessels to the eye (Fig. 13.4).

The interior eye has three chambers: anterior, posterior, and vitreous. The anterior chamber is the space between the cornea in the front and the iris and lens at the back. It contains aqueous humor, produced by the ciliary body; the amount varies to maintain pressure in the eye. The posterior chamber starts behind the iris and goes to the lens. It is also filled with aqueous humor that helps to nourish the cornea and lens. The largest vitreous chamber is adjacent to the inner retinal layer and lens. This chamber is filled with vitreous humor, which is gelatinous, holds the retina in place, and maintains the shape of the eyeball.

The retina, which is the innermost layer of the eye, receives and transmits visual stimuli to the brain for processing. The retinal structures are best viewed using an ophthalmoscope. The retina contains photoreceptors (rods and cones) that make vision possible. The rods on the outer edge of the retina are primarily responsible for vision in low light and produce images of varying shades of black and white. The cones, concentrated centrally, are adapted to bright light and produce color images and sharp fine details.

The optic disc, a well-defined round or oval area, is the opening for the optic nerve head. The macula, lateral to the optic disc, is the area with the greatest concentration of cones.

Vision

The light rays from a viewed object enter the cornea and are refracted on to the central fovea (an area on the macula). The stimulus is then inverted, reversed, and focused on the retina, which sends the stimulus through the visual pathway to the

TABLE 13.1 Eye Muscles

Muscle	Cranial Nerve Innervation	Insertion	Action: *Medial (Toward Nose)*	Action: *Lateral (Toward Temple)*
Superior rectus	CN III	Anterior, superior surface	Elevation, adduction	
Inferior rectus	CN III	Anterior, inferior surface	Depression, abduction	
Medial rectus	CN III	Anterior, medial surface	Adduction	
Lateral rectus	CN VI	Anterior, lateral surface		Abduction
Superior oblique	CN IV	Posterior, superior, lateral surface		Depression, abduction
Inferior oblique	CN III	Posterior, inferior, lateral surface		Elevation, abduction

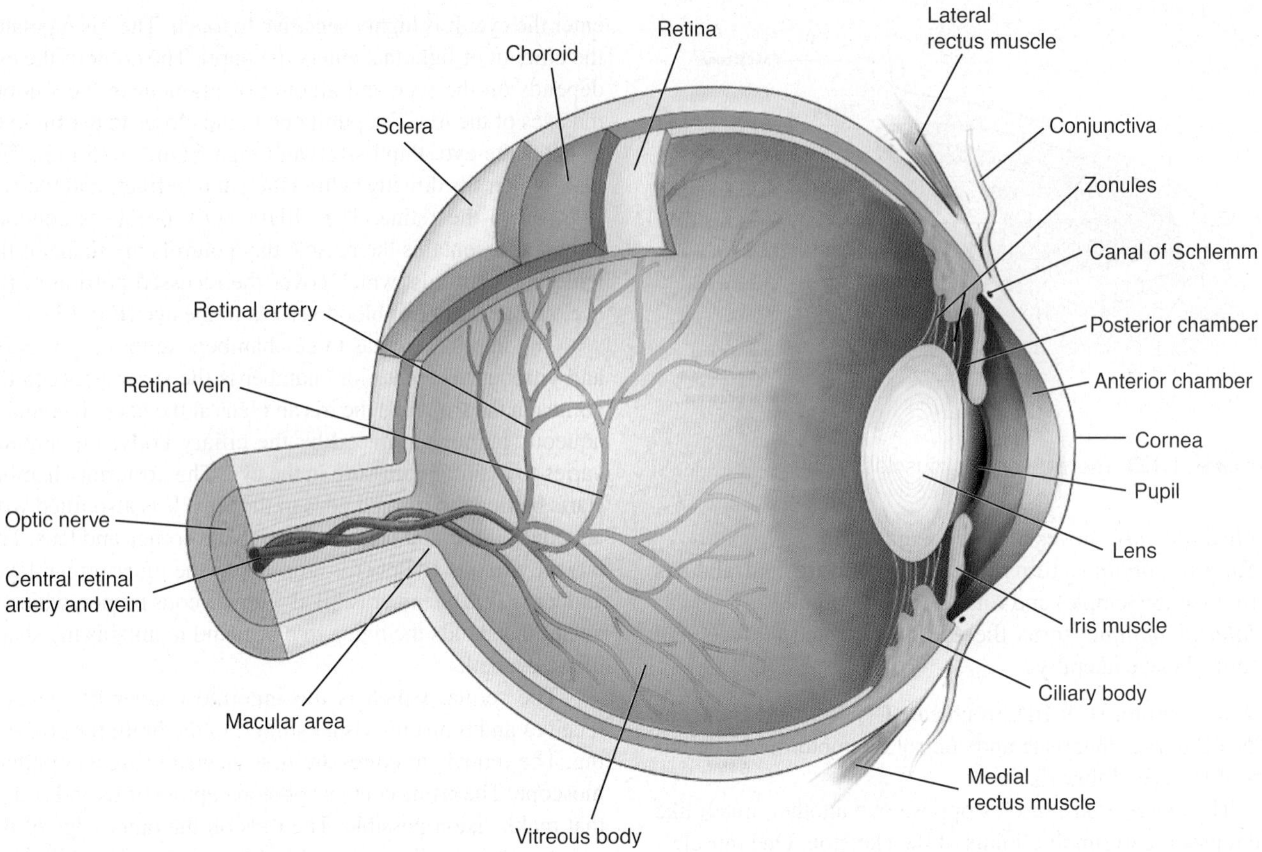

Retina
Lateral
rectus muscle
Choroid
Sclera
Conjunctiva
Zonules
Canal of Schlemm
Retinal artery
Posterior chamber
Retinal vein
Anterior chamber
Cornea
Pupil
Optic nerve
Lens
Central retinal
artery and vein
Iris muscle
Macular area
Ciliary body
Medial
rectus muscle
Vitreous body

Figure 13.4 Intraocular structures.

brain where the image returns to its original form. The neural pathway consists of the optic nerves, optic chiasm, and optic tracts that continue into the optic region of the cerebral cortex. The neural pathway is part of the central nervous system (Fig. 13.5).

Left visual
field
Right visual
field
Temporal
Temporal
Nasal
Left eye
Right eye
Optic nerve
Optic chiasm
Optic tract
Lateral
geniculate
body
1
2
3
4
Visual cortex

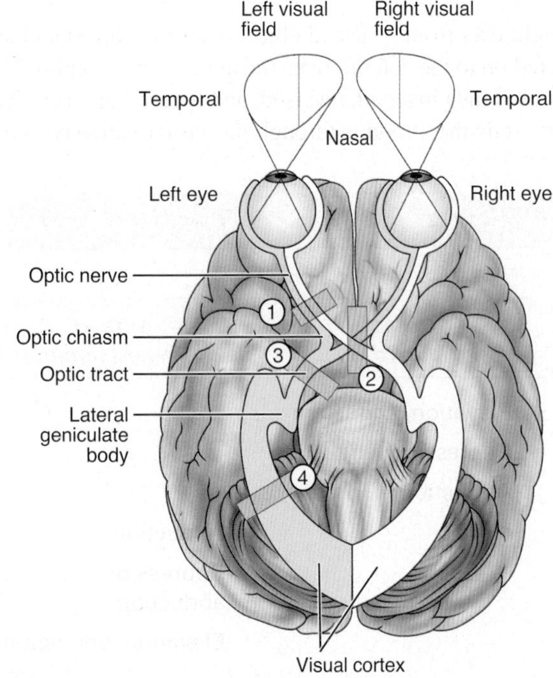

Figure 13.5 The neural pathway.

Lifespan Considerations: Older Adults

Older adults have changes both in eye structures and vision. Eyelids may droop and become wrinkled from loss of skin elasticity. The eyes sit deeper in the orbits from loss of subcutaneous fat. Eyebrows become thinner, and the outer thirds of the brows may be absent. Conjunctivae are thinner and may appear yellowish from decreased perfusion. The iris may have an irregular pigmentation. Formation of tears decreases as a result of loss of fatty tissue in the lacrimal apparatus. Vision may decline. Because the pupil is smaller, loss of accommodation, decreased night vision, and decreased depth perception occur. The lens enlarges and transparency decreases, making vision less acute (The Merck Manual for Health Care Professionals, 2013).

Cultural Considerations

Eye color differs among people of various genetic backgrounds, with lighter eyes more prevalent in more northern countries. Genetic background also influences the diameters of eyelids and eyebrows (Price, Gupta, Woodward, Stinnett, & Murchison, 2009).

Urgent Assessment

Acute assessment of the eye first involves identifying the problem and then determining whether the situation requires immediate medical attention. In the case of acute eye trauma or injury, time delay is potentially threatening to eye function.

Gradual vision loss, although significant, does not usually require an emergency referral. Furthermore, determining the source of the trauma or injury (e.g., mechanical, thermal, radiant, chemical, electrical, kinetic) helps determine whether the problem is on an emergency basis (immediate medical attention needed), urgent (medical attention needed within few hours), or nonurgent (make appointment as soon as possible). Rapid assessment of the eye involves assessing for foreign bodies, lacerations, or hyphema (blood in the anterior chamber of the eye); and testing extraocular movements. Acute glaucoma is caused by an acute blockage of the fluid at the base between the iris and cornea. This is a medical emergency and may result in permanent vision loss if untreated.

> ⚠ *SAFETY ALERT*
> *Trauma that involves a penetrating injury or suspected fracture of the orbital bone requires a referral on an emergency basis. If a patient describes loss of vision, it is critical to ascertain a timeline of vision loss. Sudden loss of vision requires an immediate referral to specialist.*

Subjective Data

Subjective data collection begins with the health history, continues with questions about specific eye conditions, and ends with detailed collection of information involving areas of concern. Health promotion goals focus on prevention of optical disease with aging and also occupational or recreational risk factors.

Assessment of Risk Factors

Eye and vision problems are common. Vision problems are the second most prevalent health problem (Centers for Disease Control and Prevention [CDC], 2013). The leading causes of blindness and impaired vision in patients in the United States are primarily age-related eye diseases such as macular degeneration, cataract, diabetic retinopathy, and glaucoma. As the nurse, you need to assess for risk factors related to eye problems, including family history, trauma, illnesses, and occupational hazards.

History and Risk Factors	Rationale
Past Medical History	
Are you having any eye problems now?	This general question opens discussion.
Eye Conditions	
• Do you have a history of cataracts, glaucoma, high blood pressure, diabetes, or thyroid disease? • Do you have any history of eye injury? • Have you ever had injuries or accidents, foreign bodies, or trauma to your eyes?	The focus is conditions that could affect vision and eye function.
Eye Surgery	
• Have you ever had any surgery on your eye(s)? • Have you ever had any facial surgery? • Have you ever had cataract removal, lens implant, or LASIK?	The focus is eye or facial surgeries, which can change the landscape of eye structures.
Allergies	
• Do you have any allergies? Are they seasonal? • Are you sensitive to pollen or animal dander, which can cause watery and itchy eyes? • How do you react to insect stings or bites? Any swelling around the eyes?	The body's response to allergens affects not only the respiratory system but also the eyes through excessive formation of tears, allergic conjunctivitis, and itching. Insect stings or bites to the eye often lead to periorbital edema and erythema. Previous occurrences increase risk of an angioedema-type allergic response with repeat exposure.
Eye Health	
• When was your last eye examination? • Were you screened for glaucoma then?	You need to determine how the patient cares for the health of the eyes.

(table continues on page 316)

History and Risk Factors	Rationale
Corrective Prescriptions • Do you wear glasses or contact lenses, or both? • Do you wear contacts for the recommended time frame only? • How do you care for your contacts? • How often do you change your contacts?	These questions address risks to reduce the number of people with uncorrected refractive errors. You can discuss the reason for not wearing prescribed glasses or contact lenses and care of contacts to prevent injuries to the eye.
Eye Protection • Are you exposed to any hazards that could affect your eyes? • Do you wear goggles or a face shield when you play sports or do home projects? • Do you wear your protective eyewear 100% of the time?	Questions address goals to reduce injuries to the eyes of people whose occupation or leisure activities put them at risk.
Nutritional Status. Do you generally eat a well-balanced diet?	Assess the diet for any vitamin deficiencies that could affect the eyes.
Medications Do you use artificial tears, decongestants, corticosteroids, antibiotics, antihistamines, or any prescribed eye drops?	Certain medications affect the eye and its functioning. Careful assessment is necessary.
Family History Do any family members have myopia, hyperopia, strabismus, color blindness, cataracts, glaucoma, retinitis pigmentosa, or retinoblastoma?	Certain conditions and diseases that affect vision have a genetic link, which increases risk for patients. Glaucoma in a first-degree relative increases the patient's risk for the same problem 200%–300% (Stein et al., 2012).
Risk Factors ***Exposure to Viruses*** • Has anyone ever told you that you were exposed to rubella in the womb? • Were you diagnosed with congenital syphilis?	Maternal exposure to rubella can lead to congenital eye problems in the fetus. Fetal exposure to rubella can cause neonatal blindness secondary to cataracts. Congenital syphilis can also cause neonatal blindness.
Environmental Exposure • Are you exposed to toxins, chemicals, infections, or allergens at work? • How would you relate your current stress level: low, moderate, or high?	Many activities can increase risk for eye injury, infections, or trauma. Stress has been linked with decreased vision.

Risk Reduction and Health Promotion

Diabetes mellitus increases risks for eye problems, including diabetic retinopathy, cataracts, and glaucoma. Sunlight exposure also increases risks, so use of sunglasses is important, especially if the patient lives in a sunny climate. Poor diet has been linked to eye problems. Foods that promote eye health include deep-water fish, fruits, and vegetables (e.g., carrots, spinach). Because the lens has no blood supply, keep it well hydrated by drinking plenty of fluids.

The goals related to visual health are

- to improve visual health through prevention
- early detection, treatment
- rehabilitation

(U.S. D.H.H.S., 2013)

Common Symptoms

In assessing the patient's health history, it is important to immediately determine whether an eye problem results from trauma, is related to changes in vision, or involves visual symptoms. Failure to obtain an accurate and complete history can lead to loss of sight.

Common Symptoms

- Pain
- Trauma or surgery
- Visual change
- Blind spots, floaters, or halos
- Discharge
- Change in activities of daily living (ADLs)

Signs/Symptoms	Rationale/Abnormal Findings
Pain Do you have any eye pain or discomfort? (Ask about location, intensity, duration, description, aggravating factors, alleviating factors, functional impairment, and pain control goal.)	Pain in the eye is never normal and should always be further explored.
Trauma or Surgery Is the problem you are having related to trauma or an injury? If so: • How was the injury/trauma sustained? • Was this a high-velocity injury? • Was this a blunt-force trauma?	High-velocity injuries are typically penetrating. Blunt force trauma often results in fracture of the orbit.
Visual Change Have you noticed any recent changes to your vision? • What is the nature of the visual change? • When did the change begin? • Was onset sudden or gradual? • Have you noticed any double vision or halos/rainbows around objects?	If the patient describes loss of vision, it is critical to ascertain a timeline. Sudden vision loss requires an immediate referral.
Blind Spots, Floaters, or Halos • Have you noticed any blind spots in your vision? • Any difficulty seeing at night? • Do you see any spots (floaters)? • Do you have any associated symptoms (e.g., flashing lights, floaters, halos around lights)?	Loss of night vision is associated with optic atrophy, glaucoma, and vitamin A deficiency. **Floaters** (translucent specks that drift across the visual field) are common in people older than 40 years of age and nearsighted patients; no additional follow-up is needed.
Discharge • Are you having any ocular discharge? • Is there any pain or grittiness, or redness, associated with the discharge? • Are one or both eyes affected? • Have you noticed any excessive tearing, dryness, or itching?	Discharge is associated with inflammation or infection.
Change in Activities of Daily Living How has your eye situation (e.g., diplopia, dry eyes) affected your ability to perform ADLs?	Assess functional limitations.

Documenting Normal Findings

Denies pain, trauma, visual changes, blind spots, floaters, halos, and discharge. No changes in ability to perform ADLs.

Lifespan Considerations: Older Adults

Additional Questions	Rationale/Abnormal Findings
Do you have a history of diabetes, glaucoma, or high blood pressure?	Aging increases risks for visual complications related to other chronic diseases that affect blood vessels in the retina and fluid in the eye (Miller, 2009).
Have you noticed any tunneling of your visual field?	This is a symptom of macular degeneration.

(table continues on page 318)

Additional Questions	Rationale/Abnormal Findings
Have you ever had your eyes checked for glaucoma, cataracts, or other eye conditions?	This provides you with an opportunity to promote eye health.
Do you have any trouble managing your usual activities because of vision changes? Have you stopped doing any activities because of vision changes?	It is important to focus on any visual impairment and how the patient functions with it.
When did you last have a test for glaucoma?	Older adults are at increased risk; glaucoma screening is not recommended by primary care providers for older adults without vision problems (U.S. Preventive Services Task Force, 2013).
Have you ever tripped or fallen because of changes in your vision?	This question assesses awareness and presence of visual impairments.

Cultural Considerations

Additional Questions	Rationale/Abnormal Findings
Have you had your eyes examined in the past year? Do you wear sunglasses when outside? Have you been tested for diabetes?	Racial groups that have higher rates of glaucoma have thicker irides. Chinese Americans have the thickest irides and have the highest rates of glaucoma (Lee et al., 2013). Certain ethnic groups are at increased risk for developing eye health problems, especially associated with diabetes-related eye disease. Ethnic populations are less likely to understand the importance of year-round ultraviolet eye protection and less likely to have access to care. Most Hispanics are unaware that the sun can damage their eyes. Some Asian Americans believe that wearing glasses may make their vision worse (Prevent Blindness America, 2012).

Therapeutic Dialogue: Collecting Subjective Data

Mr. Harris, introduced at the beginning of this chapter, is in the clinic for follow-up care related to high blood pressure, high cholesterol, and glaucoma. The following conversation is an example of a nurse's effective interview style.

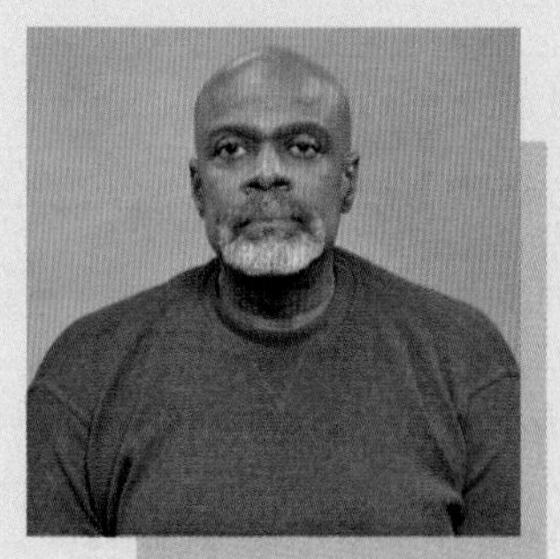

Nurse: I'm glad that you came back for your visit today. It's good to see you.

Mr. Harris: Thanks. I am really trying to take better care of myself.

Nurse: I noticed that your blood pressure is under good control.

(case study continues on page 319)

Mr. Harris: Yes, I'm really trying to make sure to eat right, get some exercise, and take my medicine. I have two beautiful grandkids that I'm helping to raise. (pauses) I'm worried about my eyesight. I have glaucoma, and I can't see as well. I'm worried that I'll go blind and won't be able to help with my grandkids.

Nurse: You've had glaucoma for about 5 years now, is that correct?

Mr. Harris: Yes. The doctor gave me some drops for it.

Nurse: Can you take them as prescribed?

Mr. Harris: Well, I ran out a bit ago and had to wait a few days until the first of the month, but I have them now.

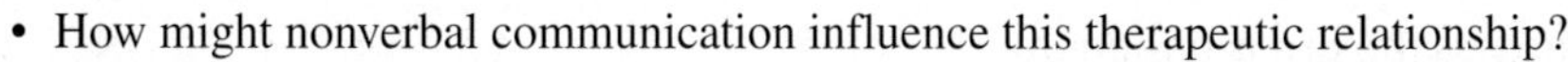

Critical Thinking Challenge

- How might nonverbal communication influence this therapeutic relationship?
- Within a culturally competent framework, how might the nurse address Mr. Harris's concern regarding being unable to help with his grandchildren?
- How might the nurse respond to Mr. Harris's not taking his eye drops as prescribed?

Objective Data

A comprehensive physical examination of the eye involves assessment of visual acuity, the external eye, eye muscle function, external ocular structures (including pupil reflexes), and internal ocular structures. The external eyes and external ocular structures are examined through inspection and palpation. The interior ocular structures are inspected with an instrument called an ophthalmoscope. Identifying anatomical landmarks of the external eye helps you document findings.

Common and Specialty or Advanced Techniques

Routine eye assessment includes the most important and common assessment techniques performed to screen for difficulties. Nurses may add specialty or advanced assessment techniques if concerns exist over a specific finding. The most common and advanced techniques used in the comprehensive assessment of the eye are summarized in the table.

Equipment

- Penlight
- Cotton wisps and cotton-tipped applicators
- Ophthalmoscope
- Snellen chart for far-vision testing
- Jaeger chart for near-vision testing
- Occlusive covers for individual eye testing
- Ishihara plates (optional for testing color vision)

Basic Versus Focused/Specialty or Advanced Techniques Related to Eye Assessment

Technique	Purpose	Screening or Registered Nurse Assessment	Focused or Advanced Practice Examination
Inspect external eyes.	To evaluate for symmetry, redness, and obvious deformities	X	
Test distance vision.	To evaluate ability to see far, drive	X	
Test near vision.	To evaluate ability to read	X	
Test cardinal fields of gaze.	To assess for movement of the eye in several planes of movement	X	

(table continues on page 320)

Basic Versus Focused/Specialty or Advanced Techniques Related to Eye Assessment *(continued)*			
Technique	**Purpose**	**Screening or Registered Nurse Assessment**	**Focused or Advanced Practice Examination**
Inspect and palpate lacrimal apparatus and conjunctiva.	To evaluate swelling, tenderness	X	
Test pupillary reflex.	To evaluate the pupil's response to direct and consensual light source	X	
Assess color vision.	To evaluate ability to differentiate color		X Color blindness
Test static confrontation.	To screen for differences in the visual field from side-to-side and inferior and superior		X Visual field deficits
Test kinetic confrontation.	To assess the gross peripheral boundaries		X Peripheral field deficits
Test corneal light reflex.	To test for strabismus		X Strabismus
Perform cover test.	To assess the presence and amount of ocular deviation		X Ocular deviation
Inspect cornea and lens.	To assess for glaucoma and cataracts		X Glaucoma and cataracts
Inspect posterior eye.	To evaluate disc, vessels, macula, and periphery		X Disc, vessels, macula and periphery

Preparation

Before you begin the examination, perform hand hygiene. If you are using hand gel, be sure that your hands are completely dry before touching the patient. If there is a complaint or signs of an infection, take measures to avoid cross-contamination: (1) wash hands, (2) don gloves, and (3) clean all equipment before you examine the first (uninfected) eye, then repeat this sequence before examining the second (infected) eye. Always examine the infected eye last.

Assessment of visual acuity, visual fields, and the retina helps you evaluate not only the function of the eye itself but also part of the central nervous system.

As you proceed with inspection and palpation of the eye, assess for sensory and motor function of cranial nerves II, III, IV, and VI (Table 13.2). As you progress through the assessment, remember not only the sensory aspects of vision but also the motor function of the eyes. Thorough examination can make the difference in identifying risks and preventing blindness.

Assessment of Visual Acuity

Visual acuity tests include testing for distance vision, near vision, peripheral vision, and color vision. Perform this first step in the eye assessment before using any type of solution to dilate the pupil.

TABLE 13.2 Cranial Nerves Associated With the Eyes

Cranial Nerve	Name of Cranial Nerve	Assessment of Cranial Nerve
II	Optic nerve	• Visual acuity • Visual fields • Funduscopic examination
III	Occulomotor	• Cardinal fields of gaze • Eyelid inspection • Pupil reaction (direct/consensual/accommodation)
IV	Trochlear	• Cardinal fields of gaze
VI	Abducens	• Cardinal fields of gaze

Technique and Normal Findings	Abnormal Findings
Distance Vision Assess distance visual acuity by having the patient read the Snellen or Allen chart (based on developmental age or reading ability). With the **Snellen test**, measure and place a mark or piece of masking tape on the floor 6 m (about 20 ft) from the chart (Fig. 13.6). With the Allen test, place the mark or piece of masking tape on the floor 4.5 m (15 ft) from the chart. The area should be well lit, and the test should be at the patient's eye level. 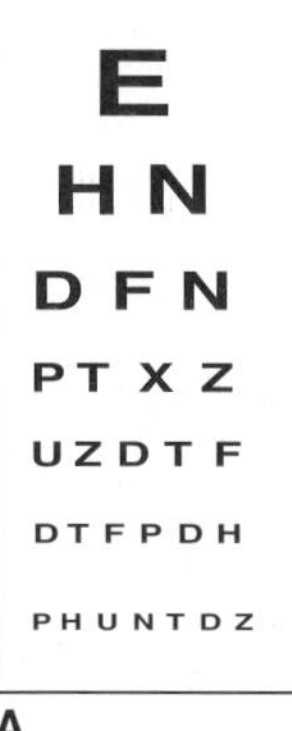 A 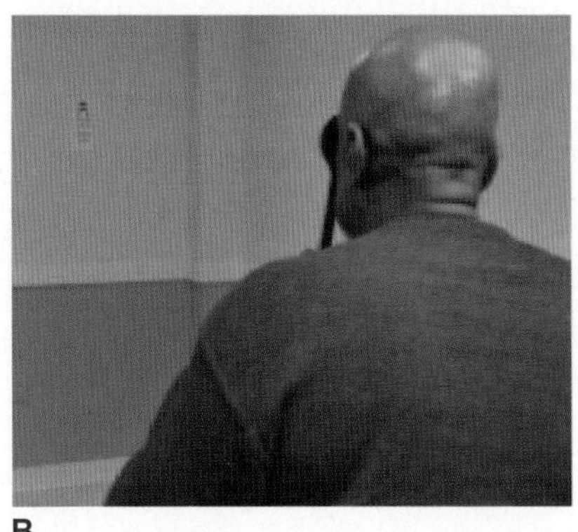 B **Figure 13.6** Assessing distance vision. **A.** The Snellen chart. **B.** The patient reads the letters of the Snellen chart from 20 ft away.	
Give the patient an opaque card or eye occluder so that he or she can cover one eye at a time during assessment. Stand by the chart and request that the patient read through it to the smallest letters possible (or the smallest pictures if using the Allen chart), occluding one eye at a time. Then request that the patient read the next smallest line. If the patient wears glasses or contacts, they should remain on; only reading glasses should be removed for the assessment.	Unexpected findings include leaning forward, squinting, hesitation, misidentification of more than three of seven objects, or more than a two-line difference between eyes. Refer to Table 13.4 at the end of the chapter.
Acuity for distance vision is documented in two numbers, with reference to what a person with normal vision sees 6 m (about 20 ft) from the test. Someone with "20/20" (normal) vision can read at 6 m (about 20 ft) what the normal eye can read at 6 m (about 20 ft). On top, mark the distance in feet the patient was from the chart (e.g., 20). On bottom, mark the number under the smallest line of letters the patient correctly identified (e.g., 40, 200). Also document the number of letters missed and whether the patient wore corrective lenses (e.g., right eye: 20/30 −2, with glasses). The larger the bottom number, the worse the visual acuity. Refractive index (emmetropia) of the eye is 20/20 bilaterally.	A larger number on the bottom (e.g., 20/60) indicates diminished distance vision. **SAFETY ALERT** *The abbreviations OD (oculus dexter—right eye), OS (oculus sinister—left eye), and OU (oculus uterque—each eye) are no longer used to document eye findings because of the potential for medical order and medication errors. Instead, it is recommended to use "right eye," "left eye," or "both eyes" to document findings.*
Near Vision Near vision is usually assessed in patients older than 40 years of age or in younger patients who report difficulty reading. When no Jaeger test (pocket screener) is available, ask the patient to read newsprint (e.g., newspaper, magazine).	Patients older than 40 years of age often have a decreased ability to accommodate; therefore, they move the card further away to read it.

(table continues on page 322)

Technique and Normal Findings (continued)	Abnormal Findings (continued)
Instruct the patient to hold the **Jaeger chart** 35 cm (about 14 in.) from the eye. Request that the person read through the chart to the smallest letters possible, occluding one eye at a time (with corrective lenses on) (Fig. 13.7). Visual acuity for near vision is 14/14 bilaterally.  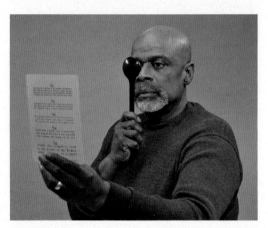 **Figure 13.7** Assessing near vision with the Jaeger chart.	
Color Vision Color vision is assessed using Ishihara cards (Fig. 13.8) or by having the patient identify color bars on the Snellen chart (specialty exam). The patient correctly identifies the embedded figures in the Ishihara cards or the colors bars on the Snellen chart.  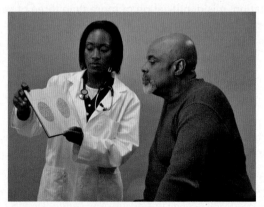 **Figure 13.8** Testing color vision.	A patient who incorrectly identifies the embedded figures or color bars may have color blindness.

Assessment of Visual Fields

The visual field refers to what in the environment is visible when the eye fixates on a stationary object. Visual injury or disease usually causes defects in the normal full visual field. The confrontation test is used to screen for visual field defects, which may not be readily apparent to the you as you examine the patient. When evaluating for visual field defects, the visual field is divided into four quadrants—inferior, superior, left, and right.

Visual field testing in the clinical setting can be performed without computerized automated perimetry; it is a gross screening of peripheral vision. You can use either the static or the kinetic technique. The static test can help you detect gross differences in all four quadrants of the visual field. You present one to four fingers in each quadrant, but you do not move your fingers in the way that you do in the kinetic test. The static test effectively screens for differences from side to side (hemianopias) and inferior and superior (attitudinal). The kinetic test assesses the gross peripheral boundaries of the patient's visual field. When using the kinetic technique, you move an object or your fingers from the periphery toward fixation at the point that the patient first becomes aware of the target. This is a specialty skill.

Technique and Normal Findings	Abnormal Findings
Static Confrontation Stand approximately 61–92 cm (2–3 ft) (an arm's length) directly in front of the patient. Your eyes and the patient's eyes should be on the same level. Ask the patient to cover the left eye with the palm of the left hand (without putting pressure on the eye). Close your right eye and instruct the patient to look only at your open eye at all times. Present one to four fingers midway between yourself and the patient in each of the four quadrants of the visual field (Fig. 13.9). Ask the patient to report the number of fingers, without looking directly at them (i.e., the patient should remain focused on your eye). Repeat the test with the other eye. Patient accurately reports the number of fingers presented in all four quadrants. 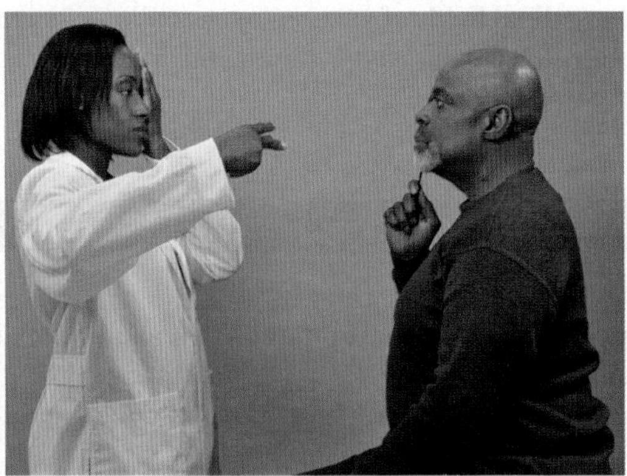 **Figure 13.9** Performing the static confrontation test.	This screening test assumes that your visual field is normal and serves as the comparison for the patient's test. Reports of an incorrect number of fingers indicate a visual field defect. Most confrontation tests are only around 60% sensitive to the identification of field loss (Prasad & Cohen, 2011).
Kinetic Confrontation As with static confrontation, your eyes and the patient's eyes must be on the same level. Instruct the patient to say "now" when the fingers first come into view. Wiggle your fingers from a far distal point and move them toward the center of each quadrant (Fig. 13.10). Your fingers should not be immediately visible (except in the inferotemporal quadrant). Patient sees the fingers at about the same time as you see them if the patient's peripheral visual field is normal in that quadrant. 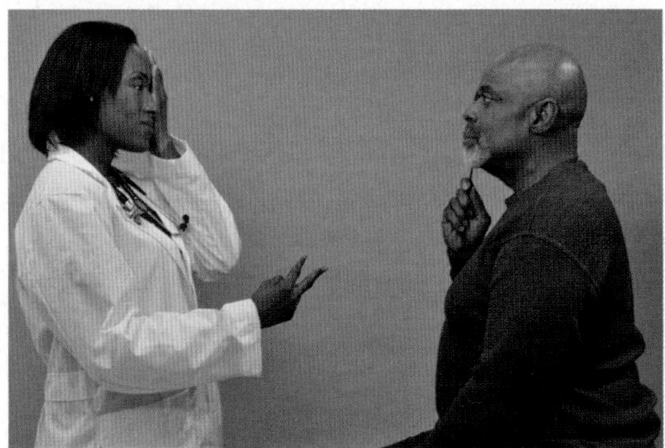 **Figure 13.10** Performing the kinetic confrontation test.	If you wave fingers on both sides, but the patient perceives motion on only one side, a hemianopic defect is suspected. If the patient sees only from an inferior or superior position, an attitudinal defect is suspected. Kinetic testing with a red target provides the highest sensitivity and specificity and, when combined with static finger wiggle testing, can achieve sensitivity of 78% and specificity of 90% (Prasad & Cohen, 2011). **SAFETY ALERT** *Defects in any quadrant in either the static or kinetic confrontation test require referral to an optometrist or ophthalmologist for more precise testing.*

> **Documenting Normal Findings**
>
> Visual acuity 20/20. Accurately reads newsprint. Identifies color bars on Snellen chart correctly. Patient sees finger at about 50 degrees superior, 90 degrees temporal, 90 degrees inferior, and 60 degrees nasal.

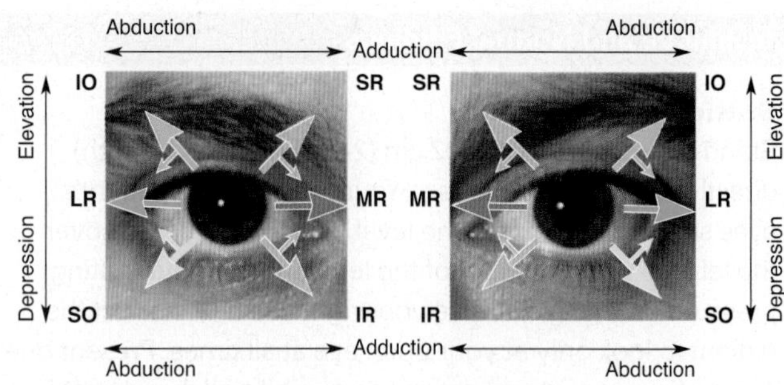

Figure 13.11 Extraocular movements.

Assessment of Extraocular Muscle Movements

Three basic tests allow examiners to assess the movement of the extraocular muscles: (1) the corneal light reflex (Hirschberg) test, (2) the cover test, and (3) the cardinal fields of gaze test. They assess movements of the eye in several planes: up and down, side-to-side, diagonally from right superior to left inferior, and diagonally from left superior to right inferior (Fig. 13.11).

- The **corneal light reflex** tests for strabismus.
- The **cover test** is for presence and amount of ocular deviation. The light level should be low, with no direct light sources shining in the patient's eyes. At rest, the extraocular muscles should have very little activity.
- The **cardinal fields of gaze** assessment allows you to detect muscle defects that cause misalignment or uncoordinated eye movements.

Technique and Normal Findings	Abnormal Findings
Corneal Light Reflex (Hirschberg) Test Instruct the patient to stare straight ahead at the bridge of your nose. Stand in front of the patient and shine a penlight at the bridge of the patient's nose. Note where the light reflects on the cornea of each eye (Fig. 13.12). Light reflection is in exactly the same spot in both eyes. 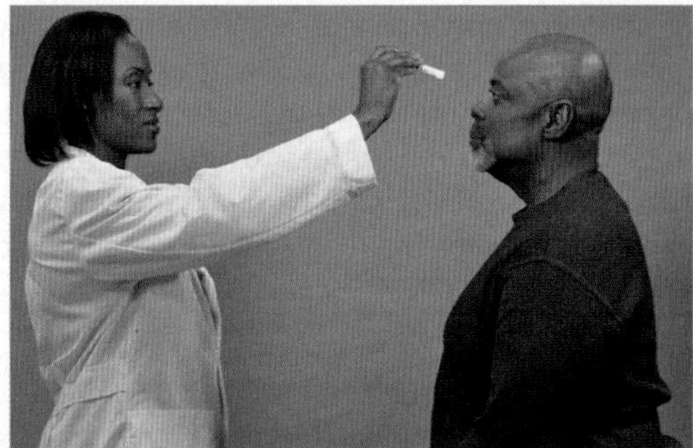 **Figure 13.12** Testing the corneal light reflex.	Unexpected findings indicate improper alignment and appear as asymmetric reflections. Document unexpected findings using the face of the clock as a guide.
Cover Test The cover test, most typically performed on children, helps with assessment of ocular alignment. Stand in front of the patient and ask the patient to focus on a near object (bridge of your nose). Place an opaque card or occluder over the eye; inspect for any movement of the uncovered eye that may indicate refixation of the gaze (Fig. 13.13). Remove the cover and observe the previously covered eye for refixation. Repeat the procedure for the other eye. Gaze is steady and fixed.	Any refixation is from muscle weakness in the covered eye (i.e., while covered, the eye drifted into a relaxed position).

(table continues on page 325)

Technique and Normal Findings (continued)	Abnormal Findings (continued)
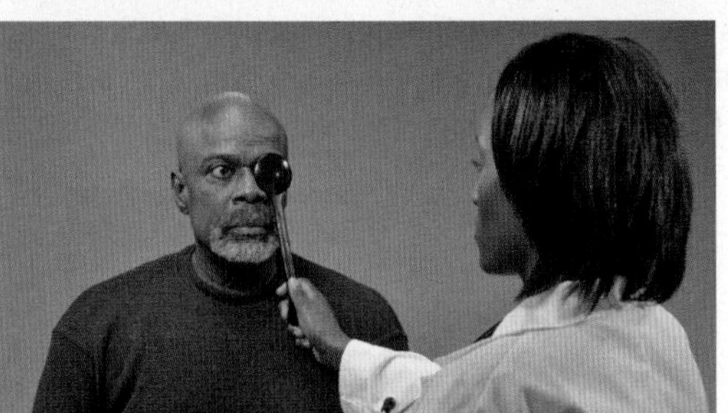 Figure 13.13 Performing the cover test.	
Cardinal Fields of Gaze Test Further testing of the extraocular muscles assesses for symmetrical movements of the eyes in all nine **cardinal fields of gaze**. Instruct the patient to hold the head steady and to follow the movement of your finger or pen with the eyes. Hold your finger or pen approximately 30–35 cm (12–14 in.) from the patient's face. Move slowly through positions 2 through 9, stopping momentarily in each, and then back to center (Fig. 13.14). Proceed clockwise. Patient's eyes move smoothly and symmetrically in all nine cardinal fields of gaze.	Document a deficit by noting in which field an abnormality is found. Mild nystagmus at the extreme lateral angles is normal; in any other position it is not. See Table 13.5 at the end of the chapter.
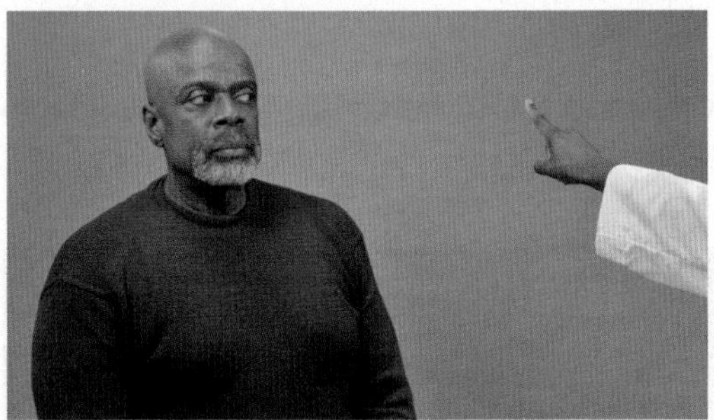 Figure 13.14 Assessing the cardinal fields of gaze.	

Documenting Normal Findings

Alignment symmetrical/corneal light reflex. Gaze fixed and steady. Extraocular movements intact (EOMI).

Assessment of External Eyes

Ensure good lighting. Wash your hands before touching the eyelids or face of the patient. Wear gloves if expecting contact with mucous membranes.

Technique and Normal Findings	Abnormal Findings
Stand directly in front of and facing the patient (who is sitting on the examination table or bed). Inspect eyebrows, lashes, and eyelids; note eye shape and symmetry. Eyebrows vary based on genetic background but show no unexplained hair loss. Lashes curve outward away from the eyes and are distributed evenly along the lid margins. Eyelids open and close completely, with spontaneous blinking every few seconds. Eye shape varies from round to almond but is symmetrical.	***Eyebrows***: unexplained hair loss; with normal aging, the outer third of the eyebrow thins ***Eyelashes***: curved inward toward the eye, distributed unevenly along lid margin, or both ***Eyelids***: incomplete opening or closing; no spontaneous blinking; improper positioning with respect to iris and limbus ***Eye shape***: asymmetry

(table continues on page 326)

Technique and Normal Findings (continued)	Abnormal Findings (continued)
Note general appearance of the eyes. Eyes are in parallel alignment.	Eyes not in parallel alignment require further assessment. Ptosis (drooping of the eyelids) is a common finding with stroke (Fig. 13.15). 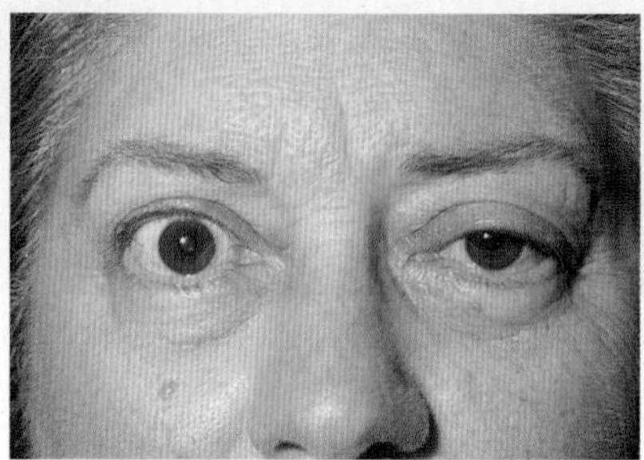 **Figure 13.15** Ptosis in a patient following stroke.
Lacrimal Apparatus Lightly slide the pad of your index finger against the client's upper orbital rim. Ask about any pain or tenderness. Palpate for the nasolacrimal duct to evaluate obstruction.	
Press against the patient's lower inner orbital rim, at the lacrimal sac. This will cause regurgitation of fluid in the puncta if obstruction exists (Fig. 13.16).	
An enlarged lacrimal apparatus is rare. If you palpate an enlarged lacrimal apparatus, evert the eyelid and inspect the gland. 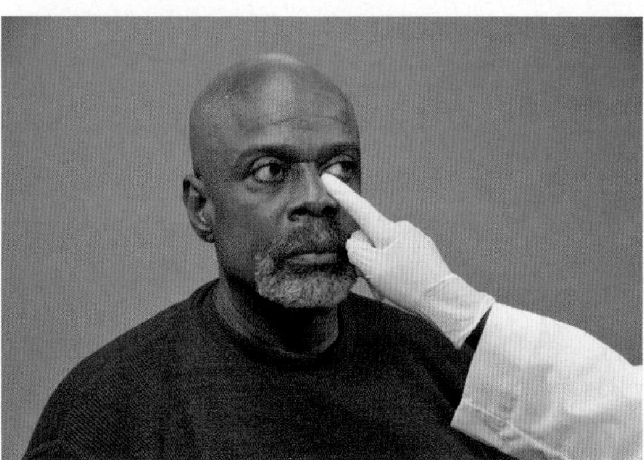 **Figure 13.16** Palpating the lacrimal apparatus.	Suspect conditions such as sarcoidosis and Sjögren syndrome (Fig. 13.17). 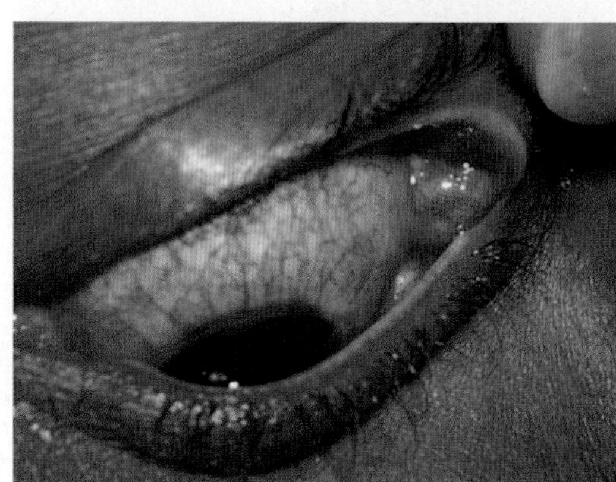 **Figure 13.17** Sjögren syndrome.
Bulbar Conjunctiva Gently lift the upper eyelid. Instruct the patient to look down and then to the right and left. Note the surface for color, injection (redness), swelling, exudates, or foreign bodies. Gently stretch down the lower lid (Fig. 13.18). Instruct the patient to look up and to the right and left. Again, examine the surface for color, injection (redness), swelling, exudates, or foreign bodies. Bulbar conjunctiva is normally transparent with small blood vessels visible.	Erythema, cobblestone appearance, or both may indicate allergy or infection. Sharply defined bright red blood indicates a subconjunctival hemorrhage (Fig. 13.19).

(table continues on page 327)

Technique and Normal Findings (continued) | **Abnormal Findings (continued)**

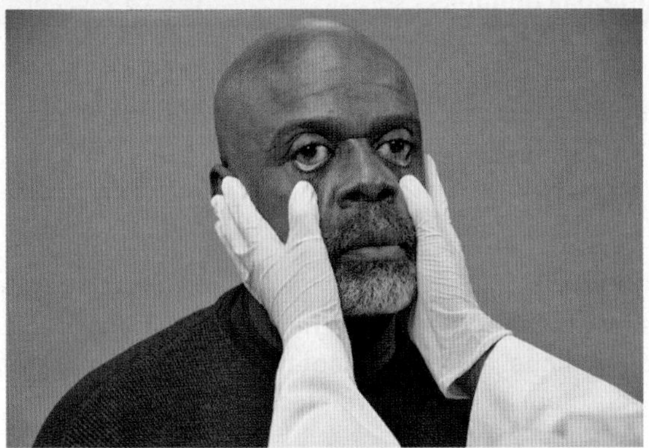

Figure 13.18 Inspecting the bulbar conjunctiva.

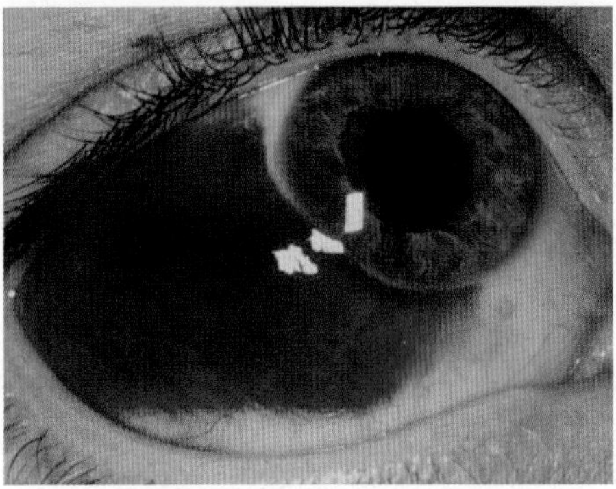

Figure 13.19 Subconjunctival hemorrhage.

An abnormal thickening of the conjunctiva from the limbus over the cornea is known as a pterygium. Pterygium is more common on the nasal side. Risk for development is heavy exposure to ultraviolet light, most commonly in equatorial areas. If pterygium advances over the pupil, it can interfere with vision (Fig. 13.20).

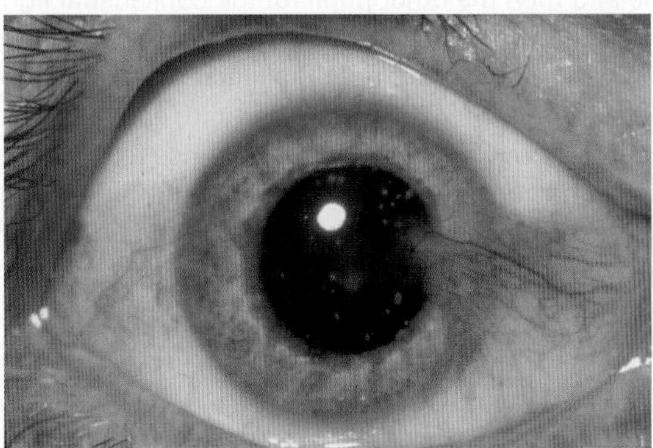

Figure 13.20 Pterygium.

Sclera

During inspection of the bulbar conjunctiva you can also inspect the sclera for color, exudates, lesions, and foreign bodies.

Sclera is clear, smooth, white, and without exudate, lesions, or foreign bodies.

Scleral abnormalities include jaundice, blueing, and drainage. Refer to Table 13.6 at the end of the chapter for abnormalities of the external eye.

Cornea and Lens

Stand in front of the patient. Use a penlight or ophthalmoscope split light to inspect the cornea. Shine the light directly on the cornea. Move the light laterally toward the bridge of the nose. Repeat on the other eye. Observe the angle of the anterior space and the clarity and translucence of the lens.

A wide angle allows full illumination of the iris. Lens is transparent.

A narrow angle indicates glaucoma.

Cloudiness of the lens can indicate a cataract, which is associated with increased age, smoking, alcohol intake, and sunlight exposure. Risk factors for cataracts are primarily environmental. See also Table 13.6.

Assessment of Exterior Ocular Structures

Technique and Normal Findings	Abnormal Findings
Iris Inspect the iris for color, nodules, and vascularity. Brown is the most common eye color in the world. Color is evenly distributed, smooth, and without apparent vascularity. A normal variation is mosaic variant.	See Table 13.6.
Pupils Examine the pupil using a direct method. Stand in front of the patient and use your light to observe the shape and size (mm) of the pupil. Pupil is black, round, and equal with a diameter of 2–6 mm (0.08–0.24 in.)	See Table 13.7 at the end of the chapter for unexpected pupil findings. Also see Chapter 22 for more information on neurological findings related to altered pupils. Describe the reaction as brisk, sluggish, fixed, pinpoint or blown.
Also test reactivity to light (see Chapter 22). Darken the room and instruct the patient to gaze into the distance to dilate the pupils. Ask him or her to keep looking ahead. Hold a light on the side (avoid pointing it into the eye). Observe for nystagmus in one or both eyes. Bringing the light in quickly from the side, observe the reaction of the same and then the other pupil for the consensual light reflex. Use a preprinted guide or scale on a penlight to identify the size. Record both the initial size and response size as R 6 → 4, L6 → 4. Pupils are round, equal, and constrict briskly (within 1 second) in response to light, both directly and consensually (when one pupil constricts to light, the other does, too). This is also recorded as PERRL (pupils equal, round, reactive to light) (Fig. 13.21). *PERRL* -pupils constrict directly and consensually. Note initial size and the reaction size. 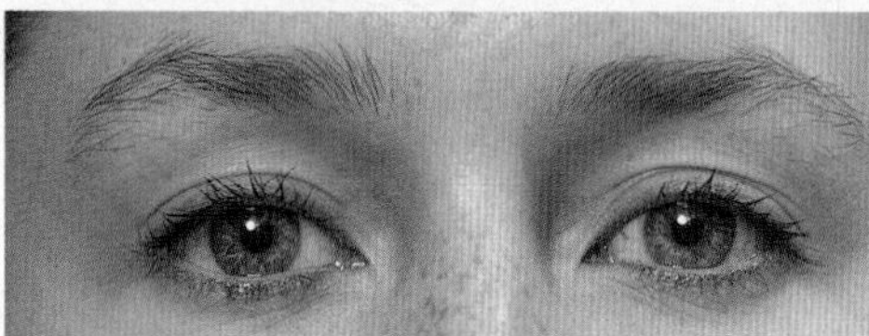 **Figure 13.21** Pupillary constriction.	Nystagmus is a jerking movement of the eye that can be quick and fluttering or slow and rolling, similar to a tremor. Causes include medications (e.g., antiseizure medications), cerebellar disease, weakness in the extraocular muscles, and damage to CN III.
To test for accommodation (CN III), instruct the patient to stare at a distant object for 30 seconds. Hold an index finger, penlight, or other safe object (e.g., pencil) about 36 cm (14 in.) in front of the nose. Ask the patient to focus on your finger as you move it toward the patient's nose (Fig. 13.22). Pupils constrict (accommodation) and eyes cross (convergence). 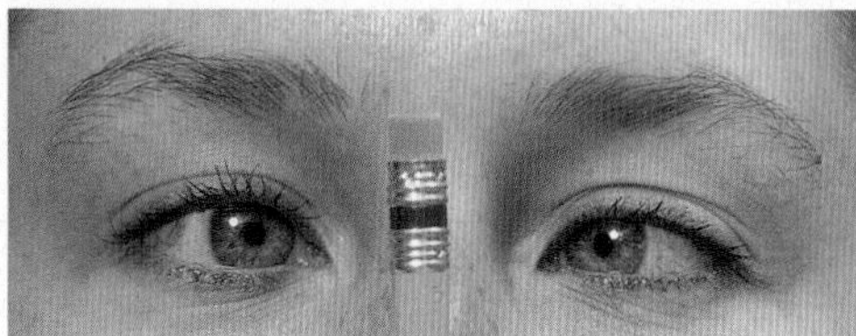 **Figure 13.22** Accommodation.	

(table continues on page 329)

Technique and Normal Findings (continued)	Abnormal Findings (continued)
Accommodation is necessary for far-to-near focus. Documentation of this sequence of assessments is easily accomplished with the following acronym: **PERRLA**, which stands for pupils equal, round, and reactive to light and accommodation.	

Documenting Normal Findings

Eyebrows full and appropriate to age. Eyelashes evenly distributed. Blinking every 2–3 seconds. Eyes round, symmetrical, and in parallel alignment. Lacrimal apparatus not enlarged or tender. Conjunctiva with small vessels visible. Sclera clear and white. Lens is transparent. Iris is brown, smooth, and without vascularity. PERRLA.

Special Techniques

Technique and Normal Findings	Abnormal Findings
Eversion of the Eyelid Eversion of the eyelid is an advanced practice skill used in specialized situations. 1. Grasp the lashes and lid margin gently between your thumb and forefinger. 2. Ask the patient to look down. 3. Pull the eyelid gently down and away from the eye. 4. Place a cotton-tipped applicator in the indentation between orbit and globe (Fig. 13.23). 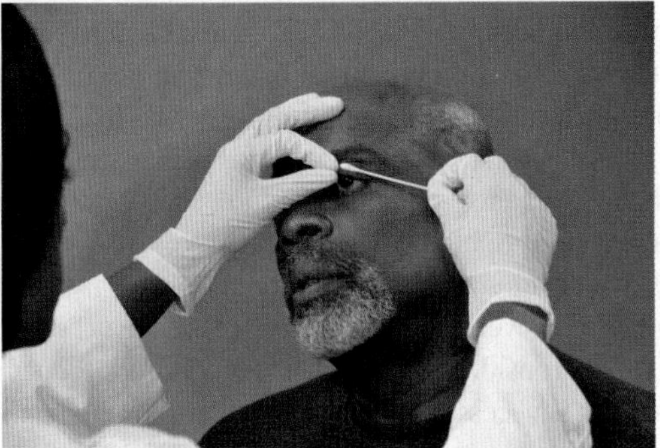 **Figure 13.23** Placement of the applicator during eyelid eversion. 5. Pull the lashes and lid margin out and upward. 6. Fold the lid back over the cotton-tipped applicator, exposing the underside of the upper eyelid. 7. Hold the eyelid in this position while you remove the applicator. 8. Assess the underside of the eyelid, inspecting for any foreign bodies, chalazia, and so on. 9. Ask the patient to blink. The eyelid will return to its normal position.	When examining the eye for a foreign body, it is important to examine the cornea, sclera, and palpebral conjunctiva. Eversion of the eyelid is essential in the assessment of an injured or red eye. Everting the upper eyelid allows for easy identification of foreign bodies. ⚠ *SAFETY ALERT* *Eversion of the eyelid should never be performed when a penetrating eye injury is suspected.*

(table continues on page 330)

Technique and Normal Findings (continued)	Abnormal Findings (continued)
10. Assess the inside of the lower lid by placing your thumb or a cotton-tipped applicator on the skin below the lower lid and pressing downward gently. 11. Ask the patient to look upward, to the right, and then to the left. There are no foreign bodies, chalazia, redness, or injuries. Tissue is pink and smooth.	
Fluorescein Examination of Cornea The advanced practitioner uses this technique to determine any abrasions or lacerations to the cornea. Fluorescein is a dye taken up by the damaged corneal epithelium. Under blue ultraviolet light (Wood lamp) it fluoresces, allowing assessment of the nature and extent of corneal injury. 1. Remove a fluorescein strip, wet it with a drop of normal saline, and apply it to the lower conjunctival sac (fluorescein drops are also available). 2. Ask the patient to blink several times to distribute the fluorescein over the cornea. Remove excess fluorescein with a gentle irrigation of normal saline. 3. Darken the room and expose the eye to blue filtered, cobalt, or "black" light.	Corneal fluorescence reveals the extent of the injury to the corneal epithelium. **SAFETY ALERT** *Fluorescein is never used if a penetrating eye injury is suspected.*

Assessment of Internal Ocular Structures

Examination of internal ocular structures is in the domain of the advance practice registered nurse (APRN).

The ophthalmoscope has some basic features that make inspecting the interior ocular structures easier: (1) a light source, (2) a viewing aperture, and (3) a lens refraction adjustment (Fig. 13.24). These features allow you to direct the light source toward the pupil by looking through the viewing aperture.

The aperture, which has a lens selector wheel, allows for adjustment of refraction to bring the internal ocular structures into sharp focus, compensating for any refractive errors you or the patient may have. The aperture is set on large for the dilated pupil or small for the constricted pupil. The slit aperture is used to examine the anterior portion of the eye and evaluate lesions at the fundal level. The grid feature is used to locate and describe fundal-level lesions. The green beam (red-free filter) is often used to evaluate retinal hemorrhaging (which appears black with this filter) or melanin spots (which appear gray).

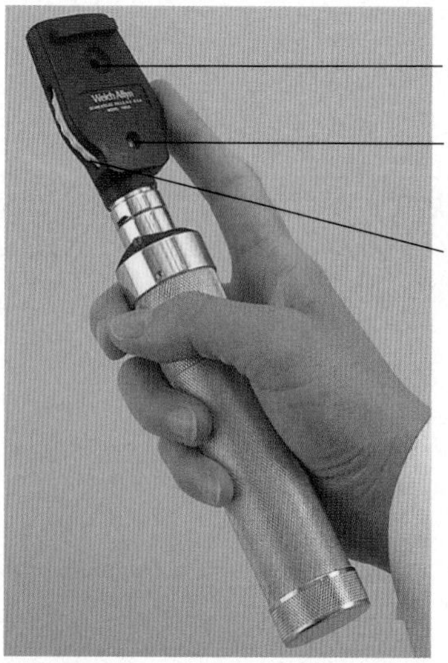

Proper inspection of the posterior ocular structures with an ophthalmoscope requires that the pupils be slightly dilated. The optometrist or ophthalmologist will often use mydriatic eye drops, which are short-acting ciliary muscle paralytics that dilate the pupil. However, accommodation reflexes may be lost with the use of eye drops. Mydriatic drops are not used if a neurological assessment is necessary because they may obscure pupil size and reactivity parameters used to determine neurological status.

Figure 13.24 The ophthalmoscope.

SAFETY ALERT

Mydriatic drops may precipitate acute angle–closure glaucoma. Those at risk include patients with a history of glaucoma and extremely farsighted patients. Additionally, the patient should be warned about blurring of vision and sensitivity to light. The patient should not drive for 1 to 2 hours following pupil dilation.

The skill of assessing the fundus of the eye is advanced and requires much practice. To assess the fundus through a partially dilated pupil, your technique must be very proficient.

In the nonophthalmic setting, conduct examination of the fundus in a darkened room to increase pupillary dilation without medications. First, set the ophthalmoscope on the

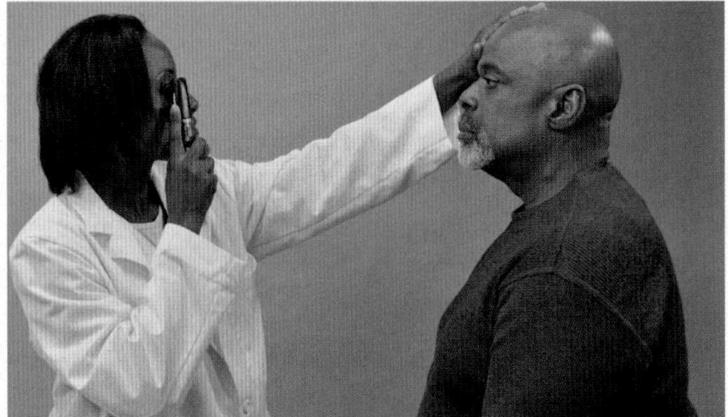

Figure 13.25 Positioning of the patient, nurse, and ophthalmoscope.

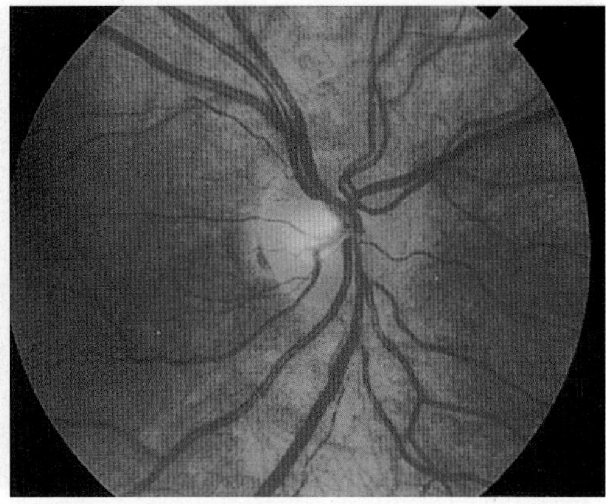

Figure 13.27 A normal optic disc.

0 lens and the aperture on small round light. When examining the right eye, grasp the ophthalmoscope in your right hand and then turn on the light source. When examining the left eye, grasp the ophthalmoscope in the left hand. This helps you to avoid bumping noses with the patient.

Ask the patient to focus on a distant object across the room. Start by placing your hand on the patient's head; this puts you 61 cm (about 2 ft) from the patient. From an angle of about 15 degrees lateral to the patient's line of vision, shine the ophthalmoscope toward the pupil of the right eye (Fig. 13.25).

Look through the ophthalmoscope's viewing hole, noting the red reflex. Continue to look through the viewing hole and focus on the red reflex. Now, move toward the patient until you are 25 cm (about 10 in.) away from the patient's forehead. Move the lens selector from 0 to the + or black numbers to focus on the anterior ocular structures. Inspect the anterior structures for transparency (Fig. 13.26). Now move the lens selector from the + black numbers to the – or red numbers to focus on structures progressively more posterior.

If the retinal structures are not in focus, adjust the focus with an index finger on the lens focus until the retina comes into focus. Look toward the nasal side of the retina. If you are having difficulty, ask the patient to look toward the right. Inspect the optic disc, which is the most prominent structure. The direct ophthalmoscope technique is difficult to master; it takes months of practice. The easiest way to find the optic disc is to find a blood vessel and then follow this vessel back to its origin at the optic disc. Inspect the shape (round or oval), color (creamy yellow-orange to pink), disc margins (distinct and sharply demarcated), and size of the disc cupping (brighter yellow-white than rest of disc) (Fig. 13.27). Cup-to-disc ratio is genetically determined and normally equal in both eyes. You may be able to pick up arteriovenous (AV) nicking from high blood pressure and retinal hemorrhages in the form of dot-blot spots or flame hemorrhages (Fig. 13.28).

The blood vessels can be directly observed in the retina. Systemic diseases of the body are often reflected in the blood vessels and can be directly observed in the eye. When examining the vascularity of the eye, make note of the number, color, artery-to-vein ratio, tortuosity, and AV crossing. Also make note of the ratio of arteries-to-veins width, which is normally 2:3 or 4:5.

The final retinal structure to assess is the macula. Move the ophthalmoscope approximately two disc diameters (2 DD) temporally to view the macula. You can also ask the patient to look at the light. The macula can be difficult to find because it is light sensitive. You may find that turning the aperture to green light (red-light filter) may make it easier to assess. The macula is a darker, avascular area with an ophthalmoscope light reflective center known as the fovea centralis (Fig. 13.29). The color of the macula varies with patients' ethnicity and age. Examine the periphery for lattice or tears.

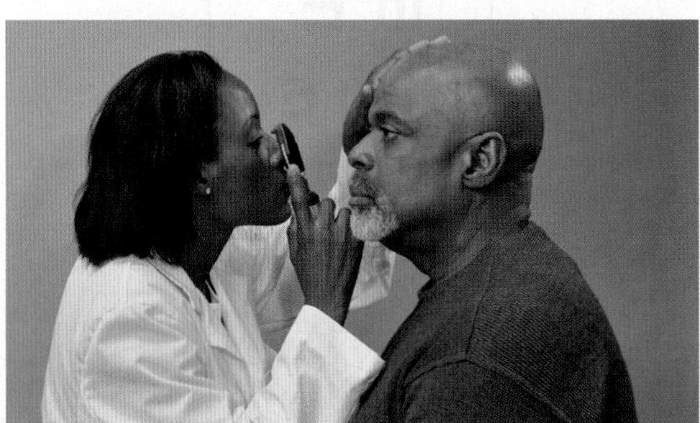

Figure 13.26 Using the ophthalmoscope to inspect the anterior ocular structures.

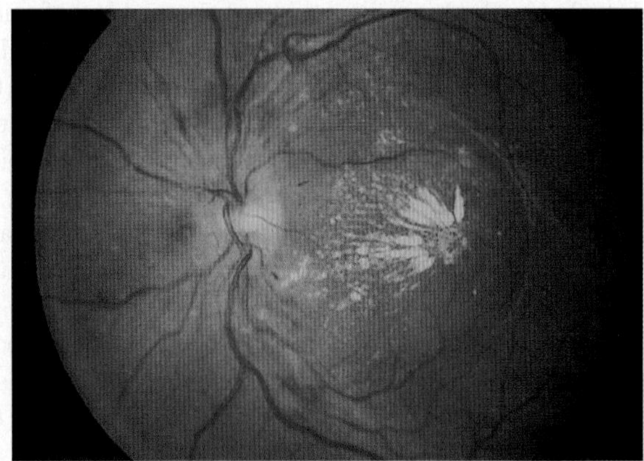

Figure 13.28 Flame hemorrhage in a patient with hypertensive retinopathy.

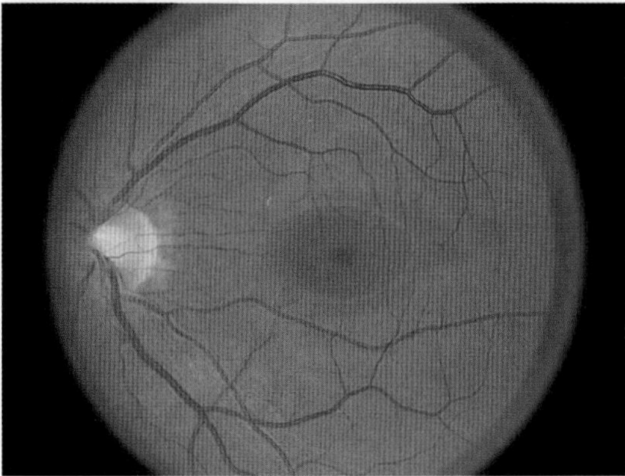

Figure 13.29 Normal macula.

To summarize, review the structures and what you are looking for:

- **Disc:** What is the cup-to-disc ratio? Do the rims look pink and healthy?
- **Vessels:** Any signs of AV nicking?
- **Macula:** Does it look flat? Is there a good light reflex off the surface?
- **Periphery:** Any lattice or tears?

See Table 13.8 at the end of the chapter for pictures.

> ⚠ *SAFETY ALERT*
>
> *A lack of* ***red reflex*** *may need urgent follow-up. If a white pupil reflex (leukocoria) is elicited, then an urgent ophthalmological referral is required. Disease or trauma (e.g., retinoblastoma, hyphema, toxocariasis, retinal detachment) often causes a white pupil reflex.*

Lifespan Considerations: Older Adults

Age-related visual changes and negative functional consequences occur slowly over time and are often overlooked. Visual impairments can begin to affect the older adult's functional capacity, decreasing ability to drive and perform usual activities. It is important to assess visual changes and how they affect lifestyle.

With aging, ability of the lens to accommodate decreases. Near vision is subsequently impaired, and thus older adults need reading glasses. Presbyopia is considered a normal part of aging.

Cataracts and age-related macular degeneration (AMD) are the two leading causes of loss of vision and blindness in the United States. In the United States, these diseases are primarily seen in the elderly (although congenital forms of cataracts exist). Glaucoma is also more common with increased age.

Loss of acuity of central vision may decrease, especially after 70 years of age. Loss of vision puts the older adult at increased risk for falls and associated hip fractures.

Additional findings related to aging include loss of adipose tissue in the orbit, decreased tear production, and decreased papillary response. Diabetic retinopathy is also increased in the elderly. Arcus senilis, a gray-white circle that circumscribes the limbus and results from deposition of lipid, is a common cloudiness that appears around the corneas (Fig. 13.30).

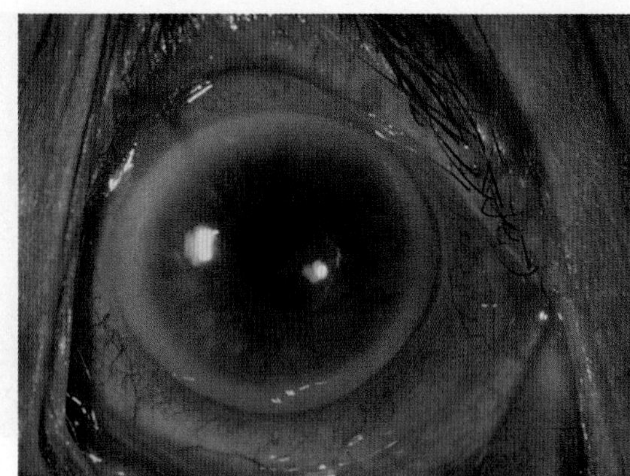

Figure 13.30 Arcus senilis.

Keep in mind that testing visual acuity in the older adult with dementia can be challenging. Provide simple, one-step directions for these patients.

Cultural Considerations

The Snellen E chart can be used for people who cannot read or speak English (see Fig. 13.31).

Ethnic variations are found in the ocular sclera, depending on skin tone. In light-skinned people, the sclera appears white with some superficial vessels. In dark-skinned people, the sclera often has tiny brown patches (patches of melanin) or is grayish-blue.

Four to five times more African Americans develop glaucoma as compared with other races. The rate of blindness from glaucoma in African Americans is seven times that of Caucasians; blindness begins 10 years earlier in African Americans (American Academy of Ophthalmology, 2013). Hispanic Americans also develop glaucoma at a much higher rate than Caucasians; the reason is unknown.

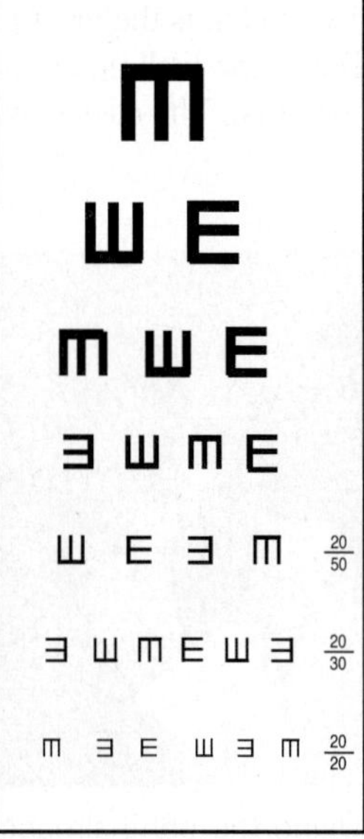

Figure 13.31 The Snellen E chart.

Documenting Case Study Findings

The nurse has just finished conducting a beginning assessment of Mr. Harris, the patient who reports worsening vision and has a history of glaucoma. Review the following important findings revealed in each of the steps of objective data collection for Mr. Harris. Consider how these results compare with the normal findings presented in the samples of normal documentation. Pay attention to how the nurse clusters data to provide a more complete and accurate understanding of the condition. Note that inspection is the major technique used in eye assessment for the RN.

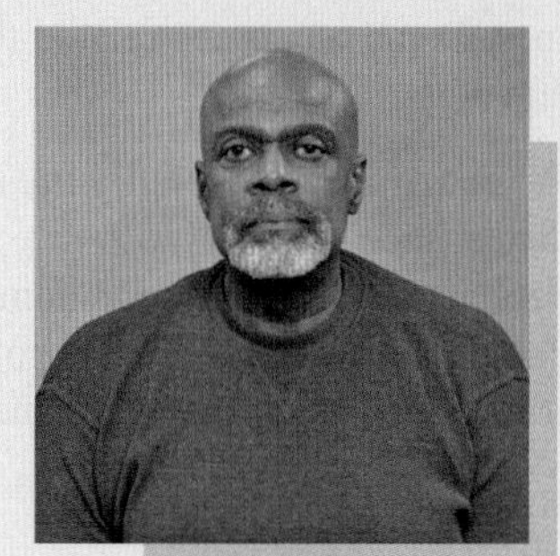

Inspection: External eyes symmetrical, no ptosis. PERRLA. EOMI. Conjunctiva clear, sclera white. Distance vision: right 20/30, left 20/50. Visual fields reduced by approximately 20% by confrontation.

Palpation: External eye lacrimal apparatus without swelling or redness, nontender.

Critical Thinking

Laboratory and Diagnostic Testing

The history and physical examination can provide information on coexisting conditions that influence eye health, such as diabetes mellitus. Vision tests are performed, as described earlier. The funduscopic examination and computerized visual examination are performed as indicated by the patient's situation. A dilated eye examination may also be performed. If an abrasion is suspected, fluorescein examination of the cornea using a Wood lamp is performed. If bacterial infection is suspected, a swab of the eye can be sent for culture and sensitivity. Tonometry may be used to measure intraocular pressure. A slit lamp exam may be performed to visualize the cornea. Gonioscopy determines the angle of the anterior chamber of the eye.

Diagnostic Reasoning

Nursing Diagnoses, Outcomes, and Interventions

When formulating nursing diagnoses, you use critical thinking to cluster data and identify patterns that fit together. You compare these data clusters with defining characteristics (abnormal findings) for the diagnosis to ensure the most accurate labeling and appropriate interventions. A nursing diagnosis is a clinical judgment about responses to health problems or life processes. Table 13.3 provides a comparison of nursing diagnoses,

TABLE 13.3 Common Nursing Diagnoses Associated With the Eyes

Diagnosis	Point of Differentiation	Assessment Characteristics	Nursing Interventions
Disturbed sensory perception	Alterations in the way the patient takes in, processes, uses, or otherwise deals with sensory (especially visual) stimuli	Wears eyeglasses, uses contacts, uses computer assistive devices	Converse with and touch patient frequently. Use lighting for reading. Use a magnifying glass for shaving or to apply makeup.
Risk for injury	At risk for physical harm and damage as a result of environmental limitations imposed by impaired vision	Near or far vision impaired, difficulty seeing in low lighting, difficulty seeing at night	Refer to optometrist for corrective lenses. Ensure that patient wears lenses and that eyeglasses are clean. Make sure that objects are out of the path. Remove hazards from room, such as razors, matches, and lighters.

unexpected findings, and interventions commonly related to the eye assessment (NANDA International, 2012).

You use assessment information to identify patient outcomes. Some outcomes related to eye problems include the following:

- Patient will plan to modify lifestyle to accommodate vision disturbance.
- Patient will remain safe in home environment.
- Patient will state measures to reduce risk of visual loss (Bulechek, Butcher, Dochterman, & Wagner, 2013).

Once outcomes are established, you implement nursing care to improve the status of the patient. You uses critical thinking and evidence-based practice to develop nursing interventions. Some examples of nursing interventions for the eye are as follows:

- Identify name and purpose of visit when entering patient's personal space.
- Keep furniture out of pathways and keep cords against walls.
- Ensure access to eyeglasses or magnifiers as needed (Moorhead, Johnson, Maas, & Swanson, 2013).

Progress Note: Analyzing Findings

The APRN has seen Mr. Harris and has performed an ophthalmoscopic examination and is concerned about Mr. Harris's worsening vision. The following nursing note illustrates how subjective and objective data are collected and analyzed and nursing interventions are developed.

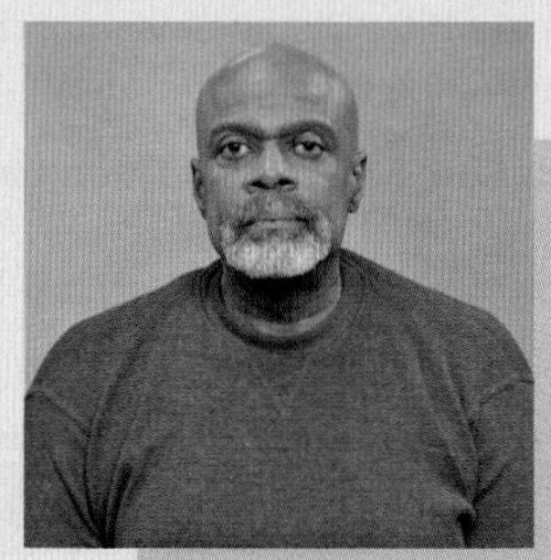

Subjective: "I'm here for my checkup to make sure that my medicines are doing what they're supposed to." Personal history of high blood pressure, high cholesterol, and glaucoma.

Objective: A 61-year-old African American man, alert and oriented, appears stated age. External eyes symmetrical, no ptosis. Conjunctiva clear, sclera white. Distance vision: right 20/30, left 20/50. Reads newsprint but says it is somewhat blurred compared with how it was 1 year ago. Visual fields reduced by approximately 20% by confrontation.

Analysis: Disturbed visual sensory perception related to loss of visual field and visual acuity.

Plan: Make referral to ophthalmologist for further testing. Additionally, refer to social work to assist with getting funding for new eyeglasses and medication. Teach about safety issues related to impaired vision, especially risk for falling. Encourage him to use magnifying devices for reading until he can get his new glasses.

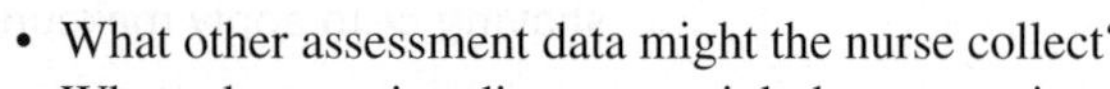

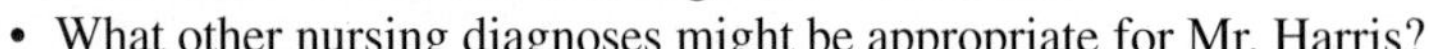

Critical Thinking Challenge

- What other assessment data might the nurse collect?
- What other nursing diagnoses might be appropriate for Mr. Harris?
- How does the role of the APRN differ from the RN role?

Collaborating With the Interprofessional Team

Because of Mr. Harris's abnormal findings, he needs referral to an ophthalmologist. The role of specialists is important in eye care because they have more advanced assessment skills and techniques. Examples include more accurate testing of the visual fields with a computerized machine and tonometry to measure pressure inside the eye.

The following conversation illustrates how the RN might organize data and make recommendations about the patient's situation to an ophthalmologist.

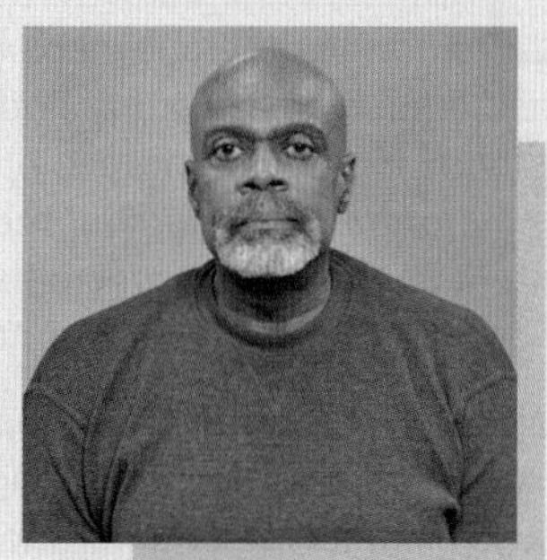

Situation: "Hello, I'm calling in a referral on a 61-year-old African American man with a change in vision."

Background: "He has a personal history of high blood pressure, high cholesterol, and glaucoma. He reads newsprint but says it is somewhat blurred compared with what he saw 1 year ago. I examined him and found that his distance vision is 20/30 on the right and 20/50 on the left. His visual fields are reduced by approximately 20% by confrontation."

Assessment: "I am concerned that he may have an underlying disease process."

Recommendations: "Would you be able to see him in the next 2 weeks to perform a more complete assessment including glaucoma testing? He also will need new prescription for eyeglasses. Thanks so much."

Pulling It All Together

The nurse uses assessment data to formulate a nursing care plan with patient outcomes and interventions. Outcomes are specific to the patient, realistic to achieve, measurable, and have a time frame for meeting the outcome. The interventions are actions that the nurse performs based on evidence and practice guidelines. After these interventions have been completed, the nurse reevaluates and documents findings to show progress toward the patient outcome. The nurse uses critical thinking and judgment to continue or revise the diagnosis, outcomes, or interventions. This is often in the form of a care plan or case note similar to the one below.

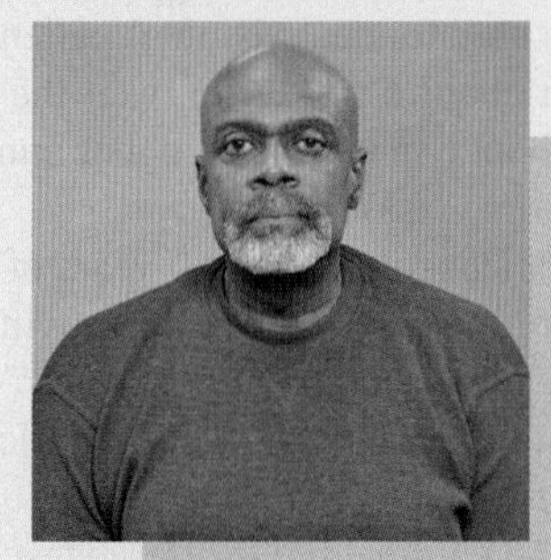

Nursing Diagnosis	Patient Outcomes	Nursing Interventions	Rationale	Evaluation
Disturbed visual sensory perception	Patient will remain free from harm resulting from a loss of vision.	Refer to ophthalmologist for further testing. Refer to social work to assist with funding for eyeglasses. Teach patient to clear cords and furniture from pathways and use good lighting.	Referral to the ophthalmologist will correct the low vision. Furniture and cords are environmental hazards that increase risk of falling. Good lighting increases visibility.	Referral made to ophthalmologist. Patient will be seen in 2 days. Patient states that his home environment is uncluttered and all furniture and cords are out of the way. He plans to get lamp for the hallway at night.

Applying Your Knowledge

Using the previous steps of diagnostic reasoning, organizing, and prioritizing, consider all the case study findings woven throughout this chapter. When answering the following questions, see how the pieces of assessment work together to create an environment for personalized, appropriate, and accurate care. As you study the content and features, consider Mr. Harris's case and how it is important to seek care for primary prevention. Begin thinking about the following points:

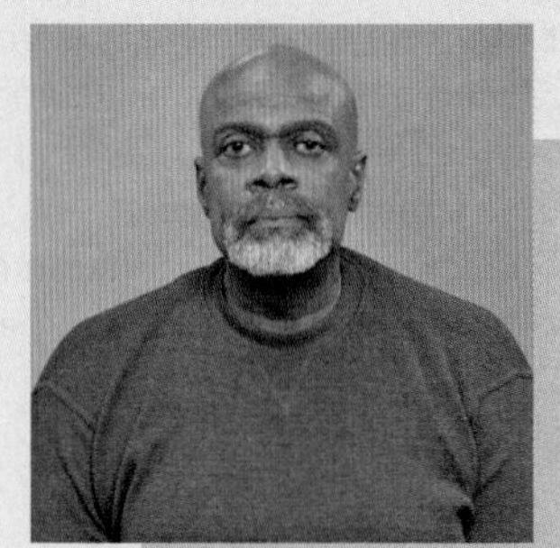

- What are the signs and symptoms of glaucoma?
- How can examination findings distinguish glaucoma from other eye conditions such as macular degeneration?
- How will you teach Mr. Harris about preventing falls associated with vision loss?
- What factors may have contributed to Mr. Harris's glaucoma?
- What recommendation for additional screening and follow-up would you recommend for Mr. Harris?
- How can you evaluate Mr. Harris's understanding of what you taught him about preventing vision loss related to falls at home?

Key Points

- Cranial nerves involved with the eyes include CN II (optic nerve), III (oculomotor), IV (trochlear), and VI (abducens).
- An important health promotion activity is the use of protective eyewear for contact sports and occupational exposure.
- Sudden visual loss is an emergency.
- Common symptoms related to the eye and vision include pain, trauma, visual change, blind spots, floaters, halos, discharge, and a related change in ADLs.
- The Snellen chart is used to assess far vision; the Jaeger test is used for near vision. A patient with 20/20 vision can read at about 6 m (20 ft) what the normal person can read at about 6 m (20 ft). A higher number at the bottom indicates worse vision.
- Patients older than 40 years of age often have a decreased ability to accommodate, moving the object further away to read.
- Static and kinetic confrontation tests measure peripheral vision.
- The cardinal fields of gaze test allows you to detect muscle defects that cause misalignment or uncoordinated movement of the eyes.
- PERRLA is documented when the pupils are equal, round, and reactive to light and accommodation.
- Assessment of the eye with an ophthalmoscope is considered an advanced skill.
- Cloudiness in the lens may indicate a cataract.
- Common unexpected findings include being nearsighted or farsighted, astigmatism, ptosis, and nystagmus.
- Cataracts, glaucoma, and macular degeneration are more common in older adults.

Review Questions

1. Which of the following patients would require immediate nursing care?
   A. An 8-year-old girl with pink conjunctivae and drainage
   B. A 20-year-old man with sudden visual loss after playing football
   C. A 52-year-old woman with clouding of vision
   D. A 77-year-old man with loss of vision in his peripheral fields

2. Which of the following teaching points would the nurse emphasize related to eye health?
   A. Always wear eye protection for occupational exposures.
   B. Eat a diet high in animal protein and dairy.
   C. Exercise five times a week for at least 20 minutes.
   D. Get at least 7 hours of sleep each night.

3. Which of the following symptoms would the nurse expect the patient to report as translucent specks that drift across the visual field?
   A. Blind spot
   B. Ptosis
   C. Halo
   D. Floater

4. When working with an older adult, what would the nurse emphasize as increased risks for the patient?
   A. Myopia and strabismus
   B. Blepharitis and chalazion
   C. Glaucoma and cataracts
   D. Exophthalmos and presbyopia

5. A public health nurse is performing annual vision screening for residents in senior housing. Which of the following charts would the nurse most likely be using?
   A. Allen chart
   B. Snellen chart
   C. Ishihara cards
   D. Confrontation cards

6. Which of the following scores for distance vision indicates the patient with the poorest vision?
   A. 200/20
   B. 18/20
   C. 24/20
   D. 20/100

7. The nurse recognizes that the 60-year-old patient may have difficulty reading fine print because of
   A. the loss of accommodation.
   B. anisocoria.
   C. amblyopia.
   D. asthenopia.

8. Peripheral vision is evaluated by the nurse using the
   A. corneal light test.
   B. cover test.
   C. confrontation test.
   D. cardinal fields of gaze test.

9. The cranial nerves involved with eye movement include
   A. II, V, and VII.
   B. III, IV, and VI.
   C. IV, V, and VIII.
   D. V, VI, and VII.

10. The nurse assesses the response of the eye to light and documents normal findings as
   A. PEERLA.
   B. PERRLA.
   C. PERLLA.
   D. PERLAA.

The Jensen suite offers these additional resources to enhance learning and facilitate understanding of this chapter:

- thePoint online resource, http://thepoint.lww.com/Jensen2e
- *Laboratory Manual for Nursing Health Assessment: A Best Practice Approach*
- *Pocket Guide for Nursing Health Assessment: A Best Practice Approach*
- *Lippincott DocuCare,* an electronic health record simulation software, http://thepoint.lww.com/docucare
- *Adaptive Learning | Powered by PrepU,* http://thepoint.lww.com/prepu

References

American Academy of Ophthalmology. (2013). *Clinical update: Glaucoma.* Retrieved from http://www.aao.org/publications/eyenet/201006/glaucoma.cfm?RenderForPrint=1&

Bulechek, G. M., Butcher, H. K., Dochterman, J. M., & Wagner, C. M. (2013). *Nursing interventions classification (NIC)* (6th ed). St. Louis, MO: Mosby.

Centers for Disease Control and Prevention. (2013). *Vision health initiative: Common eye disorders.* Retrieved from http://www.cdc.gov/visionhealth/basic_information/eye_disorders.htm

Lee, R. Y., Huang, G., Porco, T. C., Chen, Y. C., He, M., & Lin, S. C. (2013). Differences in iris thickness among African Americans, Caucasian Americans, Hispanic Americans, Chinese Americans, and Filipino-Americans. *Journal of Glaucoma, 22*(9), 673–678. doi:10.1097/IJG.0b013e318264ba68

The Merck Manual for Health Care Professionals. (2013). *Evaluation of the elderly patient.* Retrieved from http://www.merckmanuals.com/professional/geriatrics/approach_to_the_geriatric_patient/evaluation_of_the_elderly_patient.html

Miller, C. A. (2009). *Nursing for wellness in older adults* (5th ed.). Philadelphia, PA: Lippincott Williams & Wilkins.

Moorhead, S., Johnson, M., Maas, M. L., & Swanson, E. (2013). *Nursing outcomes classification (NOC): Measurement of health outcomes* (5th ed.). St. Louis, MO: Elsevier.

NANDA International. (2012). *Nursing diagnoses: Definitions and classification 2012–2014* (9th ed). Oxford, United Kingdom: Wiley-Blackwell.

Prasad, S., & Cohen, A. B. (2011). Diagnostic accuracy of confrontation visual field tests. *Neurology, 76,* 1192–1193.

Prevent Blindness America. (2012). *Focus on eye health and culturally diverse populations.* Retrieved from http://www.visionproblemsus.org/downloads/2167_MultiCultiCompanion_v08_web.pdf

Price, K. M., Gupta, P. K., Woodward, J. A., Stinnett, S. S., & Murchison, A. P. (2009). Eyebrow and eyelid dimensions: An anthropometric analysis of African Americans and Caucasians. *Plastic and Reconstructive Surgery, 124*(2), 615–623.

Stein, J. D., Niziol, L. M., Musch, D. C., Lee, P. P., Kotak, S. V., Peters, C. M., Kymes, S. M. (2012). Longitudinal trends in resource use in an incident cohort of open-angle glaucoma patients: resource use in open-angle glaucoma. *American Journal Ophthalmology, 154*(3), 452–459.

U.S. Department of Health & Human Services. (2013). *2020 Topics & objectives—Objectives A–Z.* Retrieved from http://www.healthypeople.gov/2020/topicsobjectives2020/

U.S. Preventive Services Task Force. (2013). *Screening for glaucoma.* Retrieved from http://www.uspreventiveservicestaskforce.org/uspstf13/glaucoma/glaucomasumm.htm

Tables of Abnormal Findings

TABLE 13.4 Refractive Errors

Finding	Description
Asthenopia (eye strain)	Eye strain develops after reading, computer work, or other visually tedious tasks from tightening of the eye muscles after maintaining a constant focal distance. Symptoms include fatigue, red eyes, eye strain, pain in or around the eyes, blurred vision, headaches, and, rarely, double vision.
Astigmatism 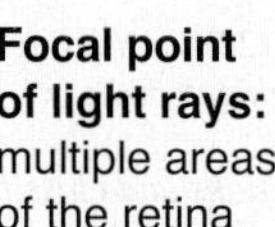 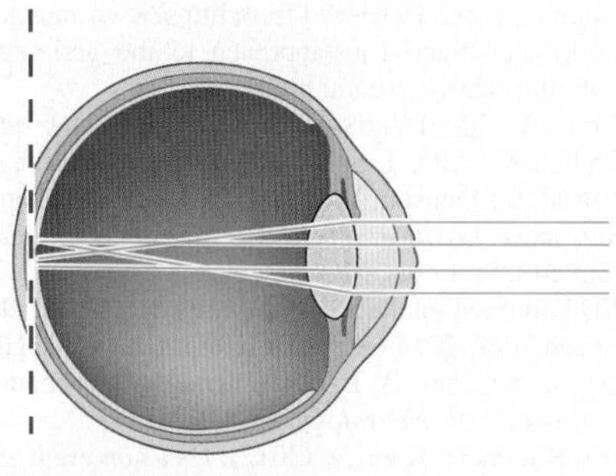	Unexpected (football-shaped) curvature of the cornea prevents light from focusing on the retina. Images appear blurred because not all optical planes are focused. This condition is corrected with a cylindrical lens that has more focusing power in one access than the other.
Myopia (nearsightedness) 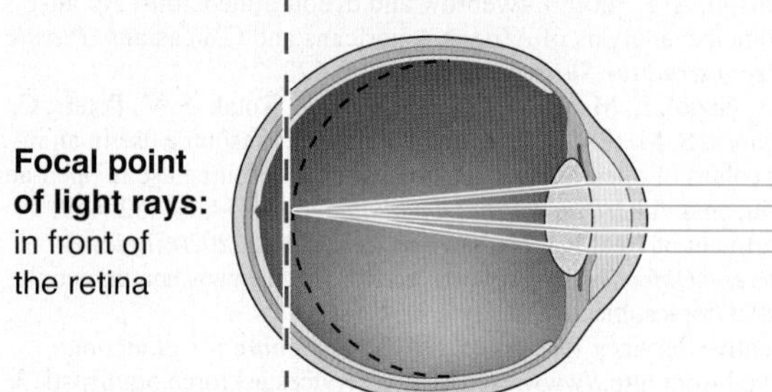	Images of distant objects focus in front of, instead of on, the retina from an imperfection in the shape of the eye or lens. Myopia occurs in approximately one quarter of the U.S. population (CDC, 2013). People with myopia can see clearly objects up close but have difficulty seeing distant objects. Myopia is corrected with a concave lens that moves the focus back to the retina.
Hyperopia (farsightedness) 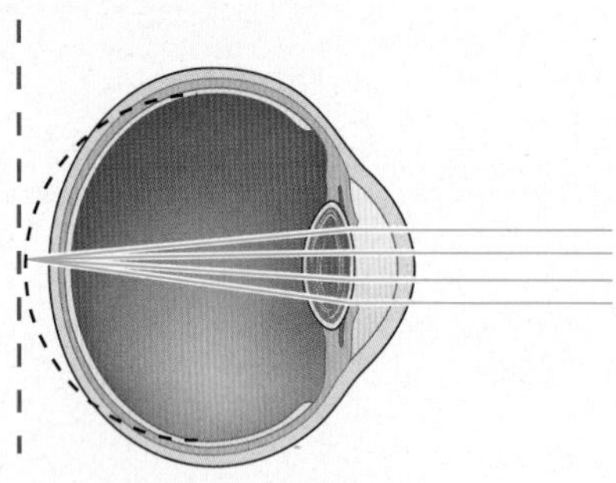	Images of near objects focus behind, instead of on, the retina from an imperfection in the shape of the eye or lens. Approximately 25% of the U.S. population has hyperopia. People with it can see distant objects clearly but have difficulty seeing objects up close. A convex lens is used to treat hyperopia, moving the focus forward onto the retina.
Presbyopia 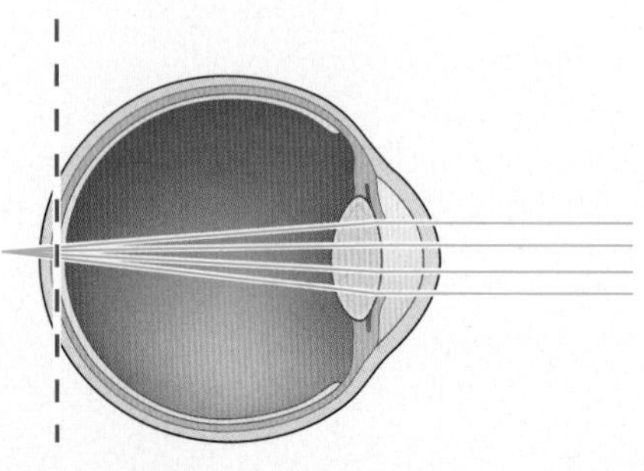	This symptom, considered a natural part of aging, is believed to result from loss of elasticity of the crystalline lens. As this happens, the ciliary muscles that bend and straighten the lens lose their power to accommodate. This condition affects near vision and therefore is corrected with a convex lens in front of the eye in the form of half-glass or as bottom of a bifocal or multifocal lens if other correction is needed for distance viewing.

(table continues on page 339)

TABLE 13.4 Refractive Errors *(continued)*

Finding	Description
Color blindness	Color blindness (inability to distinguish colors) has a genetic component. It occurs in 2%–8% of males and 0.5% of females of European descent. The cones of the eye, located in the macula, contain blue, green, and red pigments that allow color sight. Color blindness results with damage to the cones or a cone that is missing pigment. The most common form is the red/green. No effective treatment for color blindness exists. Many with it learn to compensate for the deficit and at times can discern details that a normal-sighted person would miss. Most people are not totally color blind but have deficiencies that cause some challenges, such as with discerning traffic lights, weather forecasts, and light-emitting diodes; purchasing clothes; selecting crayons; cooking; and applying makeup.
Blindness	Blindness means loss of vision or visual acuity that cannot be corrected with glasses or contact lenses. Partial blindness refers to those with very limited vision; complete blindness means an inability to see anything, including light. People with vision worse than 20/200 are classified as legally blind in most U.S. states. Numerous causes of blindness include congenital anomalies, diabetes complications, glaucoma, macular degeneration, and trauma. Worldwide, the leading causes of blindness are cataracts, river blindness (onchocerciasis), trachoma, leprosy, and vitamin A deficiency.

TABLE 13.5 Abnormal Findings of Eye Movement

Nystagmus

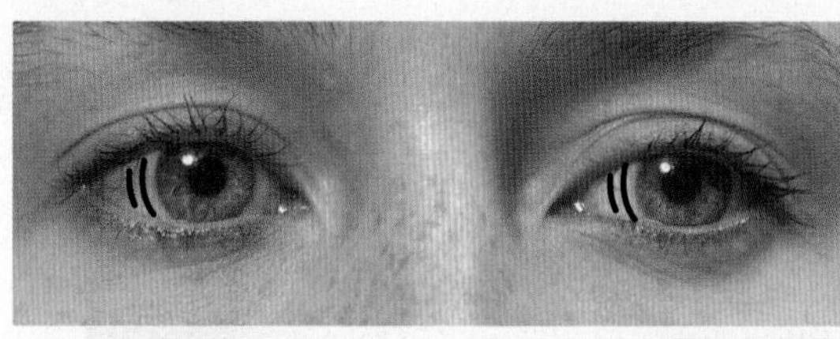

Involuntary rhythmic wobbling of the eyes; degree and direction of the movement can impair vision, with impairment varying greatly among patients.

Strabismus (cross- or wall-eyed)

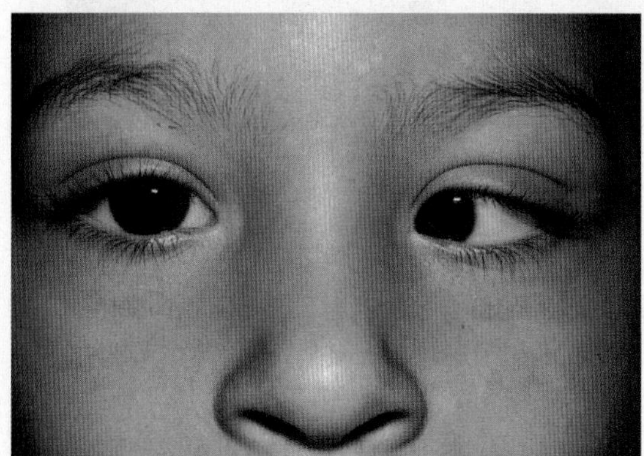

Crossed eye (esotropia)

Different forms of strabismus; appropriate evaluation and treatment required for this condition in which a person cannot align both eyes simultaneously under normal conditions. To a certain degree, strabismus occurs in 5% of all children. Strabismus is not the same as amblyopia. Children do not outgrow strabismus. Strabismus can be constant (eye turns out all the time) or intermittent (turning out only some of the time).

(table continues on page 340)

TABLE 13.5 Abnormal Findings of Eye Movement *(continued)*

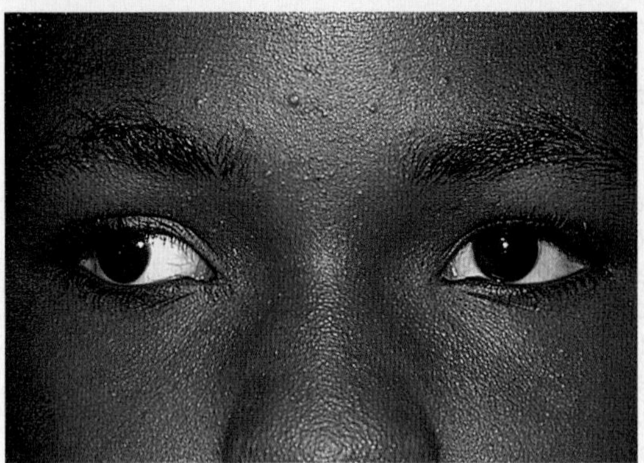

Wall eye (exotropia)

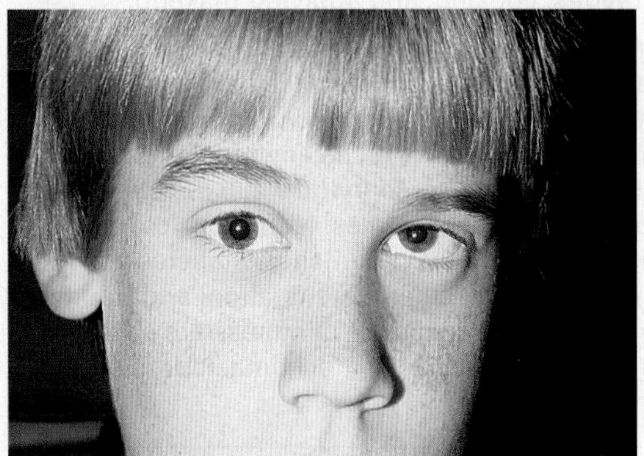

One eye pointing upward or downward (vertical deviation)

TABLE 13.6 Abnormal Findings in the External Eye

Jaundice

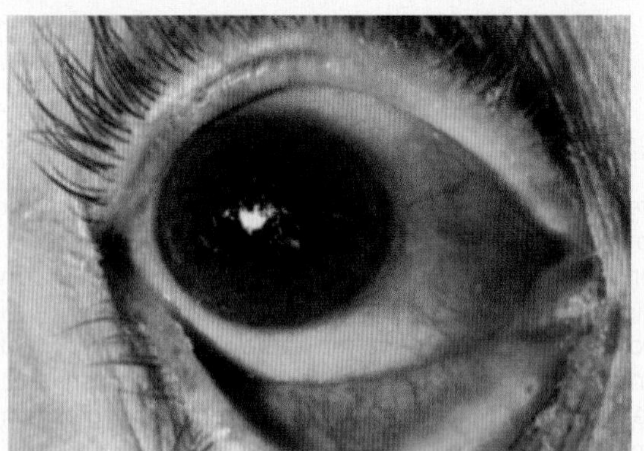

Yellowing of the sclera, which indicates liver disease

Iris Nevus

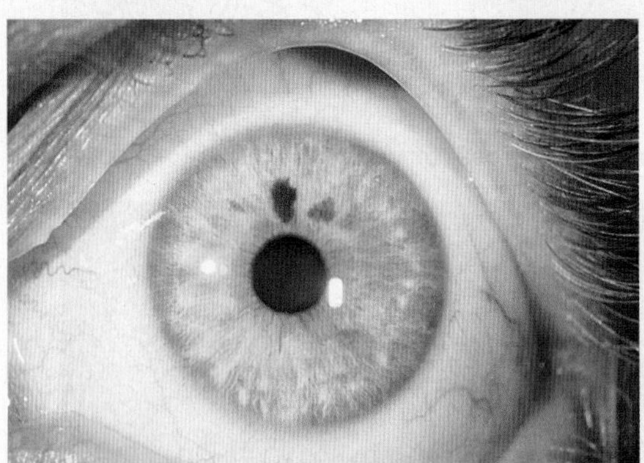

Rare condition affecting one eye, with abnormalities in appearance of the iris, pain, and decreased vision; patients may also have glaucoma on the same side

(table continues on page 341)

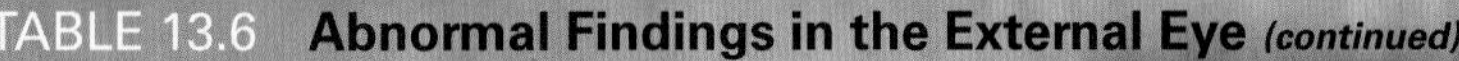

TABLE 13.6 Abnormal Findings in the External Eye *(continued)*

Hyphema

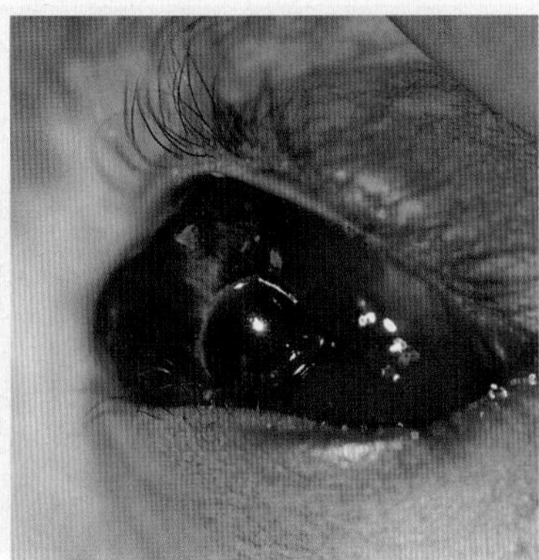

Blood in the anterior chamber of the eye, usually caused by blunt trauma

Chalazion

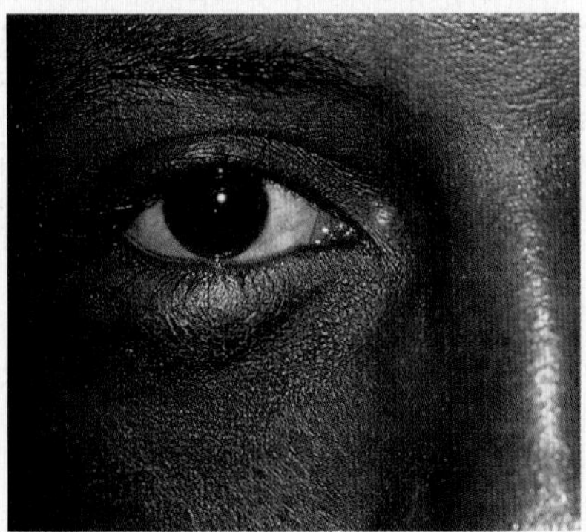

A cyst (meibomian gland lipogranuloma) in the eyelid resulting from inflammation of the meibomian gland. Most often on the upper eyelid and is sometimes confused with a hordeolum (sty); it can be differentiated because it is usually painless and tend to be larger. Rarely resolves spontaneously; usually requires treatment

Bacterial Conjunctivitis

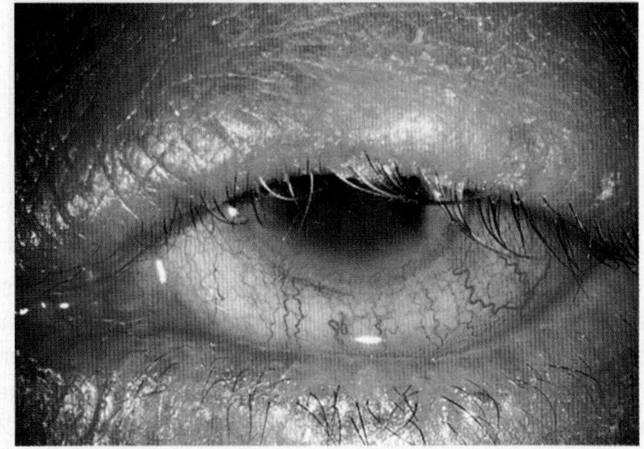

Should be suspected if there is purulent discharge (yellow or green), injected (red), and numerous follicles. Occasional blurring is common; should not be painful, constant blurring, or photophobia

Blepharitis

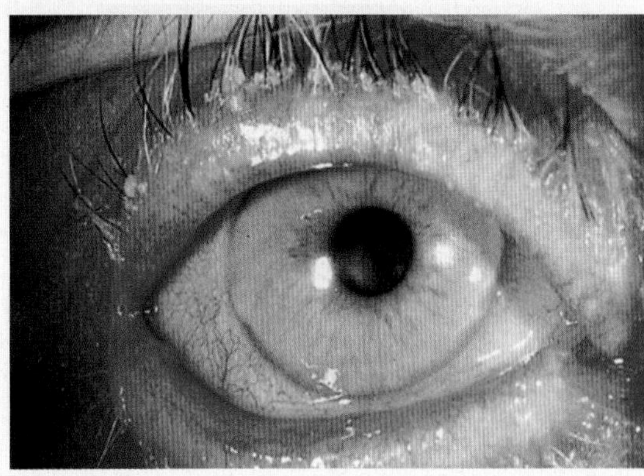

Inflammation of the margin of the eyelid; two types are anterior and posterior. Most common type is seborrheic, followed by staphylococcal, and then rosacea-associated

Viral Conjunctivitis

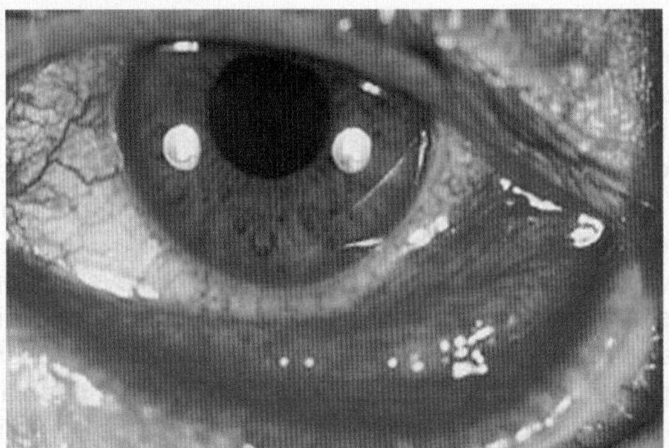

Most often associated with a watery discharge from the eye that may be accompanied by sinus congestion and rhinorrhea (runny nose), slightly injected (diffusely pink), and numerous follicles on the inferior conjunctiva

Allergic Conjunctivitis

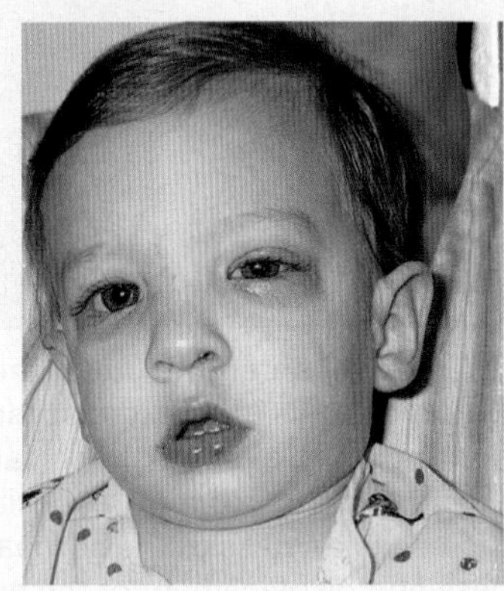

Usually bilateral and common in people with ectopic (allergic) conditions; associated with slight watery discharge and itching of the eyes

(table continues on page 342)

TABLE 13.6 Abnormal Findings in the External Eye *(continued)*

Glaucoma

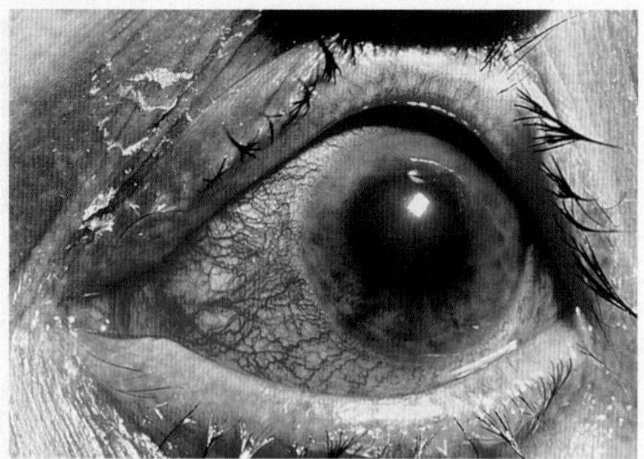

The leading cause of irreversible blindness and most common chronic optic neuropathy. Disease of the optic nerve that involves loss of retinal ganglion cells. A significant risk factor is increased intraocular pressure. Impaired flow of aqueous humor leads to increased intraocular pressure. In open-angle glaucoma, aqueous humor flows in the trabecular meshwork. In closed-angle glaucoma, the anteriorly displaced iris pushes against the trabecular meshwork, blocking fluid flow. Glaucoma has three main types: primary (primary open-angle or closed-angle); secondary (inflammatory, phacogenic, related to intraocular hemorrhage); and developmental (primary congenital, infantile). The most common type is primary open-angle glaucoma (POAG). POAG has a genetic link. Rarer are congenital eye malformations that develop in the third trimester of gestation, which cause early-angle closure and ocular hypertension, leading to optic neuropathies. Those at risk for glaucoma need an annual dilated eye examination (CDC, 2013). This photo illustrates dry eye associated with glaucoma treatment.

Amblyopia (Lazy Eye)

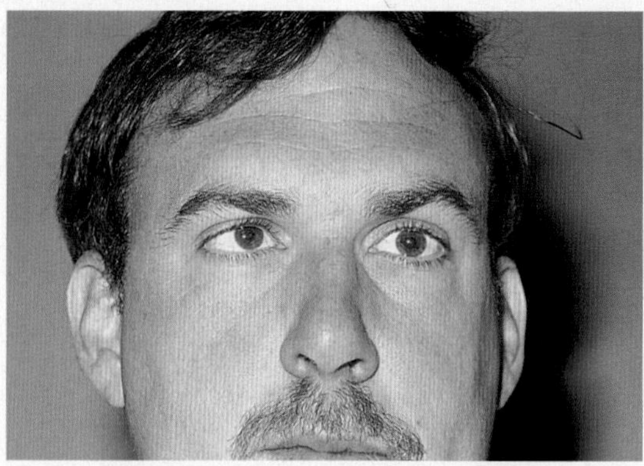

Condition in which the vision in one eye is reduced because the eye and brain are not working together. It is the most common cause of visual impairment in children (2–3:100). The eye upon examination looks normal, but vision is not normal because the brain is favoring the other eye. If amblyopia is not properly treated, it persists into adulthood, leading to monocular visual impairment. Amblyopia can be caused by strabismus, visual field discrepancies, and occasionally cataracts. The direction that the lazy eye moves is described as esotropia (medial), exotropia (lateral), hypertropia (superior), or hypotropia (inferior).

Exophthalmos

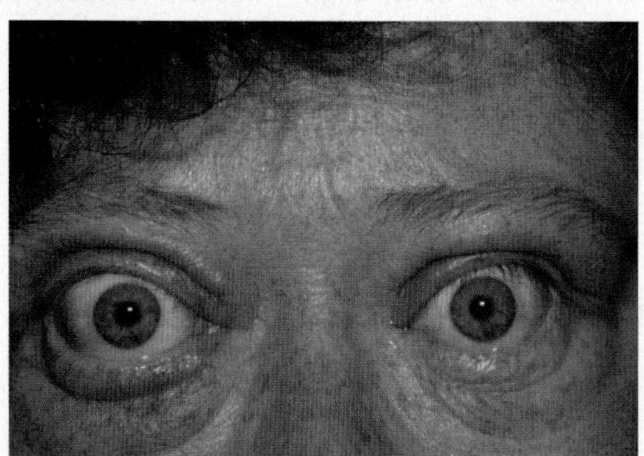

Protrusion of the eyeball anteriorly out of the socket. The most common cause is a thyroid disorder known as Graves disease. Untreated exophthalmos can impair the ability of the eyelid to close properly, especially during sleep, which increases dryness of the corneal epithelium. The process and displacement of the eye can lead to compression of the optic nerve or artery, leading to blindness.

Cataracts

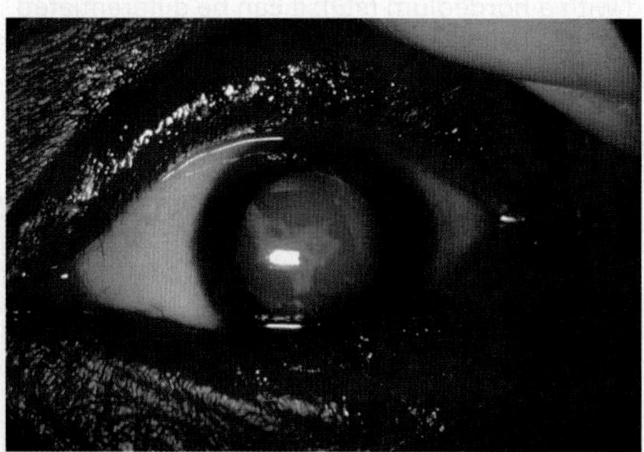

Opacity of the crystalline lens of the eye, which obstructs the passage of light. The most common causes are long-term exposure to ultraviolet light, radiation, diabetes, hypertension, and advanced age. Opacity develops from a change in the lens protein (denatured). Genetics plays a role in congenital cataracts; positive family history of cataracts seems to increase risk. Wearing ultraviolet light blocking sunglasses is believed to slow the development of cataracts.

(table continues on page 343)

TABLE 13.6 Abnormal Findings in the External Eye *(continued)*

Hordeolum (Sty)

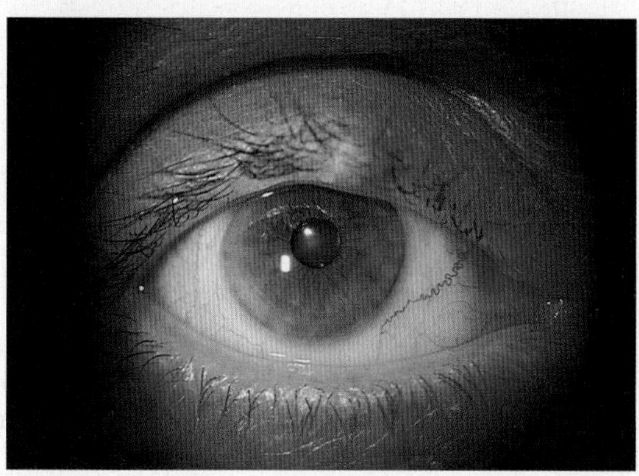

Caused by a blockage and infection of the sebaceous gland at the base of the eyelashes. Although painful and unsightly, there is generally no lasting damage.

Osteogenesis Imperfecta

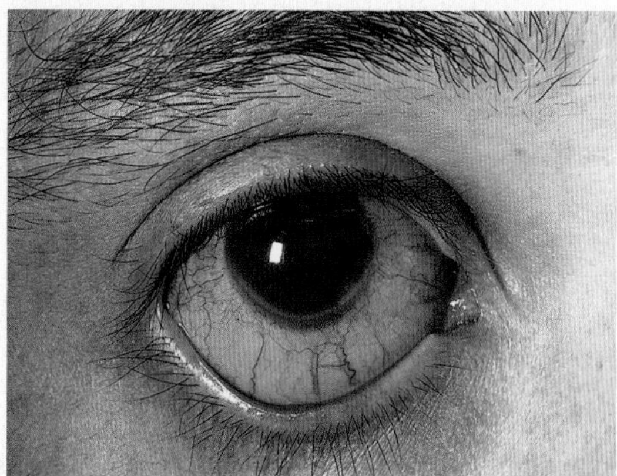

A blue sclera is due to a thinning of the sclera and is indicative of osteogenesis imperfecta.

TABLE 13.7 Abnormal Findings in the Pupil

Anisocoria (Unequal Pupils)

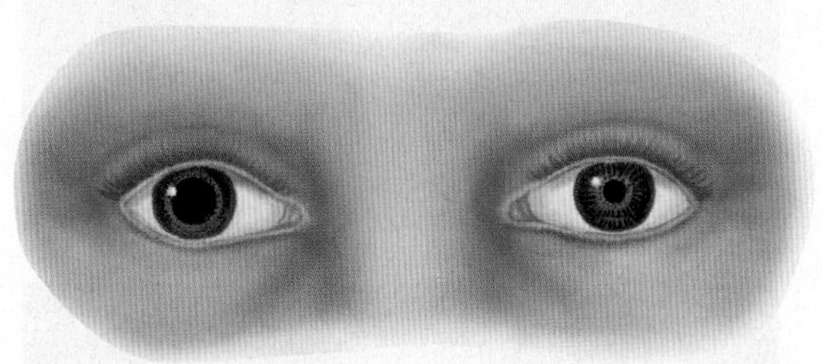

These usually result from a defect in the efferent nervous pathways controlling the oculomotor nerve. Deformities of the iris or eye must be ruled out.

Horner Syndrome

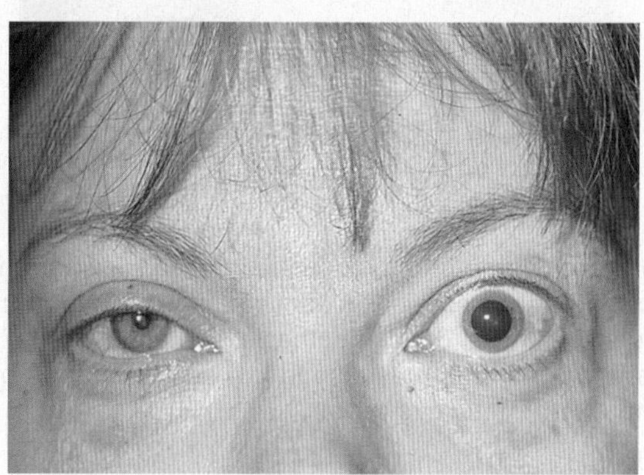

Pupillary miosis (constricted pupil) and dilation lag on the affected side. Also often present is ptosis.

Argyll Robertson Pupils

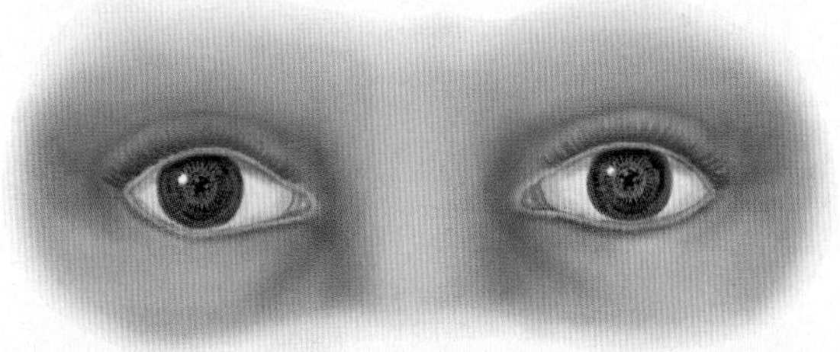

Bilateral pupils accommodate but do not dilate when exposed to bright light. Direct and consensual pupil reflexes are absent.

Adie Pupil

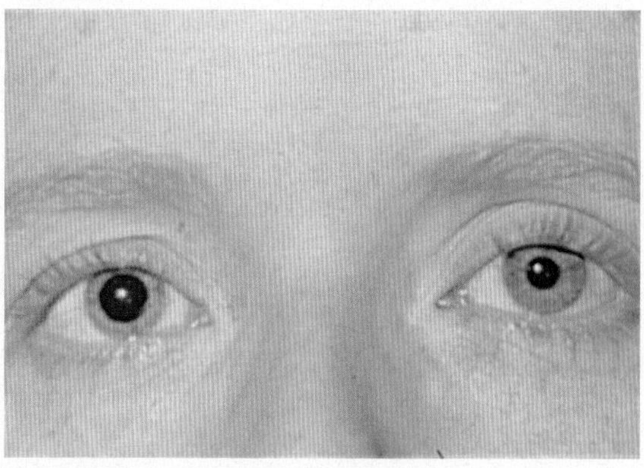

Pupils are fixed, dilated, and tonic. Direct and consensual pupil reactions are weak or absent.

(table continues on page 344)

TABLE 13.7 Abnormal Findings in the Pupil *(continued)*

Keyhole Pupil (Coloboma)

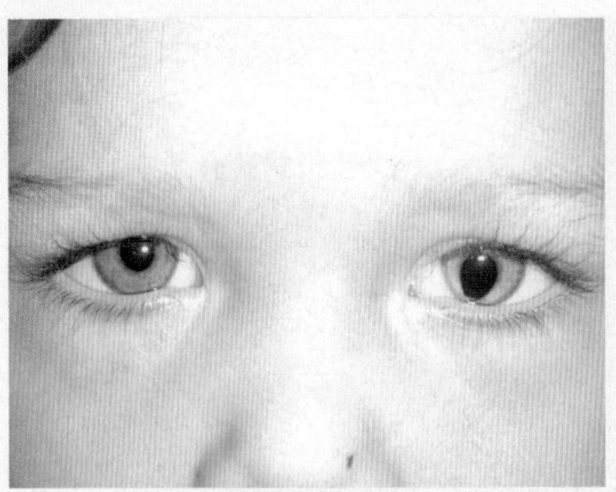

A gap appears in the iris. It can be congenital or caused during cataract or glaucoma surgery

Miosis (Small Fixed Pupil)

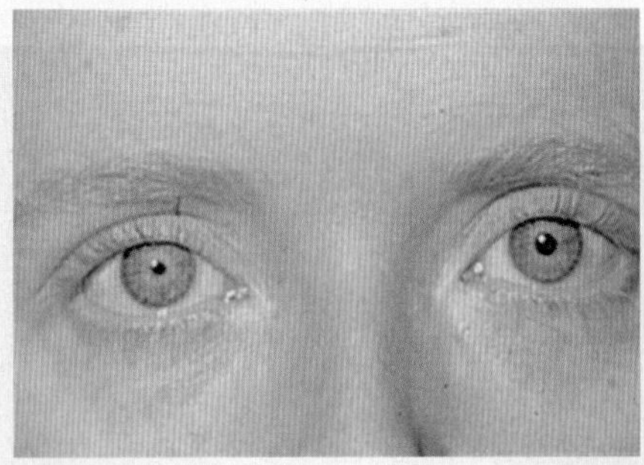

Pupils are constricted and fixed. Miosis occurs with eye drops for glaucoma, iritis, brain damage to pons, and narcotic drug use.

Mydriasis (Dilated Fixed Pupil)

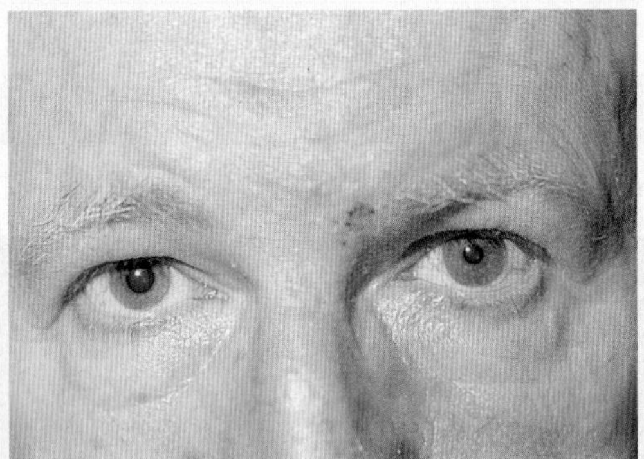

Pupils are dilated and fixed, usually from stimulation of sympathetic nerves as a consequence of CNS injury, circulatory arrest, deep anesthesia, acute glaucoma, or recent trauma. This may also follow administration of sympathomimetic eye drops.

Oculomotor (CN III) Nerve Damage

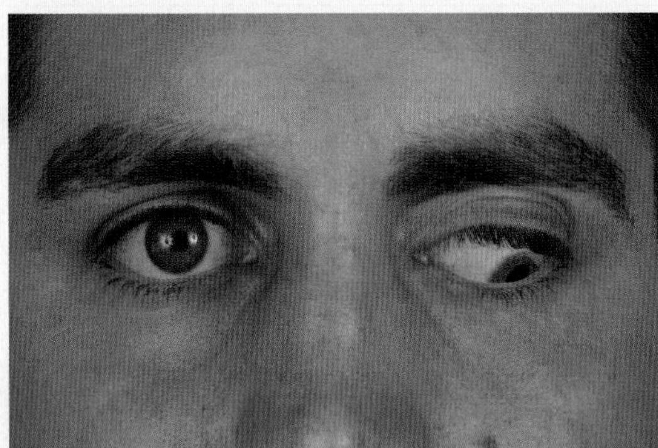

(A) Oculomotor paralysis

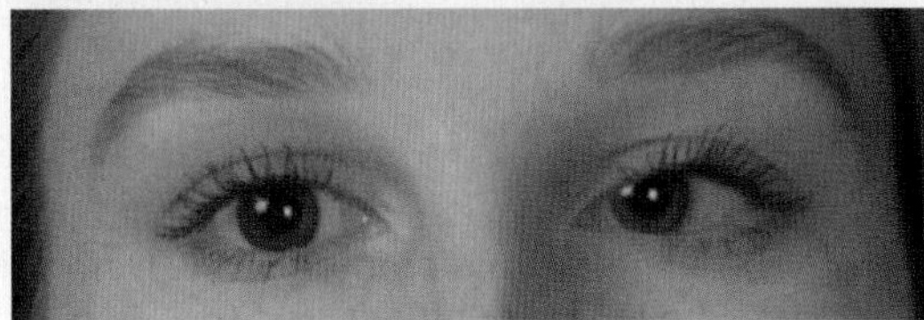

(B) Abducent paralysis

A unilateral dilated pupil has no reaction to light or accommodation.

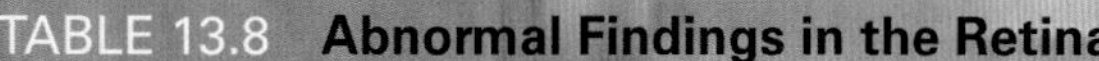

TABLE 13.8 Abnormal Findings in the Retina

Age-Related Macular Degeneration

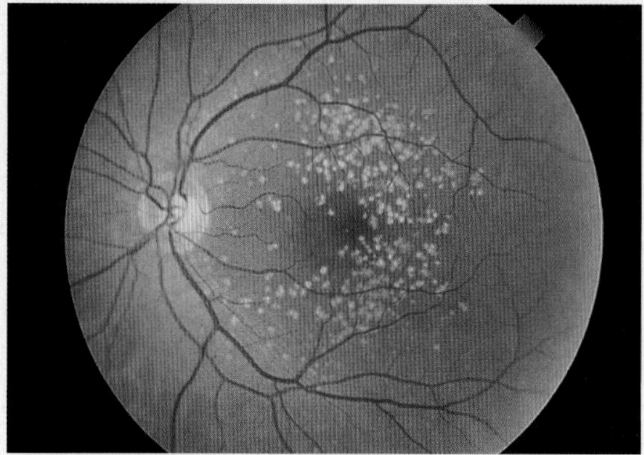

AMD gradually causes loss of sharp central vision, needed for common daily tasks (e.g., driving, reading). The macula degenerates (dry) or abnormal blood vessels behind the retina grow under the macula (wet). The more common dry AMD occurs slowly in stages: early, intermediate, and advanced. Wet AMD develops quickly without stages. The main risk factor for AMD is age, with those older than 60 years mostly affected. Other risks are smoking, obesity, European ancestry, family history, and female gender. Health education for at-risk patients includes review of a healthy diet high in leafy green vegetables and fish, smoking cessation, blood pressure and weight control, and exercise. Management options include ocular injections, laser surgery, and photodynamic therapy. None of these cure AMD, but they may slow vision loss.

Retinopathy

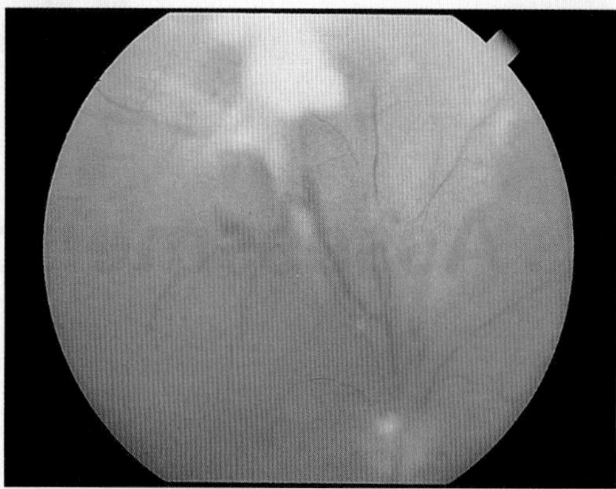

Retinopathy occurs from damage to retinal blood vessels. The two most common causes are diabetes and hypertension. *Diabetic retinopathy* is the most common cause of U.S. blindness. Its stages are (1) mild nonproliferative, (2) moderate nonproliferative, (3) severe nonproliferative, and (4) proliferative (most advanced). *Hypertensive retinopathy* presents with a dry retina (few hemorrhages, rare edema or exudate, multiple cotton wool spots), whereas diabetic retinopathy presents with a wet retina (multiple hemorrhages and exudate, extensive edema, few cotton wool spots).

Copper Wiring

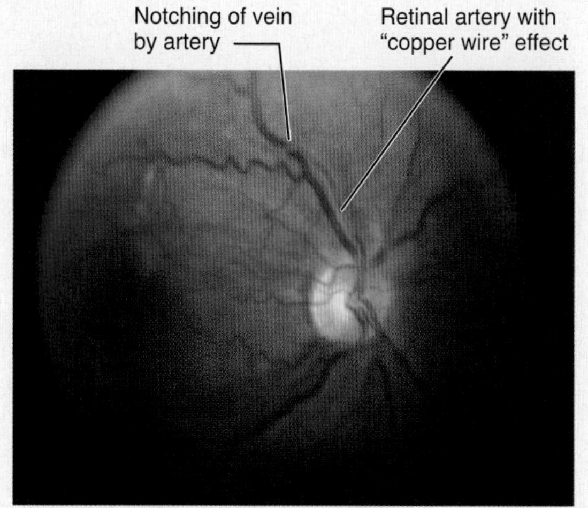

Chronic hypertension causes the retinal arterioles to thicken. The name ***copper wiring*** comes from the initial bronze appearance of the retina light reflection. As uncontrolled hypertension continues, the retina takes on a silvery or whitish appearance. The change comes from thickening of the retinal arterioles.

Retinitis Pigmentosa

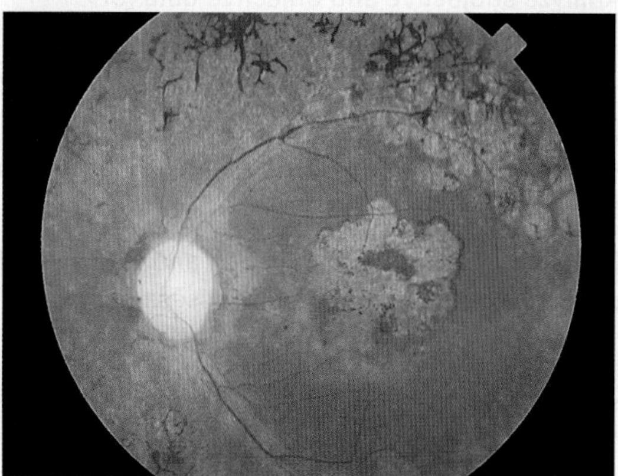

In this genetically transmitted disease, the retinas in both eyes progressively degenerate. It starts with loss of night vision, then loss of peripheral vision, progressing to tunnel vision, and finally no vision.

14

Ears Assessment

Learning Objectives

1 Demonstrate knowledge of the anatomy and physiology of the ears.

2 Identify the common landmarks of the tympanic membrane.

3 Identify important topics for health promotion and risk reduction related to the ear and hearing.

4 Collect subjective data related to the ears and hearing.

5 Collect objective data on physical structures of the ear.

6 Identify expected and unexpected findings in the inspection and palpation of the ears.

7 Identify proper techniques for otoscope use.

8 Analyze subjective and objective data for assessment of the ears and consider initial interventions.

9 Document and communicate data from ear assessment using appropriate medical terminology and principles of recording.

10 Consider age, condition, gender, and culture of the patient to individualize the ear assessment.

11 Identify nursing diagnoses and initiate a plan of care based on findings from the ear assessment.

Mrs. Garcia is a 25-year-old immigrant from El Salvador. She comes to the clinic today with concerns of ear pain, "buzzing" in her ears, and hearing loss. Mrs. Garcia has been to the clinic five times in the last 4 months for ear concerns. She was treated once for bilateral otitis media. She currently works in a tuna-packing plant as a line custodian. Her immunizations are current. Temperature is 37.4°C (99.3°F) orally, pulse 86 beats/min, respirations 16 breaths/min, and blood pressure 126/78 mmHg. Current medications include 500 mg acetaminophen taken 2 hours ago.

You will gain more information about Mrs. Garcia as you progress through this chapter. As you study the content and features, consider Mrs. Garcia's case and its relationship to what you are learning. Begin thinking about the following points:

- What are some of the possible causes of Mrs. Garcia's hearing loss?
- How will the nurse assess and document Mrs. Garcia's hearing loss?
- What information will need to be collected to assess the patient's risk for hearing loss?
- What lifestyle factors might be contributing to Mrs. Garcia's hearing loss?
- What recommendations for follow-up will the patient need?
- How will you evaluate Mrs. Garcia's understanding of her condition, treatment, and follow-up?

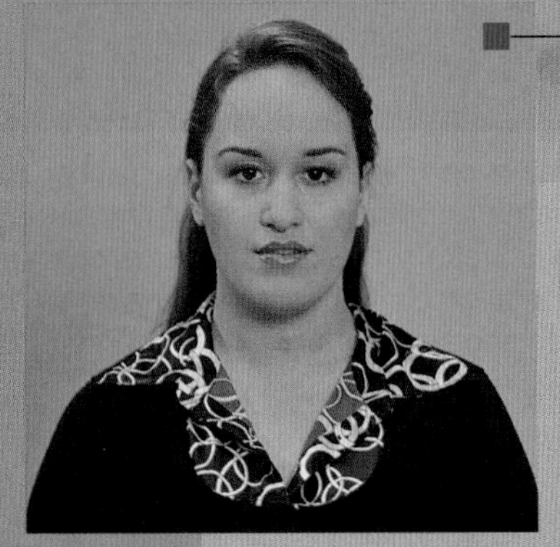

This chapter explores ear assessment. It reviews anatomy of the ear and physiology related to hearing and equilibrium, including key variations associated with lifespan, culture, and the environment. The section on subjective data collection covers family history, personal history, medications, and risk factors contributing to otitis media, loss of hearing, and vertigo. Information on collecting objective data describes methods for assessing anatomy, auditory perception, and equilibrium. A hearing screen is an essential portion of a complete physical examination. Early intervention for hearing deficit helps patients interact socially and decreases risk of injury.

Structure and Function

The ear is divided into three distinct portions: (1) the external ear, most of which is visualized easily without tools; (2) the middle ear, a small space behind the tympanic membrane (TM) extending to the pharyngotympanic (auditory) tube (formerly called the eustachian tube); and (3) the inner ear, the vestibular portion. All three portions contribute to the process of hearing. An important additional structure is the mastoid process, a bony protrusion of the skull present behind the lobule (see Fig. 14.1). The eustachian tube, although not part of the ear, affects its function. This small tube connects the anterior middle ear to the nasopharynx. The ear has two separate functions: hearing and sustaining equilibrium.

External Ear

The external ear (Fig. 14.1) is made up of flexible cartilage and skin. Its design guides sound waves into the meatus of the external auditory canal, which is a chamber that transitions from firm cartilage to bone and ends at the TM. In adults, a thin sensitive layer of skin covers the external auditory canal, which is shaped like the letter "S." Lining the canal are hairs and glands that secrete cerumen, a waxy substance. The slight S curve, hair, and cerumen help protect the canal and TM from foreign objects (Fig. 14.2).

The TM is the oblique, multilayered, translucent, pearly grey barrier between the external auditory canal and middle ear. A first layer of epidermis courses uninterrupted from the external auditory canal, a center layer, and a final mucosal layer consistent with the mucosa of the middle ear (Cohen & Clayman, 2011). The TM adheres through its concave shape to the malleus near the center. Some auditory ossicles in the middle ear can be distinguished on visualization of the translucent TM, as can portions of the malleus, umbo, manubrium, and short process (Fig. 14.3). A well-aerated middle ear allows visualization of part of the incus as well.

In the anterior quadrant of the TM, a distinct cone of light is visible, which is caused by the light of the otoscope reflecting off the posterior wall of the middle ear. The outer rim of the TM, the annulus, is thicker and more fibrous than the rest. The main part of the TM, the pars tensa, is stretched tightly and easy to see through. The pars flaccida, a small portion of the TM above the short process of the malleus, is more relaxed and opaque. (See Fig. 14.3B.)

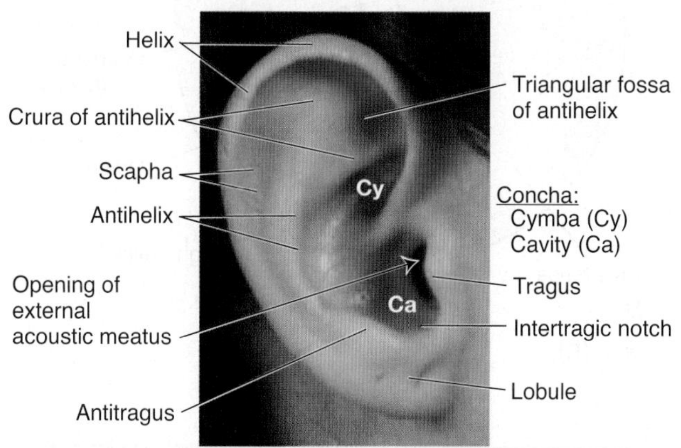

Figure 14.1 Surface anatomy of the external ear.

Middle Ear

The air-filled space behind the TM contains the malleus, incus, and stapes—tiny bones responsible for conducting sound waves to the inner ear. The middle ear acts as a volume dampener to protect the inner ear. The middle ear chamber has four openings:

1. The TM, the largest, leading to the external ear
2. The cochlear window, also called the round window, which connects the middle and inner ear
3. The oval window, on which the stapes rests to complete connection to the cochlea
4. The eustachian tube, a conduit that connects the middle ear to the nasopharynx and allows for pressure regulation of the middle ear. See Figure 14.2.

> **Clinical Significance**
>
> Ability to equalize pressure keeps the TM intact with atmospheric variances. The eustachian tube opens briefly with swallowing and yawning; otherwise, this conduit remains closed.

Inner Ear

The inner ear is responsible for the translation of sound to cranial nerve VIII (vestibulocochlear, or auditory, nerve; see Chapter 22), which transmits it to the brainstem. Although the external ear, middle ear, and inner ear all play roles in hearing, the inner ear is the only section responsible for vestibular function. The conduits of the inner ear are known collectively as the bony labyrinth, which consists of the semicircular canals, vestibule, and cochlea. The cochlea includes the portions of the inner ear responsible for hearing. **Vestibular function** is maintained in the semicircular canals and vestibule.

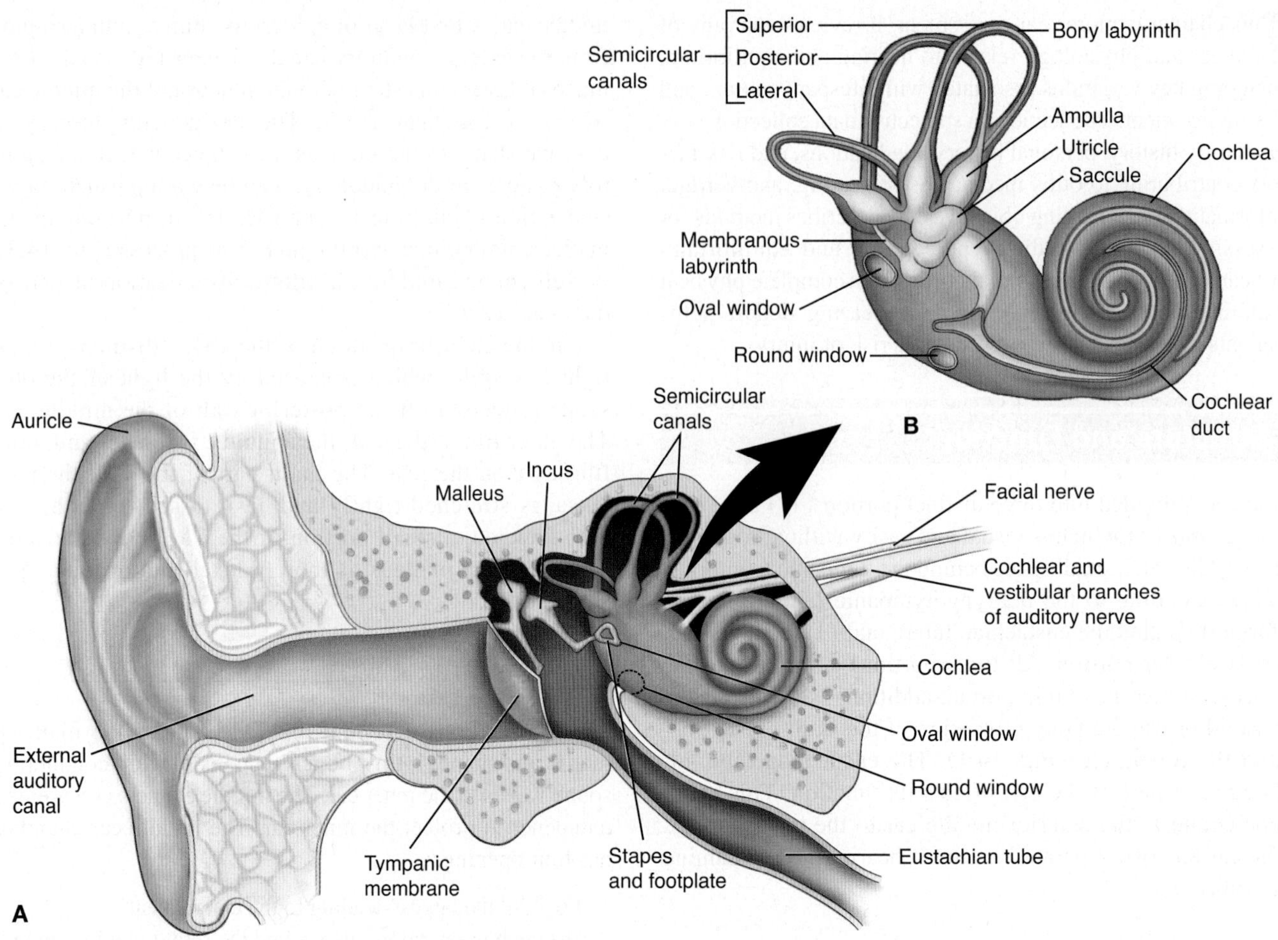

Superior
Posterior
Lateral
Semicircular canals
Bony labyrinth
Ampulla
Utricle
Cochlea
Saccule
Membranous labyrinth
Oval window
Round window
Cochlear duct
B
Auricle
Semicircular canals
Incus
Malleus
Facial nerve
Cochlear and vestibular branches of auditory nerve
Cochlea
Oval window
Round window
External auditory canal
Tympanic membrane
Stapes and footplate
Eustachian tube
A

Figure 14.2 **A.** Anatomy of the external and middle ear. **B.** Anatomy of the inner ear.

Incus
Malleus
Light source
Lens
Tympanic membrane
Stapes
A
Chorda tympani nerve
Posterior malleolar folds
Junction of incus and stapes
Pars flaccida
Short process of malleus
Anterior malleolar folds
Manubrium (handle)
Umbo
Light reflex
Pars tensa
B
RIGHT EARDRUM

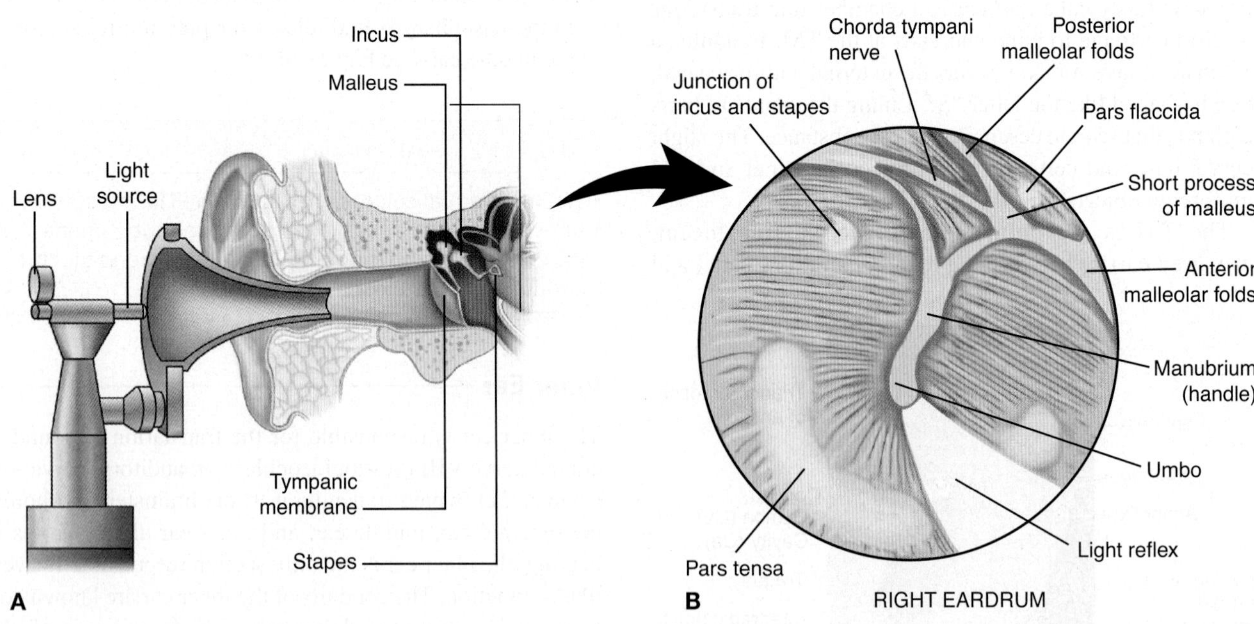

Figure 14.3 Using the otoscope **(A)** to view the tympanic membrane **(B)**.

Hearing

Hearing is a complex function. The external ear channels sound waves into the external auditory canal through the TM, to ossicles in the inner ear via the oval window, then to the cochlea. The basal membrane in the cochlea vibrates the receptor hair cells of the organ of Corti, which transfer the signal into electrical impulses for the auditory nerve. The auditory nerve then delivers those impulses to the auditory cortex in the temporal lobe of the brain (see Chapter 22), which interprets them as sound and assigns meaning to them. The brainstem detects origination of the sound and can distinguish from which ear the electrical impulses originated, even though there may be only a slight delay of sound from one ear to the other.

The cochlea interprets two components of sound: amplitude (volume) and frequency (pitch). Amplitude is the change in atmospheric pressure against the TM and is directly related to the intensity of a sound. Decibels (dB) are the measurement units of amplitude. Frequency, the number of cycles per second the sound waves make, is measured in units of hertz (Hz). A normal conversation is 60dB and 5,000 Hz. A jet engine is approximately 140 dB; a whisper is approximately 30 dB.

Air and Bone Conduction

Sound is perceived in two ways: **air conduction (AC)** and **bone conduction (BC)** (Fig. 14.4). AC, the most efficient method, is the normal pathway for sounds to travel to the inner ear. BC uses a different pathway, bypassing the external ear and delivering sound waves/vibrations directly to the inner ear through the skull. A compromise in either pathway causes hearing loss.

Hearing Difficulties

Conductive hearing loss occurs when sound wave transmission through the external or middle ear is disrupted. It may result in either blockage of the external auditory canal by cerumen or fluid in the middle ear. The health care provider can easily remedy external auditory blockage by clearing the obstruction. Fluid in the middle ear requires further investigation for pathology. Increasing the amplitude of sound will overcome conductive hearing loss.

> *SAFETY ALERT*
>
> *The most common cause of conductive hearing loss in adults is auditory trauma related to excessive noise exposure. This problem is increasing among younger people as well. Twenty-five percent of the U.S. workforce is exposed regularly to potentially damaging noise (U.S. Department of Labor, Occupational Safety & Health Administration, 2014). Because of occupational risk of noise-induced hearing loss, government standards regulate allowable noise exposure.*

Sensorineural hearing loss results from a problem somewhere beyond the middle ear, from inner ear to auditory cortex. Sites of dysfunction include the cochlea, organ of Corti, auditory nerve, and auditory cortex. **Presbycusis**, a common form of sensorineural loss, results from gradual degeneration of nerves and sensory hair cells of the organ of Corti. Such degeneration may be related to either aging or use of ototoxic drugs (e.g., gentamicin).

> **Clinical Significance**
>
> People with hearing loss are at increased risk for depression, dissatisfaction with life, reduced functional health, and withdrawal from social activities.

Tinnitus is a perception of buzzing or ringing in one or both ears that does not correspond with an external sound. It is fairly common, affecting 10% to 15% of the population (American Speech-Language-Hearing Association, 2014). The perceived sound of tinnitus may be quiet and a minor annoyance or so loud that it makes hearing normal conversation or restful sleep impossible. Little is known about what causes tinnitus, although some degree of hearing loss often accompanies it. Tinnitus may be the perception of normal sounds within the body that external noise normally blocks. Currently, very few treatments for tinnitus are available.

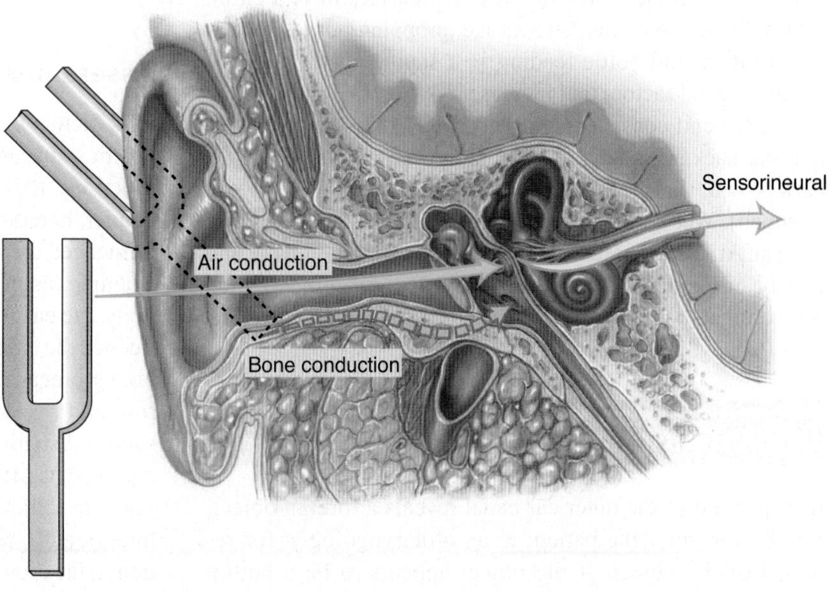

Figure 14.4 Pathways of hearing: air conduction and bone conduction.

Vestibular Function

The semicircular canals and vestibule (utricle and saccule) provide the body with proprioception and equilibrium. Each organ contains specialized epithelium for sensing position. With some diseases, the labyrinth can become inflamed and cause loss of equilibrium, which leads to a sense of **vertigo**. Symptoms of Ménière disease include vertigo along with severe nausea and vomiting. This illness has a pattern of exacerbations that often last for 24 hours followed by periods of remission (National Institute on Deafness and Other Communication Disorders, 2010).

Lifespan Considerations: Older Adults

Cartilage formation continues over the lifespan, which may make ears seem more prominent in older adults. Although it may seem that extra cartilage would help to funnel sound to the external auditory meatus, it does not. In fact, it can lead to loss of rigidity and potential collapse of the external auditory canal. In addition, fine hairs lining the ear canal become coarser and stiffer, often protruding from the external auditory meatus. This coarser hair can interfere with sound waves as they move toward the TM, decreasing hearing. With decreased hair mobility, cerumen accumulates more readily in the ear canal. This is compounded by cerumen becoming drier. This combination of factors can lead to impaction and decreased hearing in older adults. Removing mechanical blockage may restore hearing and enhance socialization. It also helps to prevent injury by preserving the sense of hearing.

Adults older than 70 years of age face greater delays in the electrical responses in the brain; thus, it takes longer for the brain to interpret input. This is one factor that contributes to the increased auditory reaction time for those in the oldest age groups.

Cultural Considerations

Socioeconomic status and environmental exposure are indicators of risk for otitis media. Lower socioeconomic status corresponds to higher rates of otitis media (Klein & Pelton, 2009). Exposure to cigarette smoke, propping bottles for babies to feed, and bottle feeding in a supine position are all environmental factors that increase risk for otitis media.

Color and consistency of **cerumen** differs according to cultural background. Most commonly, cerumen is yellow to dark brown, varying from liquid to firm paste (known as wet cerumen). Wet cerumen is most common in Caucasians and African Americans. Gray-to-white cerumen is often flaky and may be misdiagnosed as eczema. This type of cerumen, called dry cerumen, is most prevalent in Asians and Native Americans (Chang, 2014).

Urgent Assessment

If inspection of the outer ear canal reveals a foreign object, it is best to refer the patient to an otolaryngologist for removal of the object. If the object appears to be a button battery, the patient must be referred to the emergency department for immediate object removal. Button batteries can quickly erode the ear canal and extensively damage the tissues and middle ear.

Foul-smelling drainage from the ear demands immediate attention. When possible, wick the fluid from the external ear canal with either a wisp of cotton or cotton wick. Sending a culture of the fluid removed will identify the pathogen and help determine the proper antibiotic treatment. A patient with a chronically draining ear that is unresponsive to treatment requires referral to an otolaryngologist. The greatest concern with chronically draining ears is **cholesteatoma**, an abnormal accumulation of squamous epithelium within the middle ear. The growth can erode the auditory ossicles and cause great damage to the patient's hearing.

Patients with ear trauma also need evaluation for injury to nearby structures, including brain injury, basilar skull fracture, and neck injury. **Hemotympanum, otorrhea,** or **tympanic membrane** rupture may indicate barotrauma from pressure changes or a basilar skull fracture. Sudden hearing loss also can be an acute situation; the cause must be found so that appropriate treatment can be initiated.

Subjective Data

Subjective data are gathered by performing a complete and thorough health history, which begins with obtaining general information regarding the ear and its function. During the interview process, it is important to observe for any signs that the patient is having difficulty hearing. Some nonverbal cues of hearing loss include leaning forward, positioning the head or "good ear" to hear better, concentrating on lip or face movement instead of making eye contact, mumbling answers or giving answers not congruent with the question asked, asking you to repeat questions frequently, responding with a loud voice, or using a monotone conversational voice. If any of these signs is present, you need to adjust the interview and environment to facilitate communication and gather accurate data.

Assessment of Risk Factors

Risk factors play an important part in determining a patient's health status and degree of wellness related to the ear and its functions. Risk factors that cannot be controlled include age, gender, heredity, and family history. Risk factors that can be influenced are lifestyle choices and environmental risks. For example, as people age, so do the ears—like the rest of the body, the ears change with time. Nevertheless, people can influence the extent to which hearing changes and loss occur by taking precautions to guard ears from loud noises. It is your role and responsibility as a nurse to assess for risk factors such as listening to loud music or working with construction equipment. After these factors have been thoroughly assessed, you can initiate patient education during the conversational interview. To reinforce content covered, you can give the patient educational materials on how to prevent hearing loss.

History and Risk Factors	Rationale
Personal History	
How do you protect your skin from the sun? • How often do you wear a hat? • How often do you apply sunscreen? • What is the sun protection factor of the sunscreen you use? • When are you usually in the sun? • How long do you usually stay in the sun?	The ear is commonly forgotten when it comes to sun protection. For this reason, 20% of all melanomas are found in the head and neck region. The ears are the third most common site of basal cell carcinoma. The sun-exposed areas of the ear are often not protected (Skin Cancer Foundation, 2014).
What ear problems have you been diagnosed with—ear infections, hearing loss, tinnitus, vertigo? • What was the illness? • When did you have it? • How was the illness treated? • What were the outcomes?	In children, ear infections are extremely prevalent. As many as 75% of children have at least one episode by their third birthday; 50% of these have three or more episodes in their first 3 years (National Institute on Deafness and Other Communication Disorders, 2013). These children are at risk for TM rupture, scarring, and hearing loss.
What surgeries have you had? • What was the surgery? • When did you have it? • What were the outcomes? • What complications or lasting effects (sequelae) did you encounter?	Surgeries may be performed for artificial eustachian tube placement, TM repair, and cochlear implants. Cochlear implants for the hearing impaired are performed frequently. Ear surgery increases the likelihood of being exposed to ototoxic medications (e.g., aminoglycoside antibiotics).
What immunizations have you received? • What was the date of your last vaccinations? • Have you received all required doses?	Mumps (a vaccine-preventable disease and part of the measles, mumps, rubella [MMR] shot) can cause sensorineural deafness in those who have not been vaccinated, did not develop immunity with vaccination, or had decreased immunity over time. Maternal exposure to rubella (a vaccine-preventable disease and included in the MMR shot) causes deafness.
What type of loud noises have you been exposed to over your lifetime? • When were you exposed to them? • How long were you exposed to them? • What protective ear equipment did you use? • How did you monitor your exposure?	Hearing loss from loud noises is a major worldwide health issue, and disabling hearing loss affects 5% of the world's population (World Health Organization, 2014). Workers at high risk for harmful noise exposure are farmers, firefighters, police, emergency medical technicians, heavy machinery operators (e.g., construction workers), military personnel, and members of the music industry.
What exposure to cigarette, pipe, or cigar smoke have you had over your lifetime? • When were you exposed to it? • How long were you exposed to it?	Those exposed to smoke show an increased prevalence of early-onset hearing loss (Agrawal, Platz, & Niparko, 2008).
What allergies have you had? • To what are you allergic? • When did you have this difficulty? • What were the symptoms? • How were these treated? • What were the outcomes?	Allergy symptoms such as runny nose and stuffy sinuses may lead to eustachian tube dysfunction in some patients.
How often do you travel by airplane? What related ear situations have you experienced, if any?	Air pressure changes with altitude. Those who travel by plane commonly experience some middle ear discomfort during the aircraft's descent. The eustachian tubes help equalize pressure on either side of the TM. Those whose eustachian tubes may malfunction include those with colds, sinus infections, other upper respiratory infections, and other ear conditions. If the eustachian tubes cannot equalize pressure, intense middle ear and sinus pain can occur. In severe cases, the TM may rupture.

(table continues on page 352)

History and Risk Factors	Rationale
What experience with diving do you have? • How often do you dive? • What ear problems have you experienced, if any? • How do you clean your ears?	Air pressure changes with altitude; those who dive are at risk for middle ear trauma. Those at highest risk suffer from eustachian tube malfunction (as discussed under air travel). Inserting cotton-tipped applicators into the external ear canal may lead to impaction of cerumen, which can contribute to hearing loss. Cotton-tipped applicators can also cause TM perforation.
Medications What prescription and over-the-counter medications are you currently taking? • How often do you take them? • What dosage? • What route?	Several drugs have possible adverse effects on the ears (e.g., hearing loss, tinnitus, vertigo). Examples of ototoxic agents include all aminoglycosides, antiinflammatory agents (e.g., ibuprofen), antimalarials (e.g., quinine), diuretics (e.g., furosemide), nonnarcotic analgesics containing salicylates, antipyretics containing salicylates, erythromycin, quinidine sulfate, and antineoplastic drugs.
Family History Tell me about your family's history of ear or hearing problems, if any. • Who had the illness? • What was the illness? • When did the person have it? • How was the illness treated? • What were the outcomes?	Identifying a family history of possible inherited and chronic disorders (e.g., Ménière disease, otosclerosis) is important in determining the patient's risk and providing anticipatory guidance (American Hearing Research Foundation, 2012).

Risk Reduction and Health Promotion

While gathering the patient's health history, think critically about the data being gathered. The patient will reveal information about level of knowledge, health, and lifestyle. It is your role and responsibility as a nurse to analyze these data for an overall sense of the patient's wellness and to give feedback about how the patient is meeting current evidence-based health guidelines.

The health goals for the ears include the following:

- Reduce new cases of work-related noise-induced hearing loss.
- Increase access by patients who have hearing impairments to hearing rehabilitation services and adaptive devices including hearing aids, cochlear implants, or tactile or other assistive or augmentative devices.
- Increase the proportion of persons who have had a hearing examination on schedule.

(U.S. Department of Health & Human Services, 2013)

The most significant topic for patient teaching based on thorough risk assessment of the ears is general hearing loss. Although ability to hear decreases somewhat with age, much hearing loss is preventable. Patients need to be asked about their exposure to noise and what protective equipment they use. Educating patients on the types, effectiveness, and instructions for use of protective ear equipment allows them to make decisions based on their needs. Education becomes even more important if a patient cannot make changes to the environment. For example, a construction worker who works daily surrounded by loud equipment may not be able to change the amount of machinery in close proximity to the work site.

Another important topic to address is skin cancer prevention. Many melanomas are found near or on the helix of the ear. Teaching patients how to protect themselves from unnecessary sun exposure increases the likelihood of preventive behaviors (see Chapter 11).

In addition, it is important to address how the patient cleans the ears. Many people associate cerumen in the ear canal with lack of hygiene and therefore clean their ears routinely. Often, patients think cotton-tipped applicators are intended for this purpose. This self-care behavior is unsafe, placing patients at risk for cerumen impaction and TM perforation. Reinforce proper cleaning techniques such as cleaning the bowl of the helix and never introducing anything into the external auditory canal.

Common Symptoms

While taking the health history, it is important to ask about common symptoms of disorders affecting the ear. Questions about common symptoms will aid in identifying any concerns and possible problem areas related to the chief complaint or a chronic diagnosis.

Common Ear Symptoms

- Hearing loss
- Vertigo
- Tinnitus
- Otalgia

Signs/Symptoms	Rationale/Abnormal Findings
Hearing Loss Describe your hearing. What changes, if any, have you noticed? • When did this start? • Did it start suddenly or gradually? • In what situations do you find it hardest to hear? • What have you done for it? • What were the outcomes? • Do you have a family history of hearing loss? • Have you been exposed to loud noises such as machinery or gunshots?	Determining the onset of hearing loss may help uncover the cause and determine whether it can be reversed, such as with a cerumen or foreign body obstruction. Sudden hearing loss indicates trauma or obstruction. Family history of hearing loss indicates presbycusis. Environmental damage to hearing may involve consistent or one-time exposure to loud noise.
Vertigo Have you ever felt dizzy or had difficulties with balance? • Under what circumstances has this happened? • How long does this continue? • Does it feel like you are, or the room is, spinning? • How have you treated the dizziness? • What were the outcomes?	Transient vertigo and persistent vertigo have different etiologies and thus necessitate different treatments. **Vertigo**, the sensation of the room spinning, indicates dysfunction of the bony labyrinth in the inner ear.
Tinnitus Do you ever have a sensation of a buzzing or ringing that no one else can hear? • Is there any time that this seems louder? • Are you currently taking any medications, vitamins, or herbal supplements?	**Tinnitus** is thought to be an inability to filter internal noise from the external input of sound. Ototoxic agents can cause tinnitus. Stopping their use may resolve tinnitus, although some ototoxic agents cause lasting damage.
Otalgia Do you experience pain in either ear? • Is it in both ears or just in one ear? • Have you ever had this pain before? • If so, what was the cause? • Do you feel the pain deep inside or more on the outside of the ear? • Does it hurt to touch your ear? • Describe the pain. Is it persistent or intermittent? • What makes the pain better or worse? • Have you had any drainage from your ears? • What color was the drainage? • Did it have an odor? • Have you had any surgeries or illnesses recently? • How do you clean your ears?	**Otalgia** usually indicates ear dysfunction, most commonly otitis media or otitis externa. Pain in the ear can be referred from the pharynx. It is not uncommon for a patient recovering from tonsil surgery to complain of ear pain. Severe pain followed by relief and drainage indicates a ruptured TM. External ear sensitivity indicates **otitis externa**, which may result from self-induced trauma, such as inserting bobby pins, keys, or fingernails into the external ear canal. Otitis externa may also be fungal, caused by moisture in the external auditory canal. This is known as swimmer's ear.

Documenting Normal Findings

Patient alert and following conversation with no evidence of hearing loss. Denies hearing difficulty, vertigo, tinnitus, and otalgia.

Lifespan Considerations: Older Adult

Signs/Symptoms	Rationale/Abnormal Findings
Do you have hearing loss, ringing in your ears, or vertigo or dizziness?	**Otosclerosis** results from the slow fusion of any combination of the ossicles in the middle ear. The fusion leads to obstruction of the transmission of sound waves from the TM to the oval window and inner ear (American Hearing Research Foundation, 2012).

(table continues on page 354)

Signs/Symptoms	Rationale/Abnormal Findings
Do you have difficulty distinguishing sounds, especially when it is noisy? Have you noticed loss of higher pitched sounds such as the spoken "s" or "th"? Observe for garbled or mumbled speech.	Over time, some people experience a natural sensorineural loss called **presbycusis**. It happens regardless of exposure to excessive noise. Just as the hair in the external auditory canal becomes less flexible, so do the hair cells in the cochlea.

Cultural Considerations

Signs/Symptoms	Rationale/Abnormal Findings
What is the color and dryness of your ear wax? What methods do you use for cleaning the wax? Does the wax cause any problems for you?	Color and consistency of **cerumen** differs according to cultural background. Most commonly, cerumen is yellow to dark brown, varying from liquid to firm paste (known as wet cerumen). Wet cerumen is most common in Caucasians and African Americans. Gray-to-white cerumen is often flaky and may be misdiagnosed as eczema. This type of cerumen, called dry cerumen, is most prevalent in Asians and Native Americans.

Therapeutic Dialogue: Collecting Subjective Data

Remember Mrs. Garcia, introduced at the beginning of the chapter. She was admitted to the clinic today with a complaint of ear pain. She is concerned about the pain in her ears and what that might mean. The nurse uses professional communication techniques to gather subjective data.

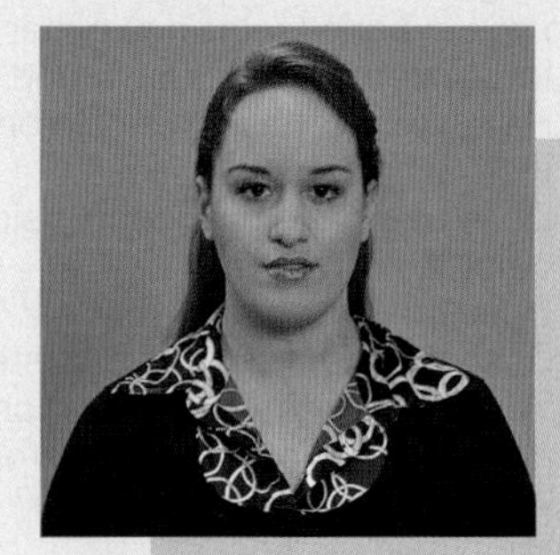

Nurse: Hello, Mrs. Garcia. I'm going to be your nurse today. My name is Lee. (smiles, pauses) How are you feeling?

Mrs. Garcia: Fine.

Nurse: Your chart says that you came in because of your ears. Is that right?

Mrs. Garcia: Yes, I have had pain. But the pain gets better with medicine and a warm cloth.

Nurse: Are you having other symptoms with your ears?

Mrs. Garcia: Yes, I have a buzzing noise in my ears. My husband says I can't hear well. My kids say I am yelling when I'm just talking. I can't understand them anymore.

Nurse: It sounds like your family is worried about you. (pauses)

Mrs. Garcia: My mom had problems hearing when she was my age, and it was hard for the family.

Nurse: This must bring back some of those memories for you. Let's talk about how your hearing has changed (smiles).

(case study continues on page 355)

Critical Thinking Challenge

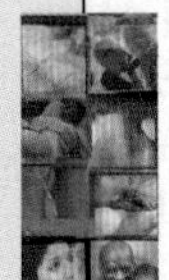

- What other assessments might the nurse perform related to the potential hearing loss?
- How might the patient's experience and culture influence her perceptions, values, and beliefs about her diagnosis and healing?
- What is the role of the nurse in giving advice versus listening to the patient's perspective?

Objective Data

Common and Specialty or Advanced Techniques

Routine head-to-toe assessment includes the most important and common assessment techniques. It is essential to learn these techniques for use in clinical practice. You may add specialty or advanced steps if concerns exist over a specific finding. Specialty techniques are used in advanced practice for diagnosis. The common and advanced techniques are summarized in the table.

The registered nurse (RN) rarely uses an otoscope to inspect the ear. An advanced practice registered nurse (APRN) completes the otoscopic examination.

Equipment Needed (for Advanced Practice Assessment)

- Otoscope
- High-pitched tuning fork

Preparation

To obtain objective data about the ears, it is best to make sure the patient is comfortable and the room is quiet. It is ideal for the patient's ears to be at your eye level to be able to inspect them without discomfort to the patient. For adults and older children, the examination can be performed with the patient sitting on the examination table.

Basic Versus Focused/Specialty or Advanced Techniques Related to Ear Assessment

Technique	Purpose	Screening or Registered Nurse Assessment	Focused or Advanced Practice Examination
Observe behavioral responses to speech.	To identify cues that might indicate hearing loss	X	
Inspect the external ear position.	To evaluate for congenital problems	X	
Inspect the size, shape, and condition of skin on external ear.	To evaluate for skin breakdown or lesions, edema, erythema, discharge	X	
Palpate external ear.	To note lumps, masses, tenderness	X	
Perform whisper test.	To evaluate for high-pitched hearing loss		X High-pitched hearing loss
Perform Rinne test.	To evaluate air conduction and bone conduction		X Air versus bone
Perform Weber test.	To evaluate unilateral hearing loss		X Unilateral loss
Inspect external canal with otoscope.	To evaluate cerumen, discharge, foreign bodies, erythema, lesions		X Foreign bodies, obstruction
Inspect TM.	To note color, characteristics, position, integrity		X Infection

Begin the examination by first washing your hands in warm water. Hand sanitizer is effective for bacteria control but leaves the hands cold and may cause discomfort for the patient.

When meeting with the patient, you will be able to move forward with the examination and intervention when you first address the problem that is most important to the patient. Often, this may not be the issue of greatest clinical significance. After you have addressed the patient's chief concern, you will find your patient is more receptive to issues of potentially greater significance such as hearing loss or **cholesteatoma**. Patient education is the primary tool to engage your patient in greater heath care and address issues that, if left unaddressed, may cause the patient harm or impair quality of life.

Comprehensive Physical Assessment

Technique and Normal Findings	Abnormal Findings
Inspection Inspect the ears (Fig. 14.5). Ears are symmetrical, equal size, and fully formed 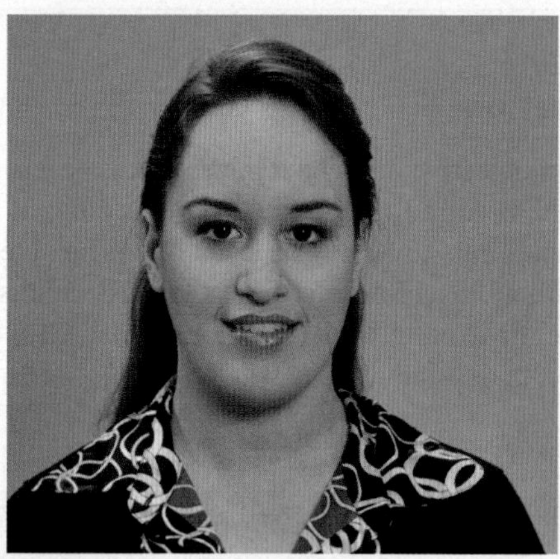 **Figure 14.5** Normal surface anatomy of the ears.	Microtia, macrotia, edematous ears, cartilaginous *Pseudomonas* infection, carcinoma on auricle, cyst, and frostbite are unexpected findings. See Table 14.2 at the end of this chapter.
Inspect the face. Facial tone is uniform with the ears. Skin is intact. Small painless nodules on the helix are a variation of normal anatomy known as darwinian tubercle (Fig. 14.6). 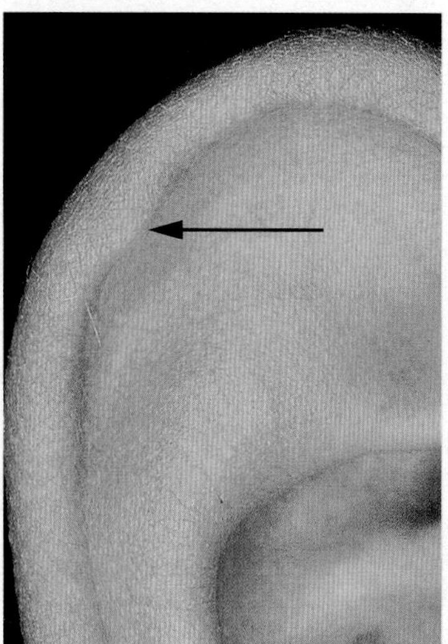 **Figure 14.6** Darwinian tubercle, a normal anatomical variation.	

(table continues on page 357)

Technique and Normal Findings (continued)	Abnormal Findings (continued)
Palpation Palpate the auricle. Ears are firm without lumps, lymph tissue is not palpable, ears are nontender, and no pain is elicited with palpation or manipulation of the auricle. No pain occurs with palpation of the mastoid process.	Enlarged lymph nodes indicate pathology or inflammation. Pain with auricle movement or tragus palpation indicates otitis externa or furuncle.
Hearing Acuity The ***whisper test*** evaluates for loss of high-frequency sounds. Instruct the patient to plug (or plug for the patient) the ear opposite to the one you are testing. With your head approximately 45 cm (18 in.) from the patient's ear and your mouth not visible to the patient, whisper a simple sentence that includes words and numbers (Fig. 14.7). Have the patient repeat what you have said. Repeat on the opposite side. Patient repeats the entire sentence to you without errors.	Not being able to repeat the sentence clearly or missing components may indicate hearing loss of higher frequencies and requires follow-up with formal testing.
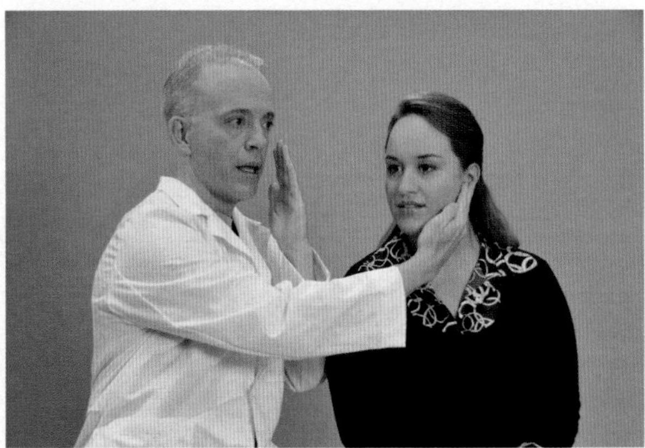 **Figure 14.7** The whisper test.	
Otoscopic Evaluation Inspect the external meatus and canal. Several sizes of speculum can be used on the otoscope; choose one that fits into the external canal without discomfort. The canal has fine hairs; some cerumen lining the wall skin is intact, with no discharge.	Redness, swelling of the external auditory canal, and discharge are signs of external otitis. Either a foreign body or cerumen can obstruct the canal.
Hold the otoscope so that your thumb is by the window and you are bracing the shaft with your fingers along the patient's cheek. This allows you to stabilize the otoscope and decreases risk of scraping the external auditory canal with the speculum. Hold the patient's ear at the helix and lift up and back to align the canal for best visualization of the TM (Fig. 14.8). After visualization of the canal, you will rotate the otoscope slightly to be able to visualize the entire TM. Visualize portions and short process of the malleus, umbo, and manubrium through the translucent membrane (Fig. 14.9).	Swelling or bulging of the TM indicates acute **otitis media** (see Table 14.3 at the end of the chapter). A diffuse cone of light indicates otitis media with effusion. Air bubbles caused by a functioning eustachian tube allow drainage of effusion and aeration of the middle ear. A perforated TM may allow for direct visualization into the middle ear.

(table continues on page 358)

Technique and Normal Findings (continued)	Abnormal Findings (continued)

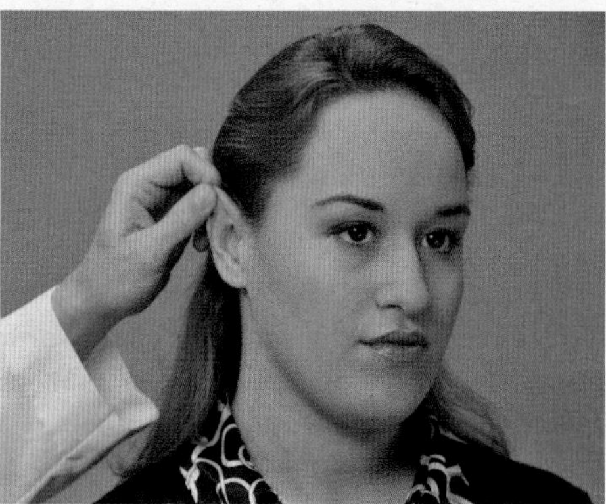

Figure 14.8 Otoscopic examination: holding the patient's ear at the helix and lifting up and back to align the canal for best visualization of the tympanic membrane.

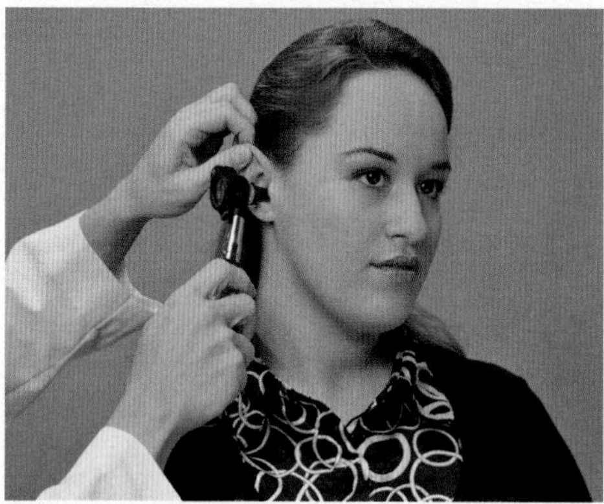

Figure 14.9 Correct placement of the otoscope.

A well-aerated middle ear allows visualization of part of the incus as well (Fig. 14.10).

TM is intact and translucent and allows visualization of the short process of the malleus. The cone of light is visible in the anterior inferior quadrant.

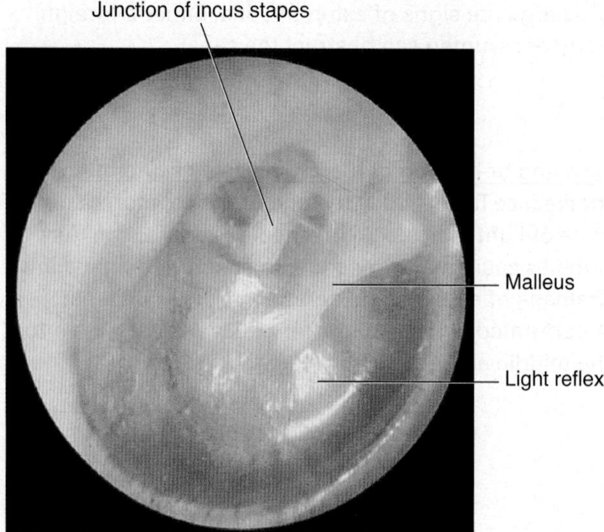

Figure 14.10 Normal tympanic membrane.

(table continues on page 359)

Technique and Normal Findings (continued)	Abnormal Findings (continued)

A variation of normal is a TM with white areas (sclerosis). These white areas are visible scars from repeated ear infections. This scarring may make the TM less flexible (Fig. 14.11).

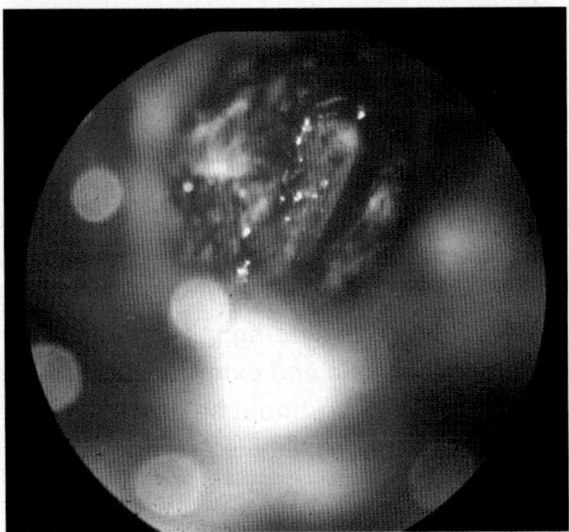

Figure 14.11 Tympanic membrane with tympanosclerosis.

After the TM has been visualized, you may use the **bulb insufflator** attached to the head of the otoscope (Fig. 14.12) to observe TM movement. First, perform gentle positive pressure that forces air into the external auditory canal and pushes down the TM. Then, release pressure quickly and note the negative pressure pulling the TM outward. The TM moves inward when inflated and outward with release.

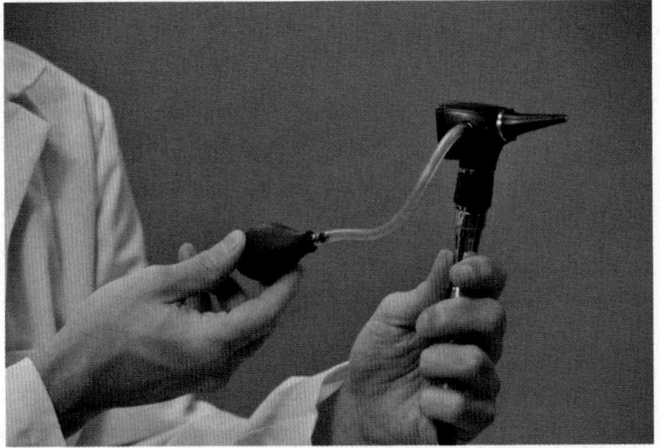

Figure 14.12 Otoscope with bulb insufflator attached.

Auditory Acuity

The most accurate way to evaluate hearing is by having an audiologist perform an **audiogram** in a soundproof room. An audiogram gives exact information about absent or diminished frequencies for the patient. It also distinguishes sensorineural from conductive loss. Including tympanometry with the audiogram will show the compliance of the TM and whether a pinhole rupture exists by providing the volume of the external ear canal. The primary care provider in an advanced practice role orders this test.

Although an audiogram provides the most accurate test, most primary clinics cannot provide it; thus, patients are referred to an otolaryngologist or audiologist.

(table continues on page 360)

Technique and Normal Findings (continued)	Abnormal Findings (continued)
Rinne Test A tuning fork is a U-shaped piece of metal with a handle attached at the apex of the U. When struck lightly against an object, it will vibrate at a specific frequency. Use of a tuning fork helps you determine whether hearing is equal in both ears and whether a conductive or sensorineural hearing loss is present by allowing you to compare the difference in BC versus AC. Remember: AC has less resistance than BC.	
The **Rinne test** examines the difference between BC and AC. 1. To begin, grasp and tap the handle of the tuning fork against the back or heel of your hand (Fig. 14.13). 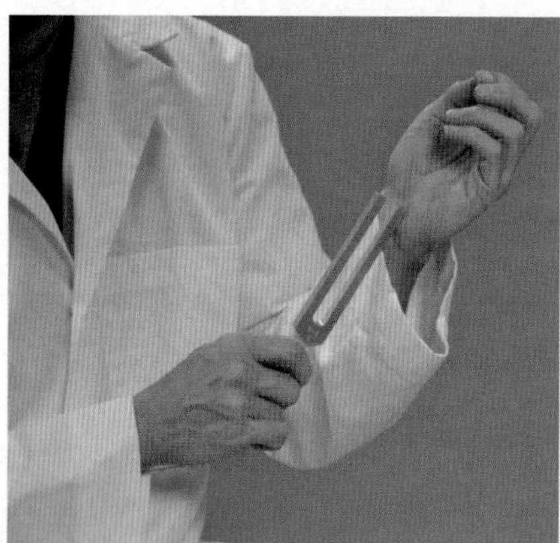 **Figure 14.13** Striking the tuning fork against the heel of the hand. 2. Place the base of the handle on the patient's mastoid process (Fig. 14.14). Note the time on the second hand of your watch. 3. Instruct the patient to tell you when he or she no longer hears the sound of the fork. Note the number of seconds. 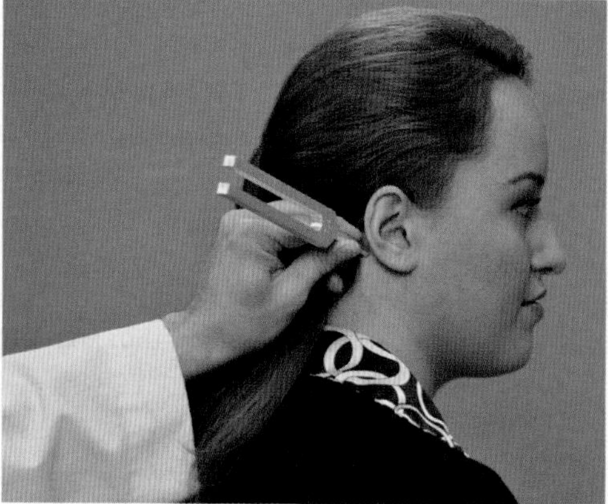 **Figure 14.14** Rinne test: placing the tuning fork on the mastoid process.	BC that is longer than or the same as AC is evidence of conductive hearing loss. Conductive hearing loss on one side may indicate external or middle ear disease. Patients with conductive hearing loss should have an assessment of the auricle and external auditory canal to look for blockage. The TM should be assessed to ensure that no middle ear abnormality is present, such as fluid or a TM perforation.

(table continues on page 361)

Technique and Normal Findings (continued)	Abnormal Findings (continued)
4. After the patient can no longer hear the sound through the mastoid process, move the tip of the tuning fork to the front of the external auditory meatus (Fig. 14.15). Again, note the time on the second hand of your watch.	
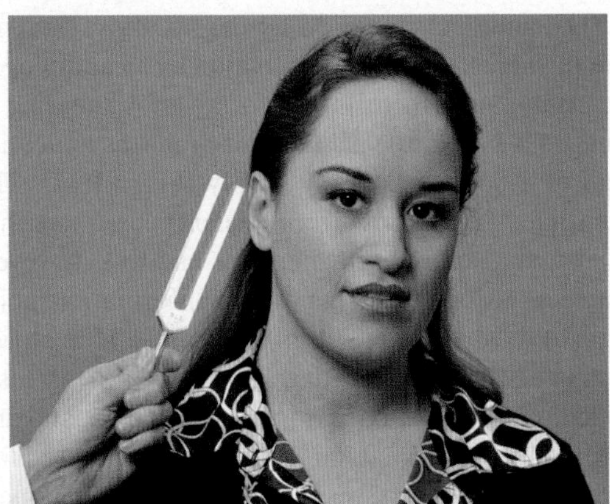 Figure 14.15 Rinne test: moving the tip of the tuning fork to the front of the external auditory meatus.	
5. Instruct the patient to inform you when he or she no longer hears the sound. AC is twice as long as BC.	
Weber Test The **Weber test** helps to differentiate the cause of unilateral hearing loss. After activating the fork, place its handle on the midline of the parietal bone in line with both ears (Fig. 14.16). The patient hears the sound in both ears and at equal intensity.	Unilateral identification of the sound indicates sensorineural loss in the ear in which the patient did not hear or had reduced perception of the sound. Sensorineural hearing loss on one side may be related to an inner ear disorder such as Ménière disease or a vestibular schwannoma (**acoustic neuroma**).
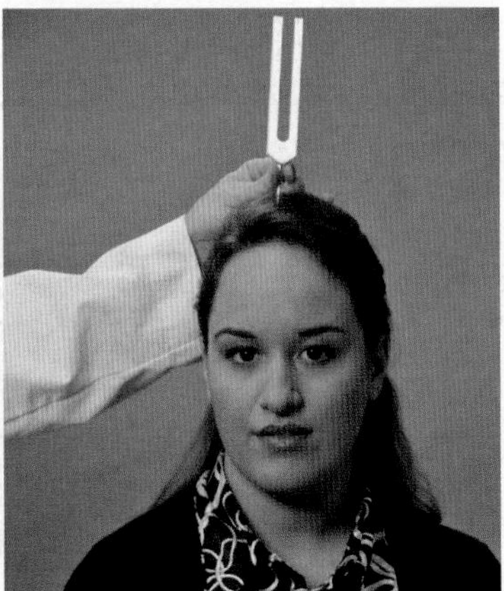 Figure 14.16 Weber test: placing the tuning fork on the midline of the parietal bone.	
Equilibrium Equilibrium can be assessed by using the **Romberg test** as described in Chapter 22.	Failure of the Romberg test may indicate dysfunction in the vestibular portion of the inner ear, semicircular canals, and vestibule.

Documenting Normal Findings:

Right pinna normal, canal well aerated, TM translucent with visible bony prominence of the malleus and sharp cone of light. Left pinna normal, canal well aerated, TM translucent with visible bony prominence of the malleus and sharp cone of light. Hearing intact bilateral with whisper test. Rinne test result normal. Weber test result normal.

Lifespan Considerations: Older Adults

The cartilage and skin around the external ear may be less pliable in older adults. The stiff hairs in the canal may require a smaller otoscope tip to separate them and increase visualization of the TM. The membrane itself may seem more opaque and less mobile. The American Academy of Family Physicians recommends screening for hearing difficulties by questioning older adults about hearing impairment.

Clinical Significance

For patients who wear hearing aids, accumulated cerumen and otitis externa can be ongoing challenges. It is important for this population to have frequent examination of their ear canals to ensure patency and health and to receive maximum benefits from their hearing aids.

Cultural Considerations

Assess carefully for hearing loss in Caucasian men older than 70 years of age. The next highest prevalence is in Caucasian women, followed by African American men and women. Expect that the rates of otitis media are highest among Native Americans, Alaskan Eskimos and Canadian Inuit, and indigenous Australian children (Klein & Pelton, 2009).

Critical Thinking

Laboratory and Diagnostic Testing

Most common hearing tests in primary care offices and schools are done with a device called an audiometer. This simple screening device consists of headphones and a box that delivers tones to each ear at variable frequencies and volumes. The audiometer is used to identify those patients who require further testing and examination by an audiologist. Audiologists use audiometers to perform various hearing tests in a soundproof booth; the audiometer produces an audiogram, a graph of a person's hearing ability (Fig. 14.17). This test differentiates conductive from sensorineural hearing loss. Audiologists also use tympanograms and tests to reveal otoacoustic emissions, which provide information about the function of the outer hair cells of the cochlea. The otoacoustic emissions test helps determine suspected hearing loss from ototoxic drugs. If a patient complains of otalgia, and drainage is present in the ear canal, this fluid may be cultured to determine the best topical treatment for either otitis externa or otitis media with TM perforation.

Diagnostic Reasoning

Nursing Diagnosis, Outcomes, and Interventions

When formulating a nursing diagnosis, it is important to use critical thinking to cluster data and identify patterns that fit together. You compare these clusters of data with the defining characteristics (abnormal findings) for the diagnosis to ensure the most accurate labeling and appropriate interventions. Table 14.1 compares nursing diagnoses, unexpected findings, and interventions commonly related to the ear assessment (NANDA International, 2012).

Documenting Case Study Findings

The nurse has just finished an initial ear examination of Mrs. Garcia, who has unexpected findings. Review the following important findings revealed in each of the steps of objective data collection for Mrs. Garcia. Consider how these results compare with the normal findings presented in the samples of normal documentation. Note that inspection is the primary technique used in ear assessment.

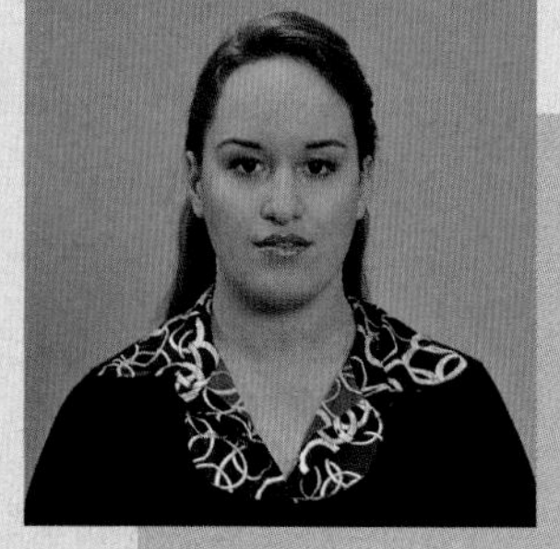

Inspection: Right ear is pink, skin is intact, external auditory canal appears clear. Left ear is pink, skin is intact, purulent drainage is noted in the external auditory canal.

Palpation: Right ear warm, no pain with palpation. Left ear is warm, painful with manipulation of the external ear and pain with pressure on the tragus.

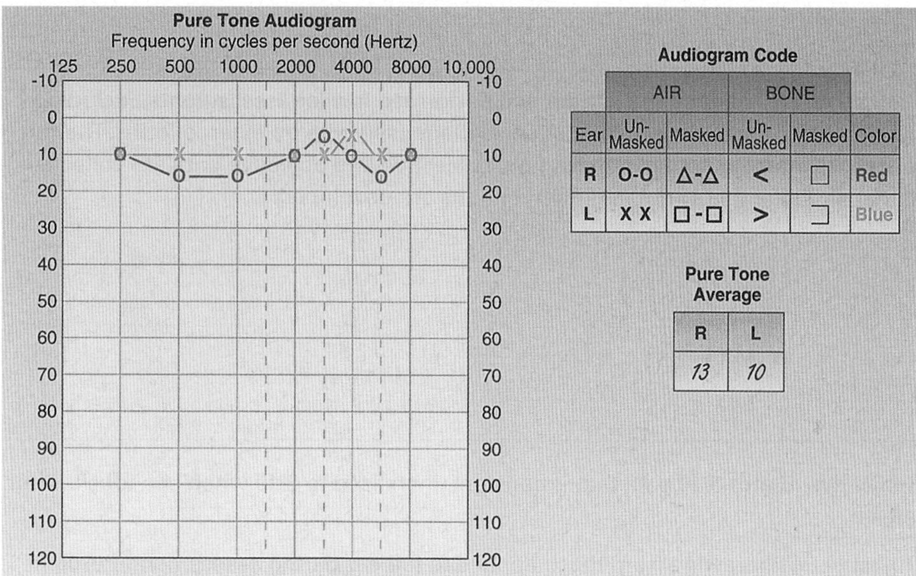

Figure 14.17 An audiogram.

You use assessment information to identify patient outcomes. Some outcomes related to ear problems include the following:

- Patient is free from ear pain.
- Patient demonstrates understanding with a verbal response.
- Patient explains plan to accommodate hearing impairment (Moorhead, Johnson, Maas, & Swanson, 2013).

After the outcomes have been established, you implement nursing care to improve the status of the patient. You use critical thinking and evidence-based practice to develop the interventions. Some examples of nursing interventions for the ear and hearing are as follows:

- Turn off televisions and radios when communicating.
- Close the door if hallway noise is loud.
- Provide a communication board and visual aids for detailed discussions (Bulechek, Butcher, Dochterman, & Wagner, 2013).

You then evaluate the care according to the patient outcomes that you developed, thus reassessing the patient and continuing or modifying the interventions as appropriate.

TABLE 14.1 Common Nursing Diagnoses Associated With the Ear

Diagnosis	Point of Differentiation	Assessment Characteristics	Nursing Interventions
Disturbed auditory sensory perception	Alterations in the way the person interprets, uses, or organizes sensory (especially hearing-related) stimuli	Change in responses to environment, impaired communication, difficulty with concentration	Minimize background noise. Sit directly in front of patient. Allow patient to see your face. Do not overenunciate or shout at patient.
Pain	Unpleasant sensory and emotional experience from skin or tissue damage	Self-report of pain is subjective. Expressions are variable and include facial grimace, guarding, muscle tension, tachycardia, tachypnea, and nausea.	Use pain scale to identify current pain intensity and effectiveness of medication. Develop pain goal collaboratively with patient. Provide pain medications as ordered.* Provide alternatives such as distraction, breathing, and relaxation.
Risk for infection	At risk for pathogenic organisms due to break in the skin or tissue, the body's primary defense	Break in skin integrity, tubes and procedures, exposure to pathogens, malnutrition, inadequate immunity, chronic disease	Follow frequent handwashing, universal precautions. Protect wound with dressing. Monitor for fever, white blood cell count, wound drainage, or erythema. Discontinue tubes as soon as possible. Encourage adequate nutrition.

*Collaborative interventions.

Progress Note: Analyzing Findings

The APRN has seen the patient and performed further assessments, including the otoscopic examination. The patient is diagnosed with an external otitis. The following RN nursing note illustrates how subjective and objective data are collected and analyzed and how nursing interventions are developed.

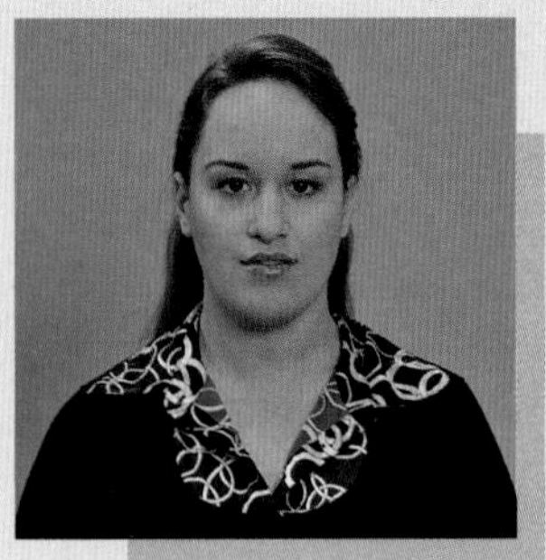

Subjective: States 5/10 pain that is constant. Increased to 8/10 when she touches her left ear.

Objective: Withdrawing from touch applied to left ear during assessment. Purulent drainage noted at the meatus of the external ear canal.

Analysis: Pain related to otitis externa of left ear.

Plan: Apply heat or cold for comfort. Encourage administration of ordered oral pain medication and adherence to antibiotic schedule to promote healing. Assess whether Mrs. Garcia has sufficient resources to obtain necessary medications. Work with the patient's family and encourage them to speak more clearly and make eye contact.

Critical Thinking Challenge

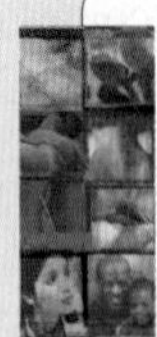

- How is the role of the RN different from that of the APRN?
- What type of ongoing assessment would you predict?
- How would you address the issue of pain assessment and management?
- What teaching should be performed related to Mrs. Garcia's otitis externa, loss of hearing, and treatment plan?

Collaborating With the Interprofessional Team

An audiology consult is indicated for evaluation of hearing loss. Audiologists are available in many specialty clinics to ensure proper evaluation. The APRN has recommended an audiology consult; the RN will make the referral.

The following conversation illustrates how the RN might organize data and make recommendations about Mrs. Garcia to the audiologist.

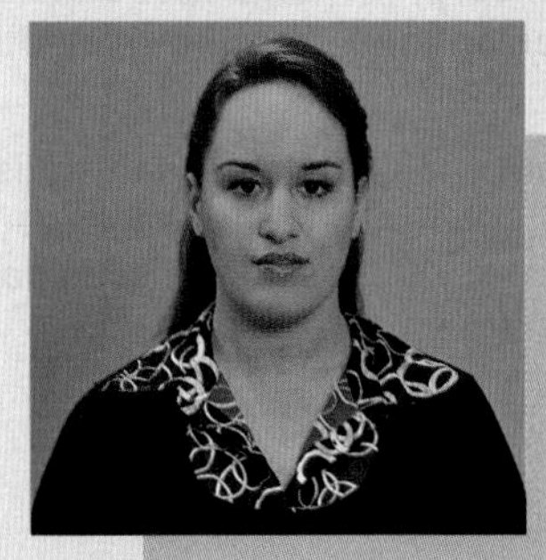

Situation: "Hello. I'm taking care of Mrs. Garcia in the clinic today. She's a 25-year-old woman with ear pain, tinnitus, and possible hearing loss."

Background: "Her mother had hearing loss at a young age. Mrs. Garcia also works in a tuna factory with many loud noises and uses ear protection. Her hearing was

(case study continues on page 365)

stable until 6 months ago when she noticed a buzzing sound in her ears. Around that time, she also required the television to be turned up to hear it clearly."

Assessment: "Her right ear is clear. She is having some drainage from her left ear, and the APRN diagnosed otitis externa. He would like her to have an audiogram to evaluate her hearing loss."

Recommendations: "When you perform your audiogram, would you please perform a tympanogram as well to check for a ruptured TM after her antibiotic treatment? What times do you have available for her? Thanks so much."

Critical Thinking Challenge

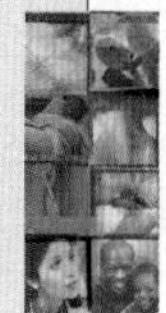

- What assessments might be performed on other body systems related to the patient's findings?
- What health promotion and teaching needs would be related to the patient's history and risk factors?
- What further assessment information might the nurse want to collect in preparation for the end of the appointment?

Pulling it All Together

The nurse uses assessment data to formulate a nursing care plan with patient outcomes and interventions. This is often in the form of a care plan or case note similar to the one below.

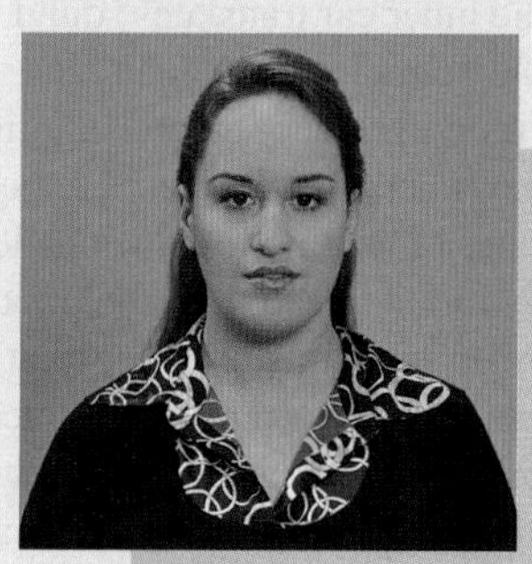

Nursing Diagnosis	Patient Outcomes	Nursing Interventions	Rationale	Evaluation
Pain related to ear infection as evidenced by stating pain 5/10 scale	Patient rates ear pain at zero or an acceptable level.	Provide warm or cool pack for comfort. Provide analgesics as prescribed.	Pain is subjective and treatment is aimed at controlling the symptoms until the cause can be resolved.	Patient states that ear pain is now 2/10 scale. Continue to provide analgesic every 4 hours.*

*Collaborative interventions.

Applying Your Knowledge

Using the previous steps of diagnostic reasoning, organizing, and prioritizing, consider all the case study findings woven throughout this chapter. When answering the following questions, begin drawing conclusions and see how the pieces of assessment must work together to create an environment for personalized, appropriate, and accurate care.

- What are some of the possible causes of Mrs. Garcia's hearing loss?
- How will the nurse assess and document Mrs. Garcia's hearing loss?
- What information will need to be collected to assess the patient's risk for hearing loss?
- What lifestyle factors might be contributing to Mrs. Garcia's hearing loss?
- What recommendations for follow-up will the patient need?
- How will you evaluate Mrs. Garcia's understanding of her condition, treatment, and follow-up?

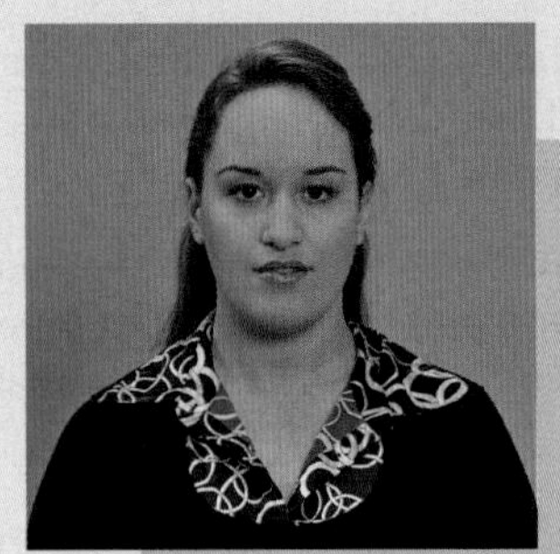

Key Points

- The ear consists of the external ear, middle ear, and inner ear.
- The TM is the barrier between the external auditory canal and the middle ear.
- The middle ear contains the malleus, incus, and stapes, which conduct sound waves to the inner ear.
- The inner ear translates sound to the nerves and brainstem.
- The semicircular canals and vestibule provide the body with proprioception and equilibrium.
- The functions of the ear are hearing and equilibrium.
- Clues of hearing loss include leaning forward to hear, positioning the head with the good ear forward, concentrating on lip movement, asking that questions be repeated, and using a loud or monotone voice.
- Risk factors for hearing loss include family history, frequent ear infections, use of certain medications, lack of immunizations, exposure to loud noises, exposure to smoke, allergies, airplane travel, diving, inappropriate cleaning of ears, and increased age.
- Common disorders of the ear include hearing loss, vertigo, tinnitus, and otalgia.
- The RN assessment includes inspection and palpation of the external ear.
- The APRN inspects the auditory meatus, canal, and TM with the otoscope.
- The most accurate evaluation of hearing is with an audiogram.
- The whisper test evaluates loss of high-frequency sounds.
- During the Rinne test, AC should be twice as long as BC. If BC is equal to or greater than AC, it is evidence of conductive hearing loss.
- The Weber test differentiates unilateral hearing loss.

Review Questions

1. The function of the ear is for
   A. hearing and equilibrium.
   B. equilibrium and perforations.
   C. perforations and balance.
   D. balance and equilibrium.

2. The inner ear
   A. contains the malleus, incus, and stapes.
   B. conducts sound waves to the external ear.
   C. translates sound to the nerves and brainstem.
   D. provides the body with proprioception.

3. Cues of hearing loss include which of the following? Choose all that are correct.
   A. Using a loud or monotonous voice
   B. Asking to repeat questions
   C. Concentrating on lip movement
   D. Leaning forward to hear

4. Risk factors for hearing loss include which of the following? Choose all that are correct.
   A. Frequent ear infections
   B. Being current on immunizations
   C. Exposure to smoke
   D. Decreased age

5. Tinnitus is described as
   A. inability to hear well.
   B. dizziness.
   C. ringing in the ear.
   D. ear pain.

6. Which of the following patients is most likely to have hearing loss?
   A. Caucasian man older than 70 years of age
   B. Hispanic woman older than 50 years of age
   C. Asian man younger than 30 years of age
   D. African American girl younger than 10 years of age

7. Which of the following differentiates the RN assessment from the APRN assessment?
   A. History and risk factors
   B. Symptom analysis
   C. Inspection and palpation
   D. Otoscopic assessment

8. A nursing diagnosis appropriate for a patient with ear problems is
   A. kinesthetic disturbed perception.
   B. disturbed sensory perception.
   C. sensory perception, gustatory.
   D. olfactory sensory perception.

9. Which of the following is an outcome appropriate for a patient with hearing impairment?
   A. Provide a communication board or picture to assist teaching.
   B. Minimize background noise and close door.
   C. Stand in front of patient and explain procedure.
   D. Patient explains plan to accommodate hearing impairment.

10. Which of the following are appropriate interventions for the patient who is at risk for ear infection? Select all that apply.
    A. Be current on immunizations.
    B. Avoid secondhand smoke.
    C. Clean only external ear.
    D. Have audiogram yearly.

The Jensen suite offers these additional resources to enhance learning and facilitate understanding of this chapter:

- thePoint online resource, http://thepoint.lww.com/Jensen2e
- *Laboratory Manual for Nursing Health Assessment: A Best Practice Approach*
- *Pocket Guide for Nursing Health Assessment: A Best-Practice Approach*
- *Lippincott DocuCare,* an electronic health record simulation software, http://thepoint.lww.com/docucare
- *Adaptive Learning | Powered by PrepU* , http://thepoint.lww.com/prepu

References

Agrawal, Y., Platz, E. A., & Niparko, J. K. (2008). Prevalence of hearing loss and differences by demographic characteristics among US adults. *Archives of Internal Medicine, 168*(14), 1522–1530.

American Hearing Research Foundation. (2012). *Otosclerosis*. Retrieved from http://www.american-hearing.org/disorders/otosclerosis/

American Speech-Language-Hearing Association. (2014). *Tinnitus*. Retrieved from http://www.asha.org/public/hearing/tinnitus/

Bulechek, G. M., Butcher, H. K., Dochterman, J. M., & Wagner, C. M. (2013). *Nursing interventions classification (NIC)* (6th ed.) St. Louis, MO: Mosby

Chang, C. (2014). *Earwax*. Retrieved from http://www.fauquierent.net/earwax.htm

Cohen, J. I., & Clayman, G. L. (2011). *Atlas of head and neck surgery*. Philadelphia, PA: Elsevier Health Sciences.

Klein, J. O., & Pelton, S. (2009). *Acute otitis media in children: Epidemiology, microbiology, clinical manifestations, and complications*. Retrieved, from http://www.uptodate.com/contents/acute-otitis-media-in-children-epidemiology-microbiology-clinical-manifestations-and-complications?source=search_result&search=Acute+otitis+media+in+children&selectedTitle=4%7E98

Moorhead, S., Johnson, M., Maas, M. L., & Swanson, E. (2013). *Nursing outcomes classification (NOC): Measurement of health outcomes* (5th ed.). St. Louis, MO: Elsevier.

NANDA International. (2012). *Nursing diagnoses: Definitions and classification* 2012–2014 (9th ed). Oxford, United Kingdom: Wiley-Blackwell.

National Institute on Deafness and Other Communication Disorders. (2010). *Meniere's disease*. Retrieved from http://www.nidcd.nih.gov/health/balance/pages/meniere.aspx

National Institute on Deafness and Other Communication Disorders. (2013). *Ear infections in children*. Retrieved from https://www.nidcd.nih.gov/staticresources/health/hearing/NIDCD-Ear-Infections-In-Children.pdf

Pratt, S. R., Kuller, L., Talbott, E. O., McHugh-Pemu, K., Buhari, A. M., & Xu, X. (2009). Prevalence of hearing loss in black and white elders: Results of the cardiovascular health study. *Journal of Speech Language and Hearing Research, 52*(4), 973–989.

Skin Cancer Foundation. (2014). *The ears: A high risk area for skin cancer*. Retrieved from http://www.skincancer.org/skin-cancer-information/basal-cell-carcinoma/the-ears-a-high-risk-area-for-skin-cancer

U.S. Department of Health & Human Services. (2013). *2020 Topics & objectives-Objectives A-Z*. Retrieved from http://www.healthypeople.gov/2020/topicsobjectives2020/

U.S. Department of Labor, Occupational Safety & Health Administration. (2014). *Occupational noise exposure*. Retrieved from https://www.osha.gov/SLTC/noisehearingconservation/

World Health Organization. (2014). *Deafness and hearing loss*. Retrieved from http://www.who.int/mediacentre/factsheets/fs300/en/

Tables of Abnormal Findings

TABLE 14.2 Abnormal Findings in the External Ear

Microtia

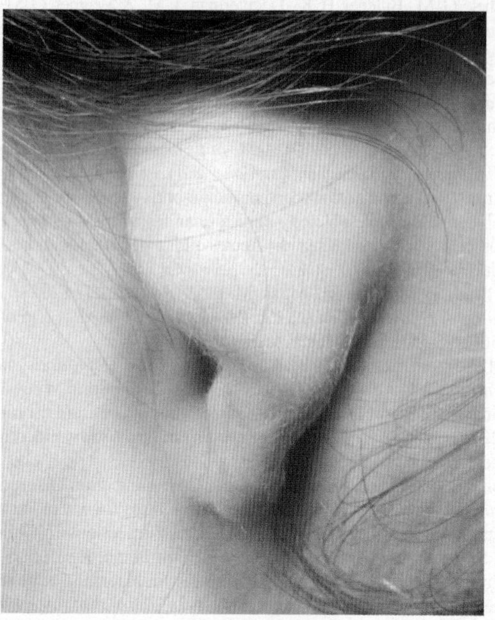

Small or deformed auricle that may be associated with a blind or absent auditory canal

Macrotia

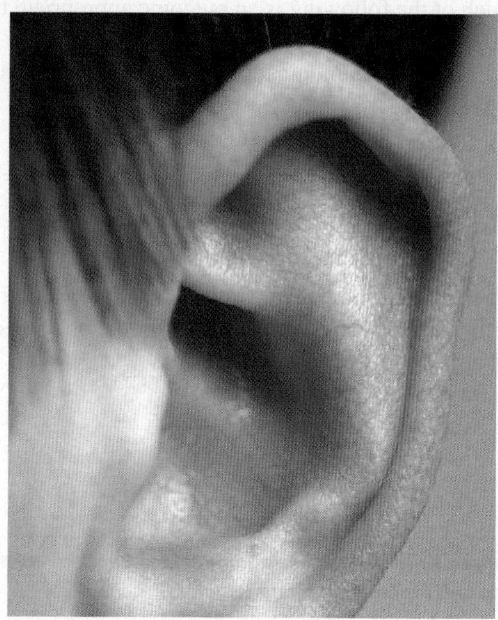

Excessive enlargement of the auricle; usually congenital

Edematous Ears

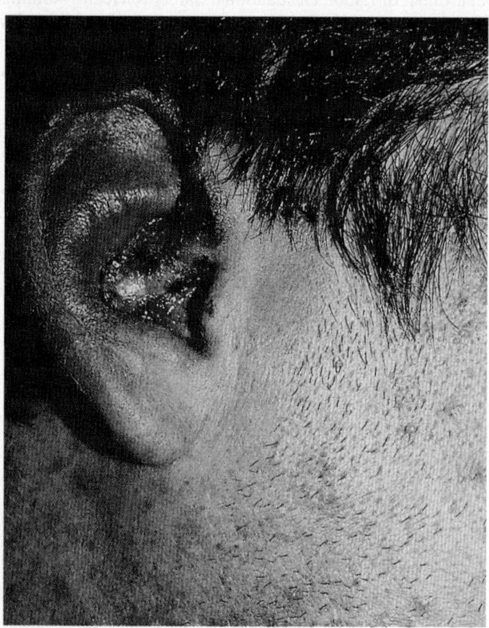

An external ear canal that is swollen with inflammation or infection

Cartilaginous *Staphylococcus* or *Pseudomonas* Infection

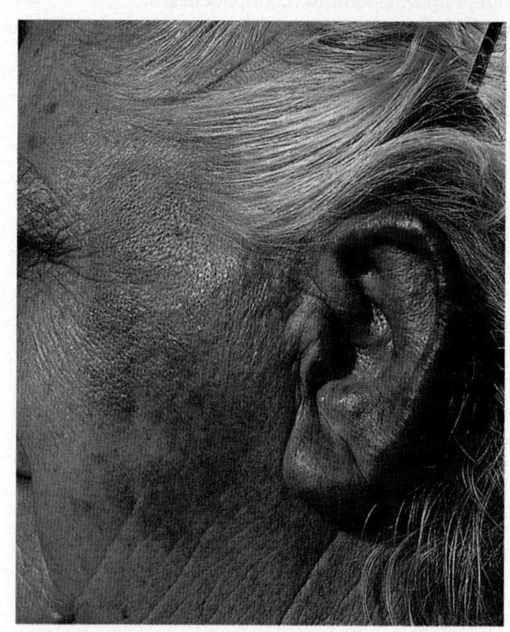

Painful, reddened ear usually surrounding incisions, ear piercing, or an area of traumatic injury

(table continues on page 369)

TABLE 14.2 Abnormal Findings in the External Ear *(continued)*

Carcinoma on Auricle

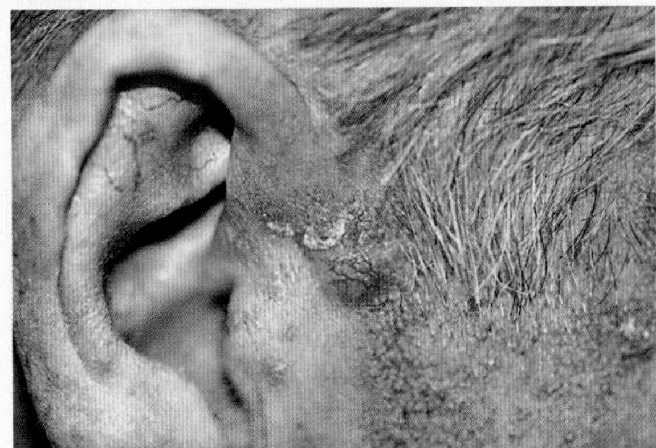

Common site of carcinoma related to sun exposure; either basal cell or squamous cell tumors may be present

Cyst

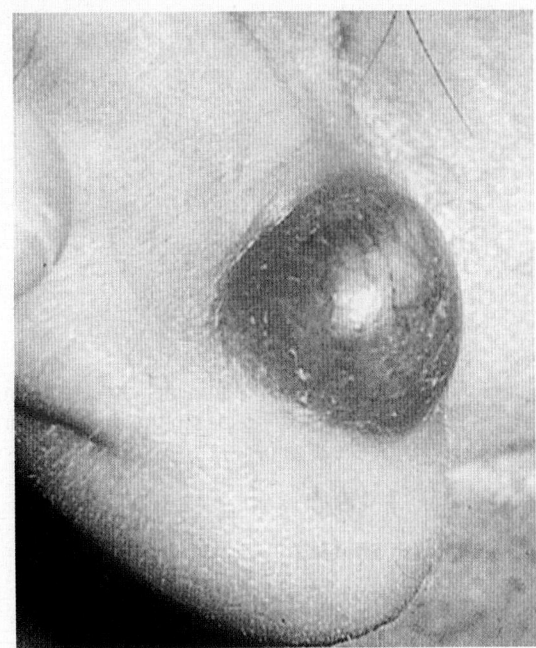

A sac or pouch with a membranous lining filled with fluid or solid material

Tophus (plural, tophi)

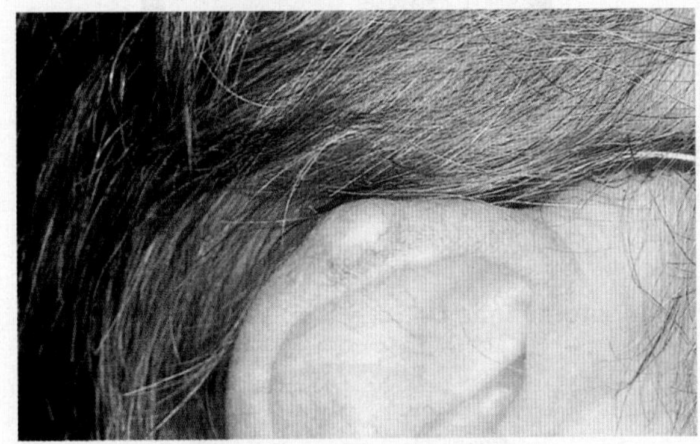

Uric acid crystals associated with gout; may appear as hard nodules on the ear surface

External Otitis Media

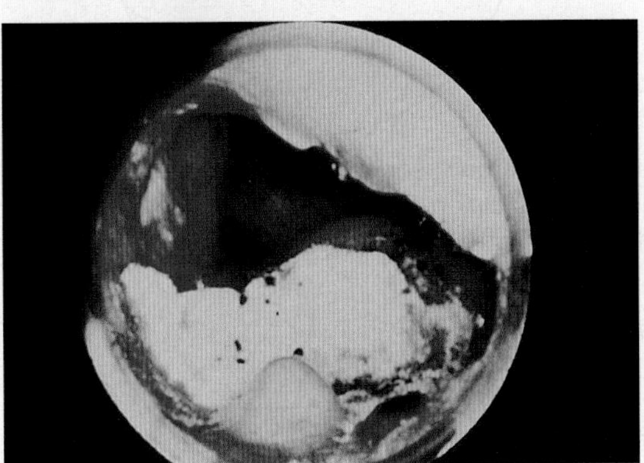

Inflammatory and infectious discharge in the external canal; associated with pain, itching, fullness, and reduced hearing

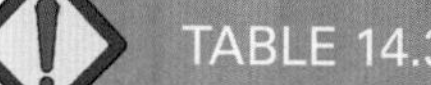

TABLE 14.3 Abnormal Findings in the Internal Ear

Tympanic Membrane Rupture

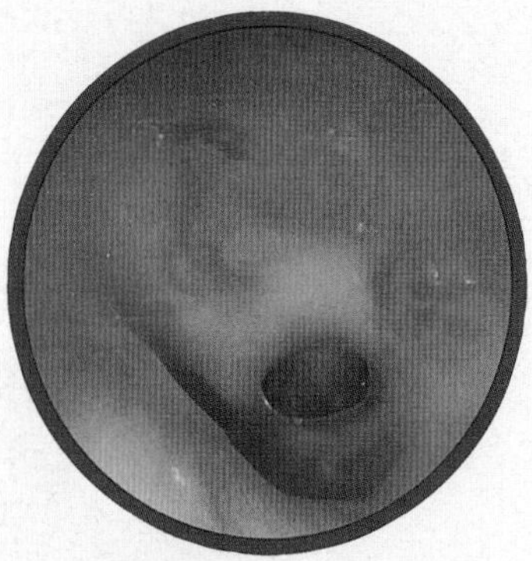

A nonintact TM; associated symptoms include clear, purulent, or bloody discharge; hearing loss in the affected ear; buzzing in the ear; and ear pain

Acute Otitis Media

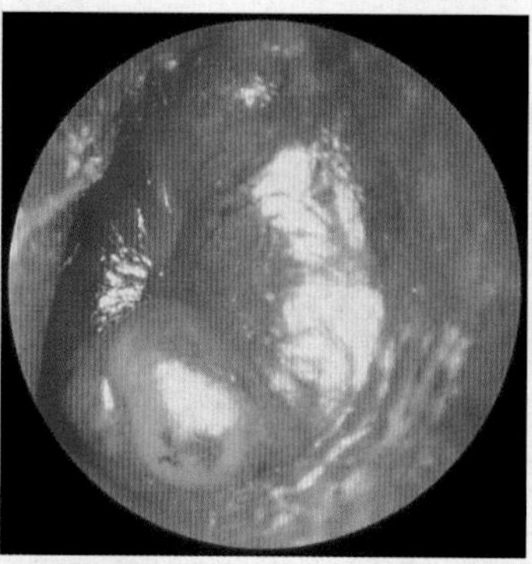

Acute infection in the middle ear. Onset is usually sudden and sometimes accompanied by fever and pain. Fluid may be in the middle ear, with signs or symptoms of middle ear inflammation. Pathogens may be viral or bacterial.

Otitis Media With Effusion

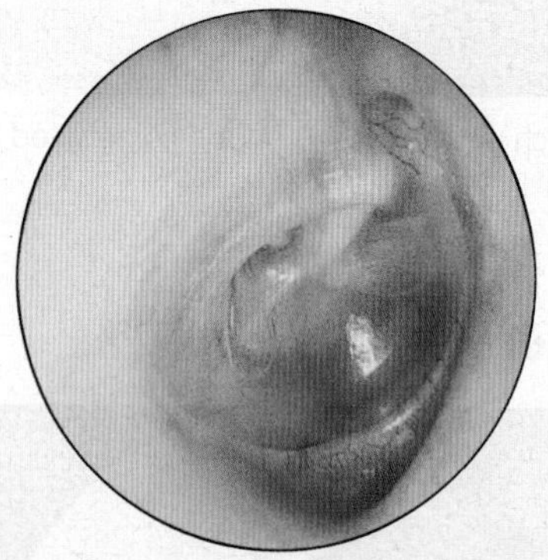

Purulent discharge associated with a bacterial infection. Redness and bulging on the TM. Onset can be sudden or gradual with increasing pain, fever, and hearing loss.

Scarred Tympanic Membrane

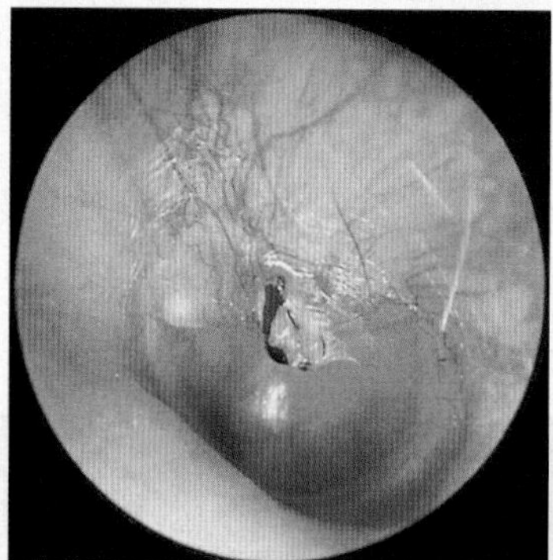

Caused by frequent ear infections with perforation of the TM. Scars are seen as dense white patches on the TM.

Foreign Body

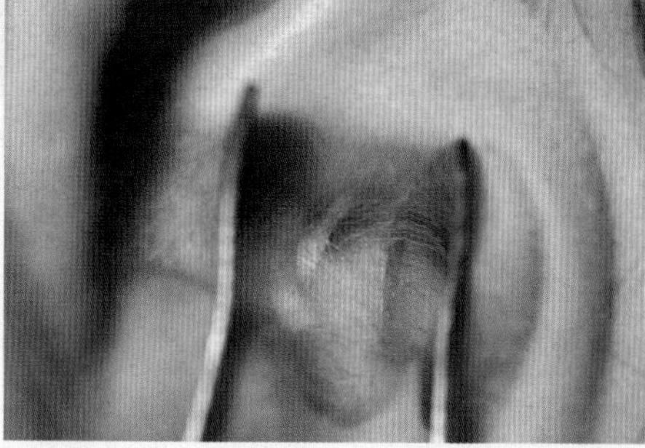

Most commonly, these are found in the canal of a child who puts a bean or bead in the ear. If the object has been in the ear for several days, the patient may present with purulent discharge, pain, or hearing loss. If an insect is in the ear, the patient may hear a bug flying around within the ear. A bean is shown here.

Tympanostomy Tube

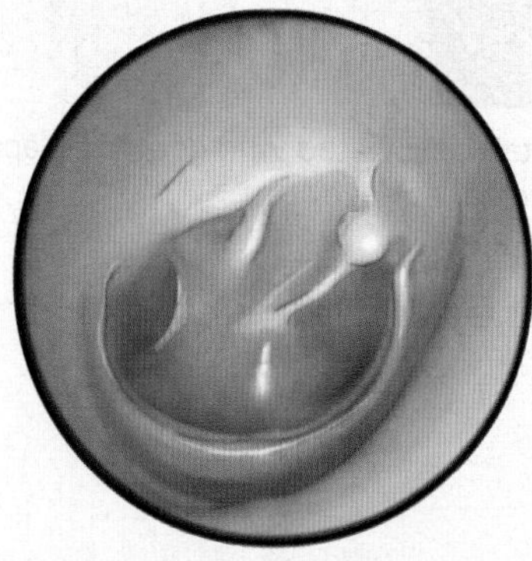

Tympanostomy tubes are indicated for chronic otitis media and its complications, recurrent acute otitis media, and antibiotic failure in children. The tubes are usually made of plastics such as silicone or Teflon. After 2–5 years, the tubes spontaneously fall out and the membrane most often closes.

15

Nose, Sinuses, Mouth, and Throat

Learning Objectives

1. Demonstrate knowledge of anatomy and physiology of the nose, sinuses, mouth, and throat.
2. Identify important topics for health promotion and risk reduction related to the nose, sinuses, mouth, and throat.
3. Collect subjective and objective data in the upper respiratory area and mouth.
4. Differentiate expected from unexpected findings in the physical assessment of the upper respiratory system and mouth.
5. Analyze subjective and objective data for assessment of the nose, sinuses, mouth, and throat and consider initial interventions.
6. Document and communicate data for the nose, sinuses, mouth, and throat assessment using appropriate terminology and principles of recording.
7. Consider age, condition, gender, and culture of the patient to individualize the nose, sinuses, mouth, and throat assessment.
8. Use assessment findings of the nose, sinuses, mouth, and throat to identify pertinent nursing diagnoses and initiate a patient care plan.

Mrs. Davis, an 89-year-old Caucasian woman, was admitted to the hospital 13 days ago with pneumonia. She had complications during her stay, was transferred to intensive care unit, and is now on the rehabilitation unit in preparation for her return home. Her temperature is 37°C (98.6°F) orally, pulse 88 beats/min, respirations 20 breaths/min, and blood pressure 138/72 mmHg. Current medications include a mild diuretic and beta-blocker for blood pressure, an inhaler to open her airways, and an antibiotic for pneumonia. Her assessment was documented on the previous shift.

You will gain more information about Mrs. Davis as you progress through this chapter. As you study the content and features, consider Mrs. Davis's case and its relationship to what you are learning. Begin thinking about the following points:

- What are some possible causes of Mrs. Davis's altered oral mucosa?
- Why is it especially important for nurses to inspect the mouth of hospitalized patients?
- The mucous membranes reflect the health of other body systems. What body systems are affecting the health of Mrs. Davis's oral mucous membranes?
- How might improvement in the patient's mouth affect her rehabilitation and functional abilities?
- What recommendations for follow-up would you make to Mrs. Davis?
- After a diagnosis has been established for Mrs. Davis, how would you evaluate her understanding of it and determine any teaching for discharge home?

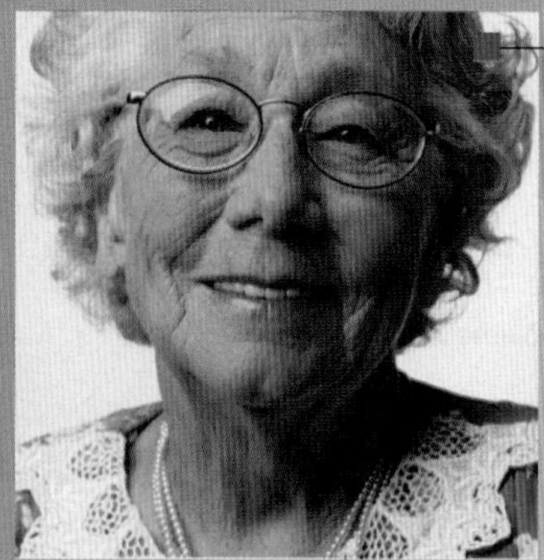

This chapter focuses on assessment of the nose, sinuses, mouth, and throat. It reviews anatomy and physiology and common variations from normal findings and discusses relevant lifespan, cultural, and environmental considerations. The chapter serves as a guide to the collection of subjective data related to upper respiratory and mouth problems, which can result from occupational exposures, recreational activities (e.g., smoking), family history of allergic rhinitis, systemic disorders, and head and neck cancer. It reviews common signs and symptoms such as nasal discharge, congestion, and obstruction; snoring; sore throat; and facial pain and pressure. Presentation of objective data collection includes examination techniques and correct documentation of expected and unexpected findings. The emphasis is a systematic, uncomplicated approach to this complex anatomical area.

Structure and Function

The upper respiratory tract (nasal cavity, pharynx, and larynx) and the mouth function as the entry point for air and food into the body. The nose, mouth, and throat serve as a common channel for air to reach the lungs and food to reach the esophagus and stomach. The upper respiratory tract warms, filters, humidifies, and transports air to the lower respiratory tract (see Chapter 16). The nose is the sensory organ for smell, whereas the mouth is the sensory organ for taste. Appreciation of the anatomy of organs along this transport passageway will help you understand why structural deviations may interfere with function.

Nose

The external nose allows air to enter the respiratory tract (Fig. 15.1). The anterior slope of the nose is the dorsum, which ends inferiorly at the tip and laterally at the ala. Bone in the upper third and cartilage in the lower two thirds of the nose support its triangular shape. The nasal bone attaches superiorly at the bridge to the frontal bone and laterally to the lacrimal and maxillary bones. The floor of the nose rests on the superior portion of the hard palate, separating it from the mouth (Fig. 15.2). The ethmoid bone (cribriform plate of ethmoid) forms and separates the roof of the nose from the brain (see Fig. 15.2). The anterior midline **columella** divides the oval nares (nostrils), which are openings that lead into the internal nose; these openings are lined with skin and ciliated mucosa. This area of the nose is known as the vestibule.

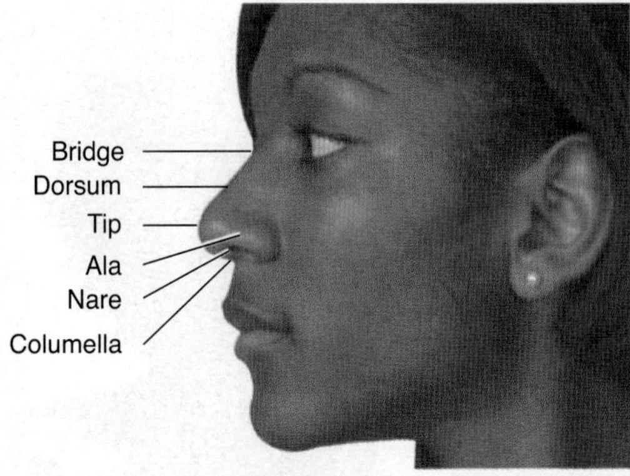

Figure 15.1 The external nose.

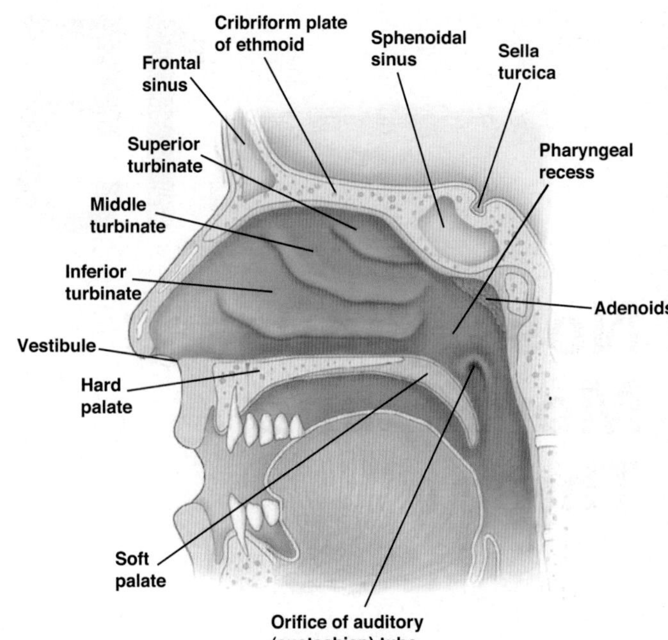

Figure 15.2 The nasal septum, left lateral wall.

> **Clinical Significance**
>
> The ciliated mucosa inside the nose warm, filter, and humidify inspired air at nearly 100% humidity and expend more than 1 L of water daily (Baroody, 2011).

The nasal septum is the central wall of bone and cartilage covered with mucosal membrane that divides the right and left nasal cavities (see Fig. 15.4). Projecting from the lateral walls of the nose are three scroll-like bones covered with erectile mucous membranes: the inferior, middle, and superior turbinates (see Fig. 15.2). The inferior turbinates, which are most anterior, are usually the first internal structures visible on nasal examination. Lateral to each turbinate is an air space: the inferior meatus, middle meatus, and superior meatus. Cilia are small hairlike structures that trap particulates and sweep them posterior to the nasopharynx, promoting mucus drainage. The nasolacrimal duct drains into the inferior meatus. The middle turbinate and middle meatus receive drainage from the frontal sinus, anterior ethmoid sinus, and maxillary sinuses. The site where the frontal, ethmoid, and maxillary sinuses empty into the nasal cavity is known as the **ostiomeatal complex**.

> **Clinical Significance**
>
> The ostiomeatal complex is the most anatomically significant area involved in chronic sinusitis.

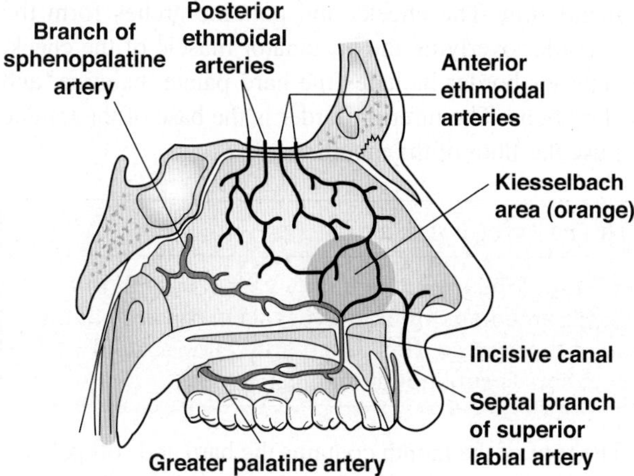

Figure 15.3 The Kiesselbach plexus.

The nose is the primary organ for smell. Air within the nasal roof stimulates the olfactory receptors of cranial nerve I (CN I). Mucosal swelling from upper respiratory inflammation such as occurs in colds, viral infections, or allergic conditions may obstruct olfactory sensory receptors, compromising the sense of smell.

> **SAFETY ALERT**
> *Patients with diminished sense of smell are at risk for decreased detection of spoiled food, smoke, and gas fumes.*

Nerve and Blood Supply

The maxillary and ophthalmic divisions of the trigeminal nerve (CN V) produce pain sensations. The facial nerve (CN VII) innervates external movement of the nose and face. The rhino-sino-brachial (sneeze) reflex results from the complex relationship of the medulla of the brain with CNs V (trigeminal nerve), VII (facial nerve), IX (glossopharyngeal nerve), and X (vagal nerve).

Branches of the internal and external carotid arteries supply blood to the nose. The anterior portion of the nasal septum has a rich vascular supply known as the Kiesselbach plexus (or area) (Fig. 15.3).

> **Clinical Significance**
> The Kiesselbach plexus is the most common site of anterior nosebleeds (Franz & Polsdorfer, 2006).

Lymph Drainage

Lymphatic drainage from the anterior nose leads to the preauricular and submandibular nodes. The deep cervical and retropharyngeal nodes drain the posterior nasal cavity.

Sinuses

The sinuses are hollow, bony, air-filled cavities within the forehead and facial cavities (Fig. 15.4). They lighten the weight of the cranium and provide timbre and resonance to the voice.

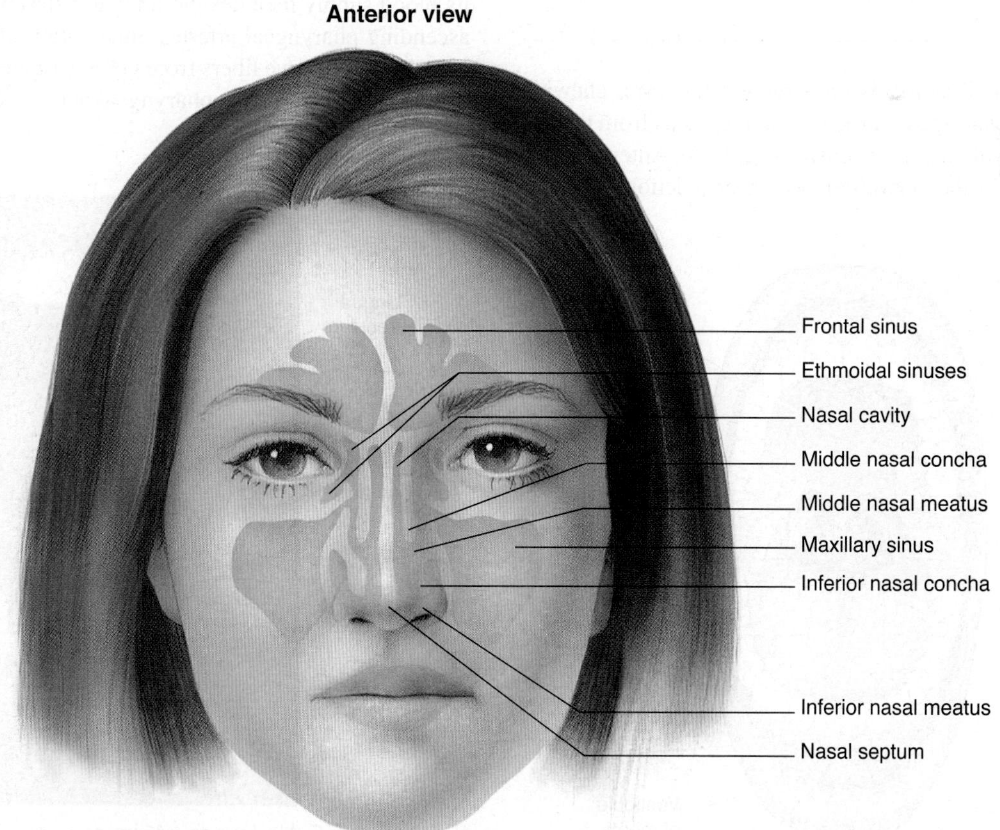

Figure 15.4 The paranasal sinuses.

The sinuses also produce mucus that empties into the nasal cavity. Three major factors are related to normal function of the nose and sinuses: patency of the sinus ostia, normal ciliary function, and normal quality and quantity of mucus.

The frontal sinus is above the eyebrows, the ethmoid sinuses are between the eyes, and the maxillary sinuses are below the eyes and above the teeth in each cheek. Sensory innervation of the sinuses is from CN V (trigeminal nerve). Lymphatic drainage from the sinuses goes to the lateral and retropharyngeal nodes.

The nasopharynx contributes to nasal resonance and assists with equilibration of middle ear pressure. Air and nasal–sinus mucus passes through the **choana** (opening) of the nose into the nasopharynx. The nasal end of the eustachian tube communicates with the middle ear by opening and closing throughout the day. This opening and closing may be noticeable during swallowing and yawning. Just posterior to the eustachian tube opening is a mound of tissue known as the torus tubarius.

> **Clinical Significance**
>
> Posterior to the torus region is the pharyngeal recess or Rosenmüller fossa, which is a common site of occult nasopharyngeal malignancies (Andresen, Hickey, Higgins, et al., 2008).

The adenoids are composed of lymphoid tissue located in the roof of the nasopharynx and laterally in the eustachian tube orifice. They have a rich blood supply from branches of the facial and internal maxillary arteries.

Mouth

The mouth (oral cavity) is the structure for taste, chewing (mastication), and speech articulation. It extends from the lips to the anterior pillars of the tonsils (Fig. 15.5). Anteriorly, the cavity begins at the **vermilion** border, or junction of the lip and facial skin. The cheeks and palatine arches form the lateral border overlying the buccinator muscle of the cheek. The superior border includes the hard palate, palatine, and maxillary bone. The inferior border is the base of the tongue and muscular floor of the mouth.

> **Clinical Significance**
>
> The floor of the mouth is highly vascular, with the largest percentage of blood vessels in the area at the base of the tongue. This vascularity allows rapid absorption of sublingual medication.

The roof of the mouth contains the hard and soft palates. The anterior hard palate comprises two thirds of the total palate. The adjacent posterior soft palate forms the uvula and separates the mouth from the pharynx. The uvula is midline at the inferior border of the soft palate.

Tongue

The tongue is muscular tissue that covers the floor of the mouth, with posterior–inferior extension into the pharynx. The median fold, also known as the **lingual frenulum**, connects the base of the tongue to the floor of the mouth (Fig. 15.6). The tongue manipulates solids and liquids in mastication and deglutition. It is also involved in speech production and taste. The anterior two thirds of the tongue surface contain taste buds known as vallate papillae, which identify sweet, sour, salty, and bitter tastes (Fig. 15.7).

The tongue is one of the body's most vascular muscles; its blood supply includes the lingual, exterior maxillary, and ascending pharyngeal arteries. Innervation of the tongue includes lingual nerve fibers from CN V (trigeminal nerve), VII (facial nerve), IX (glossopharyngeal nerve), X (vagus nerve), and XII (hypoglossal nerve).

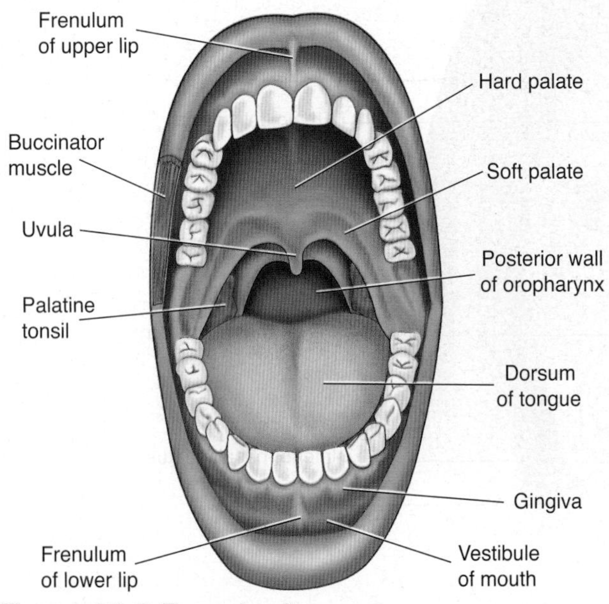

Figure 15.5 The oral cavity.

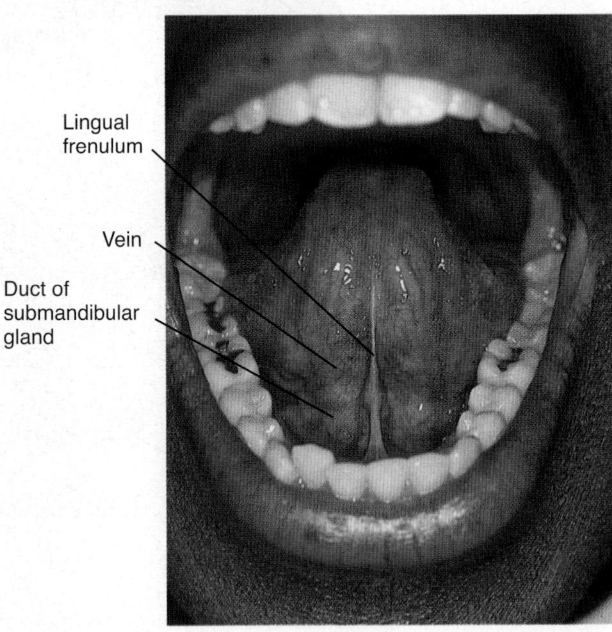

Figure 15.6 Underside of the tongue. Note the lingual frenulum.

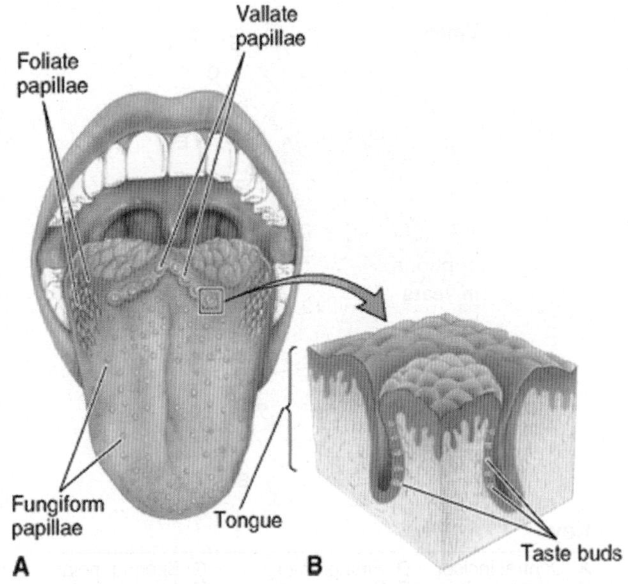

Figure 15.7 Vallate papillae.

Salivary Glands

The mouth also contains drainage ducts from three major salivary glands (Fig. 15.8). The largest, the parotid gland, is within the cheek anterior to the ear and extends from the zygomatic arch inferior to the angle of the jaw. The parotid (Stensen) duct opens into the mouth in the buccal mucosa just opposite the upper second molar. The submandibular gland is beneath the body of the mandible. Its submandibular ducts run deep to the floor of the mouth and open on both sides of the frenulum. These ducts on each side of the frenulum are known as Wharton (submandibular) ducts. The small sublingual salivary gland lies within the floor of the mouth under the tongue with many openings along the submandibular duct. In addition to these three major salivary glands, many microscopic minor salivary glands are scattered throughout the oral mucosa.

> **Clinical Significance**
>
> The major salivary glands produce 1,500 to 4,000 ml/day of saliva (Andresen et al., 2008).

Saliva begins the digestive process by releasing enzymes upon contact with food. Saliva protects the oral mucosa from heat, chemicals, and irritants. Saliva also transmits taste information, rinses the oral cavity to maintain pH, and provides lubrication for the movement of food. Salivary production increases when smelling and seeing food, tasting, chewing, swallowing, and cigarette smoking. Decreased salivary flow, called **xerostomia**, is related to emotional response, aging, disorders such as Sjögren syndrome, and damage to the glands (e.g., due to radiation therapy, obstruction, infection).

> **Clinical Significance**
>
> Blockage of the parotid duct increases the potential for periodontal disease as a result of pH imbalance, dryness, and precipitation of calcium (Andresen et al., 2008).

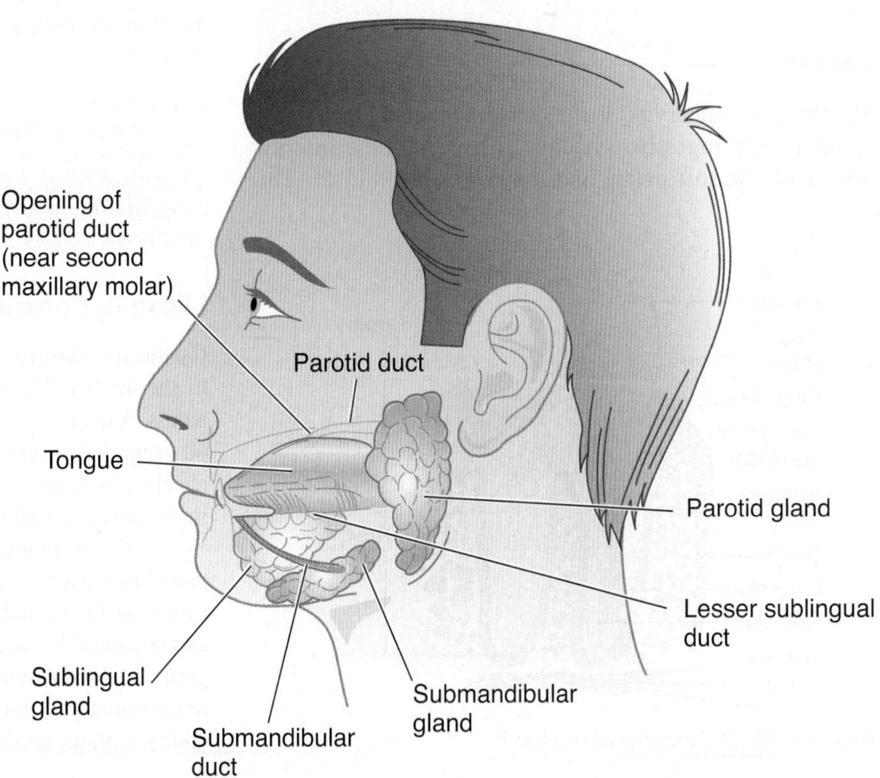

Figure 15.8 The salivary glands.

The autonomic nervous system and CN VII (facial nerve) and IX (glossopharyngeal nerve) innervate secretions of the major and minor salivary ducts. CN XII (hypoglossal nerve) innervates the submandibular glands.

Teeth and Gums

The teeth contribute to the grinding and mastication of food to prepare for swallowing. They are composed of three layers: crown, neck, and root (Fig. 15.9).

The crown is the superior surface of the tooth that is visible within the oral cavity. It consists of three layers: enamel, dentin, and pulp. The outer enamel is an avascular surface with no pain receptors; it needs saliva to maintain its hard surface. Erosion of enamel may occur without pain. Regular dental follow-up is important in detecting early dental caries. The second layer, dentin, has tubules that connect to nerve fibers. Pain is experienced if damage to the dentin occurs by trauma or erosion. The innermost layer is the pulp, which has blood vessels and lymphatics, nerve tissue, and odontoblasts (dentin-forming cells). Increased pressure secondary to inflammation within the pulp may cause necrosis of the tooth. The root is the part implanted through the gum and into the bone that holds the tooth in place. The neck is the slight indentation where the crown joins the root.

There are 32 permanent teeth (Fig. 15.10) (Andresen et al., 2008). The 8 anterior incisors have flat surfaces for biting food. The posterior teeth, the 12 molars, perform the grinding and final chewing process before swallowing. The maxillary bone supports the tissues of the upper jaw, whereas the mandibular bones support the tissues of the lower jaw. The periodontium is the gingival or gum tissue that supports the teeth.

Throat

The throat (oropharynx) is the common channel for the respiratory and digestive systems. It begins at the inferior border of the soft palate and uvula (see Fig. 15.5). The throat includes the base of the tongue, pharyngoepiglottic and glossoepiglottic folds, anterior and posterior pillars, and palatine tonsils. The tonsils are at the back of the throat between the anterior and posterior pillars. The tonsil tissue appears more granular and less smooth than the surrounding mucous membranes. Lymphatic tissue of the tonsils and adenoids contribute to immunological defense. With chronic infections, they may hypertrophy and produce chronic airway obstruction. Tonsillitis is inflammation of the tonsils. Hypertrophy of the tonsils and adenoids may develop secondary to sinusitis or otitis media (middle ear infection).

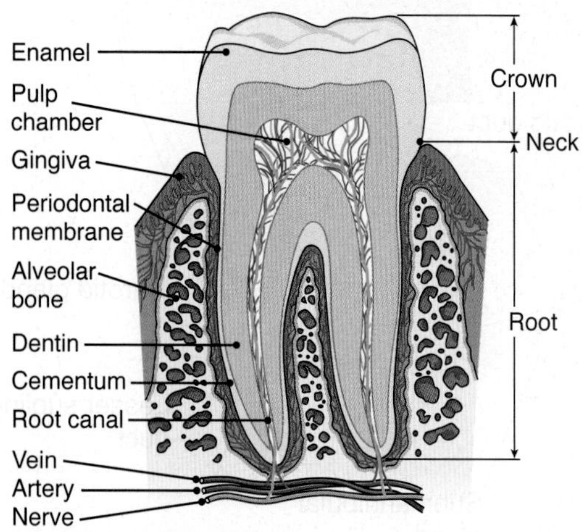

Figure 15.9 Anatomy of the tooth.

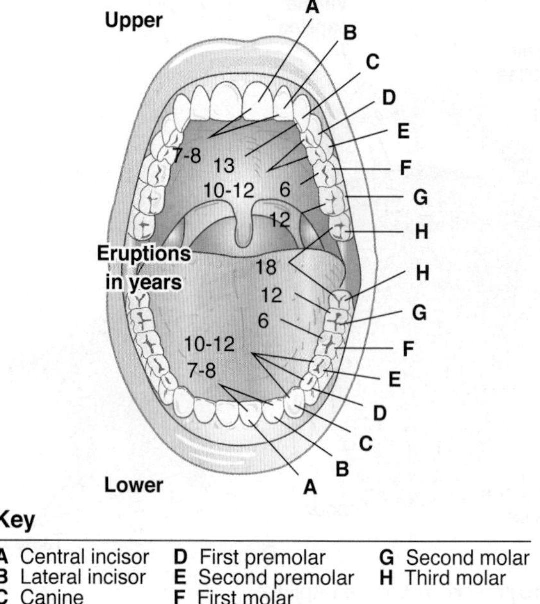

Figure 15.10 Numbers and position of the adult teeth.

> **Clinical Significance**
>
> Removal of tonsils and adenoids does not increase risk of infection (Andresen et al., 2008).

Lifespan Considerations: Older Adults

Gustatory rhinitis, which is the clear rhinorrhea stimulated by the smell and taste of food, occurs most frequently in older adults. A decrease in olfactory sensory fibers occurs after age 60 years. In the oral cavity, a thinning of the soft tissue of the cheeks and tongue results in an increased risk of ulcerations, infections, and oral cancers.

With advancing age, production of saliva and number of taste buds decrease. Resorption occurs in gum tissue, surrounding teeth, and the mandible bone. Natural tooth loss accompanies the breakdown of the tooth surface and receding gums. Malocclusion may occur with tooth loss and aggravate temporomandibular joint function. The number of older adults without teeth is declining because of an increase in reconstructive dental practices. Conversely, incidence of dental caries is rising in older adults related to retention of the teeth.

Cultural Considerations

Oral Health

Oral health of U.S. residents over the past 50 years has improved significantly. A major factor in this public health success story is community water fluoridation, benefitting about 7 out of 10 U.S. residents who get water through public systems (U.S. Department of Health & Human Services [USDHHS], 2013).

Not all U.S. residents have access to oral health care. Ability to get dental care is associated with educational level, income, and race. Incidence of dental caries varies with sociodemographic groups. Although spending for dental care has increased, the number of people who have dental insurance has not increased. The percentage of untreated dental carries is 36% in African American children, 43% in Hispanic children, and 26% in Caucasian children (USDHHS, 2013). The American Dental Association has issued evidence-based recommendation for the application of dental sealants. The U.S. Centers for Disease Control and Prevention (CDC) implemented a school-based program for the application of dental sealants, which has been shown to decrease the risk for dental decay by 60% (Bailey, 2012).

Gingivitis, or inflammation with bleeding of the gums, is prevalent among Hispanics, Native Americans, Alaskan Natives, and adults of low socioeconomic classes. It may progress to periodontal disease with a loss of connective tissue and bone (USDHHS, 2013).

Congenital Defects

Cleft lip and cleft palate occur in 1 in 1,000 births, with an increased incidence in Native Americans and Asian Americans (Dixon, Marazita, Beaty, & Murray, 2011). **Bifid uvula** is a minor cleft of the posterior soft palate and occurs in about 1 in 250 people (Langlais & Miller, 2009). **Torus palatinus**, a bony ridge running in the middle of the hard palate, is more common in Native Americans, Alaskan Natives, and Asians (Bennett, 2013).

Cancer

Oral, head, and neck cancer is the 4th most common malignancy and the 10th most common diagnosis in males worldwide (Callaway, 2011). Annually, 650,000 new cases of squamous cell carcinomas of the head and neck are diagnosed worldwide (American Cancer Society, 2012). Historically, head and neck cancer has been associated with the use of alcohol and tobacco in an estimated 85% of cases. A more recently identified cause of head and neck cancer is exposure to human papillomavirus (HPV). Prevalence in most recent studies of HPV relationship to oral, head, and neck cancers is as high as 60% (Benson, Li, Eisele, & Fakhry, 2014). People with multiple sexual partners and those who engage in oral sex are at increased risk of developing oral HPV–related cancer.

Oral head and neck cancer statistics for the United States show that men are affected twice as frequently as women. HPV-infected patients are young, Caucasian, nonsmoking, and predominantly male. Caucasians have a higher incidence, yet African Americans have a higher mortality (Farris & Petitte, 2013). Although the incidence of oral, head, and neck cancers declined worldwide consistent with the declines of the use of tobacco products, an increase in oral, head, and neck cancers has occurred in younger people in the United States, Australia, Canada, Slovakia, Denmark, and the United Kingdom (Chaturvedi et al., 2013).

Sleep-Disordered Breathing

Sleep-disordered breathing—pauses or obstructions in breathing during sleep—is another serious threat to health. Those with sleep-disordered breathing have two to four times the risk of heart attack or stroke. Obesity is a significant factor for sleep-related breathing disorders. African American children are twice as likely to develop sleep-disordered breathing as children of European descent (USDHHS, 2013).

Urgent Assessment

Severe nosebleeds need to be treated immediately. Infection in the floor of mouth may produce **Ludwig angina**, which is swelling that pushes the tongue up and back and results in eventual airway obstruction. Assessing risk for aspiration begins in the upper respiratory tract, focusing on laryngeal airway competency as well as the presence of dental prostheses or loose teeth, which may be accidentally swallowed and aspirated.

> ⚠ *SAFETY ALERT*
> *Acute airway obstruction such as in anaphylaxis, Ludwig angina, and epiglottitis may limit the opportunity for data collection other than specifics related to presentation of the patient.*

Abrupt loss of the sense of smell may indicate a brain tumor and warrants further evaluation with a magnetic resonance imaging (MRI) scan of the brain. Hard, fixed lymph nodes should be further evaluated by biopsy as well as radiological studies.

Subjective Data

Subjective data collection for this body region involves taking a detailed health history. Open-ended questions during this process help with a meaningful exchange of information. Inquire about family history that may be relevant to hereditary upper respiratory conditions. Obtain a thorough social history, including drug and alcohol exposure and consumption.

Often, opportunities arise during history taking to provide patient teaching. Such health education may help the patient avoid upper respiratory disease and exacerbation of current illnesses. One patient's history, for example, may prompt you to discuss allergen and irritant exposure and smoking, which cause upper respiratory inflammation. You can suggest strategies to manage symptoms and avoid exposures that may exacerbate symptoms as well as suggest health promotion measures such as controlling allergens at home (Table 15.1) Another patient's history may prompt dental health questions and related education. Other situations may prompt you to advise patients to avoid environmental exposures to irritants and chemicals and suggest the use of personal protective equipment when exposures may be toxic.

Assessment of Risk Factors

When exploring risk factors, the intention is to determine how likely it is that a person will develop upper respiratory disease. Questions can lead to educational opportunities and help identify areas that may require emphasis and follow-up. Teaching and interviewing can be blended.

TABLE 15.1 Controlling Allergens in the Home Setting

Allergens	Precautions in the Home
House dust mites. Mites (microscopic bugs) live and feed in carpets, upholstery, and bedding. They produce droppings, which in humans cause allergic symptoms. Concentrate cleaning efforts in the bedroom to control dust mite allergies.	• Damp-dust and vacuum weekly. • Change or clean furnace filter monthly. • Avoid feather pillows and down comforters. • Wash sheets and blankets weekly in hot water. • Avoid "dust catchers" (e.g., stuffed animals). • Consider using high-efficiency particulate air filters in the bedroom and the vacuum cleaner. • Use a smooth floor surface in the bedroom. Avoid carpeting and rugs.
Mold spores. Mold spores are found in damp, dark areas of the home.	Discourage and eliminate mold growth by • Repairing leaks • Using dehumidifiers in damp basements • Cleaning shower grouting weekly • Decreasing houseplants, removing them from bedrooms, placing fungicide in soil • Cleaning refrigerator drip pan • Meticulously cleaning or avoiding portable humidifiers • Adjusting whole house humidity to 40% or less • Avoiding wool fabrics • Avoiding foods that contain mold: fermented beverages, especially wine and beer; vinegar; cheese; foods with yeast; breads and bakery products; canned tomato products; pizza; canned, smoked, and pickled meats; mushrooms
Foods. Any food can trigger an allergic reaction.	Eliminate forever foods suspected of producing acute life-threatening symptoms; common causes are shellfish and peanuts. Eliminate for 6 months foods that cause or contribute to chronic allergies, despite cravings for them, then reintroduce the foods in a rotating manner. Common irritants include milk, egg, wheat, corn, soy, and yeast.
Pet dander. Cat dander is light and highly allergic; dog dander is heavier.	Decrease pet dander by • Having only outdoor pets • Removing pets from the bedroom • Grooming or bathing pets regularly (not by the allergic person) • Washing hands after touching pets
Pollens. Airborne pollens, present during blooming seasons, trigger allergic symptoms.	Decrease exposure to pollens by • Keeping windows closed • Grooming pets, which can carry pollens into the home • Avoiding attic fans

Adapted from Kramper, M. A. (2005). Patient education. Allergy precautions in the home. *ORL-Head and Neck Nursing, 23*, 27–28.

History and Risk Factors	Rationale
Personal History	
Describe your upper respiratory (nasal) breathing.	This question is an initial opportunity for the patient to offer an unbiased description of how his or her upper airway performs.
Have you ever been diagnosed with a mouth or upper respiratory condition? • What was the specific condition? • When did it occur? • How was the condition treated? • What were the outcomes?	Frequent upper respiratory infections suggest underlying allergy, chronic hypertrophy of the adenoids and tonsils, or chronic sinusitis. Questions about symmetry of symptoms are helpful in determining whether there is unilateral disease.
Did you have a history of chronic upper respiratory infections as a child?	Frequent upper respiratory infections in childhood raise suspicion of allergy or hypertrophy of the adenoids and tonsils. Chronic inflammation of the respiratory tract may lead to mucosal damage with resultant chronic infections (e.g., sinusitis).
Do you have a history of systemic illness or autoimmune conditions?	Conditions such as Wegener granulomatosis, sarcoidosis, or Churg-Strauss syndrome may lead to chronic inflammation and crusting of the respiratory tract. Hereditary hemorrhagic telangiectasia (HHT), also known as Rendu-Osler-Weber syndrome, is an autosomal dominant disorder that leads to the development of abnormal blood vessels. The most common clinical feature is frequent nosebleeds (Silva, Hosman, Devlin, & Shovlin, 2013).
Medications and Supplements	
What medications are you currently taking? • What are the names of all your current medications? • What dosage and how frequently are they taken?	It is helpful to know the patient's complete medication list because all medications have potential adverse effects, which may affect the mouth, nose, and sinuses. Blood pressure drugs (e.g., angiotensin-converting enzyme [ACE] inhibitors) may produce cough (Table 15.2). Anticoagulants may predispose patients to nosebleeds or exacerbate bleeding. Medication that dries the mouth may affect tooth and gum health.

(table continues on page 380)

TABLE 15.2 Medications That May Produce Symptoms in the Nose, Sinus, Mouth, and Throat

Drug Class	Possible Adverse Reaction
Antihypertensives	Cough, nasal congestion
Hormones	Nasal congestion
Anticoagulants	Epistaxis
Antihistamines	Dry mucous membranes, epistaxis
Herbal supplements	Epistaxis
Analgesics	Nasal congestion
CNS agents	Nasal congestion
Topical decongestants	Rebound nasal congestion
Antidepressants	Dry mucous membranes

Source: Lloyd, K. B., and Naclerio, R. M. (2008). Strategies for managing nasal congestion. *Post graduate healthcare education,* LLC. Philadelphia: Glaxo Smith Kline.

History and Risk Factors	Rationale
Are you taking any over-the-counter (OTC), natural, or herbal supplements? • What specific products? • How frequently are you taking them? • Do you have any allergic reactions to medications?	Patients sometimes have a false sense of safety with OTC medications. Potentially unsafe OTC medications include topical decongestant sprays. Used appropriately for a short time, they provide effective nasal decongestion. These sprays also facilitate quick vasoconstriction and are beneficial in treating acute nosebleeds. With persistent use, however, they produce rebound congestion and are addictive. Natural herbal agents (e.g., gingko biloba, garlic) may have an undesirable adverse effect of increased clotting times with resultant nosebleeds. Thus, the use of topical decongestant sprays is contraindicated in patients with frequent or chronic nosebleeds (Bent, 2008). Herbs or natural supplements may cross-react with pollen and stimulate allergic rhinitis. For example, echinacea taken to strengthen the immune system can cross-react with ragweed, increasing symptoms in sensitive patients (National Center for Complementary and Alternative Medicine [NCCAM], 2013).
Family History Do you have a family history of mouth or upper respiratory illness? • Which family member had the illness? • What was the specific illness? • What management was implemented? • What was the outcome?	Atopy (allergic disease) occurs in 25% of the U.S. population, or an estimated 18 million residents of the United States (Lloyd & Naclerio, 2008). Hereditary prevalence is strong: if one parent has allergies, a child has a 50% chance of developing them. Family history of cancer increases the patient's risk. Positive family history of genetic disorders, such as cystic fibrosis, Wegener granulomatosis, Churg-Strauss disease, sarcoidosis, and Sjögren syndrome, may put the patient at increased risk. HHT affects approximately 1 in 5,000 individuals (Silva et al., 2013).
Risk Factors Do you have any known sensitivities to inhalant allergens such as dust mites, mold, pollens, or animal dander? Have you had specific allergy testing? • What were the test results? • What were your symptoms? • When did you experience symptoms? • What treatment measures were taken?	Allergy can affect any target organ in the body. The nose and respiratory mucosa are the entry port for inhalant allergens. Thus, the nose and respiratory tract are common targets for inflammatory responses from allergen exposure.
How frequently do you experience signs of a sinus infection, including fever, facial pressure, and thick discolored nasal drainage?	Patients who have persistent symptoms of infection should be considered for immunoglobulin deficiency. With the emergence of pathogens that are resistant to antibiotic therapy, the current practice is to exhaust symptomatic management of sinus inflammatory symptoms for 1 week to 10 days before implementing antibiotic therapy for sinusitis symptoms (Temesgen, 2011).
If you have frequent complaints of tonsillitis, have you had positive cultures for strep infections?	
Dental Health • How regularly do you brush and floss? • When were your teeth last cleaned? • Have you had dental sealants applied? • Do you have any difficulties with your teeth or gums? • Do you have community-treated or well water in your home environment? Does your water supply contain fluoride?	Regular dental cleanings are important to keeping teeth and gums healthy and identifying problems early. Evidence has documented that topical fluorides and application of dental sealants can significantly reduce dental caries (Bailey, 2012).

(table continues on page 381)

History and Risk Factors	Rationale
Psychosocial History	
Do you currently smoke cigarettes, pipes, or cigars? • How many cigarettes per day do you smoke? • How many years have you smoked? • Have you ever tried to stop smoking? • Are you currently interested in stopping smoking? • Do you currently or have you ever chewed tobacco products? • Do you use smokeless tobacco, personal vaporizer, or electronic cigarette products?	Smoking increases respiratory inflammation, exacerbating allergic rhinitis and chronic sinusitis. It also increases risks for head and neck carcinoma (USDHHS, 2013). Chewing tobacco increases risk for oral cancer (Mayo Clinic Staff, 2011). See Chapter 16 for risks to the lower respiratory system related to smoking and tobacco use. Electronic cigarettes are becoming increasingly popular in the United States as an alternative "smoking" product with a positive effect on discontinuing smoking habits; however, limited safety and efficacy data for these devices are available (Zhu et al., 2013).
Are you frequently around others who smoke? What avoidance measures do you take to avoid exposure to secondhand smoke?	Secondhand smoke increases risks for head and neck cancer and exacerbates allergic rhinitis, pharyngitis, and sinusitis. Researchers have identified more than 4,000 chemicals in tobacco smoke; of these, at least 43 cause cancer in humans and animals (USDHHS, 2013).
Do you inhale, or have you ever inhaled, marijuana, cocaine, methamphetamine, heroin, glue, or spray paint? If yes, are you interested in information to reduce associated risks or to help you quit?	Inhaling these substances can irritate the lining of the upper airway. Regular marijuana use may damage the cilia, leading to airway injury and potential infection; it increases the risk of head and neck cancer. Use of cocaine may permanently damage the nasal mucosa, which can result in nasal septal perforations. Use of methamphetamines may severely damage the teeth (Padilla & Ritter, 2008).
Do you consume alcohol? How many drinks per day/week do you consume?	Head and neck cancer has been associated with the use of alcohol and tobacco in an estimated 85% of cases.
Are you sexually active? Do you have multiple sexual partners? Have you engaged in oral sex?	Exposure to HPV is common during sexual contact. Persistent infection with oncogenic HPV types has been linked to cancer of the oropharynx (Jemal et al., 2013).
Environmental Exposure	
Are you currently or have you ever been exposed to chemical substances or irritants at work? • Do you wear a mask or take other precautions to protect your respiratory tract? • Do you monitor your exposures to chemicals?	Irritating chemicals may cause inflammation of the upper airway, which predisposes patients to chronic infections. Chemical exposures may damage the cilia, affecting the natural self-cleaning ability of the mucosal lining. Repeat exposures may produce allergic reactions in atopic patients. Chemicals may also be toxic.
Do you have hobbies or employments that increase risk for upper respiratory problems, such as farming; care of or frequent exposure to animals; exposure to paint, chemical fumes, or wood dust; airplane flying; scuba diving; or swimming?	Farming may expose patients to excessive pollen, animal dander, mold, and grain smuts. Atopic patients may experience adverse reactions with persistent allergen exposure. Chemical fumes from paints and solvents may irritate or damage the respiratory mucosa. Scuba diving and flying may produce negative pressure in the ears or sinuses, leading to barotrauma. Swimming may produce or aggravate sinusitis resulting from chronic chlorine exposure. Chlorine may act as an allergen or irritant.
What type of heat do you use at home? Are you aware of any mold in your home?	Some homes may use wood or kerosene heat, which may exacerbate allergies or produce inflammation of the upper respiratory tract leading to secondary infections. Dry environments may also irritate the airway. Mold may exacerbate allergies or, in the case of toxic mold (greenish-black), act as an allergen.

Risk Reduction and Health Promotion

Major risk reduction and health promotion goals in assessment of the nose, sinuses, mouth, and throat are related to various issues, including tobacco use, obstructive sleep apnea, oral health, and cancer. In assessing for risk factors, you can identify areas to focus efforts for patient teaching and related behavior changes. The health goals include the following:

- Reduce the oropharyngeal cancer death rate.
- Reduce the proportion of children and adolescents who have dental caries in their primary or permanent teeth.
- Reduce periodontal disease.
- Increase the proportion of local health departments and community-based health centers, including community, migrant, and homeless health centers, that have an oral health component (USDHHS, 2013).

Tobacco Use

Tobacco use trends show a continued decline in use in both adults and adolescents. As a consequence, it is expected that exposure to secondhand smoke among preschool- and school-age children is also declining. In spite of the decline in tobacco use, tobacco is the single most preventable cause of death and disease in the United States (USDHHS, 2013). The use of smokeless tobacco such as snuff and dip is becoming more popular and has been linked to oral cancers, periodontitis, and tooth loss.

Smoking is a major risk to the respiratory tract and the leading cause of preventable death. At every encounter, you should question patients about smoking and their interest in stopping. Document this discussion at each visit. Offer multiple choices for discontinuing smoking and provide resources, such as support groups or individual counseling. Clinician interest can be an effective motivator in stimulating patients to quit smoking.

Sleep Disorders

Sufficient sleep is necessary for infant, child, and adolescent development. Sleep loss increases risks of heart attack and stroke in adults. Interrupted sleep negatively affect productivity and concentration in the workplace. Individuals affected by sleep-related disorders are more likely to have motor vehicle accidents (USDHHS, 2013). Obesity is a significant factor in sleep-related disorders. Counseling in sleep health and weight loss is an area for health promotion.

Cancer

Head and neck cancers have been associated with the excessive use of alcohol and tobacco products. Alcohol and drug use continue to present health concerns. As many as 95% of individuals with a chemical problem are unaware of their problem. It is estimated that 22 million Americans struggle with substance abuse problems (USDHHS, 2013).

An emergence of HPV-related oropharyngeal cancers in younger populations has been reported (Farris & Petitte, 2013). Education and early detection is essential to improving prognosis of these cancers. Make sure the patient understands the HPV-related health risks associated with sexual behaviors such as multiple sexual partners and engaging in oral sex. Promote HPV vaccination in adolescent children.

Oral Health

Visits to dental care providers are an excellent opportunity to improve oral health. Reduction of dental caries through daily oral hygiene, good dietary nutrition, community water fluoridation, and application of dental sealants after the eruption of permanent teeth are all examples of opportunities to improve oral health. Daily tooth brushing and flossing are essential to decrease dental carries as well as reduce gingivitis and periodontal disease.

Hereditary Hemorrhagic Telangiectasia

Counsel HHT patients regarding lifestyle and dietary factors that may potentially decrease the occurrence of nosebleeds, such as room humidification and the use of topical nasal creams along with nasal saline treatments. Dietary recommendations include decreasing foods high in salicylates such as red wine, spices, chocolate, coffee, and some fruits. Provide education about supplements with antiplatelet activity, such as garlic, ginger, ginseng, gingko, and vitamin E (Silva et al., 2013).

Common Symptoms

Common Mouth and Upper Respiratory Symptoms

- Facial pressure/pain/headache
- Snoring/sleep apnea
- Obstructive breathing
- Nasal congestion
- Epistaxis (nosebleeds)
- Halitosis (bad breath)
- Anosmia (decreased smell)
- Cough
- Pharyngitis/sore throat
- Dysphagia (difficulty swallowing)
- Dental aching/pain
- Hoarseness/voice changes
- Oral lesions

Signs/Symptoms	Rationale/Abnormal Findings
Facial Pressure, Pain, Headache Do you have any pain, pressure, or a headache?	Sinus pain or pressure is common with colds, influenza, and sinusitis. See also Chapters 12 and 22.
Snoring and Sleep Apnea • Do you snore? • Are you a restless sleeper? • Does anyone observe your sleep?	Snoring can be a nuisance or may be complicated by sleep apnea. All patients with sleep apnea snore, but not all who snore have sleep apnea. Patients with sleep apnea are

(table continues on page 383)

Signs/Symptoms	Rationale/Abnormal Findings
• Do you stop breathing during sleep? • Are you rested in the morning? Do you experience daytime drowsiness? • Do you drool at night?	typically unaware of nighttime arousals and are at increased risk for hypertension, stroke, heart attack, and motor vehicle accidents. Hypertrophy of the tonsils or adenoids may cause airway obstruction or sleep apnea. Children with large tonsils and adenoids may be at risk for obstructive breathing.
Obstructive Breathing	
Do you experience decreased nasal breathing? • Is this unilateral or bilateral? • Is it related to any facial trauma? • Does the congestion alternate from side to side? • Does anything aggravate or improve your nasal breathing?	Inflammation of the nose and sinuses resulting from allergen or irritant exposure may decrease nasal breathing. Structural abnormalities such as a deviated nasal septum, nasal polyp, or tumor may cause nasal obstruction. Trauma may result in a deviated nasal septum or hematoma, obstructing the nasal airway. The normal diurnal nasal cycle involves a cyclical alternating pattern of congestion and decongestion from side to side. With inflammation, this cycle may become exaggerated.
Nasal Congestion	
Do you experience excessive nasal discharge? • Is the discharge clear or cloudy? • What color is it? • Is it bilateral, from both sides, or unilateral, from one nostril?	Excessive clear rhinorrhea may represent allergic or nonallergic rhinitis. Unilateral clear discharge unresponsive to treatment may represent a rare cerebrospinal fluid leak. It can be confirmed by collection and laboratory examination of fluid for beta-2-transferrin. Cloudy or discolored discharge indicates inflammation. Persistent inflammation may result in infection.
Epistaxis	
Do you sometimes experience nosebleeds?	Nasal inflammation causes dilation of nasal blood vessels.
Do you habitually pick or remove crusts from the nose?	The most common site of nasal bleeding is the Kiesselbach plexus on the anterior septum (Andresen et al., 2008). Digital manipulation or nose picking may aggravate **epistaxis** and may result in a nasal septal perforation.
Halitosis	
Have you ever been told that your breath smells bad?	**Halitosis (foul breath)** suggests infection. Foul breath may be a factor in chronic sinusitis.
Do you have exudate or hard curds that exude from the tonsil area?	Chronic infections may result in cryptic tonsils, with collection of debris in tonsillar tissue. This exudate is sometimes referred to as tonsil stones.
Anosmia	
Do you have a decreased sense of smell? Is this a long-term or sudden change?	**Anosmia** (decreased smell) may accompany chronic inflammation of the nose and sinus. A computed tomography (CT) scan may reveal obstruction of one or more paranasal sinuses. Sudden loss of smell is an indication for CT scan or MRI of the brain to rule out a tumor or growth.
Cough	
Do you have difficulty with coughs? • Does it feel like the cough comes from your chest or upper airway? • Do you cough anything up? • If so, what does it look like? • What makes the cough worse? • What makes the cough better?	Sinus drainage, allergen or irritant exposure, or chronic sinusitis may produce cough. Persistent cough longer than 3 months or a productive cough warrants a chest x-ray to determine lung pathology. Reactive airway in asthma may produce cough. Cough may be secondary to gastroesophageal reflux disease (GERD).

(table continues on page 384)

Signs/Symptoms	Rationale/Abnormal Findings
Pharyngitis Do you experience sore throats?	Chronic hypertrophy or enlargement of the tonsils may produce sore throat or **pharyngitis**. Typically, hypertrophy of the tonsils is also associated with hypertrophy of the adenoids. Recurrent strep infections may occur with chronic tonsillitis.
Dysphagia Do you have difficulty swallowing?	**Dysphagia** (difficulty swallowing) may accompany a growth or lesion in the respiratory tract or on the thyroid gland or it may result from inflammation of the upper respiratory tract secondary to GERD.
Dental Pain Do you experience dental aching or pain? Are your teeth sensitive to cold or heat?	Sinusitis may produce dental aching, particularly of the upper teeth. Dental caries or abscess may produce tooth pain.
Voice Changes Have you experienced hoarseness or voice changes?	Common causes include sinus postnasal drainage, inflammation of the upper respiratory tract secondary to GERD, lesions of the upper respiratory tract, and inflammation from allergen or irritant exposure (e.g., chemicals, cigarette smoke).
Oral Lesions Do you have any sores in your mouth?	Smoking or chewing tobacco increases risk for oral cancer.
If so, has there been any change in the size or appearance of the sore?	Persistent or changing lesions may indicate oral cancer. Biopsy is warranted for persistent lesions. Oral examination should include a thorough investigation along the lateral borders of the tongue as well as the buccal mucosa.

Documenting Normal Findings

Patient states breathing is comfortable and quiet. Denies facial pressure, pain, headache, snoring, sleep apnea, obstructive breathing, or nasal congestion. Reports no epistaxis, halitosis, anosmia, or cough. States no pharyngitis, dysphagia, dental pain, hoarseness, or oral lesions.

Lifespan Considerations: Older Adults

Additional Questions	Rationale/Abnormal Findings
Do you experience decreased smell and taste? Do you experience increased nasal drainage at mealtime?	Diminished senses of smell and taste may produce safety risks. Gustatory rhinitis may occur in older adults with increased clear rhinorrhea at mealtime.

Cultural Considerations

Additional Questions	Rationale/Abnormal Findings
Have you recently immigrated to the United States?	Incidence of tuberculosis is approximately nine times higher among U.S. immigrants (World Health Organization, 2013).

(table continues on page 385)

Additional Questions	Rationale/Abnormal Findings
Note the patient's identified ethnicity and gender in relationship to known congenital and assessed health risks.	As discussed earlier, cleft lip and palate have increased incidence in Native and Asian Americans. African Americans and Caucasians are at higher risk for oral and pharyngeal cancers than are American Indians and Inuits. Prevalence of HPV-related oropharyngeal cancer is lower among African Americans compared with Caucasians, yet survival of these cancers is lower in African Americans (Jiron et al., 2013).

Therapeutic Dialogue: Collecting Subjective Data

Remember Mrs. Davis, introduced at the beginning of this chapter. This elderly woman has been in the hospital for 13 days with pneumonia and now is on the rehabilitation unit preparing to go home. The nurse uses professional communication techniques to gather subjective data from Mrs. Davis.

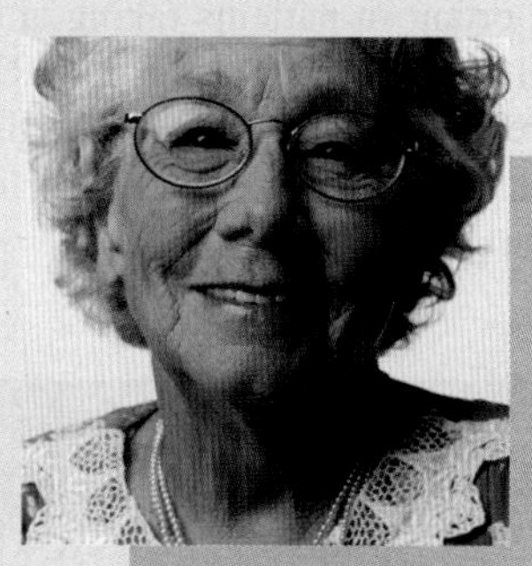

Nurse: Hi, Mrs. Davis. I'm Jen and I'm going to be your nurse today.

Mrs. Davis: Nice to meet you.

Nurse: And you, too. How are you feeling?

Mrs. Davis: (swallows with difficulty). Just fine.

Nurse: It looks like you're having a little trouble swallowing . . . (pauses)

Mrs. Davis: Well, my mouth seems so dry.

Nurse: I can see that. Let's wash your mouth out a little. Has it been awhile since you've brushed your teeth? (checks to see that there are no swallowing restrictions)

Mrs. Davis: It was yesterday. That would be so nice of you, honey.

Nurse: That's what we're here for. I'll get out your toothbrush and then we can clean things up and put on some lubricant to keep things moist. You'll feel a lot better.

Mrs. Davis: You're such a good nurse.

Critical Thinking Challenge

- Why did the nurse discuss the dry mouth instead of the pneumonia?
- Why did the nurse check for swallowing restrictions?
- How did the assessment of the nurse lead to a more effective intervention?

Objective Data

Much of the physical examination of the nose, sinuses, mouth, and oropharynx is performed by visually inspecting the area. Palpation for masses or tenderness is performed if unexpected findings are present. It is common to perform assessments in this region as focused examinations for symptoms, such as occur with nasal stuffiness or a sore throat.

Common and Specialty or Advanced Techniques

Table 15.3 summarizes common and specialized techniques used to assess the nose, sinuses, mouth, and throat.

The registered nurse (RN) primarily performs inspection of these organs. Inspection of the mouth is especially important in patients taking antibiotics who are at risk for oral candidiasis. The hospital RN also assesses the patient's nares for patency when inserting a tube into the nose for feeding; a deviated septum or obstructed nares may make insertion difficult.

The advanced practice registered nurse (APRN) uses the otoscope to visualize the nares. A flexible or rigid endoscope may be used to visualize the posterior nose, nasopharynx, or pharynx.

Equipment

- Handheld otoscope
- Nasal speculum
- Tongue blades
- Cotton gauze 4 × 4s
- Gloves
- Penlight
- Scratch and sniff test card
- Nasopharyngeal–laryngeal mirror

Preparation

Preparation involves good handwashing technique before beginning the examination. Gloves are used for the oral examination or during anticipated contact with mucous membranes. The patient is seated comfortably with the head at the examiner's eye level. If the patient wears dentures, offer a 4 × 4 gauze and ask the patient to remove them.

TABLE 15.3 Basic Versus Focused/Specialty or Advanced Techniques Related to Nose, Sinuses, Mouth, and Throat Assessment

Technique	Purpose	Screening or Registered Nurse Assessment	Focused or Advance Practice Examination
Inspect the nose.	To gather information regarding the integrity of the nose	X	
Inspect the mouth.	To gather information regarding the integrity of the oral cavity	X	
Inspect the throat.	To gather information regarding the integrity of the throat	X	
Inspect the nose with otoscope and nasal speculum.	To gather information about inflammation, infection, and structure		X Inflammation, infection, structure
Palpate the nose.	To assess for inflammation, lesions, or fractures		X Inflammation, lesions, fractures
Inspect the sinuses.	Transillumination results variable; typically assessed by CT scan; flexible or rigid fiberoptic examination allows visualization		X Infection
Palpate/percuss the sinuses.	To look for signs of infection or inflammation		X Infection
Palpate the mouth.	To look for lesions or salivary stones		X Lesions
Inspect/evaluate swallowing.	To investigate causes of complaints of dysphagia		X Dysphagia

Comprehensive Physical Assessment

Technique and Normal Findings	Abnormal Findings
External Nose ***Inspection.*** Inspect the nose. The nose appears symmetrical, midline, and proportionally shaped to facial features. Skin surface is smooth without lesions; coloration is consistent with other facial complexion.	Asymmetry, swelling, or bruising may result from trauma or accompany lesions or growths.
Palpation. Generally, the RN does not palpate the nose or sinuses unless a specific difficulty is present. The APRN gently palpates with the thumb and forefinger. There is no pain, tenderness, or break in contour.	Tenderness on palpation and crepitus suggest fracture.
Internal Nose The APRN generally inspects the internal nose with an otoscope, nasal speculum, or both (Fig. 15.11). If using a nasal speculum, insert a wide-tipped speculum gently into the nasal **vestibule** or naris and open vertically while gently lifting up on the tip of the nose. The nasal speculum may be inserted but should never be opened horizontally because this puts uncomfortable pressure on the septum. Observe the color of the mucous membranes. Inspect any mucus. Note the color and character of the nasal mucous. The inferior turbinate is the first structure visualized. The middle turbinate can be noted superior and lateral. Assess nasal airflow by asking the patient to breathe out while holding the mouth closed. Gently manipulate the external nose to assess how these changes affect airflow. Septum is midline; its mucosa is pink and moist with no prominent blood vessels or crusts. A small amount of drainage is clear. Airflow around the normal nasal structures is adequate.	Infection and inflammation of nasal mucosa may be present with viral, bacterial, or allergic rhinitis. Excessive clear watery drainage suggests allergic rhinitis. Thick discolored mucus or gross pus may accompany infection. Absence of normal structures, such as the turbinates, suggests previous surgery. **Deviation** of the nasal septum may be congenital or acquired in trauma. Note any crusting or prominence of nasal vessels with special attention to the anterior septum. A septal perforation is a hole in the midline septum. It may be secondary to trauma, surgery, or illicit drug use. **Polyps,** grapelike swollen nasal membranes, may appear white and glistening. See Table 15.6 at the end of this chapter.

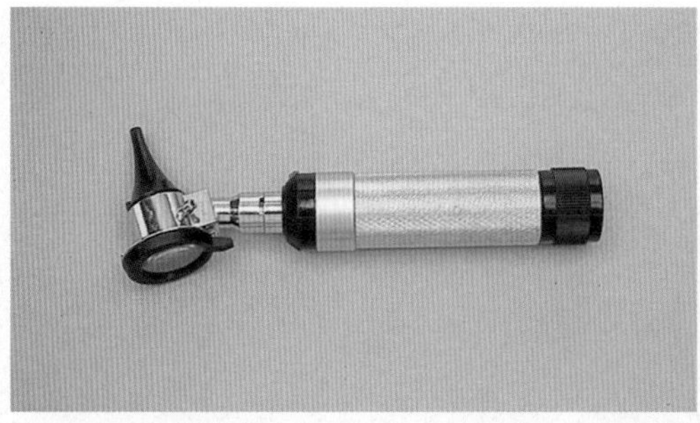

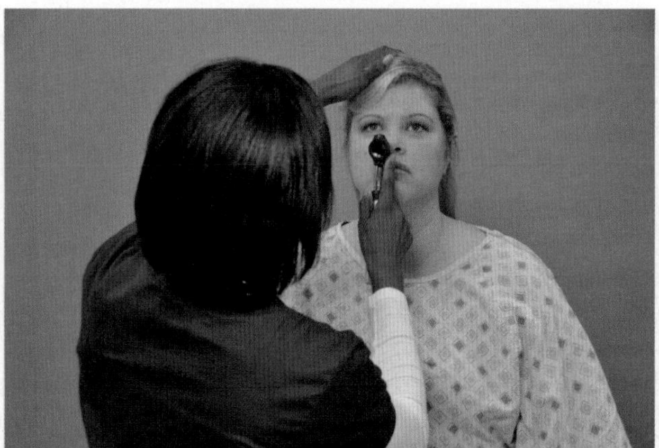

Figure 15.11 Inspecting the nasal mucosa.

Technique and Normal Findings	Abnormal Findings
If the patient notices a loss of smell, ask him or her to identify common scents. Smell testing may be performed with the use of a sniff test card. The patient correctly identifies scents.	**Anosmia** may occur with trauma, congestion, polyps, or sinus infection. Sudden loss of smell warrants consideration of radiological testing to rule out intracranial masses.

(table continues on page 388)

Technique and Normal Findings (continued)	Abnormal Findings (continued)
Sinuses	
Inspection. Inspect the sinus areas (forehead, between the eyes, and both cheeks) for redness or swelling. ■ Sinus areas are symmetrical with no redness or swelling.	Redness and swelling over the sinuses may represent acute infection, abscess, or mucocele.
Transillumination is a traditional method by which clinicians assess sinus cavities (Fig. 15.12). This method has limited clinical significance and provides inconsistent results. Flexible or rigid endoscopy is performed by the APRN. The standard diagnostic technique in evaluating sinus disease is a CT scan.	Positive findings in inspection of the sinuses warrant radiological imaging to assess involvement.

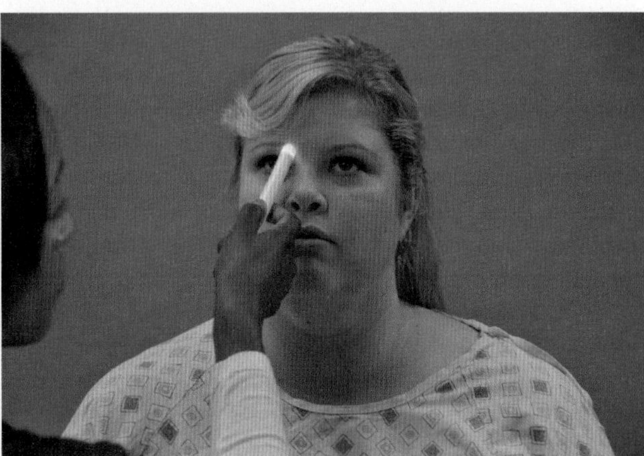

Figure 15.12 Transillumination of the sinuses.

Technique and Normal Findings (continued)	Abnormal Findings (continued)
Palpation and Percussion. Palpate and percuss the maxillary, ethmoid, and frontal sinus areas (Fig. 15.13). This technique is used by APRNs. ■ No tenderness or fullness is present.	Tenderness or fullness on palpation suggests infection or possible growth. Positive findings on palpation may warrant radiological imaging.

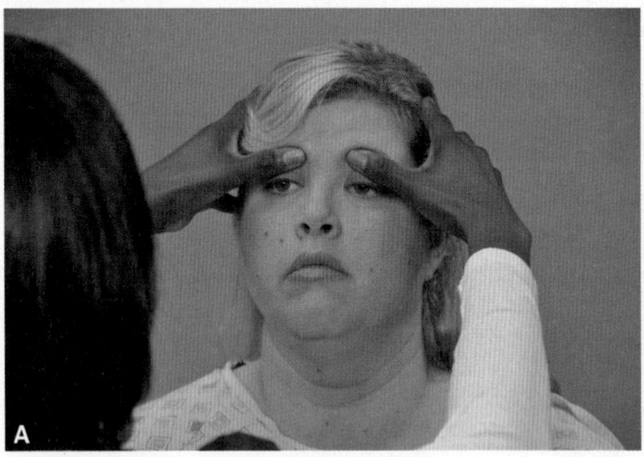

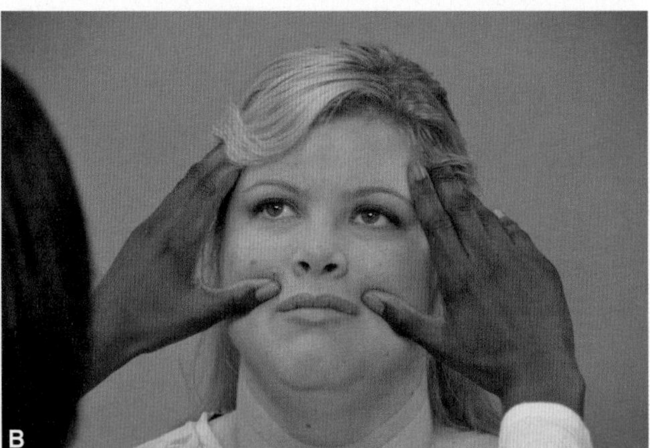

Figure 15.13 Palpating the sinus area. **A.** Palpate the frontal sinus. **B.** Palpate the maxillary sinus.

Technique and Normal Findings (continued)	Abnormal Findings (continued)
Mouth	
External Inspection. Inspect lips, noting color, moisture, lesions, and oral competence. ■ Lips are pink and moist with no lesions.	Dryness or cracking may indicate inadequate hydration. Lesions or aphthous ulcers may represent a viral infection. Swelling or edema of lips suggests allergy. Oral incompetence may occur in cleft lip or with inadequate repair. See Table 15.7 at the end of this chapter.

Technique and Normal Findings (continued)	Abnormal Findings (continued)
Internal Inspection Buccal Mucosa. Holding a light in the nondominant hand and a tongue blade in the dominant one, gently separate areas to fully inspect the buccal mucosa, noting color and pigmentation (Fig. 15.14). Inspect the entire U-shaped area in the floor of mouth. Note the parotid (Stensen) duct appearing as a small dimple just opposite the second upper molar (Fig. 15.15). Note submandibular (Wharton) ducts on either side of frenulum in the floor of the mouth. Small, isolated, white or yellow papules (**Fordyce granules**) may be noted on the cheeks, tongue, and lips (Fig. 15.16). These sebaceous cysts or salivary tissues are insignificant.	Poor oral hygiene has been linked to increased rates of pneumonia. Inflamed buccal mucosa suggests infection. White patches (**leukoplakia**) may suggest a growth or lesion. Ulceration may represent viral infection or tumor. **Petechiae** or small red spots resulting from blood, which escaped the capillaries, may occur with trauma, infection, or decreased platelet counts (Fig. 15.17). Redness or swelling of the parotid duct may represent infection or blockage of the parotid gland. Redness or swelling of the submandibular ducts on either side of frenulum in the floor of mouth may represent infection or blockage of the submandibular salivary glands.
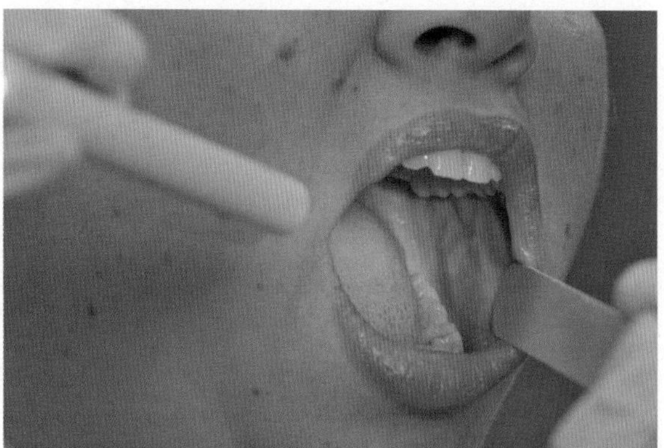 **Figure 15.14** Inspecting the buccal mucosa.	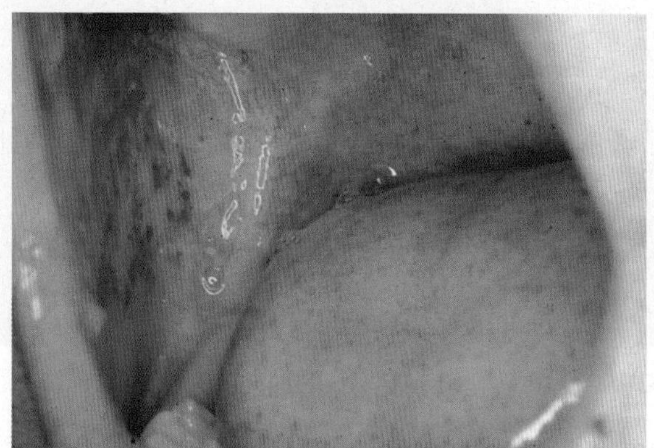 **Figure 15.17** Oral petechiae.
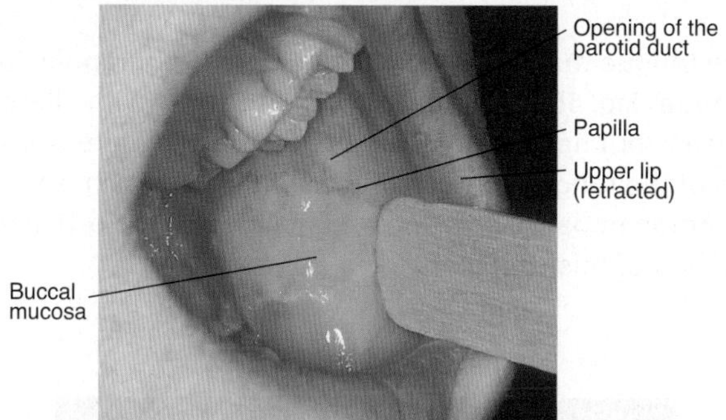 **Figure 15.15** Examination of the parotid (Stensen) duct.	
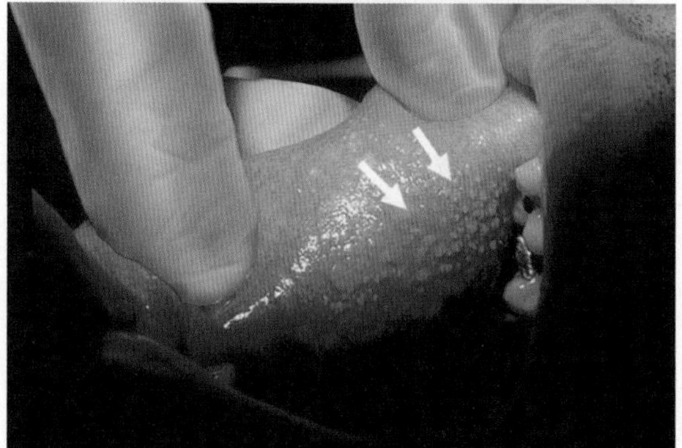 **Figure 15.16** Fordyce granules.	

(table continues on page 390)

Technique and Normal Findings (continued)	Abnormal Findings (continued)
Teeth and Gums. Inspect the teeth and gums. Note numbers and position of teeth. Note general appearance and signs of decay. Note alignment. Note the odor of the patient's breath.	Teeth may be stained or have decay. Swollen or red gums with bleeding may indicate gingivitis. Foul breath may suggest infection. Broken teeth or excessive decay may be present in methamphetamine users. See Table 15.9 at the end of this chapter.
Uvula. Note the position of the uvula (Fig. 15.18). Have the patient say "ah," noting the rise of the uvula and function of the vagus nerve (CN X). 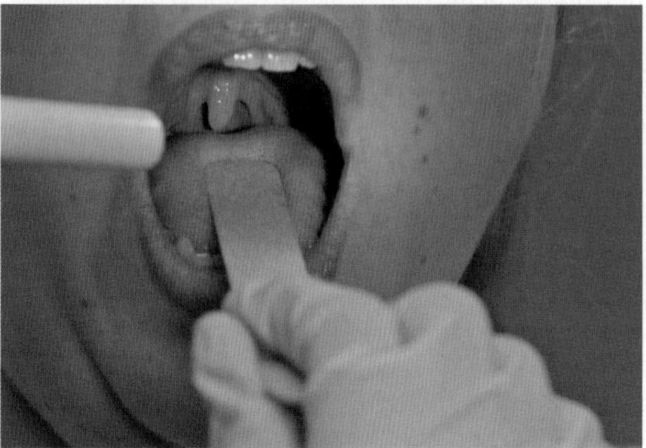 **Figure 15.18** Observing the uvula.	The uvula may be swollen with allergic reactions. It may be bifid or have a notch or cleft.
Hard and Soft Palates. Inspect the color and surface of the hard and soft palates.	With cleft palate, nasopharyngeal incompetence may be present along with resultant nasal air leak during speech.
Tongue. Inspect the tongue, including the dorsum (top surface), sides, and underneath. Note papillae on the dorsum, small anterior, and large posterior. Ask the patient to stick out the tongue (Fig. 15.19). Although generally not done during a screening assessment, the gag reflex may be tested. Gently place a tongue blade on the posterior dorsum to produce the gag reflex, which ensures function of the hypoglossal nerve (CN XII). 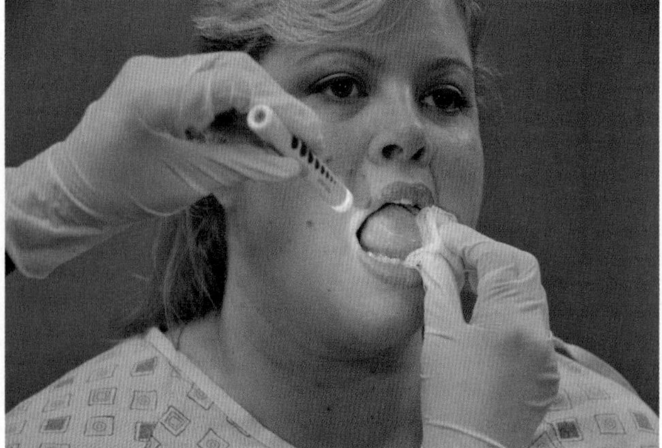 **Figure 15.19** Sticking out the tongue.	The tongue may have lesions or ulcers. **Geographic tongue** (Fig. 15.20) tends to occur in people with allergic disease but has no significant pathology. A white coating of the tongue may be **oral candidiasis**, which is very common in patients taking antibiotics. See Table 15.8 at the end of this chapter 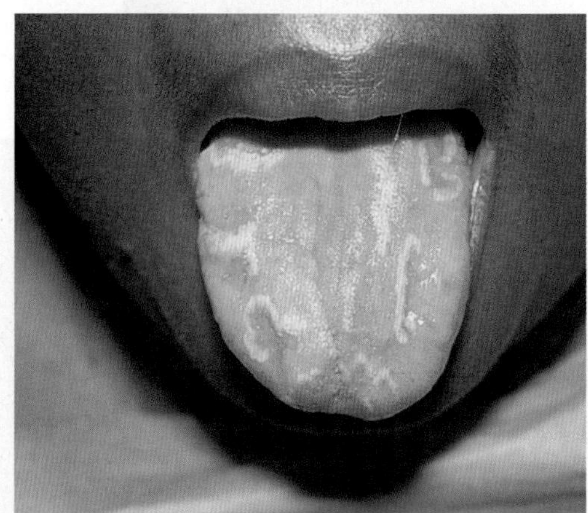 **Figure 15.20** Geographic tongue.

(table continues on page 391)

Technique and Normal Findings (continued)	Abnormal Findings (continued)
Submandibular Ducts and Salivary Flow. Inspect the submandibular ducts in the floor of the mouth. Evaluate salivary flow from the submandibular salivary gland. Buccal mucosa and soft and hard palates are pink with no lesions. Gingiva is pink and moist without inflammation. Breath has no foul odor. Tongue is smooth and midline. Teeth are well aligned with no evidence of decay. Uvula rises symmetrically with "ah." Ducts are smooth without inflammation.	Swelling or redness of the submandibular ducts suggests inflammation of the submandibular gland (Fig. 15.21). No upward movement of the uvula when the patient says "ah" indicates dysfunction of the vagus nerve. Infection in the floor of the mouth may produce Ludwig angina. 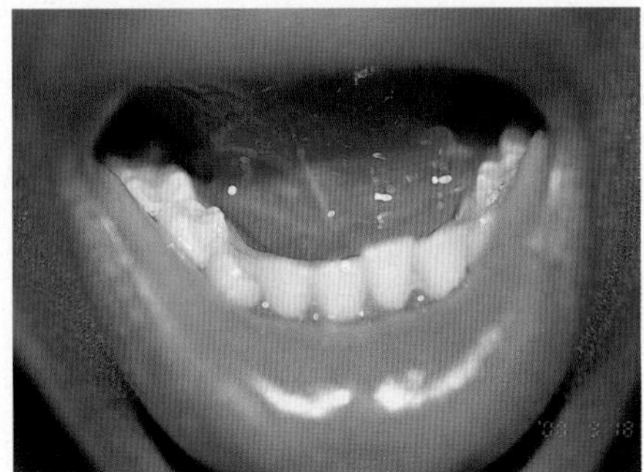 **Figure 15.21** Swollen and red Wharton ducts.
Palpation. Palpate the parotid, submandibular, and sublingual glands for swelling or tenderness. Gland size should be symmetrical. There is no swelling or tenderness.	Swelling may occur with mumps, blockage of a duct, and presence of a stone, abscess, or tumor. Duct obstruction can occur as a result of aging, dehydration, or use of anticholinergic medications.
Palpation of the mouth is usually completed as part of a specialty assessment. If performed, place a gloved hand inside the cheek to assess Stensen duct in the buccal mucosa opposite the second molars and submandibular duct. Assess these areas for a stone or growth. Palpate for any lesions. Ducts are soft and nontender without lesions.	A firm area at either parotid or submandibular ducts may be a stone or growth. Lesions of oral mucosa may indicate a growth. Examination by biopsy or with radiological films may be recommended for oral lesions. A newer technique for evaluation of the salivary gland is sialendoscopy, which can be diagnostic *and* therapeutic, facilitating locating and removing of small salivary stones (Zenk et al., 2012). When palpating masses, keep in mind that hard fixed lesions have a higher incidence of being malignant. Soft mobile lesions are more often cysts or benign disease.
Throat ***Inspection.*** Pressing down slightly with the tongue blade on the midpoint of the tongue, visualize the pharynx, tonsils, soft palate, and anterior and posterior tonsillar pillars. Note color, symmetry, enlargement, and any lesions. The tonsils are at the back of the oropharynx between the anterior and posterior pillars. The tissue appears more granular and less smooth than the surrounding mucous membranes. Grade the tonsils using the scale in Box 15.1. Tissue is pink and moist with symmetrical margins. No enlargement or lesions are noted. Tonsils are absent or 1+.	Mucosal inflammation may indicate infection or allergy. Hypertrophy of tonsils occurs with persistent recurrent infection. Frequent infections may leave superficial scars or crypts (Fig. 15.22). These crypts may collect 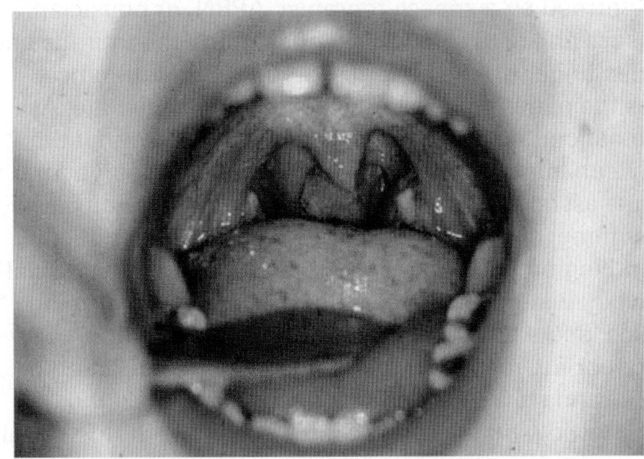 **Figure 15.22** Tonsillar crypts with debris.

(table continues on page 392)

Technique and Normal Findings (continued)

BOX 15.1 Tonsillar Grading Scale

- 1+: tonsil obstructs 0%–25% to midline
- 2+: tonsil obstructs 25%–50% to midline
- 3+: tonsil obstructs 50%–75% to midline
- 4+: tonsil obstructs 75%–100% to midline

From Pine, H. S. (2013). *Pediatric otolaryngology: An issue of pediatric clinics*. Philadelphia, PA: Elsevier.

Palpation. An APRN will find palpation of the neck helpful to assess inflammatory and other changes that may occur in the throat. Anterior and posterior cervical chain lymph nodes and submental areas are palpated as part of a normal neck examination (see Chapter 12).

Nodes are symmetrical, soft, and nontender.

Swallowing Evaluation

Evaluation of swallowing is a technique typically performed by a speech therapist, APRN, or physician. Assess ability to swallow by positioning the thumbs and index finger on the patient's laryngeal protuberance. Ask the patient to swallow; feel the larynx elevate. Ask the patient to cough. Patients can aspirate even if they have an intact gag reflex (Nettina, 2009). Observe for signs associated with swallowing difficulties, such as coughing; choking; spitting of food; drooling; difficulty handling oral secretions; double or major delay in swallowing; watery eyes; nasal discharge; wet or gurgling voice; decreased ability to move tongue and lips, chew food, or move food to the back of mouth; pocketing of food; and slow or scanning speech (Nettina, 2009).

Swallowing takes less than 1 second with no sign of aspiration.

Abnormal Findings (continued)

food and oral debris that appears as white curdlike material embedded in the tonsil mucosa. Generally, with chronic tonsillitis and hypertrophy, findings are symmetrical. Asymmetrical tonsillar enlargement raises suspicion of neoplasia. **Peritonsillar abscess**, or quinsy, may occur with collection of fluid in the anterior tonsillar pillar (Fig. 15.23). This condition presents as a sore throat with increasing unilateral pain, deviated uvula, "hot potato voice," dysphagia, and **trismus** (inability to open jaw). Tonsillar hypertrophy may lead to sleep apnea; sleep apnea is associated with an elongated palate. Strep throat presents with red and white patches in the throat, difficulty swallowing, tender or swollen glands (lymph nodes) in the neck, or red and enlarged tonsils.

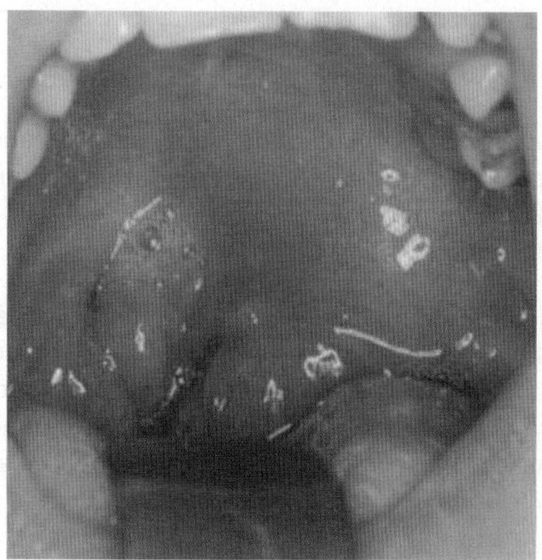

Figure 15.23 Peritonsillar abscess.

Lymph nodes are quick to respond to inflammation and slow to resolve. Inflammation causes enlargement of the anterior, posterior, or submental lymph nodes of the neck. Soft and tender enlargement may accompany minor inflammation. Hard fixed nodes should be further evaluated by biopsy or radiological films.

Patients with stroke, head injury, or other neuromuscular disorders are at risk for **dysphagia**. Swallowing difficulties are common in hospitalized patients and may prolong length of stay because of an inability to obtain adequate nutrition for healing. Dysphagia may be from a growth in the airway or enlargement of surrounding glands or tissue. Dysphagia may be secondary to GERD, which should be suspected when inflammation of the larynx is visualized on indirect or direct view. Aspiration into the larynx may be observed with incomplete closure of vocal cords or impeded movement of the epiglottis.

Documenting Normal Findings

Nose appears symmetrical, midline, and proportionally shaped to facial features. Mucosa dark pink, septum midline, nontender, intact. Turbinates pink, moist, without lesions. Sinus areas are symmetrical with no redness or swelling. Nontender on palpation bilaterally. Lips are pink and moist with no lesions. Buccal mucosa, soft and hard palates are pink and moist with no lesions. Gingivae are pink, firm and moist without inflammation. Breath has no foul odor. Tongue is smooth and midline. Teeth are intact and well aligned with no evidence of decay. Uvula rises symmetrically with saying "ah." Ducts are smooth without inflammation. Pharynx is pink and moist with no exudates bilaterally. Tonsils are absent.

Lifespan Considerations: Older Adults

Loss of subcutaneous fat may cause the nose to appear more prominent in older adults. Edentulous (without any teeth) older adults may develop a pursed-lip appearance as mouth and cheeks fold inward. Overclosure of the mouth may lead to maceration of the skin at the corners of the mouth; this condition is called **angular cheilitis** (Fig. 15.24). Teeth may appear yellow because worn enamel exposes the dentin layer. They also may appear larger as the gums recede. Teeth may loosen with bone resorption and move with palpation.

The tongue and buccal mucosa may appear smoother and shiny from papillary atrophy and thinning of the buccal mucosa. This condition is called **smooth glossy tongue** (Fig. 15.25) and may result from deficiencies of riboflavin, folic acid, and vitamin B_{12}. Fissures may appear in the tongue with increasing age. This condition, called **scrotal tongue**

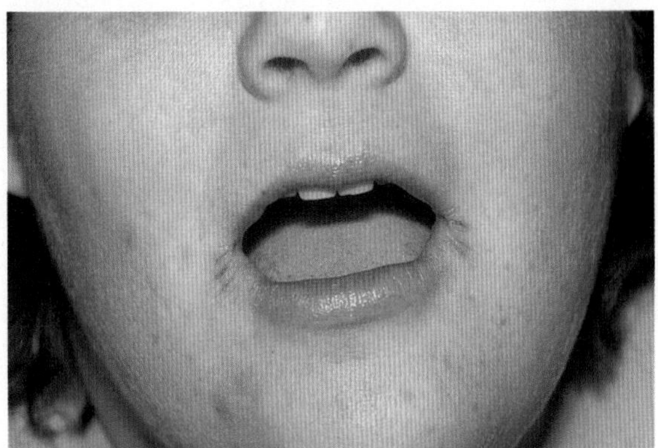

Figure 15.24 Angular cheilitis.

(Fig. 15.26), can result in the tongue becoming inflamed with the accumulation of food or debris in the fissures.

An oral health screening tool (Taub, 2012) is available that includes assessment of the lymph nodes; tissue inside the cheek, floor, and roof of the mouth; gums between the teeth or under dentures; saliva; condition of teeth; and oral cleanliness.

Cultural Considerations

The nasal bridge may be flat in African American and Asians. In dark-skinned patients, the gums are more deeply colored; a brownish ridge is often found along the gum line. Oropharyngeal cancer statistics had shown a decline consistent with decreasing use of tobacco products; however, current statistics show an increased occurrence in economically developed countries, greater in males than females. Those countries showing increased incidence include Australia, Canada, Denmark, the Netherlands, Norway, Sweden, and the United States (Chaturvedi et al., 2013).

Documenting Case Study Findings

The nurse has just finished conducting a physical examination of Mrs. Davis, the 89-year-old woman admitted with pneumonia 13 days ago. Unlike the samples of normal documentation previously charted, Mrs. Davis has unexpected findings. Review the following important findings revealed in each of the steps of objective data collection. Consider how these results compare with the normal findings presented in the samples of normal documentation. Pay attention to how the nurse clusters data to provide a more complete and accurate understanding of the condition.

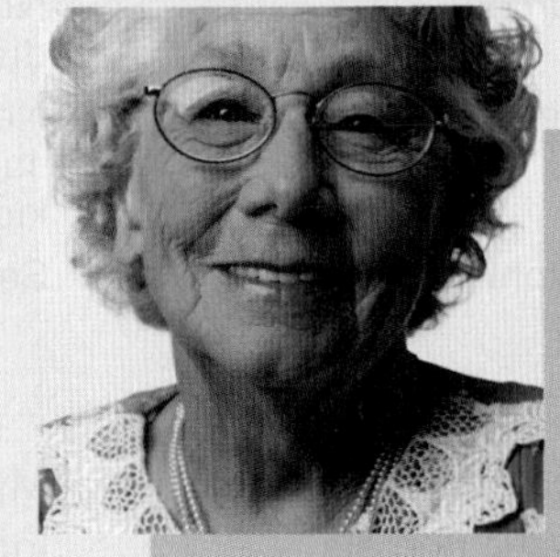

Inspection: Lips pale and dry with large amounts of crusting. No ulcers or lesions. Teeth yellowed and slightly crusted. Correct occlusion. Gums pale and intact. Tongue and buccal mucosa with cheesy white coating that scrapes off. Area under tongue is dry but smooth without lesions. Posterior palate also has white cheesy coating. Tonsils pink and smooth but not enlarged at 1+/4+ scale.

Palpation: No masses, lesions, or tenderness.

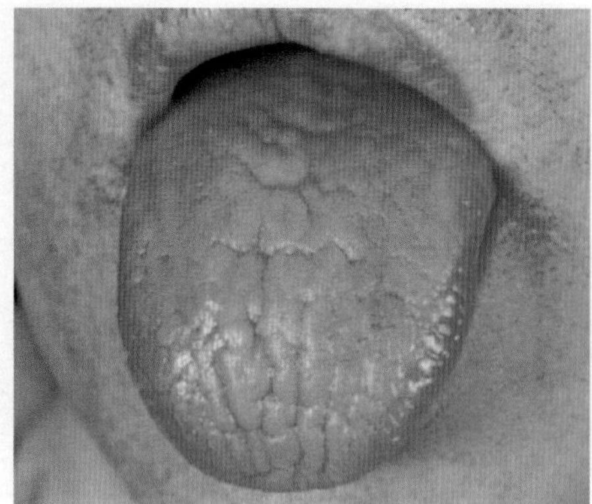

Figure 15.25 Smooth glossy tongue.

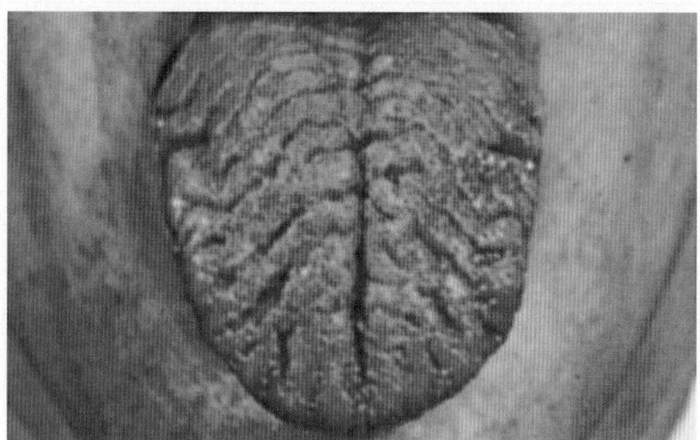

Figure 15.26 Scrotal tongue.

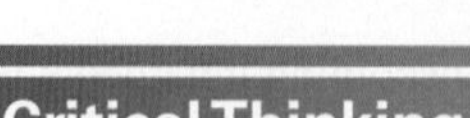

Critical Thinking

Laboratory and Diagnostic Testing

Laboratory studies of blood or other body fluids can give measures that are helpful in constructing a diagnosis. An elevated white blood cell count suggests infection, such as sinusitis or tonsillitis. Nasal–sinus cultures can help with identification of bacteria type. Biopsies provide tissue to determine whether cancer is present. Examination of clear nasal discharge for beta-2-transferrin can identify cerebrospinal fluid in the nose. Throat culture can identify the type of bacteria producing tonsillitis or pharyngitis. Nasal and oral findings also may be evidence of systemic disease (Table 15.4).

TABLE 15.4 Nasal and Oral Findings in Systemic Disease

Disease	Etiology	Nasal Findings
Churg-Strauss syndrome	Vasculitis	Nasal crusting and polyps
Sjögren syndrome	Chronic inflammatory disorder characterized by decreased lacrimal and salivary gland secretion	Atrophy and drying of oral and nasal mucosa; may lead to epistaxis
Pemphigus-pemphigoid	Autoimmune disorder	Blister formation on external nose or anterior septum
Scleroderma	Systemic sclerosis from abnormal collagen synthesis	**Telangiectasias** of nasal mucosa with no cilia
Behçet disease	Chronic inflammatory disorder	Oral ulceration, rhinorrhea, rhinalgia, aphthous ulceration of nose or nasopharynx that heals without scarring
Sarcoidosis	Noncaseating inflammatory disorder	Engorgement of turbinates with papules or nodules on septum
Wegener granulomatosis	Necrotizing granulomatous vasculitis affecting respiratory tract, kidneys, and peripheral vessels	Nasal crusting, ulcerations, epistaxis, chronic rhinosinusitis, septal perforations
Syphilis	Sexually transmitted infection	Primary 3–4 weeks after contact, ulceration in vestibule of nose or septum; secondary lesions after primary fades; tertiary nasal septal swelling may develop into perforation
Tuberculosis	Mycobacterial infection	Nasal crusting, mucosal ulcerations
Cystic fibrosis	Inherited absence of exocrine glands	Copious, thick, viscous mucus that blocks airways; chronic rhinosinusitis; nasal polyps
AIDS	HIV	Nasal ulcerations, lesions, Kaposi sarcoma
HHT; also known as Rendu-Osler-Weber syndrome	Autosomal dominant disorder that leads to abnormal blood vessel formation	Telangiectasia Most common clinical feature is nosebleeds. (Silva et al., 2013)

From Higgins, T., LeGrand, M., & Rudy, S. (2008). Nasal cavity, paranasal sinuses and nasopharynx. In L. Harris & M. Huntoon (Eds.), *Core curriculum for otorhinolaryngology and head-neck nursing* (2nd ed., p. 183). New Smyrna Beach, FL: Society of Otorhinolaryngology and Head-Neck Nurses.

Diagnostic testing for allergic sensitivity is helpful in managing persistent upper respiratory inflammation. Allergy testing may be performed by assessing skin or blood. Various approaches to allergy skin testing include percutaneous or prick testing and intradermal testing. A blending of both types of skin testing is performed typically when evaluating upper respiratory conditions. Radioallergosorbent testing (RAST) is a blood test that measures allergen-specific immunoglobulin E (IgE) antibody, which is elevated in reaction to allergens to which the patient is sensitive.

Radiographic studies are helpful in diagnosing chronic sinusitis. X-ray examination may be used in acute sinusitis, but it provides very limited information in comparison with sinus CT scan—the standard radiological film in evaluating chronic sinusitis. The detail provided by the sinus CT scan is evident when compared with plain x-ray views. CT scans and MRI films are helpful in evaluating masses and lesions of the upper respiratory tract. Routine dental x-rays improve early detection of dental carries. In patients with swelling of the salivary glands, sialendoscopy can be of diagnostic as well as therapeutic importance (Zenk et al., 2012).

Biopsy is performed on lesions of uncertain behavior for tissue diagnosis. This can be accomplished by fine-needle aspiration in some situations. Other lesions may warrant an incisional biopsy.

Sleep studies can be used to assess sleep apnea. Patients spend the night in a sleep laboratory and are monitored for breathing, heart monitoring, oxygen saturation, and excessive leg movements.

Diagnostic Reasoning

Nursing Diagnoses, Outcomes, and Interventions

When formulating a nursing diagnosis, it is important to use critical thinking to cluster data and identify patterns that fit together. You compare these data clusters with defining characteristics (unexpected findings) for the diagnosis to ensure the most accurate labeling and appropriate interventions. Table 15.5 provides a comparison of nursing diagnoses, points of differentiation, assessment characteristics, and nursing interventions commonly related to nose, mouth, sinus, and throat assessment (NANDA International, 2012).

Outcomes commonly related to nose, mouth, sinus, and throat problems include the following:

- The patient's oral mucous membranes are pink and intact.
- Patient swallows with evidence of aspiration.
- Patient states breathing is more comfortable and less congested (Moorhead, Johnson, Maas, & Swanson, 2013).

After outcomes have been established, you implement nursing care to improve the status of the patient. Use critical thinking and evidence-based practice to develop the interventions. Some examples of nursing interventions for the nose, mouth, sinuses, and throat are as follows:

- Provide oral hygiene every 8 hours.
- Consult with a speech therapist to evaluate swallowing.
- Push fluids to 2 L to liquefy secretions (Bulechek, Butcher, Dochterman, & Wagner, 2013).

TABLE 15.5 Common Nursing Diagnoses Associated With the Nose, Sinuses, Mouth, and Throat

Diagnosis	Point of Differentiation	Assessment Characteristics	Nursing Interventions
Impaired dentition	Disease, disruption, trauma, or other factors that cause problems in development, eruption, or structural integrity of teeth	Malocclusion, tooth pain, caries, plaque, halitosis, premature loss of teeth, tooth fracture	Teach toothbrushing and flossing. Provide assistance as needed. Perform mouth care if patient is unable to do so independently.
Altered oral mucous membrane	Break in the integrity of the tissues of the lips, soft tissues of the oral cavity, or both	Dry mouth, oral lesions, aphthous ulcers, coated tongue, vesicles, nodules, patches	Provide fluids and mouth care. Moisturize mucous membranes. Treat infections.*
Impaired swallowing	Associated with oral, pharyngeal, or esophageal structure or function	Delayed swallowing, gurgling voice, frequent coughing, choking or gagging, inability to clear oral cavity, food falling from mouth	Evaluate swallowing ability. Provide sips of fluids before giving dry foods. Elevate head of bed. Thicken liquids if needed.
Altered breathing pattern	Respirations that fail to produce significant ventilation	Nasal flaring, dyspnea, orthopnea	Use tissues to clear upper airway. Elevate head of bed. Give frequent fluids to liquefy secretions.

*Collaborative interventions.

Progress Note: Analyzing Findings

Remember Mrs. Davis, whose condition has been outlined throughout this chapter. Initial subjective and objective data collection is complete and the nurse has spent time reviewing the findings and other results. The following nursing note illustrates how subjective and objective data are collected and analyzed and nursing interventions are developed.

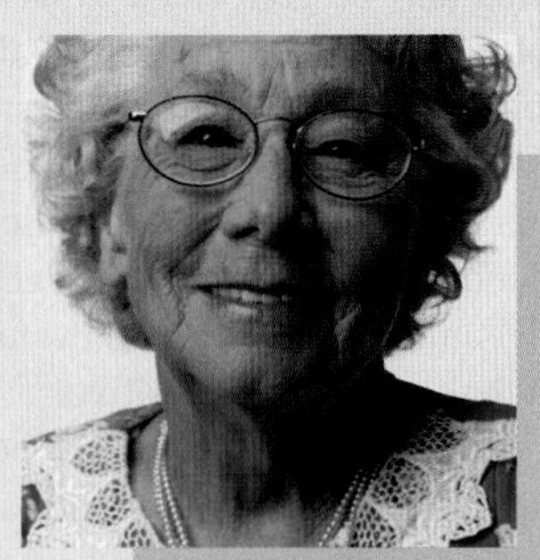

Subjective: "My mouth is dry."

Objective: Lips pale and dry with large amounts of crusting. No ulcers or lesions. Teeth yellowed and slightly crusted. Correct occlusion. Gums pale and intact. Tongue and buccal mucosa with cheesy, white coating that scrapes off. Area under tongue is dry but smooth without lesions. Posterior palate also has white cheesy coating. Tonsils pink and smooth but not enlarged at 1+/4+ scale. No masses, lesions, or tenderness palpated.

Analysis: Altered oral mucous membranes related to xerostomia, infrequent oral care, and possible infection.

Plan: Performed oral hygiene with positive results. Large reduction in crusting and mucous membranes are now pink. White coating remains on tongue and buccal mucosa. Contact primary care provider to evaluate for a possible infection. Continue oral hygiene every shift.

Critical Thinking Challenge

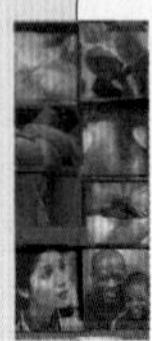

- Why did the nurse decide to focus the SOAP on the status of the patient's mucous membranes rather than on the patient's diagnosis of pneumonia?
- What other effects might poor oral hygiene have on the patient's body systems?
- What data made the nurse suspect that there might be an associated infection?

Collaborating With the Interprofessional Team

The nurse suspects that Mrs. Davis has a yeast infection (*Candida albicans*) in her mouth. Treatment requires a prescription medication. Therefore, the nurse will need to notify the primary care provider.

The following conversation illustrates how the nurse might organize the data and make recommendations about the patient's situation to the provider.

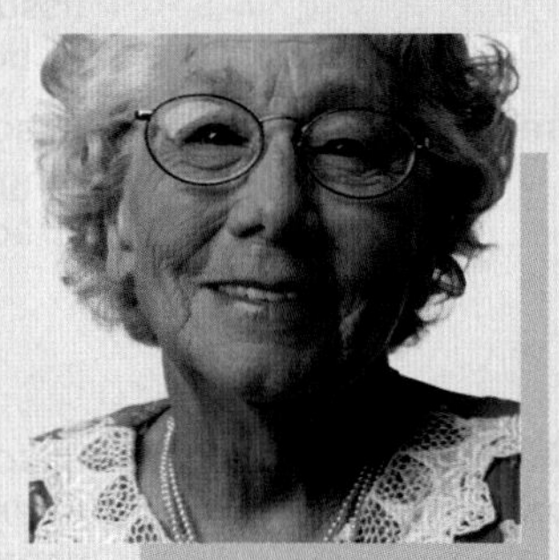

(case study continues on page 397)

Situation: "I'm Jen Tsang, and I've been caring for Mrs. Davis today. She is an 89-year-old woman admitted 13 days ago with pneumonia."

Background: "She's been on antibiotics for most of her stay here, which has been complicated with multiple infections and a 4-day stay in the ICU."

Assessment: "When I performed oral care on her today, I noticed a white coating on her tongue. I was able to clean off most of the crusts and moisturize her lips, but the white coating remains. She doesn't have any lesions but she said that her tongue is quite tender and it got quite red when I tried to scrape off the coating."

Recommendations: "I was thinking that she might have a fungal infection from the antibiotics and wonder if you could order a medication to swish and swallow in her mouth. Thanks so much."

Critical Thinking Challenge

- What information did the nurse decide not to include in the conversation and why?
- What risk factors does Mrs. Davis have for *C. albicans*?
- How can the nurse ensure that oral hygiene becomes one of the priorities in care?

Pulling It All Together

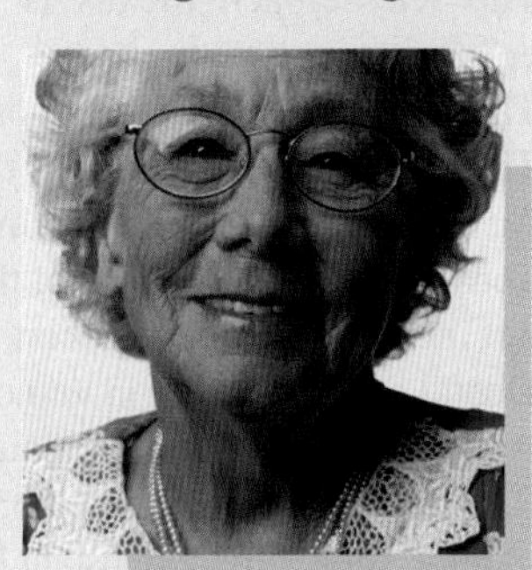

The nurse uses assessment data to formulate a nursing care plan with patient outcomes and interventions for Mrs. Davis. The nurse uses critical thinking and judgment to continue or revise the diagnosis, outcomes, or interventions. This is often in the form of a care plan or case note similar to the one below.

Nursing Diagnosis	Patient Outcomes	Nursing Interventions	Rationale	Evaluation
Altered oral mucous membrane related to *C. albicans*	Oral mucous membranes pink, moist, and without coating, lesions, or masses	Encourage fluids. Provide oral care every shift. Obtain order for medication. After oral care, have patient swish and swallow medication.*	Fluids will keep the membranes moist. Provide fluids, then oral care, and then medication last to allow the medication time in the oral cavity to work.	Patient with no crusts or dryness in mouth. States oral cavity and lips are more comfortable. Approximately half of coating on tongue is present. Continue with care.

*Collaborative intervention.

Applying Your Knowledge

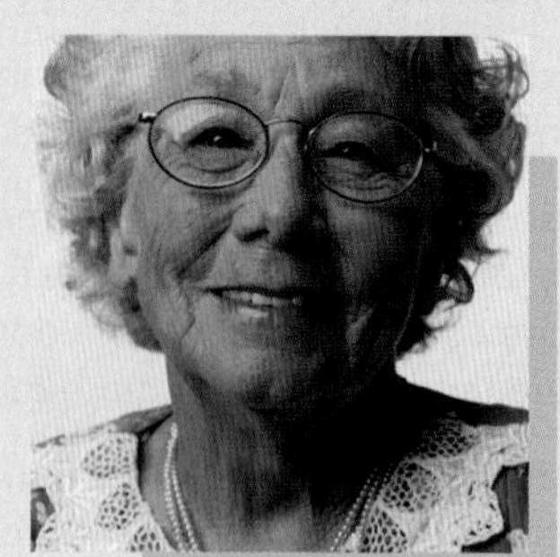

Using the previous steps of diagnostic reasoning, organizing, and prioritizing, consider all the case study findings woven throughout this chapter. When answering the following questions, begin drawing conclusions and see how the pieces of assessment must work together to create an environment for personalized, appropriate, and accurate care.

- What are some possible causes of Mrs. Davis's altered oral mucosa?
- Why is it especially important for nurses to inspect the mouths of hospitalized patients?
- The mucous membranes reflect the health of other body systems. What body systems are affecting the health of Mrs. Davis's oral mucous membranes?
- How might improvement in the patient's mouth affect her rehabilitation and functional abilities?
- What recommendations for follow-up would you make to Mrs. Davis?
- After a diagnosis has been established for Mrs. Davis, how would you evaluate her understanding of it and determine any teaching for discharge home?

Key Points

- The nose, sinuses, and throat are parts of the upper airway.
- The mouth and throat are parts of the upper gastrointestinal tract.
- The nose is the primary organ of smell.
- The mouth is the primary organ of taste.
- The Kiesselbach plexus is the most common site of epistaxis.
- The pharyngeal fossa is the most common site of oral cancer.
- The highly vascular floor of the mouth is a good location for absorption of sublingual medications.
- Tonsillitis is inflammation of the tonsils; their removal does not increase risk for infection.
- Dental care is lacking in vulnerable groups.
- Acute airway obstruction requires immediate intervention.
- Risk factors for nose, mouth, sinus, and throat problems include topical decongestant use, smoking, inhaling substances and chemicals, allergies, and dust exposure.
- Common symptoms in the nose, sinuses, mouth, and throat include facial pain, sleep apnea, obstructive breathing, nasal congestion, epistaxis, halitosis, anosmia, cough, pharyngitis, dental pain, dysphagia, hoarseness, and oral lesions.
- The nose is normally symmetrical, midline, and proportional to facial features.
- The sinuses may be tender or full due to infection.
- Fordyce granules are insignificant sebaceous cysts or salivary tissue.
- A white coating of the tongue may be a symptom of oral candidiasis and is common in patients taking antibiotics.
- Patients can aspirate even if they have an intact gag reflex.
- Fissures may appear in the tongue with increased age.

Review Questions

1. Which of the following is part of the upper gastrointestinal tract?
   A. Nasal septum
   B. Sinuses
   C. Throat
   D. Adenoids

2. The nurse is assessing the nares to evaluate the site of epistaxis. The most common site of bleeding is which of the following?
   A. Ostiomeatal complex
   B. Nasal septum
   C. Kiesselbach plexus
   D. Woodruff plexus

3. The nurse knows that the floor of the mouth is highly vascular and therefore a good location for which of the following?
   A. Absorption of sublingual medications
   B. Identification of malignancy in the pharyngeal fossa
   C. Infection with streptococcus
   D. Aspiration, even if the gag reflex is present

4. Acute airway obstruction is a situation that should be
   A. reassessed during the next visit.
   B. evaluated within 8 hours.
   C. further assessed thoroughly.
   D. quickly assessed and treated.

5. Risk factors for nose, sinus, mouth, and throat problems include
   A. topical decongestant use, smoking, and allergies.
   B. smoking, allergies, and high blood cholesterol.
   C. allergies, high blood cholesterol, and topical decongestant use.
   D. high blood cholesterol, topical decongestant use, and smoking.

6. The nurse has assessed the nose and documents expected findings as
   A. nose asymmetrical with clear drainage
   B. nose symmetrical and midline
   C. nose asymmetrical and proportional to facial features
   D. nose symmetrical with yellow drainage

7. The nurse is assessing a patient who has been taking antibiotics for 10 days. Oral assessment is important because of the increased risk for which of the following?
   A. Fordyce granules
   B. Pharyngitis
   C. Anosmia
   D. *C. albicans*

8. An adolescent male presents with complaints of nosebleeds. The nurse would further assess for
   A. hemangioma.
   B. nasal trauma.
   C. angiofibroma.
   D. cystic fibrosis.

9. The nurse assesses the child with purulent, unilateral nasal discharge. The nurse knows that the most likely causative factor is
   A. allergic rhinitis.
   B. choanal atresia.
   C. foreign body in nose.
   D. cystic fibrosis.

10. During routine physical examination of a 20-year-old woman, the nurse notes a septal perforation. This finding may be significant for which of the following causes?
   A. Illicit drug use
   B. Nose picking
   C. Nasal trauma
   D. Bifid uvula

The Jensen suite offers these additional resources to enhance learning and facilitate understanding of this chapter:

- thePoint online resource, http://thepoint.lww.com/Jensen2e
- *Laboratory Manual for Nursing Health Assessment: A Best Practice Approach*
- *Pocket Guide for Nursing Health Assessment: A Best Practice Approach*
- *Lippincott DocuCare*, an electronic health record simulation software, http://thepoint.lww.com/docucare
- *Adaptive Learning | Powered by PrepU*, http://thepoint.lww.com/prepu

References

American Cancer Society. (2012). *Cancer facts and figures 2012.* Retrieved from http://www.cancer.org/Research/CancerFactsFigures/cancer-facts-figures-2012

American College of Chest Physicians. (2013). *Chronic upper airway cough syndrome*. Retrieved from http://www.g-i-n.net/library/health-topics-collection/guidelines/chest-us/chronic-upper-airway-cough-syndrome-secondary-to

Andresen, H., Hickey, M., Higgins, T., et al. (2008). Normal anatomy and physiology. In L. Harris & M. Huntoon (Eds.), *Core curriculum for otorhinolaryngology and head-neck nursing* (2nd ed., pp. 41–77). New Smyrna Beach, FL: Society of Otorhinolaryngology and Head-Neck Nurses.

Bailey, W. (2012). Improving dental care: The intersection of public and private practice. *Journal of Evidence Base Dental Practice, 12,* 50–52.

Baroody, F. M. (2011). How nasal function influences the eyes, ears, sinuses, and lungs. *Proceedings of the American Thoracic Society*, *8*(1), 53–61.

Benson, E., Li, R., Eisele, D., & Fakhry, C. (2014). The clinical impact of HPV tumor status upon head and neck cancer. *Oral Oncology, 50,* 565–574. doi:10.1016/j.oraloncology.2013.09.008

Bennett, W. B. (2013). Images in clinical medicine: Torus palatinus. *New England Journal of Medicine, 368,* 1434. doi:10.1056/NEJMicm1205313

Bent, S. (2008). Herbal medicine in the United States: Review of efficacy, safety, and regulation: Grand rounds at University of California, San Francisco Medical Center. *Journal of General Internal Medicine*, *23*(6), 854–859.

Bulechek, G. M., Butcher, H. K., Dochterman, J. M., & Wagner, C. M., (2013). *Nursing interventions classification (NIC)* (6th ed.) St. Louis, MO: Mosby.

Callaway, C. (2011). Rethinking the head and neck cancer population: The human papillomavirus association. *Clinical Journal of Oncology Nursing*, *15*(2)165–170.

Chalmers, J. M., King, P. L., Spencer, A. J., Wright, F. A., & Carter, K. D. (2005). The oral health assessment tool—Validity and reliability. *Australian Dental Journal*, *50*(3), 191–199.

Chaturvedi, A. K., Anderson, W. F., Lortet-Tieulent, J., Curado, M. P., Ferlay, J., Franceschi, S., . . . Gillison, M. L. (2013). Worldwide trends in incidence rates for oral cavity and oropharyngeal cancers. *Journal of Clinical Oncology, 31,*1–10.

Dixon, M. J., Marazita, L., Beaty, T. H., & Murray J. C. (2011). Cleft lip and palate: Understanding genetic and environmental influences. *Nature Reviews. Genetics, 12,* 167–178. doi:10.1038/nrg2933

Epstein, J. (2007). Oral malignancies associated with HIV. *Journal of the Canadian Dental Association, 73*(10), 953–956. Retrieved from http://www.cda-adc.ca/jcda/vol-73/issue-10/953.html

Farris, C., & Petitte, D. M. (2013). Head, neck, and oral cancer update. *Home Health Nurse, 31*(6), 322–328.

Franz, J., & Polsdorfer, J. (2006). Nosebleed. In *Gale's encyclopedia of children's health: Infancy through adolescence*. Retrieved from http://www.encyclopedia.com/topic/nosebleed.aspx

Jemal, A., Simard, E., Dorell, C., Noone, A., Markowitz, L., Kohler, B., . . . Edwards, B. (2013). Annual report to the nation on the status of cancer, 1975-2009, featuring the burden and trends in human papillomavirus (hpv)-associated cancers and HPV vaccination coverage levels. *Journal of the National Cancer Institute.*, *105*(3), 175–201.

Jiron, J., Sethi, S., Rouba, A., Franceshchi, S., Struijk, L., Doorn, L., . . . Kato, I. (2013). Racial disparities in human papillomavirus (HPV) associated head and neck cancer. *American Journal of Otolaryngology, 35*(2), 147–153. doi:10:1016/jamjoto.2013.09.004

Langlais, R. P., & Miller, C. S. (2009). *Color atlas of common oral diseases* (4th ed.). Philadelphia, PA: Lippincott Williams & Wilkins.

Lloyd, K. B., and Naclerio, R. M. (2008). Strategies for managing nasal congestion. *Post graduate healthcare education,* LLC. Philadelphia: Glaxo Smith Kline.

Mayo Clinic Staff. (2011). *Chewing tobacco: Not a risk-free alternative to cigarettes*. Retrieved from http://www.mayoclinic.org/chewing-tobacco/art-20047428

Moorhead, S., Johnson, M., Maas, M. L., & Swanson, E. (2013). *Nursing outcomes classification (NOC): Measurement of health outcomes* (5th ed.). St. Louis, MO: Elsevier

NANDA International. (2012). *Nursing diagnoses: Definitions and classification 2012-2014* (9th ed). Oxford, United Kingdom: Wiley-Blackwell.

National Center for Complementary and Alternative Medicine. (2013). *Echinacea*. Retrieved from http://nccam.nih.gov/health/echinacea

Nettina, S. M. (2009). *Lippincott manual of nursing practice* (9th ed.). Philadelphia, PA: Lippincott Williams & Wilkins.

Padilla, R., & Ritter, A. (2008). *Talking with patients about meth mouth: Methamphetamine and oral health*. Chapel Hill, NC: University of North Carolina School of Dentistry.

Saxby, A., Pace-Asciak, P., Dar Santos, R., Chadha, N., & Kozak, F. (2013). The rhinological manifestations of women's health. *Otolaryngology—Head and Neck Surgery, 148*(5), 717–731

Silva, B. M., Hosman, A. E., Devlin, H. L., & Shovlin, C. L. (2013). Lifestyle and dietary influences on nosebleed severity in hereditary hemorrhagic telangiectasia. *Laryngoscope, 123*, 1092–1099.

Taub, L. F. (2012). *Oral health assessment of older adults: The Kayser-Jones Brief Oral Health Status Examination (BOHSE)*. Retrieved from http://consultgerirn.org/uploads/File/trythis/try_this_18.pdf

Temesgen, Z. (2011). Introduction to the symposium on antimicrobial therapy. *Mayo Clinic Proceedings, 86*(2), 86–87.

U.S. Department of Health & Human Services. (2013). *2020 Topics & objectives - Objectives A-Z*. Retrieved from http://www.healthypeople.gov/2020/topicsobjectives2020/

World Health Organization. (2013). *Global tuberculosis report 2013*. Retrieved from http://www.who.int/tb/publications/global_report/en/

Zenk, J., Koch, M., Klintworth, N., Konig, B., Konz, K., Gillespie, M., & Iro, H. (2012). Sialendoscopy in the diagnosis and treatment of sialolithiasis: A study on more than 1000 patients. *Otolaryngology—Head and Neck Surgery, 147*(5), 858–863.

Zhu, S., Gamet, A., Lee, M., Cummins, S., Yin, L., & Zoref, L. (2013). The use and perception of electronic cigarettes and snus among the U.S. population. *PLos ONE, 8*(10), e79332. doi:10.1371/journal.pone.0079332

Tables of Abnormal Findings

TABLE 15.6 Common Assessment Findings: Nose and Sinuses

Condition	Description and Risk Factors	Findings and Diagnostic Testing
Epistaxis (Nosebleed) 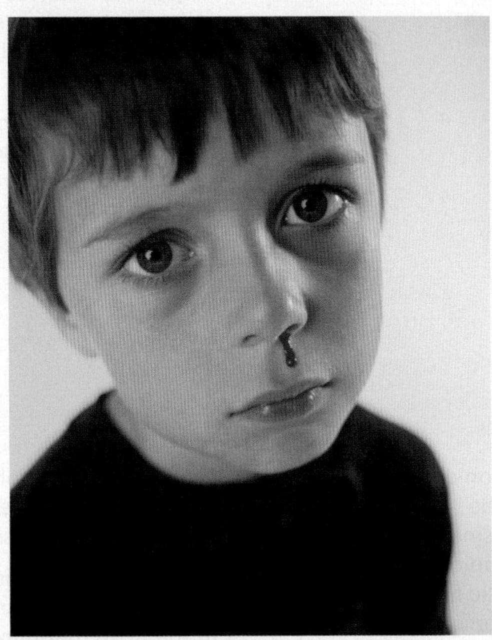 Most commonly involve the Kiesselbach plexus in the anterior septum (Little area), which is vulnerable to trauma, and also the Woodruff plexus under the posterior portion of the inferior turbinate	Increased nasal congestion, dry mucosa, digital manipulation or nose picking, trauma, anticoagulants, foreign bodies, tumors, infection, inflammation, blood or coagulation disorders such as HHT	*Subjective:* Dry sensation or crusting in nose *Objective:* Prominent vessels, scabs, or crusts on anterior septum; blood in nasal vestibule *Testing:* Consider hemoglobin and hematocrit levels with recurrent nosebleeds. Balloon angiography may locate and treat posterior bleeds; intravascular embolization can occlude vessels.
Rhinitis 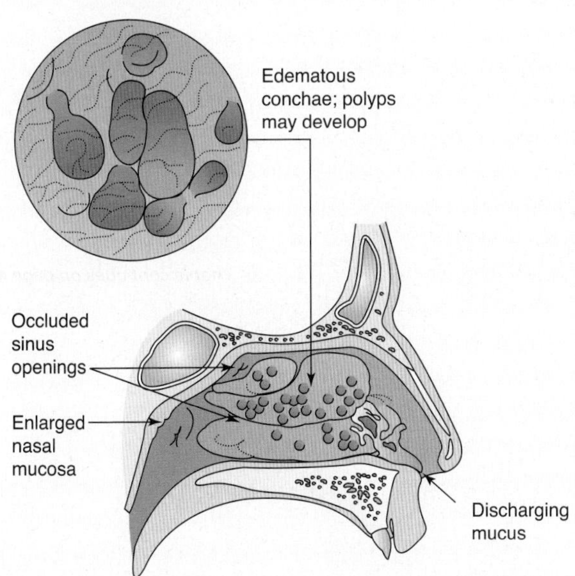 Inflammation of the nasal mucosa; may be subdivided as allergic and nonallergic	Familial or personal atopic disease, exposure to allergens (e.g., pollens, dust, mold, animal dander, food) or chemical irritants (e.g., smoke), use of illicit drugs, overuse of topical decongestant sprays	*Subjective:* Watery, itchy nose with frequent sneezing and congestion *Objective:* Excessive clear watery nasal drainage; pale blue, boggy mucosa or redness and inflammation *Testing:* Specific skin or blood testing (i.e., RAST) measures IgE antibody, which is elevated in atopic disease

(table continues on page 402)

TABLE 15.6 **Common Assessment Findings: Nose and Sinuses** *(continued)*

Condition	Description and Risk Factors	Findings and Diagnostic Testing
Sinusitis 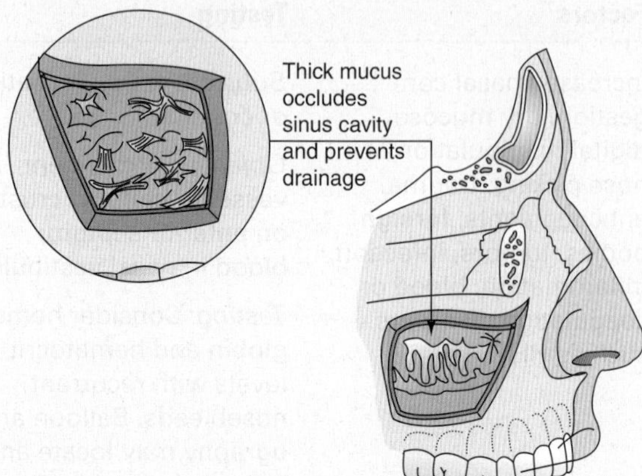 Infection of one or more paranasal sinuses; may be acute or chronic; chronic sinusitis may result in fungal pathology.	Chronic mucosal swelling from allergy, irritants, or chemicals; inflammation secondary to GERD	*Subjective:* Facial pain or pressure, thick nasal discharge, fever, cough, halitosis *Objective:* Redness and inflammation of nasal mucosa; thick purulent drainage *Testing:* Endoscopic examination of nose; CT scan (standard radiographic tool)
Nasal Polyps 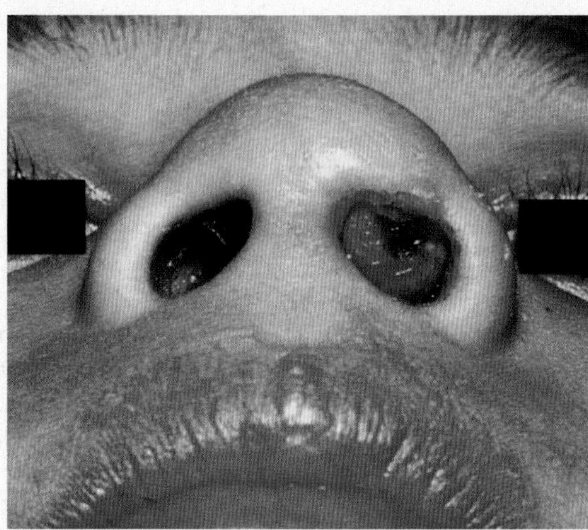 Grapelike swelling of the nasal and sinus mucosa leading to nasal obstruction; often associated with other inflammatory conditions of the nasal mucosa	Chronic inflammation of the nose and paranasal sinuses, allergic or chronic rhinitis, asthma, cystic fibrosis, and chronic sinusitis	*Subjective:* Nasal obstruction and congestion, facial pain and pressure *Objective:* White glistening grapelike structures in the nose that may also fill the sinus cavities *Testing:* Nasal/sinus endoscopy, CT scan

(table continues on page 403)

TABLE 15.6 Common Assessment Findings: Nose and Sinuses *(continued)*

Condition	Description and Risk Factors	Findings and Diagnostic Testing
Deviated Septum 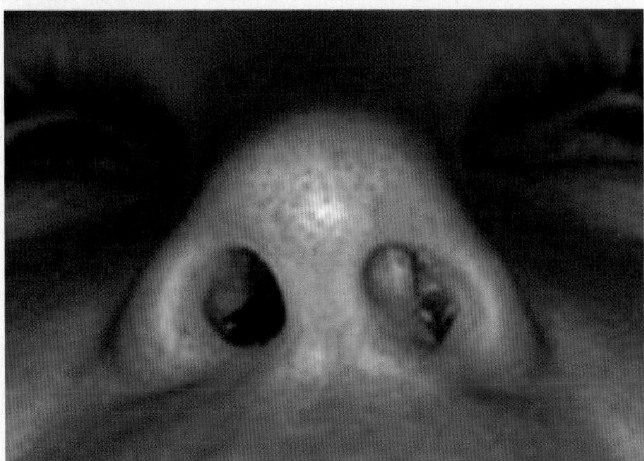 Deflection of the center wall of the nose (septum)	May be congenital or occur due to trauma to the nose	*Subjective:* A unilateral decreased ability to breathe through the nose; pressure or headache *Objective:* Narrowing of the nasal chamber *Testing:* Endoscopy of the nose; x-ray or CT scan
Perforated Septum 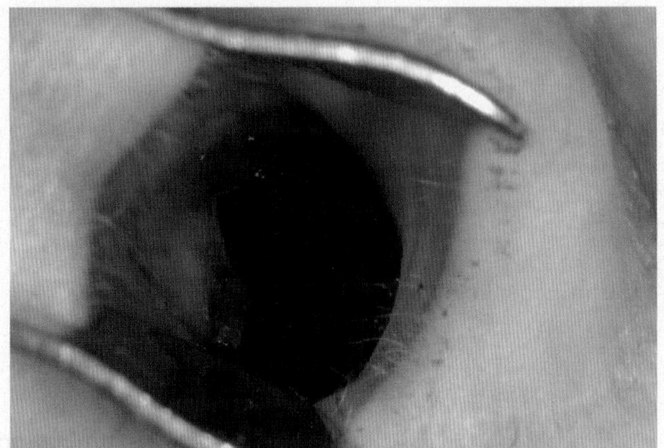 A hole in the nasal septum	Illicit drug use (e.g., snorting cocaine), nasal trauma, nasal septal surgery, digital manipulation or nose picking, chronic epistaxis	*Subjective:* Foul odor, whistling sound, recurrent crusting or bleeding from the nose *Objective:* A hole in the septum, which may have crusting or purulent drainage *Testing:* Endoscopy, direct visualization, or CT scan
Foreign Body 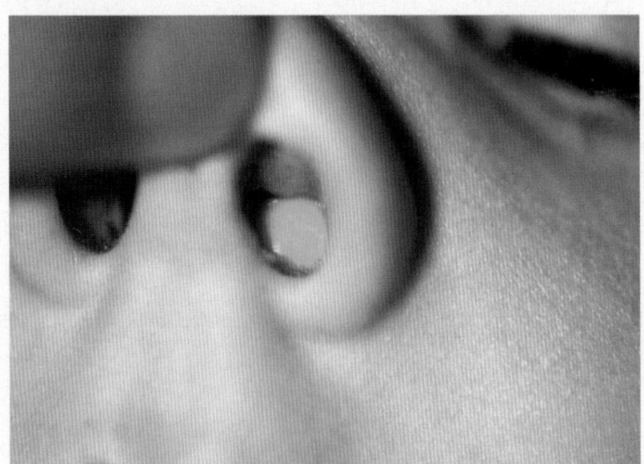 Any object not commonly found in the upper aerodigestive tract	Nasal piercing; deliberately placed objects in nose (as with small children); postsurgical remnant of cotton or gauze	*Subjective:* Unilateral nasal congestion or obstruction *Objective:* Unilateral purulence or thick nasal drainage *Testing:* Endoscopic examination; x-ray of the nose—in small children, examination under anesthesia is typically performed with removal of the foreign body

(table continues on page 404)

TABLE 15.7 **Common Assessment Findings: Palate and Throat**

Condition	Risk Factors	Findings and Diagnostic Testing
Cleft Lip/Palate 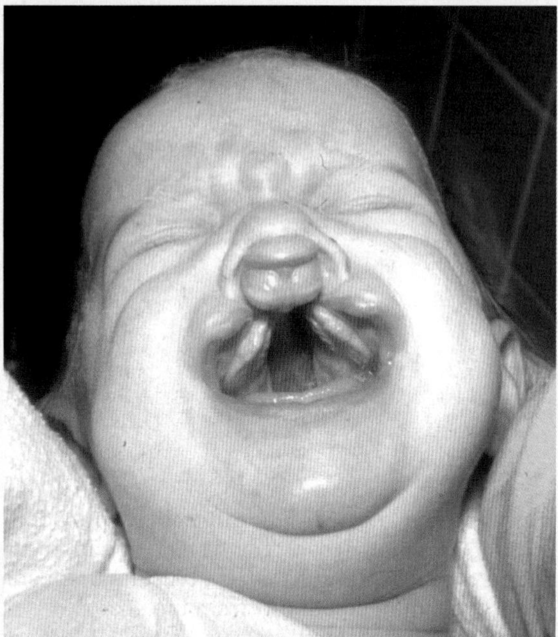 Most common congenital malformation of oral cavity (1 in 1,000 births); an opening or fissure of the lip/alveolus and palate; represents a fusion abnormality of the midfacial skeleton and soft tissues	Native American and Asian ancestry; maternal exposure to phenytoin, methotrexate, and cigarette smoke and maternal alcohol abuse	*Subjective:* Recurrent middle ear and sinus infections; feeding difficulties *Objective:* Cleft lip apparent at birth; notch or full opening on hard palate, soft palate, or both *Testing:* Oral/facial examination
Bifid Uvula 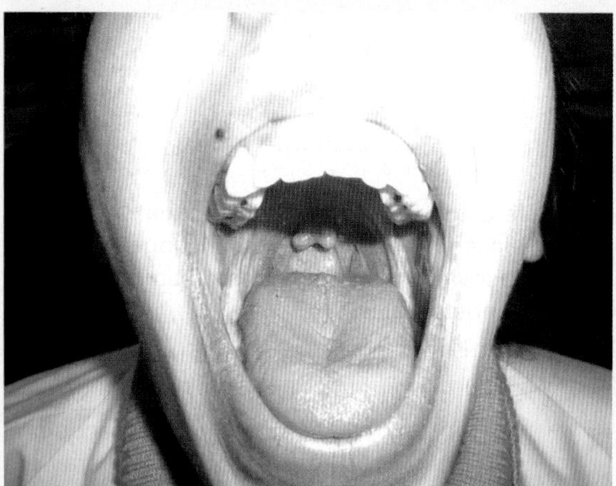 Congenital complete or partial split of uvula; adenoidectomy may be contraindicated	Submucosal cleft palate	*Subjective:* Usually asymptomatic *Objective:* A split or fork visible in uvula *Testing:* Oral examination

(table continues on page 405)

Condition	Risk Factors	Findings and Diagnostic Testing
Kaposi Sarcoma 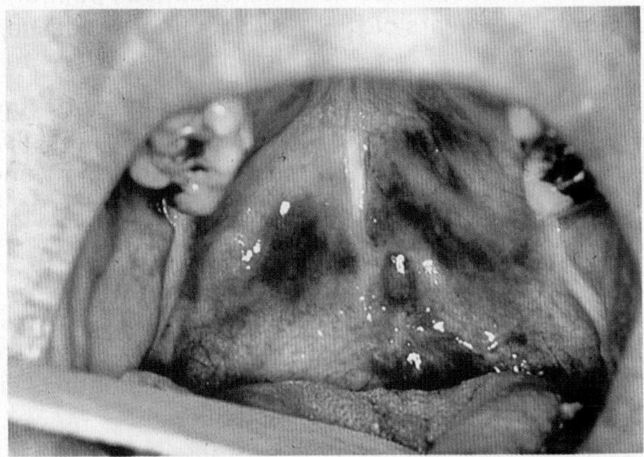 Rapidly proliferating malignancy of the skin or mucous membranes; oral involvement includes the tongue, gingiva, and palate	HIV; 5–10 times greater in male homosexuals infected with HIV than others with the illness (Epstein, 2007)	*Subjective:* Nonhealing oral lesions; may complain of facial lymphedema *Objective:* Bruiselike lesions that form plaques and progress into nodular, red-purple, nonblanching firm lesions *Testing:* Endoscopic examination of nose; chest x-ray, CT scan, or MRI for disease surveillance
Acute Tonsillitis or Pharyngitis 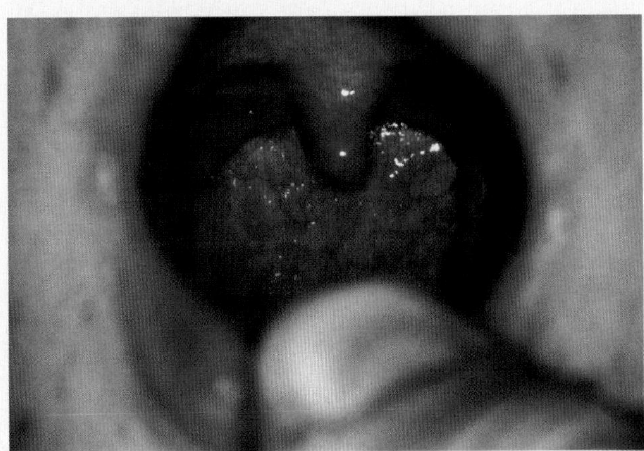 *Pharyngitis*: inflammation of the pharyngeal walls; may include tonsils, palate, uvula *Tonsillitis:* inflammation in lymphoid tissue of oropharynx including Waldeyer ring, palatine or lingual tonsils, pharyngeal bands, nasopharynx, adenoids	Beta-hemolytic streptococcus; may be viral; smoking; mouth breathing	*Subjective:* Sore throat, malaise, anorexia, headache, dysphagia, increased postnasal secretions *Objective:* Infection, redness of pharyngeal walls, exudate, fever, rash; in severe cases, airway obstruction *Testing*: Throat culture; complete blood count (CBC) with differential to determine whether pathogen is viral or bacterial

(table continues on page 406)

TABLE 15.7 Common Assessment Findings: Palate and Throat *(continued)*

Condition	Risk Factors	Findings and Diagnostic Testing
Strep Throat 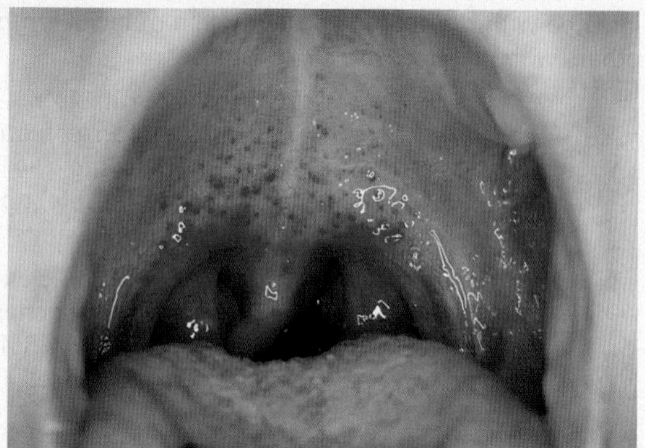 Infection of the tonsils involving *Streptococcus* bacterium	Exposure to infected individuals; most common in children 5-15 years old	*Subjective:* Sore throat, chills, difficult painful swallowing, headache, laryngitis *Objective:* Infection and enlargement of tonsils; enlargement of jaw and neck lymph nodes *Testing:* Rapid strep swab, throat culture, monospot test, CBC with differential to determine whether pathogen is viral or bacterial
Torus Palatinus 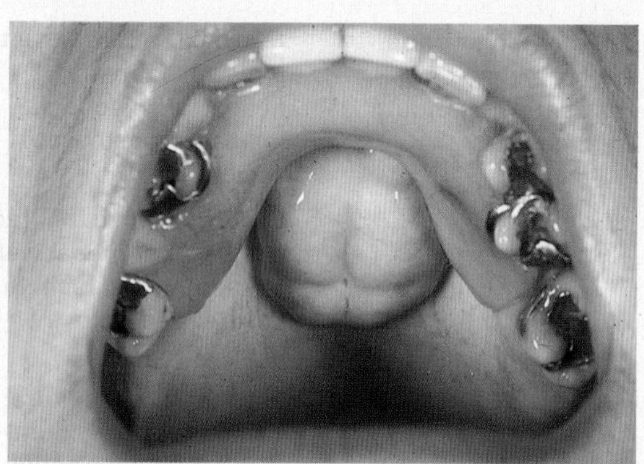 A bony prominence in the middle of the hard palate	Congenital; no clinical significance	Presence of a hard raised bump on palate

TABLE 15.8 Common Assessment Findings: Lips and Tongue

Condition	Risk Factors	Findings and Diagnostic Testing
Herpes Simplex Virus 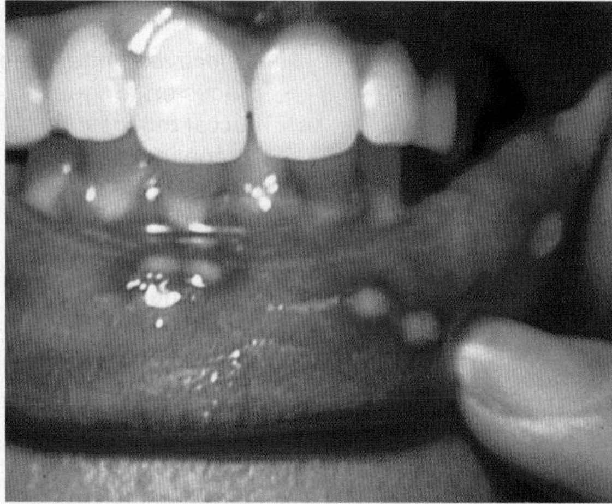 Clear vesicular lesions with indurated base caused by herpes simplex 1 virus	Direct contact with infected person, fever, colds, allergies; may be precipitated by sunlight exposure	*Subjective:* Painful oral lesions; frequently appears at lip–skin juncture *Objective:* Lesions evolve into pustules that rupture, weep, and crust; typical course is 4–10 days *Testing:* Typically none recommended, but may culture persistent lesions
Aphthous Ulcers (Canker Sores) 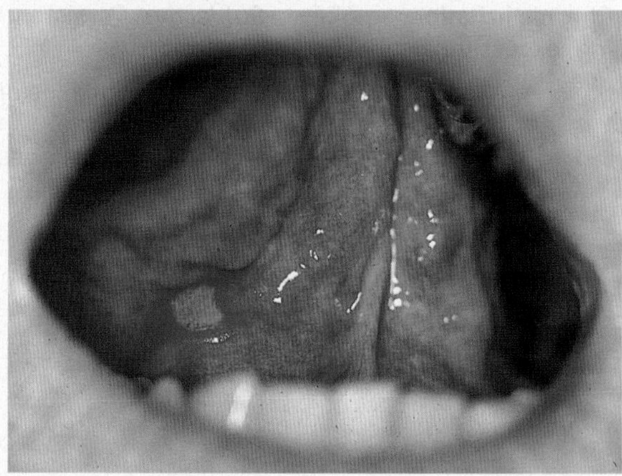 Vesicular oral lesion that evolves into a white ulceration with a red margin	Stress, fatigue, allergies, autoimmune disorders	*Subjective:* Pain at and around site *Objective:* Visible oral lesion(s) *Testing:* Typically not recommended, but may culture persistent lesions

(table continues on page 408)

TABLE 15.8 **Common Assessment Findings: Lips and Tongue** *(continued)*

Condition	Risk Factors	Findings and Diagnostic Testing
Candidiasis 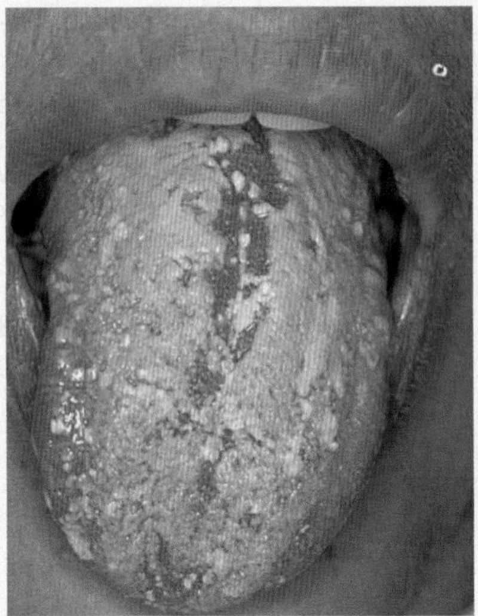 Opportunistic yeast infection of the buccal mucosa and tongue	May occur in newborns; antibiotic or corticosteroid therapy; immunosuppression	*Subjective:* White sticky mucus on tongue or oral mucosa *Objective:* White, cheesy mucus on tongue or buccal mucosa; may scrape mucus off but tissue is raw and vascular beneath *Testing:* No specific recommendation; consider immune compromise workup in recurrent infections
Leukoplakia 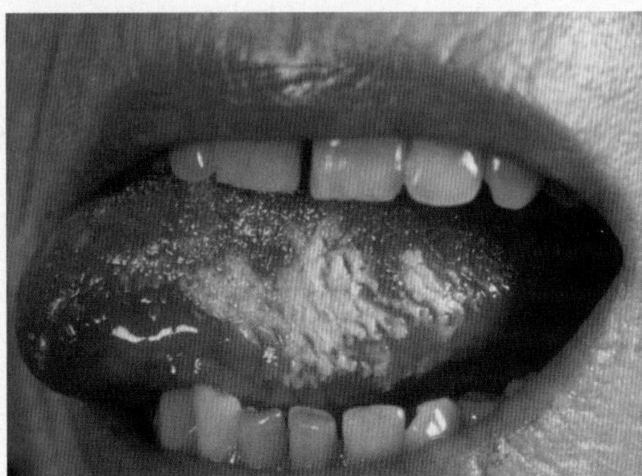 White patchy lesions with well-defined borders	Chronic irritation, smoking, excessive alcohol use	*Subjective:* Persistent oral lesion *Objective:* White lesion firmly attached to mucosal surface; does not scrape off *Testing:* May require biopsy

(table continues on page 409)

TABLE 15.8 Common Assessment Findings: Lips and Tongue *(continued)*

Condition	Risk Factors	Findings and Diagnostic Testing
Black Hairy Tongue 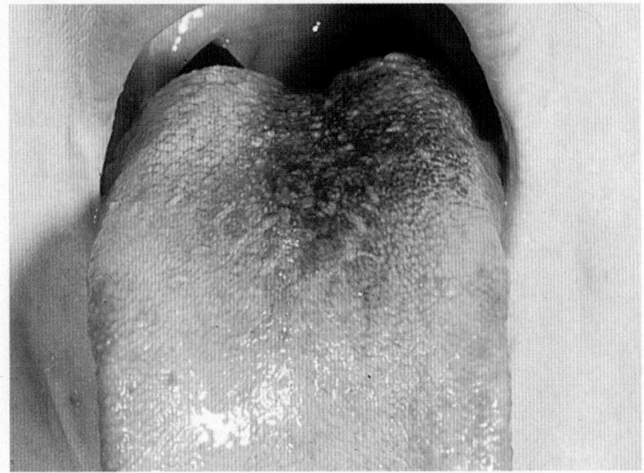 Fungal infection of the tongue involving elongation of the papillae	May follow antibiotic therapy; immunocompromised status	*Subjective:* Brown/black hairy coating on tongue *Objective:* Black/brown hairy appearance from elongation of papillae with a painless overgrowth of fungus *Testing:* None recommended
Carcinoma 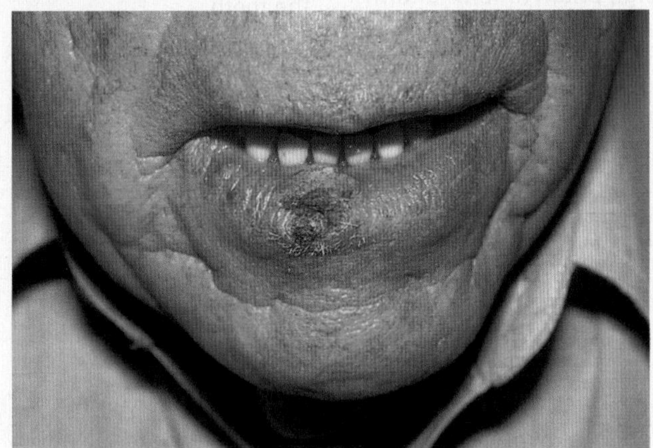 An initially indurated lesion with rolled irregular edges; later may crust or scab but does not heal	Tobacco use, heavy alcohol consumption, chemical exposure	*Subjective:* A lesion that may be painful or limit mobility of the tongue *Objective:* Initially, indurated lesion with rolled irregular edges; later appears crusty; possible swelling in adjacent lymph nodes *Testing:* Biopsy

(table continues on page 410)

TABLE 15.9 Common Assessment Findings: Gums and Teeth

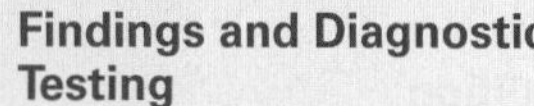

Condition	Risk Factors	Findings and Diagnostic Testing
Dental Caries 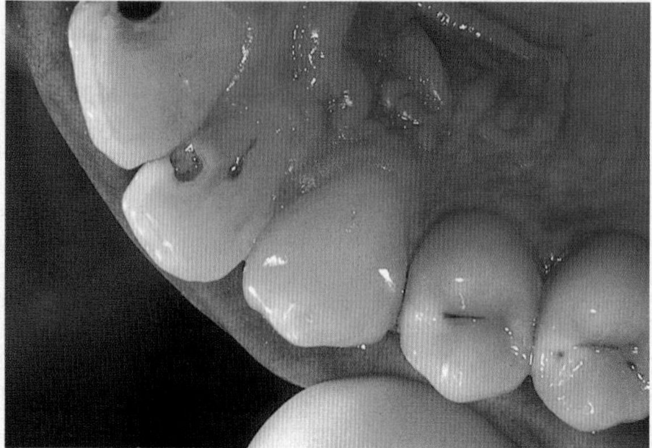 Progressive destruction of tooth	Poor oral hygiene	*Subjective:* Early, no complaints; with further destruction, pain with hot and cold substances *Objective:* Early, may appear chalky white; later becomes brown or black and forms a cavity *Testing:* Dental x-ray
Gingival Hyperplasia 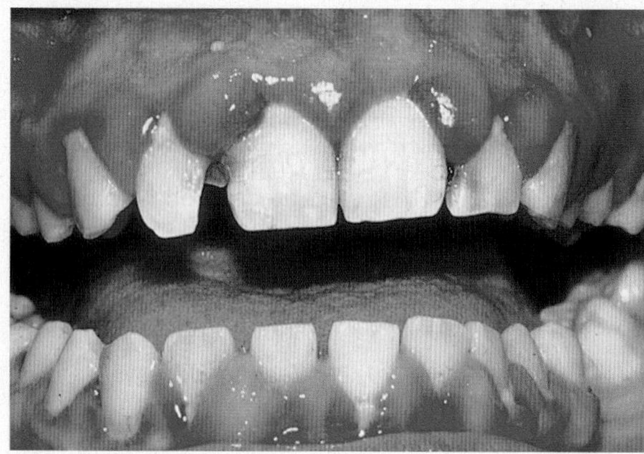 Painless enlargement of the gums	May accompany states of hormonal fluctuation (e.g., puberty, pregnancy); leukemia; adverse effect of drugs (e.g., phenytoin [Dilantin])	*Subjective:* Swelling of gums *Objective:* Enlargement of gum tissue; may overreach the teeth *Testing:* Dental x-ray
Gingivitis 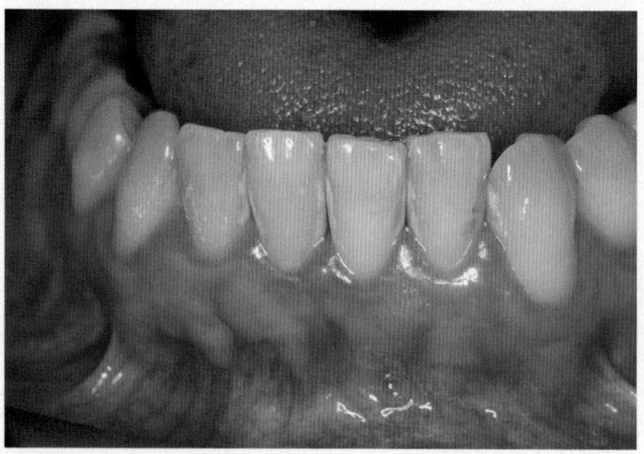 Painful, red, swollen gums	Poor oral hygiene, hormonal fluctuations, vitamin B deficiency	*Subjective:* Sore, bleeding gums *Objective:* Red, swollen, possibly bleeding gums; may involve desquamation of gingival tissue *Testing:* Dental x-ray

(table continues on page 411)

TABLE 15.9 Common Assessment Findings: Gums and Teeth *(continued)*

Condition	Risk Factors	Findings and Diagnostic Testing
Ankyloglossia (Tongue-tie) 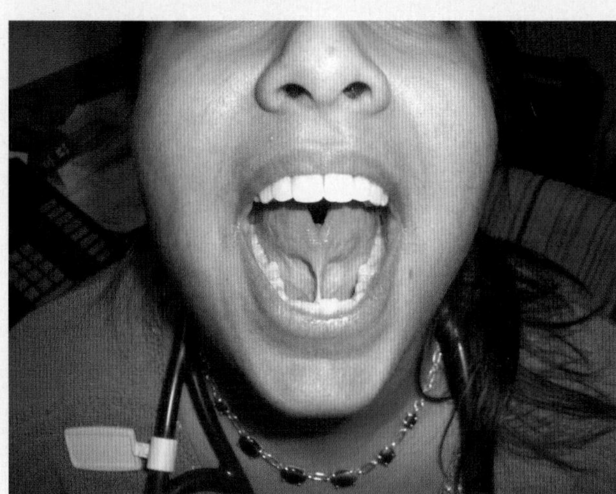 A shortened lingual frenulum	Congenital defect	*Subjective:* Limited movement of tongue; speech disruption, particularly with a, d, and n sounds *Objective:* A tight frenulum fixing the tongue to the floor of mouth *Testing:* None recommended

16

Thorax and Lung Assessment

Learning Objectives

1. Demonstrate knowledge of the anatomy and physiology of the respiratory system.
2. Identify important topics for health promotion and risk reduction related to the respiratory system.
3. Collect subjective data related to the respiratory system using appropriate interviewing techniques.
4. Collect objective data related to the respiratory system using accurate physical examination techniques.
5. Identify expected and unexpected findings related to the respiratory system.
6. Identify expected and unexpected breath sounds including crackles, wheezes, gurgles, and stridor.
7. Analyze subjective and objective data from assessment of the respiratory system, consider need for immediate intervention, and cluster the data to identify patterns.
8. Document and communicate data from the respiratory system assessment using appropriate terminology and clinical reasoning.
9. Consider age, condition, gender, and culture of the patient to individualize the respiratory assessment.
10. Identify nursing diagnoses and initiate a plan of care based on findings from the respiratory assessment.

Mr. Lee, a 65-year-old Chinese man, has come to the clinic today reporting increasing shortness of breath and fatigue. Mandarin is his first language; however, he speaks English with only a slight accent and has a well-developed vocabulary and fluent pacing. He has smoked two packs of cigarettes a day for 49 years. Mr. Lee has a history of chronic obstructive pulmonary disease (COPD), congestive heart failure (CHF), and high blood pressure. He states that he has been using his prescribed albuterol and ipratropium inhalers, but for the last few days, his breathing has gotten worse.

You will gain more information about Mr. Lee as you progress through this chapter. As you study the content and features, consider Mr. Lee's case and its relationship to what you are learning. Begin thinking about the following points:

- Why is the sternal angle (angle of Louis) an important landmark for assessment of the thorax?
- What subjective data collected are cause for concern?
- What health promotion and teaching needs are identified for Mr. Lee?
- Is Mr. Lee's condition stable, urgent, or something requiring immediate attention?
- How will the nurse individualize assessment to meet Mr. Lee's specific needs, considering his condition, age, and culture?
- How will the nurse evaluate the success of patient teaching for Mr. Lee?

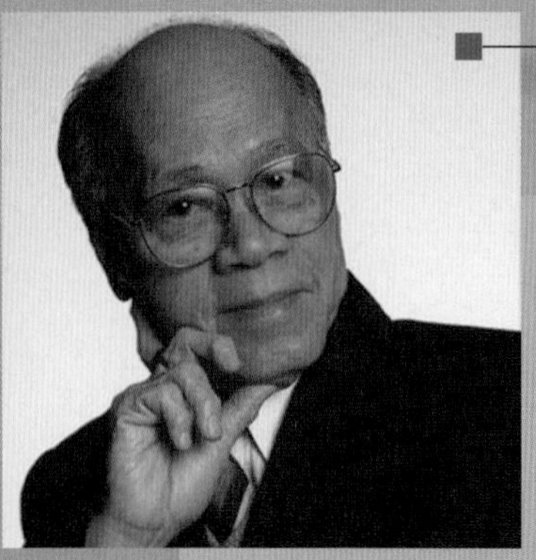

This chapter explores assessment of the thorax and lungs. It reviews pertinent anatomy and physiology related to respiratory and pulmonary function as well as key variations based on lifespan, culture, and environment. The chapter explores methods for collecting subjective data about risks for pulmonary disease, such as cigarette smoking, environmental and occupational exposures, and family history of respiratory-related disorders. It reviews specific respiratory symptoms, such as shortness of breath, coughing, and chest discomfort. Content about objective data describes the correct techniques for assessing breathing patterns, identifying expected and unexpected breath sounds, and labeling findings so you can document them accurately.

Auscultation of the lungs is performed during a complete physical examination and in ongoing assessment of patients with diagnosed respiratory disorders or diseases. Although challenging, lung auscultation provides important information to assist you in identifying accurate nursing diagnoses, patient outcomes, and nursing interventions. Auscultation of the lungs can also help you to identify life-threatening problems requiring immediate interventions.

Structure and Function

Structurally, the respiratory system is divided into upper and lower portions. The upper portion warms, moisturizes, and transports air to the lower portion, where oxygenation and ventilation occur (Moini, 2012).

Understanding the anatomy of the thoracic cage and how to use its landmarks to identify underlying structures is essential when conducting a physical examination and documenting your findings for the respiratory system. In addition, this knowledge is required for you to accurately document your findings when examining the heart as well as the anterior, lateral, and posterior thoracic areas of the integumentary system. Thorough knowledge of the location and lobes of the lungs and other vital structures within the pulmonary system, along with understanding the physiology of respiration, enhances your ability to accurately assess and interpret findings of the thoracic and lung regions.

The Thorax

The thorax is one of the most dynamic regions of the body because it is constantly in motion (Moore, Dalley, & Agur, 2014). See Figure 16.1 for the surface anatomy of the thorax in men and women.

The bony thoracic cage includes the sternum and clavicle anteriorly, scapulae and 12 vertebrae posteriorly, and 12 pairs of ribs encircling the thoracic cage. The thoracic cavity contains three main compartments. The mediastinum is the central compartment, located in the middle of the thoracic cavity, and contains the heart, great vessels, lymph nodes, nerves, and fat (see Fig. 16.9). Other structures within the thoracic cavity include the thymus, the distal part of the trachea, and most of the esophagus. The other two compartments contain the lungs (Moore et al., 2014). The thoracic nerves (T1–T12) each supply a surrounding area of skin horizontally, following dermatome patterns (see Chapter 22). The phrenic nerve innervates the diaphragm, and the intercostal nerves innervate the intercostal muscles (Moini, 2012). The thoracic muscles include the intercostals, transverse thoracic, subcostal, levator costarum, and serratus posterior

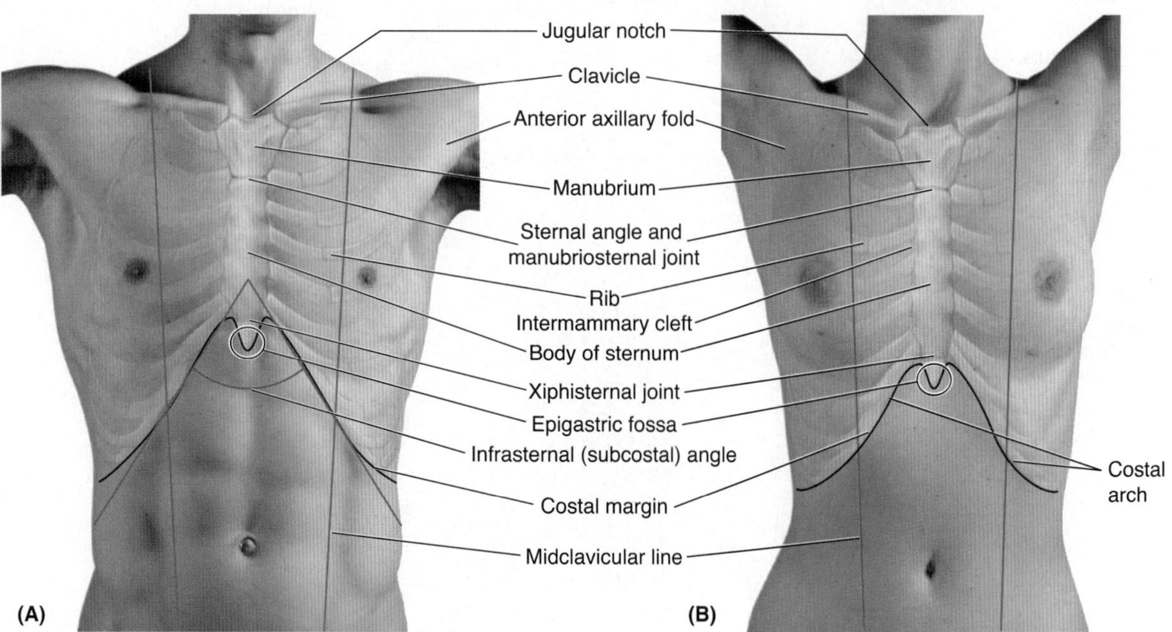

Figure 16.1 Surface anatomy of the thorax in adult men **(A)** and women **(B)**. Note how the lines go from the center of the clavicle to the middle of the chest. This is nonspecific and varies among gender, age, and characteristics of the patient. Every patient has a unique chest and is always interesting to assess because there are so many important body structures contained in it.

(Moore et al., 2014). Arterial blood supply to the chest comes from the thoracic aorta and from the subclavian, brachial, and axillary arteries; numerous veins return blood to the heart. The two pulmonary arteries carry deoxygenated blood from the right side of the heart to each lung, where gas exchange occurs, whereas two pulmonary veins return oxygenated blood to the left side of the heart for circulation to the rest of the body (Moore et al., 2014).

Accurate documentation of findings for the thorax and lungs requires the use of both vertical and horizontal landmarks. The ribs provide vertical reference points, whereas a series of lines provide horizontal reference marks.

Anterior Thoracic Landmarks

The anterior vertical landmarks are the ribs and their associated interspaces. The easiest location to begin is the suprasternal (jugular) notch (Fig. 16.2). This U-shaped depression lies just above the sternum and between the clavicles. To locate the suprasternal notch, place your fingers on your sternum and walk them up until you feel the notch. An alternate method is to lightly place your fingers on your trachea and move them down until you feel the notch. From the suprasternal notch, walk your fingers down approximately 4 to 5 cm to the bony ridge where the manubrium attaches to the sternum. This ridge, called the **sternal angle** (also known as the **angle of Louis** or **sternomanubrial angle**), varies in prominence and is usually easier to locate in thinner people. The sternal angle is continuous with the 2nd rib. It also marks the site of the apex of the heart as well as the location where the trachea branches (bifurcates) into the right and left main stem bronchi (Moore et al., 2014). This area of bifurcation is known as the **carina** (Porth, 2011).

> **Clinical Significance**
>
> The carina is also the site of the cough reflex. Patients who need nasotracheal suctioning will cough when the nasotracheal tube reaches the carina (approximately the 2nd rib space).

Landmarks on the rib cage are identified by the **intercostal space** (ICS) below each rib. Slide your fingers from the sternal angle laterally to the 2nd rib and then down where you will feel an indentation; this is the 2nd ICS. Each ICS is named for the rib directly above it (Moore et al., 2014). Take a moment to make sure that you can identify the bony raised rib and sunken rib space. From the second ICS, walk another finger approximately 3 cm down the chest wall to the 3rd ICS. Continue to "walk" your fingers down, keeping one finger in the rib space and using a second to locate the next rib space (see Fig. 16.2). In women, it may be necessary to displace the breast laterally (or ask the patient to displace it) or stay closer to the sternum to avoid breast tissue. Avoid pressing tender breast tissue too hard.

The 2nd through 6th ribs are easy to count because they articulate directly with the sternum. However, below the

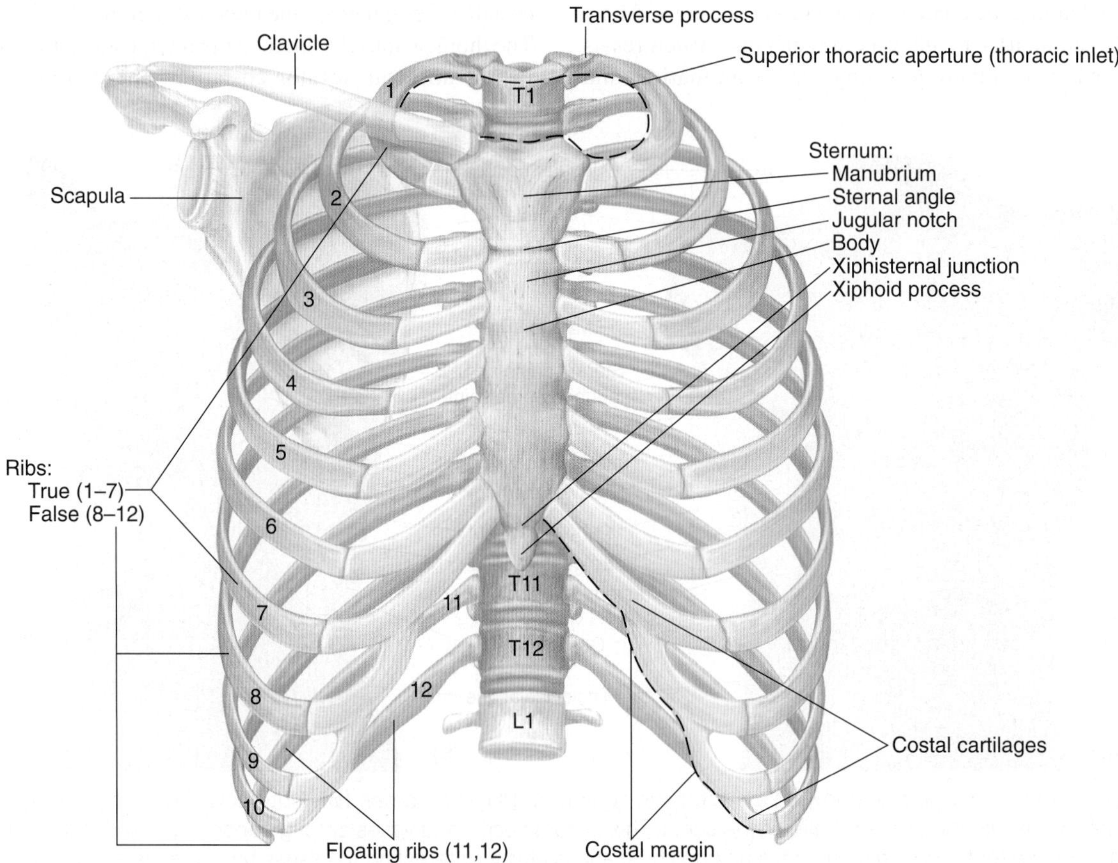

Figure 16.2 Landmarks of the thoracic cage, anterior view.

6th rib, it becomes more difficult to count them. This is because the 6th and 7th ribs lie side by side, articulating at the lowest area of the sternum, so the 6th ICS is not palpable near the sternum. Another factor making it difficult to count ribs below the 6th and 7th is that the costal cartilages of the 8th through 10th ribs each articulate with the rib above it rather than the sternum. Therefore, you must slide your fingers laterally below the 6th rib until you feel the 6th ICS (see Fig. 16.2). For example, if you slide your fingers laterally on the right side of the chest, you can easily feel the 6th ICS midway between the sternal area and the right axilla. At this point, you can walk your fingers down, laterally on an oblique line, to the 10th rib anteriorly. The 11th and 12th ribs, known as the "floating ribs," do not articulate with any structure anteriorly (Hogan-Quigley, Palm, & Bickley, 2012).

The angle between the ribs at the costal margins forms the **costal angle**, located at the bottom of the sternum at the xiphoid process. The costal angle is usually 90 degrees or less.

> **Clinical Significance**
>
> During cardiorespiratory resuscitation (CPR), hands are placed above the xiphoid process to avoid breaking it off from the sternum and causing complications, such as pneumothorax, hemothorax, or liver injury.

Posterior Thoracic Landmarks

It is more difficult to palpate the ribs posteriorly because of the overlying musculature. On the posterior thorax, the ribs articulate with their respective thoracic vertebrae. Therefore, the ribs are located indirectly by palpating the spinous processes of their vertebrae (Weber & Kelley, 2014).

Flex your neck forward to feel the vertebral spinous processes. The spinous process that protrudes the most is usually C7, the 7th cervical vertebra (Fig. 16.3). If two are protruding, the upper one is C7, and the lower one is T1 (Moore et al., 2014). The spinous process of T1 usually correlates with the 1st rib. However, the spinous processes correlate with their respective ribs only to the level of T4 because starting at the level of T5, each spinous process angles down, overlapping the vertebral body below it. An alternate method for identifying the ribs posteriorly is to locate the lower tip of the scapula, which is generally between the 7th and 8th. The tip of the 11th floating rib can be palpated laterally, whereas the tip of the 12th floating rib can be palpated posteriorly (Moore et al., 2014).

Reference Lines

To describe and document findings horizontally on the chest, a series of vertical reference lines is used. On the anterior chest, the midsternal, midclavicular, and anterior axillary lines are used as landmarks and are named for the structural areas they describe (Fig. 16.4). The **midsternal line** runs vertically down the center of the sternum. The bilateral **midclavicular lines** (MCL) are parallel to the midsternal line and extend down from each clavicle midway between the sternoclavicular and acromioclavicular joints. The bilateral **anterior axillary lines** extend down from the top of the anterior axillary fold when the arms are at the sides.

On the posterior thorax, the vertebral and bilateral scapular lines provide landmarks for documenting assessment findings (Fig. 16.5). The **vertebral line** runs vertically down the center of the vertebral spinous processes. The **midscapular lines** are parallel to the vertebral line and run vertically through the middle of each scapula (Bickley & Szilagyi, 2013).

In addition to the previously mentioned anterior axillary line, other lines from a lateral view are identified by their location in the axillary region. The **posterior axillary lines** run vertically along the posterior edge from the top of each axilla down to the lower thoracic area (Moore et al., 2014). The **midaxillary lines** drop from the middle of the axilla running parallel between the anterior and posterior axillary lines (see Fig. 16.6).

Other areas that may be referenced when identifying findings include supraclavicular (above the clavicle), suprascapular and subscapular (above and below the scapula, respectively), and sites medial or lateral to the reference lines.

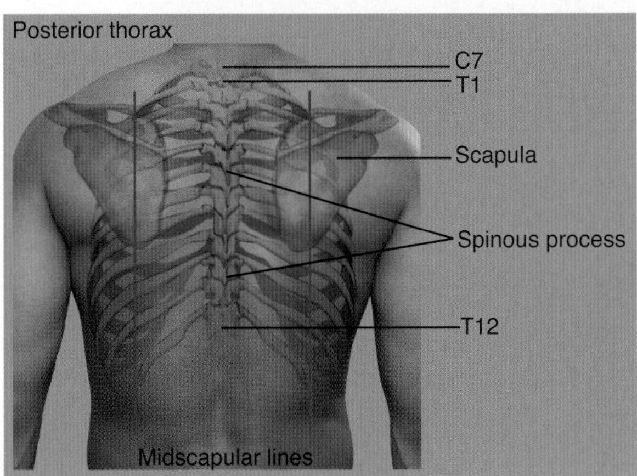

Figure 16.3 Posterior thoracic landmarks.

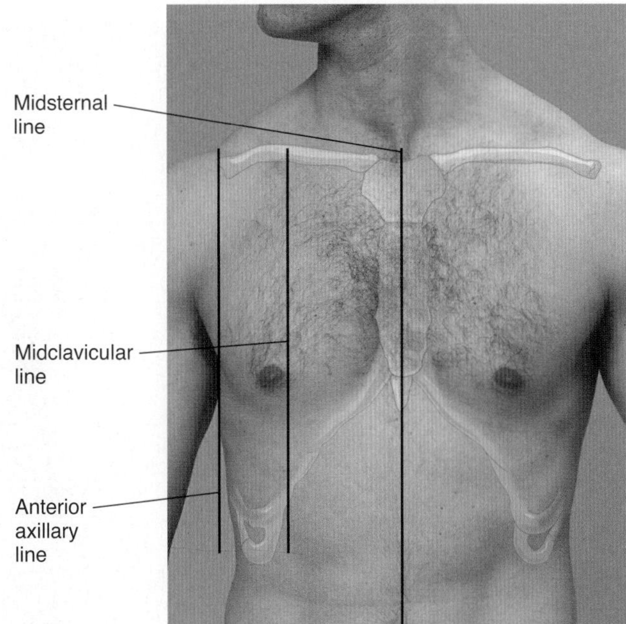

Figure 16.4 Reference lines of the chest, anterior view.

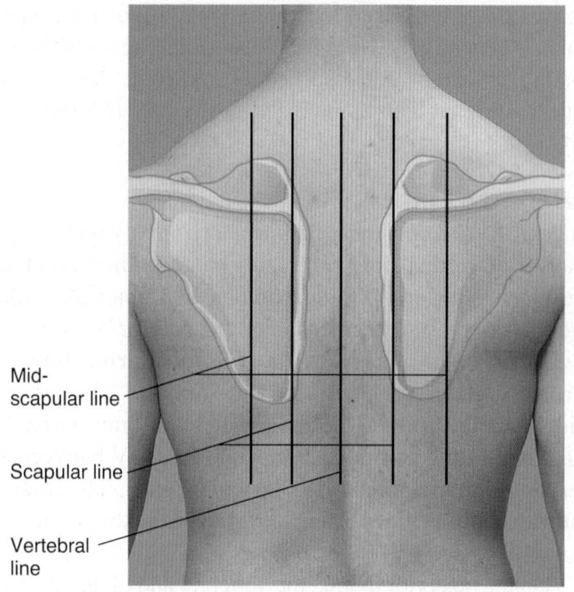

Figure 16.5 Reference lines of the chest, posterior view.

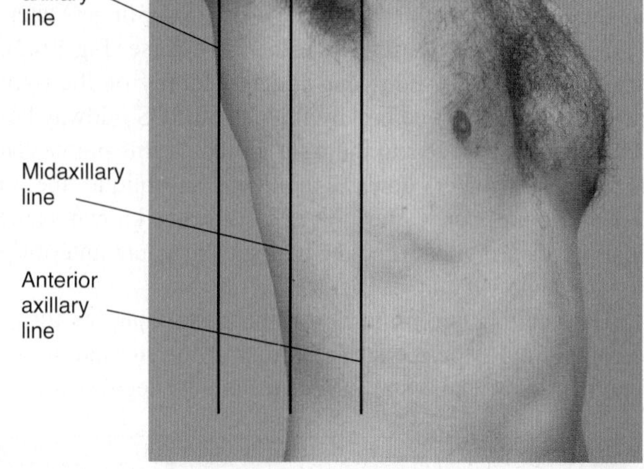

Figure 16.6 Reference lines of the chest, lateral view.

Lobes of the Lungs

The previously described landmarks help identify the approximate location of the lobes of the lungs on the chest wall. Each lung is divided almost in half by an oblique fissure that runs from the 6th rib MCL anteriorly to the T3 spinous process posteriorly (Figs. 16.7A and B). The left lung has two lobes; the right lung has three. The horizontal (minor) fissure divides the right upper and middle lobes of the lung. The right upper lobe (RUL) and right middle lobe (RML), together, are approximately the size of the left upper lobe (LUL). The RML extends from the 4th rib at the sternal border to the 5th rib at the midaxillary line (Fig. 16.8) (Moore et al., 2014). The right lower lobe (RLL) and left lower lobe (LLL) are approximately the same size.

> **Clinical Significance**
>
> It is important to note that the RML is auscultated using an anterior approach, although a small portion of it can be auscultated laterally. Accurate auscultation of the RML can be challenging in women, however, because of its location underlying the right breast.

The lower border of the right lung is approximately 2.5 cm (1 in.) higher than the left because the liver displaces the lung tissue upward. The left lung is narrower than the right because the heart and pericardium bulge to the left, displacing

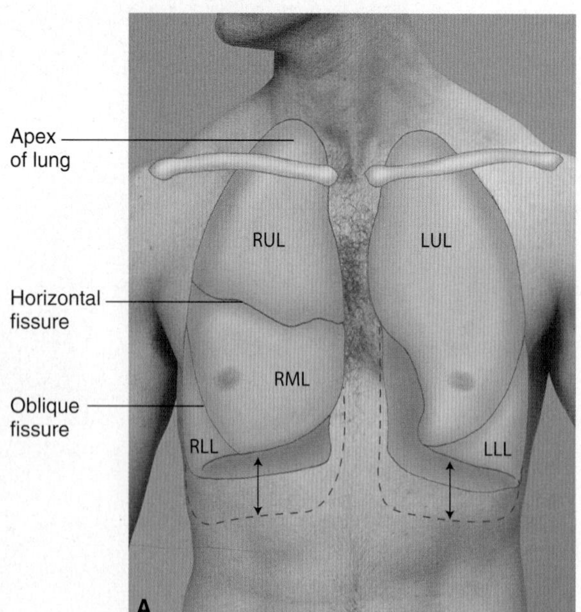

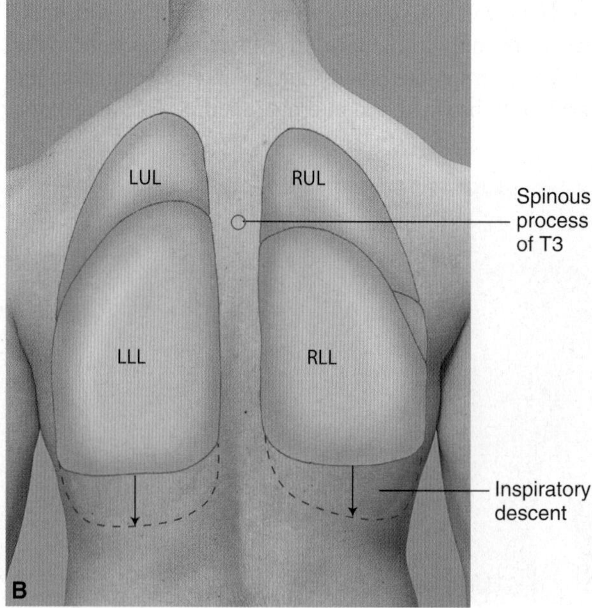

Figure 16.7 Views of the lungs. **A.** Anterior. **B.** Posterior.

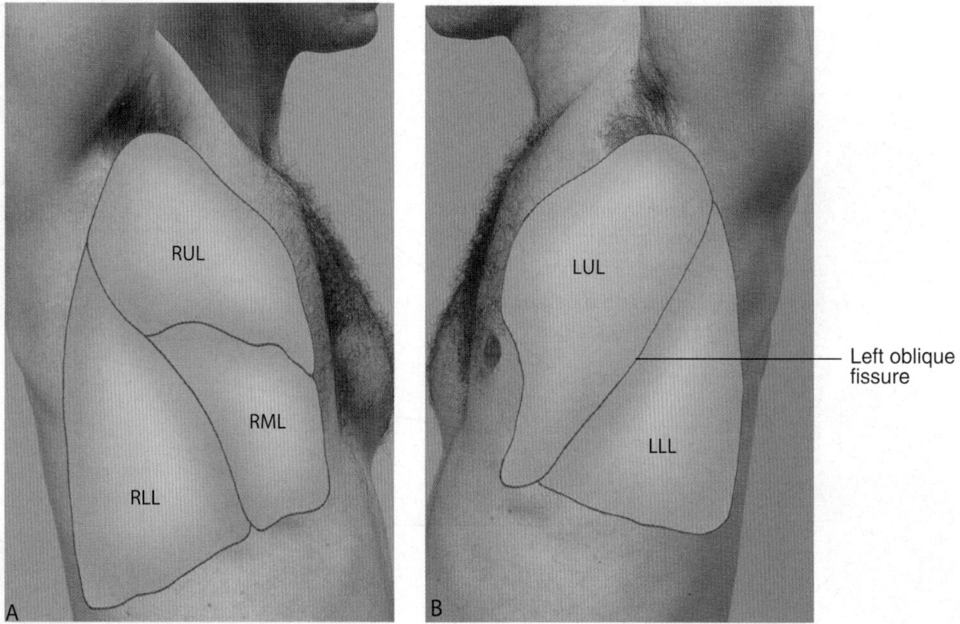

Figure 16.8 Views of the lungs. **A.** Right. **B.** Left.

the lung tissue. You can see from Figures 16.7 and 16.8 why you use an anterior approach when examining the upper lobes and the RML and a posterior approach primarily when assessing the lower lobes of the lung. Portions of all lobes can be evaluated using a lateral approach. These descriptions only approximate the location of the lung lobes, however, so it is more accurate to document findings using chest wall landmarks.

Upper, middle, and lower lung fields are generally separated into approximately equal thirds. The **base** refers to the very bottom of the lung fields; the **apex** is the very top (opposite of the labeling of the heart). Lungs should be auscultated from apex to base. Anteriorly, the apex of each lung rises approximately 2 to 4 cm (about ¾ to 1 ½ in.) above the inner third of the clavicle. Each lung base rests on the diaphragm at the level of the 6th rib in the MCL and the 8th rib in the midaxillary line. Posteriorly, the apex of each lung is near C7, whereas the lower border of each base is near the level of the T10 spinous process (three rib spaces below the inferior tip of the scapula). With deep inspiration, the base descends to about the T12 level (Moore et al., 2014).

> **Clinical Significance**
>
> The apex of each lung rises above the clavicle, where lung sounds may be audible during auscultation of the anterior thorax. When a central venous catheter is being inserted through the chest wall, the needle may accidentally nick the lung apex, causing pneumothorax. Therefore, it is essential to auscultate and compare lung sounds in each apex following this procedure.

Lower Respiratory Tract

The trachea bifurcates at the carina into the right and left mainstem bronchi, and these in turn branch into smaller bronchi one for each lobe of the lungs. These smaller bronchi continue to separate like branches on a tree until they eventually become terminal bronchioles, which give rise to alveolar sacs lined by alveoli (Fig. 16.9). The right mainstem bronchus is shorter, wider, and more vertical than the left (Moore et al., 2014).

> **Clinical Significance**
>
> The structure of the right mainstem bronchus makes it more susceptible to aspiration and unsuccessful endotracheal intubation. This occurs when the tube is inserted too far and enters the right bronchus, essentially blocking off the left lung. This is why lungs sounds are always auscultated after a patient is intubated; if sounds are heard only on the right side, the tube is slowly withdrawn until sounds are heard equally on both sides, confirming correct placement.

Breath sounds over the trachea and mainstem bronchi are louder and harsher than over the other lung fields because these airways have larger diameters, and thus more airflow, than the smaller airways. Breath sounds become softer, finer, and more difficult to auscultate as the bronchioles get narrower.

Gas exchange occurs in the alveoli of the lungs. When fluid fills the alveoli, fine crackles may be audible on auscultation. Excessive fluid in the alveoli interferes with gas exchange, resulting in decreased or absent breath sounds in that portion of the lung.

The pleurae are two continuous membranes within the thorax. The visceral pleura lines the outer surface of the lungs,

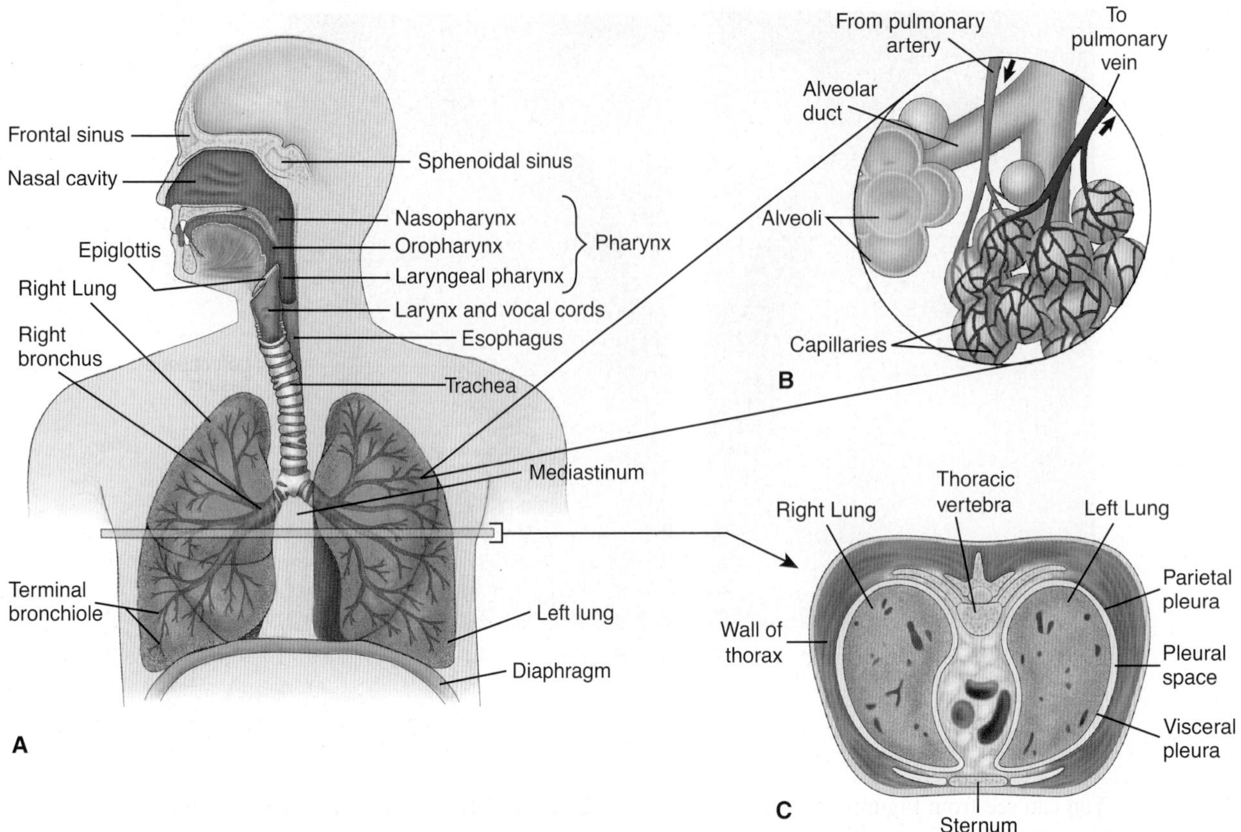

Figure 16.9 **A.** Structures of the upper and lower respiratory tract. **B.** Alveoli. **C.** Horizontal cross section of the lungs.

whereas the parietal pleura lines the thoracic wall, mediastinum, and diaphragm (see Fig. 18.9C). The space between the visceral and parietal pleura contains a thin layer of pleural fluid that lubricates the two surfaces, enabling a smooth sliding movement of the lungs during respiration. The surface tension of the pleurae keeps the lungs in contact with the chest wall, maintaining a negative pressure that enables full lung expansion.

Upper Respiratory Tract

The upper respiratory tract is responsible for moisturizing inhaled air and filtering noxious particles.

Mechanics of Respiration

Respiration is primarily an automatic process initiated by the respiratory center of the brainstem (pons and medulla) based on cellular demands (Moini, 2012). The main trigger for breathing is increased level of carbon dioxide in the blood. Decreased oxygen or increased acidity also may stimulate breathing. Some medications (e.g., opiates) may reduce the ability of the brain to trigger breathing, causing hypoventilation (slow breathing). Anxiety or brain injury may stimulate breathing, causing hyperventilation (fast breathing).

When breathing is triggered, the diaphragm contracts and flattens, pulling the lungs down. The thorax and lungs elongate, increasing the vertical diameter. The external intercostal muscles open the ribs and lift the sternum and the anteroposterior diameter of the thorax increases. With increased thoracic size, pressure within the thorax is less than pressure in the atmosphere. As a result, approximately 500 to 800 ml of air enters the lungs with each breath in adults (Moore et al., 2014).

Expiration is primarily a passive process. As the diaphragm, internal intercostal muscles, and abdominal muscles relax, pressure in the lungs is greater than in the atmosphere. Subsequently, air is pushed out and the chest and abdomen return to their relaxed position.

Sufficient nerve innervation, muscle excursion, and strength are needed for effective breathing. Patients with conditions affecting the spinal cord, especially injuries above the level of C3–C5, may require ventilator support. Extreme obesity can limit chest wall expansion (and thus compromise breathing). Progressive loss of muscle function (e.g., muscular dystrophy) can limit ability to ventilate and cough (Moini, 2012).

Lifespan Considerations: Older Adults

With aging, respiratory strength declines. Lungs lose elasticity, flexibility decreases in the cartilage of the ribs, and bone density decreases. The anterior-to-posterior depth of the chest widens, causing the thorax to become more rounded or barrel shaped. Although this occurs to a much greater degree in smokers, even nonsmokers older than age 50 years have some evidence of these thoracic changes. When the thorax is rounded, it is harder to inhale deeply. The ultimate result of all these changes is diminished respiratory volume, making it more difficult for the elderly to exercise as long or as hard as they could earlier in life (Moini, 2012).

Cultural Considerations

Cultural variations in the size of the thoracic cavity occur, which in turn affects lung volumes. In general, Caucasians have the largest chest size, followed closely by African Americans. In comparison, Asians and American Indians have smaller chest cavities and decreased lung volumes.

Prevalence of certain diseases also varies across cultures within the United States. For example, asthma, a relatively common chronic lung disease, is most common in African American and American Indian adults and least common in Asian and Hispanic adults (Gorman & Chu, 2009). In the United States, asthma is the most common chronic disease in children, and evidence suggests that the extent to which the disease is controlled varies among cultural groups. Indicators of poorly controlled asthma, such as increased use of emergency room services, decreased use of inhaled corticosteroids, and more frequent need for rescue inhalers, are higher in African American and Hispanic children as compared with Caucasian children (Crocker et al., 2009).

Cultural and ethnic variability is also noted in the risk of developing tuberculosis (TB), an infection that primarily affects the respiratory system. Compared with Caucasians, TB rates are approximately 7 times higher among Hispanics, 8 times higher among African Americans, and 25 times higher among Asians/Pacific Islanders (Centers for Disease Control and Prevention [CDC], 2013a, p. 150). TB screening should be provided for immigrants, those who are travelling to high-risk areas, and those at risk for other reasons, including drug and alcohol abuse and HIV infection.

Genetic patterns of inheritance increase risks for respiratory disorders such as cystic fibrosis and alpha-1 antitrypsin deficiency (associated with early onset emphysema). Cystic fibrosis occurs most often in Caucasians and is rare in African Americans and Asians. Emphysema associated with the most severe form of inherited alpha-1 antitrypsin deficiency is most common among persons of Scandinavian heritage, whereas it is rare in African Americans and persons of Jewish and Japanese descent (Porth, 2011).

Urgent Assessment

It is absolutely critical that you accurately prioritize assessments and interventions in urgent or emergency respiratory situations. If a patient has acute shortness of breath, immediately assess respiratory and pulse rates, blood pressure, and oxygen saturation. Auscultate the lungs to identify significant abnormalities, such as diminished or absent breath sounds, or evidence of fluid in the lungs. Simultaneously, administer oxygen; you may also give the patient a bronchodilating inhaler. If the patient is in bed, elevate the head of the bed to reduce the effect of gravity on the effort of breathing.

Patients who are short of breath become anxious, and because anxiety increases the work of breathing, it becomes a worsening cycle. Remain with the patient and encourage relaxation techniques to decrease the patient's anxiety. As the oxygen level in the blood and body tissues decreases, patients become more dyspneic and may become cyanotic. Insufficient oxygen supply to the brain results in confusion and decreasing level of consciousness. If the situation does not improve rapidly, you may need to alert the emergency response team.

A patient may be clinically stable but be unable to fully cooperate in the assessment process because of fatigue. For example, thorough auscultation of all lung fields may not be possible because deep breathing generally worsens the level of fatigue in patients with pulmonary disorders. The effect of gravity increases the likelihood of significant findings in the lower areas of the lungs, so listen to lung sounds in the bases first; you can delay further auscultation to allow patient rest. Consider clustering care. Auscultate the lungs when turning the patient or getting the patient up in a chair. Prioritize the subjective data collected; ask only questions most relevant to the current situation. Even simple tasks, such as eating and toileting, may be physically taxing to the patient, so it is important to cluster interventions and schedule assessments for times when the patient is more rested.

Subjective Data

Begin subjective data collection with the health history, continue with questions about specific respiratory conditions, and end with detailed collection of information involving areas of concern. If the patient is short of breath, you will need to conduct the interview in segments over a period of time, with frequent breaks for the patient to rest. In such instances, prioritize the data to collect the most essential information first. For example, ask important questions about the patient's primary symptoms to enable a relevant physical examination and obtain a list of current medications and any allergies—a necessary step before any medications can be administered.

> ⚠ *SAFETY ALERT*
>
> *If the patient is having extreme difficulty breathing, stop the assessment and get help. A decreased level of consciousness, respiratory rate above 30 breaths/min, O_2 saturation less than 90%, and cyanosis may indicate hypoxia (a medical emergency).*

Assessment of Risk Factors

When questioning patients about risk factors, your intent is to identify how likely patients are to develop or to already be experiencing symptoms of respiratory disorders.

Such investigation creates an environment in which health care providers can implement necessary interventions to manage symptoms, provide essential patient teaching, and document in the patient record concerns needing ongoing follow-up. For example, smoking contributes to the development and worsening of COPD. Thus, you must thoroughly assess the patient's smoking history and give educational materials to patients willing to begin a smoking-cessation program. Unless the patient is in acute distress, you can provide pertinent education as soon as you identify a risk factor.

History and Risk Factors	Rationale
Past Medical History	
Have you ever been diagnosed with a respiratory disease or condition, such as asthma, bronchitis, emphysema, pneumonia, or lung cancer? • When did the condition first occur? • How was the condition treated? • What were the outcomes (e.g., full recovery, recurrences, persistent or progressive disease)?	A history of respiratory disorders in childhood increases the risk for subsequent respiratory disorders. Chronic diseases, such as COPD, often have long-term effects that result in a slow but progressive decline in function. Asthma symptoms may occur at any age and improve or worsen over time. Pneumonia usually has an acute course that resolves with appropriate treatment (Damjanov, 2012).
Have you ever had an allergic reaction to a medication, something in the environment, or a food product? (If yes, ask the following): • What allergen(s) have you reacted to? • When did the reaction(s) occur? • What were the symptoms and how severe were they? • How were the allergies treated? • What were the outcomes (e.g., any subsequent exposure to the allergen? If yes, did the symptoms recur)?	Exposure to known environmental, food, or medication allergens may precipitate bronchoconstriction. Common allergens include pollens, dust mites, grasses, molds, animal dander, beestings, peanuts, shellfish, certain antibiotics, and latex. Exercise can also induce bronchoconstriction in some people (e.g., exercise-induced asthma) (Weatherspoon & Weatherspoon, 2012).
Have you ever been told that you had a positive TB skin test result? (*If yes, ask:*) • When did this happen? • Have you ever received any treatment for TB? • When was your most recent (TB) skin test or chest x-ray? • What was the result? • Have you had close contact with anyone with active TB?	Risk factors for TB include having close contact with an infected person and immigration from a country with a high prevalence of TB. Certain groups of people are at higher risk for developing TB. These include homeless persons, substance abusers, prisoners, persons with HIV infection, and people who work with these high-risk groups. Health care workers should be screened annually (CDC, 2013d).
When did you receive your last influenza and/or pneumococcal vaccine? Are you interested in being immunized this year?	Influenza vaccine is recommended annually for everyone older than 6 months of age. Pneumococcal vaccine is recommended every 5 years for immunocompromised adults, people older than 65 years of age, people with HIV infection, and children older than 2 years of age with chronic illnesses or HIV infection (CDC, 2013b, 2013c).
Lifestyle and Personal Habits	
Do you smoke, or have you ever smoked, cigarettes, pipes, or cigars? • How many packs per day do you smoke? • How many years have you smoked? • Have you ever tried to stop smoking? • Are you interested in quitting?	Smoking history is documented as the number of **pack years** (number of years smoked × average number of packs per day). For example, a patient who has smoked half a pack per day for 30 years has a 15-pack-year smoking history. As the number of pack-years increase, the risk for and severity of smoking-related conditions also increases (Weatherspoon & Weatherspoon, 2012). For example, the risk of developing lung cancer increases as the number of smoking pack-years increases (Khan & Pelengaris, 2013).
Are you frequently around people who smoke in the home or car? What measures do you take to control this exposure?	Secondhand smoke increases the risk of developing emphysema and lung cancer (Boardman, 2013).
Do you currently, or have you ever inhaled recreational drugs such as marijuana, cocaine, methamphetamine, or glue or spray paint? Are you interested in information about how to quit or reduce your risk?	These inhaled substances can irritate the linings of the upper or lower airway. Airway irritation can induce an inflammatory response, causing bronchoconstriction and wheezing. People with history of injection drug use are at high risk for HIV infection and respiratory complications associated with it (Foster, Gilbert, & Long, 2012).

(table continues on page 421)

History and Risk Factors	Rationale
Are you involved in any activities that might increase your risk for developing respiratory conditions, such as exposure to wood dust, bird breeding, or growing mushrooms?	Exposure to these products may cause lung injury. Exposure over time to bird droppings or feathers may cause hypersensitivity pneumonitis and respiratory fibrosis. (Damjanov, 2012).
Occupational History Are you currently, or have you ever been, exposed to asbestos or substances, including fumes, which cause irritation in your throat or difficulty breathing at work? • What is (or was) your occupation? • Do you wear a mask or take other precautions to protect your lungs? • What steps do you take to monitor your exposure?	Coal miners have an increased risk of pneumoconiosis, or black lung disease. Silicosis is increased in glassmakers, stonecutters, miners, cement workers, and semiconductor manufacturers. Occupational asthma may develop in 2%–5% of workers exposed to grain dust, wood dust, soldering flux, and dyes. Industrial bronchitis is found in textile workers. Shipyard and construction workers, pipefitters, and insulators may develop asbestosis (Damjanov, 2012).
Environmental Exposures Have you ever been, or are you now, exposed to substances or irritants at home such as pollen, dust, pet dander, cockroaches, or cooking smoke particles? Is there any history of exposure to radon or to asbestos in heating/cooling systems?	Common household irritants can contribute to asthma as well as itchy eyes, sneezing, and runny nose. Radon and tobacco smoke can cause even more dangerous health effects, including lung cancer (Bailey, 2013).
Have you recently traveled to any high-risk areas for respiratory conditions such as other areas in the United States, Asia, or southern Africa? • Where? • How long were you there? • Were you exposed to people with a cough, cold, or the flu?	Histoplasmosis, a fungal infection, is common in the midwestern United States and endemic in Ohio, Missouri, and the Mississippi River valley. Another fungal infection, coccidioidomycosis, is found in the southwestern United States and Central and South America (Damjanov, 2012). High-risk areas for TB include Asia and southern Africa (CDC, 2013a). Prompt identification and treatment of these contagions is essential.
Medications Are you taking any medications for respiratory conditions? • What are the medications and dosages? • How often are you taking them? • How well are you following your prescribed medication regimen?	Many respiratory medications, such as bronchodilating inhalers, are used as needed. Trends of increased use may indicate a worsening condition. Glucocorticosteroids are also commonly used during times of airway inflammation, such as during an acute asthma attack.
Are you taking any natural supplements or over-the-counter medications? • What are they? • How often are you taking them?	Over-the-counter medications that block beta-2 receptors may exacerbate bronchoconstriction. Sensitivity to nonsteroidal antiinflammatory drugs (NSAIDs) (e.g., ibuprofen, naproxen) may cause wheezing in patients with asthma (Weatherspoon & Weatherspoon, 2012).
Family History Do you have any family history of respiratory conditions or disorders? • Who had the condition? • What was the condition? • When did the person have it? • How was the condition treated? • What were the outcomes?	A positive family history of lung-related conditions, especially inherited diseases such as cystic fibrosis, increases the patient's risk for respiratory illness. Note any infectious diseases and the possibility for familial transmission. Also consider whether the condition is chronic (e.g., COPD) or episodic (e.g., common cold). Mounting evidence supports a genetic predisposition for lung cancer in some families. This may help explain the fact that although 85% of people diagnosed with lung cancer are current or previous smokers, only 15% of smokers develop lung cancer. Also, smoking is a major risk factor for cardiovascular disease (the first leading cause of death in the United States) and COPD (the fourth leading causes of death in the United States). Smokers may die from these conditions before lung cancer can develop or be identified (Weatherspoon & Weatherspoon, 2012).

Risk Reduction and Health Promotion

An important reason for obtaining a patient's health history is to gather information to individualize health promotion teaching and interventions. Health promotion activities focus on preventing disease from developing (primary prevention), screening to identify conditions at an early curable stage (secondary prevention), and reducing complications of existing or established medical diagnoses (tertiary prevention). Recognizing and reinforcing healthy habits the patient is already practicing is another important component of health promotion.

People in the United States rate nurses as the most trusted professionals, and nurses are uniquely qualified to influence health-related lifestyle behaviors (Gallup Polling, 2013). In your role as a nurse, it is important that you promote a healthy lifestyle through role-modeling healthy behaviors and teaching patients specific strategies they can use to reduce their risk for injury and disease. Introduce relevant topics at appropriate intervals while conducting the initial health history, and then discuss in more depth during subsequent interactions with the patient.

The following are health goals related to the respiratory system:

1. Increase the proportion of adults vaccinated against influenza and pneumococcal infections.
2. Reduce the number of missed school or work days due to asthma exacerbations.
3. Reduce the proportion of adults whose activity level is limited by symptoms associated with chronic lung disease and reduce mortality from respiratory-associated disorders.
4. Reduce the proportion of previous smokers and never smokers (defined as people who have smoked 100 or fewer cigarettes in their lifetime) exposed to secondhand tobacco smoke.
5. Increase the number of smoking cessation attempts by adolescent and adult smokers and during pregnancy.
6. Establish laws prohibiting indoor smoking; alternately, limit indoor smoking to separately ventilated areas in public buildings and worksites.

(U.S. Department of Health & Human Services [USDHHS], 2013)

Smoking Cessation

All patients who smoke should be asked at every appointment about their readiness to stop. Smoking has been linked to lung cancer, emphysema, chronic bronchitis, cardiovascular disease, and oropharyngeal cancer; it is considered the leading cause of preventable death (Leahy & Rosof-Williams, 2012). Patients who smoke should be counseled about quitting and assessed for readiness to quit at every visit (Swartz, 2010). Patients can be given several choices to assist with quitting, such as individual or group counseling, medical treatment, or nicotine replacement.

Prevention of Occupational Exposure

Another focal point is modification of the work environment to limit exposure to irritants. In some cases, consultation with employees at the work site may be recommended. Occupational health and safety guidelines should be followed. For example, people exposed to dust should have the opportunity to wear respirator masks (Weatherspoon & Weatherspoon, 2012).

Prevention of Asthma

Asthma triggers include tobacco smoke, dust, dust mites, molds, furred and feathered animals, and cockroaches and other pests. For patients with allergies, recommend modification of the home environment. Examples include covering the bed and pillows and ensuring that pets sleep separately from owners (i.e., outside the bedroom).

Immunizations

The CDC recommends that all children older than 6 months of age and all adults receive the influenza vaccine on an annual basis. Therefore, you should discuss and counsel patients about this recommendation. It is especially important that all health care providers receive this vaccine annually. In addition to being at increased risk for contracting influenza from patients, health care providers who do not receive the vaccine unnecessarily place their patients at risk, especially older adults and patients with compromised immune systems (CDC, 2013b, 2013c).

Common Symptoms

When conditions involving the respiratory system are present, ask the patient which symptoms occur most often. If the patient reports experiencing any of these common symptoms, further assess for important characteristics of each symptom. You will use information obtained during the interview to determine the focus of the physical examination. A thorough history of the patient's symptoms is also necessary for identifying accurate nursing diagnoses and developing an optimal plan of care.

Common Respiratory Symptoms

- Chest pain or discomfort
- Dyspnea
- Orthopnea or paroxysmal nocturnal dyspnea
- Cough
  - If present: any sputum or phlegm produced from cough, including amount, appearance, color, odor, and viscosity (e.g., watery vs. thick)
- Wheezing or tightness in chest
- Change in functional ability

Signs/Symptoms	Rationale/Abnormal Findings
Chest Pain Do you have any chest pain or discomfort? • Where is it? Can you point to where it hurts? Does the pain go anywhere else? Can you describe the pain (e.g., sharp, shooting, burning, aching)? • When did it start? How long has it lasted? What were you doing when it started (e.g., walking, climbing stairs, resting)? Did anything happen before the pain started (e.g., an injury or fall)?	⚠ *SAFETY ALERT* *Health care providers should assume that chest pain is due to cardiac ischemia until proven otherwise. (Inadequate oxygen delivery to the heart leads to damage and eventual death of heart muscle cells if not urgently identified and treated.) Chest pain is an emergency requiring immediate help (see Chapter 17). Pain brought on by exertion and relieved by rest is more likely to be coming from the heart.*
• How bad is it on a scale from 1 to 10, with 10 being the worst pain you can imagine? Has the intensity of the pain changed in any way since it started? • Have you noticed a pattern to the pain? Has it been continuous since it started? Does it come and go? Does it occur at certain times of the day? Does it wake you up at night? • Have you ever had this kind of pain before? If so, when? • Have you noticed anything that makes the pain better? Have you tried any type of medicine or treatment? Did it help? Does anything make the pain worse? • Do any other symptoms come with the pain (e.g., shortness of breath, cough, fever)? • What do you think is causing the pain? • What is your goal for the pain? What would you like to be able to do that you can't because of the pain?	Lung tissue has no pain fibers, but many pain fibers are present in the pleurae. Pleuritic chest pain (pleurisy) can be caused by inflammation of the parietal pleura. Patients usually describe such pain as sharp or stabbing, worsening with deep breathing (as the lung comes in contact with the inflamed pleura) or coughing, and is often located in the lateral or posterior area of the chest. Antiinflammatory drugs often relieve pleuritic pain. Tracheobronchitis can cause pain starting in the area of the trachea and large bronchi; patients usually describe this as a burning sensation in the upper sternum. It is usually associated with a cough. Chest wall pain can be due to muscle strain caused by frequent and/or forceful coughing. Presence of productive cough and fever suggests an infectious cause, such as bronchitis or pneumonia. It is important to be aware of particular fears the patient may have, such as a heart attack or cancer, and also to determine whether, and how much, the pain is affecting function.
Dyspnea Have you had any difficulty or problems breathing? • How bad is it on a scale from 1 to 10, with 10 being the worst? • When did it start? How long has it lasted? • What activities make it worse? What makes it better? • Do you have other symptoms? • How has this limited your activities? • Is the breathing difficulty associated with anxiety?	**Dyspnea,** or feeling "short of breath," is a subjective term used when patients report labored breathing and breathlessness. This response to exercise or heavy activity is expected if it rapidly disappears upon return to rest. Patients with lung disease, however, may experience dyspnea with certain activities or even at rest. Dyspnea associated with chest pain, especially brought on by activity, is an emergency requiring immediate help. Note what causes dyspnea, such as climbing two flights of stairs, walking one block, or walking uphill. Also note whether onset was gradual (e.g., COPD) or sudden (e.g., pneumonia) and whether the patient suffered any injury or trauma (e.g., pneumothorax). Anxiety can precipitate dyspnea and hyperventilation or can occur as a result of dyspnea. Anxious patients may describe dyspnea as smothering; they also may report tingling around the lips from a low carbon dioxide level. Patients with COPD or CHF may describe dyspnea as scary, hard to breathe, shortness of breath, cannot get enough air, or gasping (Murphy, 2013).

(table continues on page 424)

Signs/Symptoms	Rationale/Abnormal Findings
Orthopnea and Paroxysmal Nocturnal Dyspnea Do you have difficulty breathing when you sleep? • On how many pillows do you sleep? • Do you have difficulty breathing when lying flat? • Do you wake up suddenly at night short of breath? • Has anyone told you that you snore or stop breathing when you sleep? • Do you have night sweats, weight loss?	Gravity increases the work of breathing when lying flat. Patients with **orthopnea** (difficulty breathing when lying flat) often sleep on two or more pillows or even in recliners. Patients who awaken at night with sudden shortness of breath have **paroxysmal nocturnal dyspnea**. The cause is fluid overload resulting from elevation of the legs, which shifts the fluid present there to the body's core. The excess fluid cannot be pumped through the heart and suddenly accumulates in the lungs, causing dyspnea. Sleep apnea commonly interrupts sleep and can lead to respiratory complications over time. Night sweats and weight loss are associated with TB.
Cough • Do you have a cough? • Where does the cough feel like it's coming from (e.g., sinuses, runny nose, throat, or lungs)? • What does it feel or sound like? • How bad is it? • How often do you cough? When is it worse? • When did it start? How long has it lasted? • Is it worse in any particular setting? • What makes it worse? What makes it better? • Do you have any other symptoms? • Does the cough interfere with your sleep? • What do you think has caused the coughing?	Cough can originate in the upper or lower airway. With sinus congestion or allergic rhinitis, mucus or watery fluid can drip into the throat and cause coughing. A tickle in the throat can also trigger coughing. A cough that accompanies laryngeal irritation is croupy, barking, or brassy. Alternatively, lung irritation can trigger coughing, such as with a cold, bronchitis, or other infection. These coughs are usually dry and hacking. Such coughs usually are productive (wet or moist). Coughs upon waking are associated with pooled secretions secondary to smoking, allergies, or bronchitis. Coughs at night may be from sinus drainage, heart failure, or asthma. Dry irritating coughs, especially following a meal, may be related to gastroesophageal reflux disease (GERD) or a hiatal hernia (Smith & Houghton, 2013). A cough is generally a symptom of an underlying condition, so an accurate description of the cough can help identify its cause and direct treatment.
Sputum Do you cough up any mucus or phlegm? How much? Has the amount increased or decreased? • What color is it? • Is it thick or thin? • Do you notice an odor?	Quantifying the amount of sputum (e.g., teaspoon, tablespoon, ¼ cup, ½ cup) may provide clues about the cause and severity of the condition. Sputum color may suggest a specific cause. The **mucoid** sputum of bronchitis is clear or white. **Purulent** yellow or green sputum, or creamy sputum, especially with a foul odor, indicates the presence of white cells and bacterial infection. Rust-colored sputum is found with TB and pneumococcal pneumonia. Other colors may be green, yellow, brown, or tan. An increase in amount or quality of sputum, especially when accompanied by worsening dyspnea, in a patient with chronic bronchitis (a form of COPD) indicates an acute exacerbation requiring antibiotics. Sticky **tenacious** sputum may be thick from dehydration or cystic fibrosis; sputum resulting from heart failure is thin and frothy and may be slightly pink. Sputum may also be described as copious if a large amount is present. Sputum may be bloody or blood-tinged with lung cancer or TB (Weatherspoon & Weatherspoon, 2012). Examine such sputum carefully to see whether blood is integrated or just coats the outside. An irritated throat or sinus may bleed and contact the sputum during expectoration. **Hemoptysis** is the term for coughing up frank blood. Sputum may also be serous or serosanguineous with inflammation or irritation. Some patients may expectorate from the mouth; this is not considered sputum but instead oral secretions.

(table continues on page 425)

Signs/Symptoms	Rationale/Abnormal Findings
Wheezing Do you have any wheezing or chest tightness? • How severe is wheezing compared to your expected function? • Do you use a peak flow meter? What are your usual/current values? • When did the situation start? How long has it lasted? • Is wheezing associated with allergies? If so, what are they? Do you notice that the situation is worse in a particular environment? • What makes it worse? What makes it better? How often do you use your inhalers? • Do you have other symptoms? • What do you think is causing this? What will make it better?	Wheezing is associated with asthma, CHF, and bronchitis. It occurs in response to narrowed bronchioles. Wheezing with asthma is worse in response to offending allergens, at night, and in the early morning (Weatherspoon & Weatherspoon, 2012). Patients with asthma are taught to use a peak flow meter to provide objective data about how much they can inhale with each breath. If airways are greatly constricted, breaths will be small, and patients may need to use their inhalers (Weatherspoon & Weatherspoon, 2012). ⚠ *SAFETY ALERT* *In an acute asthma attack, auscultate lung sounds frequently for presence and degree of wheezing. If wheezing is audible or auscultated, some air is squeezing through the narrowed airways. Previous wheezing that is no longer heard on auscultation in a patient with obvious signs of respiratory distress (e.g., use of accessory muscles; rapid, irregular breathing pattern; O_2 saturation below 88%) is an ominous sign, indicating a worsening condition.*
Functional Abilities Have breathing difficulties changed any of your expected activities? How do you plan the day and pace your activities? (Along with assessing the patient's ability to perform activities of daily living [ADLs], such as eating, grooming, and dressing; also consider the patient's ability to perform household chores, such as vacuuming, laundry, and bed making, as well as the ability to provide for his or her own nutritional needs, such as cooking and buying groceries.)	Patients with respiratory diseases or conditions, especially those with chronic disorders such as COPD, commonly have more energy in the morning and need frequent rest during the day. Some are short of breath even at rest or with speech, needing to pause after a few words. Others become breathless when eating, grooming, or dressing. Patients with declining health may need plans for assistance. Ask which activities they like to do and whether they can do these things. Patients with respiratory problems may be able to engage in sexual activity and exercise if they plan to do them during high-energy times.

Documenting Normal Findings

Patient denies chest pain or discomfort, dyspnea, orthopnea, paroxysmal nocturnal dyspnea, cough, sputum, wheezing or tightness in chest, or any change in functional ability.

Lifespan Considerations: Older Adults

Additional Questions	Rationale/Abnormal Findings
Have you noticed any shortness of breath or fatigue when doing your usual daily activities?	Older adults have lower tolerance for performing ADLs than younger patients (Moini, 2012). Assess how any respiratory disorders are affecting ability to function. Assess energy level and activities that cause patients to tire more easily. Consider recommendations for pacing activities, allowing for rest, and performing higher energy tasks during time of day when well rested.
Have you had any recent respiratory infections or worsening of your current condition?	Counsel high-risk patients to avoid exposure to people with infections and to plan modifications for weather variations, such as walking in a shopping mall instead of outside on a cold day. Educate about lifestyle changes to increase health and prevent chronic disease (e.g., not smoking).

Cultural Considerations

Additional Questions	Rationale/Abnormal Findings
Have you recently immigrated to the United States? Have you been immunized with the bacille Calmette-Guérin (BCG) vaccine?	Incidence of TB is higher in immigrants from countries with high incidence of TB (CDC, 2013a). Multiple countries vaccinate against TB using the BCG vaccine. However, because there are multiple strains of TB, including multidrug resistant (MDR) strains, the vaccine does not provide adequate protection against infection. Furthermore, people who have received the BCG vaccine often test positive when tested for TB. Therefore, it becomes difficult to evaluate patients with symptoms of TB who have received the vaccine. Chest x-ray is recommended; evaluation and treatment is the same regardless of BCG status (Bailey, 2013).
Do you have concerns about exposure to environmental pollution?	Children in urban environments are more likely to have asthma. Air pollution contributes to COPD and lung cancer (Braun & Anderson, 2011).
Are there any concerns about exposure to dust, fumes, or mold in your home?	Recent immigrants may cook or heat with kerosene or wood. Make sure proper ventilation is adequate to avoid carbon monoxide poisoning. Also consider quality of housing, including density of residents, ventilation systems, and presence of black mold (Weatherspoon & Weatherspoon, 2012).
	Asthma is more common in females, those in poverty, and multiracial people (Braun & Anderson, 2011). Hispanics, African Americans, and Asians have TB rates 7–19 times higher than Caucasians (CDC, 2013d). Globally, cigarette smokers, persons of African or Asian descent, and women (especially those who smoke) are more likely to develop lung cancer than persons who do not belong to the above groups (Steward and Thomas, 2013).

Therapeutic Dialogue: Collecting Subjective Data

The nurse's role in subjective data collection is to gather information to improve the patient's health status and to help determine the cause of current symptoms. Remember Mr. Lee, who was introduced at the beginning of this chapter. He was diagnosed with COPD 15 years ago. Today, he is visiting the clinic because of increasing dyspnea and fatigue. Because Mr. Lee is fatigued, efficient questioning is essential. Thus, questions must be prioritized, with the most important issues addressed first.

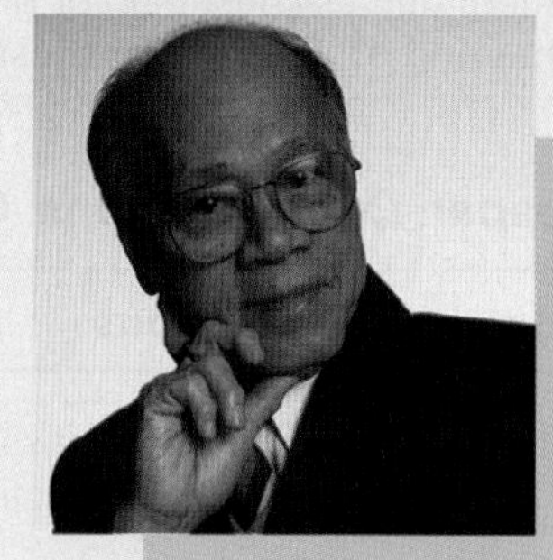

Nurse: *(Before beginning, the nurse reads the chart and notes that Mr. Lee has a 98 pack-year history of smoking, continues to smoke, and has a diagnosis of COPD for 15 years. The record states that Mr. Lee is allergic to pollen, which causes symptoms of red teary eyes and sinus congestion.)* It looks like your last visit was 2 weeks ago, Mr. Lee. How do you feel now?

(case study continues on page 427)

Mr. Lee: I'm still not feeling well. When I came in last time, they said I had bronchitis, but it feels like it's getting worse.

Nurse: It feels like it is getting worse. . .? (pause)

Mr. Lee: Last time I felt wheezy. This time I'm coughing more.

Nurse: Are you coughing anything up?

Mr. Lee: Yes.

Nurse: What does it look like?

Mr. Lee: It's yellow.

Nurse: And is it thick or thin?

Mr. Lee: It's quite thick.

Nurse: How much would you say you're coughing up in a day; a few teaspoons, a half cup, a cup, or another amount?

Mr. Lee: I probably cough something up three to four times an hour. Maybe in a day about a cup.

Critical Thinking Challenge

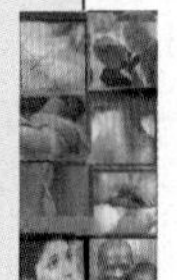

- What makes the therapeutic dialogue effective?
- Could the nurse have done anything differently to improve data collection and communication with Mr. Lee?
- Does the patient's childhood and family history require further exploration? Provide rationale.
- Is this an appropriate time to discuss risk factor modification and smoking cessation? Provide rationale.

Objective Data

Common and Specialty or Advanced Techniques

Routine assessment includes the most important and common techniques. Examiners may add specialty or advanced steps if concerns exist over a specific finding. The table summarizes the most common techniques for thoracic and lung assessment, which are therefore essential to master in clinical practice. Although all registered nurses (RNs) must be proficient at performing a physical examination of the thorax, percussion for diaphragmatic excursion is usually performed by advanced practice nurses. All other physical examination techniques described in this chapter can and should be learned and performed by RNs in any practice setting.

Equipment Needed

- Examination gown
- Stethoscope and alcohol swab
- Marking pen and small ruler for diaphragmatic excursion (optional)

Preparation

Make sure that the room is a comfortable temperature. Take measures to facilitate a private and quiet setting. Wash and warm your hands to avoid spreading infection and to facilitate patient comfort.

For inspection, expose only the area of the chest that you will be examining. Cover the anterior chest when inspecting posteriorly. Explain the rationale for the need to expose the chest to ease the patient's anxiety.

Lung auscultation is easiest to perform with the patient sitting. If sitting is not possible, the anterior lungs can be auscultated when the patient is lying down and the posterior lungs can be auscultated with the patient turned from side to side. When possible, it is best for a second person to help the patient to sit. It is never acceptable to omit auscultation of the posterior chest because the effect of gravity makes it more likely to hear significant abnormal breath sounds in the lower lobes, which can only be auscultated posteriorly.

Your stethoscope can be a source of bacterial transmission across patients (Hogan-Quigley et al., 2012). Thus, be sure to use an alcohol swab to clean the diaphragm of the stethoscope before bringing it into contact with the patient. You also may warm the diaphragm of the stethoscope with your clean hands before placing it on the patient's chest.

Basic Versus Focused/Specialty or Advanced Techniques Related to Thorax and Lung Assessment

Comprehensive Assessment Technique	Purpose	Screening or Registered Nurse Assessment	Focused or Advanced Practice Examination
Inspection of patient	Assists to determine the acuity of the situation	X	
Inspection of chest	Provides information on chest shape and breathing pattern	X	
Palpation of chest	Assessed when tenderness, masses, or lesions are present	X	
Chest expansion	Assessed in cases of physical or neuromuscular limitations	X	
Tactile fremitus	Assessed when consolidation or hyperinflation is anticipated	X	
Percussion of chest	Assessed when consolidation or hyperinflation is anticipated	X	
Auscultation	Performed to accurately identify breath and adventitious sounds	X	
Diaphragmatic excursion	Assessed in cases of physical or neuromuscular limitations		X Neuromuscular function
Auscultation of voice sounds	Assessed when consolidation is anticipated		X Suspected pneumonia

Comprehensive Physical Assessment

Technique and Normal Findings	Abnormal Findings
General Closely observe the patient's body positioning and posture. 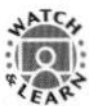 Posture is relaxed and upright with the arms at the sides.	Patients in respiratory distress or with COPD often assume a **tripod** position, leaning forward on a stationary object such as a table or with their elbows on their knees (Fig. 16.10). This position increases the size of the thoracic cavity, facilitating airflow. 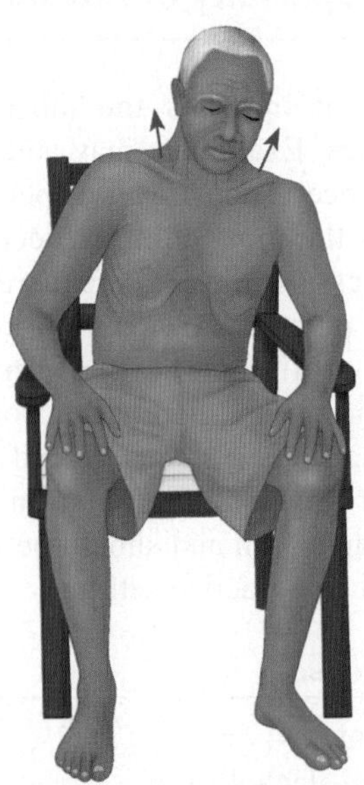 **Figure 16.10** A patient with chronic obstructive pulmonary disease assuming the tripod position.

(table continues on page 429)

Technique and Normal Findings (continued)	Abnormal Findings (continued)
Observe for **pursed lip breathing** and **nasal flaring**. ▮ Facial expression is relaxed.	Patients in **respiratory distress** may have an anxious expression. Patients with COPD may breathe with their lips pursed, providing some positive pressure in the bronchial tree to prevent airway collapse. Respirations may be described as irregular, labored, gasping, grunting, or retracting. Nasal flaring may accompany respiratory distress, which is noted more often in children.
Evaluate level of consciousness. ▮ Patient is alert, cooperative, and oriented to person, place, time, and situation.	The patient with hypoxemia may be irritable, drowsy, somnolent, restless, confused, combative, or disoriented.
Inspect skin color; pay special attention to the face, mucous membranes (oral cavity), and nail beds. Document the absence of cyanosis or pallor. ▮ Skin color is an appropriate tone for the patient's racial background. ▮ *Observe the undertone of the skin rather than the amount of melanin. Expected skin color is pink.*	With hypoxemia, **cyanosis** (bluish discoloration) may be noted around the mouth (circumoral), in the oral mucous membranes, and in the nail beds. **Pallor** (pale whitish color) and grayish tones indicate poor oxygenation or anemia. Patients who smoke and those with chronic respiratory diseases may have a **ruddy**, or **reddish-purple**, facial color due to increased red blood cells (polycythemia), a compensatory mechanism to maintain oxygenation of tissues.
Observe chest movement as the patient breathes. Note which portion of the chest moves more during respiration (upper, lower, or equal) and the length of inspiration time relative to expiration. *Normally, expiration is twice as long as inspiration (inspiration: expiration = 1:2).*	Patients with disorders that impair outflow (e.g., COPD) may have **forced expiration**. **Guarding** may accompany pleuritic or postoperative pain. **Effort or work of breathing** is less efficient with use of upper chest muscles.
As you observe the patient's respiratory movements, listen for audible sounds and also count the respiratory rate. Do not tell the patient that you are doing this because he or she may subconsciously alter the rate. If it is difficult to see the chest moving, gently rest your hand on the patient's shoulder to feel the rate. *Normal respiratory rate is 12–20 breaths/min for adults. Rhythm is regular, and breathing appears easy and quiet. This is labeled* eupnea. *An occasional sigh is common and not a cause for concern.*	**Wheezing** may be audible in severe asthma or bronchitis. **Tachypnea** is breathing greater than 24 breaths/min; **bradypnea** is less than 10 breaths/min. See Table 16.4 at the end of this chapter for other unexpected respiratory patterns. ⚠ *SAFETY ALERT* ***Stridor**, a high-pitched crowing sound from the upper airway, results from tracheal or laryngeal spasm or constriction. In severe laryngospasm, the larynx may completely close off. This life-threatening emergency requires immediate medical intervention.*
Assess oxygen saturation level (pulse oximetry; see Chapter 5). *Normal O_2 saturation is 95% or more.*	Many pulmonary disorders cause hypoxemia. For example, pulmonary embolism produces hypoxemia because blockage of a pulmonary vein prevents oxygenated blood from returning to the heart and the rest of the body. ⚠ *SAFETY ALERT* *Oxygen saturation less than 92% requires immediate supplemental oxygen and assistance.*

(table continues on page 430)

Technique and Normal Findings (continued)	Abnormal Findings (continued)
Observe nails for color and shape. Nail beds are pink, and the angle between the nail base and proximal skin is around 160 degrees.	Pallor or cyanosis of the nail beds indicates hypoxia. An angle of 180 degrees or more is called **clubbing** of the fingers, which indicates long-term (chronic) hypoxia (see Chapter 11).
Posterior Chest ***Inspection.*** **NOTE:** As you move around the side of the patient to inspect the posterior chest, inspect and compare the anteroposterior (AP) (front to back) diameter to the transverse (side to side) diameter and assess the overall shape and configuration of the thoracic cage. Observe spontaneous chest expansion. Spinous processes of the vertebrae are midline; scapulae are symmetrical in each hemithorax. Chest wall is cone-shaped (narrower at the bottom than the top), symmetrical, and oval (narrower from front to back than from side to side). The AP-to-transverse ratio is between 1:2 and 5:7. Although ribs are not visible in most people, they can be visible in very thin people and they slope at approximately 45 degrees. Chest expansion is symmetrical.	Skeletal scoliosis and kyphosis can limit respiratory excursion. In **barrel chest**, which can accompany COPD, the AP-to-transverse ratio approximates 1:1, giving the chest a round appearance. Also with COPD, the expanded ribs slope more horizontally, inverting the chest's expected cone shape. Asymmetry and paradoxical respirations occur in pneumothorax and flail chest. See Table 16.5 at the end of the chapter.
Assess for use of accessory muscles to breathe. Respirations are quiet with regular rhythm, using only the diaphragm and external intercostal muscles.	Patients experiencing respiratory distress require additional muscles for breathing. Generally, the *sternomastoid*, *scalene*, and *trapezius* muscles are considered **accessory muscles** for inspiration; however, in very severe respiratory distress, occasionally the *latissimus dorsi* and *pectoralis* muscles can assist. Expiration or exhalation is generally a passive process, but patients with COPD require the *rectus abdominis* and *internal intercostal* muscles to facilitate exhalation.
Assess for any supraclavicular or intercostal retractions during respirations. No retractions are noted.	**Retractions** appear as indentations in the supraclavicular fossa and ICSs. They are noted in conditions of airflow resistance, such as occurs in severe asthma.
Palpation. Palpate the chest for tender areas. Using the fingertips, start above the scapula over the lung apex and progress from side to side to compare findings bilaterally, ending at the base of the lung and moving laterally to the midaxillary line (Fig. 16.11). Note any lesions, lumps, or masses; use gloves if there are lesions or open areas. Palpate for crepitus if the patient has had rib fractures, recent chest surgery, or chest tubes. Thorax is nontender without any lesions, masses, or crepitus.	Tender areas may indicate muscle strain, rib fracture, or soft tissue damage. In chest trauma, air can enter the lungs to escape into subcutaneous tissue. This free air creates a crackling sensation similar to bubble wrap or crispy rice cereal under the skin (**crepitus**). Because air floats, subcutaneous emphysema migrates, so it may be found in the head and neck. If there is a large amount, mark the borders with a pen so that changes can be noted. Note any skin lesions or masses. If present, note their size, depth, borders (round, smooth, or irregular), color, tenderness, consistency (firm, soft, or spongy), mobility, and whether skin over lesion or mass is intact (if not, is the open area dry or is there drainage?)

(table continues on page 431)

Technique and Normal Findings (continued)	Abnormal Findings (continued)
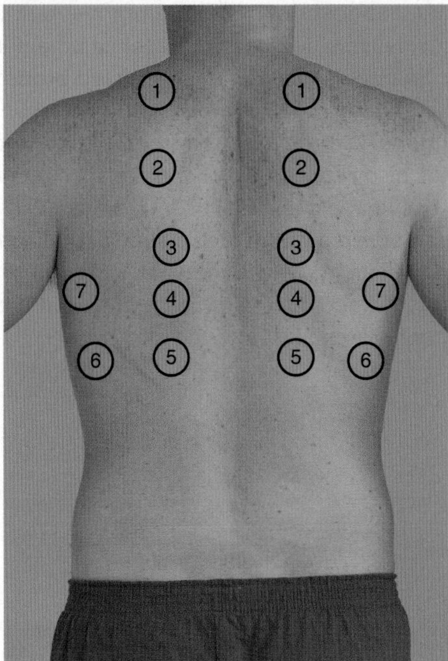 **Figure 16.11** Sites for and sequence of palpation and percussion of the posterior thorax.	
Test for symmetrical chest expansion when concerns about reduced lung volumes arise. With the thumbs at the level of T9–T10, wrap the palmar surface of the hands laterally and parallel to the rib cage (Fig. 16.12). Slide the thumbs and hands medially to pinch up a small fold of skin between the thumb and vertebra. Ask the patient to inhale deeply and observe the thumbs. The thumbs move apart symmetrically.	**Asymmetrical movements** indicate collapse or blockage of a significant portion of the lung such as with pneumothorax, rib fracture, severe pneumonia, pleural effusion, or atelectasis. Patients with localized lung disease may have asymmetrical chest expansion (one side of the chest moves less than the opposite side) (Swartz, 2010).
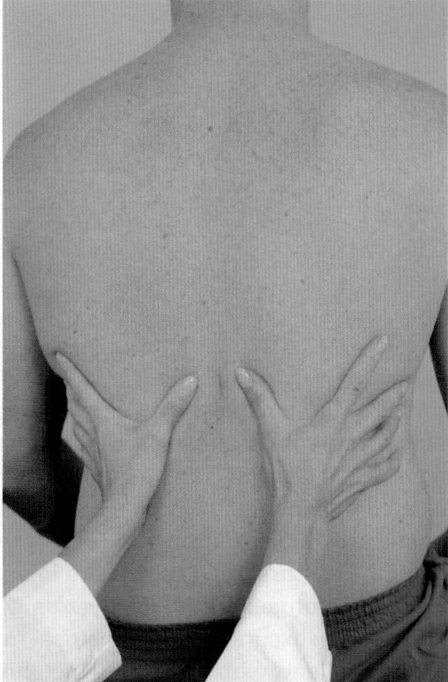 **Figure 16.12** Testing for chest expansion.	

(table continues on page 432)

Technique and Normal Findings (continued)	Abnormal Findings (continued)
Tactile Fremitus. This assessment is made to evaluate the density of lung tissue. Following the sequence for palpation but avoiding the scapula, place the palmar base or ulnar surface of the hand on the patient's chest above the scapula. Ask the patient to say "ninety-nine." Vibrations of air in the bronchial tree are transmitted to the chest wall when the patient speaks. Assess for intensity and symmetry of fremitus from one side of the chest to the other at the same level. If fremitus is difficult to palpate, ask the patient to speak louder. As you become more experienced with the technique, you should be able to palpate tactile fremitus more accurately and efficiently by using both hands simultaneously, one on each side at the same level. *Tactile fremitus is normally felt more intensely in the upper lung fields between the scapulae, where the trachea bifurcates, and gradually diminishes as you move your hands down toward the bases, where more porous tissue reduces the transmission of vibrations. The most important consideration is that the vibrations are felt equally well at the same level from side to side.*	Conditions that obstruct or block air movement through lung tissue cause a decrease or absence of tactile fremitus. Examples include an obstructed bronchus (e.g., foreign body or large mucus plug), pleural effusion, pulmonary fibrosis, solid tumor, or pneumothorax. Fremitus is also reduced when the distance between the lung tissue and chest wall is increased, such as is found in an obese patient. Tactile fremitus is increased when lung tissue density increases or becomes more solid; this is termed consolidation, which can occur with localized pneumonia (Swartz, 2010).
Percussion. As with fremitus, percussion is a technique used to assess the density of underlying tissue. Percussion can help establish whether the tissue is air-filled, fluid-filled, or solid. Use the percussion technique described in Chapter 3. On the posterior chest wall, begin at the apex of the lungs (C7 bilaterally) and percuss from side to side to compare symmetry (see Fig. 16.11). Working toward the bases, side to side in the ICSs, move fingers approximately 5 cm (2 in.) apart. When the fingers are placed below the level of lung tissue, the sound changes from resonant to dull (around T10); from this point, move laterally to percuss near the anterior axillary line and the 7th and 8th ICSs. Avoid the area over the ribs and scapulae because the sound of normal bone is flat. Percussion penetrates only 5–7 cm (about 2–2¾ in.) into the thorax, so abnormalities must be close to the surface and large enough (at least 2–3 cm [about ¾–1¼ in.]) to be detected. Thus, percussion is usually interpreted in combination with other exam techniques and diagnostic tests (e.g., chest x-ray). *Healthy lung tissue sounds resonant. In obese patients and those with extremely large chests, percussion sounds may become dull because the sound does not penetrate deep enough to the lung tissue.*	Percussion sounds are dull when fluid or solid tissue replaces the normally air-filled spaces in the lungs, such as with pneumonia, hemothorax, or tumor. If fluid is in the pleural space (e.g., empyema, pleural effusion), the sound may also be dull. Generalized hyperresonance (a low-pitched, louder sound with a hollow quality, sounding very close to tympany) may be heard over hyperinflated lungs found in patients with emphysema. Unilateral hyperresonance may be found with a large pneumothorax.
Percussing for **diaphragmatic excursion** helps estimate the degree to which the diaphragm descends as the lungs expand. Ask the patient to exhale deeply and hold it; then, percuss in the ICSs down the scapular line (Fig. 16.13).	Diaphragmatic excursion may be reduced in emphysema (in which the diaphragm is already flat) or atelectasis (in which lung tissue is collapsed at the base). Extreme ascites, advanced pregnancy, and extreme obesity also limit diaphragmatic excursion. Neuromuscular paralysis or weakening of the diaphragm in spinal cord injury, stroke, Guillain-Barré syndrome, or muscular dystrophy can also decrease respiratory excursion. Asymmetrical excursion can be found in patients with damage to the phrenic nerve, splenomegaly, or unilateral pleural effusion.

(table continues on page 433)

Technique and Normal Findings (continued)	Abnormal Findings (continued)

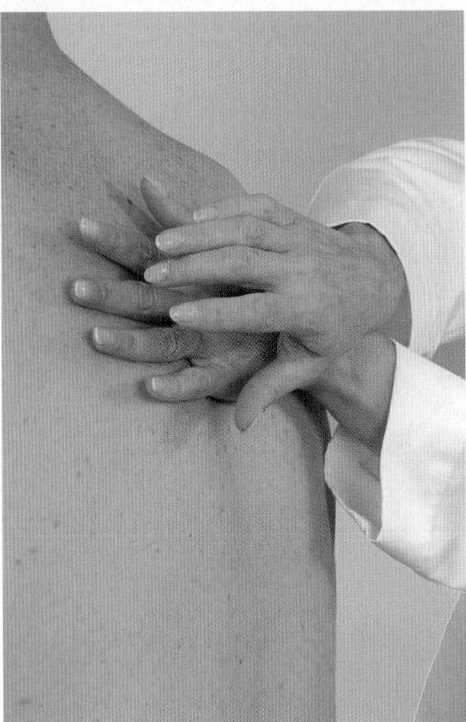

Figure 16.13 Assessing diaphragmatic excursion: percussing in the ICSs.

A strategy to increase patient tolerance and safety is for the nurse to hold his or her breath at the same time as the patient; this will remind the nurse to tell the patient to breathe, limiting the time breath is held.

Mark the location where the sound changes from resonant to dull, which indirectly identifies the level of the diaphragm on full expiration (Fig 16.14). Allow the patient to take several slow breaths, then ask the patient to breathe in as deeply as possible and hold it. Percuss downward, starting just above the mark made where resonance turned to dullness, until the sound becomes dull again; mark this location, then measure the distance between the two marks. *The diaphragmatic excursion normally measures around 3–5 cm (about 1–2 in.), but in well-conditioned people, it may measure up to 8 cm (about 3 in.). The most important factor, though, is that the measurement is approximately the same on both sides. Note that the markings will be slightly higher on the right side because the liver displaces the diaphragm upward, but the measurements will be equal on both sides.*

Auscultation of Breath Sounds. Auscultation of the lung fields is the most important physical examination technique for assessing air flow through the respiratory passages and alveoli. In the larger airways, breath sounds are louder and coarser, whereas sounds in the smaller airways are softer and finer. Auscultate by listening from the top down, alternating between left and right sides.

SAFETY ALERT

Deep breathing can be especially exhausting for patients with respiratory disease; it can also cause some patients to hyperventilate and become dizzy. Monitor the patient closely, and move your stethoscope slowly from one location to the next to allow adequate rest for the patient.

(table continues on page 434)

Technique and Normal Findings (continued)	Abnormal Findings (continued)
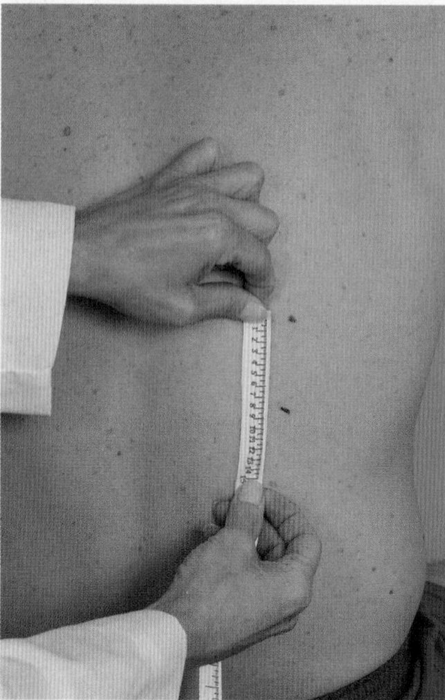 **Figure 16.14** Assessing diaphragmatic excursion: marking the location of lung tissue.	
It is very important to make sure that the stethoscope is in direct contact with the skin. If the patient is wearing a gown or other clothing, place the stethoscope underneath, either from the top or bottom, directly on the chest wall. Avoid listening through any type of clothing, which can generate additional sounds, mimicking adventitious sounds or muffling actual sounds. In addition, take care that the tubing does not rub against bed rails, the patient, or yourself, which can create additional noise.	
Ask the patient to breathe deeply, in and out, through the mouth each time the stethoscope is felt on the skin. Place the diaphragm of the stethoscope firmly on the chest wall to block extraneous noise. Listen to one full breath in each location, moving from side to side to compare symmetry. Be careful not to interpret chest hair sounds as crackles; if this occurs, press more firmly or moisten the chest hair. Stand behind the patient and listen from the lung apices to the bases, then move from side to side, listening in the axillary areas, using the same sequence as percussion (see Fig. 16.15). Be sure to compare each lateral lung field at the same level. If breath sounds are too soft to hear, ask the patient to try to breathe deeper.	
Although the usual sequence is to auscultate from the apices down to the bases, if your patient is very dyspneic or fatigued, it is prudent to begin listening where abnormal sounds are most likely to be present. This means starting at the bases and moving up the chest wall, while closely assessing your patient for signs of excessive fatigue. If this occurs, stop auscultation and allow the patient to rest. As you listen, note any abnormal (adventitious) sounds, such as crackles, wheezes, or rhonchi.	Careful auscultation of the bases is important because they are often the first area to collapse with atelectasis when a patient is immobile. This is also where fluid collects in a pleural effusion (outside the lungs) or with pulmonary edema (in the lungs) in heart failure.

(table continues on page 435)

Technique and Normal Findings (continued)	Abnormal Findings (continued)

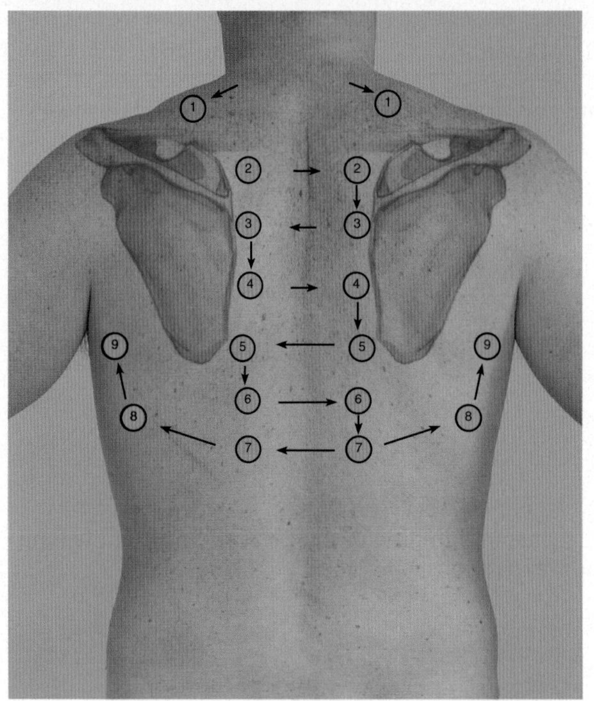

Figure 16.15 Sites and sequence for posterior auscultation.

Identify the breath sounds by listening for their intensity, quality, pitch, and duration of inspiration compared with expiration:

- **Vesicular breath sounds** are soft, low-pitched, and found over fine airways near the site of air exchange (the lung periphery).
- **Bronchovesicular breath sounds** are found more centrally, over major bronchi that have fewer alveoli.
- **Bronchial breath sounds** are loud, high-pitched, and found over the trachea and larynx.

Expiration is longer than inspiration, similar to expected breathing. As auscultation progresses down to the smaller airways, it takes time for air to move in, so inspiration is longer than expiration in vesicular sounds. See Table 16.1 for a thorough description of normal breath sounds.

Breath sounds are considered abnormal when heard outside their expected location, such as bronchial breath sounds heard in the bases. Bronchial or bronchovesicular sounds in the lung periphery are labelled as **coarse breath sounds.**

Decreased or diminished lung sounds are heard in areas of emphysema, atelectasis, or pleural effusion (Bickley & Szilagyi, 2013). Auscultating sounds in obese patients or in those with large chests may be difficult because the lungs are at a greater distance from the chest wall. The breath sounds may be very soft, so a quiet room and a good seal with the stethoscope and the patient's skin are especially important.

Absent breath sounds may be noted over areas where air transmission through the bronchioles is completely blocked, such as in a lung portion blocked by a tumor, or when a pleural effusion is present.

> ⚠ *SAFETY ALERT*
> *Absent breath sounds over a large portion of the lung, such as with a large pleural effusion or mucus plug, when accompanied by respiratory distress, constitutes an emergency. Get help immediately.*

(table continues on page 436)

TABLE 16.1 **Characteristics of Normal Breath Sounds**

	Intensity and Pitch	Quality	Duration	Locations
Bronchial	Loud and high	Coarse or tubular	Inspiration less than expiration	Larynx and trachea
Bronchovesicular	Intermediate and intermediate	Intermediate	Inspiration = expiration	Anteriorly between 1st and 2nd ICSs; between scapula
Vesicular	Soft and low	Whispering undertones	Inspiration greater than expiration	Over most of the lung fields

Technique and Normal Findings (continued)	Abnormal Findings (continued)
Normal breath sounds are vesicular without adventitious sounds (e.g., crackles, wheezes, rhonchi). It is not uncommon, however, to hear crackles on inspiration with the first deep breath, especially when the patient awakens from sleep, or needs to cough. These crackles are the sound of collapsed alveoli opening, which is a common consequence of immobility. If you hear crackles, ask the patient to cough. Normally, these sounds will disappear after cough. It is important to note the absence of adventitious sounds when documenting.	**Adventitious** (added) **breath sounds** are not normally heard. These extra sounds are overlying normal breath sounds. If extra sounds are heard, listen for their volume, pitch, duration, number, timing in the respiratory cycle (inspiration versus expiration), location on the chest wall, variation from breath to breath, and any change after a cough or deep breath. It may be necessary to listen in the same area for a few cycles of breathing to differentiate the timing in the respiratory cycle and note changes that occur with breathing. If crackles, wheezes, or rhonchi are heard, ask the patient to cough to determine whether these sounds resolve. • **Crackles** are discontinuous sounds that are caused by fluid in the airways or alveoli or that result from the opening of collapsed airways and alveoli as they reinflate during deep breathing. They sound like hairs rubbing together near the ear or Velcro opening and are most often heard on inspiration, although they can occasionally be heard during expiration. • **Wheezes** are continuous,high-pitched, musical sounds caused by air squeezing through narrowed airways, as occurs in asthma. Wheezes are generally heard during the expiratory phase in mild-to-moderate airway narrowing. In severe asthma attacks, however, they can be heard during both inspiration and expiration. It is important to document if you hear wheezes during inspiration, expiration, or both (Weber & Kelley, 2014).

(table continues on page 437)

Technique and Normal Findings (continued)	Abnormal Findings (continued)
	• **Rhonchi** are continuous, low-pitched, snoring sounds resulting from secretions moving around in airways. Although they are often louder during the expiratory phase, they can be heard throughout the respiratory cycle. Rhonchi may clear with coughing and are heard most commonly in patients with chronic bronchitis. See Table 16.2 for a complete description of adventitious sounds.
Transmitted voice sounds are evaluated when abnormal breath sounds are auscultated, either sounds heard in abnormal locations, or adventitious sounds noted. Voice sounds do not need to be assessed when thorough percussion and auscultation reveal normal findings.	**Bronchophony**, **egophony**, and **whispered pectoriloquy** (described next) are all found with consolidation or compression, as with pneumonia and pulmonary edema.
To assess bronchophony, ask the patient to repeat "ninety-nine" as you auscultate in the usual locations on the chest wall with a stethoscope, comparing sides. *Bronchophony is negative or absent when sounds are muffled and difficult to distinguish.*	The word "ninety-nine" is clear and louder over denser areas. It sounds as if the patient is speaking directly into the stethoscope. This is documented as positive **bronchophony**. Pneumonia is present 96 to 99% of the time in patients with bronchophony, but patients with pneumonia seldom have it (McGee, 2012)

(table continues on page 27)

TABLE 16.2 Adventitious Breath Sounds

Abnormal Sound	Description	Mechanism	Associated Conditions
Crackles (fine)	High-pitched, soft, brief crackling sounds that can be simulated by rolling a strand of hair near the ear or stethoscope	Deflated small airways and alveoli will pop open during inspiration. In early CHF, small amounts of fluid in the alveoli may cause fine crackles.	Late inspiratory crackles are associated with restrictive disease (e.g., fibrosis and heart failure). Early inspiratory crackles occur with obstructive diseases (e.g., asthma and COPD).
Crackles (coarse)	Low-pitched, moist, longer sounds that are similar to Velcro slowly being separated	Small air bubbles flow through secretions or narrowed airways.	Respiratory fibrosis, respiratory edema, COPD
Wheeze (high-pitched or sibilant)	High-pitched musical sounds heard primarily during inspiration	Air passes though narrowed airways and creates sound, similar to that of a vibrating reed. Note if inspiratory or expiratory.	Asthma, bronchitis, emphysema
Rhonchi (low-pitched wheeze, snoring)	Low-pitched snoring or gurgling sound that may clear with coughing	Airflow passes around or through secretions or narrowed passages.	Pneumonia
Pleural friction rub	Loud, coarse, and low-pitched grating or creaking sound similar to a squeaky door during inspiration and expiration; more common in the lower anterolateral thorax	Inflamed pleural surfaces lose their normal lubrication and rub together during breathing.	Pleuritis
Stridor	Loud, high-pitched, crowing or honking sound louder in upper airway	Laryngeal or tracheal inflammation or spasm can cause stridor, as can aspiration of a foreign object.	Epiglottitis, croup, partially obstructed airway; can indicate an emergency requiring immediate attention

Technique and Normal Findings (continued)	Abnormal Findings (continued)
To assess for egophony, ask the patient to repeat "e e e" while you are auscultating the chest in the usual locations, comparing sides. *Egophony is negative when the sound is muffled and difficult to hear.*	In **egophony**, the "e e e" sounds like a loud "a a a." This finding is often documented as **"Egophony: e → a changes"** or positive egophony.
Whispered pectoriloquy is evaluated by asking the patient to whisper "one-two-three" while you are listening to the chest, comparing sides. *Normal sounds are faint, muffled, and difficult to hear.*	Sounds are louder and clearer than the whispered sounds, as if the patient is directly whispering into the stethoscope. This is documented as positive **whispered pectoriloquy**.
Anterior Chest Inspect the anterior chest using the same techniques as for the posterior chest. Inspect the chest wall for deformities or asymmetry between the right and left sides. Assess the size (degree) of the costal angle. ■ There is no deformity or asymmetry. The costal angle is within 90 degrees.	Asymmetry across sides indicates unequal air entry, which can occur in pneumothorax or flail chest. Deformities of the chest wall could be due to trauma or congenital malformations, such as **pectus excavatum** (also known as funnel chest), which is when the sternum and adjacent cartilages are significantly sunken inward or indented, or **pectus carinatum** (commonly referred to as pigeon chest), when the sternum protrudes outward, resulting in the attached ribs sloping backward. Although these congenital malformations may have no clinical significance, the patient can be very self-conscious about his or her appearance. If the deformity is severe, though, it can restrict lung expansion, thereby decreasing lung capacity (Weber & Kelley, 2014). Widening of the costal angle (i. e., greater than 90 degrees) that occurs when the lungs are chronically hyperinflated is called barrel chest; if mild, it could be a result of aging, but moderate to severe widening indicates COPD. (See Tables 16.6 and 16.7 at the end of the chapter).
Observe for use of accessory muscles to breathe. ■ There is no use of accessory muscles.	Patients in respiratory distress may require the use of accessory muscles to increase the amount of air they inhale. During inspiration, these are primarily the *sternomastoid*, *scalene*, and *trapezius* muscles, but additional chest muscles can also be used when respiratory distress is severe. During forced expiration, which occurs in patients with COPD, the *rectus abdominis* and *internal intercostal* muscles are used.
Inspect ICSs for retractions or bulging. ■ No retractions or bulging are observed.	Intercostal retractions indicate increased inspiratory effort, which can occur in any severe pulmonary condition, such as asthma, pulmonary embolism, or COPD. Retractions appear as indentations in the spaces between the ribs. When **intercostal bulging** is noted, it indicates that trapped air is present, as in an acute asthma attack or emphysema (Weber & Kelley, 2014).
Palpation. Palpate the anterior chest for tenderness, masses, or lesions. Begin at the lung apices and move from side to side, ending below the costal angle and moving laterally to the midaxillary line. See Fig. 16.16. *Normally there is no tenderness, masses, or lesions.*	Tenderness on palpation could indicate musculoskeletal injury, rib fracture, or soft tissue damage. See palpation of posterior chest for other unexpected findings.

(table continues on page 439)

Technique and Normal Findings (continued)	Abnormal Findings (continued)
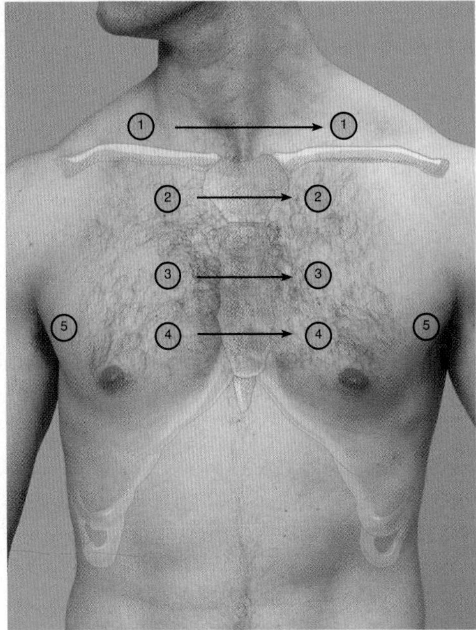 **Figure 16.16** Sites for anterior chest palpation, percussion, and auscultation.	
Assess anterior chest expansion by palpating with the thumbs along each costal margin near the sternum and with the palmar surface laterally on the rib cage (Fig. 16.17). Slide the thumbs medially so that they raise a small skinfold between them. Ask the patient to inhale deeply; observe the thumb movement. Feel for the extent of symmetrical chest expansion. *Anterior chest expansion is greater than posterior because the rib cage has more anterior mobility.* Lateral movement of the thumbs is symmetrical.	Asymmetrical lateral movement of the thumbs indicates unequal airflow between the sides, as in pneumothorax or pleural effusion.
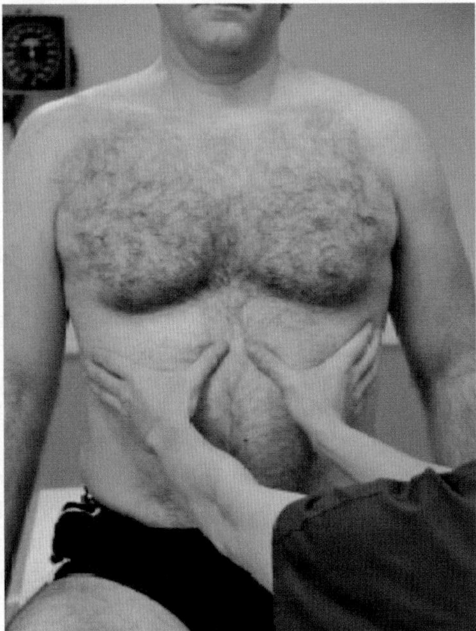 **Figure 16.17** Assessing anterior chest expansion.	

(table continues on page 440)

Technique and Normal Findings (continued)	Abnormal Findings (continued)
Palpate for tactile fremitus, using the same technique identified in the "Posterior Chest" section, beginning at the lung apices and continuing to the bases and laterally, comparing bilateral symmetry. It may be necessary to ask female patients to lift or to displace their breasts to the sides because fremitus is decreased over this soft tissue. *Fremitus is decreased or absent over the precordium because of the heart. Fremitus is greatest over large airways in the 2nd and 3rd ICSs near the sternum and is equal bilaterally.*	Refer to section on assessing the "Posterior Chest" for abnormal tactile fremitus findings.
Percussion. Percuss the anterior and lateral chest in the ICSs, comparing bilateral findings. Use the percussion technique described in Chapter 3. Women may need to displace their breasts to avoid percussion over tender breast tissue, which produces a dull sound. Avoid percussing over bone, which produces a flat tone. *Percussing over lung tissue produces resonance. Percussing over the heart produces dullness from the 3rd–5th ICS to the left of the sternum. The upper border of liver dullness is percussed in the 5th ICS in the right MCL. Tympany is percussed over the stomach in the 5th ICS in the left MCL.*	Dullness percussed over lung tissue indicates consolidation (or solidification, usually from fluid), as in pneumonia.
Auscultation. Auscultate the trachea and anterior and lateral lung fields, beginning at the trachea. Listen to the lung apices, moving the stethoscope from side to side to evaluate symmetry. Place the stethoscope around the breasts in female patients. Listen down to the 6th ICS bilaterally or when breath sounds become absent, signaling the end of the lung fields. *Breath sounds are usually louder in the upper chest, where the larger airways are closer to the chest wall. Bronchial breath sounds are audible over the trachea; bronchovesicular sounds are heard over the 2nd–3rd ICSs to the right and left of the sternum over the bronchi. Vesicular sounds are heard in other areas of the lung fields. No adventitious sounds are heard (see Table 16.2).* If indicated, auscultate for transmitted voice sounds using the same pattern and technique as for the posterior chest.	See Table 16.2 for abnormal lung sounds.

Lifespan Considerations: Older Adults

Immobility in older adults creates a risk for airway collapse (**atelectasis**), reduced air exchange, hypoxia, hypercapnia, and acidosis. Reduced gag and cough reflexes can place older people at risk for aspiration of secretions and, potentially, aspiration pneumonia. Postoperative respiratory complications are another possibility because of impaired cough reflex, weaker muscles, and decreased inspiratory capacity.

Older adults are at increased risk for respiratory complications during stress. Pay attention to maintaining effective ventilation, keeping lung volumes high, clearing secretions, and positioning to prevent aspiration. Respiratory assessment may be tiring for people of this age group, so allow frequent rest periods. Postpone activities that can wait until strength has returned so the patient can use energy for breathing.

Cultural Considerations

Providing culturally competent care is an essential component of high-quality patient care. As previously noted, a considerable variability exists among different cultures with respect to health care practices and conditions involving the respiratory system. It is important to be aware of any biases you may have about other cultural groups and their practices. For example, you may have a negative condescending attitude toward cigarette smokers. Smoking rates vary across cultural groups; if you care for a patient from a culture with a high rate of smoking who has just been diagnosed with lung cancer, your attitude could affect all aspects of that patient's care. This is less likely to occur if you are aware of your bias and have developed a strategy of working to understand the patient's world view.

Documenting Case Study Findings

The nurse has just finished conducting a physical examination of Mr. Lee. Review the following significant findings revealed during objective data collection for this patient. Pay attention to how the nurse clusters data to provide a more complete and accurate understanding of Mr. Lee's condition. This information is collected before initiating the SBAR conversation.

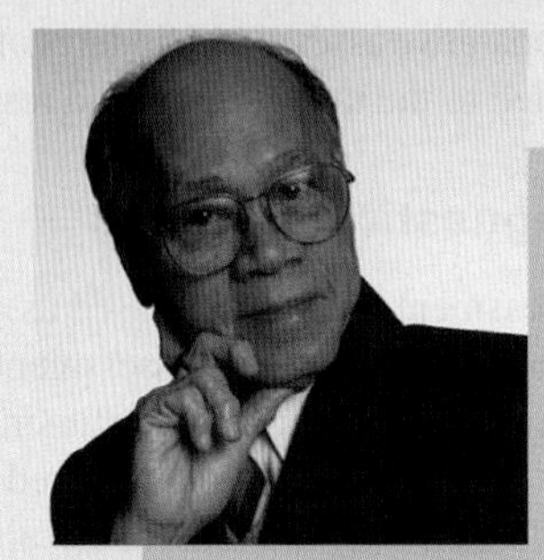

Inspection: T 38°C (100.4°F) oral, P 102 beats/min, R 24 breaths/min, BP 156/78 mm Hg, SaO_2 90%. Alert and oriented. Patient sitting in tripod position in chair with increased respiratory effort. Pursed lip breathing noted. Needs to pause for breath while saying brief sentences. Skin color pale, using neck muscles to breathe, no intercostal retractions noted. Clubbing present in fingers bilaterally. Coughing up moderate amounts of thick yellow sputum. Chest wall nontender to palpation. Increased dyspnea and respirations 32 breaths/min when ambulated to bathroom.

Palpation: Tactile fremitus increased in right base.

Percussion: Right base dull to percussion.

Auscultation: Few wheezes scattered through lung fields. Decreased breath sounds noted in right base. Bronchophony, egophony, and whispered pectoriloquy present over right base.

Critical Thinking

Laboratory and Diagnostic Testing

Laboratory data taken from samples of blood or other body fluids provide indirect measures of disease. For example, an elevated white blood cell count may indicate infection (e.g., pneumonia). Analysis of a sputum sample may help identify the causative microorganism. Arterial blood gas sampling is a direct measure of blood levels of oxygen, carbon dioxide, and acid balance. Radiographic studies can provide objective evidence of a disease process within the thorax and lungs. Positron emission tomography (PET) scans measure the metabolic rate of various body tissues, providing valuable information about the presence and stage of a malignancy. Evaluation of PET scan results helps the surgeon and patient make an informed evidence-based decision about the potential benefit compared with possible mortality risk of undergoing a thoracotomy to remove a lung cancer. If the PET scan revealed adrenal metastasis, for example, the potentially lethal surgery would not provide benefit to the patient.

Chest x-rays are commonly performed in patients with conditions involving the respiratory system. Radiography can identify an area of consolidation suggesting pneumonia, or a cavitary lesion suggesting TB. Chest x-rays can also identify lung masses, although not necessarily at an early curable stage. When more accurate testing is needed to identify the size and shape of lesions, a computed tomography (CT) scan or magnetic resonance imaging (MRI) scan may be indicated. These methods, however, are expensive and not without risk.

Advances in diagnostic testing enable more definitive diagnoses. A spiral (helical) CT scan allows for direct visualization of the cardiac and pulmonary vasculature in cases of suspected pulmonary embolism (PE). Physical findings may include pleuritic chest pain, dyspnea, orthopnea, cough, calf or thigh swelling, and crackles or decreased breath sounds (Stein, et al., 2007). The American Thoracic Society reported that both sensitivity and specificity of spiral CT for PE was greater than 95%; consequently, it has become the most frequent study performed for diagnosing PE (Thompson, 2012).

Pulmonary function tests (PFTs) provide information about the patient's ability to move air into and out of the lungs. PFTs provide objective measurement of a patient's lung function, including the total vital capacity, inspiratory volume, forced expiratory volume in 1 second (FEV1), and the ratio of the FEV1 to the forced vital capacity (FVC). The FEV1-to-FVC ratio has become an important value in diagnosing COPD. Measuring these values is also essential when considering a patient for lung cancer surgery as well as determining if the lungs are healthy enough to tolerate certain chemotherapy agents. In addition, PFTs help determine a patient's need for home oxygen therapy and how reversible a patient's obstructive disease is with bronchodilators. All of this data enhances the ability of health care providers to deliver high-quality care to patients with respiratory disorders (Weatherspoon & Weatherspoon, 2012).

Refer to Tables 16.6 and 16.7 at the end of this chapter for comparative assessment findings of common medical diagnoses related to the thorax, lung, and respiratory functioning.

Diagnostic Reasoning

Assessment findings are used as a basis for nursing care. An accurate and complete assessment provides a firm foundation for identifying appropriate nursing and collaborative diagnoses, developing patient-centered outcomes, providing individualized interventions, and evaluating the patient's progress toward outcome achievement.

You use assessment data to identify desired patient outcomes. Some outcomes related to respiratory disorders are as follows:

- Demonstrate improved ventilation and adequate oxygenation.
- Maintain clear lung fields.
- Remain free of signs of respiratory distress.
- Verbalize understanding of therapeutic interventions.
- Demonstrate correct use of home supplemental oxygen equipment.
- Demonstrate effective coughing.
- Maintain a patent airway at all times.
- Explain methods useful to enhance removal of secretions (Ackley & Ladwig, 2014).

After you have established patient-centered outcomes, you can implement nursing care to improve the patient's clinical condition. You use critical thinking and evidence-based practice to develop appropriate interventions. The following are examples of nursing interventions for patients with respiratory disorders:

- Auscultate breath sounds every 2 to 4 hours.
- Position the patient to optimize respirations.
- Teach and encourage correct use of incentive spirometer every 2 hours.
- Monitor oxygen saturation level using pulse oximetry every 4 hours (Ackley & Ladwig, 2014).

Evaluate the patient's progress toward outcome achievement on an ongoing basis through frequent focused assessments. Use the data obtained from these assessments to modify the plan, as necessary.

An accurate and complete nursing assessment is an essential foundation for provision of holistic nursing care. Even novice nursing students can use patient assessment findings to implement new interventions, evaluate the effectiveness of the interventions, and influence the quality of patient care.

Nursing Diagnoses, Outcomes, and Interventions

Difficulty breathing could be a manifestation of many underlying situations. The patient may be unable to tolerate activity, or there may be thick, tenacious secretions the patient is unable to expectorate. Interventions for each of these problems are very different. If the problem is ineffective airway clearance, interventions to liquefy and mobilize secretions are required. However, if activity intolerance is identified, interventions to achieve balance between oxygen demand and supply are indicated. When formulating a nursing diagnosis, it is important to use critical thinking skills. However, good critical thinking will not compensate for incomplete or inaccurate history and physical examination findings to identify correct nursing diagnoses. Note that the diagnoses are supported by abnormal assessment findings. See Table 16.3 for nursing diagnoses commonly related to thorax, lung, and respiratory assessment (Ackley & Ladwig, 2014).

TABLE 16.3 Common Nursing Diagnoses Associated With the Respiratory System

Diagnosis	Point of Differentiation	Assessment Characteristics	Nursing Interventions
Impaired gas exchange	Describes changes at the capillary level and film/fluid impairing movement across the alveolar wall	Low SaO_2, confusion, cyanosis, fatigue, tachycardia, use of accessory muscles	Administer oxygen,* deep breathing, incentive spirometer, inhalers*
Ineffective airway clearance	Describes situations related to thick tenacious sputum that the patient is too fatigued and weak to expectorate	Weak, ineffective cough; thick secretions; wheezes; rhonchi; cyanosis	Cough and deep breathe, increase fluids, expectorants,* postural drainage*
Ineffective breathing pattern	Describes changes in respiratory rate, rhythm, or depth	Decreased chest excursion, dyspnea, nasal flaring, increased rate, decreased depth, accessory muscles	Position to decrease workload of breathing, pace activity, provide rest, reduce fever
Activity Intolerance	Describes an imbalance between oxygen supply and demand	Dyspneic with minimal activity, SaO_2 decreases and respiratory rate increases with activity	Teach energy-conserving measures, evaluate need for supplemental oxygen, teach slow and steady walking with gradual increase in distance

*Collaborative interventions.
SaO_2, arterial oxygen saturation.

Progress Note: Analyzing Findings

Remember Mr. Lee, whose condition has been outlined throughout this chapter. The initial subjective and objective data collection is complete; the nurse has spent time reviewing the findings and other results. The following nursing note illustrates how subjective and objective data are analyzed, nursing diagnoses are identified, patient-centered outcomes are determined in collaboration with the patient and caregivers, and nursing interventions are developed as part of the nursing process described earlier. The subjective and objective data provide evidence supporting the nursing diagnoses.

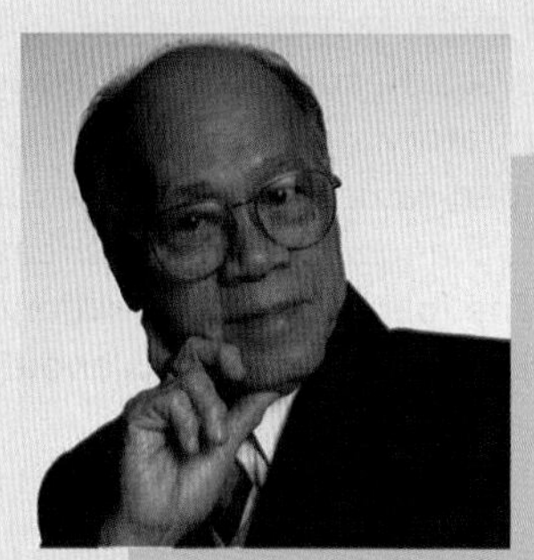

Subjective: "I'm still not feeling very well. When I came in last time, they said that I had bronchitis, but it feels like it's getting worse. Last time I felt wheezy; this time, I'm coughing more." Denies chest pain, complains of increasing fatigue and shortness of breath, coughing up approximately ½ cup thick yellow sputum daily.

Objective: Alert and oriented to person, place, time, and situation. Sitting in tripod position in chair with increased respiratory effort. T 38°C (100.4°F) oral, P 102 beats/min, R 24 breaths/min, BP 156/78 mm Hg, SaO_2 90% in room air. Skin pale. Using sternomastoid and scalene muscles to assist breathing, but no intercostal retractions noted. Breath sounds decreased in base of right lung; few scattered expiratory wheezes in all lung fields. Respirations increased to 32 breaths/min after ambulating about 6 m (20 ft) to bathroom. Required 10 minutes of rest for respirations to return to baseline of 24 breaths/min.

Analysis: Increasing dyspnea, cough, sputum, and fatigue. Impaired gas exchange related to fluid in alveoli as evidenced by SaO_2 90%, decreased breath sounds right base. Activity intolerance related to imbalance between oxygen supply and demand as evidenced by increased respirations of 24–32 breaths/min after walking 20 ft, pallor, complaints of dyspnea and fatigue.

Plan: Contact primary care provider (PCP) with assessment findings, discuss need for sputum culture and chest x-ray, and obtain medication orders; assess effect of dyspnea on patient's sleep pattern and ability to do ADLs; teach correct technique for coughing and deep breathing; teach energy-conserving measures; consult with respiratory therapy team about need for nebulizer treatments, then contact PCP for orders, as indicated. Discuss concerns with patient and his wife.

Critical Thinking Challenge

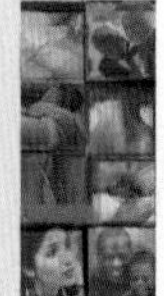

- Critique the objective data that were documented. How will the nursing data collection differ from that of the PCP?
- What additional data might be collected to identify problems affecting other body systems or functional status?
- How will the nurse work collaboratively with the PCP to evaluate interventions?

Collaborating With the Interprofessional Team

In many facilities, nurses initiate referrals for respiratory care based on assessment findings. Results that might trigger a respiratory therapy consult include worsening respiratory status, increased wheezing, absent breath sounds, sudden decrease in oxygen saturation, accessory muscle use, respiratory rate greater than 30 breaths/min, change in pattern of breathing, cyanosis, and/or increasing dyspnea.

The following conversation illustrates how the nurse might organize data and make recommendations about the patient's care to the respiratory therapist.

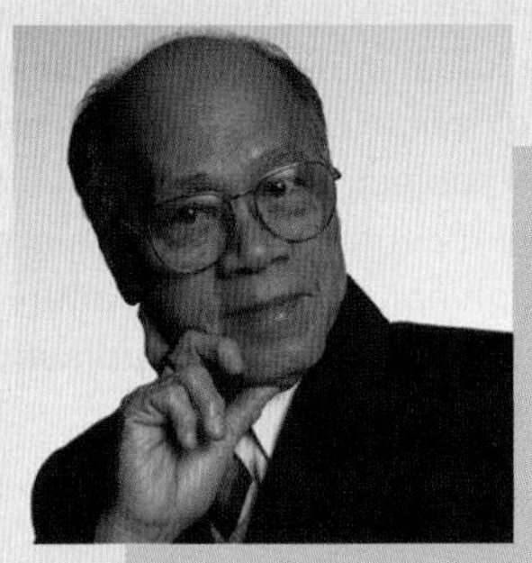

Situation: "Hi, I'm June Nguyen, a nurse working with Mr. Lee. He is 65 years old with a history of COPD, CHF, and hypertension."

Background: "He came in 2 weeks ago for acute exacerbation of his chronic bronchitis and returned to the clinic today with increasing productive cough of thick yellow sputum and fatigue. His temperature is 38°C (100.4°F), respirations are 24 breaths/min, and pulse is 112 beats/min. His oxygen saturations have decreased from his usual level of 92%–94% to 90%. He is short of breath and his respirations increased to 32 after walking only 6 m (20 ft). He usually has scattered wheezes but has a new finding of decreased breath sounds in the right base."

Analysis: "I'm concerned about his low oxygen saturation and ability to handle his increased sputum."

Recommendations: "He is continuing to use his inhalers and he says that they help. I was wondering if you could come to assess his need for supplemental oxygen and evaluate his use of inhalers to make sure that he is using them properly. Could you also listen to his lungs and see whether you think that he might benefit from some chest physiotherapy to assist with mobilizing his secretions?"

Critical Thinking Challenge

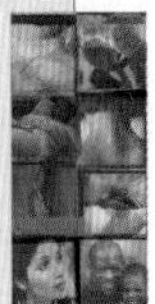

- How did the nurse prioritize which subjective information to share?
- Critique the objective data. Is the organization logical? Would adding or removing any information make it clearer?
- Critique the analysis and recommendations. What is the nurse's role in coordinating collaborative care with respiratory therapy?

Pulling It All Together

The nurse uses assessment data to formulate a nursing care plan for Mr. Lee. The nurse may independently perform teaching on appropriate inhaler use, teach cough and deep breathing techniques, and teach the need for increased fluids to liquefy secretions. The nurse also may initiate a referral to respiratory therapy about inhaler use and possible chest physiotherapy and may consult with the PCP about the patient's potential infection. The assessment data are included as the "as evidenced by" part of the nursing diagnostic statement. Outcomes and interventions are established collaboratively with the patient. After the interventions have been implemented, the nurse will reevaluate (or reassess)

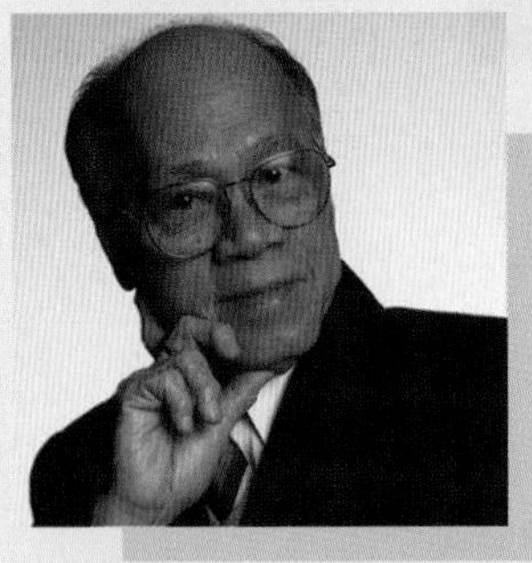

(case study continues on page 445)

Mr. Lee and document the findings in the patient record to show the patient's progress toward meeting outcomes. Although all patients require documented nursing care plans, the formats differ among facilities. Here is an example of a nursing care plan for Mr. Lee:

Nursing Diagnosis	Patient Outcomes	Nursing Interventions	Rationale	Evaluation
Impaired gas exchange related to fluid in alveoli as evidenced by SaO_2 90%, decreased breath sounds right base	Patient will: • Demonstrate correct technique for coughing and deep breathing by 24 hours • Expectorate 25% less sputum by 24 hours • Have SaO_2 of 92% or greater by 48 hours	Contact PCP with assessment findings, discuss need for sputum culture and chest x-ray, and obtain medication orders; encourage oral fluids of 2 L/day.	PCP is responsible for medical plan. Patient has fever and thick yellow sputum, so he may have infection. Increased fluids may liquefy secretions and improve gas exchange.	• Met: Demonstrated accurate cough and deep breathing techniques. • Met: Sputum decreased in viscosity and volume since yesterday. • Not met: SaO_2 today 91% in room air
Activity intolerance related to imbalance between oxygen supply and demand as evidenced by increased respirations of 24–32 breaths/min after walking 20 ft; pallor; complaints of dyspnea and fatigue	Patient will: • Walk 20 ft without increase in respiratory rate by 48 hours • State two strategies to conserve energy for enjoyable activities by 24 hours	Teach energy conservation measures. Consult respiratory therapy about evaluating need for supplemental oxygen. Assist patient to ambulate at tolerable pace; gradually increase distance walked.	• Pacing events throughout the day will allow patient to do enjoyable activities. • SaO_2 90% room air; patient may need supplemental oxygen	• Not met: Respiratory rate increased from 22 to 28 after walking 20 ft. • Met: Patient stated two effective strategies to conserve energy and pace activities.

Applying Your Knowledge

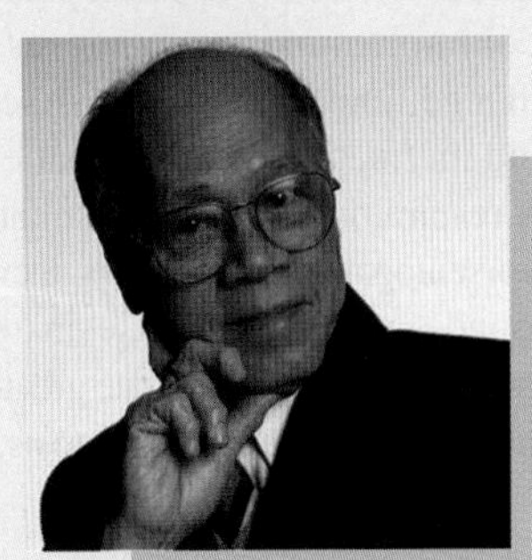

You have reviewed how subjective and objective assessment data are used in developing a diagnosis, planning care, and evaluating progress toward established outcomes. Using the nursing process and your critical thinking skills, consider all the case study findings woven throughout this chapter. While answering the following questions, begin drawing conclusions to see how the pieces of assessment work together to create an environment for individualized, evidence-based, high-quality nursing care.

- Why is the sternal angle (angle of Louis) an important landmark for assessment of the thorax?
- What subjective data collected are cause for concern?
- What health promotion and teaching needs are identified for Mr. Lee?
- Is Mr. Lee's condition stable, urgent, or something requiring immediate attention?
- How will the nurse individualize assessment to meet Mr. Lee's specific needs, considering his condition, age, and culture?
- How will the nurse evaluate the success of patient teaching for Mr. Lee?

Key Points

- Anterior and posterior landmarks are used to document the location of assessment findings.
- Reference lines include the midsternal, midclavicular, anterior axillary, midaxillary, posterior axillary, vertebral, and scapular lines.
- On the anterior chest, the apex of the lung extends approximately 2 to 4 cm (¾ to 1 ½ in) above the inner third of the clavicle, and on the posterior chest wall, the lung base is near T10.
- With aging, the lungs lose elasticity, respiratory muscle strength decreases, cartilage loses flexibility, and bones lose density.
- Dyspnea, decreased level of consciousness, respirations greater than 30 breaths/min, oxygen saturation less than 90%, intercostal retractions, and accessory muscle use may indicate an acute or emergency situation.
- Health promotion includes recommending influenza and pneumococcal vaccines and teaching avoidance of smoking, occupational exposure to irritants, recreational drug use, and high-risk travel.
- Common respiratory symptoms include chest pain, dyspnea, orthopnea, paroxysmal nocturnal dyspnea, cough, sputum, audible wheezing, and change in functional ability.
- The initial survey includes evaluating patient position, pursed lips, nasal flaring, level of consciousness, skin color, respiratory movement and rate, oxygen saturation level, accessory muscle use, and intercostal retractions.
- Abnormal breathing patterns include tachypnea, hyperventilation, bradypnea, hypoventilation, Cheyne-Stokes respiration, Biot breathing, agonal breathing, and apnea.
- Objective assessment includes inspection, palpation, chest expansion, tactile fremitus, percussion, diaphragmatic excursion, and auscultation.
- Breath sounds are auscultated and labeled as vesicular, bronchial, or bronchovesicular.
- Adventitious lung sounds include crackles, wheezes, rhonchi, pleural friction rub, and stridor.
- Auscultate transmitted voice sounds for bronchophony, egophony, and whispered pectoriloquy.
- Common nursing diagnoses include impaired gas exchange, ineffective airway clearance, activity intolerance, and ineffective breathing pattern.
- A respiratory therapy consultation may be indicated with a worsening respiratory status, increased wheezing, absent breath sounds, sudden decrease in oxygen saturation, accessory muscle use, respiratory rate greater than 30 breaths/min, change in pattern of breathing, cyanosis, and increasing dyspnea.

Review Questions

1. When the nurse assesses a 78-year-old patient with pneumonia, what is the priority assessment?
   A. Breath sounds
   B. Airway patency
   C. Respiratory rate
   D. Percussion sounds

2. A 45-year-old man has been admitted to the hospital with suspicion of pulmonary embolism. Which of the following symptoms should the nurse report to the primary health practitioner *immediately*?
   A. Chest pain
   B. Shortness of breath
   C. Respirations 20 breaths/min
   D. Productive cough

3. A 62-year-old woman comes to the clinic with an exacerbation of asthma. Which of the following findings indicate worsening status of her asthma?
   A. Increased wheezing
   B. Sustained rhonchi
   C. Decreased respirations
   D. Pulse oximetry 94%

4. A 3-year-old boy is brought to the emergency department with stridor, nasal flaring, intercostal and supraclavicular retractions, and respiratory rate of 40 breaths/min. What type of situation is this?
   A. Stable
   B. Acute
   C. Urgent
   D. Emergency

5. A 92-year-old woman with a history of COPD presents with increasing shortness of breath, decreased lung sounds in the bases, increased ankle edema, and 5-lb weight gain in 1 week. What is the most likely problem?
   A. Impaired gas exchange
   B. Ineffective airway clearance
   C. Activity intolerance
   D. Excess fluid volume

6. Which of the following factors is the most significant risk factor for COPD?
   A. Increased age
   B. Immune suppression
   C. Tobacco smoking
   D. Occupational exposure

7. When the nurse assesses the client with respiratory symptoms, which of the following complaints should be evaluated first?
   A. Chest pain
   B. Dyspnea
   C. Cough
   D. Sputum

8. When assessing the patient with atelectasis, what assessment findings are expected? Choose all that apply.
   A. Shortness of breath
   B. Decreased breath sounds
   C. Decreased oxygen saturation
   D. Increased tactile fremitus
   E. Hyperresonance

9. Which assessment findings would indicate that inhaled bronchodilators have been effective?
   A. Expiratory wheezing, O_2 saturation 94%, pallor
   B. Vesicular breath sounds, O_2 saturation 96%, pink
   C. Bronchial breath sounds, O_2 saturation 100%, erythema
   D. Crackles, O_2 saturation 90%, circumoral cyanosis

10. The nurse auscultates bronchovesicular breath sounds in the second ICS near the sternum. The nurse interprets this as
    A. a normal finding over the trachea.
    B. a normal finding over the bronchi.
    C. an abnormal finding over the lung.
    D. an abnormal finding over the trachea.

The Jensen suite offers these additional resources to enhance learning and facilitate understanding of this chapter:

- thePoint online resource, http://thepoint.lww.com/Jensen2e
- *Laboratory Manual for Nursing Health Assessment: A Best Practice Approach*
- *Pocket Guide for Nursing Health Assessment: A Best Practice Approach*
- *Lippincott DocuCare,* an electronic health record simulation software, http://thepoint.lww.com/docucare
- *Adaptive Learning | Powered by PrepU*, http://thepoint.lww.com/prepu

References

Ackley, B. J., & Ladwig, G. B. (2014). *Nursing diagnosis handbook: An evidence-based guide to planning care* (10th ed.). Maryland Heights, MO: Mosby Elsevier.

Bailey, P. P. (2013). Tuberculosis. In T. M. Buttarro, J. Trybulski, P. P. Bailey, & J. Sandberg-Cook (Eds.), *Primary care: A collaborative practice* (4th ed., pp. 1283–1291). St. Louis, MO: Elsevier Mosby.

Bickley, L. S., & Szilagyi, P. G. (2013). *Bates' guide to physical examination and history taking* (11th ed.). Philadelphia, PA: Lippincott Williams & Wilkins.

Boardman, M. B. (2013). Chronic obstructive pulmonary disease. In T. M. Buttarro, J. Trybulski, P. P. Bailey, & J. Sandberg-Cook (Eds.), *Primary care: A collaborative practice* (4th ed., pp. 445–454). St. Louis, MO: Elsevier Mosby.

Braun, C. A., & Anderson, C. M. (2011). *Pathophysiology: A clinical approach* (2nd ed.). Philadelphia, PA: Lippincott Williams & Wilkins.

Centers for Disease Control and Prevention. (2013a). CDC Health Disparities and Inequalities Report—United States, 2013. *Morbidity and Mortality Weekly Report, 62*(Suppl. 3), 1–186. Retrieved from http://www.cdc.gov/tb/topic/populations/HealthDisparities/default.htm

Centers for Disease Control and Prevention. (2013b). *Immunization schedule recommendations for adults (ACIP).* Retrieved from http://www.cdc.gov/vaccines/schedules/hcp/imz/adult.html

Centers for Disease Control and Prevention. (2013c). *Immunization schedule recommendations for children (ACIP).* Retrieved from http://www.cdc.gov/vaccines/schedules/hcp/child-adolescent.html

Centers for Disease Control and Prevention. (2013d). *Tuberculosis: Basic TB facts*. Retrieved from http://www.cdc.gov/tb/topic/basics/risk.htm

Crocker, D., Brown, C., Moolenaar, R., Moorman, J., Bailey, C., Mannino, D., & Holguin, F. (2009). Racial and ethnic disparities in asthma medication usage and health-care utilization: Data from the National Asthma Survey. *Chest, 136*(4), 1063–1071.

Damjanov, I. (2012). *Pathology for the health professions* (4th ed.). St. Louis, MO: Elsevier Saunders.

Foster, J., Gilbert, T., & Long, R. (2012). Immune problems. In J. M. Foster & S. S. Prevost (Eds.), *Advanced practice nursing of adults in acute care* (pp. 652–692). Philadelphia, PA: F. A. Davis.

Gorman, B. K., & Chu, M. (2009). Racial and ethnic differences in adult prevalence, problems, and medical care. *Ethnicity & Health, 14*(5), 527–552.

Gallup Polling. (2013). *Nurses rated highest in honesty and ethical standards in 2013.* Retrieved from http://www.gallup.com/video/166502/nurses-rated-highest-honesty-ethical-standards-2013.aspx

Hogan-Quigley, B., Palm, M. L., & Bickley, L. (2012). *Bates' nursing guide to physical examination and history taking.* Philadelphia, PA: Wolters Kluwer Health/Lippincott Williams & Wilkins.

Khan, M., & Pelengaris, S. (2013). Nature and nurture in oncogenesis. In S. Pelengaris & M. Khan (Eds.), *The Molecular biology of cancer: A bridge from bench to bedside* (2nd ed., pp. 67–110). West Sussex, United Kingdom: John Wiley & Sons

Leahy, L. G., & Rosof-Williams, J. (2012). Psychosocial health problems. In J. M. Foster & S. S. Prevost (Eds.), *Advanced practice nursing of adults in acute care* (pp. 98–173). Philadelphia, PA: F. A. Davis Company.

McGee, S. (2012). *Evidence-based physical diagnosis.* Philadelphia, PA: Elsevier.

Moini, J. (2012). *Anatomy and physiology for health professionals.* Sudbury, MA: Jones & Bartlett Learning.

Moore, K. L., Dalley, A. F., & Agur, A. M. (2014). *Clinically oriented anatomy* (7th ed.). Philadelphia, PA: Lippincott Williams & Wilkins.

Murphy, D. P. (2013). Dyspnea. In T. M. Buttarro, J. Trybulski, P. P. Bailey, & J. Sandberg-Cook (Eds.), *Primary care:A collaborative practice* (4th ed., pp. 454–458). St. Louis, MO: Elsevier Mosby.

Porth, C. M. (2011). *Essentials of Pathophysiology: Concepts of altered health states* (3rd ed.). Philadelphia, PA: Wolters Kluwer Health/Lippincott Williams & Wilkins.

Smith, J. A., & Houghton, L. A.(2013). The oesophagus and cough: Laryngo-pharyngeal reflux, microaspiration and vagal reflexes. *Cough, 9*(1), 12. doi:10.1186/1745-9974-9-12

Stein, P. D, Beemath, A., Matta, F., Weg, J. G., Yusen, R. D., Hales, C. A., . . . Woodard, P. K. (2007). Clinical characteristics of patients with acute pulmonary embolism: data from PIOPED II. *American Journal of Medicine, 120*(10), 871–879.

Steward, W. P., & Thomas, A. L. (2013). The burden of cancer. In S. Pelengaris & M. Khan (Eds.), *The Molecular biology of cancer: A bridge from bench to bedside* (2nd ed., pp. 43–66). West Sussex, United Kingdom: John Wiley & Sons.

Swartz, M. H. (2010). *Textbook of physical diagnosis: History and examination* (6th ed.). Philadelphia, PA: Saunders Elsevier.

Thompson, C. J. (2012). Cardiovascular problems. In J. M. Foster & S. S. Prevost (Eds.), *Advanced practice nursing of adults in acute care* (pp. 239–397). Philadelphia, PA: F. A. Davis.

U.S. Department of Health & Human Services. (2013a). *2020 Topics & objectives – Objectives A-Z.* Retrieved from http://www.healthypeople.gov/2020/topicsobjectives2020/

Weatherspoon, D. L., & Weatherspoon, C. A. (2012). Pulmonary problems. In J. M. Foster & S. S. Prevost (Eds.), *Advanced practice nursing of adults in acute care* (pp. 398–443). Philadelphia, PA: F. A. Davis.

Weber, J. R., & Kelley, J. H. (2014). *Health assessment in nursing* (5th ed.). Philadelphia, PA: Wolters Kluwer Health/Lippincott Williams & Wilkins.

Tables of Abnormal Findings

TABLE 16.4 Abnormal Respiratory Patterns

Visual Pattern	Description	Associated Conditions
Expected Inspiration Expiration	Rate of 10–20 breaths/min Ratio of respiration to pulse is approximately 1:4 500–800 ml/breath Regular rhythm	Expected findings
Tachypnea	Rate greater than 24 breaths/min Less than 500 ml/breath, shallow Regular rhythm	Anxiety, fear, elevated metabolic rate, fever, exercise, respiratory diseases in which rate must be increased to maintain oxygenation
Hyperventilation	Rate greater than 24 breaths/min Greater than 800 ml/breath, deep Regular rhythm	Extreme anxiety or fear, exercise, increased intracranial pressure Kussmaul respirations are seen with diabetic ketoacidosis because the body is attempting to remove carbon dioxide to normalize pH.
Bradypnea	Rate less than 10 breaths/min 500–800 ml/breath, shallow Regular rhythm	Conditions in which the breathing center in the medulla is depressed, such as narcotic overdose; diabetic coma and increased intracranial pressure
Hypoventilation	Rate less than 10 breaths/min Less than 500 ml/breath, shallow Irregular rhythm	Narcotic or anesthetic overdose, increased intracranial pressure
Cheyne-Stokes respiration Hyperpnea Apnea	Rate variable Depth variable Regular irregular rhythm that cycles from deep and fast to shallow and slow, with some periods of apnea	Expected in children and the elderly; also, terminal illness, renal failure, drug overdose, increased intracranial pressure, and heart failure. Count the rate for 1 full minute and record the length of apnea.
Biot respiration	Rate variable Depth variable Irregular rhythm	Severe brain damage, commonly at the level of the medulla. Count the rate for 1 full minute and record the length of apnea.
Agonal	Rate intermittent Depth variable	Finding in patients at end of life. Count the rate for 1 full minute and record the length of apnea.
Apnea	No breaths	Cardiac arrest and brain death

TABLE 16.5 Abnormal Thoracic Configurations

Normal Adult

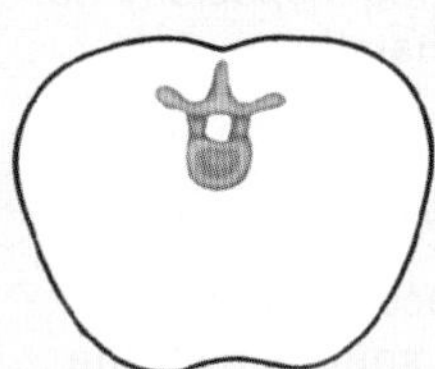

Anteroposterior (AP)-to-lateral: ratio is 1:2, wider than it is deep, oval shaped. Cone-shaped from head to toe.

Kyphoscoliosis

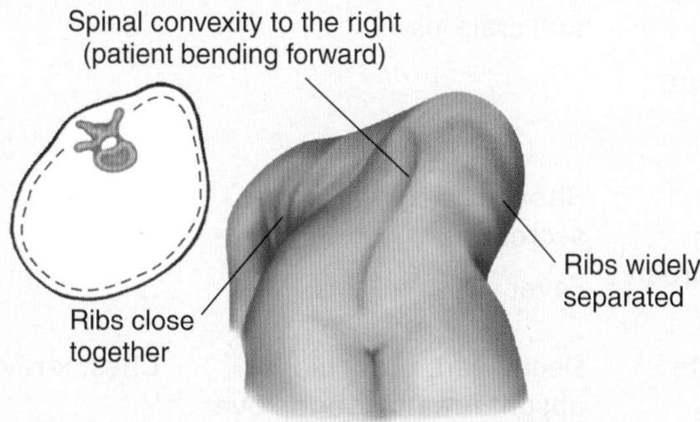

With kyphosis, the thoracic spine curves forward, compressing the anterior chest and reducing inspiratory lung volumes. With scoliosis, a lateral S-shaped curvature of the spine causes unequal shoulders, scapulae, and hips. In severe cases, asymmetry may impede breathing.

Pectus Carinatum (pigeon chest)

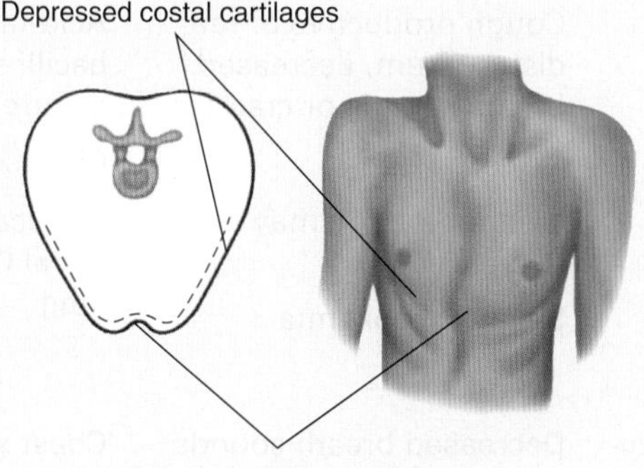

Sternum is displaced anteriorly, depressing the adjacent costal cartilages. Congenital condition with increased AP diameter.

Pectus Excavatum (funnel chest)

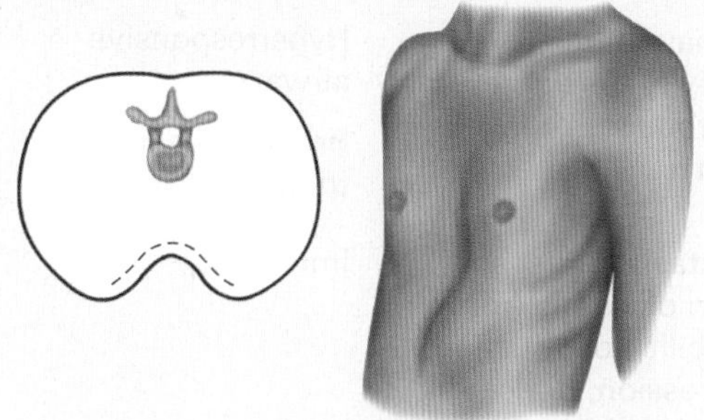

Depression in lower part of sternum. Congenital condition may compress the heart or great vessels and cause murmurs.

Barrel chest

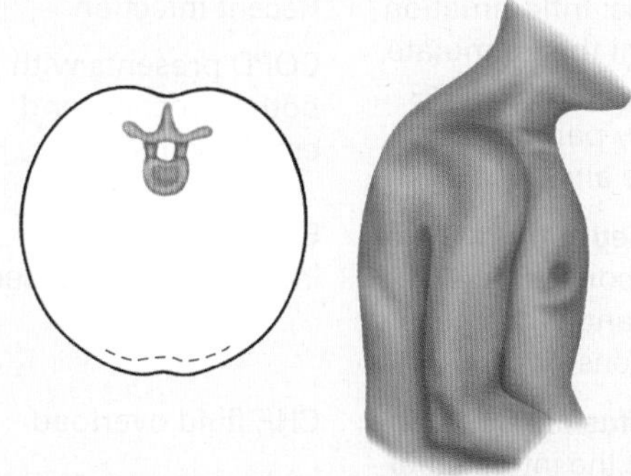

AP-to-lateral ratio near 1:1, round shaped. Ribs are more horizontal and costal margin is widened. Associated with COPD, chronic asthma, and normal aging.

Flail chest

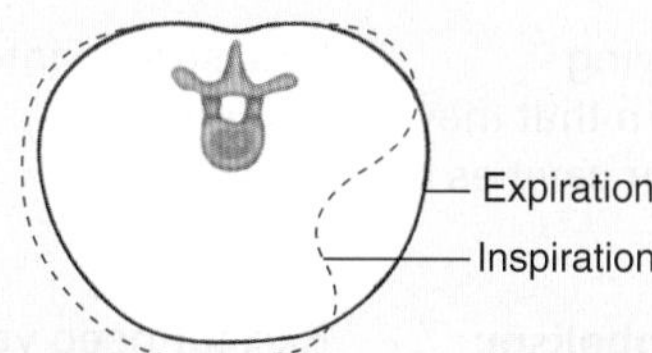

When multiple ribs are fractured, paradoxical movements of the chest may occur. As the diaphragm pulls down during inspiration, negative pressure causes the injured area to cave inward; during expiration, it moves out.

TABLE 16.6 Common Respiratory Conditions

Condition	Risk Factors	History and Subjective Data	Objective Data	Diagnostic Tests
Asthma: Allergic hypersensitivity to allergens that produces bronchospasm	Hyperresponsive airways Bronchospasm triggers	Cough worse at night and early morning	Wheezing, especially during exhalation Diminished lung sounds Clear sputum	Respiratory function with short-acting bronchodilator
Atelectasis: Collapsed section of alveoli from immobility, obstruction, compression, or decreased surfactant	Immobility	Dyspnea Fever possible No sputum	Decreased or absent breath sounds over the atelectasis area, reduced inspiratory capacity	Chest x-ray
Emphysema: Destruction of respiratory capillary bed and alveoli creating large air sacs and bullae	Smoking Occupational exposure	Shortness of breath Chronic cough	Cough, shortness of breath, decreased breath sounds, barrel chest	Respiratory function tests
Bronchitis: Inflammation of bronchi that stimulate mucous glands. Secretions may partially obstruct the airways	Recent infection COPD presents with both bronchitis and emphysema	Chest tight or wheezy Clear sputum	Occasional wheezing or fine crackles	Chest x-ray
Lobar pneumonia: Alveoli become congested with bacteria and white cells causing consolidation	Elderly, immunocompromised	Productive cough with yellow or green sputum	Rhonchi resulting from secretions Fever	Sputum culture
Pleural effusion: Collection of fluid in the intrapleural space that compresses the lung tissue	CHF, fluid overload	Frothy white sputum	Decreased, bronchial or absent breath sounds over effusion	Chest x-ray
Pneumothorax or hemothorax: Collapsed or blood-filled lung	Trauma, central line placement	Dyspnea	Absent breath sounds over area of collapse or bleeding	Chest x-ray
CHF: Fluid overload and respiratory congestion	High blood pressure, renal disease	Dyspnea, edema, weight gain	Decreased breath sounds, fine late inspiratory crackles	Chest x-ray
TB: Slow growing mycobacterium that may form lesions or cavities in the lung	Exposure to infected person	Night sweats	Cough productive of reddish sputum, decreased breath sounds or crackles	Acid-fast bacilli sputum culture Chest x-ray
Pulmonary embolism: Blood clot in the pulmonary vein that causes shunting of blood to atelectasis area	Risk for deep vein thrombosis	Severe dyspnea, no sputum	Clear or if large may be decreased. Severe hypoxemia	V/Q scan or spiral CT of lung
***Pneumocystis jiroveci* pneumonia:** Pathogenic infection that is common in immunosuppressed people	HIV/AIDS	Dry nonproductive cough	Decreased breath sounds	Chest x-ray Sputum culture

TABLE 16.7 Common Respiratory Diagnoses

Condition	Auscultation	Sputum	Percussion
Asthma	Wheezes Diminished lung sounds	Clear	Occasional hyperresonance
Atelectasis	Diminished lung sounds in lower lobe	None	Dullness over affected lung
Bronchitis	Occasional wheezing or fine crackles	Clear	Resonance
COPD	Wheezes	Clear	Hyperresonance
Pneumothorax	Absent sounds	Absent	Hyperresonance over affected area
Hemothorax	Absent sounds	Bloody	Dull over affected area
Pneumonia	Wheezes, crackles, or gurgles	Purulent	Dull over affected area
CHF	Absent bases	Frothy	Dull bases
Pleural effusion	Absent over affected lung	None	Dull over affected lung
Respiratory embolism	Clear or mild wheezes	None	Tympanic

17

Heart and Neck Vessels Assessment

Learning Objectives

1 Identify the structures and functions of the heart.

2 Identify the location of the heart and common auscultatory areas on the precordium.

3 Identify teaching opportunities for cardiovascular health promotion and risk reduction.

4 Collect subjective data about common cardiovascular symptoms: chest pain, dyspnea, orthopnea, cough, diaphoresis, fatigue, edema, and nocturia.

5 Collect objective data about the carotid artery, jugular veins, and heart.

6 Identify normal and abnormal findings from the inspection, palpation, and percussion of the precordium.

7 Auscultate normal and abnormal heart sounds, including S1, S2, split sounds, extra sounds, murmurs, and rubs.

8 Analyze subjective and objective data and then plan interventions related to the cardiovascular system.

9 Document and communicate data about the cardiovascular system using appropriate medical terminology.

10 Individualize cardiovascular health assessment considering the condition, age, gender, and culture of the patient.

Mrs. Lewis, a 77-year-old Caucasian woman, has been admitted to the hospital with chest pain and myocardial infarction (MI, commonly known as a heart attack). She has been on the cardiac unit for 4 hours. Nurses from the previous shift documented their admitting assessment data. The patient's current vital signs are oral temperature 37°C (98.6°F), pulse 112 beats per minute (bpm), respirations 20 breaths/min, and blood pressure 148/78 mmHg. Current medications include a thiazide diuretic and beta-blocker for high blood pressure and a cholesterol-lowering drug. She has nitroglycerin tablets ordered as needed for chest pain.

You will gain more information about Mrs. Lewis as you progress through this chapter. As you study the content and features, consider Mrs. Lewis's case and its relationship to what you are learning. Begin thinking about the following points:

- What might be causing the change in Mrs. Lewis's condition?
- Is Mrs. Lewis's condition stable, urgent, or an emergency?
- What immediate health promotion and teaching needs are evident?
- What lifestyle factors might be contributing to Mrs. Lewis's situation?
- How will the nurse focus, organize, and prioritize objective data collection?
- How will the nurse evaluate the effectiveness of patient teaching?

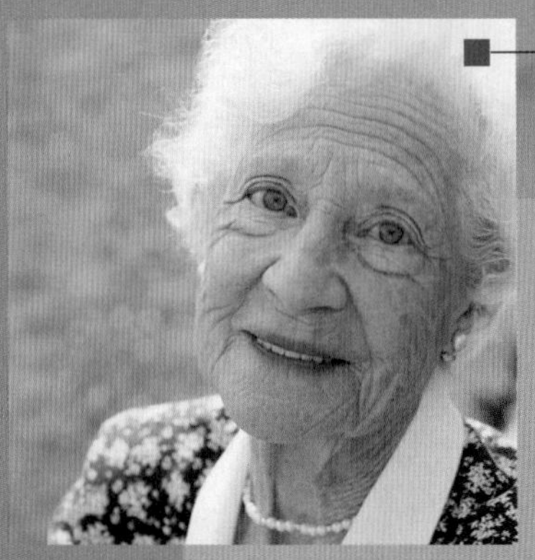

The human cardiovascular system is complex. Disorders in structure or function can affect the entire body. Thus, it is important to understand the many factors that contribute to performing an accurate and complete assessment of this region for each patient.

Thorough knowledge of pertinent anatomy and physiology, especially the cardiac cycle, is essential in order to conduct an accurate assessment and understand normal and abnormal findings. Along with other health care providers, you will assess cardiovascular risk factors and common symptoms as part of subjective data collection. During the interview and health history, you will gather information about current risk factors, such as a diet high in fat and cholesterol, high blood pressure, physical inactivity, and smoking. Auscultation of the heart will help you verify the presence of normal sounds heard upon closure of the heart valves as well as identify any abnormal and extra sounds, including murmurs and gallops. You will document and communicate assessment information to appropriate health care providers. You will also plan care to promote healthy heart habits, prevent cardiovascular disease, and treat identified conditions.

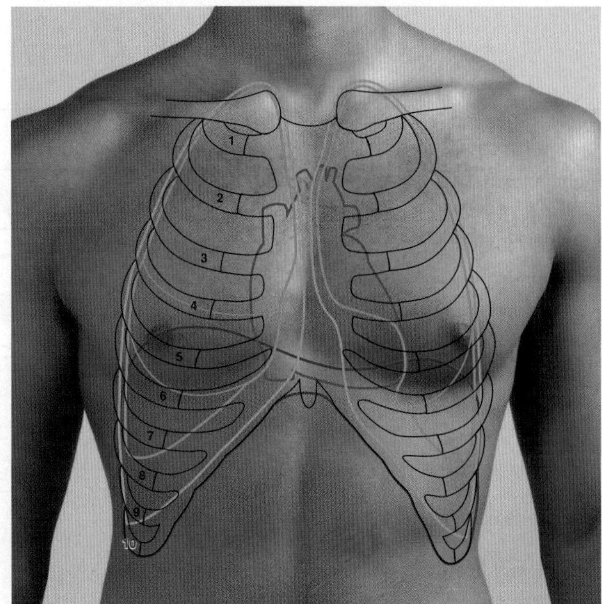

Figure 17.1 Surface anatomy of the thoracic contents. Note the outline of the heart's placement in relation to the thoracic cage.

Structure and Function

The cardiovascular system includes the heart and blood vessels (great vessels and peripheral vascular system). It delivers oxygen and nutrients to the cells and tissues and returns waste products to the central circulation for excretion. This chapter concentrates on the heart and great vessels; see Chapter 18 for a detailed discussion of the peripheral vascular system.

Anatomy

The heart and great vessels are located in the mediastinum between the lungs and above the diaphragm from the center to the left of the thorax (Fig. 17.1). The total size of the heart is approximately that of a clenched adult fist. The female heart is normally smaller and weighs less than the male heart across all age groups (Woods, Sivarajan Froelicher, Motzer, & Bridges, 2010).

The locations for auscultating heart sounds are identified by landmarks on the anterior thoracic wall. The intercostal spaces (ICSs), sternal lines, and midclavicular line (MCL) are used to describe the location of heart sounds and impulses.

The top of the heart is referred to as the base because it is broad; the bottom of the heart is referred to as the apex. This is the opposite of the lungs, where the top is the **apex** and the bottom is the base. The base of the heart is found at the 2nd ICS, spanning from the left to right sternal border, whereas the apex is located in the fifth ICS, 7 to 9 cm (2¾ to 3½ in.) left of the midsternal line.

The **point of maximal impulse (PMI)** is used to describe the area where the apical pulsation can be seen or palpated. In most adults, this impulse can commonly be found at the intersection of the 5th ICS and the left MCL.

The inferior border of the heart lies at the junction between the xiphoid process and the sternum to the left 5th ICS in the MCL laterally. The precordial area on the anterior chest overlies the heart and great vessels, between the 2nd and 5th ICS at the right sternal border to approximately the 2nd and 5th ICS at the left MCL (Fig. 17.2).

The arterial great vessels include the carotid arteries, aorta, and pulmonary veins. The venous great vessels are the jugular veins, superior vena cava, inferior vena cava, and pulmonary arteries. The great vessels originate from the base (top) of the heart and then turn in the direction of the body part that they supply (Fig. 17.3).

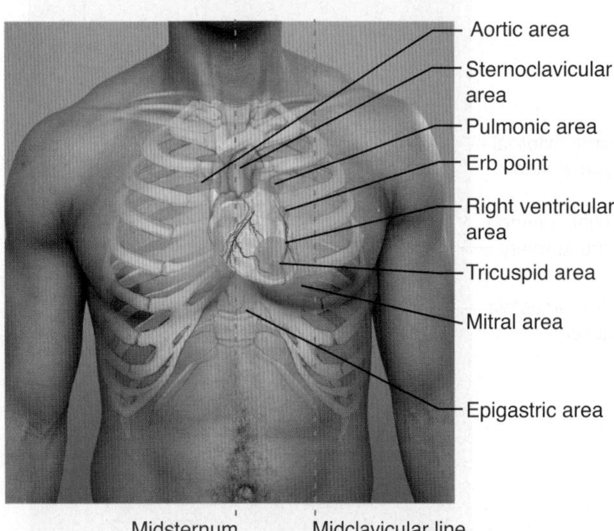

Figure 17.2 The anterior chest and cardiac landmarks.

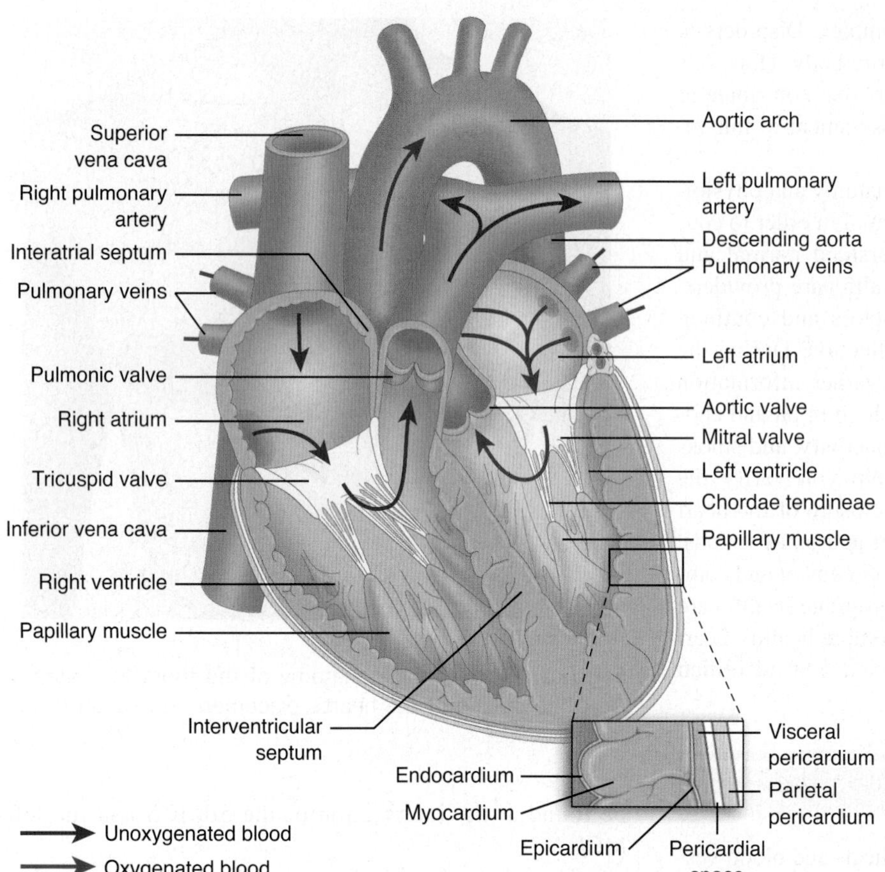

Figure 17.3 Interior anatomy of the heart. The *arrows* show the direction of blood flow through the heart chambers.

Neck Vessels

The neck vessels include the carotid arteries and internal and external jugular veins (Fig. 17.4).

The carotid arteries are located in the depression between the trachea and sternomastoid muscle in the anterior neck and run parallel to the trachea from clavicle to jaw bilaterally. Palpation of the carotid arteries normally reveals a strong pulsation.

The internal and external jugular veins are named for their position in the neck. The internal jugular vein is deeper and nearer the carotid artery. Because of its location, it usually is not visible; because it is a vein, it is not palpable.

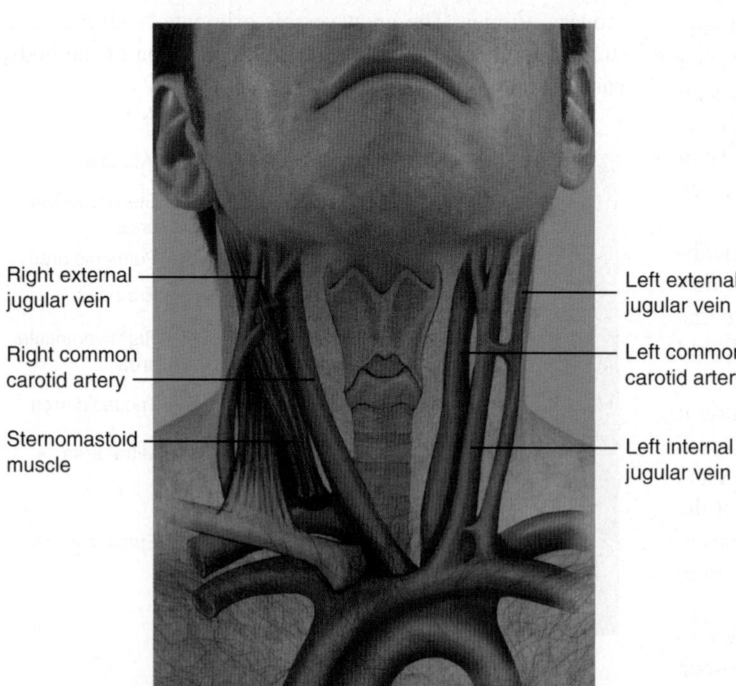

Figure 17.4 Anatomy of the neck vessels. Note how the jugular vein rises above the middle of the clavicle lateral to the carotid artery.

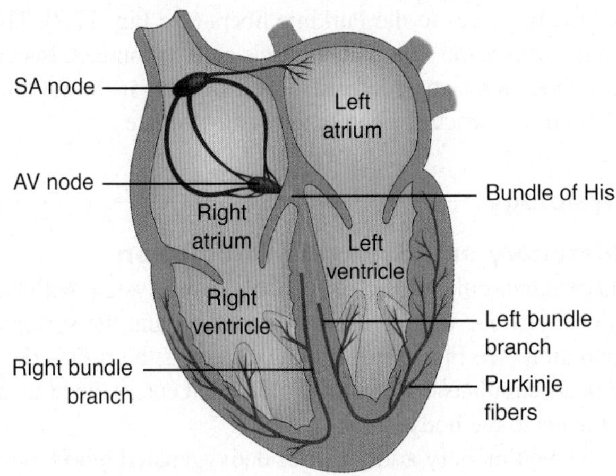

Figure 17.5 The heart wall, chambers, and valves.

The more superficial external jugular vein is visible in the depression above the middle of the clavicle. It is lateral instead of anterior to the sternomastoid muscle and travels from the clavicle up to the jaw line.

Heart Chambers

Two main walls divide the heart into two upper and two lower chambers (Fig. 17.5). The upper chambers, or atria, collect and pump blood into the ventricles. The ventricles pump blood out to the lungs and body. The septum separates the left and right sides of the heart. The left side is larger and more muscular; it circulates blood farther (to the entire body) and against a higher pressure (the blood pressure). The right side circulates blood to the lower pressure pulmonary system; it is thinner walled and smaller.

Valves

The heart has four valves that open and close to permit blood to flow forward in one direction and prevent blood from flowing backward during contraction (see Fig. 17.3).

The two atrioventricular (AV) valves separate the atria from the ventricles. The tricuspid valve separates the right atrium and ventricle, whereas the mitral valve separates the left atrium and ventricle.

The two semilunar valves separate the ventricles from the great vessels. The pulmonic valve lies between the right ventricle and pulmonary artery, whereas the aortic valve lies between the left ventricle and aorta. These valves are named after the vessel that they fill.

Heart Wall

The wall of the heart consists of three layers:

1. The thin endocardium lines the inside of the heart's chambers and valves.
2. The thick muscular myocardium is the middle layer responsible for the pumping action of the heart.
3. The thin epicardium is a muscle layer on the outside of the heart.

The tough fibrous pericardium encloses and protects the heart. Its two layers contain a small amount of fluid for lubrication during pumping. The pericardium adheres to the great vessels, esophagus, sternum, and pleurae and is anchored to the diaphragm.

Coronary Arteries and Veins

The muscular part of the heart needs its own blood supply. The coronary arteries arise from the base and branch out to the apex of the heart. The more muscular left side has a greater blood supply, with two main arteries instead of one (Fig. 17.6). The left coronary and circumflex arteries supply the left side; the right coronary artery supplies the right side. The arteries fill when the heart relaxes. Cardiac veins empty deoxygenated blood into the coronary sinus at the base.

> **Clinical Significance**
>
> The coronary arteries may develop atherosclerotic plaques that narrow them, leading to MI (heart attack) or angina.

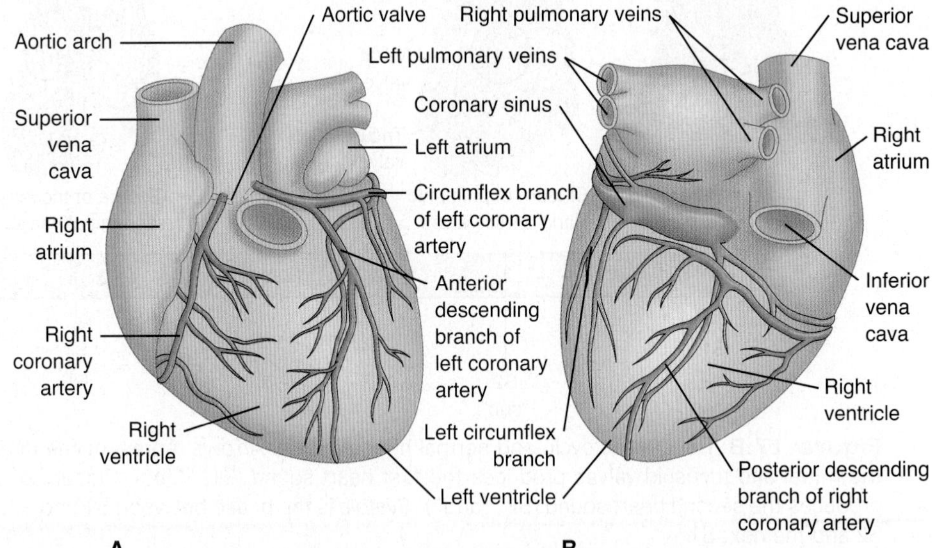

Figure 17.6 The coronary arteries adjust the flow of oxygenated blood to the heart muscle according to metabolic needs. **A.** Anterior view. **B.** Posterior view.

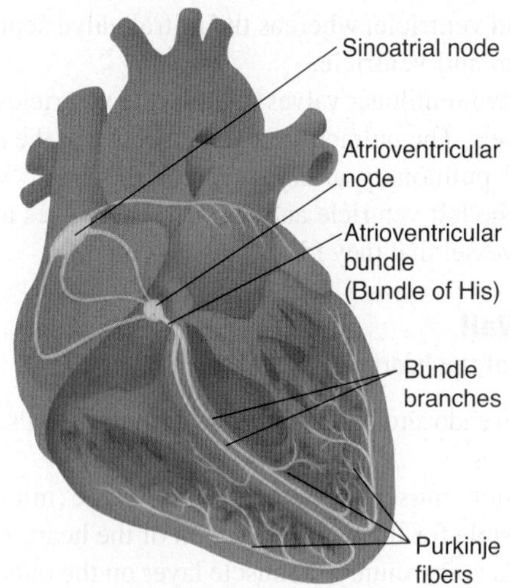

Figure 17.7 Outline of the path and involved structures of the cardiac conduction system.

Conduction System

A small electrical impulse that fires in the sinoatrial (SA) node in the right atrium generates the normal heartbeat. The SA node functions as the "pacemaker" of the heart (Fig. 17.7). Cells in the SA node possess automaticity (a property that enables the cardiac cells to generate their own impulses). Other cells in the heart also possess automaticity but generally have a slower intrinsic rate than the SA node, causing their impulses to be suppressed by the faster SA node.

After an impulse has been generated, it moves through an electrical "wiring" pathway through the left and right atria (via intraatrial pathways). The electrical impulse causes the atrial muscle cells to contract. Then, the impulse pauses briefly at the AV junction, travels through the electrical pathways in the bundle of His and bundle branches in the left and right ventricles, and finally moves to the Purkinje fibers (see Fig. 17.7). This impulse causes the ventricular muscle cells to contract. In people without conduction defects, the rate of firing in the SA node determines ventricular contraction and pulse rate.

Physiology

Pulmonary and Systemic Circulation

The cardiovascular system is a double pump system with two major divisions: the pulmonary circulation and the systemic circulation (see Fig. 17.6). Blood that enters the right side of the heart circulates to the lungs; blood that enters the left side circulates to the body.

The pulmonary artery carries deoxygenated blood to the lungs. At the lungs, the blood picks up oxygen and releases carbon dioxide. The pulmonary vein delivers oxygenated blood to the left atrium, which circulates the blood to the left ventricle and then out to the systemic circulation. Note that this process is the opposite of other body areas, where arteries carry oxygenated blood and veins carry deoxygenated blood.

The systemic circulation supplies the tissues with oxygen and nutrients and returns waste to the central circulation for excretion. The jugular veins and carotid arteries perfuse the brain, the superior vena cava and subclavian arteries perfuse the upper limbs, and the inferior vena cava and thoracic aorta perfuse the lower limbs.

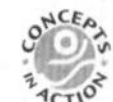 Cardiac Cycle

The continuous rhythmic movement of blood during contraction and relaxation of the heart is the cardiac cycle. Squeezing of the heart during contraction is referred to as **systole**; relaxing of the heart is called **diastole** (Fig. 17.8).

Deoxygenated blood enters the right atrium from the superior and inferior vena cava. The right and left atria fill with blood until the SA node initiates atrial contraction by

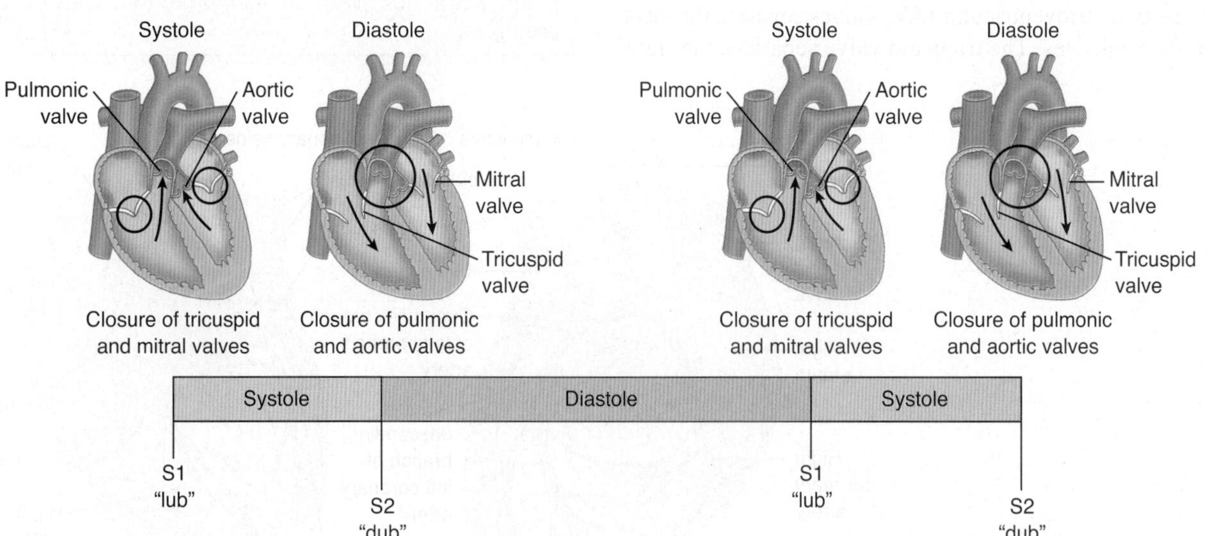

Figure 17.8 The cardiac cycle and normal heart sounds. *Arrows* represent the direction of blood flow. Closure of the mitral and tricuspid valves produces the first heart sound (S1, "lub"). Closure of the aortic and pulmonic valves produces the second heart sound (S2, "dub"). *Systole* is the phase between S1 and S2. *Diastole* is the phase between S2 and the next S1.

firing its pacemaker cells. When atrial contraction begins, the mitral and tricuspid valves open in response to the increased pressure. Blood moves from the atria into the ventricles.

As the impulse begins traveling down the bundle branches, it initiates ventricular contraction, leading to increased ventricular pressure. This increased pressure causes the mitral and tricuspid valves (between the atria and ventricles) to close. The closure of the valves is the first heart sound (S1).

The aortic and pulmonic valves open to allow blood to flow to the lungs and body, producing the pulse. Opening of these valves is normally silent (i.e., no sounds are heard). As the ventricles finish contracting and start relaxing, pressure in the ventricles drops, and the aortic and pulmonic valves close (between the ventricles and great vessels). This causes the second heart sound (S2).

To summarize, S1, or "lub," results from closure of the mitral and tricuspid valves; S2, or "dub," results from closure of the aortic and pulmonic valves. Understanding this basic physiology is essential to understand normal and abnormal heart sounds. If an abnormal sound is heard, knowledge of normal physiology will assist with the identification of its cause.

Systole. During systole, the ventricles contract and eject blood to the lungs and body. The beginning of systole correlates with the pulse as blood is being circulated. During systole, the closed mitral and tricuspid valves prevent regurgitation (backflow) of blood into the atria. The aortic and pulmonic valves are open as blood moves forward.

Diastole. Diastole is twice as long as systole to allow time for the ventricles to fill. As the heart rate increases, however, length of diastole shortens and becomes approximately equal to systole. The coronary arteries are also perfused during diastole.

During diastole, the aortic and pulmonic valves are closed to prevent regurgitation of blood from the aorta and pulmonary artery into the ventricles. The open mitral and tricuspid valves allow filling from the atria to the ventricles. The three phases of ventricular filling are early filling, slow passive filling, and finally, atrial systole, also called "atrial kick." An additional 5% to 30% of blood volume is squeezed into the ventricles during the atrial kick.

Relation to Heart Sounds (S1 and S2). As mentioned, closure of the heart valves during the cardiac cycle causes healthy sounds. The lub sound of S1 signals the beginning of ventricular systole, whereas the dub sound of S2 signals the end of systole and beginning of diastole. Systole occurs between S1 and S2, whereas diastole occurs between S2 and the next S1. When the heart rate is faster than 100 bpm, it may be necessary to identify S1 by palpating the radial pulse or by visualizing the carotid upstroke, which occurs just prior to S2.

Cardiac Output. Volume in the right atrium at the end of diastole is called **preload**, an indicator of how much blood will be forwarded to and ejected from the ventricles. With increased blood in the right ventricle, force of contraction (**contractility**) will be stronger. The heart has to pump against the high blood pressures in the arteries and arterioles. This pressure in the great vessels is termed **afterload**.

To review, preload is the amount of blood in the right atrium to be squeezed out. Contractility is the ability of the heart to shorten its muscle fibers, producing a contraction during systole. Afterload is the amount of pressure the heart has to work against, similar to the resistance in the arterioles with the blood pressure. These three factors influence how much blood is ejected with each beat or stroke, called **stroke volume**.

Cardiac output is the amount of blood ejected from the left ventricle each minute. In addition to stroke volume, the other factor that influences how much blood is circulated is heart rate. The formula is

$$\text{cardiac output} = \text{heart rate} \times \text{stroke volume}$$

A normal cardiac output is 6 to 8 L/min, or approximately 80 bpm with 80 ml in each beat. Ways to increase circulating blood (cardiac output) are by increasing heart rate, increasing stroke volume, or both. The stress hormones epinephrine and norepinephrine increase both heart rate and stroke volume during exercise, trauma, or anxiety. The heart is continually adjusting heart rate and stroke volume during daily activities to supply needed oxygen and nutrients to active tissues.

> **Concepts in Action — Clinical Significance**
>
> Reduced cardiac output is associated with the medical diagnosis of heart failure. In this clinical syndrome, reduced contractility causes preload to increase. Blood backs up, causing congestion. Congestion on the left backs blood into the lungs, whereas congestion on the right backs blood into the body, especially the legs and feet. Signs and symptoms of heart failure are shortness of breath, weight gain, and swollen ankles with decreased cardiac output.

Control of Heart Rate. The sympathetic and parasympathetic divisions of the nervous system control heart rate in response to stress and other variables. Overstimulation of the sympathetic division can cause a heart rate that is too fast, whereas overstimulation of the parasympathetic division can cause a rate that is too slow.

Stimulation of the sympathetic nervous system, or "fight-or-flight" reactions, triggers the release of epinephrine (adrenaline) and norepinephrine. These neurotransmitters increase heart rate, contractility (to increase cardiac output), and blood pressure. The sympathetic division acts indirectly through baroreceptors and chemoreceptors. Baroreceptors in the aortic arch and carotid sinus regulate heart rate. Reduced baroreceptor stimulation (as with dehydration) increases sympathetic stimulation and, subsequently, heart rate. Chemoreceptors in the aortic arch and carotid body sense the body's pH, carbon dioxide, and oxygen levels. Accumulated acid or depleted oxygen levels stimulate the chemoreceptors, thus increasing heart rate.

The parasympathetic division, or "rest-and-digest" reaction, triggers a decreased heart rate by stimulating the vagus nerve that innervates the SA node to slow the natural pacemaker. The vagus nerve also slows conduction through the AV junction, which in turn slows the heart rate.

Relation to Electrocardiogram. As previously described, the heart has a pacemaker (SA node) and electrical conduction system that transmits signals for the cardiac muscle cells to contract at 60 to 100 bpm. This specialized "wiring" is a pathway similar to an electrical cord, by which signals travel quickly and efficiently to muscle cells. After the signal has been delivered, the muscle cells depolarize, causing filaments within to slide over one another and contract. Depolarization occurs when there is an exchange of electrolytes, including sodium, potassium, and calcium. This shift in electrolytes causes electrical changes that can be detected by electrocardiography and recorded on an electrocardiogram (ECG).

The electrical changes in the heart are measured through special patches connected to the ECG that are placed in specific areas on the chest, arms, and legs. The ECG records cellular depolarization primarily when sodium is released from the inside to the outside of cells. The ECG also records repolarization when sodium shifts back into cells at the end of contraction. The ECG records the electrical changes that produce cardiac contraction (depolarization) and relaxation (repolarization) as specific waves and intervals on the ECG (Fig. 17.9):

- *P wave:* represents the spread of depolarization in the atria that causes atrial contraction (note that atrial repolarization is not seen because it is hidden when the ventricles contract in the QRS complex)
- *PR interval:* represents the time from the firing of the SA node to the beginning of ventricular depolarization (includes a slight pause at the AV junction)
- *QRS complex:* represents the spread of depolarization and sodium release in the ventricles that causes ventricular contraction
- *T wave:* represents cellular repolarization, or the restoration of the ventricular resting state, caused by the return of intracellular sodium

Reading the ECG is an advanced skill used by nurses in cardiac and intensive care units. It takes practice and repetition to learn the normal variations and abnormal findings. Health care providers use information from the ECG to analyze assessment data and plan care (see later discussion).

Heart Rhythm. The heart rhythm is an important element to assess in addition to the heart rate. **Arrhythmias** are abnormal heart rhythms with early (premature), delayed, or irregular beats which can arise from the atria, AV junction, or ventricles. Although an irregular heart rhythm can be identified with auscultation, an analysis of the ECG is necessary to classify the arrhythmia.

A type of rhythm common in older adults is called atrial fibrillation. In this situation, many sites in the atria send signals to the ventricles. The ventricles contract very irregularly, causing an irregular heart rhythm.

Cardiac arrhythmias are diagnosed by the location of impulse origination, rate, and regularity. Additionally, the clinician evaluating the ECG tracing will use intervals and the presence or absence of waves to identify the arrhythmia. An irregular pulse indicates a need to test with an ECG to diagnose the type of arrhythmia.

Jugular Pulsations

The venous neck vessels reflect the pressure in the right atrium because no valve exists between the right atrium and jugular veins. The jugular pulse has five pulsations resulting from the backward effects of activity in the heart. The waves reflect atrial contraction and relaxation, ventricular contraction, and passive atrial and ventricular filling. Refer to Figure 17.10.

Lifespan Considerations: Older Adults

With aging, the left ventricular wall becomes thicker and stiffer, even in the absence of increased arterial hypertension or left ventricular afterload (Borlaug et al., 2013). The left atrial size increases and the mitral valve closes more slowly. The heart fills more slowly in early diastole but compensates by filling more quickly in late diastole during atrial contraction. In young hearts, approximately twice as much blood enters the ventricle during early diastolic filling compared with late diastole; in

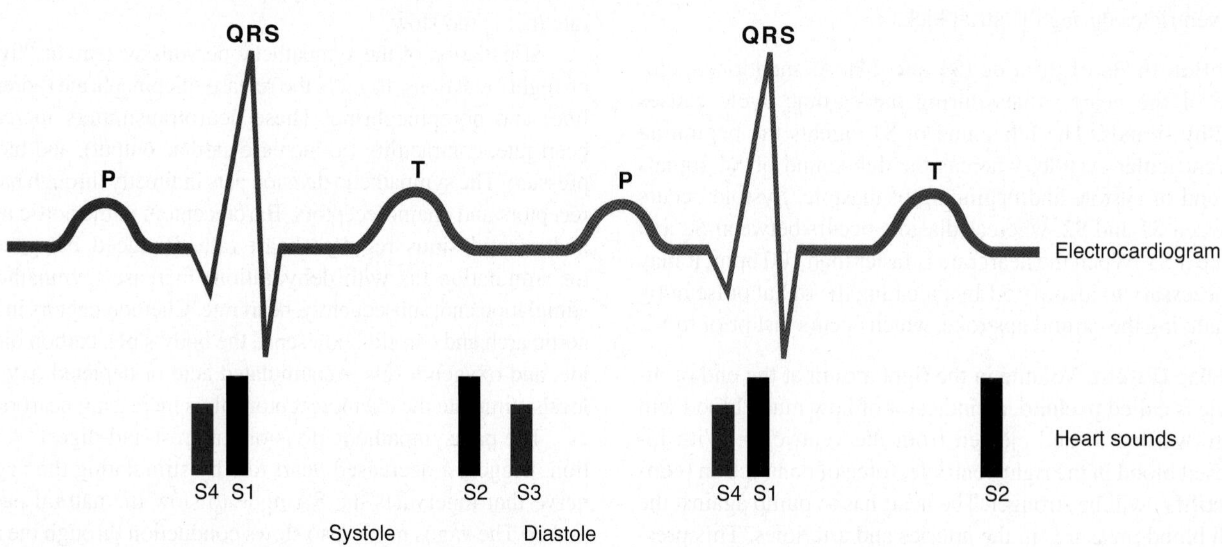

Figure 17.9 Correlation of the waves of the electrocardiogram with the cardiac cycle.

Jugular venous pulsations

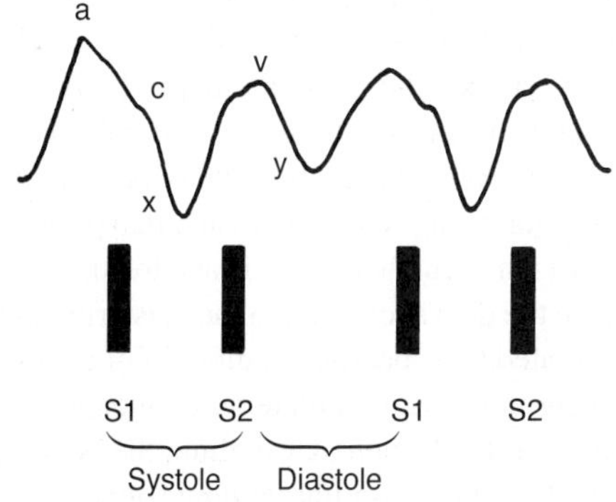

Jugular venous pressure curves
a = atrial contraction
c = carotid transmission not visible clinically
x = descent in right atrium following *a*
v = passive venous filling of atria from the venae cavae
y = descent during atrial resting phase before contraction

Figure 17.10 Jugular venous pressure curves.

older hearts, blood flow is approximately equal during early and late diastole. Consequently, the volumes in the heart remain about the same as in younger people. During stress or exercise, younger people pump out more blood in the ventricle (ejection fraction); in older adults, there are only slight increases in the ejection fraction, possibly causing exercise intolerance (Karavidas, Lazaros, Tsiachris, & Pyrgakis, 2010).

Because of fibrotic changes and fat deposits on the SA node, older adults have less heart rate variability than younger adults. Additionally, their hearts respond less to the sympathetic nervous system, so older adults have reduced maximum heart rates. A 20-year-old person can increase heart rate to 180 bpm, whereas an 80-year-old person has a maximum heart rate of 140 to 150 bpm. Receptors for stress hormones also may become less sensitive in older adults (Block & Jablonski, 2010), making them less able to respond to stressors.

Cultural Considerations

Heart disease is the leading cause of death in high-income countries; coronary heart disease (CHD) contributes to approximately 50% of deaths from heart disease (National Heart, Lung, and Blood Institute [NHLBI], 2011). Heart disease is the leading killer across most of the United States's racial and ethnic minority communities, accounting for 32% of all deaths in 2010.

The prevalence of CHD is greatest among people aged 65 years and older (20%), followed by those aged 45 to 64 years (7%) and those aged 18 to 44 years (1%). CHD prevalence is greater among men (8%) than women (5%). CHD prevalence is greatest among American Indians/Alaska Natives (12%), followed by African Americans (7%), Hispanics (6%), Caucasians (6%), and Asians or Native Hawaiians/other Pacific Islanders (4%) (Centers for Disease Control and Prevention [CDC], 2011). From 1999 to 2009, the death rate from CHD declined by one-third; however, African American men and women have a 30% to 40% higher risk of dying from CHD than Caucasians (CDC, 2011). The reasons for this disparity are still being investigated, but current research suggests that it is correlated with an increase in risk factor burden present in the African American population (Safford et al., 2012).

One in three adults in the United States has hypertension, with 20% of this population being unaware of their high blood pressure. African Americans are 1.5 times more likely to have high blood pressure than Caucasians (Yoon, Burt, Louis, & Carroll, 2012). African American women are 80% more likely to be obese than are non-Hispanic white women (U.S. Department of Health & Human Services, Office of Minority Health [USDHHS OMH], 2013b). Although African American women have higher rates of heart disease with earlier onset and more severe consequences, they are less aware of their susceptibility to and the seriousness of the disease than are other groups (Darlow, Goodman, Stafford, Lachance, & Kaphingst, 2012).

Mexican Americans, who make up the majority of the U.S. Hispanic population, suffer in greater percentages than Caucasians from overweight and obesity, two of the leading risk factors for heart disease. Premature death is higher for Hispanics (24%) than non-Hispanics (17%). Although Hispanic women believe that the best way to prevent heart disease is exercise, procrastination and culture-related issues are barriers to physical activity as well as not seeing a doctor on a regular basis. Perceived self-efficacy, having a concern for one's own and family health, social support and norms for physical activity, serving as a role model to others, and perceived neighborhood resources are factors that promote health maintenance.

In the Asian and Pacific Islander community, heart disease causes one third of deaths, ranking as the overall leading contributor to mortality. Overall, Asian/Pacific Islander adults are less likely than non-Hispanic white adults to have and to die from heart disease (American Heart Association, 2013).

The number of premature deaths from heart disease (i.e., younger than 65 years of age) is greatest among American Indians or Alaska Natives and lowest among Caucasians. American Indian/Alaska Native adults are twice as likely as Caucasians to have heart disease and 1.4 times as likely to be current cigarette smokers. American Indian/Alaska Native adults are 1.6 times as likely as Caucasians to be obese and 1.3 times as likely as Caucasians to have high blood pressure (USDHHSS OMH, 2013a).

Urgent Assessment

⚠ SAFETY ALERT

If a patient is experiencing chest pain, dyspnea, cyanosis, diaphoresis, or dizziness, focus assessment on collecting data to resolve the discomfort. Gather information while performing treatments (such as administration of oxygen and nitroglycerine tablets sublingually as ordered) and diagnostic tests (such as electrocardiography). If chest pain continues, ask for help because more than one clinician may be necessary to collect data and to intervene appropriately.

Cardiac emergencies that necessitate rapid assessment and intervention include acute coronary syndromes, acute decompensated heart failure, hypertensive crisis, cardiac tamponade, unstable cardiac arrhythmias, cardiogenic shock, systemic or pulmonary embolism, and aortic dissection. Patients with these conditions may have chest pain, shortness of breath, abnormal (too high or too low) blood pressure, or inadequate tissue perfusion. Initial assessment includes a brief exploration of the presenting symptom (location, onset, intensity, alleviating and aggravating factors, associated symptoms), a focused physical examination of the cardiovascular and respiratory systems, an ECG, and a chest x-ray. Selected laboratory and diagnostic tests are done on an emergency basis to evaluate for cardiac muscle damage, embolism, and electrolyte imbalance. Team members perform interventions while gathering assessment data because prompt treatment is essential.

Accurate assessment of patients with cardiovascular conditions is vital because nurses are often the health care providers who first identify abnormal findings. As the nurse, you play a key role in assessment of chest pain and assisting in gathering data so that the source of the chest pain is quickly identified and treated. Differential diagnosis of chest pain is important because ischemic cardiac pain involves loss of muscle cells that can cause further damage if left untreated. An accurate description of the pain and alleviating or aggravating factors is helpful in identifying the source.

Other priority assessments relate to arrhythmias. Quickly assess the effects of the arrhythmia by checking level of consciousness and obtaining the blood pressure to evaluate peripheral perfusion. If level of consciousness, blood pressure, or both are decreased, page the rapid response team. You must think quickly when working with patients who have cardiac problems because the status of such patients often changes rapidly.

Assessing for fluid volume overload and decompensated heart failure (which leads to pulmonary edema) is also a priority. You can identify the presence of pulmonary edema by auscultating lung sounds, measuring respiratory rate, and obtaining an oxygen saturation level. Assess for infectious or inflammatory disorders (e.g., endocarditis, pericarditis) by looking for related findings, such as fever, heart sounds, and pain. Patients with cardiac disease are often aware of subtle symptoms that indicate improving or worsening status; they can often provide valuable data that assists in accurate diagnosis and treatment.

Organize the data according to the clustering of signs and symptoms related to a specific condition. For example, if you identify a new murmur, complete assessments that relate to fluid volume overload, such as weighing the patient, evaluating intake and output, auscultating lung sounds for fluid, and inspecting the extremities for edema. Then, analyze the findings to determine the effects of the murmur on the patient's physical and functional status.

Subjective Data

Assessment of Risk Factors

When questioning patients about risk factors, the goal is to identify how likely the patients are to develop or to already be experiencing consequences of cardiovascular diseases. Such investigation creates an environment in which health care providers can implement necessary interventions to control symptoms, direct education to prevent new problems or complications, and document areas needing ongoing follow-up and emphasis. For example, in the interview, you assess for smoking, high blood pressure, physical inactivity, and diabetes mellitus—all major contributors to heart disease (Roger et al., 2011). After assessment, you identify focused teaching areas and evaluate the patient's ongoing progress in controlling modifiable risks.

The following screening questions are important to establish the patient's risks for cardiovascular disease.

History and Risk Factors	Rationale
Biographical Information Obtain the following information from the patient's chart: • Age • Ethnic background • Gender • Date and result of last blood pressure measurement • Date and result of last cholesterol level • Date and result of last C-reactive protein level • Date and result of B-type natriuretic peptides (BNPs) • Thyroid levels	Advanced age, hypertension, male gender, and particular ethnic heritages (African American, Mexican American, American Indian, Native Hawaiian, and Asian American) are risk factors for cardiovascular disease. Risk of a cardiovascular event more than doubles with elevated cholesterol and C-reactive protein levels (Ridker, 2009). BNP is both sensitive and specific to heart failure (Jensen, Ma, Bjurman, Hammarsten, & Fu, 2012). Hyperthyroidism has been linked to atrial fibrillation and may increase the likelihood of cardiovascular disease and risk of mortality in patients with other morbidities (Yang, Jiang, Zhang, Feng, & Gao, 2012).
 **Past Medical History** Have you ever been diagnosed with a cardiac condition such as chest pain, syncope, heart attack, heart failure, or irregular rhythm?	A history of past problems provides information that can assist with anticipating future needs.

(table continues on page 461)

History and Risk Factors	Rationale
Has anyone ever told you that you have high blood pressure? • What is the normal range of your blood pressure? • Do you take anything for it?	In untreated hypertension, the risk of dying from cardiac disease or any other cause is 40% higher. Increases in systolic blood pressure are more likely than increases in diastolic pressure to be associated with mortality (Gu, Dillion, Burt & Gillum, 2009).
Has anyone ever told you that you have high blood cholesterol? • What is the usual level? • Do you take anything for it?	Patients with an elevated low-density lipoprotein (LDL) (bad) cholesterol level are twice as likely to develop cardiovascular disease (Deedwania & Volkova, 2013).
Do you have a history of diabetes mellitus? • What is your usual glucose level? • Do you take anything for it? • What was your last hemoglobin A1C assessment?	Patients with diabetes mellitus are approximately twice as likely to develop cardiovascular disease (Deedwania & Volkova, 2013).
Medications Are you taking any medications for cardiac conditions? • What are they? • How often are you taking them? • Why were they prescribed? • How well are you following your prescribed medication regimen?	Note the drug, dosage, and frequency. Obtaining the reason for the medication is important because some drugs have several purposes. It is also essential to review compliance with medications because many cardiac medications have adverse effects that cause patients to stop taking them.
Are you taking any natural supplements or over-the-counter medications? • What are they? • How often do you take them?	Some supplements, such as ephedrine, may have cardiac adverse effects. Also note any potential drug interactions between prescribed and over-the-counter medications.
Family History Do you have any family history of cardiovascular conditions? • Who had the illness? • What was the illness? • When did the relative have it? • How was the illness treated? • What were the outcomes? • Any family history of high blood pressure, high cholesterol, diabetes, or obesity?	Premature coronary artery disease in a first- or second-degree relative increases the patient's risk for the same condition. Premature onset is before 55 years of age in men and before 65 years of age in women. Evidence suggests that premature coronary artery disease in siblings is a stronger risk factor than is disease in parents or grandparents (Naghavi, 2010; Taraboanta, Hague, Mancini, Forster, & Frohlich, 2012).
Risk Factors Do you smoke cigarettes or use other tobacco products? • How long? • How many packs per day?	Smokers are two to four times more likely to develop CHD and are twice as likely to have sudden cardiac arrest (CDC, 2013b).
What is your usual weight? What is your height?	Being overweight or obese is associated with an increased risk for cardiovascular disease as well as an increased risk for the development of cardiovascular risk factors, including hypertension, hyperlipidemia, and diabetes mellitus. (Roger et al., 2011).
What is your usual level of physical activity? • Do you exercise? • What type? • How often and for what duration?	A low level of activity is associated with an increased risk for cardiovascular disease (Roger et al., 2011). Physical activity can help control blood cholesterol, diabetes, and obesity as well as help lower blood pressure. Assess occupational activities, commuting patterns, and recreational exercise to determine how much these factors contribute to overall physical activity.

(table continues on page 462)

History and Risk Factors	Rationale
What is your typical diet?	A diet low in fruits and vegetables and high in fat and cholesterol is associated with an increased risk of cardiovascular disease (Roger et al., 2011).
How much alcohol do you usually drink per day? Week? Month? Do you use any recreational drugs such as cocaine?	Drinking more than two drinks of alcohol per day for men or one drink of alcohol per day for women can raise blood pressure and contribute to heart failure. It also can elevate triglyceride levels, contribute to obesity, and produce irregular heartbeats (Roger et al., 2011). Cocaine and other amphetamines increase the risk of MI and coronary vasospasm.

Risk Reduction and Health Promotion

As mentioned, the completion of a risk assessment helps to identify potential conditions so that health care providers can give patients information to positively influence behavioral choices. Both primary prevention, in those without evidence of cardiovascular disease, and secondary prevention, to detect early disease through blood pressure and cholesterol screening, are priorities for public health. The most important cardiovascular focus areas are the modifiable risk factors of smoking, high blood pressure, and high cholesterol level. Additionally, a high-fat diet, overweight or obesity, and physical inactivity contribute to cardiovascular disease. Nurses work with patients over time to modify lifestyle choices that reflect healthy behaviors. The most important are stopping smoking, reducing high blood pressure, and reducing high cholesterol. The overall goals for cardiovascular health are as follows:

- Reduce CHD deaths.
- Increase the proportion of adults aged 20 years and older who are aware of the early warning symptoms and signs of a heart attack and the importance of accessing rapid emergency care by calling 911.
- Increase the proportion of eligible patients with heart attacks who receive timely electrical shock and artery-opening therapy.
- Increase the proportion of adults with high blood pressure whose blood pressure is under control.
- Reduce the mean total blood cholesterol levels and LDL cholesterol levels among adults.
- Increase the proportion of physician office visits made by patients with a diagnosis of cardiovascular disease, diabetes, or hyperlipidemia that include counseling or education related to diet and nutrition.
- Increase the proportion of adults who engage in vigorous physical activity that promotes the development and maintenance of cardiorespiratory fitness 3 or more days per week for 20 or more minutes per occasion (U.S. Department of Health & Human Services, 2013).

Smoking Cessation

Ask patients who smoke about their willingness to quit at every visit. Patients who quit reduce their risk of cardiac events by 50% after the first year (CDC, 2010). You can give patients choices about tools to help them quit, such as referral to behavioral therapy, information about support groups, and information about medication.

Control of Blood Pressure and Cholesterol Level

High blood pressure should be controlled with medication if diet, exercise, and weight reduction are unsuccessful. Patients may not adhere to prescribed medications because of adverse effects or difficulty following the schedule. You might suggest a dosing regimen simplified to improve adherence (Flack & Nasser, 2011).

High cholesterol can also be modified by eating a low-cholesterol diet with reduced animal fat. Lean cuts of grilled or roasted meat are better than deep-fried fatty cuts. Dietary changes can usually lower cholesterol by 9% to 12% or up to 30% when combined with regular exercise (Kelly, 2010). If diet and exercise are unsuccessful, the physician may prescribe a statin, which reduces the risk of cardiovascular events by approximately 20% (Cholesterol Treatment Trialists' Collaboration, 2010).

Common Symptoms

Assess for common cardiovascular symptoms in all patients to screen for early signs of cardiac disease. If a patient is concerned about a cardiac condition, you can use this concern to identify focused areas of assessment. A thorough history of cardiovascular symptoms assists with identifying the current condition or diagnosis.

Common Cardiovascular Symptom

- Chest pain
- Dyspnea, orthopnea, and cough
- Diaphoresis
- Fatigue
- Edema
- Nocturia
- Palpitations

Signs/Symptoms	Rationale/Abnormal Findings
⚠ *SAFETY ALERT* *All health care providers should assume that a patient's chest pain is cardiac pain until another cause can be determined. If chest pain is ischemic, rapid treatment is necessary to prevent the death of cardiac cells. If medication or angioplasty can open the artery, the severity of the MI can be reduced.*	Cardiac pain indicates ischemic heart tissue which, if unrelieved after 20 minutes, can cause cell death and MI.
Chest Pain Do you have any chest pain or discomfort? • Where is the pain? Can you point to where it hurts? Does it go anywhere? • When did you first notice the pain? Is it constant or does it come and go? How long has it lasted? • How bad is it on a scale from 0 to 10, with 10 being the worst? • Describe the pain or discomfort. What does it feel like? • What makes it worse? What makes it better? Have you taken any nitroglycerin? How many tablets and how far apart? • What were you doing when you noticed it? Does anything consistently bring it on? • Do any other symptoms accompany the pain? • Have you tried any treatments for the pain? Did they help? • What is your goal for the pain? What would you like to be able to do that you are unable to do because of the pain?	The pain of MI typically is on the left side of the chest, radiates down the left arm or into the jaw, and is diffused rather than localized. Onset can be sudden or gradual. Patients often describe the pain as crushing or viselike. Others may not identify ischemia as pain but rather as pressure or discomfort, like "having an elephant on the chest." Some patients become nauseated and vomit; others describe indigestion resulting from cardiac ischemia. Associated symptoms include diaphoresis, pallor, anxiety, and fatigue. Palpitations, tachycardia, and dyspnea may also be present. About 43% of women and patients older than 65 years of age do not complain of chest pain with an acute MI (Navis, Goss, and Roach, 2010). Angina pectoris is temporary heart pain, resolving in less than 20 minutes. It can be aggravated by physical activity and stress, or there may be no triggers (unstable angina). Chest pain may also result from pulmonary, musculoskeletal, or gastrointestinal causes. Factors that aggravate or alleviate the pain may help identify the cause. Nitroglycerin often relieves angina, whereas an antacid may relieve pain from reflux. Refer to Table 17.1 for the differential diagnosis of chest pain.
Dyspnea Have you had any shortness of breath? • How bad is it on a scale from 0 to 10, with 10 being the worst? • When did it start? How long has it lasted? • What makes it worse? What makes it better? • Do any other symptoms accompany the shortness of breath? • Have you tried any treatments for the shortness of breath? Did they help? • Is it better or worse when compared with how you felt 6 months ago?	Patients with heart failure may be short of breath from fluid accumulation in the pulmonary bed. About 85% of patients with heart failure have dyspnea, but only about half with dyspnea have heart failure. Onset may be sudden with acute or chronic pulmonary edema. It is important to assess how much activity brings on dyspnea, such as rest, walking on a flat surface, or climbing. **Dyspnea on exertion** is common with physical activity. Note the amount of activity that elicits dyspnea—for example, four stairs or one city block. Fatigue, chest pain, or diaphoresis may accompany dyspnea. Typically, resting alleviates it; if not, there may be another cause such as worsening heart failure, pulmonary embolism, or MI. Women are more likely to have dyspnea than chest pain as an acute symptom of MI.
Orthopnea and Paroxysmal Nocturnal Dyspnea Have you had difficulty sleeping? • How many pillows do you sleep on at night? • Do you wake in the night short of breath?	Patients with heart failure may have fluid in their lungs, making it difficult to breathe when lying flat **(orthopnea)**. Fluid backs up into the pulmonary veins, the heart cannot keep up with the volume, and fluid leaks into the lungs. Patients also may wake up suddenly as the fluid is redistributed from edematous legs into the lungs **(paroxysmal nocturnal dyspnea [PND])**, typically after a few hours of sleep. They may waken feeling tired, anxious, or restless. Approximately 50% of women report difficulty sleeping 1 month prior to an acute MI.

(table continues on page 464)

TABLE 17.1 Differential Diagnosis of Chest Pain

Condition	Significant Findings in the History	Symptoms	Aggravating Factors	Alleviating Factors
MI	Cardiac risk factors	Chest pain or discomfort in men; fatigue and shortness of breath in women lasting more than 20 minutes Accompanied by nausea and diaphoresis	Anxiety, physical exertion	Nitroglycerin; thrombolytic medication or angioplasty is necessary to prevent damage
Stable angina	Cardiac risk factors	Discomfort lasting less than 20 minutes	Cold, fatigue, physical exertion	Nitroglycerin and rest
Unstable angina	Cardiac risk factors	Discomfort lasting less than 20 minutes	Occurs at rest	Nitroglycerin; no relation to activity
Gastrointestinal disease: esophageal, gastritis, biliary	History of ulcer, reflux, or gallbladder disease	Described as indigestion, difficulty swallowing, burning, acid stomach; biliary pain may be colicky or cramping	Food intolerances, large or fatty meals	Antacids
Pulmonary disease/pleural chest pain	History of lung disease, pneumonia	Stabbing or grating pain, typically at the bases of the lungs	Worse with deep inhalation or coughing	Splinting chest, nonsteroidal anti-inflammatory medications
Musculoskeletal	History of trauma, such as cardiopulmonary resuscitation, musculoskeletal history	Muscle tenderness with palpation, located near joints or costochondral cartilages, chronic	Increased movement	Rest
Aortic dissection	Cardiovascular disease	Middle or upper abdominal pain, ischemic pain in legs	Not relieved until treated	Measures to increase perfusion
Pericardial pain	History of cardiac inflammation such as with MI	Described as stabbing	Position changes, such as leaning forward	Nonsteroidal antiinflammatory medications

Signs/Symptoms	Rationale/Abnormal Findings
Cough Have you noticed a cough? • When did it start? How long has it lasted? • What makes it worse? What makes it better? • What brings it on? • Do any other symptoms accompany the cough? • Have you tried any treatments for the cough? Did they help? • Is it better or worse when compared with how you felt 6 months ago?	Coughing occurs for the same reason as dyspnea. The cough may produce white or pink blood-tinged mucus. Mild wheezing also may occur. Treatment with an angiotensin-converting enzyme inhibitor also can cause the adverse effect of a dry, hacking cough.
Diaphoresis Have you noticed any excessive sweating? • When? Is it during any particular activities? • Are any associated symptoms such as heart pounding or chest pain present?	Nighttime diaphoresis, commonly known as night sweats, is associated with other diseases, such as tuberculosis. Diaphoresis in response to exercise or activity may be related to cardiac stress. Diaphoresis associated with chest pain or palpitations is an autonomic response of the body to stress.

(table continues on page 465)

Signs/Symptoms	Rationale/Abnormal Findings
Fatigue Have you been especially fatigued or tired? • When did it start? How long has it lasted? • What makes it worse? What makes it better? • Do any other symptoms accompany the fatigue? • Have you tried any treatments for the fatigue? Did they help?	Fatigue occurs because the heart cannot pump enough blood to meet the needs of tissues. The body diverts blood away from less vital organs, particularly limb muscles, and distributes it to the heart and brain. Common activities that might cause fatigue include shopping, climbing stairs, carrying groceries, and walking. Women are more likely to report unusual fatigue 1 month before acute MI.
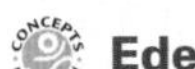 **Edema** Have you noticed any swelling in your feet, legs, or hands? • When did it start? How long has it lasted? • What makes it worse? What makes it better? • Do any other symptoms accompany the swelling? • Have you tried any treatments for the swelling? Did they help?	When blood flow out of the heart is reduced, blood returning to the heart through the veins backs up, causing fluid to accumulate in the organs and dependent areas of the body. Blood flow to the kidneys is also reduced, decreasing excretion of sodium and water and causing further fluid retention in the tissues. Usually, standing exacerbates leg edema, whereas elevating the legs above heart level reduces it. Patients who retain fluid may also notice weight gain. About 75% of patients with heart failure have edema.
Nocturia Do you need to get up at night to use the bathroom? • How often? • Have you made any changes because of this?	**Nocturia** is a common symptom associated with redistribution of fluid from the legs to the core when lying. As the fluid shifts, the kidneys are better perfused, increasing urine production. Nocturia may also be caused by prescribed diuretics administered later in the day. Patients may avoid drinking water after dinner if nocturia is present.
Palpitations Do you notice that your heart is beating faster? Are you having skipped or extra beats? • When did it start? How long has it lasted? • What makes it worse? What makes it better? • Do any other symptoms accompany the heartbeats? • Have you tried any treatments? Did they help?	Patients with cardiovascular disease may have tachycardia from decreased contractile strength of the heart muscle. With reduced stroke volume, the pulse increases to maintain cardiac output. **Palpitations** experienced as a rapid throbbing or fluttering of the heart may be associated with arrhythmias. Patients tolerate these arrhythmias differently, ranging from a mild awareness of the sensation to more severe dizziness or loss of consciousness. Women are more likely to present with palpitations during acute MI than are men (Berg, Bjorck, Dudas,Lappas, & Rosengren, 2009). ⚠ *SAFETY ALERT* *Patients with a history of loss of consciousness should have a complete workup to diagnose the cause. They are at risk for falling and require fall precautions.*

Documenting Normal Findings

No chest pain or discomfort. Denies dyspnea, orthopnea, PND, cough, fatigue, edema, nocturia, and palpitations.

Lifespan Considerations: Older Adults

Additional Questions	Rationale/Abnormal Findings
• Have you noticed any changes in your ability to tolerate activity? • Have you had any periods where you felt dizzy or faint or actually passed out? • Have you been short of breath or had trouble breathing at night?	Age-related changes may decrease activity tolerance. Arrhythmias and heart failure are common symptoms for nurses to assess with people of this age group. Syncope can be caused by orthostatic hypotension or arrhythmias.

Cultural Considerations

Additional Questions	Rationale/Abnormal Findings
• What do you do to keep your heart healthy? • How would you describe your general health? • Do you ever worry about heart disease?	Asking general questions may identify areas in which people of various cultural groups have different perceptions of heart health and risk for disease. Such questions may also provide an opportunity to educate patients and clarify misperceptions. For example, although heart disease is the number one cause of mortality in African American women, studies have shown that they generally do not perceive this condition as a threat and are less likely to modify risk factors (Mosca, Mochari, Dolor, Newby, & Robb, 2010).

Therapeutic Dialogue: Collecting Subjective Data

Remember Mrs. Lewis, introduced at the beginning of this chapter. She was admitted to the hospital 4 hours ago for chest pain and is experiencing some anxiety about a diagnosis of MI. The nurse is meeting Mrs. Lewis for the first time at the start of the shift. In addition to obtaining an assessment, the nurse must provide support and listen to the patient's responses to reduce anxiety.

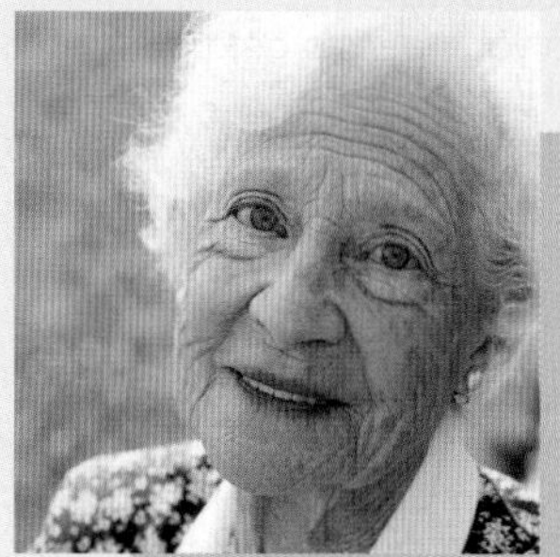

Nurse: Tell me a little about what brought you to the hospital today.

Mrs. Lewis: I was taking a walk in my neighborhood and all of a sudden it felt like there was an elephant sitting on my chest. I couldn't breathe and had to stop. I was close to home, and when I got there, my husband knew that something was wrong. He was the one who called 911.

Nurse: Tell me more about what you were feeling.

Mrs. Lewis: I've never felt anything like it before. It was right in the middle of my chest, and it didn't go away until the medics gave me a nitroglycerin tablet. It must have lasted about 20 minutes. I was so glad that they came fast. It was the worst pain that I've ever had. I felt all clammy and kind of dizzy.

Nurse: That must have been very scary for you.

Mrs. Lewis: I'm still scared. Do you think that I had a heart attack?

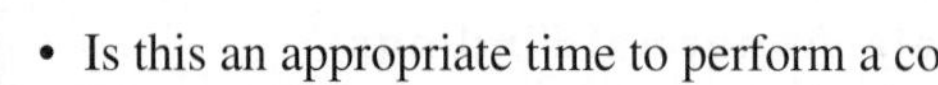

Critical Thinking Challenge

- Is this an appropriate time to perform a complete health history and review of systems? Provide rationale.
- What therapeutic communication techniques did the nurse use?
- How will the nurse balance the need for patient education and expressing her fear and anxiety?
- How would the nurse respond to Mrs. Lewis's question about the diagnosis of heart attack? Provide rationale.

Objective Data

Common and Specialty or Advanced Techniques

The focused examination mainly involves the neck vessels and precordium. A complete cardiovascular assessment incorporates additional data. The blood pressure, peripheral vascular system, neck vessels, and heart sounds are all indicators of adequate circulation and tissue perfusion.

The routine head-to-toe assessment includes the most important and common cardiovascular assessment techniques. You may add specialty or advanced steps if you have a concern about a specific finding. The table summarizes the most essential techniques for clinical practice. Additional techniques that are used more regularly in advanced practice may be necessary if indicated by the clinical situation.

Equipment

- Stethoscope with bell and diaphragm
- Watch with second hand indicator
- Penlight or examination light for visualizing neck veins

Preparation

Evaluation of the neck vessels and heart requires exposure of and contact with the thorax. If possible, the patient should wear a gown. Provide a drape to cover the patient when exposure of the chest is necessary. Ensure that the room is at a comfortable temperature and take measures to facilitate a private and quiet setting. Wash and warm your hands to avoid spreading infection and to facilitate patient comfort.

For inspection, expose only the area of the chest that needs examination, especially for women. When visualization is required, gather the gown from the bottom in the direction

Basic Versus Focused/Specialty or Advanced Techniques Related to Heart and Neck Vessels Assessment

Technique	Purpose	Screening or Registered Nurse Assessment	Focused or Advanced Practice Examination
Inspect the jugular veins.	Helps determine jugular venous pressure	X	
Palpate the carotid arteries.	Helps indicate the strength of the pulse	X	
Auscultate the carotid artery.	Enables the hearing of bruits	X	
Inspect the precordium.	Identifies abnormalities	X	
Palpate the PMI.	Assesses for cardiac enlargement	X	
Palpate the precordium.	Assesses for masses, tenderness	X	
Auscultate the pulse.	Determines rate, rhythm	X	
Auscultate extra heart sounds S3 and S4.	Identifies ventricular filling sounds	X	
Auscultate systolic and diastolic murmurs.	Identifies presence of sounds through valves	X	
Palpate and inspect for hepatojugular reflex.	Identify liver congestion with heart failure		X Liver congestion
Percuss the precordium.	Evaluates heart size		X Hypertrophy
Auscultate and grade, identify location of, and identify whether murmurs are related to regurgitation or stenosis.	Determines rate, rhythm, and valves affected		X Specific diagnosis of valve dysfunction
Auscultate specific split sounds, rubs, snaps, and clicks.	Determines timing and valves affected		X Specific valves and timing

of the shoulders so that the patient feels less exposed anteriorly. Cover the anterior chest when inspecting posteriorly. To ease the patient's anxiety, explain the rationale for the need to expose the chest.

If an abnormality is suspected, it may be necessary to listen to the heart in several different positions. Alert the patient that he or she will need to lean forward, turn to the left, or sit up to improve the volume and quality of the sounds. Also alert the patient that you will be listening for a longer period than usual and that doing so does not mean you have found abnormalities. Provide reassurance by saying, "I'm going to listen to your heart sounds carefully, but it doesn't mean that anything is wrong. I will let you know what I hear when I am finished."

Patient positioning is important for the cardiac examination. The patient may be sitting during auscultation of the carotid arteries. To evaluate the jugular pulses, lower the head of the bed to a 45-degree angle to allow for visualization of the softer impulses (Fig. 17.11). (Most beds and examination tables have an indicator of the degree of elevation to identify 45 degrees.) The jugular pulse on the right side is usually easier to identify, so it may be most efficient and accurate for the examiner to stand on the patient's right. When auscultating the heart sounds, the patient may be sitting or lying (supine). Additionally, if auscultation of heart sounds is difficult, or if concerns exist about cardiac conditions, the heart can be auscultated with the patient supine, in the left lateral position, or leaning forward.

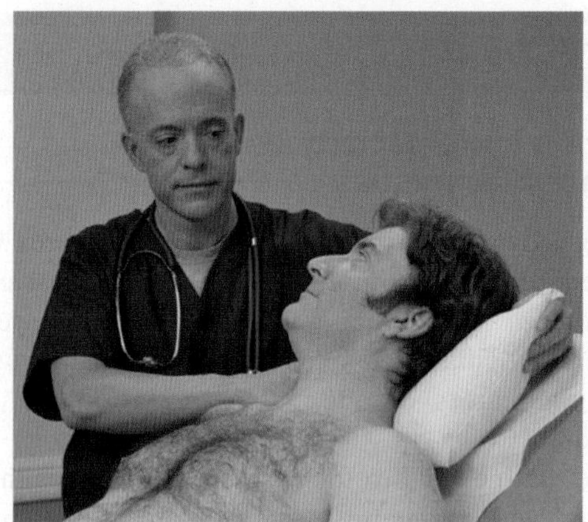

Figure 17.11 The head of the bed is at a 30- to 45-degree angle to better visualize the soft jugular venous pulses.

Studies have shown that a stethoscope can transmit bacteria among patients (Alothman, Bukhari, Aljohani, & Muhanaa, 2009). Thus, be sure to clean the diaphragm of the stethoscope with an alcohol swab before bringing the diaphragm into contact with the patient. Also, warm the diaphragm of the stethoscope with your clean hands before placing it on the chest.

 Comprehensive Physical Assessment

Jugular Vein

Technique and Normal Findings	Abnormal Findings
Jugular Venous Pulses. The jugular venous pulses are subtle, making their inspection challenging to learn. Accurate inspection requires practice and visualization with several patients because chest size and shape and appearance of the jugular veins vary greatly.	If severe heart failure is suspected, invasive hemodynamic monitoring may be used. The waveform is examined for specific pressures and characteristics that indicate the severity of the heart failure. This advanced technique is used primarily in the intensive care setting.
Rather than identify all the waves, nurses in clinical settings more commonly observe the pattern and rhythm of the jugular venous pulse.	
Position the patient with the head of the bed at 30–45 degrees to promote visibility of the pulsation (see Fig. 17.11). Place a folded pillow under the patient's head to relax the sternocleidomastoid muscle and improve visualization. Keep the patient's shoulders on the mattress. Move any long hair away from the patient to enhance visibility. The right side is easiest to see; it may help the patient to turn the head slightly away from the side being examined and elevate the jaw slightly. Light the area to emphasize the shadows of the pulsations; indirect lighting from a 45-degree angle is usually best rather than a bright direct light (Chua, Parikh, & Fergusson, 2013). The external veins are lateral to the sternomastoid muscles, and the pulsations are best observed in the groove near the middle of the clavicle.	Patients with dehydration or volume depletion have barely visible neck veins (described as **flat neck veins**), even when lying flat. If the patient is unusually dehydrated, it may be necessary to lower the head of the bed to visualize the vein. The patient with fluid overload may need to have the head of the bed elevated. At times, the neck veins may be so distended that they extend all the way to the ear; in this case, raise the head of the bed until the pulsation is visible.

(table continues on page 469)

Technique and Normal Findings (continued)	Abnormal Findings (continued)
The internal jugular veins can easily be confused with the carotid artery pulsation. The internal vein is not visible, but the pulsations are transmitted to the soft tissue and are usually most prominent in the suprasternal notch, the supraclavicular fossa, or just below the earlobe. If the pulsation is not visible, it may be necessary to lower the head of the bed.	
When learning to distinguish between the more subtle pulsations of the jugular veins, it may help to use a hand to shield the more prominent carotid pulsations and isolate the fluttery venous pulsations. *There are usually two pulsations with a prominent descent as compared with the carotid pulse, which has one pulsation and a prominent ascent with systole.*	
Jugular Venous Pressure. After locating the internal jugular vein in the sternal notch, identify the top height of the pulsation. If the internal vein is difficult to visualize, use the more prominent external vein (Chua et al., 2013). Locate the sternal angle in the 2nd ICS. Using a line parallel to the horizon, from the sternal angle, estimate the difference between the parallel line and the top of the pulsation in the external jugular vein (Fig. 17.12). Because of wide differences in chest shape and location of the sternal angle, exact measurement varies widely among patients (Chua et al., 2013). Most commonly, nurses identify that normal veins appear about halfway up the neck. Note whether neck veins appear distended, normal, or flat.	**Jugular venous distention (JVD)** is associated with heart failure, tricuspid regurgitation, and fluid volume overload. The neck veins appear full, and the level of pulsation may be have elevated jugular venous pressure greater than 3 cm (about 1 1/4 in.) above the sternal angle. About 75% of patients with elevated JVD have heart failure.
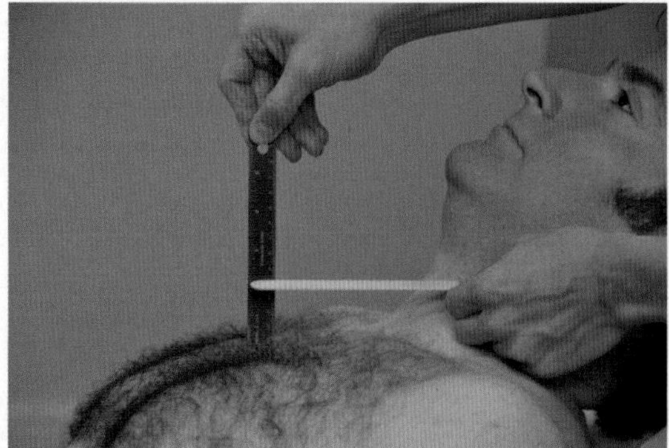 **Figure 17.12** Estimate the jugular venous pressure. Measurement is illustrated as a visual cue for the learner.	
Findings are up to 3 cm above the sternal angle, which is equivalent to a central venous pressure of 8 mmHg. If exact levels are not measured, document findings as "JVP normal," "JVP not elevated," "neck veins not distended," or "no JVD."	

Documenting Normal Findings

Heart rate and rhythm regular. No gallops, murmurs, or rubs.

Carotid Arteries

Technique and Normal Findings	Abnormal Findings
Inspection. Inspect the carotid artery for a double stroke seen with S1 and S2. The contour is smooth with a rapid upstroke and slower downstroke.	The pulse may be bounding and prominent with hypertension, hypermetabolic states, and disorders with a rapid rise and fall of pressure (e.g., patent ductus arteriosus) (Woods et al., 2010). It may be low in amplitude and volume and have a delayed peak in aortic stenosis (from decreased cardiac output). If it is diminished unilaterally or bilaterally (often associated with a systolic bruit), the cause may be carotid stenosis from atherosclerosis (Woods et al., 2010).
Palpation *⚠ SAFETY ALERT* *Palpate the carotid arteries one at a time. Palpating them together poses a risk for obstructing both arteries, reducing blood flow to the brain, and potentially causing dizziness or loss of consciousness.*	
Palpate the carotid artery medial to the sternomastoid muscle in the neck between the jaw and the clavicle (Fig. 17.13).	A diminished or thready pulse may accompany decreased stroke volume, found with reduced fluid volume. If the heart's ability to pump is decreased and cardiac output is low, as in heart failure, pulse strength may be reduced. Another cause of decreased pulse strength is a narrowed carotid artery from atherosclerosis. Pulse strength may increase during exercise or stress.

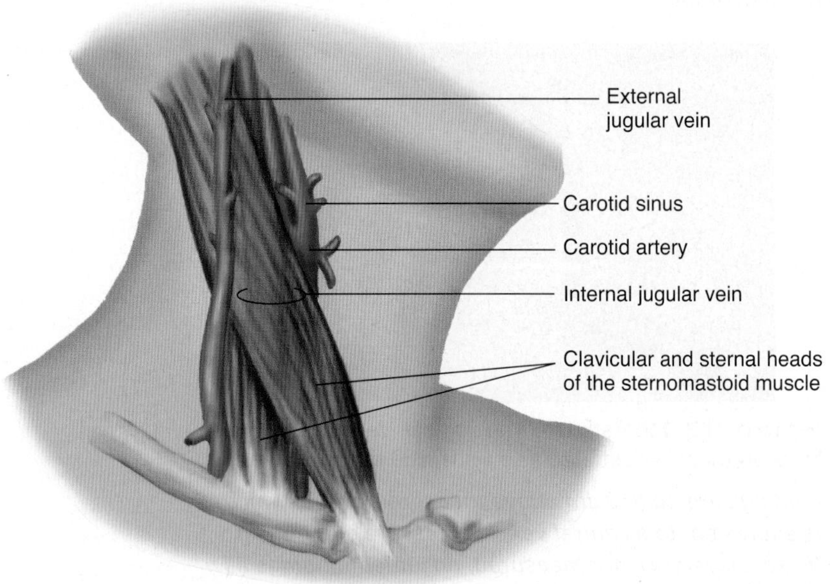

Figure 17.13 Palpate each carotid artery medial to the sternomastoid muscle in the neck one at a time and avoiding the carotid sinus.

(table continues on page 471)

Technique and Normal Findings (continued)	Abnormal Findings (continued)
⚠ SAFETY ALERT *Avoid compressing the carotid sinus. Stimulation of the sinus causes parasympathetic stimulation, which may lead to reduced pulse rate and bradycardia. Older adults and patients sensitive to this stimulation may develop periods of life-threatening asystole.*	
Palpate the strength of the pulse and grade it, as with peripheral pulses (see Chapter 18). Strength is 2+ or moderate. Pulses are equal bilaterally.	
Auscultation. Auscultation of the carotid arteries is performed in cases of suspected narrowing. Use the bell to hear the higher pitched sound of the bruit. Lightly apply the bell over the artery medial to the sternomastoid muscle at three locations: near the jaw, in the middle of the neck, and near the clavicle. Avoid compressing the artery because doing so causes a bruit, similar to the compression from the cuff when taking blood pressure. No bruits are heard.	**Bruits** are swooshing sounds similar to the sound blood pressure makes. They result from turbulent blood flow related to atherosclerosis. A bruit is audible when the artery is partially obstructed. With complete obstruction, no bruit is audible because no blood gets through. Bruits have been associated with an increased risk of stroke (Pickett, Jackson, Hemann, & Atwood, 2010). Distinguishing a murmur from a bruit can be challenging. Murmurs originate in the heart or great vessels and are usually louder over the upper precordium and quieter near the neck. Bruits are higher pitched, more superficial, and heard only over the arteries (Woods et al., 2010).

Documenting Normal Findings

Without JVD, hepatojugular reflux negative. Carotid pulses 2+ bilaterally without bruits.

Precordium

Technique and Normal Findings	Abnormal Findings
Inspection. Inspect the anterior chest for any lesions, masses, or areas of tenderness (see Chapter 16). Observe for the PMI in the apex at the 4th–5th ICS at the left MCL. It is easier to observe in children, men, and adults with a thin chest wall. *Impulses are absent or located in the 4th–5th left ICS at the MCL with no lifts or heaves.*	The enlarged heart of cardiomegaly displaces the PMI laterally and inferiorly. Observe for a heave or lift, which appears as a forceful thrusting on the chest and is the result of an enlarged ventricle. A right ventricular heave is observed at the lower left sternal border; a left ventricular heave is observed at the apex.
Palpation. Palpate the anterior chest for any lesions, masses, or tender areas (see Chapter 16). When palpating for sensations related to the heart, use the palmar surface of the hand. Beginning at the apex of the heart, feel for the pulse in the location in which you observed it during inspection. To localize the impulse, it may help to use the finger pads and depress in the left 5th ICS at the MCL (Fig. 17.14). If present, the PMI is usually felt as a light tap that lasts from S1 to halfway through systole and is less than 1–2 cm. It may or may not be palpable in adults. Also palpate in the sternoclavicular area, right and left upper sternal borders, right and left lower sternal borders, apical area, and epigastric area. Palpate all areas of the chest using the fingertips, heel, or ulnar surface of the hand. *The PMI is in the 5th left ICS at the MCL when present. No pulsations are palpated in other areas.*	An abnormal PMI is displaced left or downward, may raise a larger-than-normal area, and may be sustained throughout systole. It may result from heart failure, MI, left ventricular hypertrophy, or valvular heart disease. Abnormal sensations palpated on the chest include lifts and heaves. Thrills are vibrations detected on palpation. A palpable, rushing vibration (thrill) is caused from turbulent blood flow with incompetent valves, pulmonary hypertension, or septal defects. This vibration is usually in the location of the valve in which it is associated. With chest pain that increases with movement, palpate the costochondral junction to determine whether the pain is of musculoskeletal origin.

(table continues on page 472)

Technique and Normal Findings (continued)	Abnormal Findings (continued)
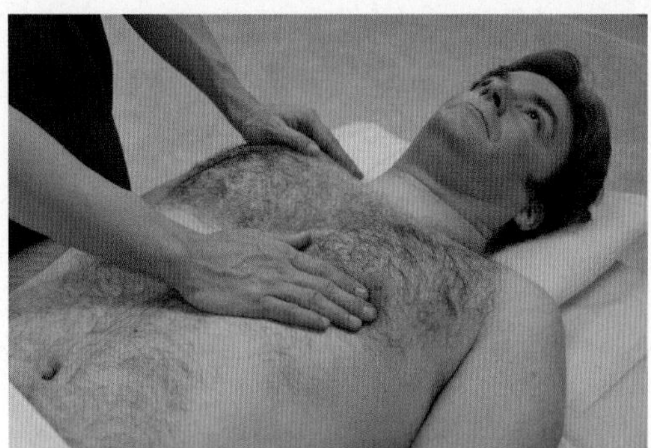 Figure 17.14 Location of the apical impulse.	

Documenting Normal Findings

PMI observed and palpated in 5th left ICS at the MCL. No thrills, heaves, or lifts.

Auscultation

Auscultation is the most important technique of cardiovascular examination. It is essential for the room to be quiet and for the stethoscope to be free of distracting noise. Chest hair, bumping of the stethoscope, or shivering may cause sounds that interfere with accuracy. Make sure that the patient is calm, warm, and draped as previously described.

Identify the locations for auscultation by accurately identifying the rib spaces and landmarks (Fig. 17.15). The most important landmark is the sternal angle at the 2nd rib space. There are two methods of identifying it. The first is to begin at the sternal notch and palpate to the right for the clavicle. Below the clavicle is the 1st rib; below the 1st rib is the 1st ICS. Feel the 2nd rib and then below it to the 2nd rib space. This is the first location for cardiac auscultation (aortic area). Recheck that this is the 2nd ICS by palpating the sternum for the indentation caused from the manubrium joining it (also called the sternal angle or angle of Louis).

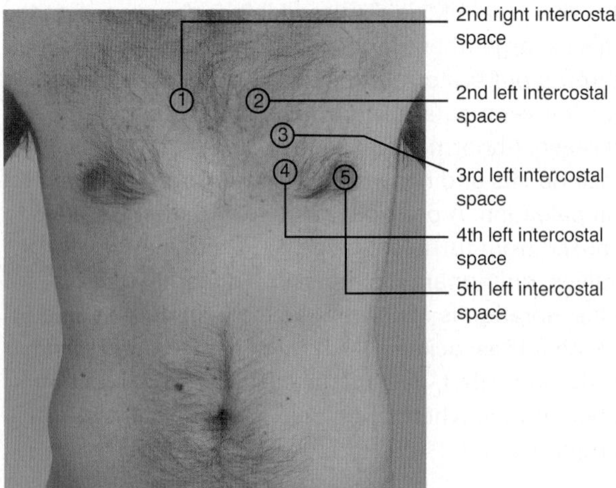

Figure 17.15 Sites for cardiac auscultation.

The second method is to first locate the angle of Louis on the sternum. A vertical motion is usually best for palpating this depression. Palpate directly across in the 2nd ICS at the left sternal border; this is the second location for auscultation (pulmonic area).

The method used depends on the comfort of the nurse and the body structure of the patient; sometimes both methods are necessary to validate correct position. Walk the fingers one rib space at the left sternal border (approximately 1 in. apart) to locate the 3rd left rib space; this is the third site for auscultation (Erb point). Walk the fingers to the 4th ICS, this is the fourth site for auscultation (tricuspid area). Move the fingers to the 5th ICS, follow the ribs down and over to the MCL; this is the fifth location for auscultation (mitral area).

These auscultatory areas are near, but not directly over, the locations of the valves because the sounds radiate in the direction in which blood flows. Note that although the pulmonic valve is on the right side of the heart, the valve is heard on the left sternal border. Not only does the sound radiate in this direction but also the right side is more forward in the chest so the pulmonic valve is turned more anteriorly and laterally. Also note that the aortic valve on the left side of the heart is heard best on the right side. It is more posterior in the chest and the vessel branches to the right side before descending inferiorly. This flow of blood causes the aortic valve sound to radiate to the right. The tricuspid valve sound radiates to the left and is heard at the sternal border; the mitral sound is heard at the MCL. The **Erb point** is where the valves usually are equally audible; this site is especially effective for taking an apical pulse.

When listening to heart sounds, begin by listening for the rhythm of the beat and the characteristic "lub-dub." Usually, the first heart sound is followed by the second with a pause before the next lub-dub. The lub, which correlates with the beginning of systole, is called S1 (see Fig. 17.8). The dub correlates with the end of systole and beginning of diastole (see Fig. 17.8). Each lub-dub is one pulse; when learning the heart sounds, it may help to palpate and feel how the pulse (ventricular systole) occurs at the same time as S1.

In general, the health care provider should stand to the patient's right, extending the length of the stethoscope across the patient's thorax. In patients with diminished heart sounds due to obesity, increased anteroposterior (AP) diameter, or pathological findings, auscultation may be improved by placing the patient in the left lateral decubitus position or asking the patient to lean forward. This displaces the heart more closely to the thoracic wall, allowing for improved transmission of sounds.

First, auscultate the heart rate and rhythm in one area (Fig. 17.16). Usually, Erb point is a good location to hear both S1 and S2 equally. Listen for a regular versus irregular rhythm. Count the heart rate for 30 seconds if regular and for 60 seconds if irregular. Then listen to each auscultatory area, usually beginning at the aortic area and proceeding laterally and inferiorly along the sternal border in each rib space. Listen first with the diaphragm and then with the bell to hear both high- and low-pitched sounds.

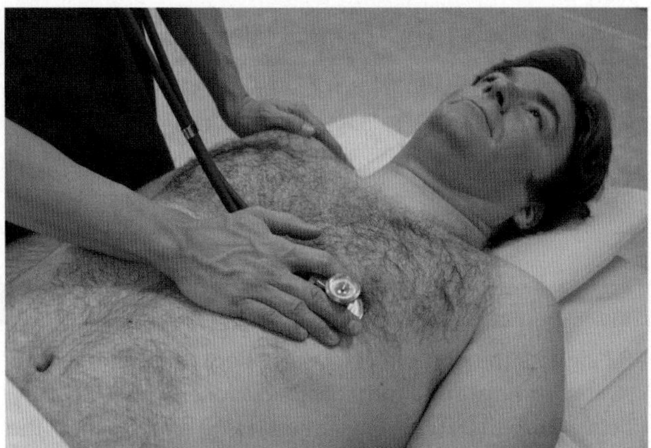

Figure 17.16 Auscultating the heart.

In all auscultatory areas:

1. Isolate the lub-dub rhythm, listening for a regular rhythmic cadence.
2. Listen first to S1 and then to S2 for a single sound or split sound. Identify if S1 or S2 is louder or softer, depending on the area being auscultated.
3. Listen for extra heart sounds (then identify if before or after S1 or S2).
4. Listen for murmurs (then identify if in systole or diastole).

Technique and Normal Findings	Abnormal Findings
Identify Rate and Rhythm. Using the diaphragm, listen to the Erb point to identify S1, S2, heart rhythm, and heart rate as described. Rhythm may vary with respiration in some patients, especially children and young adults. Rate increases at the peak of inspiration and slows at the peak of expiration. This normal variation is referred to as a **sinus arrhythmia**. *Heart rate is 60–100 bpm and regular in adults.*	If the rhythm is irregular, identify whether the irregularity has a pattern or is totally irregular. For example, every third beat missed would be described as a regular irregular rhythm. No detectable pattern is characteristic of atrial fibrillation, common in older adults. If the rhythm is irregular, take the radial pulse while listening to the apical pulse. Count the apical and radial heart rate at the same time. The easiest way to do so is to count the apical pulse while counting the number of missed beats; the difference is referred to as the **pulse deficit**. Refer to Chapter 5 for rate variations.
Identify S1 and S2. After identifying S1 as lub and S2 as dub, listen to each sound separately (Table 17.2). Normally, they are each heard as one sound. S1 signals the beginning of systole as the mitral and tricuspid valves close. Because the right side of the heart may contract slightly more slowly than the left, the tricuspid valve may close slightly after the mitral, causing a split S1. A split S1 is heard in the tricuspid area.	The rare split S1 is constant, does not vary with respiration, and so is referred to as a fixed split. Wide splitting occurs when bundle branch block delays activation of the right ventricle or when stenosis of the pulmonic valve or pulmonary hypertension delays emptying of the right ventricle. A paradoxical split is the opposite of what is expected. When closure of the aortic valve is delayed (as in left bundle branch block, right ventricular pacing, aortic stenosis, or left ventricular failure), the pulmonic valve closes before the aortic. The split is heard during expiration and disappears with inspiration (Chatterjee, 2010). See also Table 17.4 at the end of this chapter.

(table continues on page 474)

TABLE 17.2 Characteristics of Normal Sounds

Visual Representation	Intensity and Pitch	Quality	Duration	Locations
S1	Louder at apex	Lub	Correlates with carotid pulse	Mitral tricuspid
S2	Louder at base	Dub	Correlates with beginning of diastole	Aortic pulmonic

Technique and Normal Findings (continued)	Abnormal Findings (continued)
S2 signals the end of systole and beginning of diastole as the aortic and pulmonic valves close. A split S2 may occur from the pulmonic valve closing slightly after the aortic; it may be heard in the pulmonic valve area during inspiration in children (see Table 17.4). Split sounds are very close together and difficult to auscultate. S1 is louder than S2 in the mitral and tricuspid areas because those valves close at the beginning of systole (signaled by S1). S2 is louder than S1 in the aortic and pulmonic areas because those valves close at the beginning of diastole (signaled by S2). *S1 is greater than S2 in the mitral and tricuspid areas; S2 is greater than S1 in the aortic and pulmonic areas; S1 is equal to S2 at the Erb point.*	

Extra Sounds. Extra heart sounds occur from vibrations during rapid ventricular filling. They include **S3 and S4** (Fig. 17.17).

The third heart sound (S3) occurs during the early rapid diastolic filling phase immediately after S2. Blood rushes into ventricles abnormally resistant to filling, distending the ventricular walls and causing vibration. S3 is quiet, low-pitched, and often difficult to hear. It usually is audible in patients with heart failure who are fluid overloaded (Heart Failure Society of America, 2010). At the end of ventricular diastole, the atria contract (this is called atrial kick) and push an additional 25% to 30% of stroke volume into the heart. Abnormal resistance to filling during this phase also causes vibrations. S4 is heard late in diastole immediately before S1. Both S3 and S4 sound similar to S1 or S2. They are commonly referred to as ventricular "gallops." Presence of both S3 and S4 is referred to as a "summation gallop." S3 may be normal in children, young adults, and pregnant women in the third trimester.

Murmurs. **Murmurs** may result from intrinsic cardiovascular disease or circulatory disturbances (e.g., anemia, pregnancy). Some murmurs have no underlying pathology (these are referred to as "innocent murmurs"). Correlating the clinical situation with the murmur is necessary to better determine whether the murmur is insignificant or abnormal.

An innocent flow murmur may originate from higher blood flow velocities in the left ventricular outflow tract and

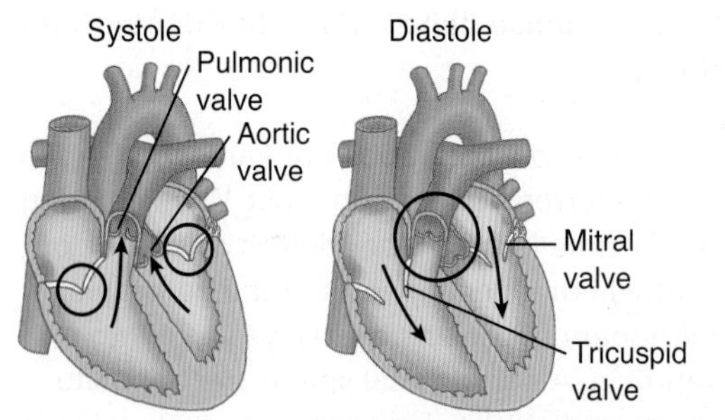

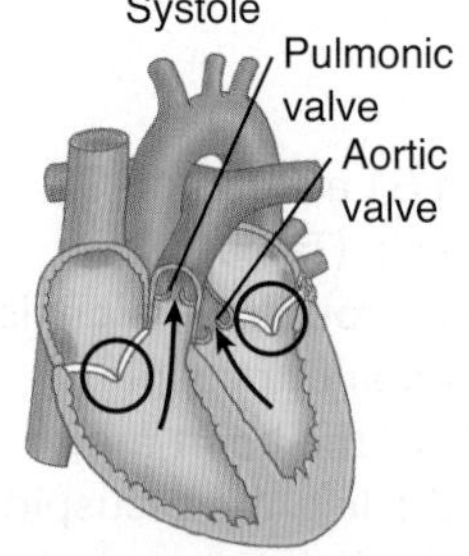

Figure 17.17 Extra heart sounds. Arrows represent the direction of blood flow. An S3 (DUB) is an abnormal sound heard immediately following S2 (closure of the semilunar valves). S3 is generated very early in diastole as blood flowing into the right or left ventricle is met with resistance. S4 (LUB) is an abnormal sound created during atrial systole as blood flowing into the right or left ventricle is met with resistance.

aortic valve. The increased flow velocity results from a larger stroke volume passing through the relatively narrow left ventricle and aortic valve in children (Moller, 2012). Innocent murmurs are usually systolic. Functional murmurs in pregnancy usually result from increased circulating fluid volumes.

Murmurs in adults usually indicate disease. If the heart valve fails to totally close, during systole, the blood leaks back through the valve and causes a whooshing sound (similar to the Korotkoff sounds heard during assessment of blood pressure). Similarly, a valve may fail to totally open, causing turbulence during diastole as the blood rushes against a partially closed valve to fill the heart. Therefore, these murmurs may occur during either systole or diastole. Murmurs also may result from vibration of tissue or excessive flow, as in pregnancy. They may occur in any of the four valves.

Murmurs usually are heard best over the precordial area where the affected valve is loudest. To identify murmurs accurately, listen for the timing in systole or diastole, loudness versus softness, and location on the chest wall. Follow-up studies, such as an echocardiogram, will identify structural abnormalities when a new murmur is detected.

Clinical Significance

Systolic murmurs occur during contraction between S1 and S2 when the mitral and tricuspid valves are closed and the aortic and pulmonic valves are open. Diastolic murmurs occur during filling from the end of S2 to the beginning of the next S1, when the mitral and tricuspid valves are open and the aortic and pulmonic valves are closed.

Technique and Normal Findings	Abnormal Findings
Listen for Extra Sounds.	⚠ *SAFETY ALERT* *Auscultation of a new extra sound may indicate a change in the patient's condition or worsening heart failure. A new S3 or S4 requires investigation and consultation with a physician for further diagnostic testing.*
S3 and S4 are commonly called **"gallops."** When S3 exists, it follows S2 and sounds like "lub dub-dub." It usually is heard best in the apex with the patient lying on the left side. This may be normal in young patients.	S3 is abnormal in patients older than 40 years of age and results from increased atrial pressure related to systolic heart failure or valvular regurgitation. Almost all patients with gallops have some degree of heart failure. Using the bell of the stethoscope, listen for a left ventricular S3 over the apex of the heart. Listen for a right ventricular S3 over the lower left sternal border. Have the patient move to the left lateral position to bring the cardiac apex closer to the chest wall, making the left ventricular S3 easier to hear.
S4 in late diastole, right before S1, sounds like "lub-lub dub." It is usually abnormal.	S4 results from a noncompliant ventricle as a consequence of hypertension, hypertrophy, or fibrosis (Chatterjee, 2010). A left ventricular S4 is heard best at the apex with the patient lying in the left lateral position; a right ventricular S4 is loudest over the left sternal border in the 5th ICS.
Listen to Murmurs. In clinical practice, nurses are more concerned with recognizing changes in murmurs than with diagnosing and labelling them. Describe murmurs according to timing in the cardiac cycle, loudness, pitch, pattern, quality, location, radiation, and position. When learning murmurs, it is helpful to identify how other health care professionals have labeled them and attempt to hear how they have been described (see Table 17.6 at the end of this chapter). The advanced practice health care provider may listen with the patient lying in the left lateral position and leaning forward. *Normally no murmurs are heard.*	The most common systolic murmurs in adults are produced by aortic stenosis, mitral insufficiency, and ventricular septal defect. In older adults, the murmur of aortic sclerosis (thickening of aortic valve leaflets with age) is common. The most common diastolic murmurs are aortic insufficiency and mitral stenosis. Nurses are often the first to identify the onset of murmurs related to papillary muscle dysfunction associated with MI. This high-pitched, crescendo decrescendo–shaped, systolic murmur must be recognized immediately so that interventions can be instituted to prevent rupture, which poses a high mortality rate (see Table 17.7 at the end of the chapter).

Additional Techniques

Technique and Normal Findings	Abnormal Findings
Hepatojugular Reflux. Pressing gently on the liver increases venous return (Fig. 17.18). Apply gentle pressure (30–40 mmHg) over the right upper quadrant or middle abdomen for at least 10 seconds (some studies suggest up to 1 minute) (Kauffman, 2013). ■ The pulsation increases for a few beats and then returns to normal less than 3 cm (about 1 1/4 in.) above the sternal angle. 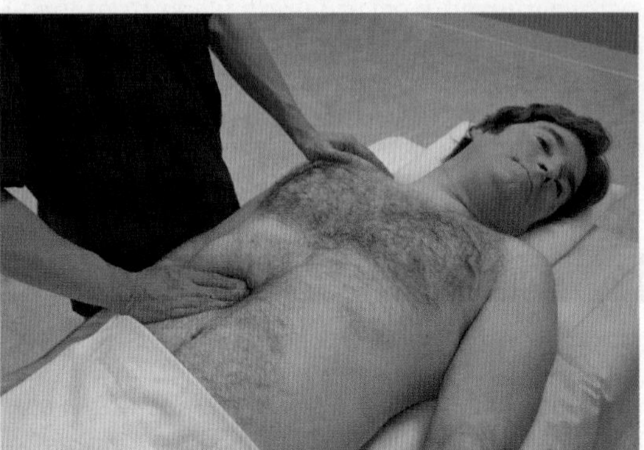 **Figure 17.18** To assess hepatojugular reflux, press gently on the liver.	A positive result is when the highest level of pulsation stays above 3 cm for more than 15 seconds. The pulsation remains elevated in disorders that cause a dilated and poorly compliant right ventricle or in obstruction of the right ventricular filling by tricuspid stenosis (Woods et al., 2010). A positive result of the **hepatojugular reflux** test is highly sensitive and specific for right ventricular fluid overload (Goel & Stewart, 2012).
Percussion of the Precordium. Chest x-ray has largely replaced chest percussion. Detecting percussion sounds over an obese or muscular chest or female breast tissue can be difficult. If x-ray is not available, percussion may be useful in identifying the left border if the heart is enlarged (as in cases of suspected heart failure). Identification of the right border is rarely useful. If heart failure or cardiomegaly is suspected, cardiac dullness may be percussed in the ICSs. Beginning at the anterior axillary line in the 4th ICS, percuss medially toward the sternum. Note the point at which the note changes from resonant (lung tissue) to dull (cardiac tissue). Repeat the procedure in the 5th and 6th ICSs. *The left border of the heart is percussed from the apex in the 4th–5th left ICS at the MCL.*	When the heart is enlarged, the left lateral border of the heart is percussed laterally and inferiorly to the normal location.

Variations in Heart Sounds

Split Heart Sound. One normal variation in heart sounds is the split heart sound. When the valves close at the same time, one S2 is heard for both valves. If the valves close at slightly different times, however, two discernible components of the same sound are heard, a situation referred to as a **split heart sound**. The right-sided pressures are lower than the left, and with inspiration, the intrathoracic pressures are even lower. The right heart can fill with more blood, which takes longer, and the closure of the pulmonic valve (on the right) is delayed.

The split S2 is more commonly heard during inspiration and disappears during expiration. S1 can also be split because the tricuspid valve closes slightly after the mitral valve during systole. Splitting of S1 is usually constant and does not vary with respiration because the AV valves are less sensitive to changes in intrathoracic pressures than are the semilunar valves. See Table 17.4 at the end of this chapter.

Systolic Ejection Click. Systolic ejection **clicks** may occur early or in the middle of systole (see Table 17.4 at the end of this chapter). The early systolic sound occurs quickly after S1. Causes are either a sudden bulging of an abnormal aortic or pulmonic valve or the sudden distention of the associated great artery. Aortic stenosis, pulmonic stenosis, and a bicuspid aortic valve can all produce this sound, with or without a murmur. Pulmonic ejection sounds often decrease in intensity with inspiration and are best heard at the left sternal border. Aortic ejection sounds are best heard at the apex.

The midsystolic click is associated with mitral valve prolapse (see Table 17.5 at the end of this chapter). There may or may not be an associated late systolic murmur, which is caused by mitral regurgitation. The click is produced by systolic prolapse of the mitral valve leaflets into the left atrium. If present, the Valsalva or squatting-to-standing maneuver should be performed to assess for increases in the click or murmur (Chatterjee, 2010).

Snap. The opening **snap** is an early diastolic sound associated with mitral stenosis (see Table 17.5). It is audible shortly after S2 and may or may not be associated with a late diastolic murmur. It results from rapid opening of the anterior mitral valve leaflet during diastole with high left atrial pressures. The opening snap is challenging to differentiate from either S3 or split S2 (Chatterjee, 2010).

Pericardial Friction Rub. The pericardial friction **rub** is an important physical sign of acute pericarditis. It may have up to three components during the cardiac cycle and is high pitched, scratching, and grating (see Table 17.5). It can best be heard with the diaphragm of the stethoscope at the left lower sternal border. The pericardial friction rub is heard most frequently during expiration and increases when the patient is upright and leaning forward (Buss & Thompson, 2010). The examiner may need to ask the patient to hold his or her breath briefly to determine whether the rub is pleural or cardiac in origin.

Lifespan Considerations: Older Adults

In the older adult, changes in the heart and blood pressure are primarily due to age-related stiffening of the vasculature and decreased responsiveness to stress hormones. Blood and pulse pressures increase as a result of the stiffened blood vessels. Additionally, body mass index increases, causing the heart to work harder. Elevated late diastolic filling increases the volume of atrial contraction, which may be associated with the S4 gallop of late diastolic filling.

The ventricles hypertrophy, increasing the risk for heart failure and resultant atrial fibrillation. Approximately 2.7 million Americans live with this chronic condition, which causes an irregular heartbeat and increases the patient's risk for stroke (CDC, 2013a). Assess older adults for symptoms of heart failure, including weight gain, shortness of breath, and edema. Symptoms of atrial fibrillation include fatigue, palpitations, and heart failure with loss of the atrial kick that supports ventricular filling.

Older adults are also more likely to develop atherosclerosis and cardiovascular disease. The vasculature is undergoing constant remodeling, forming new capillaries and collateral circulation (Brock & Jablonski, 2010). Older adults, however, are more prone to atherosclerosis because they are more sensitive to the effects of lifestyle choices, such as smoking and high-fat diets (NHLBI 2011). Assess these patients carefully for chest pain, fatigue, and dyspnea associated with symptoms. Ideally, interventions are targeted toward primary prevention of disease. Counseling is effective in reducing risk factors.

Cultural Considerations

Women and men present with heart disease differently. Women with diabetes mellitus have a significantly higher cardiovascular mortality rate than men with that disease. In addition, women with atrial fibrillation are at greater risk for stroke than are their male counterparts. The incidence of clinically significant heart failure is increasing in women. Women are also more likely to live with more cardiovascular disabilities and have a lower health-related quality of life than are men. Historically, women have been underrepresented in clinical trials studying heart disease. The lack of complete evidence concerning gender-specific outcomes in heart disease has led to assumptions about treatment in women that may have resulted in inadequate diagnoses, suboptimal treatment, and less favorable outcomes. Mortality rates in men have steadily declined, whereas mortality rates in women have remained stable over the past decade. The incidence of cardiovascular disease increases with age for both men and women.

Documenting Case Study Findings

The nurse has just finished a physical examination of Mrs. Lewis, the 77-year-old woman admitted with chest pain. Unlike the samples of normal documentation previously noted, Mrs. Lewis has abnormal findings. Review the following important findings revealed by the objective data collection. Consider how these results compare with the normal findings presented in the samples of normal documentation. Begin to think about how the data cluster and what additional data might be needed. Think critically about Mrs. Lewis's conditions, and anticipate appropriate nursing interventions. Pay attention to how the nurse clusters the data to provide a more accurate and complete understanding of the condition.

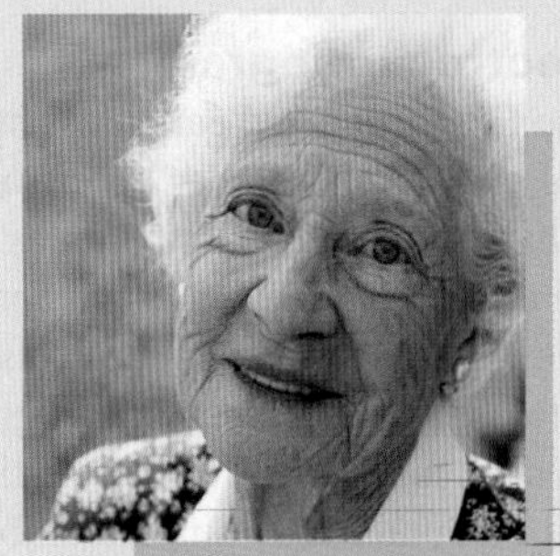

Inspection: Sitting with head of bed at 45-degree angle, appears comfortable but somewhat anxious. BP 122/62 mmHg, P 112 bpm, R 16 breaths/min, T 37°C (98.6°F),

(case study continues on page 478)

oxygen saturation 94%. Skin color pale, some diaphoresis. Chest shape symmetrical without visible apical impulse. Respirations without dyspnea. No neck vein distention.

Palpation: Apical impulse not palpated. Peripheral pulses 3+ without edema.

Percussion: Not performed.

Auscultation: Heart rate 112 with 3–5 premature bpm. Pulse deficit of 5. S1 greater than S2 at apex and S2 greater than S1 at base. No murmurs, rubs, or gallops.

Critical Thinking

Laboratory and Diagnostic Testing

Laboratory and diagnostic testing helps confirm and expand information obtained through subjective and objective data collection. All tests require explanation to the patient; some require special preparation (e.g., a period of fasting), and some require special monitoring by nurses during and after the test (e.g., exercise tolerance testing). Cardiac testing ranges from low-risk ECG to more invasive cardiac catheterization. Results from such tests help identify patterns of data that indicate areas for care planning and interventions.

Lipid Profile

Elevated levels of blood lipids are a risk factor for cardiovascular disease. A lipid profile includes total cholesterol, high-density lipoprotein (HDL), LDL, and triglyceride levels. For the general population, the guidelines designate a desirable cholesterol level less than 200 mg/dl, an optimal LDL level less than 100 mg/dl, an HDL level less than 40 mg/dl, and triglyceride level less than 150 mg/dl (National Cholesterol Education Program Expert Panel, 2013).

Cardiac Enzymes and Proteins

The myocardium releases cardiac enzymes and proteins in response to cell damage. These enzymes and proteins are measured in blood samples to diagnose or rule out MI. Creatine kinase-MB (CK-MB) and troponin-I are intracellular proteins specific to the myocardium; their values are elevated with MI.

Electrocardiogram

The ECG discussed earlier assists with diagnosis of myocardial ischemia, chamber hypertrophy, pericarditis, electrolyte imbalances, cardiac arrhythmias, and heart block. Electrodes are attached to the limbs and anterior chest wall using adhesive pads; the electrical changes in the heart are transferred onto a paper or computerized graph. Nurses with additional training may perform ECG testing. Home ECG monitoring can be conducted using an ambulatory ECG monitor or an event recorder.

Chest X-ray

A chest x-ray film helps determine the size, contour, and position of the heart; alterations in the pulmonary circulation; and acute or chronic lung disease.

Echocardiogram

An echocardiogram uses high-frequency sound waves and the Doppler effect to evaluate the size, shape, and motion of cardiac structures and the direction and velocity of blood flow through the heart. A gel (often cold) is placed on the patient's chest wall and the transducer is moved around the anterior chest wall.

The echocardiogram may also be done with the transducer inserted through the mouth into the esophagus (transesophageal echocardiogram or TEE). Compared with the simple echocardiogram, this invasive procedure provides superior images when compared with traditional transthoracic echocardiography but requires fasting and sedation, with potential complications such as a perforated esophagus or impaired swallowing.

Hemodynamic Monitoring

Bedside hemodynamic monitoring includes measurement of central venous pressure, pulmonary artery pressures, and systemic interarterial pressures using a catheter placed in the heart. Systemic intraarterial pressure monitoring provides access to direct and continuous blood pressures in critically ill patients; this catheter is usually placed in the radial artery. Hemodynamic monitoring requires the advanced training and skill of nurses in critical care areas.

Stress Test

Stress testing compares cardiac function and perfusion at rest versus during stress. A simple exercise stress test consists of ECG monitoring for signs of ischemia or arrhythmia while the patient walks on a treadmill or rides a stationary bicycle. A radionuclide ventriculogram, also known as a multiple-gated acquisition (MUGA) scan, is a test in which a small amount of a patient's blood is withdrawn, mixed with a radionuclide, and reinjected. This study is most commonly used to monitor the effects of potentially cardiotoxic chemotherapeutic agents. Both of these tests are performed in dedicated settings.

Cardiac Catheterization and Coronary Angiography

Cardiac catheterization and coronary angiography are invasive diagnostic procedures that delineate coronary anatomy and CHD using fluoroscopy, usually in the radiology department. Right-sided heart catheterization is performed to measure right-sided heart pressures and structures. Left-sided heart catheterization involves placing a catheter through the femoral or radial artery to the coronary arteries where dye is used for visualization. Following the procedure, the patient is on bed rest (if a femoral approach is used), and the puncture site and distal circulation must be monitored frequently. Nursing staff also monitor blood pressure and cardiac rhythm.

Cardiac Electrophysiology

Cardiac electrophysiology studies are used in the diagnostic investigation of arrhythmias and syncope. Flexible catheters with multiple electrodes are placed within the heart to stimulate arrhythmias. The patient fasts for several hours before the study; usually, he or she is sedated during the procedure. Complications include the inability to induce arrhythmias, cardiac perforation and pericardial effusion, venous thrombosis or infection from the catheter site, and intractable ventricular fibrillation and death (Fogoros, 2012). Patients are monitored closely following this procedure.

Diagnostic Reasoning

Nursing Diagnoses, Outcomes, and Interventions

Table 17.3 compares nursing diagnoses commonly related to cardiovascular assessment (NANDA International, 2012). From the assessment information and established nursing diagnoses, you then work to identify patient outcomes. Some outcomes related to cardiovascular problems are the following:

- The patient demonstrates adequate circulation status with strong peripheral pulses, normal blood pressure, and adequate urinary output.
- The patient demonstrates cardiac pump effectiveness with normal heart rate, negative JVD, no S3 or S4, and no arrhythmias.
- The patient maintains fluid balance with no edema, clear lung sounds, stable body weight, and balanced intake and output (Moorhead, Johnson, Maas, & Swanson, 2013).

After outcomes have been established, you can implement care to improve the patient's status. Critical thinking and evidence-based practice are essential to develop effective interventions. Examples of nursing interventions for cardiovascular care are as follows:

- Teach the patient the signs of cardiac ischemia and when to call 911.
- Assess for chest pain, shortness of breath, and edema; document cardiac arrhythmias.
- Weigh the patient daily; monitor trends. Maintain accurate intake and output recordings.

You then evaluate care according to the developed patient outcomes, reassessing the patient and continuing or modifying the interventions as appropriate. An accurate and complete nursing assessment is an essential foundation for holistic nursing care. Even beginning nursing students can use assessment data to implement new interventions, evaluate the effectiveness of those interventions, and make a difference in the quality of patient care.

You also collect assessment data to assist physicians in identifying medical diagnoses so that appropriate treatment may be ordered. You must understand the association of assessment findings with underlying conditions in order to gather data to support or discount medical diagnoses. For example, chest pain may result from MI, pulmonary embolism, or musculoskeletal tenderness. First, you assess the patient's history to determine whether the pain is acute or chronic. Then you assess heart sounds for S3, S4, or murmurs, which may accompany MI. Oxygen desaturation may be associated with pulmonary embolism, whereas chest wall tenderness may be due to musculoskeletal problems. An ECG helps with diagnosis of MI. As you can see, you need to use critical thinking to know which data to collect. Then you will need to organize findings to assist physicians to arrive at a medical diagnosis.

TABLE 17.3 Common Nursing Diagnoses Associated with Cardiovascular Conditions

Diagnosis	Point of Differentiation	Assessment Characteristics	Nursing Interventions
Decreased cardiac output	The heart pumps inadequate blood to meet the body's metabolic demands.	Arrhythmias, palpitations, ECG changes, increased fluid volume, decreased blood pressure, dyspnea, S3 or S4, murmur	Monitor for symptoms of heart failure. Observe for chest pain or discomfort. Place patient on cardiac monitor. Assess blood pressure carefully.
Impaired tissue perfusion, cardiac	Decreased oxygen results in failure to nourish tissues at the capillary level.	Chest pain, ECG changes, elevated CK-MB or troponin-I, diaphoresis, dyspnea, low oxygen saturation	Place patient on cardiac monitor. Administer nitroglycerin with MD order.* Place oxygen.* Ensure the IV is in place for emergency use.* Notify physician.
Excess fluid volume	Increased fluid retention and edema	Jugular vein distention, weight gain, dyspnea, orthopnea, PND, S3 or S4, edema	Monitor edema, intake, and output. Weigh patient daily. Auscultate lung and heart sounds. Administer diuretic with order.* Elevate head of bed for dyspnea.

*Collaborative interventions.

Progress Note: Analyzing Findings

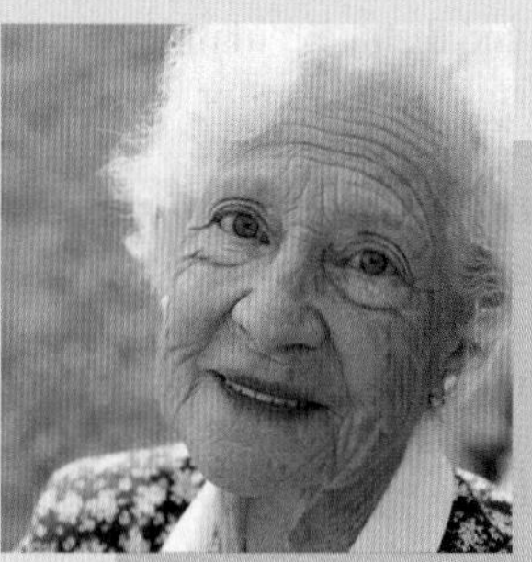

Mrs. Lewis's issues have been outlined throughout this chapter. The initial collection of subjective and objective data is complete. Mrs. Lewis expressed concerns about her new diagnosis of MI; additionally, she developed an irregular rhythm with some pallor and diaphoresis.

Unfortunately, Mrs. Lewis also develops a new onset of chest pain, so the nurse must reassess her and document findings. The following nursing note illustrates how the nurse collects and analyzes subjective and objective data and begins to develop nursing interventions.

Subjective: "I'm having chest pain again." States chest pain 8/10 scale. Describes pain as a heavy weight at the center of her chest that radiates down her left arm. Started approximately 5 minutes ago and has been increasing. Is similar to the pain that she had earlier in the day, although this pain began at rest.

Objective: BP 100/66 mmHg, P 122 with 3–5 premature bpm, R 28 breaths/min, oxygen saturation 94%. Increased diaphoresis, dizziness, and nausea. Skin pale, appears anxious. Peripheral pulses 2+ and thready.

Analysis: Impaired cardiac tissue perfusion related to possible myocardial ischemia.

Plan: Stay with patient and continue to monitor vital signs. Give nitroglycerin tablets as ordered by physician. Page rapid response team for assistance. Obtain 12-lead ECG and bedside monitor. Place oxygen as ordered and assess lung sounds. Elevate head of bed. Ensure that IV site is patent and suction is at bedside if needed. Provide calm reassurance that the patient will not be left alone and that treatment will be given for the chest pain. Use therapeutic touch as appropriate. Inform family of new onset of chest pain.

Critical Thinking Challenge

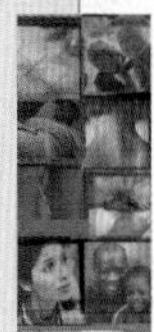

- What type of assessment is this? Would you further investigate any subjective data?
- Critique the documented objective data. Is the organization logical? Would you add any data?
- Why did the nurse prioritize impaired cardiac tissue perfusion as the diagnosis to document?
- How is the nurse using assessment information to organize and plan nursing interventions?

Collaborating With the Interprofessional Team

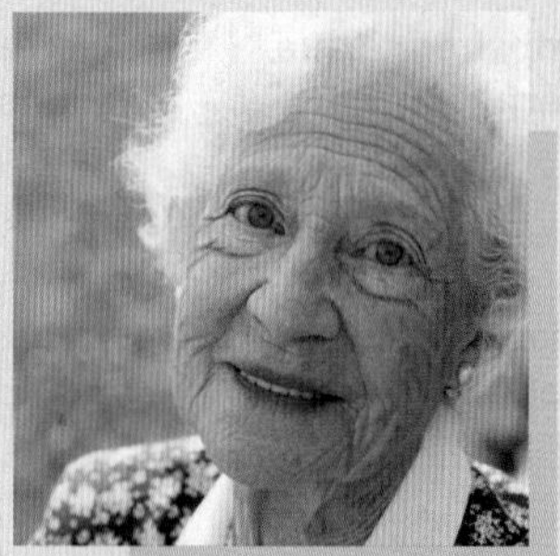

The Agency for Healthcare Research and Quality (AHRQ, 2012) has recommended the formation of rapid response teams to provide prompt assistance to patients with early warning signs of deterioration. Intervening before the patient's condition further declines has been proven to improve patient outcomes. The role of the team is to assess, stabilize, assist with communication, support, and assist with transfer if needed. Results that might trigger a page to the rapid response team are as follows:

- Any staff member is worried about the patient.
- The patient has an acute change in heart rate of less than 40 or more than 130 bpm.
- Systolic blood pressure changes acutely to less than 90 mmHg.
- Respiratory rate changes acutely to less than 8 or more than 28 breaths/min.

(case study continues on page 481)

- Saturation falls below 90% despite oxygen administration.
- Conscious state changes acutely.
- Urinary output falls below 50 ml in 4 hours (Institute for Healthcare Improvement, 2011)

Mrs. Lewis was admitted 6 hours ago with chest pain and is having new chest pain. Rapid response is indicated because the nurse is worried about the patient's new chest pain. The following conversation illustrates how to organize data and make recommendations about the patient's situation to team members when they arrive. Usually, several people on the team come to assist with care at the bedside. Assessments and interventions occur simultaneously to resolve chest pain, which indicates cardiac ischemia and is an urgent issue.

Introduction: "I'm Galen Indigo and I'm the nurse for Mrs. Lewis."

Situation: "She was admitted with chest pain 6 hours ago and a diagnosis of MI. She has a new onset of chest pain that she rates as 8 out of 10."

Background: "Her medical history includes hypertension. She is taking a beta-blocker and a thiazide diuretic and also a statin to lower her cholesterol. Her blood pressure is 100/66 mmHg, which is down from 148/78 mmHg. Her pulse is 122 beats/min, respirations 28 breaths/min, and oxygen saturation is 94%. She's having 3–5 premature bpm and had a pulse deficit earlier. Her peripheral pulses are 2+ and thready. I have given her one nitroglycerin tablet, and she's still rating her pain as a 7 on a 1–10 scale."

Assessment: "I called for you because I'm worried that she might be having some cardiac ischemia and I can use some help in getting her treated."

Recommendations: *To a member of rapid response:* "It's time for her to have another nitroglycerin, so I can do that if you can get the ECG and then set up the bedside monitor. If someone else could hook up the oxygen, that would be great. She has an IV in place already." *To the charge nurse:* "Could you page the physician and let her know the situation?" *To Mrs. Lewis:* "I'll stay with you because I know you're a little anxious." *To an assisting nurse:* "Her husband is in the waiting room—could you let him know that she's having chest pain? If he would like to come in, that's OK. Let him know that we're working closely with her." *To the patient:* "Mrs. Lewis, let me know if your pain is any better after this second nitroglycerin. How are you doing?"

Critical Thinking Challenge

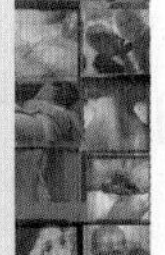

- How will the nurse conduct assessments and nursing care while considering Mrs. Lewis's anxious state?
- Which part of the nursing process is highest priority during this time?
- What is the nurse's role in coordinating collaborative care with the rapid response team?
- What will be the frequency of assessment for Mrs. Lewis after this event? What items will be assessed?

Pulling It All Together

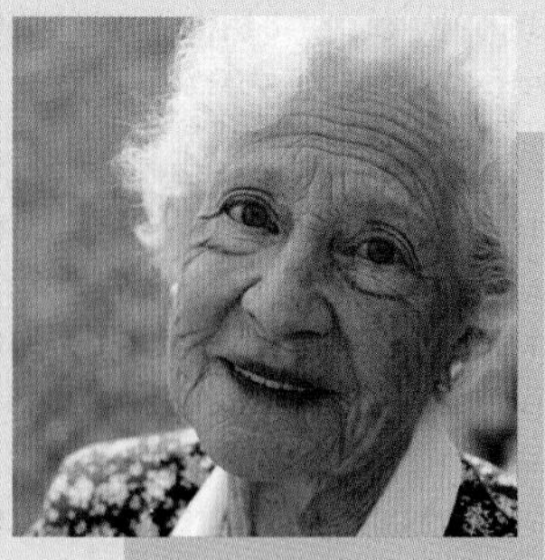

Nurses use assessment data to formulate a nursing care plan for Mrs. Lewis. After completing the outlined interventions, they reevaluate and document findings in the chart. This is often in the form of a care plan or case note similar to the one below.

Nursing Diagnosis	Patient Outcomes	Nursing Interventions	Rationale	Evaluation
Impaired cardiac tissue perfusion related to possible cardiac ischemia	Blood pressure is stable within 30 minutes. Chest pain resolves within 5 minutes.	Monitor vital signs every 5 minutes until stable. Ensure IV access. Encourage patient to rest and reduce anxiety. Monitor for cardiac arrhythmias. Administer nitroglycerin and oxygen prn according to orders. Elevate head of bed.	IV access is essential in case the patient's condition deteriorates and IV medications are needed. Rest reduces the demand for oxygen. Arrhythmias may accompany ischemia. Nitroglycerin causes coronary arteries to dilate, relieving chest pain and increasing oxygen delivery to the myocardium. Oxygen improves supply to the heart tissue.	Blood pressure has improved to 132/78 mmHg. Chest pain has resolved with the third nitroglycerin dose. Patient is resting comfortably with head of bed elevated. Heart rate 102 bpm and rhythm with no premature beats. Transfer to coronary intensive care for unstable chest pain.

Applying Your Knowledge

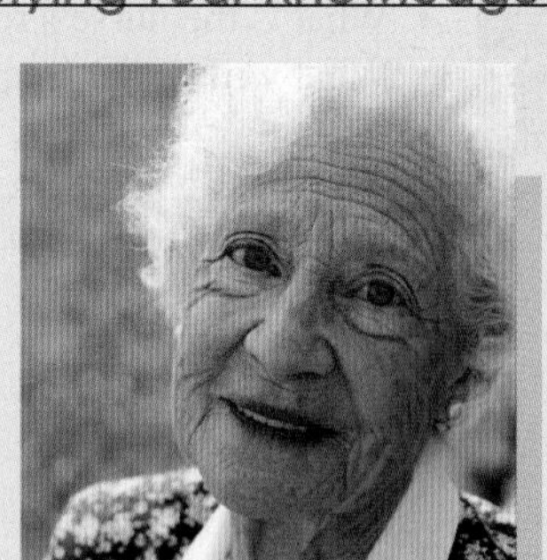

Using the previous steps of diagnostic reasoning, organizing, and prioritizing, consider all the case study findings woven throughout this chapter. When answering the following questions, begin drawing conclusions and see how the pieces of assessment must work together to create an environment for personalized, appropriate, and accurate care.

- What might be causing the change in Mrs. Lewis's condition?
- Is Mrs. Lewis's condition stable, urgent, or an emergency?
- What immediate health promotion and teaching needs are evident?
- What lifestyle factors might be contributing to Mrs. Lewis's situation?
- How will the nurse focus, organize, and prioritize objective data collection?
- How will the nurse evaluate the effectiveness of patient teaching?

Key Points

- Knowledge of cardiac anatomy and physiology is essential to understanding cardiac assessment.
- The cardiovascular system is a double pump with pulmonary and systemic circulation.
- The cardiac cycle consists of rhythmic movements of systole (ventricular contraction) and diastole (relaxation).
- The S1 or first heart sound results from closure of the mitral and tricuspid valves; this sound signals the beginning of systole.
- The S2 or second heart sound results from closure of the aortic and pulmonic valves; this sound signals the beginning of diastole and end of systole.
- Health care providers assume that chest pain is cardiac in origin until another diagnosis is established. Chest pain is an acute situation that requires intervention in addition to assessment.
- Risk factors for cardiovascular disease include increasing age, family history, male gender, high blood pressure, high blood cholesterol level, smoking, diabetes mellitus, overweight and obesity, decreased activity, high-fat diet, excessive alcohol intake, elevated C-reactive protein, and elevated BNP.
- Common symptoms of CVD are chest pain, dyspnea, orthopnea, cough, diaphoresis, fatigue, edema, and nocturia.
- Inspection and palpation of the PMI should be at the 4th to 5th left ICS in the MCL.
- The nurse auscultates heart sounds in specific areas on the precordium: aortic, pulmonic, tricuspid, and mitral.
- A split heart sound is audible when the valves close at slightly different times: the S1 is split from the mitral and tricuspid and the S2 is split from the aortic and pulmonic.
- Murmurs are identified by their location, intensity, quality, timing in the cardiac cycle, and radiation.
- S3 and S4 are extra sounds that result from ventricular filling; the S3 follows the S2 and the S4 precedes the S1.
- The nursing diagnoses most commonly associated with cardiac problems are decreased cardiac output, ineffective cardiac tissue perfusion, and excess fluid volume.

Review Questions

1. Which of the following statements describes the cardiovascular system most accurately?
   A. It is a double pump with pulmonary and systemic elements.
   B. It has a heart with six chambers and valves.
   C. It includes concepts of precontractility, aftercontractility, and load.
   D. It functions with a conduction system that starts in the ventricles.

2. In a healthy patient, the myocardial cells in the ventricle depolarize and contract during
   A. prediastole.
   B. diastole.
   C. systole.
   D. postsystole.

3. When the nurse listens to S1 in the mitral and tricuspid areas, the expected finding is
   A. S1 greater than S2.
   B. S1 is equal to S2.
   C. S2 greater than S1.
   D. No S1 is heard.

4. The nurse assesses the neck vessels in the patient with heart failure to determine which of the following?
   A. The strength of the carotid pulse
   B. The presence of bruits
   C. The highest level of jugular venous pulsation
   D. The strength of the jugular veins

5. The nurse is caring for a patient with a sudden onset of chest pain. Which assessment is highest priority?
   A. Auscultate heart sounds.
   B. Inspect the precordium.
   C. Percuss the left border.
   D. Obtain a blood pressure reading.

6. A patient who visits the clinic has the controllable risk factors of smoking, high-fat diet, overweight, decreased activity, and high blood pressure. What concept should the nurse use when performing patient teaching?
   A. Teach the patient the most serious information.
   B. Give the patient brochures to review before the next visit.
   C. Discuss risk factors that the patient is interested in modifying.
   D. Describe consequences of risk factors to motivate the patient.

7. Which of the following clusters of symptoms are common in women preceding an MI?
   A. Chest pain, nausea, diaphoresis
   B. Weight gain, edema, nocturia
   C. Dizziness, palpitations, low pulse
   D. Fatigue, difficulty sleeping, dyspnea

8. The nurse auscultates a medium-loud whooshing sound that softens between S1 and S2. The nurse documents this finding as which of the following?
   A. Grade III decrescendo systolic murmur
   B. Grade IV crescendo systolic murmur
   C. Grade II crescendo diastolic murmur
   D. Grade I decrescendo diastolic murmur

9. The nurse auscultates an extra sound on a patient 1 week after an MI. It is immediately after S2 and is heard best at the apex. Which of the following does the nurse suspect?
   A. S3 gallop
   B. S4 gallop
   C. Systolic ejection click
   D. Split S2

10. A patient has dyspnea, edema, weight gain, and liquid intake greater than output. These symptoms are consistent with which nursing diagnosis?
   A. Ineffective cardiac tissue perfusion
   B. Decreased cardiac output
   C. Impaired gas exchange
   D. Excess fluid volume

The Jensen suite offers these additional resources to enhance learning and facilitate understanding of this chapter:

- thePoint online resource, http://thepoint.lww.com/Jensen2e
- *Laboratory Manual for Nursing Health Assessment: A Best Practice Approach*
- *Pocket Guide for Nursing Health Assessment: A Best Practice Approach*
- *Lippincott DocuCare*, an electronic health record simulation software, http://thepoint.lww.com/docucare
- *Adaptive Learning | Powered by PrepU*, http://thepoint.lww.com/prepu

References

Alothman, A., Bukhari, A., Aljohani, S., & Muhanaa, A. (2009). Should we recommend stethoscope disinfection before daily usage as an infection control rule? *The Open Infectious Disease Journal, 3,* 80–82

Agency for Healthcare Research and Quality. (2012). *Patient safety primers: Rapid response systems.* Retrieved from http://psnet.ahrq.gov/primer.aspx?primerID = 4

American Heart Association. (2013). *Asian and Pacific Islanders and cardiovascular diseases.* Retrieved from https://www.heart.org/idc/groups/heart-public/@wcm/@sop/@smd/documents/downloadable/ucm_319570.pdf

Berg, J., Bjorck, L., Dudas, K., Lappas, G., & Rosengren, A. (2009). Symptoms of a first acute myocardial infarction in women and men. *Gender Medicine, 6*(3), 454–462

Bonow, R., Mann, D. L., Zipes, D. P., & Libby, P. (2014). *Braunwald's heart disease: A textbook of cardiovascular medicine* (9th ed). Philadelphia, PA: Elsevier.

Borlaug, B., Redfield, M., Melenovsky, V., Kane, G., Karon, B., Jacobsen, S., & Rodeheffer, R. J. (2013). Longitudinal changes in left ventricular stiffness: A community based study. *Circulation. Heart Failure, 6*(5), 944–952.

Brock, A., & Jablonski, R. (2010). Physiology of aging: Impact on critical illness and treatment. In M. Foreman, K. Milisen, & Fulmer, T. (Eds.), *Critical Care Nursing of Older Adults: Best Practices* (3rd ed., pp. 241–266). New York, NY: Springer Publishing.

Buss, J., & Thompson, G. (2010). *Auscultation skills: Breath and heart sounds.* Ambler, PA: Lippincott Williams & Wilkins.

Canto, J. Rogers, W., Goldberg, R. J., Peterson, E. D., Wenger, N. K., Vaccarino, V., . . . Zheng, Z. J. (2012). Association of age and sex with myocardial infarction symptom presentation and in-hospital mortality. *The Journal of the American Medical Association, 307*(8), 813–822.

Centers for Disease Control and Prevention. (2010). 2010 Surgeon General's Report—How tobacco smoke causes disease: The biology and behavioral basis for smoking-attributable disease. Retrieved from http://www.cdc.gov/tobacco/data_statistics/sgr/2010/index.htm

Centers for Disease Control and Prevention. (2011). Prevalence of coronary heart disease: United States, 2006-2010. *Morbidity and Mortality Weekly Report, 60*(40), 1377–1381. Retrieved from http://www.cdc.gov/mmwr/preview/mmwrhtml/mm6040a1.htm?s_cid= mm6040a1_w

Centers for Disease Control and Prevention. (2013a). *Atrial fibrillation fact sheet.* Retrieved from http://www.cdc.gov/dhdsp/data_statistics/fact_sheets/fs_atrial_fibrillation.htm

Centers for Disease Control and Prevention. (2013b). *Health effects of cigarette smoking.* Retrieved from http://www.cdc.gov/tobacco/data_statistics/fact_sheets/health_effects/effects_cig_smoking/

Chatterjee, K. (2010). Physical examination. In K. Chatterjee (Ed.), *Cardiology: An illustrated textbook* (pp. 151–173). New Delhi, India: Jaypee Medical.

Cholesterol Treatment Trialists' Collaboration. (2010). Efficacy and safety of more intensive lowering of LDL cholesterol: A meta-analysis of data from 170,000 participants in 26 randomised trials. *Lancet, 376,* 1670

Chua, J., Parikh, N., & Fergusson, D. (2013). The jugular venous pressure revisited. *Cleveland Clinic Journal of Medicine, 80*(10), 638–644

Darlow, S., Goodman, M. S., Stafford, J. D., Lachance, C. R., & Kaphingst, K. A. (2012). Weight perceptions and perceived risk for diabetes and heart disease among overweight and obese women, Suffolk County, New York, 2008. *Preventing Chronic Disease, 9,* 110185.

Deedwania, P., & Volkova, N. (2013). Metabolic syndrome and cardiovascular disease: Epidemiology, pathophysiology, and therapeutic considerations. In P. Shah (Ed.), *Risk factors in coronary artery disease.* New York, NY: Taylor and Francis

Flack, J., & Nasser, S. (2011). Benefits of once-daily therapies in the treatment of hypertension. *Vascular Health and Risk Management, 7,* 777–787

Fogoros, R. (2012). *Electrophysiologic testing.* Hoboken, NJ: Wiley-Blackwell.

Goel, S., & Stewart, W. (2012). Key clinical findings. In S. Anwaruddin, J. Martin, A. Askari, & J. Stephens (Eds.), *Cardiovascular hemodynamics: An introductory guide* (pp. 77–98). New York, NY: Springer Publishing.

Gu, Q., Dillion, C., Burt, V., & Gillum, R. (2009). Association of hypertension treatment and control with all-cause and cardiovascular mortality among US adults with hypertension. *American Journal of Hypertension, 23*(1), 38–45

Heart Failure Society of America. (2010). *Evaluation of patients for ventricular dysfunction and heart failure: HFSA 2010 comprehensive heart failure practice guideline.* Retrieved from http://www.guideline.gov/content.aspx?id = 23900

Institute for Healthcare Improvement. (2011). *Establish criteria for activating the rapid response team.* Retrieved from http://www.ihi.org/knowledge/Pages/Changes/EstablishCriteriaforActivatingtheRapidResponseTeam.aspx

Jensen, J., Ma, L., Bjurman, C., Hammarsten, O., & Fu, M. (2012). Prognostic values of NTpro BNP/BNP ratio in comparison with NTpro BNP or BNP alone in elderly patients with chronic heart failure in a 2-year follow up. *International Journal of Cardiology, 155*(1), 1–5.

Karavidas, A., Lazaros, G., Tsiachris, D., & Pyrgakis, V. (2010). Aging and the cardiovascular system. *Hellenic Journal of Cardiology, 51,* 421–427.

Kauffman, M. (2013). *History and physical exam: A common sense approach.* Burlington, MA: Jones and Bartlett.

Kelly, R. (2010). Diet and exercise in the management of hyperlipidemia. *American Family Physician, 81*(9), 1097–1102.

Moller, J. (2012). History and physical examination. In J. Moller & J. Hoffman (Eds.), *Pediatric cardiovascular medicine* (2nd ed., pp. 81–101). Hoboken, NJ: Wiley-Blackwell

Moorhead, S., Johnson, M., Maas, M. L., & Swanson, E. (2013). *Nursing outcomes classification (NOC): Measurement of health outcomes* (5th ed.). St. Louis, MO: Elsevier.

Mosca, L., Mochari, H., Dolor, R., Newby, K., & Robb, K. (2010). Twelve-year follow up of American women's awareness of cardiovascular disease risk and barriers to heart health. *Circulation, 3,*120–127.

Naghavi, M. (2010). *Asymptomatic atherosclerosis: Pathophysiology, detection and treatment.* New York, NY: Springer Publishing.

NANDA International. (2012). *Nursing diagnoses: Definitions and classification 2012-2014* (9th ed). Oxford, United Kingdom: Wiley-Blackwell.

National Cholesterol Education Program Expert Panel. (2013). *Blood cholesterol in adults: Systematic evidence review from the Cholesterol Expert Panel.* Retrieved from http://www.nhlbi.nih.gov/guidelines/cholesterol/atp4/index.htm

National Heart, Lung, and Blood Institute. (2011). *Who is at risk for atherosclerosis?* Retrieved from http://www.nhlbi.nih.gov/health/health-topics/topics/atherosclerosis/atrisk.html

National Heart, Lung, and Blood Institute. (2012). NHLBI fact book. *Chapter 4: Disease statistics.* Retrieved from http://www.nhlbi.nih.gov/about/factbook/chapter4.htm

Navis, C., Goss, J., & Roach, L. (2010). Anything but typical: Recognize and treat everyday cardiac complaints. *Journal of Emergency Medical Services, 35*(7), 84–87

Pickett, C., Jackson, J., Hemann, B., & Atwood, J. (2010). Carotid bruits and cerebrovascular disease risk: A meta-analysis. *Stroke, 41,* 2295–2302.

Ridker, P. (2009). The JUPITER trial: Results, controversies, and implications for prevention. *Circulation: Cardiovascular Quality and Outcomes, 2,* 279–285.

Roger, V. L., Go, A. S., Lloyd-Jones, D. M., Adams, R. J., Berry, J. D., Brown, T. M., . . . Wylie-Rosett, J. (2011). Heart disease and stroke statistics—2011 update: A report from the American Heart Association. *Circulation, 123,* e18–209.

Safford, M., Brown, T., Muntner, P., Durant, R., Glasser, S., Halanych, J., . . . Howard, G. (2012). Association of race and sex with risk of incident of acute coronary heart disease. *The Journal of the American Medical Association, 308*(17), 1768–1774.

Taraboanta, C., Hague, C., Mancini, J., Forster, B., & Frohlich, J. (2012). Coronary artery calcium findings in asymptomatic subjects with family history of premature coronary artery disease. *British Cardiovascular Disorders, 12,* 53.

U.S. Department of Health & Human Services. (2013). *2020 Topics and objectives - Objectives A-Z.* Retrieved from http://www.healthypeople.gov/2020/topicsobjectives2020/

U.S. Department of Health & Human Services, Office of Minority Health. (2013a). *Heart disease and American Indians/Alaska Natives.* Retrieved from http://minorityhealth.hhs.gov/templates/content.aspx?ID =3025

U.S. Department of Health & Human Services, Office of Minority Health. (2013b). Obesity and African Americans. Retrieved from http://minorityhealth.hhs.gov/templates/content.aspx?ID=6456

Woods, S. L., Sivarajan Froelicher, E. S., Motzer, S. A., & E. J. (2010). *Cardiac nursing* (6th ed.). Philadelphia, PA: Lippincott Williams & Wilkins.

Yang, L., Jiang, D., Qi, W., Zhang, T., Feng, Y., & Gao, L. (2012). Subclinical hyperthyroidism and the risk of cardiovascular events and all-cause mortality: An updated meta-analysis of cohort studies. *European Journal of Endocrinology, 167,* 75–84

Yoon, S. S., Burt, V., Louis T., & Carroll, M. D. (2012). *Hypertension among adults in the United States, 2009–2010* [NCHS Data Brief No. 107]. Hyattsville, MD: National Center for Health Statistics.

Tables of Abnormal Findings

TABLE 17.4 Variations in S1 and S2

Heart Sound	Description
Accentuated S1 S1 S2 S1 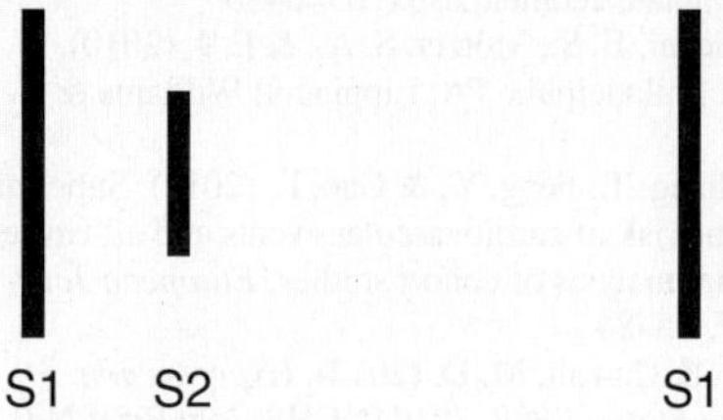	S1 is louder when mitral valve leaflets are recessed into the ventricle, as with rapid heart rate, hyperkinetic states, short PR interval, atrial fibrillation, or mitral stenosis.
Diminished S1 S1 S2 S1	S1 is softer with long PR interval, depressed contractility, left bundle branch block, obesity, or a muscular chest.
Varying Intensity of S1 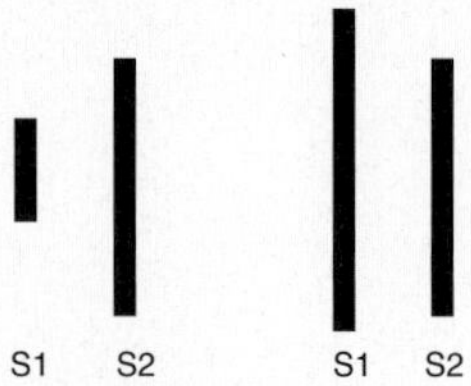 S1 S2 S1 S2	S1 varies in atrial fibrillation and complete heart block when the valve is in varying positions before closing.
Split S1 S1 S2 S1 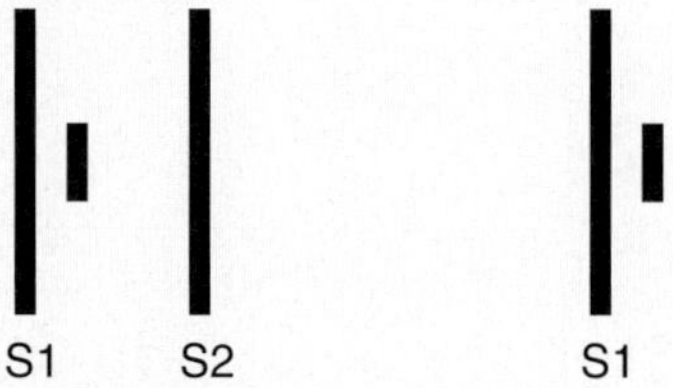	The first component is heard at the base; the second component is heard at the lower left sternal border. Split S1 accompanies right bundle branch block.
Accentuated S2 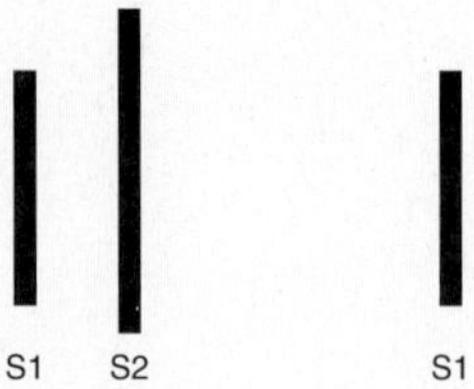 S1 S2 S1	S2 is increased in systemic hypertension or when the aorta is close to the chest wall. Another cause is pulmonary hypertension.

(table continues on page 487)

TABLE 17.4 Variations in S1 and S2 *(continued)*

Heart Sound	Description
Diminished S2 	S2 may be decreased from aortic calcification, pulmonic stenosis, and aging, with reduced mobility of the valves.
Fixed Split 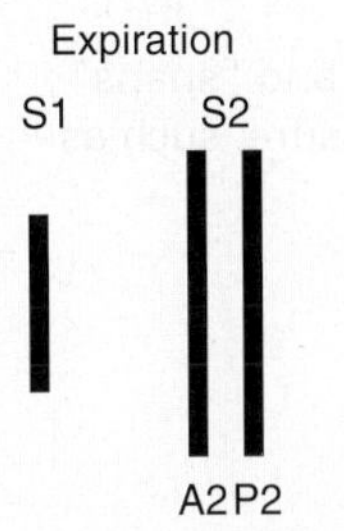 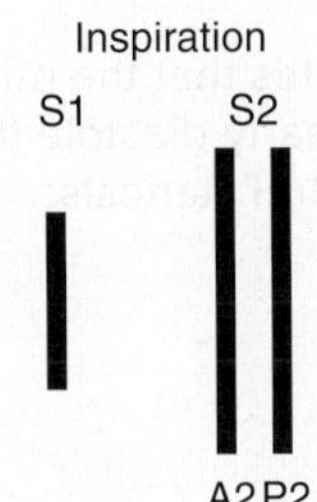	The two components are heard during both inspiration and expiration. The split is wide and results from right bundle branch block or early opening of the aortic valve.
Paradoxical Split 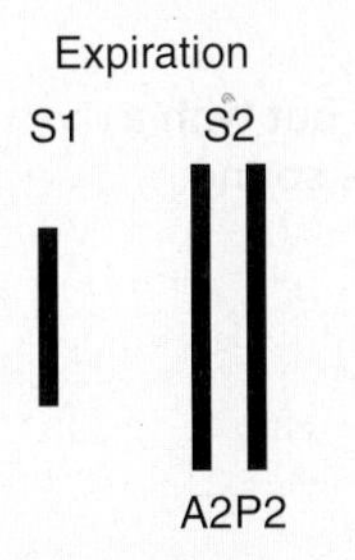 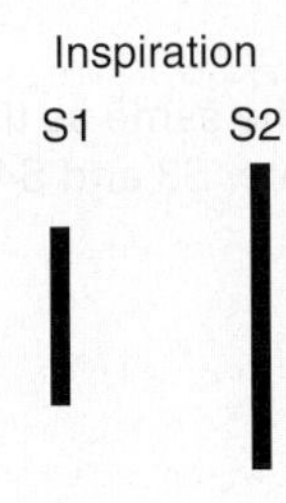	The pulmonic valve closes before the aortic from left bundle branch block, right ventricular pacemaker. The sounds usually fuse during inspiration.
Wide Split 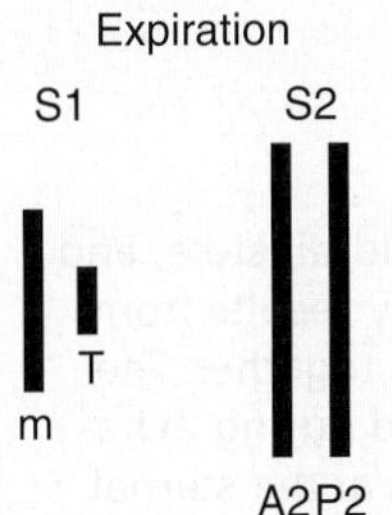 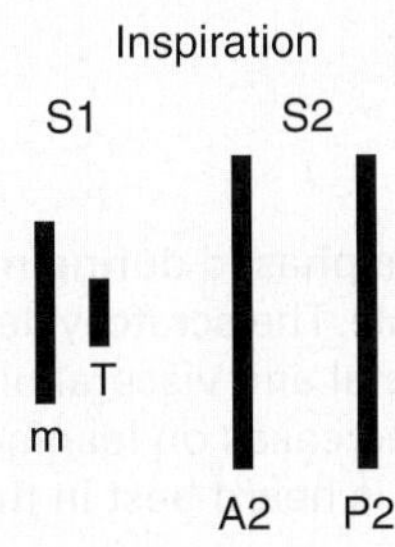	A wide split is found with right bundle branch block from delayed depolarization of the right ventricle.

TABLE 17.5 Identifying Extra Sounds

Heart Sound	Description
Ejection Click 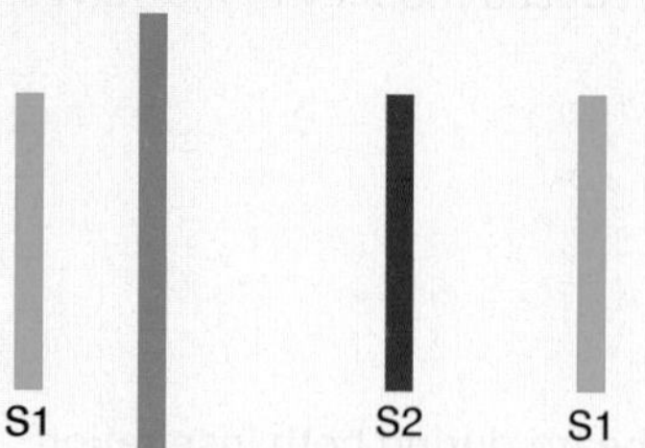 	This sound results from an open valve that moves during the beginning of systole. It is heard best with the diaphragm of the stethoscope and may be audible over the aortic or pulmonic areas.
Opening Snap 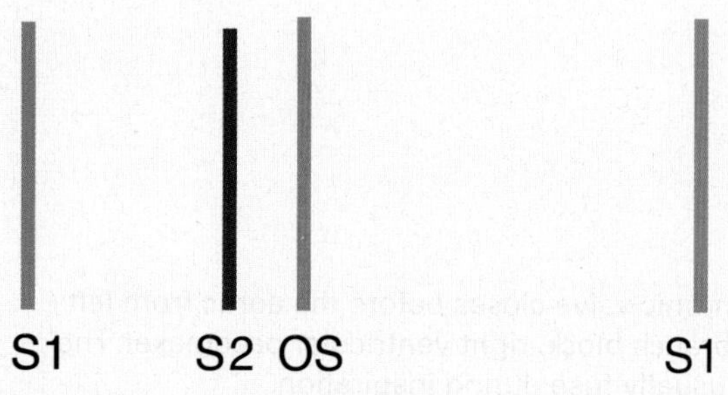 	It indicates that the mitral valve is mobile and "snaps" during early diastole from high atrial pressure, such as with mitral stenosis.
Summation Gallop 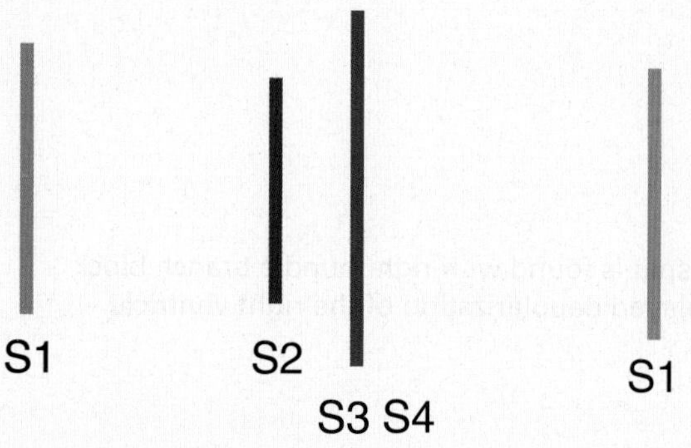 	This is the same as the quadruple rhythm but with a faster rate. S3 and S4 merge to create one sound.
Pericardial Friction Rub 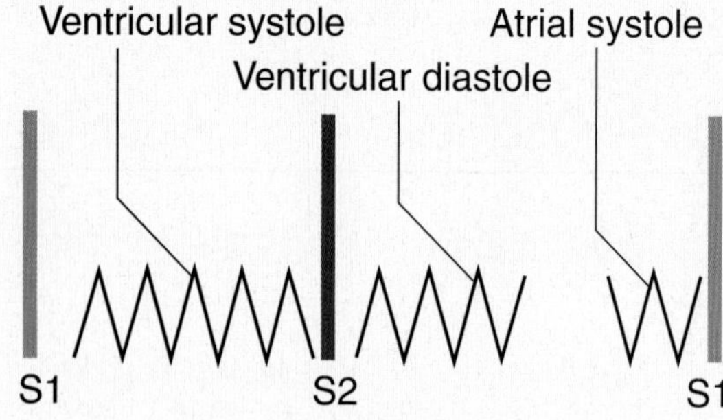 	It is triple phased during midsystole, mid-diastole, and presystole. The scratchy, leathery quality results from the parietal and visceral pleura rubbing together. The sound increases on leaning forward and during exhalation. It is heard best in the 3rd left ICS at the sternal border.

(table continues on page 489)

TABLE 17.5 Identifying Extra Sounds *(continued)*

Heart Sound	Description
Venous Hum 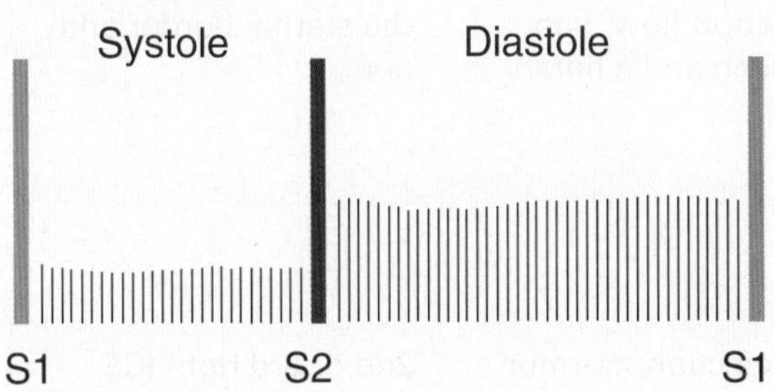	This continuous sound is normal in children and during pregnancy. It is rough, noisy, and occasionally accompanied by a high-pitched whine. It may be louder during diastole. It is low pitched and heard best with the bell above the medial third of the clavicles.
Quadruple Rhythm with S3 and S4	S3 is generated during early diastolic filling; S4 is generated during atrial contraction late in diastole. Both are present. It is heard best with the bell of the stethoscope over the apex of the heart.

TABLE 17.6 Description of Murmurs

Intensity: Loudness	**I.** Faint; heard only with special effort **II.** Soft but readily detected **III.** Prominent but not loud **IV.** Loud; accompanied by thrill **V.** Very loud **VI.** Loud enough to be heard with stethoscope just removed from contact with the chest wall (Bonow et al., 2014).
Timing: Point in the cardiac cycle	**Systolic:** Sounds like "swish-dub"; falls between S1 and S2 **Diastolic:** Sounds like "dub-swish," falls after S2 and before the next S1 More specifically, murmurs may be labeled as early, middle, or late systolic and early, middle, or late diastolic. **Holosystolic murmurs:** Occur during all of systole **Holodiastolic murmurs:** Occur during all of diastole **Continuous murmurs:** Begin in systole and continue through S2 into part but not necessarily all of diastole
Pitch: High or low tone	**High:** Heard best with diaphragm **Medium** **Low pitch:** Heard best with bell
Pattern: Increasing or decreasing in volume	**Crescendo:** Increasing intensity **Decrescendo:** Decreasing intensity **Plateau:** Remain constant
Quality: Type of sounds	Harsh, blowing, raspy, musical, rumbling
Location: Site on the precordium	Area of maximum intensity using either the valvular areas or thoracic landmarks
Radiation: Direction it travels	Where the sound radiates, usually in the direction of blood flow in the vessel
Position: Changes with patient position	If the murmur changes depending on patient position, the patient may be turned to the left and right, lie down, sit up, and lean forward. Children may squat.

TABLE 17.7 Distinguishing Murmurs

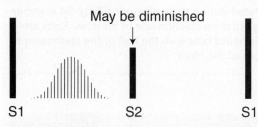

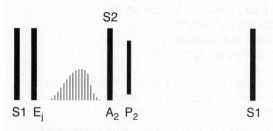

Heart Sound	Description	Optimal Site for Auscultation
Physiological Murmur S1 S2 S1	This murmur, caused by a temporary increase in blood flow, has a soft, medium pitch and a harsh quality.	2nd–4th left ICS between the sternal border and apex
Aortic Stenosis May be diminished S1 S2 S1	This midsystolic ejection murmur begins after S1, crescendos, and then decrescendos before S2. It radiates upward to the right 2nd ICS and into the neck. It is soft to loud, with a medium pitch and harsh quality. It is associated with ejection click, split S2.	2nd or 3rd right ICS
Pulmonic Stenosis S2 S1 E_j A_2 P_2 S1	This midsystolic ejection murmur may radiate toward the left shoulder and neck. It is soft-loud, medium pitch, harsh quality, and associated with ejection click, split S2.	2nd or 3rd left ICS
Mitral Stenosis S1 Accentuated S1 S2 OS	This mid-diastolic murmur is associated with an opening snap and has a low-pitched, rumbling quality.	Heard best with the bell over the apex with the patient turned to the left
Mitral Regurgitation Diminished S1 S2 S3 S1	This midsystolic ejection murmur is soft to loud, medium to high pitch, with a blowing quality. It radiates to the left axilla and is associated with a thrill and lift at the apex.	Apex

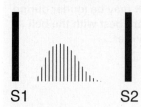

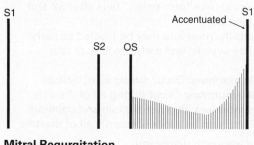

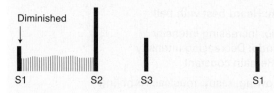

(table continues on page 491)

TABLE 17.7 Distinguishing Murmurs *(continued)*

Heart Sound	Description	Optimal Site for Auscultation
Tricuspid Regurgitation Diminished S1 S2 S3 S1	This midsystolic ejection murmur can be holosystolic with elevated right ventricular pressure. It increases with inspiration, with a medium pitch and blowing quality.	Lower left sternal border
Aortic Regurgitation S1 S2 S1	This early diastolic murmur is decrescendo, soft, high pitched, and blowing.	2nd–4th left ICS; heard best with the diaphragm of the stethoscope when the patient leans forward during exhalation
Pulmonic Regurgitation	This early diastolic murmur may begin with a loud S2. It is a high-frequency blowing murmur with a crescendo–decrescendo pattern.	
Tricuspid Stenosis	The loudness of this mid-diastolic murmur increases with inspiration. It has a rumbling quality and is louder during inspiration.	Heard at the lower left sternal border

TABLE 17.8 Congenital Heart Disease

Heart Sound	Description	Optimal Site for Auscultation
Patent Ductus Arteriosus 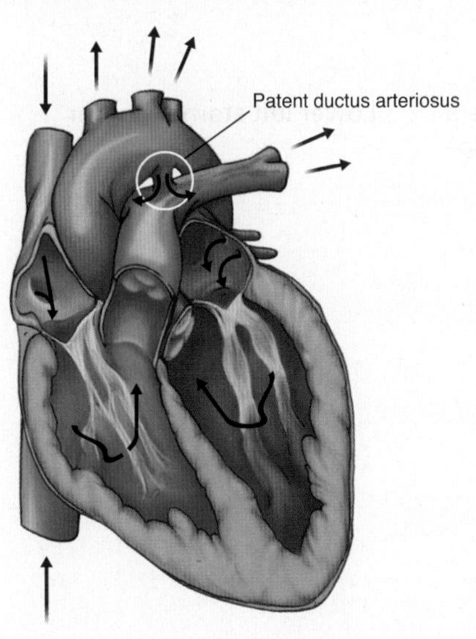 	The continuous murmur peaks just before and after S2. It has a rough, harsh, mechanical quality with a palpable thrill.	2nd left ICS

(table continues on page 492)

TABLE 17.8 Congenital Heart Disease *(continued)*

Heart Sound	Description	Optimal Site for Auscultation
Atrial Septal Defect 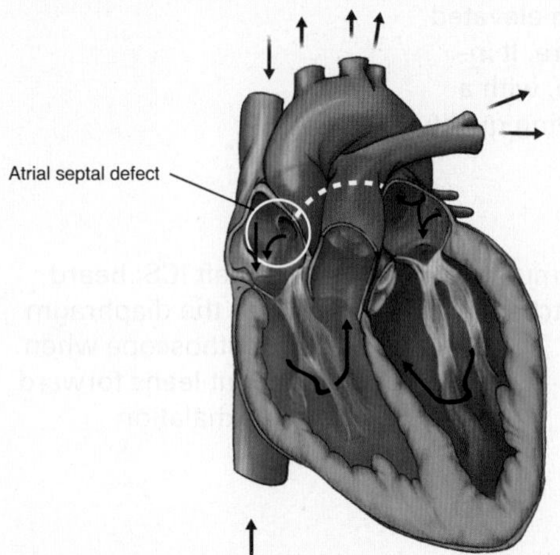	This continuous murmur is altered by the Valsalva maneuver. It is a systolic ejection murmur with medium pitch.	Base in the 2nd left ICS
Ventricular Septal Defect 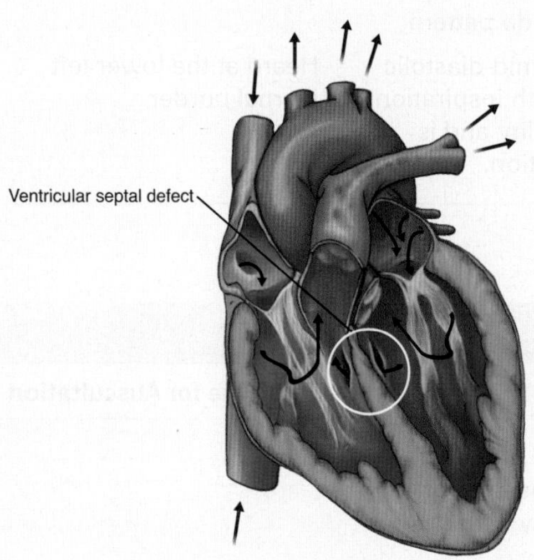	This murmur is holosystolic because left ventricular pressures exceed right ventricular pressures. It radiates, often loudly with a thrill. The quality is high-pitched and harsh.	3rd–5th left ICS
Tetralogy of Fallot 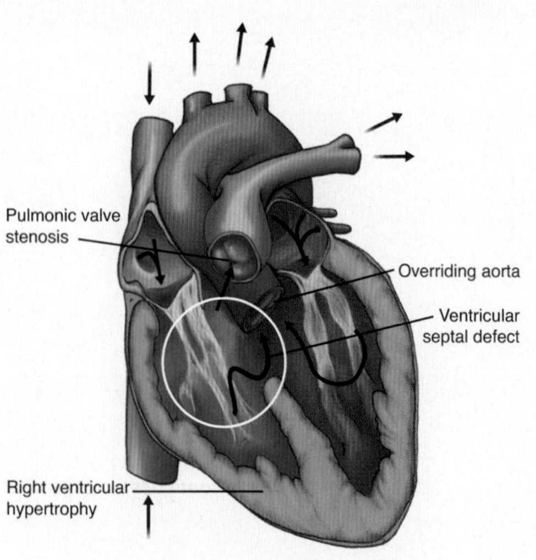	This early diastolic murmur has a thrill. It is loud, with a crescendo–decrescendo pattern.	Lower left sternal border

(table continues on page 493)

TABLE 17.8 Congenital Heart Disease *(continued)*

Heart Sound	Description	Optimal Site for Auscultation
Coarctation of the Aorta	This systolic murmur radiates to the back.	Left sternal border

18

Peripheral Vascular and Lymphatic Assessment

Learning Objectives

1. Identify the structures and functions of the arterial, venous, and lymphatic systems.
2. Identify teaching opportunities for health promotion and risk reduction related to the arterial, venous, and lymphatic systems.
3. Collect subjective data related to peripheral vascular symptoms, including pain, numbness or tingling, skin changes, edema, cramps, and decreased functional ability.
4. Collect objective data about the peripheral vascular system, including color, temperature, pulses, capillary refill, and edema.
5. Identify normal and abnormal findings from the general survey, inspection, palpation, and auscultation of the peripheral vascular and lymphatic systems.
6. Identify the locations of the peripheral pulses.
7. Use subjective and objective data to analyze findings of and plan interventions for the peripheral vascular and lymphatic systems.
8. Document and communicate data from peripheral vascular and lymphatic assessments using appropriate medical terminology.
9. Individualize peripheral vascular and lymphatic assessment considering the condition, age, gender, and culture of the patient.
10. Use assessment findings of the peripheral vascular and lymphatic systems to identify diagnoses and to initiate a plan of care.

Mr. Rossi, an 88-year-old Caucasian man, lives in a long-term care facility. His medical diagnoses include a myocardial infarction 15 years ago, high blood pressure, high cholesterol level, chronic renal failure, and peripheral arterial disease (PAD). He is taking a statin for his cholesterol and an antiplatelet medication for the PAD. He also is slightly confused, with impaired recent memory.

You will gain more information about Mr. Rossi as you progress through this chapter. As you study the content and features, consider Mr. Rossi's case and its relationship to what you are learning. Begin thinking about the following points:

- List the six "Ps" used to assess for arterial occlusion.
- How does Mr. Rossi's health history relate to his current health status?
- What assessment findings might the nurse note if Mr. Rossi's PAD worsens?
- What assessment data will the nurse want to collect related to other body systems?
- How might the nurse modify history taking and physical examination based on Mr. Rossi's age and present state of confusion?
- How will the nurse evaluate the effectiveness of health teaching with Mr. Rossi?

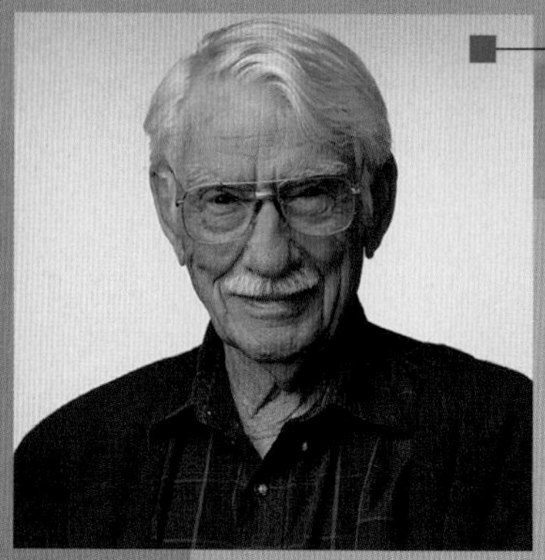

This chapter focuses on comprehensive assessment of the peripheral vascular and lymphatic systems. You must understand the independent roles of the arterial, venous, and lymphatic systems as well as their integrated functioning as the circulatory system. Doing so enables you to develop holistic plans for circulatory well-being in your patients. A review of pertinent anatomy and physiology provides the basis for the collection of subjective and objective information. The section on subjective data collection gives details that will help you evaluate history, risk factors, and symptoms associated with peripheral vascular health. The content on objective assessment outlines a methodical approach to assessing peripheral pulses, extremity temperature, skin condition, perfusion, and fluid status and describes alterations from normal. The chapter presents advanced assessment techniques as well.

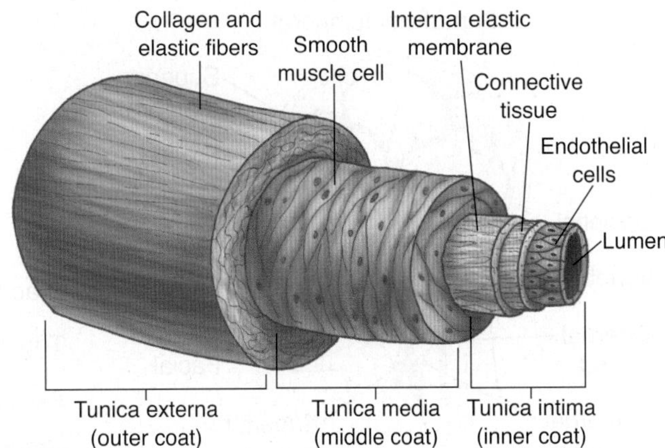

Figure 18.1 Structure of an artery.

Structure and Function

The organs and tissues of the body depend on a healthy intact peripheral vascular system, which consists of a complex network of arteries, veins, and lymphatic vessels. The vascular network transports oxygenated blood throughout the body and returns deoxygenated blood to the heart and lungs for reoxygenation. The lymphatic system supports the vascular system by returning excess fluid from the tissues to the vascular network. Disruption of the peripheral vascular or lymphatic system can have debilitating and, in some cases, fatal consequences. Thus, comprehensive and accurate assessment of the arterial, venous, and lymphatic systems provides an essential foundation for holistic and thorough nursing care. Such assessment depends on a solid understanding of the anatomy and physiology of these systems.

Arterial System

The arterial system consists of arteries, arterioles, and capillaries that deliver oxygenated blood from the heart to the rest of the body. The walls of the arteries and arterioles have three layers: the tunica intima or inner layer; the tunica media, which is the middle layer; and the tunica externa (adventitia) or outer layer (Fig. 18.1). Arteries have many elastic fibers, which allow them to constrict and recoil with systole and diastole.

> **Clinical Significance**
>
> Arterioles have more smooth muscle, and it is here that blood pressure is controlled (Grossman & Porth, 2014).

The largest vessel of the arterial system is the aorta. The subclavian arteries branch off the aorta to feed the vessels of the upper extremities (Fig. 18.2). The largest arteries of the upper extremities are the brachial arteries. They bifurcate into the radial and ulnar arteries, which further divide into two arterial arches that supply the hands.

The aorta bifurcates distally into the iliac arteries. The iliac arteries continue into the femoral arteries, which go to the lower extremities. At the popliteal fossa, the femoral artery becomes the popliteal artery, which bifurcates into the dorsalis pedis and posterior tibial arteries. These arteries form a connecting arch at the foot.

Smooth endothelial cells line the inner layer of all blood vessels and play a critical role in the prevention of platelet adhesion and thrombus formation. Injury to the endothelial layer thus contributes significantly to the pathogenesis of atherosclerosis (Grossman & Porth, 2014). Interruption of arterial flow results from narrowing of the arteries, rupture or dissection of the layers of an artery, or thrombus formation (Grossman & Porth, 2014).

Venous System

The venous system consists of veins, venules, and connecting veins called perforators, which collect unoxygenated blood from the body and return it to the heart (Fig. 18.3). In contrast to arteries, veins are thin-walled. The venous system is a low-pressure system. Veins often are referred to as capacitance vessels because they can stretch and accommodate large volumes of fluid.

The veins of the upper extremities, upper torso, head, and neck drain into the superior vena cava and then the right atrium. Those of the lower extremities and lower torso drain into the inferior vena cava and right atrium. Veins in the upper and lower extremities are either superficial or deep. The superficial system includes the greater and lesser saphenous veins. The deep system includes the common femoral, femoral, profunda femoris, popliteal, and anterior, posterior, and peroneal tibial vessels.

A pressure gradient created by respiration, skeletal muscle contraction, and intraluminal valves regulates blood flow in the venous system (Grossman & Porth, 2014). During inspiration, the diaphragm drops and abdominal pressure increases. During expiration, abdominal pressure decreases, creating a suction effect that promotes venous return. Because veins do not have the same muscular walls that arteries do, they also rely on the calf muscle pump to combat the pull of gravity and promote venous return. For example, as a person walks, the contraction of the calf muscles promotes venous

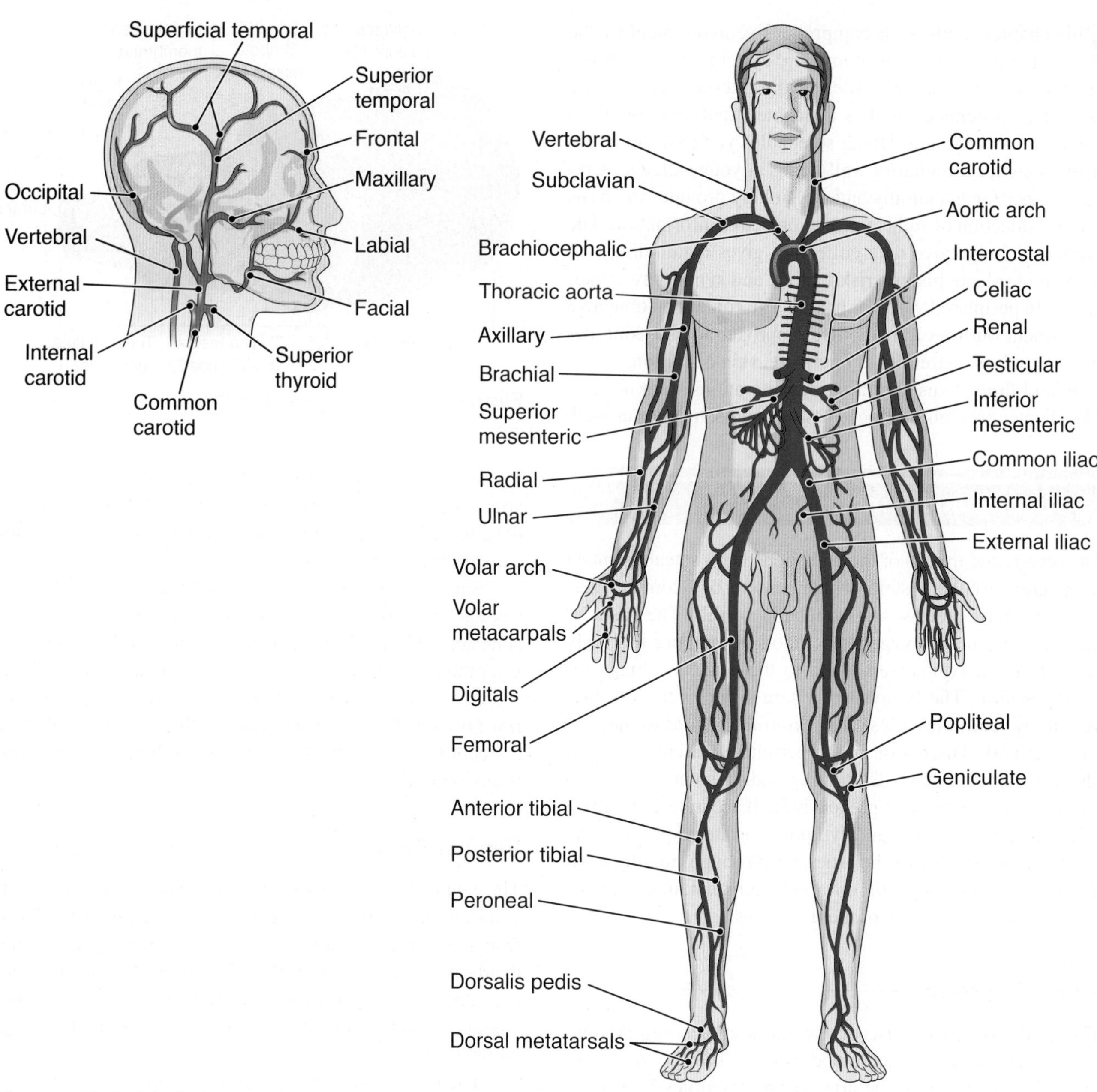

Figure 18.2 Principal systemic arteries.

flow. Additionally, veins contain bicuspid valves that prevent the retrograde flow of venous blood, thus maintaining unidirectional flow. The more distal a vein is, the greater the number of valves because the pull of gravity is stronger (Grossman & Porth, 2014). Interruption of venous flow results from obstruction, valve incompetence, or trauma.

> **Clinical Significance**
>
> Because veins are capacitance vessels and are less muscular than arteries, blood tends to collect in them. When moving from lying to standing or when standing suddenly, dizziness may result until the calf and leg muscles contract to increase the venous return to the central part of the body and brain.

Capillaries

The exchange of nutrients, gases, and metabolites between blood vessels and tissues occurs in the capillary beds. Oxygen-rich blood delivers nutrients from the arterioles to the capillaries. Venules then return metabolites from the capillary beds to the venous system (Grossman & Porth, 2014).

Lymphatic System

The lymphatic system consists of the lymph nodes and lymphatic vessels (Fig. 18.4) as well as the spleen, tonsils, and thymus (Fig. 18.5). It maintains fluid and protein balance and functions with the immune system to fight infection. The lymphatic vessels carry lymph in the tissues back

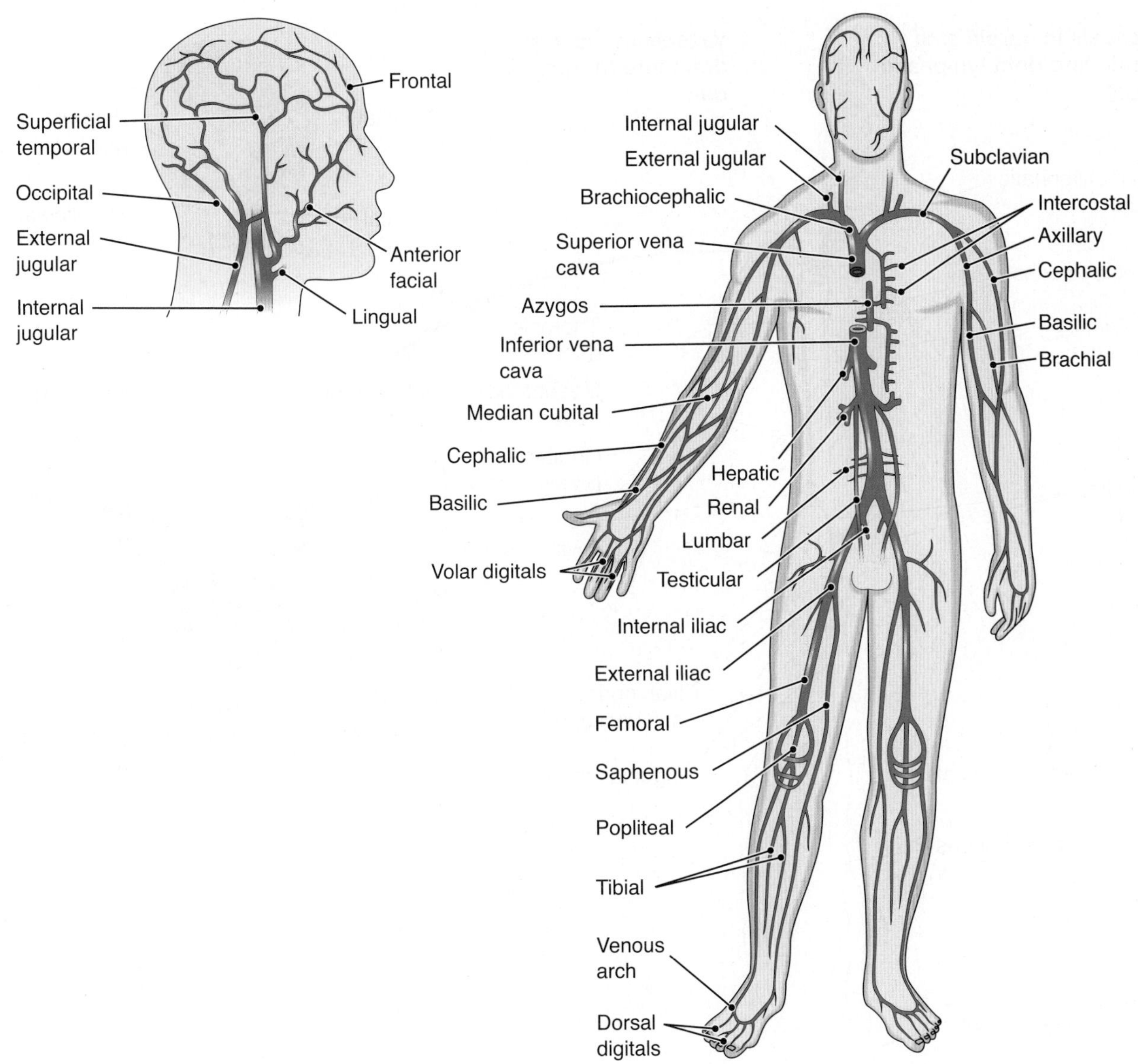

Figure 18.3 Principal systemic veins.

to the bloodstream. The pathways of lymphatic vessels often run parallel to the arteries and veins (Grossman & Porth, 2014). The thoracic ducts at the junctions of the subclavian and internal jugular veins return the lymph fluid to the circulation. The lymphatic vessels contain valves to maintain unidirectional flow. Skeletal muscle contraction, passive movement, and increases in heart rate all support lymph flow.

Only the superficial lymph nodes are accessible for palpation. Lymphatic flow in the arms drains into the epitrochlear, axillary, and infraclavicular nodes. In the lower extremities, the lymph drains primarily into the inguinal nodes.

When the amount of lymph in interstitial tissue exceeds the capacity of the lymphatic vessels, **lymphedema** occurs. Edema high in protein fills the tissue and is ultimately replaced by fibrous tissue and collagen. If untreated, the fibrosis may progress and result in irreversible tissue enlargement. Lymphedema may be congenital or it may result from a scarring injury, removal of lymph nodes, radiation therapy, or chronic infection (Lee, Bergan, & Rockson, 2011).

Lifespan Considerations: Older Adults

Calcification of the arteries, or arteriosclerosis, causes them to become more rigid in older adults. Less arterial compliance results in increased systolic blood pressure (Grossman & Porth, 2014). This is often compounded by the coexistence of atherosclerotic disease in the arteries supplying the brain, heart, and other vital organs. The incidence of **PAD** increases dramatically in the seventh and eighth decades of life (Al Mahameed, 2009; Grossman & Porth, 2014). The prevalence of PAD in men and women is equal at this stage. The population burden of PAD in women in the United States, as indicated by financial cost, morbidity, and mortality, may actually be greater than that of men (Hirsch et al., 2012).

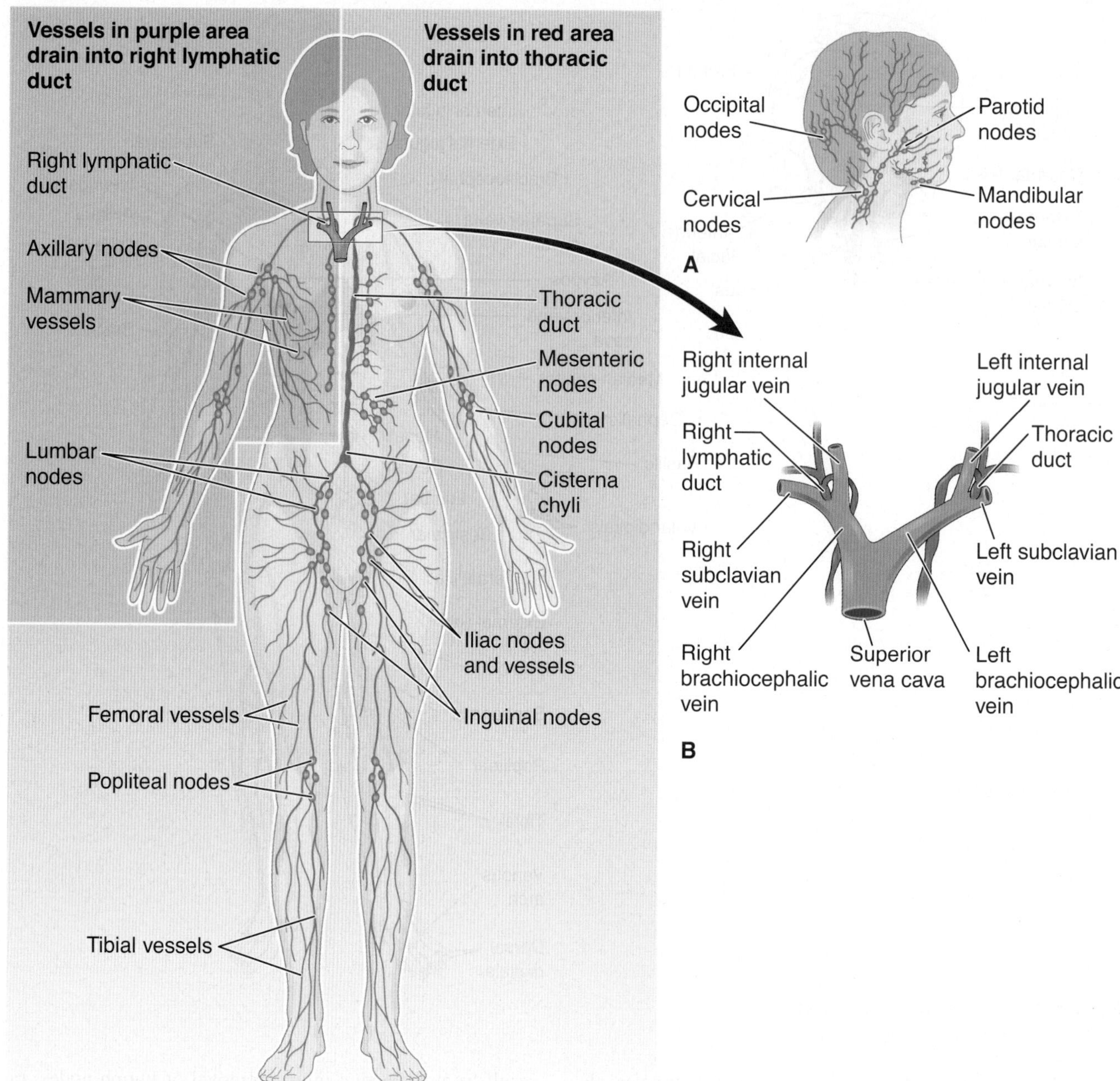

Figure 18.4 The lymphatic vessels and nodes. **A.** Lymph nodes and vessels in the head. **B.** The right lymphatic duct and thoracic duct drains into the subclavian veins.

Cultural Considerations

Incidence of PAD, the most prevalent vascular disease, is highest in African Americans of both sexes. Rates of PAD in Mexican American women are also slightly higher (Centers for Disease Control and Prevention [CDC], 2013). An increase in cardiovascular disease (CVD) exists among African Americans and Hispanics as well. Hypertension, a significant risk factor for PAD, is increased in African Americans (CDC, 2013; Wierzbicki, 2012). Smoking, another primary risk factor, also may have hazardous environmental effects, such as in the case of secondary smoke inhalation. Genetics plays a prominent role in atherosclerosis development, as do many of the cardiovascular risk factors. Hypertension, diabetes, and hyperlipidemia are cardiovascular risk factors with strong genetic components (Leeper, Kullo, & Cooke, 2012).

Primary **varicose veins** are seen more often in people older than 50 years of age and in those with obesity (Grossman & Porth, 2014). Varicose veins are more common in women, which may be related to the increased venous stasis that accompanies pregnancy. An increase in varicose veins in those who stand for most of the day also exists (Grossman & Porth, 2014). Varicose veins and lymphedema may be familial (Lee et al., 2011; Zoller, Sundquist, & Sundquist, 2011).

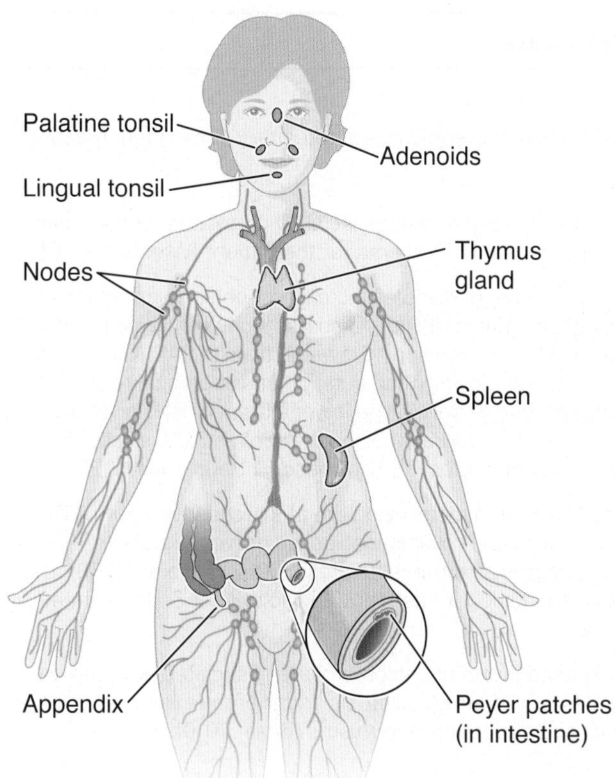

Figure 18.5 Lymphoid tissues.

Urgent Assessment

If the patient is experiencing symptoms of complete arterial occlusion such as pain, numbness, coolness, or color change of an extremity, stop the assessment and get help. This is a limb-threatening situation (Grossman & Porth, 2014). If the patient is experiencing symptoms of **deep vein thrombosis (DVT)** such as pain, edema, and warmth of an extremity, stop the assessment and get help. Immediate intervention to start anticoagulants is necessary. A **pulmonary embolism (PE)** may result from a DVT. Be alert for any signs of a PE, including acute dyspnea, chest pain, tachycardia, diaphoresis, and anxiety (see Chapter 16). This life-threatening emergency requires immediate intervention (Grossman & Porth, 2014).

It is essential that you prioritize assessment and interventions based on urgently acute rather than chronic situations. The patient with PAD and symptoms of acute occlusion needs immediate intervention to avoid the threat of limb loss (Wennberg, 2013). Focus your assessment on the **six Ps (pain, pallor, poikilothermia, paresthesias, pulselessness, and paralysis)**. Collect past cardiovascular history as you proceed with the physical assessment. You may then prepare the patient for interventional radiology, surgery, or both in situations of medical emergency. You may need to shave and cleanse the physical area, establish an intravenous access, and have consent forms signed. Carry out patient education simultaneously with preparation.

Subjective Data

The subjective portion of the health assessment includes identification of cardiovascular risk factors and history related to those symptoms that are frequently associated with arterial, venous, and lymphatic disorders. Evaluation of the subjective portion of the assessment should include analysis of the information for the development of health promotion measures. If the patient is having any critical symptoms of complete arterial occlusion or DVT, take only critical history information as you prepare the patient for emergency intervention.

Assessment of Risk Factors

The World Health Organization (2011) identifies CVDs, including PAD, as the leading cause of death globally. In the United States, CVD mortality has declined among middle-aged people but is the leading cause of death for those older than 75 years of age. In developing countries, however, CVD mortality remains high for middle-aged persons (Berra, Fletcher, Hayman, & Miller, 2013). Patients who have PAD are at a much higher risk of morbidity and mortality from CVD—namely myocardial infarction and stroke—than are people without PAD (Aponte, 2011; Baas, 2010; Kim, Wattanakit, & Gornik, 2012).

The cardiovascular risk factors for the development of atherosclerosis are well defined (Box 18.1). They may be categorized as modifiable (e.g., smoking) and nonmodifiable (e.g., hereditary factors). The risk factors that are most strongly associated with PAD are advancing age, smoking tobacco, and diabetes mellitus. It is essential that you identify these risk factors, the patient's understanding of them, resources available to the patient, and the patient's support network. You and the patient can then work together to develop a comprehensive plan to improve the patient's cardiovascular risk profile. Many of these cardiovascular risk factors also pose a risk for **venous thromboembolism (VTE)**—DVT and PE—in which a blood clot travels from the legs to the lungs. The shared risk factors for PAD and VTE include cigarette smoking, hypertension, diabetes, and obesity (Goldhaber & Bounameaux, 2012).

BOX 18.1 Cardiovascular Risk Factors

- Smoking
- Hypercholesterolemia
- Diet high in saturated fats
- Sedentary lifestyle
- Hypertension
- Diabetes
- Obesity
- Genetics

History and Risk Factors	Rationale
Personal and Family History	
Do you have a family history of cardiovascular problems? • Who had the illness? • Was the illness arterial, venous, or lymphatic? • How was it treated? • What was the outcome?	CVD has a well-established hereditary component (Baas, 2010). A family history of premature CVD correlates with a much greater risk of CVD events for the patient (Wierzbicki, 2012).
Do you have a family or personal history of diabetes? • Who had/has the illness? • How is it treated? • How well is it controlled? • Have there been any complications related to diabetes?	Family history of diabetes increases a person's risk of developing the same condition. Diabetes significantly increases a patient's risk of developing lower extremity PAD (Gibbons & Shaw, 2012). Severity and duration of diabetes correlate with the likelihood of developing lower extremity PAD and how quickly it may progress (Gibbons & Shaw, 2012). Diabetes is also a risk factor for VTE (Goldhaber & Bounameaux, 2012).
Do you have a family or personal history of hypertension? • Who had/has the illness? • How is it treated? • How well is it controlled? • Have there been any complications related to hypertension?	Patients with hypertension are at increased risk for CVD, especially cerebrovascular disease, lower extremity PAD, and abdominal aneurysms (Baas, 2010; Robbins, 2010). They are also at a higher risk for VTE (Goldhaber & Bounameaux, 2012).
Do you or does anyone in your family have an elevated cholesterol level? • Who had/has the elevated cholesterol level? • How is it treated? • How well-controlled is it?	Increased levels of cholesterol are associated with the development of atherosclerosis and therefore lower extremity PAD and abdominal aneurysms (Baas, 2010).
Have you had any recent trauma to any of your extremities? • If so, what was the trauma? • What was the treatment? • Have you had any long-term effects?	Monitor for VTE, a possible adverse effect of trauma (Goldhaber & Bounameaux, 2012). Arterial damage can also result from trauma such as penetrating or blunt force injuries (Asongwed, Chesbro, & Karavatas, 2009).
Do you have a family history of lymphedema? • Who in your family had/has lymphedema? • How was it treated? • What was the outcome? • Have you ever had any lymph nodes removed? • Why were the lymph nodes removed? • From what part of your body were they removed? • When were they removed? • Have you had any problems with swelling since they were removed?	Lymphedema may be familial (Lee et al., 2011). It also may result from trauma, the excision of lymph nodes, or infection (Lee et al., 2011).
Personal Behaviors and Lifestyle	
Do you smoke cigarettes, pipes, or cigars? • How many cigarettes per day do you smoke? • How many years have you smoked? • Have you ever tried to stop smoking? • Are you interested in quitting now? • Does anyone living with you smoke cigarettes, pipes, or cigars? • Are you frequently around people who smoke cigarettes, pipes, or cigars? • What measures do you take to control your exposure to people who smoke cigarettes, cigars, or pipes? • Do you use vaporizers or electronic cigarettes?	Smoking is considered the most significant risk factor for lower extremity PAD; it increases the risk for abdominal aneurysms as well. The number of cigarettes smoked per day and the number of years the patient has smoked directly affect the degree of risk for developing lower extremity PAD and the rate of progression (Fritschi et al., 2013; Hennrikus et al., 2010). Exposure to secondary smoke may affect risk as well (Baas, 2010). In addition, smoking is a risk factor for the development of VTE (Goldhaber & Bounameaux, 2012). There is lack of scientific evidence on vaporizers and electronic cigarettes (Etter, et al., 2011). Current recommendations from the American College of Cardiology Foundation/American Heart Association (ACCF/AHA) (Rooke et al., 2011) include assisting patients with counseling and pharmacological therapies to quit smoking, if appropriate for the patient.

(table continues on page 501)

History and Risk Factors	Rationale
Do you exercise regularly? • What type of exercise? • How often and for how long do you exercise? • Do you sit or stand for long periods? • Do you have any problems with swelling in your legs because of this?	The AHA (2013) recommends regular exercise of at least 30 minutes, a minimum of 5 days a week, with additional muscle strengthening exercises at least 2 days a week to promote cardiovascular health and to decrease the risk of CVD. The World Health Organization (WHO, 2011) has similar recommendations. Regular exercise also promotes the well-being of the venous system.
Do you use oral contraceptives or take estrogen? • If so, for how long have you used them? • Have you experienced any adverse effects from them?	Oral contraceptives and estrogen replacement therapy may contribute to VTE and possibly increase blood pressure (Goldhaber & Bounameaux, 2012; Grossman & Porth, 2014).

Risk Reduction and Health Promotion

The subjective portion of the assessment lends itself well to incorporating patient education into the discussion. The setting of a private one-on-one meeting with the patient focusing on risk factors and symptoms provides the ideal opportunity to initiate the patient education process, which is an integral component of nursing care.

The health history includes key information for the development of health promotion measures, including the educational needs of the patient. During the subjective assessment, identify cardiovascular risk factors and evaluate the patient's understanding of them; you and the patient can then develop a plan to eliminate modifiable risk factors and to control as much as possible the severity of those that cannot be changed. Using this approach, you and the patient may prevent disease through early intervention or lessen disease progression and complications.

The health goals for peripheral vascular disease relate to controlling risk factors for heart disease and stroke. These include the following:

- Treating high blood pressure and high cholesterol
- Reducing cigarette smoking
- Controlling diabetes mellitus
- Improved nutrition and physical inactivity
- Reducing overweight and obesity

(U.S. Department of Health & Human Services, 2013).

These issues are covered more completely in Chapter 17.

Atherosclerosis is a progressive systemic disease. Initially, it manifests in one area of the body but it is likely to also be found in other vessels (Olin et al., 2010). Risk assessment is essential in order to determine areas for focused teaching. You can then provide the patient with the necessary information to make behavioral choices that may prevent future health concerns or improve the outcome of current health problems.

Patients With Peripheral Arterial Disease

Identifying options for the modification of risk factors can significantly improve the outcome for patients with PAD. The most modifiable risk factors are smoking, a high-fat diet, and limited activity level. Of these, smoking has been found to be one of the most devastating risk factors. PAD is twice as likely to occur in people who smoke cigarettes; smoking is a very strong risk factor for abdominal aortic aneurysms as well (Fritschi et al., 2013; Robbins, 2010). Ask patients about their readiness to quit smoking. Suggest various resources to assist patients with smoking cessation, including individual and group counseling, support groups, medical treatment, and pharmacological agents such as varenicline, bupropion, and nicotine replacement therapy (Rooke et al., 2011).

Diet modification can also improve the outcome of patients with PAD and includes weight management and decreasing the consumption of foods high in saturated fats. Monitoring and management of cholesterol and triglyceride levels is important for patients with PAD. They should have a thorough understanding of the relationship that diet, activity, and genetic factors have to cholesterol levels and the development of atherosclerosis. If applicable, educate the patient about lipid-lowering medications he or she may be taking (Baas, 2010). You can also discuss the preventive role of exercising at least five times a week as recommended by the AHA (2013) and the WHO (2011).

Daily assessment of the feet is essential for patients with PAD. With decreased arterial blood supply, minor cuts or areas with excessive pressure may quickly develop into arterial ulcers. Because of the decreased blood supply, these ulcers may be difficult to heal, leading to gangrene and limb amputation; in the worst cases, they may lead to death (Olin & Sealove, 2010).

Hypertension, diabetes, and heredity are also risk factors for PAD. Although they may not be eliminated, hypertension and diabetes are modifiable by close monitoring and tight control (Aponte, 2011; Olin & Sealove, 2010). Patients with diabetes are significantly more likely to develop PAD than the general population (Gibbons & Shaw, 2012). Maintaining glycemic control and blood pressure within the guidelines of the AHA and the ACCF is critical to slowing the progression of PAD (Smith et al., 2011).

Patients With Venous Disease

Patients with venous disease should receive education on methods of decreasing venous pressure. Advise these patients to avoid standing and sitting for long periods and to elevate the legs periodically to help combat the chronic edema that may accompany venous disease (Grossman & Porth, 2014). For patients with minor swelling or varicose veins, it is appropriate to recommend compression stockings. Patients at risk for or with a history of VTE need thorough education on the signs and symptoms of DVT and PE and, in some cases, anticoagulant therapy (Baas, 2010; Goldhaber & Bounameaux, 2012).

Patients With Lymphatic Disorders

Patients with lymphatic disorders have several issues that you must address. As with venous disease, edema in the extremities is the primary symptom of lymphedema. Suggest that the patient avoid sitting or standing for long periods. Patients with chronic lymphedema may experience disfigurement that affects their body image and self-esteem (Grossman & Porth, 2014). It is essential that you address these issues because they affect the patient's quality of life.

Common Symptoms

Common symptoms of vascular disease should be part of the assessment of all adults. As discussed previously, underdiagnosis of vascular problems and lack of aggressive treatment of risk factors have been identified as major areas of concern in primary care (Rooke et al., 2011). The AHA/ACCF guidelines recommend lowering the age of ankle-brachial index (ABI) testing for PAD and now suggest that it be 65 years of age. At-risk populations should be evaluated earlier (Rooke et al., 2011). Some providers now recommend that all adults age 40 years and older with one CVD risk factor or more be screened for PAD in particular (Aponte, 2011). Consistent evaluation of vascular and lymphatic wellness is necessary to better serve the adult population. Common symptoms associated with particular vascular disorders are listed in Box 18.2.

Common Peripheral Vascular and Lymphatic Symptoms

- Pain
- Numbness or tingling
- Edema
- Cramping
- Skin changes
- Decreased functional ability

BOX 18.2 Common Symptoms of Vascular Disorders

Peripheral Arterial Disease
- Claudication
- Rest pain

Acute Arterial Occlusion

The six Ps:
- Pain
- Poikilothermia
- Paresthesia
- Paralysis
- Pallor
- Pulselessness

Abdominal Aortic Aneurysm
- Bruit
- Laterally pulsating abdominal mass

Abdominal Aortic Aneurysm Dissection or Rupture
- Chest pain
- Abdominal pain
- Back pain
- Shortness of breath

Raynaud Phenomenon and Disease
- Numbness
- Tingling
- Pain
- Coolness
- Extreme pallor

Chronic Venous Insufficiency
- Edema of the extremity

Deep Vein Thrombosis
- Unilateral edema
- Pain or achiness
- Erythema
- Warmth

Thrombophlebitis
- As with DVT
- Palpable mass or cord along the vein

Neuropathy
- Burning pain
- Numbness
- Paresthesias

Lymphedema
- Unilateral edema

Signs/Symptoms	Rationale/Abnormal Findings
Pain Do you have any pain in your arms or legs?	⚠ *SAFETY ALERT* *It is critical to determine whether pain is acute or chronic before proceeding with the interview.*

(table continues on page 503)

Signs/Symptoms	Rationale/Abnormal Findings
• Where is the pain? • Can you point to where it hurts? • Does it radiate to other parts of your body?	The location of pain in PAD usually closely approximates the affected vessel (Wennberg, 2013).
• Describe it. • What does it feel like? • How bad is it on a 0–10 scale, with 0 being no pain and 10 being the worst possible pain that you can imagine?	Chronic pain is described as dull or aching. Acute pain is often described as sharp and stabbing. Acute pain of the extremities is a symptom of acute arterial occlusion as well as DVT.
• What brings on the pain? How long does it last? • What would you like to be able to do that you can't do because of the pain? • Do other symptoms accompany it?	Pain brought on by exertion and relieved by rest is called **intermittent claudication (IC)**. It is important to quantify the claudication time as much as possible—for example, "one-block claudication." Research supports the use of clinical rehabilitation programs to decrease these symptoms (Simmons, Sinning, Pearson, & Hendrix, 2013).
• Does the pain wake you up at night? • What do you think that the problem is?	The patient with PAD often describes feeling the need to hang the foot of the affected extremity over the side of the bed. Pain that awakens patients from sleep is termed **rest pain.**
Numbness or Tingling Have you experienced any changes in sensation in your arms or legs? • Do you experience any numbness or tingling in your hands or feet? • What makes it worse? • What makes it better?	Peripheral neuropathies often develop as a complication of diabetes. They may manifest as numbness, tingling, or pain and may result in a loss of sensation, increasing the patient's risk for injuries. The potential exists for subsequent damage to skin, which further increases the risk for wounds that are difficult to heal (Wennberg, 2013).
Cramping Do you have any cramping in your legs? • Do cramps come on suddenly or gradually? • Are cramps associated with walking or activity? • How many blocks can you walk without cramping? • What makes the cramps better?	The area of cramping or claudication in arterial disease closely approximates the level of arterial occlusion. It should be noted that many patients with PAD are asymptomatic (Olin & Sealove, 2010).
Skin Changes Have you had any changes in your skin, hair, or nails? • Do you have hair loss on your arms or legs? • Have your arms or legs become pale or cool? • Have your nails changed? Have they become thicker? • Have you had any color changes in your fingers or toes related to cold weather?	Decreased arterial blood supply may lead to changes on the lower extremities, such as loss of hair, pallor, or cool temperature. Another potential consequence is **hypertrophic nail changes** (Grossman & Porth, 2014). Chronic venous disease may result in a **brownish discoloration** in the "gaiter" or ankle area. Raynaud disease is characterized by color changes in cold weather (Grossman & Porth, 2014).
Edema Have you experienced any swelling in your arms or legs? • Does it go away when you put your legs up? • Is it worse at night or in the morning? • Have you experienced any swelling in your arms or legs that is accompanied by redness or tenderness?	Vascular causes of swelling in the arms or legs may result from venous occlusion or incompetence of the valves of the venous system, which often results in venous insufficiency (Grossman & Porth, 2014). DVT, often the precursor to venous insufficiency, is characterized by unilateral acute pain, swelling, and erythema (Grossman & Porth, 2014). **Postthrombotic syndrome** often results from DVT and is characterized by chronic pain and swelling at the site (Machlus, Aleman, & Wolberg, 2011).
Functional Ability Have difficulties with your arms or legs affected your daily life in any way? Can you continue activities without fatigue or pain in your arms or legs?	Decreased functional ability may result from arterial insufficiency. It is a symptom that is often overlooked (Fritschi et al., 2013).

Documenting Normal Findings
Patient denies upper or lower extremity pain; no claudication, coolness, numbness, pallor, hair loss, or nail changes in the extremities; no color changes related to cold temperatures, edema, or redness in fingers or toes. Patient states there is no change in functional ability.

Lifespan Considerations: Older Adults

Additional Questions	Rationale/Abnormal Findings
Have you experienced any fatigue, cramping, or aching in your legs? How have these symptoms affected your activities of daily living?	Many older adults have general, sometimes vague symptoms of arterial disease that primary care providers frequently overlook. It is being recommended that all individuals aged 65 years and older be assessed for PAD by **ABI** and that younger patients with risk factors be monitored as well (Kim et al., 2012; Rooke et al., 2011).
Have you noticed any swelling in your legs? Is it on one side or both sides?	Because older adults often have multisystemic problems, it is important for health care providers to clearly differentiate vascular disease from other sources.

Cultural Considerations

Additional Questions	Rationale/Abnormal Findings
Note the patient's self-identified ethnic group and gender.	African Americans have the highest incidence of PAD, with Hispanics also having a slightly higher incidence than Caucasians (CDC, 2013). The rate of PAD in women is thought to be higher than appreciated statistically because they are often asymptomatic and are underrepresented in research studies (Aponte, 2011; Hirsch et al., 2012).

Therapeutic Dialogue: Collecting Subjective Data

The nurse's role in subjective data collection is to gather information to improve the patient's health status and to help determine the cause of the patient's current symptoms. Remember Mr. Rossi, introduced at the beginning of this chapter. His long problem list includes PAD and confusion. His risk factors include 50 years of smoking a pack of cigarettes a day (50-pack-year history), high cholesterol level, and hypertension.

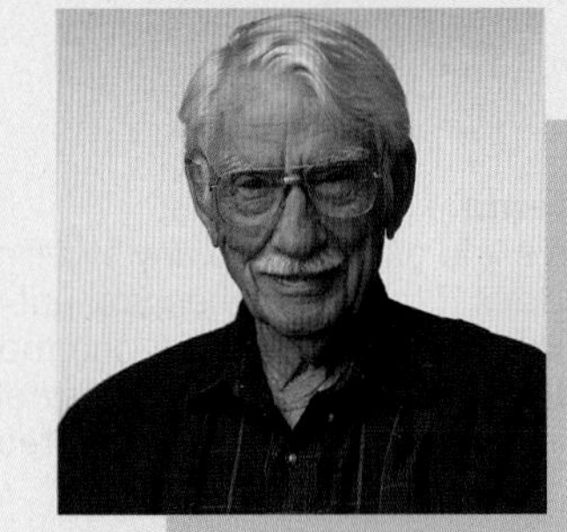

The long-term care nurse is working with Mr. Rossi today. Because the patient is confused, simple questioning is essential. Thus, the nurse must arrange questions with the simplest first, leading to more complex questions as the interview progresses. Cueing Mr. Rossi during the interview is another technique that can help keep him focused on the topic of the conversation.

Nurse: Mr. Rossi, I'm your nurse and I want to ask some questions about the circulation in your legs (pauses). I want to talk about the circulation in your legs.

Mr. Rossi: You want to ask me some questions about my circulation. It's pretty bad.

(case study continues on page 505)

Nurse: So you don't think the circulation in your legs is very good? Do you have any pain in your legs or feet?

Mr. Rossi: Just when I walk. But I don't walk very much because the nurses make me stay in this wheelchair. I fall sometimes.

Nurse: You fall because of your bad circulation in your legs. Sometimes people with bad circulation have tingling in their legs. Do you ever have tingling?

Mr. Rossi: No. You sure are asking me a lot of questions about my legs.

Nurse: I want to know how good the circulation is and I think that you've helped me understand that. How's the feeling in your legs? (pauses 10 seconds) (touches him) How's the feeling in your legs?

Mr. Rossi: Sometimes I can't feel my feet and then I fall.

Critical Thinking Challenge

- What issues did the nurse perceive and validate during the interview?
- What additional data about other body systems did the nurse gather during this interview?
- Is this an appropriate time to discuss risk for falling and safety issues? Provide rationale.

Objective Data

Common and Specialty or Advanced Techniques

The head-to-toe physical examination focuses on both the most common and most important assessment techniques. The examiner may incorporate advanced techniques to collect additional data for a special concern. The table summarizes the most common techniques for peripheral vascular and lymphatic assessment, which are therefore essential to master in clinical practice.

Equipment

- Examination gown
- Nonstretchable measuring tape
- Ultrasonic Doppler stethoscope
- Ultrasonic gel
- Sphygmomanometer
- Tourniquet

Basic Versus Focused/Specialty or Advanced Techniques Related to Peripheral Vascular and Lymphatic Assessment

Technique	Purpose	Screening or Registered Nurse Assessment	Focused or Advanced Practice Examination
Inspect arms and legs.	To identify symmetry, range of motion, color, hair, nails	X	
Palpate arms and legs.	To identify tenderness, warmth, erythema	X	
Palpate peripheral pulses.	To assess for effectiveness of peripheral circulation	X	
Auscultate blood pressure.	To compare circulation in both arms	X	
Auscultate Doppler stethoscope signals.	Performed when unable to palpate peripheral pulses	X	
Assess for edema.	To evaluate effectiveness of venous return	X	
Perform Allen test.	To assess for blood flow in radial and ulnar arteries		X For ABG draws

(table continues on page 506)

Basic Versus Focused/Specialty or Advanced Techniques Related to Peripheral Vascular and Lymphatic Assessment *(continued)*

Technique	Purpose	Screening or Registered Nurse Assessment	Focused or Advanced Practice Examination
Perform ABI assessment	Performed if arterial insufficiency is suspected		X Arterial insufficiency
Assess for color change	To assess for arterial insufficiency		X Arterial insufficiency
Perform manual compression	To evaluate competence of valves in the patient with varicose veins		X Varicose veins
Perform Trendelenburg test	To evaluate the saphenous vein valves and retrograde filling of the superficial veins		X Varicose veins

Preparation

Objective assessment of the peripheral vascular and lymphatic systems should take place in a quiet and private setting. Vasoconstriction accompanies cool temperatures, which may affect the peripheral vascular examination. Thus, the room should be at a comfortable temperature before the assessment begins.

Wash and warm your hands as an infection control measure and for the patient's comfort. The patient will need to wear a gown for the examination. He or she may leave on undergarments. The arms and legs must be accessible for inspection, palpation, and auscultation because side-to-side visualization and palpation for comparison is essential.

The examination requires the patient to be supine, sitting, and standing. Take safety precautions while helping the patient change positions. Pay attention to mobility constraints as well as the effects of position changes on respiratory effort as they apply to the patient. Cleanse the ultrasonic **Doppler stethoscope** before and after use to prevent the spread of infection. Use soap and water only because alcohol is damaging to the transducer.

Comprehensive Physical Assessment

Technique and Normal Findings	Abnormal Findings
Arms ***Inspection.*** Note the size and symmetry of the arms and hands as well as muscle atrophy or hypertrophy. ■ Arms and hands are symmetrical with full joint movement.	PAD may result in muscle atrophy. Hypertrophy may result from activity in which the patient uses one arm more than the other, such as tennis.
Assess the color of the arms and hands; evaluate for venous pattern. ■ Color is pink, symmetrical, and consistent without prominent venous pattern.	**Pallor** indicates arterial insufficiency. **Erythema** may accompany thrombophlebitis or DVT.
Evaluate the nail beds for color and angle. ■ Nail beds are pink. Nail base angle is at least 160 degrees without clubbing.	Capillary refill may be decreased with arterial disease.
Note any edema of the arms and hands. Evaluate for pitting by pressing the tissue with your fingers. ■ Pitting edema absent *When no indentation remains after you remove your fingers, that means that pitting edema is absent.*	Lymphedema results in unilateral edema. Use the scale in Box 18.3 to document degree of pitting edema. **BOX 18.3 Pitting Edema Scale** +1: Slight pitting, 2-mm depression +2: Increased pitting, 4-mm depression +3: Deeper pitting, 6-mm depression; obvious edema of extremity +4: Severe pitting, 8-mm depression; extremity appears very edematous

(table continues on page 507)

Technique and Normal Findings (continued)	Abnormal Findings (continued)
Evaluate for any ecchymosis or lesions of the upper extremities. ■ Ecchymosis and lesions are absent.	Be alert for signs of abuse (see Chapter 9) or falls. Delayed wound healing occurs with arterial disease and should be carefully assessed for.
Palpation. Palpate the arms and hands for temperature. Use the dorsal aspect of the hands and assess the extremities simultaneously. ■ Arms and hands are warm and equal in temperature.	**SAFETY ALERT** *Coolness of an extremity may indicate arterial occlusion. Assess quickly for the other six Ps (see Box 18.2) and determine whether condition constitutes an emergency*
Assess skin texture and turgor by pinching the skin to evaluate elasticity and hydration. With aging, elasticity decreases. ■ Skin texture is firm, even, and elastic. Turgor is intact, as shown by rapid return of skin after pinching.	Rough or dry texture and poor turgor may be noted with dehydration.
Assess capillary refill by depressing and blanching the nail bed then releasing and noting the time it takes for the color to return (Fig. 18.6). ■ Capillary refill is less than 3 seconds.	Capillary refill taking 3 seconds or longer may indicate vasoconstriction, decreased cardiac output, impaired arterial circulation, significant edema, or anemia.

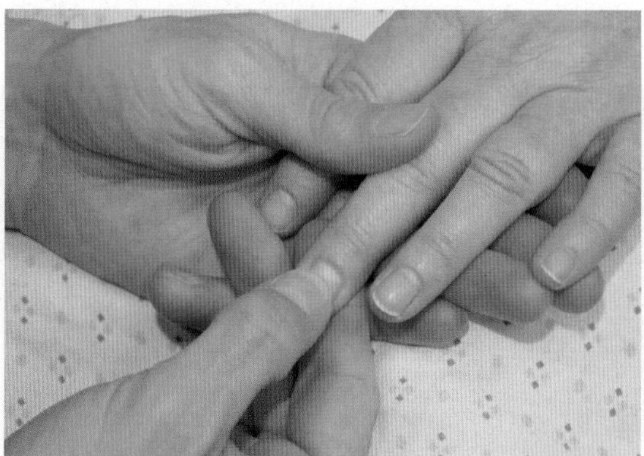

Figure 18.6 Testing capillary refill.

Technique and Normal Findings (continued)	Abnormal Findings (continued)
Palpate the brachial and radial pulses. Grade the pulses based on the scale in Box 18.4. Use the radial pulse site when assessing the pulse for vital signs (Fig. 18.7). The brachial pulses are located at approximately the inner third of the antecubital fossa when the palm is held upward. (Fig. 18.8). It is not usually necessary to palpate the ulnar pulse, which is difficult to locate. ■ A normal pulse is graded 2+/4 on the scale shown. The denominator indicates the scale being used and should always be indicated when documenting pulses because two scale variations exist.	**SAFETY ALERT** *Evaluate any pulse that cannot be palpated with the Doppler stethoscope for an arterial signal. If pulselessness persists, quickly evaluate the remaining of the six Ps to determine whether this problem constitutes an emergency (see Box 18.2).* See Table 18.3 at the end of the chapter.

BOX 18.4 Grading of Pulses

0: Nonpalpable or absent
1+: Weak, diminished, and barely palpable
2+: Normal, expected
3+: Full, increased
4+: Bounding
Document a normal pulse as 2+/4.

(table continues on page 508)

Technique and Normal Findings (continued)	Abnormal Findings (continued)
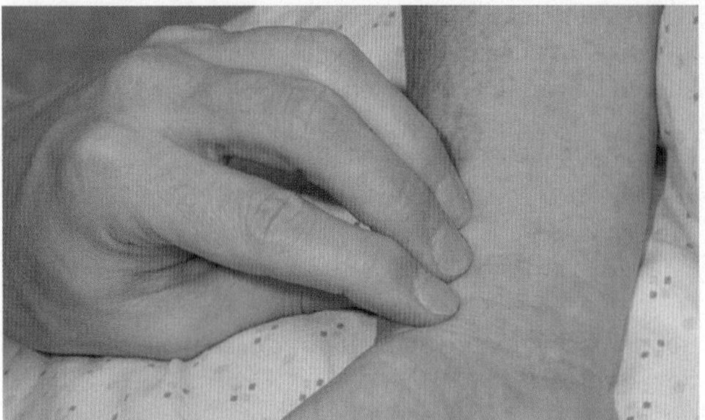 **Figure 18.7** Assessing the radial pulse.	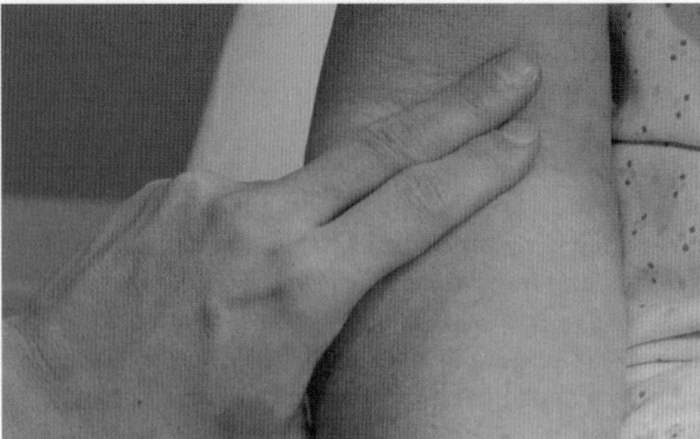 **Figure 18.8** Assessing the brachial pulse.
When indicated, perform the **Allen test** to assess the patency of the collateral circulation of the hands (Fig. 18.9). Ask the patient to make a fist. Occlude the radial and ulnar arteries of the same hand. Have the patient open the hand; release pressure on the ulnar artery. Color returns within 2–5 seconds, indicating adequate collateral circulation.	**SAFETY ALERT** *The Allen test is done prior to radial cannulation, such as for the drawing of arterial blood gases (ABGs) or the insertion of an arterial line. Lack of color return indicates inadequate collateral circulation. Do not draw ABGs or insert an arterial line in this hand—doing so will impede blood flow and ischemia may result.*

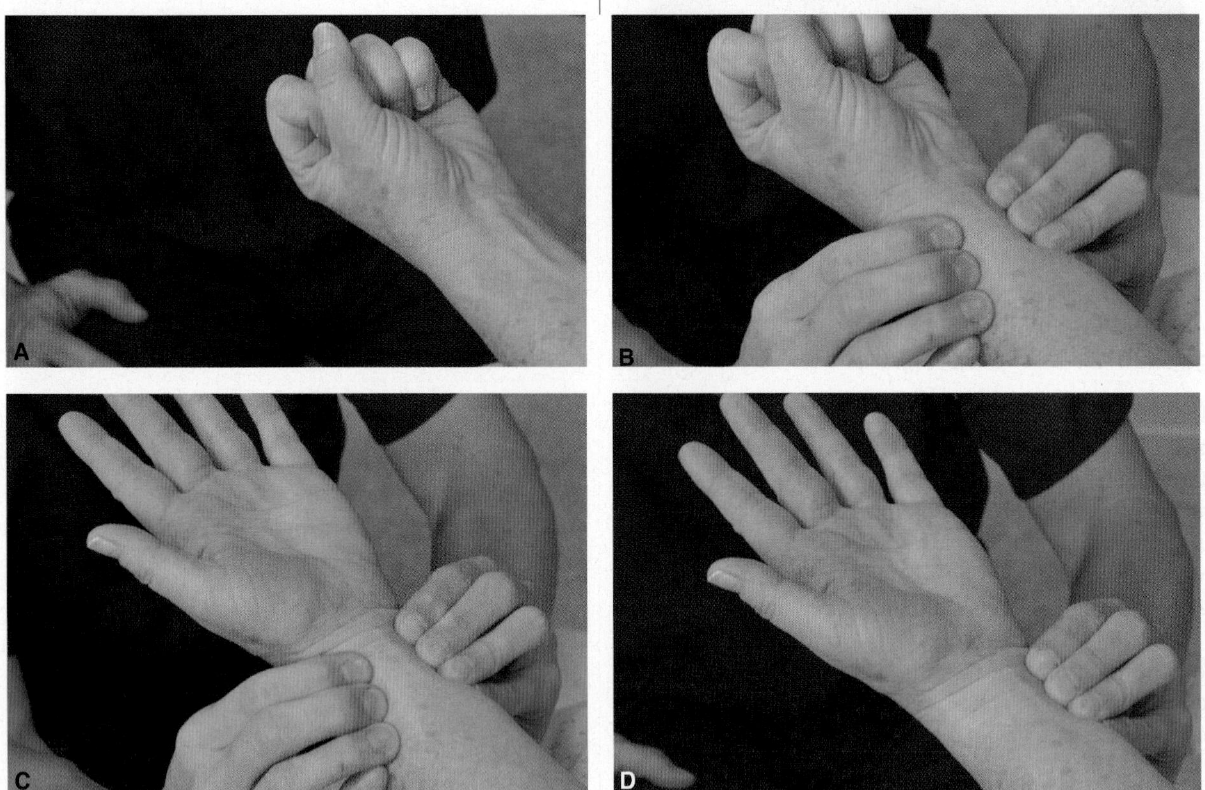

Figure 18.9 The Allen test. **A.** Ask the patient to make a fist. **B.** Occlude the radial and ulnar arteries. **C.** Ask the patient to open the hand. **D.** Release pressure on the radial artery to evaluate patency of the radial artery; the ulnar artery may also be released.

Palpate for the epitrochlear nodes. Flex the patient's arm and palpate in the groove between the biceps and triceps muscles just proximal from the medial epicondyle. *Normally, the epitrochlear nodes are not palpable.* If palpated, note size, consistency, mobility, and tenderness. *Normal palpable nodes are 2 cm or less.*	Enlarged nodes may be noted with regional inflammation, generalized lymphadenopathy, and some types of cancers such as lymphomas.

(table continues on page 509)

Technique and Normal Findings (continued)	Abnormal Findings (continued)
Auscultation. Evaluate the blood pressure in both arms. Document the arm with the higher pressure and take subsequent blood pressures in that arm. *A normal adult blood pressure is 100–120 mmHg systolic and 60–80 mmHg diastolic.*	A difference greater than 10 mmHg may indicate arterial disease. A palpatory pressure should be taken first to avoid missing an **auscultatory gap** (see Chapter 5).
Legs ***Inspection.*** Note the size and symmetry of the legs as well as muscle atrophy or hypertrophy. Legs are symmetrical with full joint movement.	**Atrophy** may occur with arterial disease. See Table 18.3 at the end of the chapter.
Assess the color of the legs; evaluate for venous pattern. Color is symmetrical and consistent without predominant venous pattern.	⚠ *SAFETY ALERT* *Pallor may indicate arterial insufficiency. Evaluate the other five Ps (Box 18.2) to determine whether the pallor represents a condition mandating emergency therapy. Erythema, edema, and tenderness may indicate DVT, which may also represent an emergency.* Color change to white in the toes may indicate one of the Raynaud syndromes. Venous insufficiency may result in dilated and tortuous veins. See Table 18.4 at the end of this chapter.
Evaluate the nail beds for color and capillary refill. Blanch the nail bed, release, and observe the time it takes for color to return. Nail beds are pink, with capillary refill less than 3 seconds.	Delayed capillary refill may be the result of arterial disease or vasoconstriction.
Note any **edema** of the legs. Evaluate for pitting by pressing the tissue with your fingers. Press firmly with thumb for at least 5 seconds over dorsum of each foot, over each medial malleolus, and over the pretibial area. No indentation should remain when you remove your thumbs (Fig. 18.10). See Box 18.3 for the grading scale for pitting edema. No edema is found. 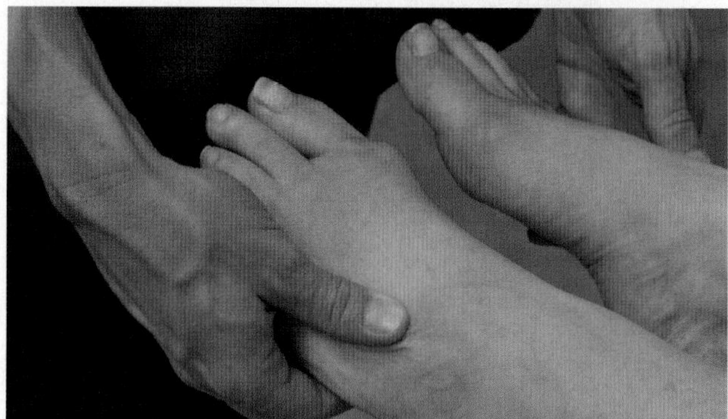 **Figure 18.10** Assessing for pitting edema.	Chronic venous insufficiency, DVT, and lymphedema result in edema. Asymmetry of the legs should be further investigated. Calf or leg swelling, pain, and unilateral pitting edema are associated with a DVT.
Evaluate for any **ecchymosis** or lesions of the lower extremities. Ecchymosis and lesions are absent.	Differentiate ulcers as **arterial** or **venous** in cause (Hinkle & Cheever, 2014). See Table 18.5 at the end of this chapter. Assess for gangrene.

(table continues on page 510)

Technique and Normal Findings (continued)	Abnormal Findings (continued)
Palpation. Palpate the legs for temperature. Use the dorsal aspect of the hands and assess the extremities simultaneously. Legs and feet are warm and equal in temperature.	⚠ *SAFETY ALERT* *One extremity cooler than the other indicates arterial occlusion. A warm, edematous, and tender extremity indicates DVT. Evaluate whether either of these conditions constitute an emergency.*
Assess the texture and turgor of the skin by pinching the skin. Texture is firm, even, and elastic. Turgor is intact when skin rapidly returns after pinching (indicating elasticity and hydration).	Rough or dry texture and poor **turgor** are found in dehydration. Thin shiny skin is found in PAD.
Palpate the femoral, popliteal, dorsalis pedis, and posterior tibial pulses. The femoral pulse is about halfway between the symphysis pubis and anterior iliac spine, just below the inguinal ligament (Fig. 18.11). The popliteal pulse is often difficult to locate. With your fingers braced on the knee, curl your hands around the back and press against the lower edge of the femur (Fig. 18.12). It may be felt immediately lateral to the medial tendon. The posterior tibial pulse is located in the groove between the medial malleolus and Achilles tendon (Fig. 18.13). A light touch is important to avoid obliterating the dorsalis pedis pulse. It is normally about halfway up the foot immediately lateral to the extensor tendon of the great toe (Fig. 18.14). Grade the pulses based on the scale in Box 18.4. *A normal pulse is 2+/4 on the scale shown. The denominator indicates the scale being used and should be indicated when documenting pulses because two scale variations exist. Evaluate any pulse that cannot be palpated with the Doppler stethoscope for an arterial signal. Document a Doppler signal as present or absent.*	⚠ *SAFETY ALERT* *If pulselessness and no Doppler signal are present, quickly assess the other of the **six Ps** to determine whether the emergent nature of the condition constitutes an emergency.* ⚠ *SAFETY ALERT* *The dorsalis pedis pulse may be absent in up to 12% of the population (Olin & Sealove, 2010). In such cases, assess for a Doppler signal and, if evidence of insufficient circulation exists, notify the primary care provider.*
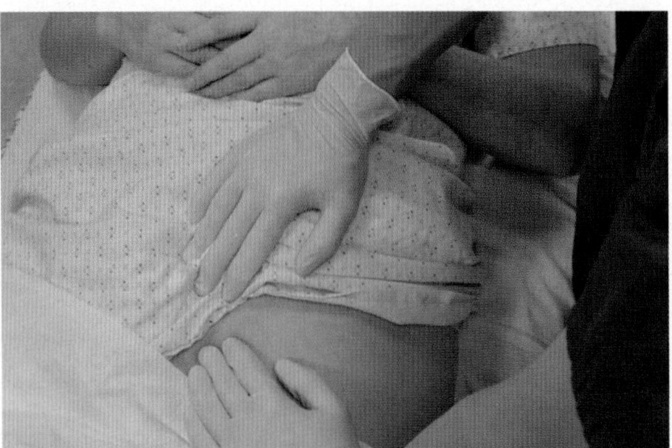 **Figure 18.11** Assessing the femoral pulse.	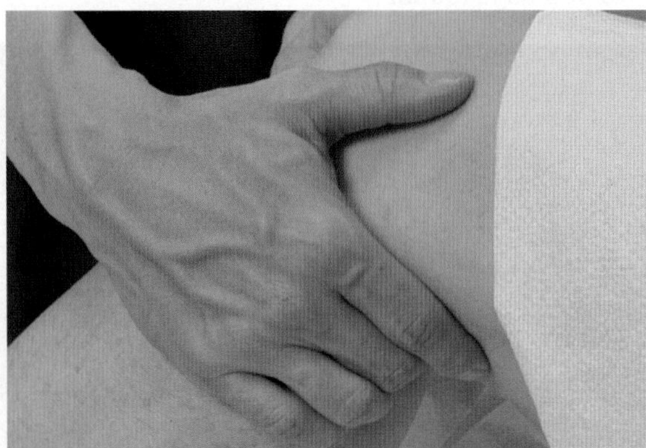 **Figure 18.12** Assessing the popliteal pulse.
Palpate the upper and medial thigh for the superficial **inguinal lymph nodes**. *They may be palpable and up to 1–2 cm, movable, and nontender.*	Nodes greater than 2 cm may be caused by either local or generalized conditions. Local causes include inflammation from trauma or wounds.

(table continues on page 511)

Technique and Normal Findings (continued)	Abnormal Findings (continued)

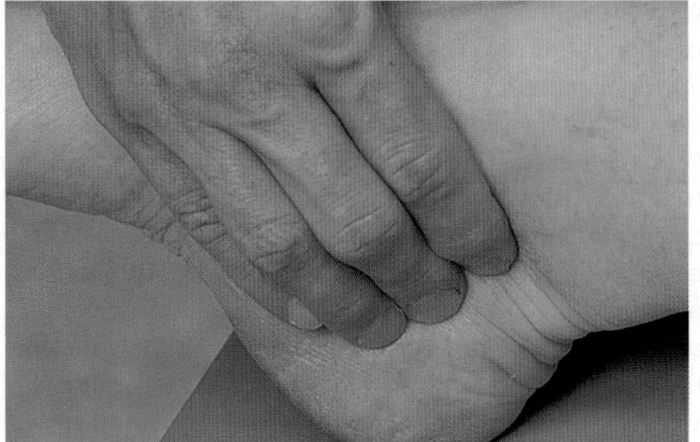

Figure 18.13 Assessing the posterior tibial pulse.

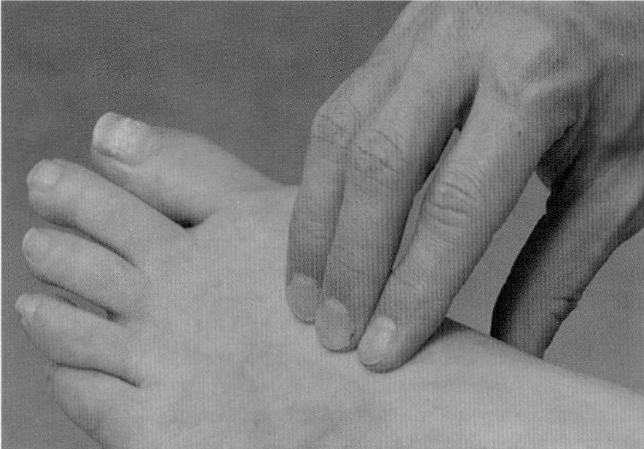

Figure 18.14 Assessing the dorsalis pedis pulse.

Auscultation. The Doppler ultrasonic stethoscope can assess weak peripheral pulses (Fig. 18.15). It magnifies pulsatile sounds from the heart and blood vessels as an arterial signal. The arterial signal is a rhythmic, triphasic, whooshing sound. To use the Doppler, apply a drop of ultrasonic gel to the transducer, and then place the transducer slightly angled to point in a proximal direction over the artery and turn on the volume. *The Doppler signal is present or absent; a scale is not used to grade the signal.*

The arterial signal is rhythmic and should not be mistaken for the sound of venous flow, which sounds more like a "windstorm" and is not rhythmic.

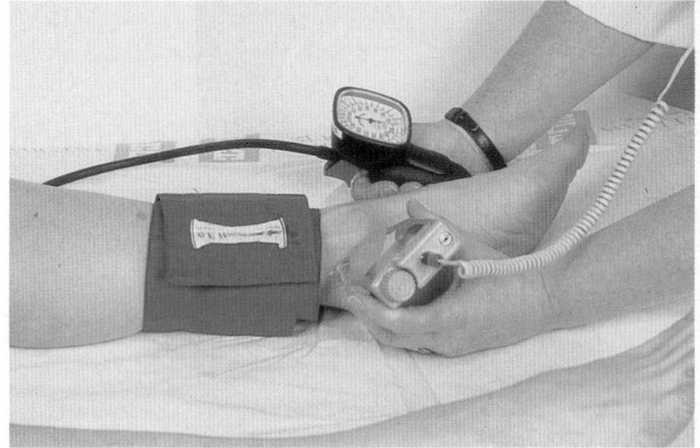

Figure 18.15 Doppler ultrasonic stethoscope.

To assess the **ABI**, assist the patient to a supine position. Take the systolic pressure of the brachial arteries using the Doppler. Use the higher of the two brachial systolic pressures as the denominator for both ankle pressures. Then apply a blood pressure cuff to the ankle and obtain either a dorsalis pedis or posterior tibial artery systolic blood pressure using the Doppler. *The ankle pressure is slightly higher or equal to the brachial pressure.* Divide both ankle pressures by the highest brachial pressure to get an ABI for the left leg and an ABI for the right leg:

$$\frac{\text{134 systolic ankle pressure}}{\text{128 systolic brachial pressure}} = 1.04 \text{ or } 104\%$$

The result is 1.0 (100%) or greater. Refer to Box 18.5 for a reference scale.

An ABI of 0.90 or less is considered to indicate arterial insufficiency. See Box 18.5 for delineation of approximate degree of occlusion based on ABI. Because of calcification of the arterial wall and subsequent arteries that are not compressible, patients with diabetes, renal failure, or both and some obese patients may have false-high results, so results greater than 1.40 are considered to be due to noncompressible arteries (Kim et al., 2012). The same may be true for patients with prosthetic bypass grafts. The ABI is considered to have a high degree of sensitivity for assessing PAD (Kim et al., 2012).

(table continues on page 512)

Technique and Normal Findings (continued)	Abnormal Findings (continued)

BOX 18.5 Interpretation of Ankle-Brachial Index (Values)

1–1.40:	Normal
0.91–0.99:	Borderline
Less than 0.90:	Abnormal
Greater than 1.40:	Noncompressible arteries

From Rooke, T. W., Hirsch, A. T., Misra, S., Sidawy, A. N., Beckman, J. A., Findeiss, L. K., . . . Zierler, R. E. (2011). 2011 ACCF/AHA focused update of the guideline for the management of patients with peripheral artery disease (updating the 2005 guideline): A report of the American College of Cardiology Foundation/American Heart Association Task Force on Practice Guidelines. *Journal of the American College of Radiology, 58*, 2020–2045.

New guidelines suggest that the ABI should be done on all patients who are aged 65 years or older and on younger patients who have one or more cardiovascular risk factors as a primary care screening assessment (Rooke et al., 2011). In addition to its use as a screening tool, the ABI is also used to monitor patients who have undergone peripheral extremity arterial intervention or surgery (Kim et al., 2012). The ABI is important in assessing PAD, but it is also a valuable marker for other cardiovascular events (Aboyans et al., 2012). Note that the systolic blood pressure of the lower extremities is typically higher than that of the lower extremities.

Additional Techniques

Color Change. This test is to check for arterial insufficiency. With the patient supine, elevate the legs about 30 cm (12 in.) above the level of the heart and have the patient pump his or her feet to drain off the venous blood (Fig. 18.16A). Have the patient then sit up and dangle the legs over the side of the table (Fig. 18.16B). Color returns to the feet and toes within 10 seconds. The superficial veins of the feet fill within 15 seconds.

Return of color taking longer than 10 seconds or persistent dependent **rubor** indicates arterial insufficiency.

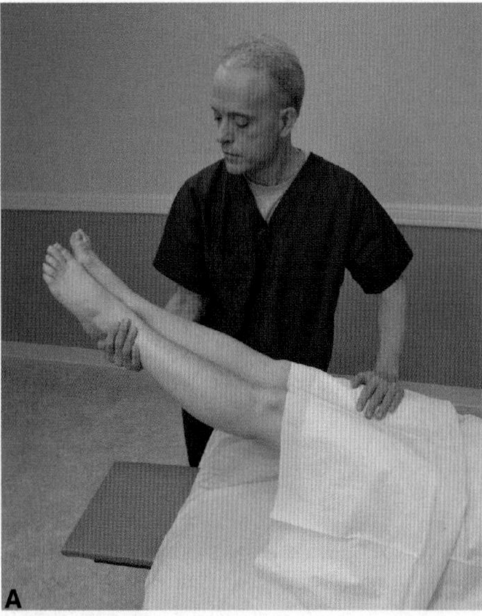

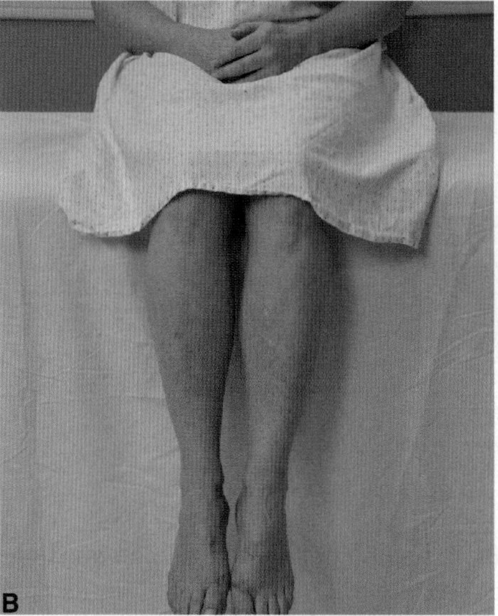

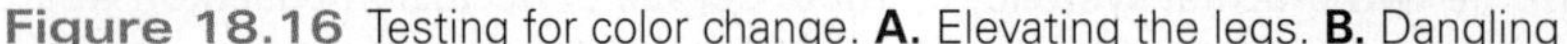

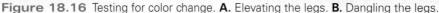

Figure 18.16 Testing for color change. **A.** Elevating the legs. **B.** Dangling the legs.

Manual Compression Test. This test evaluates the competence of the valves in the patient with varicose veins. Have the patient stand. Compress the lower portion of the vein with one hand and place your other hand 15–20 cm (6–8 in.) higher (Fig. 18.17). If the valves are competent, a wave transmission is not palpable. This is considered a negative–negative result.

A transmission wave indicates that the valves are incompetent.

(table continues on page 513)

Technique and Normal Findings (continued)	Abnormal Findings (continued)
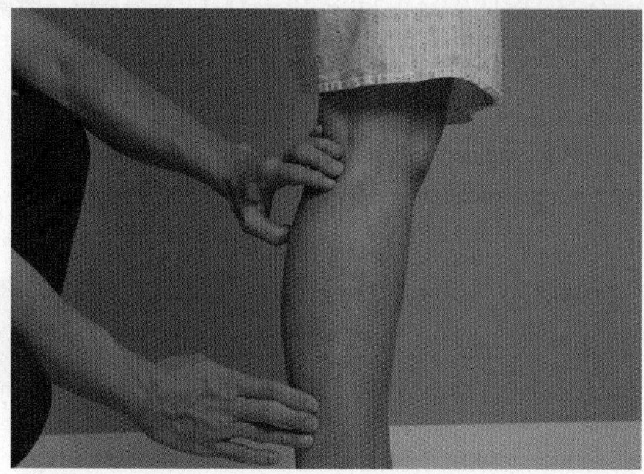 **Figure 18.17** Manual compression test.	
Trendelenburg Test. For the patient with varicose veins, this test evaluates the saphenous vein valves and retrograde filling of the superficial veins. With the patient supine, elevate the leg 90 degrees for 15 seconds. Apply a tourniquet to the upper thigh. Assist the patient to stand and inspect for venous filling. After 30 seconds, release the tourniquet. The saphenous veins fill from the bottom up while the tourniquet is on.	Filling from above while the tourniquet is on or rapid retrograde filling when the tourniquet is removed indicates that the valves are incompetent.

Documenting Normal Findings

The arms and legs are symmetrical with full joint movement. Upper and lower extremities pink and smooth with no ecchymosis or lesions. Skin is warm, dry, and supple with turgor intact bilaterally. Capillary refill is 2 seconds on all four extremities. Radial, brachial, dorsalis pedis, and posterior tibial pulses 2+/4 bilaterally. No edema. No tenderness or pain. ABI 1.03 bilaterally.

Lifespan Considerations: Older Adults

Arterial disease is common in older adults as a result of arteriosclerotic changes that are often coupled with atherosclerosis. The literature suggests that PAD is frequently underdiagnosed in the older population (Smith et al., 2011; Stephens, Hagler, & Clark, 2011). Intimal changes in the arteries begin at birth and progress throughout life. The thickening of the arterial walls decreases nourishment of the tissue, often resulting in classic findings of trophic nail changes, thin shiny skin, and hair loss of the lower extremities. Decreased functional ability such as fatigue with walking may be an indication of PAD that providers overlook or attribute to other factors (Fritschi et al., 2013; Wennberg, 2013). Evidence-based parameters suggest the integration of the ABI, a very simple and noninvasive tool, into the assessment of patients who have exertional leg pain or poorly healing wounds; those who are 50 years of age or older with clinical histories, smoking, or diabetes; as well as all patients who are 65 years of age or older regardless of whether they have risk factors (Rooke et al., 2011).

Systolic hypertension often increases with age as the arterial vessels become less compliant. Taking a palpatory blood pressure before taking the brachial blood pressure is essential in this population to avoid missing an **auscultatory gap** caused by decreased compliance.

Older adults often become less active over time, which can result in an increase in venous stasis and the development of DVTs. The incidence of VTE is highest in the elderly (Zoller et al., 2011).

A regular walking program is important and will improve quality of life. Inactivity may be an overlooked symptom in patients with undiagnosed PAD and may worsen the disease's progress (Wennberg, 2013). Venous insufficiency and chronic lymphedema may eventually decrease joint mobility (Grossman & Porth, 2014). Inclusion of an evaluation of joint mobility is therefore an essential component of the peripheral vascular assessment.

Cultural Considerations

Ethnic minorities, women, and the elderly are underrepresented in clinical research on PAD, but it is hoped that this will change and add a greater focus to strategies for the care of PAD in these populations (Smith et al., 2011).

Documenting Case Study Findings

The nurse has just finished conducting a physical examination of Mr. Rossi. Review the following important findings that each of the steps of objective data collection revealed for this patient. Consider how these results compare with the expected findings presented in the samples of normal documentation. Pay attention to how the nurse clusters data together to provide a more complete and accurate understanding of the condition.

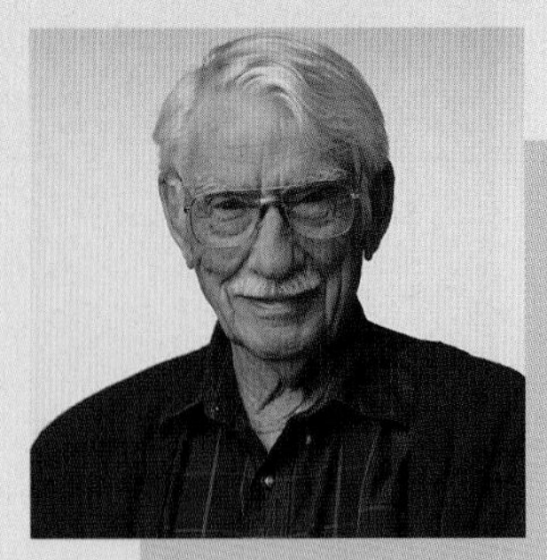

Inspection: Skin thin, shiny, and taut. Hair growth absent bilaterally distal to the knees. Toenails are hypertrophied. Dependent rubor on lower leg when limbs are dependent. Foot becomes pale when elevated. Able to wiggle toes slowly. Integument intact, no lesions.

Palpation: 1+/4 dorsalis pedis and posterior tibial pulses bilaterally. Feet cool. Capillary refill 7 seconds. No pedal edema. Unable to differentiate sharp versus dull sensations on feet and lower legs.

Critical Thinking

Research has shown that risk assessment and intervention have significant effects on outcomes for patients with CVD. Modification of risk factors significantly slows disease progression (Smith et al., 2011). Because of the systemic nature of CVDs, you must critically investigate far beyond the initial reason for which the patient sought care. After you have analyzed the history, physical assessment, laboratory data, and diagnostic study results, you can develop a plan of care. Determining and prioritizing nursing diagnoses are the basis for the plan, in collaboration with the patient and family. Patient education to facilitate modification of risk factors is paramount in this patient population. You must educate the patient and family and coordinate support resources for effective care. A collaborative plan with the health care team is the most effective way to manage patient care.

In the past, the **Homan sign** was used to test for DVT. The test was performed by dorsiflexing the foot; pain was suggested as a positive result, indicating DVT. However, because this test is neither sensitive nor specific, it is now recommended that the Homan sign be omitted from the assessment of patients with suspected DVT. In addition to misinterpretation of results and poor testing efficacy, it has the potential for mobilizing a clot (Grant, 2012). Instead, the **Wells Score System** (Box 18.6) is often used, in conjunction with the D-dimer and venous duplex scan, to make the diagnosis of DVT.

In most patients with a DVT, the focus is initiation of intravenous anticoagulant therapy (Goldhaber & Bounameaux, 2012). Document baseline assessment of calf size at the widest point in addition to any findings of pain, warmth,

BOX 18.6 Wells Score for Deep Vein Thrombosis

Clinical Characteristic*	Score†
Active cancer (treatment ongoing, administered within previous 6 months or palliative)	1
Paralysis, paresis, or recent plaster immobilization of the lower extremities	1
Recently bedridden longer than 3 days or major surgery within previous 12 weeks requiring general or regional anesthesia	1
Localized tenderness along the distribution of the deep venous system	1
Swelling of entire leg	1
Calf swelling greater than 3 cm larger than asymptomatic side (measured 10 cm below tibial tuberosity)	1
Pitting edema confined to the symptomatic leg	1
Collateral superficial veins (nonvaricose)	1
Previously documented DVT	1
Alternative diagnosis at least as likely as DVT	−2

*In patients who have symptoms in both legs, the more symptomatic leg is used.

†A score of 2 or higher indicated that the probability of DVT is "likely"; a score of less than 2 indicates that the probability is "unlikely."

Information from Scarvelis, D., & Wells, P. S. (2006). Diagnosis and treatment of deep vein thrombosis. *Canadian Medical Association Journal*, *175*(9), 1087–1092; Bates S. M., Jaeschke R., Stevens S. M., Goodacre, S., Wells, P. S., Stevenson, M. D., . . . Guyatt, G. H. (2012). Diagnosis of DVT: Antithrombotic therapy and prevention of thrombosis, 9th ed: American College of Chest Physicians evidence-based clinical practice guidelines. Chest, 141(Suppl. 2), e351S–e418S. doi:10.1378/chest.11-2299

or tenderness. Past history of DVTs or other thrombus formation as well as family history are important to risk stratification (Zoller, 2011). The possibility of PE is always a concern in the patient with a DVT. Ongoing assessments should include consideration of the signs and symptoms of a PE (see Chapter 16).

Laboratory and Diagnostic Testing

Accurate data collection is essential for the patient to receive the appropriate care. The primary care provider relies on your accurate assessment of the patient to determine the appropriate medical interventions. For example, it is important to differentiate between problems that are arterial rather than venous. An **arterial ulcer** has a deep necrotic base, whereas a **venous ulcer** is superficial and pale. The treatment for these ulcers is quite different. An acute arterial occlusion will be painful with accompanying symptoms of pallor, pulselessness, poikilothermia, paresthesias, and/or paralysis. A venous occlusion will result in pain, edema, erythema, and warmth of the affected extremities (Grossman & Porth, 2014). For an arterial occlusion, the primary provider will order that the patient be prepared for an arteriogram, whereas for a venous occlusion, the provider will order serum D-dimer, venous ultrasonography, and anticoagulation. Your critical thinking skills in assessment, prioritization, and organization will facilitate the arrival at a medical diagnosis so that intervention will be immediate.

Laboratory testing related to the peripheral vascular and lymphatic systems includes serum evaluation for known risk factors as well as cholesterol and triglyceride levels. Patients with diabetes require monitoring of blood glucose levels and hemoglobin A1C (Smith et al., 2011). Research has led to the evaluation of C-reactive protein and homocysteine levels often being included in the cardiovascular evaluation (Baas, 2010). The serum **D-dimer** is assessed in the patient with a possible DVT (Goldhaber & Bounameaux, 2012).

Diagnostic **ultrasonography** is noninvasive and can evaluate anatomic and hemodynamic functions. At the bedside, the continuous wave Doppler is a common tool to evaluate arm and ankle pressures. In the vascular laboratory, ultrasonic imaging and plethysmography provide detailed anatomical and flow information. Postexercise ABIs as well as the toe ABI are also tools used in the diagnosis of arterial disease (Kim et al., 2012). These noninvasive diagnostic tests are used to evaluate the degree of venous obstruction and location and degree of arterial disease as well as provide follow-up postoperatively. In the patient with arterial disease or aneurysm, the angiogram remains the test for definitive diagnosis (Wennberg, 2013).

Diagnosis of lymphedema may include magnetic resonance imaging and computerized tomography to identify features of lymphedema or obstruction. Lymphangiography has the drawback of possibly causing acute lymphangitis. Rarely, a lymph node biopsy may be needed. Lymphoscintigraphy is a safe alternative (Lee et al., 2011).

Diagnostic Reasoning

The different vascular systems have some separate and some shared nursing diagnoses. Tissue perfusion is altered in arterial disease; interventions are specific to increasing arterial blood flow and preventing further progression of atherosclerosis through modification of risk factors and use of antiplatelet medications such as clopidogrel and aspirin (Rooke et al., 2011).

In patients with venous disorders, the focus is promotion of venous flow. With DVT, interventions seek to prevent increased thrombus size and pulmonary embolism with the use of anticoagulants (Goldhaber & Bounameaux, 2012). In chronic venous and lymphatic disease, interventions are similar to promote venous and lymphatic return. Recommendations include the use of compression devices, avoiding long periods of sitting or standing, increasing exercise, and elevating the affected extremity (Baas, 2010; Shannon, Hawk, Navaroli, and Serena, 2013).

Nursing Diagnoses, Outcomes, and Interventions

When formulating a nursing diagnosis, it is important to use critical thinking to cluster data and identify patterns that fit together. Table 18.1 provides a comparison of nursing diagnoses, abnormal findings, and interventions commonly related to the peripheral vascular system assessment (NANDA, 2012). Additionally, pain, fatigue, impaired skin integrity, risk for infection, knowledge deficit, activity intolerance, and a disturbance in body image may affect all vascular patients.

Critical assessment of the data gathered leads to a plan with the goal of achieving specific patient outcomes. Outcomes that are related to vascular problems include the following:

- Peripheral pulses are strong and symmetrical.
- Capillary refill is less than 3 seconds.
- Patient states treatment regimen including exercise, medications, and healthy behaviors.
- Patient senses sharp and dull sensations accurately.
- Peripheral edema is decreased.
- Patient verbalizes an understanding of risk factors and risk modification.
- Patient verbalizes a decrease in pain.

To achieve desired outcomes, you apply evidence-based interventions. Examples include the following:

- Monitor peripheral pulses every 4 hours or more often.
- Assess and document degree of edema using scale every 4 hours.
- Evaluate pain on 10-point scale.
- Provide patient education on risk factors and modifications.
- Keep limbs warm and have patient wear skid-free slippers.
- Perform meticulous foot care once a day (Ralph & Taylor, 2014).

Periodically evaluate the effectiveness of interventions and modify them as appropriate. For the continual process of reevaluation and modification to achieve desired outcomes, you need a thorough knowledge of assessment and accurate application.

TABLE 18.1 Common Nursing Diagnoses Associated With the Peripheral Vascular System			
Diagnosis	**Point of Differentiation**	**Assessment Characteristics**	**Nursing Interventions**
Altered tissue perfusion, arterial	Decrease in oxygen resulting in failure to nourish tissues at the capillary level	Reduced hair, thick nails, dry skin, weak or absent pulses, pale skin, cool, reduced sensation, prolonged capillary refill	Assess dorsalis pedis and posterior tibial pulses bilaterally. If pulses reduced or you are unable to find them, assess with a Doppler stethoscope. If no arterial signal picked up using Doppler, notify physician.
Risk for peripheral neurovascular dysfunction	Potential for one or more extremities to experience negative changes in circulation, sensation, or motion	Trauma, fractures, surgery, mechanical compression, burns, immobilization, obstruction	Perform assessment: pain, pulses, pallor, paresthesia, paralysis. Contact physician if present.
Activity intolerance	Energy that is compromised and cannot facilitate endurance for completion of daily activities	Report of pain or claudication, fatigue, weakness	Gradually increase activity. Refer to physical therapy or peripheral arterial disease rehabilitation program as indicated. Allow rest periods before and after activity.

Progress Note: Analyzing Findings

Remember Mr. Rossi, whose problems have been outlined throughout this chapter. The initial subjective and objective data collection is complete. The nurse has spent time reviewing the findings and other results. The following nursing note illustrates how subjective and objective data are analyzed and nursing interventions are developed.

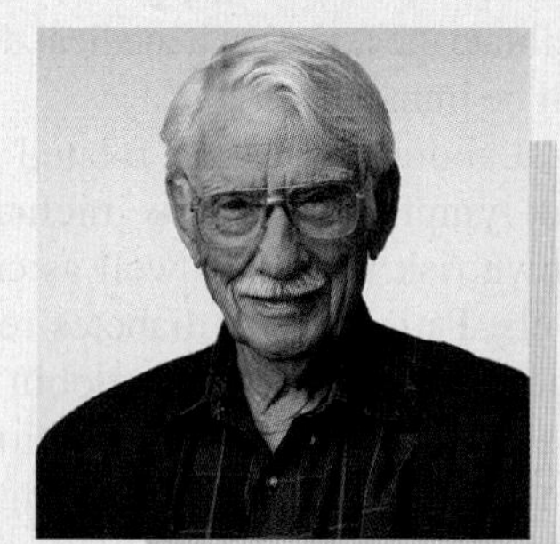

Subjective: "Sometimes I can't feel my feet and then I fall."

Objective: 1+/4 dorsalis pedis and posterior tibial pulses bilaterally. Dependent rubor bilaterally. Elevational pallor bilaterally. Feet cool. Capillary refill 7 seconds. Able to wiggle toes slowly. Cannot differentiate sharp versus dull sensations on feet and lower legs. Skin thin, shiny, and taut. Hair absent bilaterally distal to knees. No pedal edema. Toenails hypertrophied. Integument intact, no lesions.

Analysis: Altered peripheral tissue perfusion related to PAD

Plan: Keep lower extremities in a dependent position. Keep socks and shoes or slippers on feet during the day and loose socks at night. Remind patient to change positions frequently and provide range-of-motion exercises twice daily. Assist with walking twice daily and begin use of a walker to increase safety. Have the patient stop when pain develops. Apply skin moisturizer to legs every morning. Inspect feet daily for injuries and pressure points. Consult with physical therapy team to develop a daily walking program.

(case study continues on page 517)

Critical Thinking Challenge

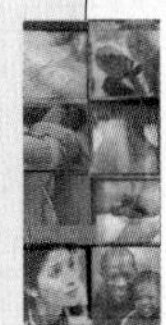

- What might be included when writing another SOAP note focusing on Mr. Rossi's confusion?
- What overlap is present between the peripheral vascular assessment and other body systems?
- What assessments are highest priority based on his health history and current problems?

Collaborating With the Interprofessional Team

In many health care facilities, nurses initiate referrals for physical therapy based on assessment findings. Results that might trigger a consultation with physical therapy include musculoskeletal injury, reduced functional status, impaired balance, mobility issues, sensorimotor loss, assistance with techniques on seating or transfers, low endurance, impaired safety awareness, impaired strength or flexibility, use of adaptive equipment, and training for body mechanics.

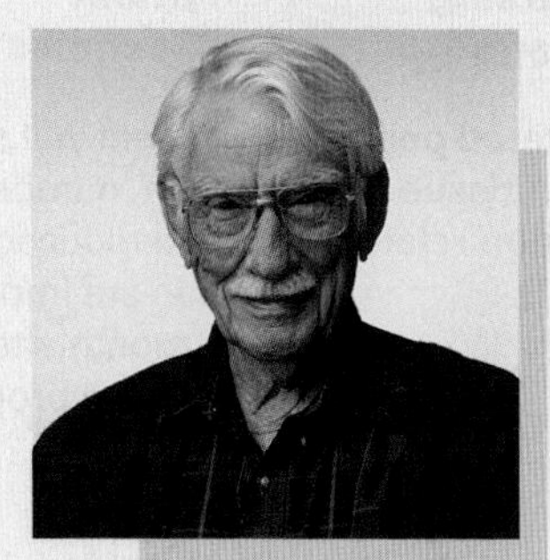

Mr. Rossi has been experiencing many of the problems noted earlier; therefore, a physical therapy consult might be indicated. The following conversation illustrates how the nurse might organize data and make recommendations about the patient's care to the physical therapy department.

Situation: "I'm Ronald, the nurse who is taking care of Mr. Rossi, an 88-year-old man with multiple diagnoses, including peripheral arterial disease in his legs."

Background: "He has been falling because of reduced sensation in his feet and legs. He's also a bit confused."

Assessment: "His peripheral pulses are decreased bilaterally. His feet are cool and his capillary refill is prolonged. He has slower and reduced range of motion in his feet and legs also."

Recommendations: "I think that a more structured walking program might help him improve his circulation and the use of a walker in addition might reduce his risk of falling. We are ambulating him twice daily, but it doesn't seem to be helping much. Could you come to evaluate whether a program like this might be helpful for him? If you have other ideas about things that the nursing staff could do to reduce his pain and increase his circulation, that would be helpful, too."

Critical Thinking Challenge

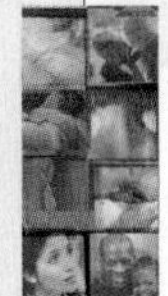

- How will the nurse organize information before initiating the call for the consult?
- Comment on the reliability of the historian. How will the nurse collect assessment data based on the patient's reliability?
- How will Mr. Rossi be reassessed to evaluate the effectiveness of therapy? How frequently?

Pulling It All Together

The nurse uses assessment data to formulate a nursing care plan for Mr. Rossi. He or she may independently perform teaching, give reminders to get assistance for transfers, and set up environmental cues for the patient to remember to call for those transfers. Because Mr. Rossi is confused and his memory is poor, the nurse will need to take more initiative to remind him to keep his legs dependent and change position often. The nurse also may initiate a referral to physical therapy about use of a walker and a daily walking program. After completing such interventions, the nurse will reevaluate Mr. Rossi and document the findings in the chart to show the nursing critical thinking. This is often in the form of a care plan or case note similar to the one below.

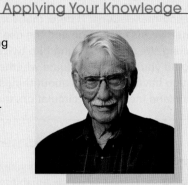

Nursing Diagnosis	Patient Outcomes	Nursing Interventions	Rationale	Evaluation
Altered peripheral tissue perfusion related to PAD	Patient will state that pain, numbness, and reduced sensation are improved 1 month after starting walking program.	Keep lower extremities in a dependent position. Provide range-of-motion exercises twice daily. Teach use of walker and assist with walking twice daily and stop when pain develops. Consult with physical therapy and develop a walking program.	Keeping legs in a dependent position uses gravity to assist flow toward the feet. Range of motion prevents loss of mobility. Walking programs stimulate improved arterial perfusion and prevent further loss of function.	Patient states that pain, numbness, and sensation remain about the same. He reports keeping his legs dependent except when in bed. Continue plan and reevaluate in another 2 weeks.

Applying Your Knowledge

Using the previous steps of diagnostic reasoning, organizing, and prioritizing, consider all the case study findings woven throughout this chapter. When answering the following questions, begin drawing conclusions and see how the pieces of assessment must work together to create an environment for personalized, appropriate, and accurate care.

As you study the content and features, consider Mr. Rossi's case and its relationship to what you are learning. Begin thinking about the following points:

- List the six "Ps" used to assess for arterial occlusion.
- How does Mr. Rossi's health history relate to his current health status?
- What assessment findings might the nurse note if Mr. Rossi's PAD worsens?
- What assessment data will the nurse want to collect related to other body systems?
- How might the nurse modify history taking and physical examination based on Mr. Rossi's age and present state of confusion?
- How will the nurse evaluate the effectiveness of health teaching with Mr. Rossi?

Key Points

- Arterioles have smooth muscle and are primarily responsible for blood pressure.
- Veins are thin-walled capacitance vessels that stretch and accommodate large volumes of fluid.
- The lymphatic system maintains fluid and protein balance and fights infection.
- Pain, paresthesia, paralysis, poikilothermia, pallor, and pulselessness (the six Ps) are signs of acute arterial occlusion.
- Pain, edema, and erythema may be signs of a DVT.
- Risk factors for peripheral vascular disease include family history, diabetes mellitus, hypertension, elevated cholesterol levels, smoking, lack of exercise, oral contraceptive use, and estrogen replacement therapy.
- Common symptoms of peripheral vascular disease include pain, numbness or tingling, cramping (IC), skin changes, edema, and reduced functional ability.
- Edema is graded on a scale from 0 or absent to 4+ deep pitting.
- A normal pulse is 2+ on a 4-point scale.
- The Allen test is performed prior to radial cannulation.
- A difference of more than 10 mmHg in BP in limbs may indicate arterial disease.
- Venous insufficiency may result in dilated and tortuous veins.
- Lymph nodes larger than 2 cm may be caused by local or generalized conditions.
- The Homan sign is not sensitive or specific for DVT.
- The Doppler ultrasound is used to locate an arterial signal when pulses are not palpable.
- An ABI of 0.90 or less indicates arterial insufficiency.

Review Questions

1. Which of the following is a normal ABI?
   A. 56
   B. 87
   C. 1.0
   D. 24

2. Which of the following peripheral vascular diseases is not known to have a hereditary component?
   A. Lymphadenopathy
   B. Raynaud disease
   C. Abdominal aortic aneurysm
   D. PAD

3. When assessing the lower extremities, it is critical that the examiner
   A. starts at the feet.
   B. compares side to side.
   C. evaluates the venous system and then the arterial system.
   D. starts at the femoral area.

4. The six Ps of an acute arterial occlusion include
   A. polythermia.
   B. popliteal edema.
   C. pain.
   D. polycythemia.

5. A history of smoking has an extremely significant role in the development of which of the following?
   A. Venous insufficiency
   B. DVT
   C. PAD
   D. Raynaud disease

6. A dorsalis pedis of +1/4 may indicate
   A. DVT.
   B. PAD.
   C. Raynaud disease.
   D. lymphadenopathy.

7. During history taking, a patient reports cramping in his calf when walking a few blocks. He states that it goes away when he sits down for a few minutes. How would the nurse document this symptom?
   A. Intermittent claudication
   B. Rest pain
   C. Poikilothermia
   D. Venous stasis

8. A patient reports swelling in her ankles. How would the nurse proceed with physical examination?
   A. Have the patient elevate her feet to better visualize her ankles.
   B. Measure her ankles at their widest point.
   C. Evaluate further for the brown hyperpigmentation associated with venous insufficiency.
   D. Press the fingers in the edematous area evaluating for a remaining indentation after the nurse removes his or her fingers.

9. While evaluating the inguinal lymph nodes of a patient, the nurse palpates a 1-cm (about ½-in.) soft and freely movable node. What action should the nurse take next?
   A. Nothing—this finding is normal.
   B. Refer this patient to a specialist.
   C. Immediately check the patient's dorsalis pedis pulse.
   D. Refer the patient for immediate management of a life-threatening condition.

10. A patient with diabetes mellitus who closely monitors and controls her blood glucose level is very interested in preventing complications of her illness. The nurse would emphasize the following consideration in patient teaching:
    A. How to count calories
    B. How to assess her feet daily
    C. What are good carbohydrates
    D. The signs of venous insufficiency

The Jensen suite offers these additional resources to enhance learning and facilitate understanding of this chapter:

- thePoint online resource, http://thepoint.lww.com/Jensen2e
- *Laboratory Manual for Nursing Health Assessment: A Best Practice Approach*
- *Pocket Guide for Nursing Health Assessment: A Best Practice Approach*
- *Lippincott DocuCare,* an electronic health record simulation software, http://thepoint.lww.com/docucare
- *Adaptive Learning | Powered by PrepU*, http://thepoint.lww.com/prepu

References

Aboyans, V., Criqui, M. H., Abraham, P., Allison, M. A., Creager, M. A., . . . , C., and Treat-Jacobson, D. (2012). Measurement and interpretation of the ankle-brachial index: A scientific statement from the American Heart Association. *Circulation, 126,* 2890–2909. doi:10.1161/CIR.0b013e318276fbcb

Al Mahameed, A. (2009). *Peripheral arterial disease.* Retrieved from http://www.clevelandclinicmeded.com/medicalpubs/diseasemanagement/cardiology/peripheral-arterial-disease/

American Heart Association. (2013). American Heart Association Recommendations for Physical Activity in Adults. Retrieved from http://www.heart.org/HEARTORG/GettingHealthy/PhysicalActivity/StartWalking/American-Heart-Association-Guidelines_UCM_307976_Article.jsp#

Aponte, J. (2011). The prevalence of asymptomatic peripheral arterial disease risk factors in the US population. *Holistic Nursing Practice*, *25*(3), 147–161. doi:20.1097/HNP.0b013e3182157c4a

Asongwed, E. T., Chesbro, S. B., & Karavatas, S. G. (2009). Peripheral vascular disease and the ankle-brachial index: What home health care clinicians need to know. *Home Healthcare Nurse*, *27*(3), 160–167. Retrieved from http://www.homehealthcarenurseonline.com

Baas, L. S. (2010). *Cardiac vascular nursing* (3rd ed.). Silver Spring, MD: American Nurses Credentialing Center.

Bates S. M., Jaeschke R., Stevens S.M., Goodacre, S., Wells, P. S., Stevenson, M. D., . . . Guyatt, G. H. (2012). Diagnosis of DVT: Antithrombotic therapy and prevention of thrombosis, 9th ed: American College of Chest Physicians evidence-based clinical practice guidelines. *Chest*, 141(Suppl. 2), e351S–e418S. doi:10.1378/chest.11-2299.

Berra, K., Fletcher, B., Hayman, L. L., & Miller N. H. (2013). Global cardiovascular disease prevention: A call to action for nursing executive summary. *The Journal of Cardiovascular Nursing*, *28*(6), 505–513. doi 10.1097/JCN0b-13e3182b6822

Caboral, M. F. (2013). Update on cardiovascular disease prevention in women. *The American Journal of Nursing,, 113*(3), 26–33.

Centers for Disease Control and Prevention. (2013). *Peripheral arterial disease (PAD) fact sheet.* Retrieved from http://www.cdc.gov/dhdsp/data_statistics/fact_sheets/docs/fs_PAD.pdf

Etter, J. F., Bullen, C., Flouris, A. D., Laugesen, M., & Eissenberg, T. (2011). Electronic nicotine delivery systems: A research agenda. *Tobacco Control, 20*(3):243–248. doi: 10.1136/tc.2010.042168. Epub 2011 Mar 17.

Fritschi, C., Collins, E. G., O'Connell, S., McBurney, C., Butler, J., & Edwards, L. (2013). The effects of quality of life in patients with peripheral arterial disease. *Journal of Cardiovascular Nursing*, *28*(4), 380–386. doi:10.1097/JCN.0b-13e31824a1587

Gibbons, G. W., & Shaw, P. M. (2012). Diabetes vascular disease: Characteristics of vascular disease unique to the diabetic patient. *Seminars in Vascular Surgery*, *25*(2), 89–92.

Goldhaber, S. Z., & Bounameaux, H. (2012). Pulmonary embolism and deep vein thrombosis. *The Lancet, 379(9828)*, 1835–1846.

Grant B. (2012). *Diagnosis of suspected deep vein thrombosis of the lower extremity*. Retrieved from http://www.uptodate.com/contents/diagnosis-of-suspected-deep-vein-thrombosis-of-the-lower-extremity

Grossman, S. C., & Porth, C. M. (2014). *Porth's pathophysiology* (9th ed.). Philadelphia, PA: Lippincott Williams & Wilkins.

Hennrikus, D., Joseph, A. M., Lando, A. Duval, S., Ukestad, L., Kodl, M., & Hirsch, A. T. (2010). Effectiveness of a smoking cessation program for peripheral artery disease patients. *Journal of the American College of Cardiology*, *56*(225), 2105–2112.

Hinkle, J. L., & Cheever, K. H. (2014). *Brunner & Suddarth's textbook of medical-surgical nursing* (13th ed.). Philadelphia, PA: Wolters Kluwer Health | Lippincott Williams & Wilkins.

Hirsch, A. T., Allison, M. A., Gomes, A. S., Corriere, M. A., Duval, S., Ershow, A.G., . . . Treat-Jacobson, D. (2012). A call to action: Women and peripheral artery disease: A scientific statement from the American Heart Association. *Circulation*, *125,* 1449–1472.

Kim, E. S. H., Wattanakit, K., & Gornik, H. L. (2012). Using the ankle-brachial index to diagnose peripheral artery disease and assess cardiovascular risk. *Cleveland Clinic Journal of Medicine*, *79*(9), 651–661.

Lee, B. B., Bergan, J. J., & Rockson, S. G. (2011). *Lymphedema: A concise compendium of theory and practice.* London, United Kingdom: Springer-Verlag

Leeper, N. J., Kullo, I. J., & Cooke, J. P. (2012). Genetics of peripheral artery disease. *Circulation*, *125,* 3220–3228

Machlus, K. R., Aleman, M. M., & Wolberg, A. S. (2011). Update on venous thromboembolism: Risk factors, mechanisms, and treatments. *Arteriosclerosis, Thrombosis, and Vascular Biology*, *31,* 476–478

NANDA International. (2012). *Nursing diagnoses: Definitions and classification 2012-2014* (9th ed). Oxford, United Kingdom: Wiley-Blackwell.

Olin, J. W., Allie, D. E., Belkin, M., Bonow, R. O., Casey, Jr., D. E., Creager, M.A., . . . Zheng, Z. J (2010). ACCF/AHA/AcR/SCAI/SIR/SVM/SVN/SVS 2010 Performance measures for adults with peripheral artery disease: A report of the American College of Cardiology Foundation/American Heart Association task force on performance measures, the American College of Radiology, the Society for Cardiac Angiography and Interventions, the Society for Interventional Radiology, the Society for Vascular Medicine, the Society for Vascular Nursing, and the Society for Vascular Surgery (Writing Committee to Develop Clinical Performance Measures for Peripheral Artery Disease). *Circulation*, *122,* 2583–2618.

Olin, J. W., & Sealove, B. (2010). Peripheral artery disease: Current insight into the disease and its diagnosis and management. *Mayo Clinic Proceedings*, *85*(7), 678–692.

Robbins, D. A. (2010). Current for abdominal aortic aneurysm repair: Implications for nurses. *Journal of Vascular Nursing*, *28*(4), 136–146. doi:10.1016/j.jvn.2010.09.002

Rooke, T. W., Hirsch, A. T., Misra, S., Sidawy, A. N., Beckman, J. A., Findeiss, L. K., . . . Zierler, R. E. (2011). 2011 ACCF/AHA focused update of the guideline for the management of patients with peripheral artery disease (updating the 2005 guideline): A report of the American College of Cardiology Foundation/American Heart Association Task Force on Practice Guidelines. *J Journal of the American College of Radiology*, *58*, 2020–2045.

Scarvelis, D., & Wells, P. S. (2006). Diagnosis and treatment of deep vein thrombosis. *Canadian Medical Association Journal, 175*(9), 1087–1092.

Shannon, M. M., Hawk, J., Navaroli, L., & Serena, T. (2013). Factors affecting patient adherence to recommended measures for prevention of recurrent venous ulcers. *Journal of Wound, Ostomy and Continence Nursing*, *40*(3), 268–274.

Simmons, K. R., Sinning, M. A., Pearson, J. D., & Hendrix, C. (2013). Implementing a home-based exercise prescription for older patients with peripheral arterial disease and intermittent claudication: A quality improvement project. *Journal of Vascular Nursing*, *31*(1), 2–8.

Smith, S. C., Jr., Benjamin, E. J., Bonow, R. O., Braun, L. T., Creager, M. A., Franklin, B. A., . . . Taubert, K. A. (2011). AHA/ACCF Secondary prevention and risk reduction therapy for patients with coronary and other atherosclerotic vascular disease: 2011 update: A guideline from the American Heart Association and American College of Cardiology Foundation. *Circulation, 124,* 2458–2473

Stephens, J., Hagler, D., & Clark, E. (2011). Got PAD? Hidden dangers revealed with ABI. *Journal of Vascular Nursing, 29*(4), 153–157. doi:10.1016/j.jvn.2011.08.002

U.S. Department of Health & Human Services. (2013). *Healthy people 2020:Topics & objectives – Objectives A-Z.* Retrieved from http://www.healthypeople.gov/2020/topicsobjectives2020/

Wennberg, P. W. (2013). Approach to the patient with peripheral arterial disease. *Circulation, 128,* 2241–2250

Wierzbicki, A. S. (2012). New directions in cardiovascular risk assessment: The role of secondary risk stratification markers. *International Journal of Clinical Practice*, *66*(7), 622–630.

World Health Organization. (2011). *Global atlas on cardiovascular disease prevention and control.* Geneva, Switzerland: Author. Retrieved from http://whqlibdoc.who.int/publications/2011/9789241564373_eng.pdf?ua=1

Zoller, B., Sundquist, J., & Sundquist, K. (2011). Age- and gender-specific familial risks for venous thromboembolism: A nationwide epidemiological study based on hospitalization in Sweden. *Circulation, 124,* 1012–1020.

Tables of Abnormal Findings

TABLE 18.2 Variations in Arterial Pulses

Pulse	Characteristics	Causes
Weak Pulse	Decreased pulse pressure, weak on palpation and easily obliterated, slow upstroke with prolonged systolic peak	Decreased cardiac output, as with congestive heart failure, hypovolemia, and severe aortic stenosis; peripheral arterial disease
Bounding Pulse	Increased pulse pressure, strong and bounding, rapid rise and fall, brief systolic peak	Increased stroke volume such as with exercise and fever, hyperthyroidism, decreased aortic compliance as with atherosclerosis or aging
Pulsus Alternans	Alternating small and large amplitude, regular rate	Left ventricular failure, may be accompanied by S3
Pulsus Bigeminus *Premature contractions*	Alternating irregular beats; one normal beat and then one premature beat with alternating strong and weak amplitude	Premature ventricular or atrial contractions
Pulsus Bisferiens	Double systolic peak	Aortic regurgitation, combined aortic regurgitation and stenosis, less often hypertrophic cardiomyopathy
Pulsus Paradoxus *Expiration* — *Inspiration*	Palpable decrease in amplitude on quiet inspiration; with blood pressure cuff, systolic decreases of more than 10 mmHg during inspiration	Pericardial tamponade, constrictive pericarditis and obstructive lung disease

TABLE 18.3 Abnormal Arterial Findings

Peripheral Arterial Disease

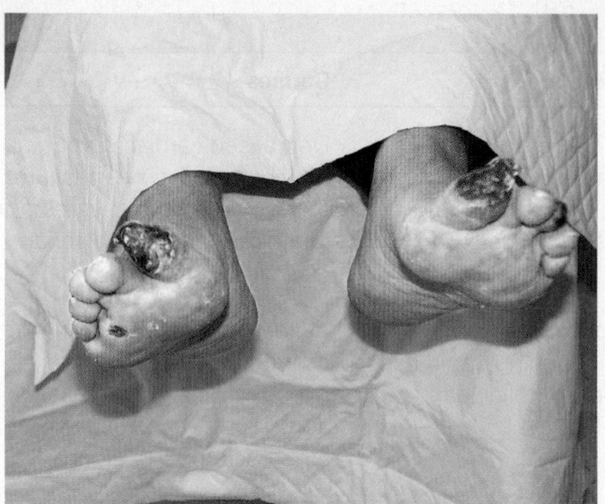

Chronic atherosclerotic occlusion may develop anywhere in the arterial system. As with coronary artery disease (CAD), peripheral arteries narrow from plaque, which limits oxygenated blood from reaching the tissues. Resulting ischemia causes cramping pain, which in the lower extremities is called *intermittent claudication*. It is usually exertional and the pain occurs in relation to arterial blockage. Lower arterial blockage may lead to calf claudication. Blockage at the sacroiliac bifurcation may cause hip claudication. Rest generally relieves claudication. As the disease progresses, rest pain may occur, awakening patients from sleep. At this point, dorsalis pedis and posterior tibial pulses are decreased significantly compared to the opposite leg. Also, the diseased leg has a cool temperature and pale or blue color. ABI is decreased. Severe occlusion is chronically painful and may cause ulcers, which in turn may lead to gangrene and amputation. Total occlusion, often from thrombus, is limb threatening. Any combination of the six Ps (see Box 18.2) constitutes a clinical emergency requiring immediate intervention. Well-refined assessment skills are paramount. Modification of risk factors is critical. Smoking cessation is of utmost importance. Stringent control of unmodifiable risk factors (e.g., blood glucose level in patients with diabetes mellitus) is essential. Pain assessment and management are also issues.

Acute Arterial Occlusion

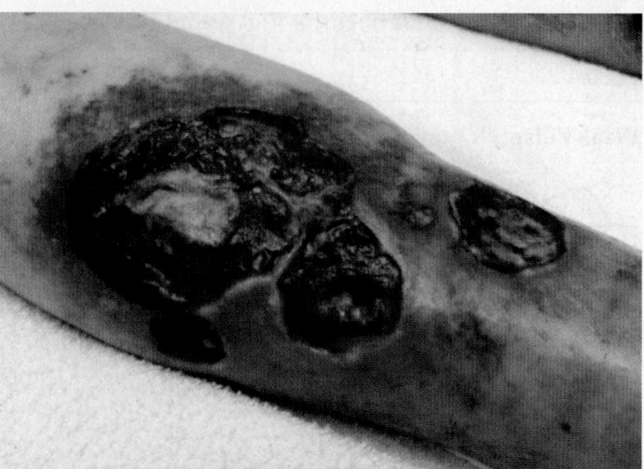

Acute arterial occlusion may result from progression of peripheral arterial disease (as discussed) or thrombus from another source (e.g., cardiac catheterization puncture site). In the latter case, a thrombus may break off and travel through the arterial system to a smaller vessel that is then occluded. The six Ps would again be assessment findings. As with deep vein thrombosis, this is a clinical emergency.

(table continues on page 523)

TABLE 18.3 Abnormal Arterial Findings *(continued)*

Abdominal Aortic Aneurysm

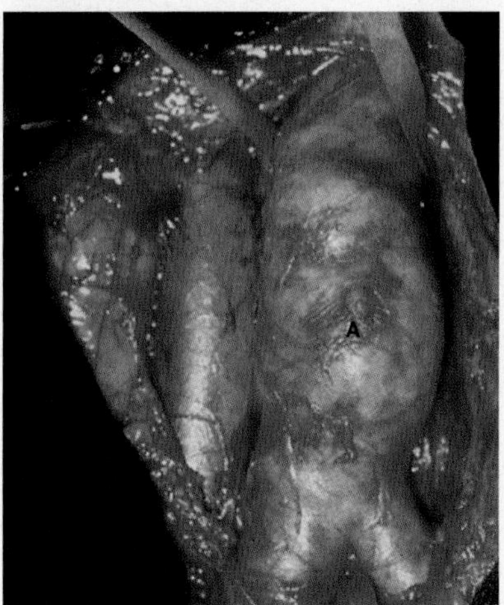

An aneurysm is an outpouching of an arterial wall, which results from a weakened or damaged medial arterial layer. Aneurysms may occur in any artery but are most common in the aorta. Aortic aneurysms may be thoracic, below the renal arteries, or abdominal. The predominant cause of aortic aneurysm is atherosclerosis. Hypertension may accelerate aneurysm development in an already damaged aortic wall. Aortic aneurysms are also seen with Marfan syndrome, a congenital disorder. In addition to smoking and hypertension, family history of aortic aneurysm is a risk factor. Aortic aneurysms affect men up to nine times more than women (Caboral, 2013). Aortic aneurysms may rupture or dissect, in which the layers of the artery separate and fill with blood. Either situation results in compromised blood supply to major arteries and therefore to organs and tissues. These critical emergencies are often fatal. Assessment findings include chest pain, abdominal pain, back pain, shortness of breath, laterally pulsatile mass on palpation, and a bruit. Patients with an abdominal aortic aneurysm are usually asymptomatic.

Raynaud Phenomenon and Raynaud Disease

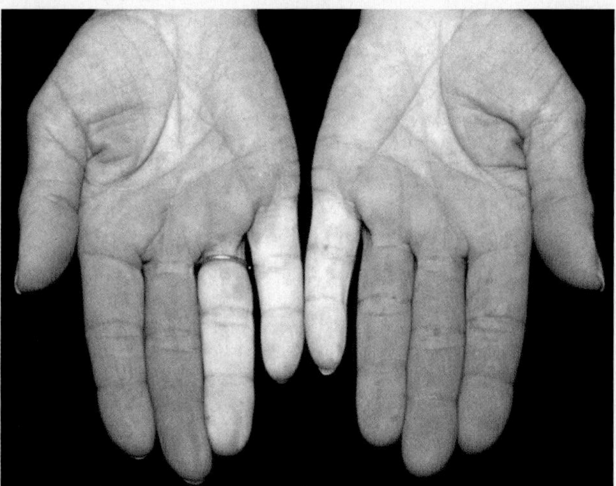

These vasospastic disorders primarily affect women. Raynaud phenomenon is the term used when the cause is attributed to a connective tissue disorder (e.g., lupus erythematosus, rheumatoid arthritis, scleroderma). When the etiology is unknown (most cases), it is called Raynaud disease. Symptoms include numbness, tingling, sometimes pain, extreme pallor progressing to cyanosis, and coolness of the hands. The symptoms usually begin in the fingers and are symmetrical. When the ischemic episode is over, hyperemia, erythema, and burning pain may follow. Smoking, emotional stress, and exposure to cold often precipitate vasospasm. Management includes smoking cessation, avoiding cold temperatures, wearing thermal socks and gloves in cool temperatures, and stress management. In patients with Raynaud phenomenon, treatment of the underlying cause may offer relief. Tissue injury is rare, but with repeated ischemic episodes, skin over the fingertips may develop small ulcers. The nails may become brittle. In rare cases, gangrene of the fingers may occur.

Arterial diseases involve narrowing of the vessels, weakening of the vessel walls, and thrombus formation. Risk factors are the same as for CAD: smoking, diabetes, hypertension, hypercholesterolemia, and family history of arterial problems. Atherosclerosis is the most common cause.

TABLE 18.4 Abnormal Venous Findings

Chronic Venous Insufficiency

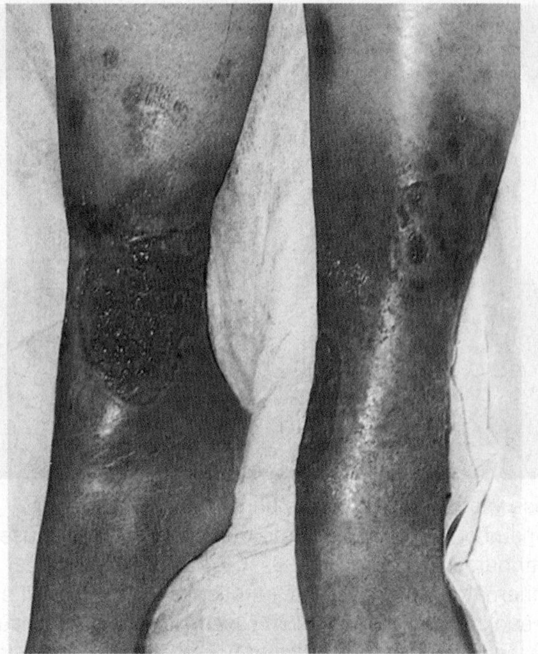

Malfunctioning of the unidirectional valves impairs venous blood return to the affected extremity. Causes are primary valvular incompetence (which may be from a congenital absence of valves), sequelae of DVT, or both. DVT permanently damages the valve leaflets, which cannot close. The veins then cannot empty, leading to edema. Venous insufficiency from dysfunctional valves causes tissue congestion, which eventually impairs nutrition to the tissue. Brown hyperpigmentation may develop from hemosiderin deposits remaining after the breakdown of red blood cells. Lymphatic insufficiency follows venous insufficiency, compounding tissue congestion. Patients complain of edema and aching pain. As venous insufficiency progresses, stasis dermatitis (characterized by dry, scaling skin) may lead to superficial and relatively painless venous ulcers. Chronic pressure from edema makes these ulcers difficult to heal (see Table 18.5). Long periods of standing promote edema. Elevating the legs above the heart promotes venous return, providing some relief. Compression stockings are recommended to prevent increasing edema and recurrence of venous ulcers.

Deep Vein Thrombosis

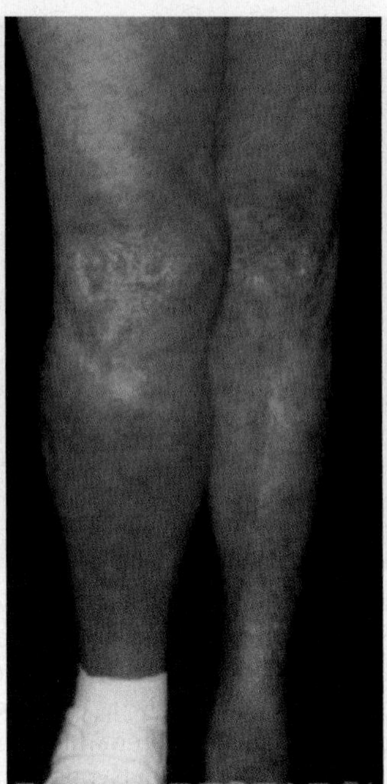

DVT results from thrombus formation in the deep veins. They are more common in the lower extremities, but increasing use of venous access catheters is contributing to more upper extremity DVTs. The Virchow triad identifies risk factors for venous thrombosis: blood stasis, vessel wall injury, and increased blood coagulability. Immobility and decreased mobility, both more common in older adults, pose risks for stasis. Trauma or surgery may damage vessel walls. Increased blood coagulability may stem from the prolonged sitting and dehydration associated with airplane travel, cancer, use of oral contraceptives and estrogen replacement therapy, and inherited or acquired coagulation disorders. Treatment is anticoagulation; for some patients with chronic problems or postthrombotic syndrome, anticoagulation may offer long-term prophylaxis. Presenting symptoms of DVT are unilateral edema of the extremity, redness, pain or achiness, and warmth. The leg is measured daily at the same place throughout treatment. Unrecognized DVTs are responsible for most deaths from PE. Acute care patients often have at least one risk factor for venous thrombosis or venous thromboembolism, so knowledge of the features of DVT and PE is critical.

(table continues on page 525)

TABLE 18.4 Abnormal Venous Findings *(continued)*

Thrombophlebitis

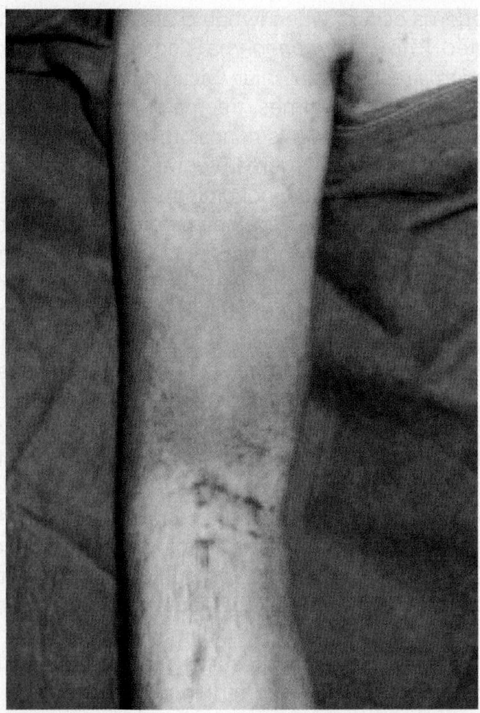

Superficial thrombophlebitis results from thrombus formation in the superficial veins. The same risk factors apply as with DVT. Assessment findings are unilateral localized pain or achiness, edema, warmth, and redness. In superficial veins, a palpable mass or cord may also be present along the vein.

Neuropathy

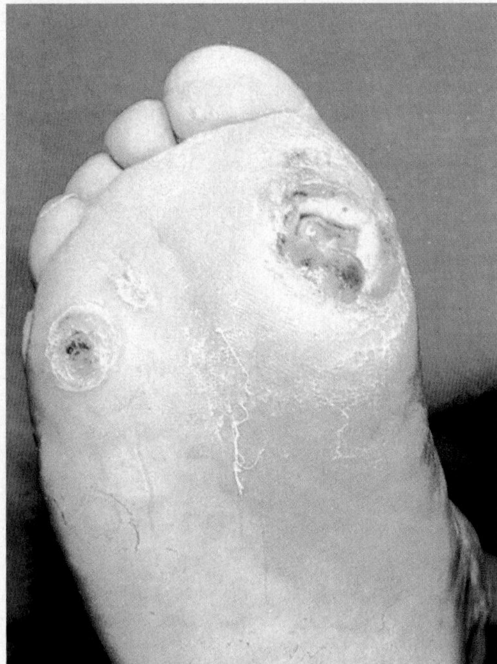

Peripheral neuropathies, most common in patients with diabetes mellitus and chronic hyperglycemia, are classified as somatic or autonomic. *Somatic neuropathies* typically affect lower extremities. Paresthesias, burning sensations, and numbness may occur along with decreased senses of vibration, pain, temperature, and proprioception. These symptoms increase risks for tissue injury and falls. Daily foot assessment is critical because these patients may not feel a break in the skin or a burn and develop subsequent foot lesions, which are challenging to heal. For some patients, peripheral neuropathies cause chronic lower extremity pain. Pain assessment and management are crucial to their quality of life. A pharmacological approach to management is often employed.

(table continues on page 526)

TABLE 18.4 Abnormal Venous Findings *(continued)*

Lymphedema

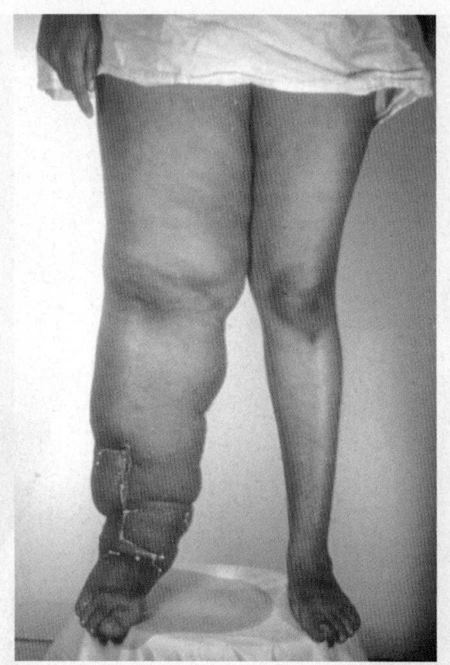

Lymphedema occurs when lymph channels or nodes are obstructed. *Primary lymphedema* is congenital. *Secondary lymphedema* results from injury, scarring, excision of lymph nodes, or, sometimes, trauma or chronic infection. Assessment initially reveals nonpainful pitting edema of the extremity. As lymphedema progresses, the skin may thicken, redden, and show nonpitting edema. Small vesicles with lymphatic fluid may develop in more advanced stages. Cellulitis is a frequent complication. Management begins with treating the cause. Bed rest with the leg elevated 45 degrees at night and frequently during the day for several days is usually very effective in reducing edema. Compression pumps, manual lymphatic drainage, and massage may also be used. Patients should wear elastic compression wraps or stockings when the extremity is dependent to combat gravity-related pooling. Patients should apply these devices in the morning when edema is lowest. Exercise enhances treatment as do weight control and decreased salt intake. Ongoing skin assessment is essential because breaks in the skin occur more easily in edematous extremities and are difficult to treat. Diuretics may also promote fluid elimination. Chronic lymphedema can be disfiguring and limit joint mobility. Psychosocial support for body image and self-esteem is very important in care.

The structure of veins and their reliance on a unidirectional valve, the skeletal muscle pump, and changes in abdominal and intrathoracic pressures lend them to problems of stasis and insufficiency.

TABLE 18.5 Arterial Versus Venous Ulcers

	Arterial	Venous
Location	Toes, metatarsals, malleoli, heels	Ankle, medial malleolus, distal third of leg
Borders	Regular	Irregular
Ulcer base	Pale, yellow	Red, pink
Drainage	Minimal	Moderate to large amount
Gangrene	May be present	Not present
Pain	Painful; decreased with dependency	Aching pain, feeling of heaviness; decreased with elevation
Skin	Pale, inflamed, necrotic	Stasis dermatitis, pigmentation changes
Pulses	Decreased or absent	Normal, may be difficult to palpate because of edema

19

Breasts and Axillae Assessment

Learning Objectives

1. Demonstrate knowledge of anatomy and physiology of the breast structures and axillae.
2. Identify important topics for health promotion and risk reduction related to the breasts and axillae.
3. Collect subjective data related to conditions of the breast and axillae.
4. Collect objective data related to the breasts and axillae.
5. Identify expected and unexpected findings related to the breast and axillae during the general survey and when performing inspection and palpation.
6. Use subjective and objective data from assessment of the breasts and axillae and consider initial interventions.
7. Document and communicate data from the assessment of the breasts and axillae using appropriate medical terminology and principles of recording.
8. Individualize health assessment of the breasts and axillae considering the condition, age, gender, and culture of the patient.
9. Identify nursing diagnoses and initiate a plan of care based on findings from the assessment of the breasts and axillae.

Mrs. Randall, a 66-year-old African American woman, is receiving a home care visit for the management of Stage III breast cancer. She recently had preoperative chemotherapy and a mastectomy; she is currently undergoing radiation treatments. Medications include oxycodone for moderate to severe pain, acetaminophen (Tylenol) for mild to moderate pain, senna (Senokot) as a laxative, and metoclopramide (Reglan) for nausea. Mrs. Randall can get out of bed for meals, but she has not been eating much because of a lack of appetite and fatigue. The nurse performed and documented an assessment of Mrs. Randall last week. Temperature was 37°C (98.6°F) orally, pulse 78 beats/min, respirations 24 breaths/min, and blood pressure 138/70 mmHg.

You will gain more information about Mrs. Randall as you progress through this chapter. As you study the content and features, consider Mrs. Randall's case and its relationship to what you are learning. Begin thinking about the following points:

- What age group of women has the highest risk for breast cancer?
- Why is cancer in the upper outer quadrant of the breast at such high risk?
- Are Mrs. Randall's psychosocial or physical needs in this case more important?
- What lifestyle factors might be contributing to Mrs. Randall's risk for breast cancer?
- What recommendations for screening and follow-up would you suggest for Mrs. Randall and her daughters?
- How would you evaluate the success of interventions for Mrs. Randall?

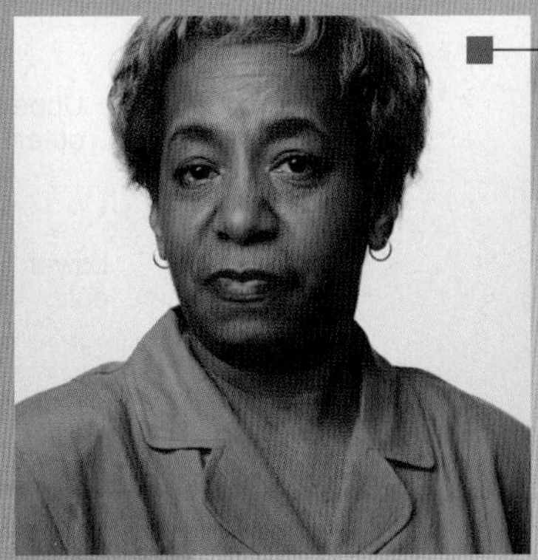

This chapter discusses the assessment of the breasts and regional lymphatics. It reviews pertinent anatomy and physiology as well as key variations based on pregnancy, lifespan, sex, and culture. This chapter explores methods for collecting subjective data related to the risk of breast disease (cancerous and benign). It also presents specific unexpected findings, such as color changes, nipple discharge, retraction, heat, warmth or redness, and lumps.

Structure and Function

Breasts are paired mammary glands found in both sexes. Male breasts, which remain rudimentary, have a thin layer of breast tissue with a centrally located small nipple and surrounding areola. Mature female breasts are accessory reproductive organs that respond to cyclical changes in sex hormones and provide nourishment for infants through milk production. Many cultures associate the breasts with female sexuality.

Landmarks

Female breasts are located on the anterior chest wall extending from the second intercostal space superiorly to the sixth or seventh intercostal space inferiorly (Lemaine & Simmons, 2013, p. 23). They extend from the sternal margin to the midaxillary line, with the tail of each breast extending into its respective axilla. The pectoral muscles and superficial fascia provide support.

To describe clinical findings, it is best to divide each breast into four quadrants by imagining horizontal and vertical lines that intersect at the nipple. The tail of Spence, which extends from the upper outer breast quadrant into the axilla, can be described separately (Fig. 19.1). An alternative method is to compare the breast to the face of a clock and describe findings based on their distance from the nipple (e.g., [R] breast at 8:00, 3 cm [about 1¼ in.] from nipple). Most breast cancers occur in the upper outer quadrant, so examiners must pay close attention to this area.

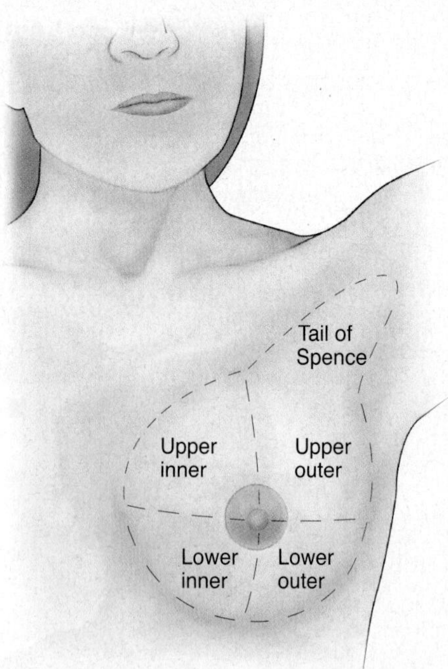

Figure 19.1 Breast with four quadrants and tail of Spence delineated.

> **Clinical Significance**
>
> Breast cancer is the leading cause of cancer in females, but males also can develop the disease (approximately 1% of all cases). In 2010, 2,039 men were diagnosed with breast cancer and 439 men died from it in the United States (Centers for Disease Control and Prevention [CDC] 2013).

Breast Structures

On the surface, the breasts lie anterior to the serratus anterior and pectoralis major muscles (Fig. 19.2A). Each breast has a nipple with a surrounding areola as well as Montgomery glands, fibrous tissue, glandular tissue, and lymph nodes (Fig. 19.2B). The nipple is at the center of the breast. It is darkly pigmented, round, rough, and usually protuberant; it is composed of smooth muscle fibers. Autonomic, sensory, or

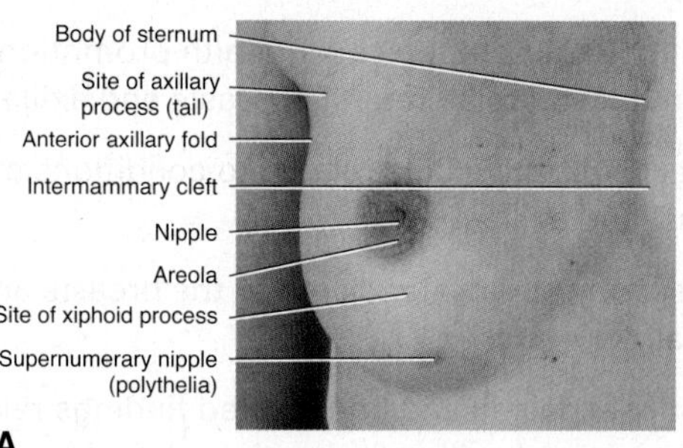

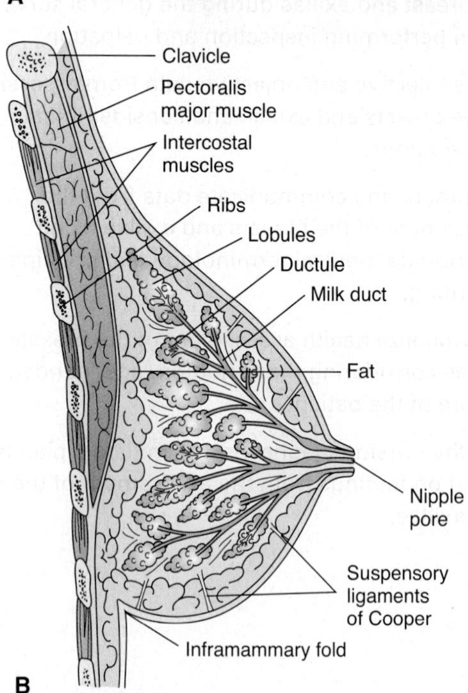

Figure 19.2 **A.** Surface anatomy of the breast. **B.** Internal structures of the breast.

tactile stimulation produces nipple erection and emptying of lactiferous ducts during breastfeeding. Surrounding the nipple is a 1- to 2-cm (about ¼ to ¾ in.) areola, which is also darkly pigmented. Within the areola are small sebaceous glands called Montgomery glands. During lactation, these glands secrete a protective lubricant.

Breasts consist of two types of tissue, fibrous and glandular, and two types of fat, subcutaneous and retromammary. The fibrous tissue is supportive. Suspensory ligaments of Cooper (fibrous bands) extend from the connective tissue to the muscle fascia, providing additional support. The glandular tissue consists of 15 to 20 glandular lobes in each breast that extends from the nipple in a radial fashion. Within each lobe, 20 to 40 lobules contain milk-producing acini cells. When milk is produced, it drains into the lactiferous ducts; the milk from each lobe empties into one sinus that terminates at the nipple. During lactation, milk is stored in these sinuses until it is released. This ductal system may be noticeable in pregnant or lactating women.

Most of the breast consists of subcutaneous and retromammary fat surrounding the glandular tissue. Actual breast size and the proportions of each tissue component vary with age, genetic predisposition, pregnancy, lactation, and nutritional status.

Branches of the internal mammary and lateral thoracic arteries provide most of the blood supply to the deep breast tissues and nipple. The superficial tissues receive blood from the intercostal, subscapular, and thoracodorsal arteries (Lemaine & Simmons, 2013).

Axillae and Lymph Nodes

Each breast has an extensive lymphatic network for drainage that includes pathways to the axillary, internal mammary, interpectoral, intraparenchymal, anterior and posterior intercostal, and supraclavicular nodes (Hassiotou & Geddes, 2013). Most drainage is channeled to the axillary lymph nodes on the same side (ipsilateral lymph nodes; Fig. 19.3). Axillary nodes are relatively superficial, so they are more accessible than deep lymph nodes (e.g., internal mammary nodes) and fairly easy to palpate when enlarged.

- The *lateral axillary* (*brachial*) *nodes* are located inside the upper arm along the humerus.
- The *central axillary* (*midaxillary*) *nodes* are palpable high up in the axilla at the top of the ribs. These nodes receive lymph from the lateral, posterior, and anterior axillary nodes.
- The *posterior axillary* (*subscapular*) *nodes* lie inside the posterior axillary fold along the lateral edge of the scapulae.
- The *anterior axillary* (*pectoral*) *nodes* are located inside the lateral axillary fold along the pectoralis major muscle.

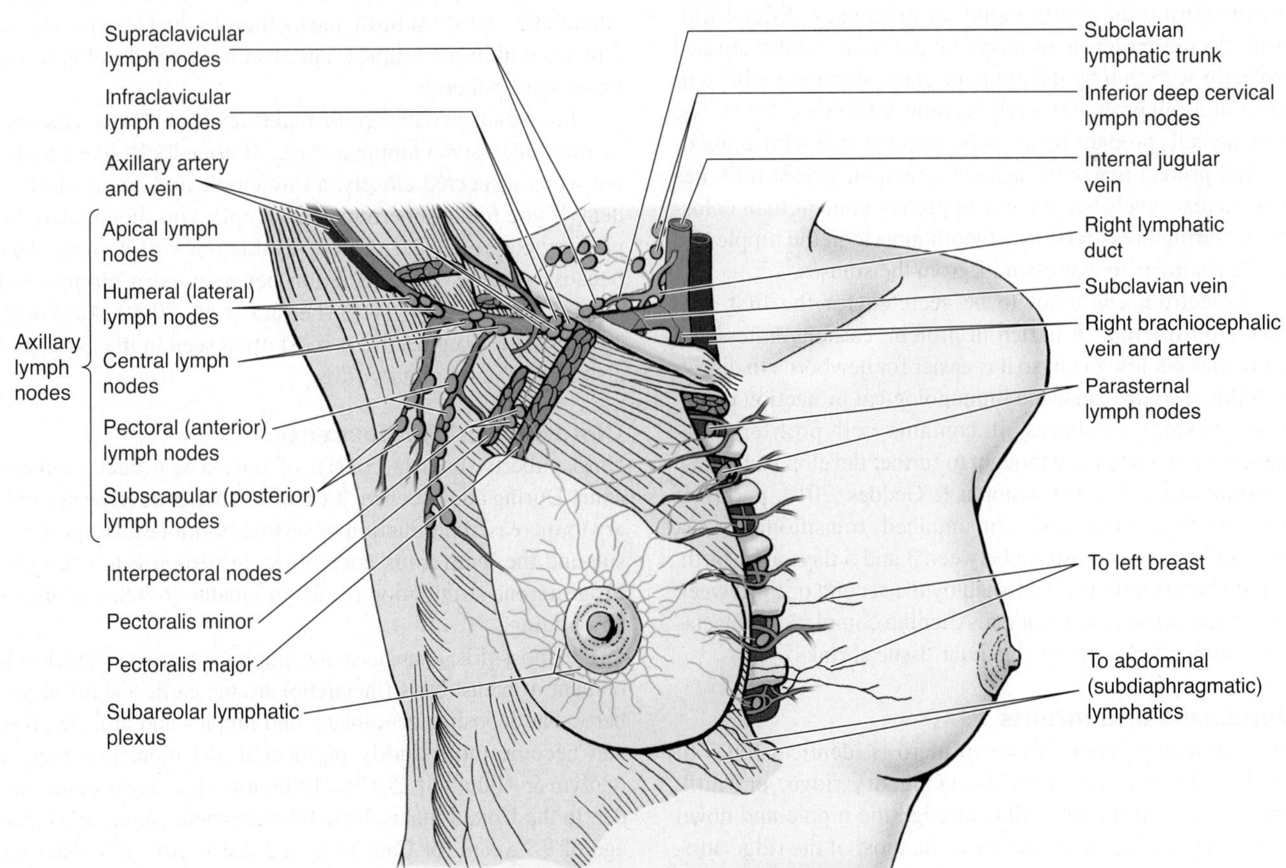

Figure 19.3 Location of lymph nodes in relation to breasts.

> **Clinical Significance**
>
> Lymphatic spread of breast carcinoma cells may lead to enlargement of the axillary lymph nodes as well as the infraclavicular and supraclavicular lymph nodes. Enlargement of these nodes may be noted during physical assessment and warrants further evaluation. Tenderness or enlargement of any of these nodes also may be related to infection or clinical blockage.

Lifespan Considerations

Women Who Are Pregnant

During pregnancy, women's breasts become fully functional under the influence of estrogen, progesterone, prolactin and other hormones, and growth factors (e.g., placental lactogen, epidermal growth factor, stromal paracrine factors) (Hassiotou & Geddes, 2013, p. 29). Women experience breast changes as early as the first 2 months of pregnancy. The ductal system expands, secretory alveoli develop, and breasts enlarge, often feeling nodular as a result of the mammary alveoli hypertrophy that occurs. Nipples darken, enlarge, and become more erect. As pregnancy progresses, areolae also become larger, darker, and more prominent. Small, scattered Montgomery glands develop within the areolae. Because of increased blood flow, a bluish venous pattern is often evident in the breast tissue.

The breasts may begin to express **colostrum** (milk precursor) during the fourth month of pregnancy. After childbirth, decreased levels of placental hormones and increased prolactin secretion by the pituitary gland stimulate milk synthesis and cell proliferation (Hassiotou & Geddes, 2013). The alveolar cells produce breast milk, which is rich with antibodies that protect newborns against infection. Breast milk has high lactose levels but is lower in protein content than colostrum. During breastfeeding, smooth muscle in the nipple and areola contracts to express milk from the sinuses.

Colostrum continues to be secreted for the first 3 to 5 days postpartum. It is rich in protein, carbohydrates, and antibodies but low in fat, so it is easier for newborns to digest. In addition to the enhanced immunological protection colostrum provides newborns, it contains cell proliferation–inducing factors that are thought to further develop newborns' gastrointestinal tracts (Hassiotou & Geddes, 2013, p. 32). If breastfeeding occurs and is maintained, transitional breast milk will replace colostrum between 3 and 5 days after birth. Mature breast milk is established by the second or third week postpartum in lactating women. After the completion of lactation, women's mammary glandular tissue shrinks.

Newborns and Infants

Development of breast tissue in utero is identical for both genders. During this time, the mammary ridge, or "milk line," extends from the axillae through the nipple and down to the inguinal ligament. Before birth, most of the ridge atrophies, leaving two bilateral breasts along the ridge over the thorax.

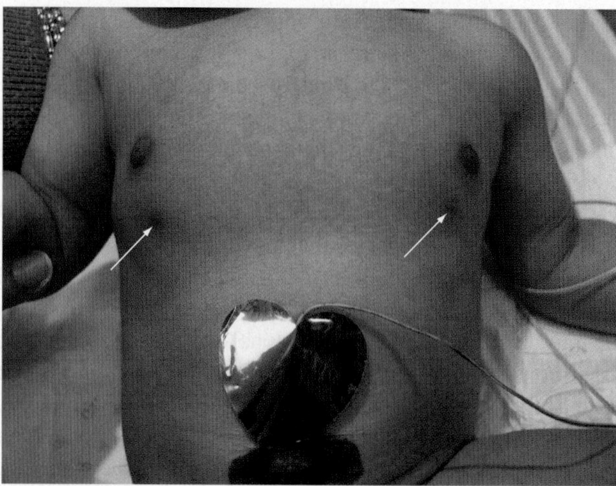

Figure 19.4 Supernumerary nipples (*arrows*) in a newborn.

Enlarged breast tissue and white discharge (commonly called "witch's milk") in newborns of either gender may occur for the first few weeks of life, secondary to the effects of maternal estrogens (Colvin & Abdullatif, 2013). If breast enlargement, witch's milk, or both are present, it is important to reassure the newborn's parents/caregivers that nothing is wrong and the conditions will resolve spontaneously. Uncommonly, complete resolution of the breast enlargement may not take place over several months; however, by the age of 2 years, resolution should be evident and breast enlargement is not observed again until the onset of puberty (Colvin & Abdullatif, 2013). At birth, the lactiferous ducts are present in females within the nipples, but alveoli do not develop in females until puberty.

In a small percentage of males and females, a supernumerary (accessory) nipple persists. It often looks like a mole, but when inspected closely, a tiny nipple and areola are evident. If you find a supernumerary nipple, you should alert the primary care provider; kidney evaluation will be necessary because there is an association between extra nipples and renal anomalies (Fig. 19.4) (Ferrara et al., 2009). Accessory breast tissue (polymastia) is most often seen in the axilla and also along the mammary ridge.

Children and Adolescents

Until puberty, breasts consist of only a few ducts without acini. During adolescence, breasts in females develop secondary to increased production of several hormones. Adipose tissue and the lactiferous ducts grow in response to estrogen. Progesterone stimulation results in lobular growth and alveolar budding.

In most girls, changes in the nipples and areolae and development of breast buds (thelarche) are the earliest signs of puberty. Fat deposits accumulate, and nipples and areolae grow and become more darkly pigmented and more protuberant (Colvin & Abdullatif, 2013). The breasts also may become tender. In the United States, breast development begins at a mean age of 9.7 years for Caucasian and Asian girls, 8.8 years for African American girls, and 9.3 years for Hispanic girls (Herman-Giddens, 2013). The average age of breast development

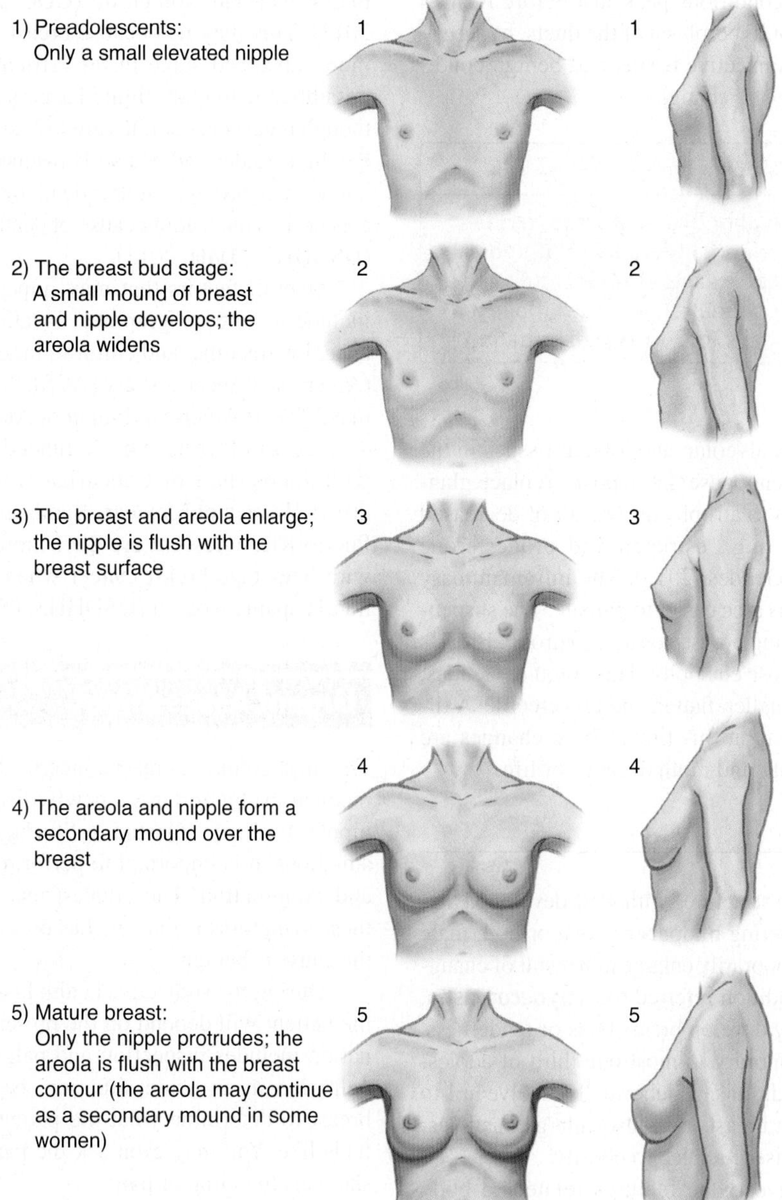

1) Preadolescents:
Only a small elevated nipple
1
1
2) The breast bud stage:
A small mound of breast and nipple develops; the areola widens
2
2
3) The breast and areola enlarge; the nipple is flush with the breast surface
3
3
4) The areola and nipple form a secondary mound over the breast
4
4
5) Mature breast:
Only the nipple protrudes; the areola is flush with the breast contour (the areola may continue as a secondary mound in some women)
5
5

Figure 19.5 Tanner staging of breast development.

has decreased over the past century in the developed world as a result of improvements in nutrition, sanitation, and infection control; this decrease has not occurred in countries where children are malnourished or have high rates of disease (de Onis, Garza, Victora, Bhan, & Norum, 2004). Full breast development occurs on average over a 3-year period. Breast development is described by **Tanner staging** (Fig. 19.5).

Breast growth over this 3-year period is usually not steady or symmetrical. It may occur rapidly and then subside, changing with an uneven pace. It is not uncommon for one breast to grow more quickly than the other, but with time, breast size may equalize. These changes in the breasts are linked to body image and self-esteem, especially during a developmental stage in which the peer group assumes increasing importance. Additionally, the breasts often symbolize the development of sexuality and reproductive capacity. The adolescent girl often will compare her growth to that of others. Early maturing girls may experience more dissatisfaction with their physical appearance because most of their peers have the slim body shape that cultural norms perpetuate. Late-maturing girls may worry that they will be "flat-chested." Timing of breast development in girls has a social stigma; girls who mature either early or late may be concerned. Reassure the adolescent that the rate of breast growth is uniquely individual, as are the size and shape of the mature breast.

Menarche (the beginning of menstruation) occurs during late puberty or Tanner Stage 3 or 4, which coincides with the peak of the adolescent growth spurt (Melmed, Polonsky, Larsen, & Kronenberg, 2011). During menstruation, the glandular tissues of the breasts change in response to cyclical hormonal fluctuations. At the start of the cycle, the ductal cells grow, interstitial fluid increases, and the tissue may become slightly inflamed. These conditions peak just before menses and may lead to dilation or hyperplasia of the ducts, hypertrophy of the surrounding connective tissue, and benign conditions referred to as fibrocystic changes.

> **Clinical Significance**
>
> In adult women, unilateral or bilateral breast tenderness and changes in size and nodularity (lumpiness) may accompany menses. Breasts often feel full, sore, or heavy just before menstruation and are smallest and least tender in the days following menstruation.

Older Adults

As women age, glandular, alveolar, and lobular tissues in the breasts decrease. After menopause, fat deposits replace glandular tissue that continues to atrophy as a result of decreased ovarian hormone levels (e.g., estrogen and progesterone secretion) (Hassiotou & Geddes, 2013). The inframammary ridge thickens, making this area easier to palpate. The suspensory ligaments relax, causing breasts to sag and droop. Breasts also decrease in size and lose elasticity (Hassiotou & Geddes, 2013). Nipples become smaller, flatter, and less erectile. Axillary hair may stop growing at this time. These changes are more apparent in the eighth and ninth decades of life.

Male Breasts

Male breasts are immature structures with well-developed areolae and small nipples. During midpuberty, one or both male breasts commonly and temporarily enlarge as a result of changing hormone levels, a condition referred to as **gynecomastia**. Pubescent males also may develop breast buds or tenderness, which also is usually temporary. Almost one third of adolescent males have these conditions, which usually resolve in 1 to 2 years (Rakel, 2011). The breasts may also enlarge in adolescent males from adipose tissue related to obesity.

It is important to investigate feelings related to body image and sexual identity in adolescent males with enlarged breasts. Gynecomastia is physically benign but can cause emotional distress. Reassurance that this is temporary and normal may help alleviate the distress. As males age, gynecomastia (enlarged breasts) may recur from decreases in testosterone levels, causing the female hormones to predominate.

Cultural Considerations

As a nurse, you should be aware of variations in breast development related to ethnicity. For example, African American females mature earlier than Caucasians (U.S. Department of Health & Human Services, Office of Minority Health [USDHHS, OMH], 2013). Variations in the color of the skin and nipple relate to ethnic background. Differences exist in the incidence and outcomes of breast cancer. Hispanic, Asian, and American Indian women have a lower risk for developing breast cancer. African American women experience a lower incidence but a 40% higher mortality rate from breast cancer than Caucasian women do (CDC, 2013; USDHHS, OMH, 2013). This may be because breast cancer is diagnosed at a more advanced stage in the African American population, possibly due to more limited access to breast health care. Although breast cancer rates are lowest among Asian American/Pacific Islander and Native Hawaiian women, Native Hawaiian women have the highest death rates associated with breast cancer; it is the leading cause of death among Filipino women (USDHHS, OMH, 2013).

Overall factors that may impede access to health care include remote geographical location, lack of health insurance, low income, and cultural, racial, and language barriers (American Cancer Society [ACS], 2013). It has been reported that 3.5% of American Indian or Alaska Native women aged 40 years or older have had a funded mammogram compared with almost half of Caucasian women (USDHHS, OMH, 2013). Women of Mexican, South and Central American, and Puerto Rican descent are 20% more likely to be diagnosed with late-stage breast cancer when compared with rates in non-Hispanic women (USDHHS, OMH, 2013).

Urgent Assessment

The most common breast concerns that cause women to seek medical evaluation are a newly discovered lump, pain, and nipple discharge (Onstad & Stuckey, 2013). In any of these situations, it is important to perform a focused health history and examination. The greatest fear a woman has related to these symptoms is that she has breast cancer, although often, the cause is benign.

During the subjective health history, the questions to ask the patient will depend on the presenting symptoms. Examination includes inspection and palpation. When performing palpation in an acute situation, begin with the unaffected breast to determine what the patient's normal breast tissue feels like. You may even ask the patient to show you where she feels the lump or pain.

> ***SAFETY ALERT***
>
> *Conditions requiring further investigation to determine a need for tests to rule out cancer include the following:*
>
> - *A new breast lump*
> - *A lump that has changed in size, shape, texture, or tenderness*
> - *A lump in the axilla, supraclavicular, or intraclavicular regions*
> - *Bloody nipple discharge*
> - *Swelling, reddening, or thickening of breast skin*
> - *Dimpling or retraction of an area of the breast (ACS, 2013)*

Nipple discharge alone is not a reliable sign of cancer, but its presence is associated with cancer in approximately 15% of women (Onstad & Stuckey, 2013). Therefore, this symptom should be considered with other symptoms and the clinical presentation. Mammary duct ectasia (dilation of the mammary ducts) is a benign condition that may cause bilateral green, brown, or other colored discharge from multiple ducts. It may occur in women and men (Onstad & Stuckey, 2013, p. 462).

Subjective Data

Subjective data collection begins with the current health history related to the breast (such as breast discomfort, masses or lumps, nipple discharge) and continues with questions related to past history (previous breast disease; positive result for breast cancer antigen [BRCA1 or BRCA2] mutation; surgeries; menstrual, pregnancy, and lactation history; and past hormone replacement therapy), personal history (breast trauma, surgery, and self-care behaviors), and family history (of breast cancer, other breast disease, confirmed BRCA1 or BRCA2 mutation) (ACS, 2013). It is important to ask questions sensitively when obtaining data because conditions related to the breast may be difficult or embarrassing for some women to discuss.

Assessment of Risk Factors

The most common type of cancer in U.S. women is breast cancer, accounting for about 30% of newly diagnosed cancer cases (ACS, 2013). The probability of developing breast cancer increases with age, but breast cancer also occurs in young women and (rarely) in men. The National Cancer Institute (NCI, 2013) estimated that in 2013, 232,340 women and 2,240 men will be diagnosed with breast cancer and that 39,620 women and 410 men will die of the disease. A woman's risk for breast cancer is as follows (NCI, 2013):

- From age 30 to 39 years, 0.4% (often expressed as "1 in 227")
- From age 40 to 49 years, 1.5% (often expressed as "1 in 68")
- From age 50 to 59 years, 2.4% (often expressed as "1 in 42")
- From age 60 to 69 years, 3.6% (often expressed as "1 in 28")
- From age 70 years and older, 3.8% (often expressed as "1 in 26")

During the last half of the 20th century, incidence of breast cancer in the United States doubled, with early-stage and in situ discoveries being most prevalent. More diligent screening may be a factor in the increased cases; however, other factors—such as fewer pregnancies, menopausal hormone use, increase in obesity rates, improved nutrition, and increased life expectancy—may also be contributing to the increased rates of breast cancer (ACS, 2013).

The good news is that U.S. breast cancer death rates have decreased overall by 34% from 1990 to 2010. Annual declines in the death rates have been observed in all racial and ethnic groups of women except for American Indian/Native Alaskan women, where the rates have remained unchanged (ACS, 2013). Nevertheless, long-term differences in mortality rates among racial/ethnic groups remain evident. In 2010, the death rates for African American women with breast cancer were 41% higher than those for Caucasian women (ACS, 2013, p. 9). Possible reasons for the observed differences in deaths in some groups of women are that less frequent mammogram screenings have been documented in some groups of women (e.g., African American women) and, as a result, breast cancers are discovered at a more advanced stage. In addition, the use of and response to some newer treatments (e.g., tamoxifen to treat hormone receptive positive breast cancers) may not be an option for some women who are less likely to have these types of cancers (e.g., African American women) (ACS, 2013, p. 9).

The purpose of assessing risk factors is to identify a patient's likelihood of developing breast cancer and to work with him or her to modify controllable factors. Refer to Box 19.1 for breast cancer risk factors that you should review with patients. These include increased age, prior history of breast cancer, family history, genetics, reproductive history, having children, history of breastfeeding, alcohol consumption, tobacco use, and ethnicity (ACS, 2013).

If a patient already has a breast condition, it is important to gather more information about its effects and how it is being treated. This information provides needed information to implement appropriate interventions that will control or improve symptoms and prevent complications. Additionally, these discussions illuminate areas in which patients need further follow-up or education. Questioning and education can occur simultaneously.

History and Risk Factors	Rationale
Personal History Have you ever been diagnosed with breast cancer? • If yes, what kind of breast cancer? • When was it diagnosed? • Any treatment? What and when? • At what age were you diagnosed? • How were you treated?	To encourage diligent breast examinations and medical follow-up, it is important to evaluate the patient's previous breast conditions, especially those that may increase risk for breast cancer (i.e., personal history of previous breast cancer or cancer in situ; previous atypical epithelial hyperplasia found on biopsy; personal history of endometrial, colon, ovarian, or thyroid cancer; or family history of breast cancer). Previous history of breast cancer increases risk for a new mass being cancerous by two to four times (ACS, 2013).

(table continues on page 534)

History and Risk Factors	Rationale
Have you ever been diagnosed with any breast conditions such as cysts or benign breast disease (BBD), fibroadenoma, or breast abscess?	**Cysts** (due to BBD) are common lumps that are usually elliptical or round, soft, and mobile. Size may vary, and they often occur in multiple numbers, usually in both breasts, and frequently in the upper outer quadrants (Katz & Dotters, 2012). They occur during the childbearing years and are most tender just before menses. BBD with a positive biopsy for atypical hyperplasia (increased abnormal cells) or lobular carcinoma in situ carries an increased risk for breast cancer later in life (Katz & Dotters, 2012). **Fibroadenoma** is a well-defined, usually single (may be multiple), nontender, firm or rubbery, round or lobular mass that is freely movable. It does not change in size with menses as BBD does and occurs most commonly in patients in their 20s–40s (Katz & Dotters, 2012). **Breast abscess** (infection) may occur after **mastitis** (inflammation from a blocked duct that may develop with lactation), traumatic injury, or chest/breast surgery.
Have you ever had breast surgery? • If yes, what kind (e.g., breast biopsy, reduction, augmentation, mammoplasty, mastectomy)? • What was the result of the surgery?	Surgery of the breast is very personal; patients may have difficulty talking openly about it. A relaxed but professional demeanor is especially important when obtaining this information. A patient who has had breast augmentation (enlargement) could have the complication of a ruptured implant.
Have you been tested for the BRCA1 or BRCA2 mutation?	It is important to determine whether and why a patient has been tested for BRCA1 and/or BRCA2 mutations. If the patient *has* been tested, it is essential to ask about the results and the follow-up plan of care (e.g., genetic counseling, evaluation by breast oncologist).
Have you been treated for a breast infection recently?	Recent breast infection may block ducts, causing a change in breast tissue.
When was your last period?	Breast tissue may be tender in the days before the onset of menses.
Have you ever been pregnant? • If so, did you give birth? • What age did you give birth? • Did you breastfeed your child/children? • If so, for how many months?	Pregnancy before age 30 years has been associated with an overall decreased risk of breast cancer (ACS, 2013). Breastfeeding children for at least a year or longer has been associated with a slight reduction in breast cancer (ACS, 2013).
Lifestyle and Personal Habits	
Do you jog or run? If so, do you wear a sports bra?	Jogging or running increases breast movement, which may put strain on the shoulders or back. The effects of running in a regular or sports bra is uncertain (Scurr, White, & Hedger, 2010).
Do you drink alcohol? If so, how often and how much do you drink per day or per week?	Consumption of 10 g of alcohol (i.e., one drink per day) has been associated with a 7%–12% increased risk of breast cancer (regardless of the type of drink consumed) (ACS, 2013, p. 16)
Do you smoke tobacco? If so, for how long and how many cigarettes a day do you smoke?	Tobacco use has been associated with an increased risk of developing breast cancer (ACS, 2013).

(table continues on page 535)

History and Risk Factors	Rationale
Breast Examination Have you ever had a clinical breast examination? If so, how often? Have you been taught how to perform self-breast examinations (SBEs)? • If yes: How often do you perform them? Can you show me how you perform your SBEs? • If no: Would you like me to show you how to perform an SBE?	Monthly SBE coupled with yearly clinical breast examinations (CBE) by a medical professional increase the chances of detecting cancer in early stages. To optimize health maintenance, women should familiarize themselves at a young age with how their breasts normally feel to detect even slight changes. Women who perform SBE are more likely to discover cancer at an earlier stage (Katz & Dotters, 2012). For this reason, it is important to guide patients through SBE that emphasizes timing, inspection, and palpation.
Have you ever had a mammogram, ultrasound, or magnetic resonance imaging (MRI)? If yes, when was it done and what were the results?	Annual mammograms should begin at age 40 years; ultrasounds should begin at an earlier age if indicated; MRIs are only recommended in certain circumstances and are not routine (ACS, 2013).
Medications Are you taking any medications? • What medications? What is the dose and schedule?	Some medications that can affect breasts are listed in the following chart:

	Female	Male
Androgens	Decreased breast size	Gynecomastia
Antidepressants	Engorgement	Gynecomastia
Antipsychotics	Engorgement, mastalgia, galactorrhea	Gynecomastia
Cardiac glycosides	—	Gynecomastia
Progestins	Galactorrhea, breast tenderness	—
Menopause hormone therapy (estrogens, progestins)	Galactorrhea, breast tenderness. Long-term use of menopause hormone therapy has been associated with increased risk of breast cancer (ACS, 2013).	—

Are you taking any natural supplements or over-the-counter medications? • Which ones, and how often?	Although over-the-counter supplements are not known to affect breast lumps or pain, they may interfere with concurrent medications and contribute to adverse effects.
Family History Do you have a family history of breast cancer? • If so, who had it? • What type of breast cancer was it? • How old was she (he) when it was diagnosed? • How was it treated? • Has anyone in your family been tested for the BRCA1 or BRCA2 mutation? If so, who, why, and what was the result of the test (if you know it)?	The patient's risk for breast cancer increases if one or more first-degree blood relatives (e.g., mother, sister, daughter, brother) had breast cancer (especially if it was diagnosed before the affected person was 40 years old). Breast cancer in second-degree relatives (e.g., grandmother, aunt) also may increase the patient's risk.

Risk Reduction and Health Promotion

As a nurse, you are often the primary patient educator. The promotion of healthy behaviors and teaching about risk reduction are very important nursing roles. A person's educational level and financial situation influence his or her ability to practice healthy behaviors. For example, women who have less than a high school education, those who are without health insurance, and those who recently immigrated to the United States are least likely to have had a recent mammogram (ACS, 2013).

BOX 19.1 Risk Factors for Breast Cancer

Modifiable

- **History of childbirth:** Nulliparity or having first child after age 30 years slightly increases risk.
- **Oral contraceptive use:** Controversial; findings suggest that women currently using oral contraceptives have a slightly increased risk, which declines when they stop use.
- **Combined and estrogen-alone postmenopausal hormone therapy (PHT):** Long-term combined (estrogen and progesterone) PHT increases risks of breast cancer and death from it; risks return to that of the general population within 5 years of stopping use of combined PHT. Long-term estrogen alone (estrogen replacement therapy [ERT]) increases risk of ovarian and breast cancer.
- **Breastfeeding:** Nursing children for 1.5–2 years may decrease risk.
- **Alcohol:** Risk is slightly higher for those who consume one alcoholic drink per day; risk increases to 1½ times that of non-drinkers in those who consume two to five drinks per day.
- **Overweight or obesity, especially after menopause:** Prior to menopause, the ovaries produce most of a woman's estrogen, and fat produces a small amount. After menopause, fat produces estrogen because the ovaries stop doing so. Estrogen levels can increase post-menopause with increased fat (which increases breast cancer risk).
- **Physical inactivity:** The ACS recommends 45–60 minutes of exercise at least 5 days/week to reduce breast cancer risk.

Non-modifiable

- **Gender:** Women are at a much greater risk of developing breast cancer than are men.
- **Aging:** Approximately two of three diagnoses of invasive breast cancer occur in women older than 55 years of age, whereas one out of eight occurs in those younger than 45 years of age.
- **Genetic risk factors:** Women with BRCA1 or BRCA2 genes have up to an 80% chance of developing breast cancer at some point in their lives. These mutations are most common in Jewish women of Ashkenazi origin, but they also occur in African American and Hispanic women. Other less common genes, such as ATM, CHEK2, p53, and PTEN, may also increase the risk of breast cancer.
- **Family history:** Having one or more first-degree relatives (i.e., mother, sister, daughter) with breast cancer doubles risk. Having two first-degree relatives with breast cancer increases risk fivefold.
- **Personal history of breast cancer:** Those with previous incidence have a three- to fourfold increased risk of developing breast cancer in another part of the same breast or in the other breast.
- **Race:** Caucasian women are slightly more likely to develop breast cancer, but African American women are slightly more likely to die from it. Risk is lowest in Asian, Native American, and Hispanic women.
- **Abnormal breast biopsy results:** Proliferative lesions (overgrowth of breast tissue) without atypia (abnormal cells) increase risk 1.5–2 times that of normal; proliferative lesions with atypia increase risk 4–5 times that of normal.
- **Menstrual periods:** Women who begin menstruating before 12 years of age or stop after 55 years of age have a slightly increased risk.
- **Previous chest radiation:** Those who underwent such treatment for another cancer are at a significantly increased risk.
- **DES exposure:** Patients exposed to diethylstilbestrol (DES) have a slightly increased risk of developing breast cancer.

Controversial Possibilities

High-fat diets
Antiperspirants
Bras
Induced abortion
Breast implants
Environmental pollution
Tobacco
Night work

Adapted from American Cancer Society. (2007). *Detailed guide: Breast cancer. What are the risk factors for breast cancer?* Retrieved from http://www.cancer.org/docroot/CRI/content/CRI_2_4_2X_What_are_the_risk_factors_for_breast_cancer_5.asp

The health goals for breast health include the following:

- Increase the proportion of mothers who breastfeed their babies.
- Increase the proportion of women who receive breast cancer screening according to current guidelines to 80%.
- Reduce the female breast cancer death rate by 10%.
- Reduce late stage female breast cancer.

(USDHHS, 2013)

It is important for women to be aware of their specific risk factors for breast cancer. Although many factors are not modifiable, some are. When a patient is aware of her own specific risk factors, she may be more diligent in practicing healthy habits, such as monthly SBEs, yearly physical examinations, and mammograms if indicated. She may also adjust other personal behaviors, such as physical inactivity and obesity. Recommendations should be based on the patient's individual risk factors, such as age, heritage and family history, and number of relatives with breast or ovarian cancer at an early age (U.S. Preventive Services Task Force, 2009).

Primary care providers should discuss the potential benefits and risks of screening tests and develop a plan for early detection. The chief benefit is early detection and the chief risk is false-positive findings, causing unnecessary worry and further testing, such as surgical biopsies. Conflicting recommendations exist for SBE and mammography in some age groups. This text is following the American Cancer Society and American College of Gynecology screening recommendations as general guidelines for testing (ACS, 2013; American College of Obstetricians and Gynecologists, 2011). For further information, refer to Table 19.1.

As a nurse, you will teach patients how to perform SBEs and alert them to the importance of performing them monthly beginning in their early 20s. Recognizing what her normal breast tissue feels like alerts the patient to changes if they develop. Between ages 20 and 39 years, women should also have CBEs performed by a health professional every 3 years; from age 40 years onward, patients should have CBEs yearly.

TABLE 19.1 Partial List of Recommendations for Breast Cancer Screening

	Age 20–39 Years	Age 40–49 Years	Age 50–74 Years	Age 75 Years or Older	High Risk*
Self-breast exam	Against[†] Optional[**††]	Not routine[‡] Annual[**]	Every 2 or 3 years[†‡] Annual[**††‡‡]	Annual[**]	Annual[**††]
Clinical breast exam	Every 1–3 years[††]	Not routine[‡] Annual[††]	Not routine[‡] Annual[††]	Not routine[‡] Annual[††]	Annual[**††]
Mammography	Not routine[†] Every 2 or 3 years[‡]	Not routine[‡] Annual[**††] Annual[**††‡‡]	Annual[**††] Every 2 years[†] Annual[**††‡‡]		

*Consider genetic testing, contrast-enhanced MRI, and ultrasound

[†]U.S. Preventive Services Task Force. (2009). *Screening for breast cancer.* Retrieved from http://www.uspreventiveservicestaskforce.org/uspstf/uspsbrca.htm

[‡]Canadian Task Force on Preventive Health Care. (2011). Recommendations on screening for breast cancer in average risk women. *Canadian Medical Association Journal,* 183(17), 1991.

**American Cancer Society. (2012). Cancer screening in the United States: 2012. *CA: A Cancer Journal for Clinicians,* 62(2), 129.

[††]American College of Obstetricians and Gynecologists. (2011). *Breast cancer screening. Obstetrics and Gynecology,* 118(2, Pt. 1), 372.

[‡‡]American College of Radiology & Society of Breast Imaging. (2010). Guideline on imaging screening for breast cancer. *Journal of American College of Radiology,* 7(1), 18.

They also should begin yearly (or every other year) mammograms at age 40 years. Women at high risk should have an MRI and a mammogram every year. Women at moderately increased risk should talk with their care providers about the benefits and limitations of adding MRI screening to their yearly mammogram (ACS, 2013). Refer to SBE instructions later in the chapter.

Common Symptoms

When conditions associated with the breasts are present, ask the patient about symptoms that occur most often. If the patient reports experiencing any of these common symptoms, further assess for important characteristics of each symptom. You will use information obtained during the interview to determine the focus of the physical examination. A thorough history of the patient's symptoms is also necessary for identifying accurate nursing diagnoses and developing an optimal plan of care.

Common Breast and Axillary Symptoms

- Breast pain
- Rash
- Lumps
- Swelling
- Nipple discharge
- Trauma

Signs/Symptoms	Rationale/Abnormal Findings
Breast Pain Do you have any pain or discomfort in either or both breasts?	When asking questions about the symptom (pain in this case), it is important to gather all the relevant information.
• *Location:* Where is the pain? Can you point to where it hurts? Does it stay in the one spot or move around?	
• *Intensity:* Can you rate the pain using a 0–10 scale?	Severe pain (mastalgia) is more likely to result from trauma or infection.
• *Duration:* How long have you had the pain? When did the pain start? How long has it lasted? Does it fluctuate (or is it worse at certain times of the month)? Have you ever had this pain before? If so, when? Does the pain occur at the same time every month?	Breast pain is common at some point during a woman's life, especially during menstrual years. Pain may occur in one or both breasts and may be cyclical (same time each month). Cyclical pain is very common in women who take oral contraceptives or have BBD (Katz & Dotters, 2012). Typically, cyclical pain is worst in the days preceding menstruation and spontaneously disappears during or immediately after a period. It is often generalized, whereas pain from trauma is usually localized to one spot.

(table continues on page 538)

Signs/Symptoms	Rationale/Abnormal Findings
• *Quality/description:* Can you describe the pain (e.g., sharp, dull, throbbing, shooting, burning, tingling)?	Patients may describe noncyclic pain as sharp or burning; they tend to describe cyclic pain as heaviness.
• Do you have any other symptoms along with the pain (e.g., warmth or redness, fever, muscle aches, nausea, vomiting)?	Pain associated with warmth or redness at the site may indicate a localized infection. Fever, muscle aches, nausea, and vomiting may indicate a systemic infection.
• *Aggravating factors:* Does anything make the pain worse?	Pressure or trauma will make the pain worse.
• *Alleviating factors:* Have you tried anything to make it feel better (e.g., heat, ice, acetaminophen [Tylenol], or other medications)? If so, did it work?	Determining what treatments or remedies the patient has tried will help determine future treatments.
Rash Do you have a rash? If so, when and where did it start?	Rashes from contact dermatitis or eczema usually start on the breast tissue and move toward the nipple. Paget disease produces scaly lesions that begin at the nipple and progress to a lump behind the nipple well. Axillary rashes may result from allergy to deodorant or soaps.
Lumps Have you noticed any lumps in your breasts or axillae? • Where is the lump? • When did you notice it? • Has it changed at all (in size, is it more painful)? • If you have had previous lumps, does this feel the same or different? • Do you have a history of cystic breast changes or "lumpy" breasts?	Lumps can have many causes (e.g., BBD, fibroadenoma, cancer). It is important to investigate any lump, especially if it is new or if patients have noticed changes. You must also include information about the axillae because breast tissue and many lymph nodes extend to this area. Single breast masses can indicate benign conditions (e.g., cysts, fibroadenoma, fat necrosis, lipoma) or more serious conditions (e.g., cancer).
Swelling Do you notice any swelling of the breasts? • Is it cyclical (or are you breastfeeding)? • Is it in one area or does it involve your entire breast? • Has your bra size increased from the swelling?	Cyclical swelling and tenderness on a continuum corresponding with the menstrual cycle are common and benign. Patients experiencing this often complain of a "full" feeling in their breasts during menstruation, most often affecting both breasts.
Discharge Do you have any discharge from your nipple? • What is the color? • Could you be pregnant?	Nurses must evaluate spontaneous nipple discharge. Milky discharge in the absence of pregnancy or lactation (nonpuerperal galactorrhea) may result from hyperprolactinemia (caused by a prolactin-secreting tumor) or adrenergic medications (e.g., methyldopa). ⚠ *SAFETY ALERT* *Nipple discharge can be associated with a benign papilloma, ductal ectasia, and, less commonly, cancer. Early diagnosis and treatment are needed.*
• What medications are you taking?	Clear discharge may rarely occur from ingestion of steroids, calcium channel blockers, or oral contraceptives. Tranquilizers may also cause nipple discharge. When the medication is discontinued, the discharge will cease.
Trauma Have you had any injuries or trauma to your breasts? • When/how did it occur? • Did it cause any break in the skin (or any residual lumps, swelling, or discoloration)?	Injuries to the breast may cause a patient to feel a previously undetected lump or mass. A break in the skin could lead to an infection.

Documenting Normal Findings

Patient states she is without breast pain, lumps, nipple discharge, rashes, swelling, or trauma; no axillary lymph node enlargement or tenderness. Negative history of breast disease or breast surgery. Reports performing monthly breast exams; routine mammogram 9/10/10, which was "normal."

Lifespan Considerations

Additional Questions	Rationale/Abnormal Findings
Women Who Are Pregnant	
Do you feel that your breasts are getting larger or feel "full?"	Breast changes are expected during pregnancy. Providing reassurance and answering questions is beneficial.
Are you planning to breastfeed or bottle-feed your baby?	Breastfeeding provides antibodies that protect infants against illnesses and allergies and promotes bonding between mother and child. It has also been associated with a slight decrease in overall breast cancer risk if it is continued for 1 year or longer (ACS, 2013).
Are your nipples inverted (go inward) or everted (go outward)?	Reassure the pregnant woman that breastfeeding is possible with inverted nipples.
Adolescent Girls	
Have you noticed any changes in your breasts (e.g., are they getting larger or are they tender)? If yes, when did you first notice any changes?	It is important to assess the adolescent girl's perception of her own development and to provide appropriate teaching and reassurance.
Many changes occur as you grow up. Have you noticed any other changes? If yes, how do you feel about them?	This is a time when girls often compare themselves with other girls their age and body image is important to address.

Cultural Considerations

Additional Questions	Rationale/Abnormal Findings
At what age did you notice breast development?	African American females mature earlier than Caucasians (USDHHS, OMH, 2013).
Have you noticed variations in the color of your skin and nipple?	Variations in the color of the skin and nipple relate to ethnic background.
Are you eligible for a funded mammogram? What obstacles prevented you from obtaining it?	Overall factors that may impede access to health care include remote geographical location, lack of health insurance, low income, and cultural, racial, and language barriers (ACS, 2013).

Therapeutic Dialogue: Collecting Subjective Data

The nurse's role in subjective data collection is to gather information to improve the patient's health status and to help determine the cause of the patient's current symptoms. Remember Mrs. Randall, who was introduced at the beginning of this chapter. She was diagnosed with breast cancer 6 weeks ago, had a mastectomy, and is currently undergoing radiation. Some risk factors that the nurse assessed during subjective data collection were a family history of breast cancer in first-degree relatives (patient's mother and grandmother), early onset of menstruation (age 11 years), bottlefeeding of her children, obesity, a high-fat diet, and lack of exercise. In addition to obtaining a health history and physical assessment, the nurse also assesses the patient's coping skills. She is being seen at home by the visiting nurse.

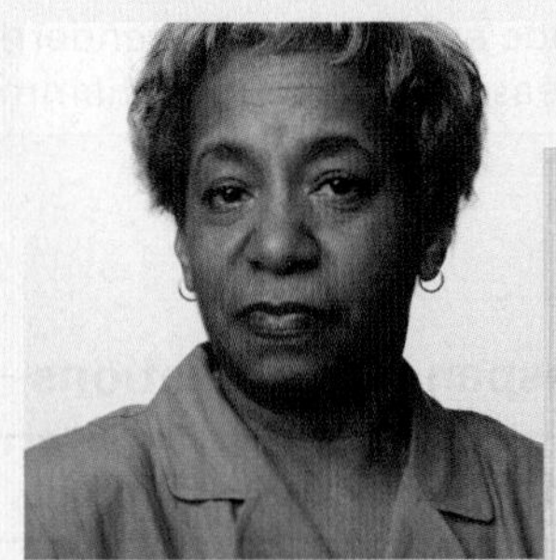

Nurse: Good morning, Mrs. Randall. How are you doing today?

Mrs. Randall: I'm feeling tired, real tired. (5-second pause) I can hardly get myself out of bed to eat. Why am I so tired?

Nurse: You sound a little discouraged.

Mrs. Randall: It's just been that after all of this happened, here I am feeling worse than when I started. (Begins to cry)

Nurse: (Silent. Touches Mrs. Randall on the arm, gives her a tissue.)

Mrs. Randall: I'm just tired of all of these treatments. And I'm worried that my breast won't heal. It's still all red and weepy (continues to cry).

Nurse: I'm sorry that you're not feeling well. Would this be a good time for me to look at it with you?

Critical Thinking Challenge

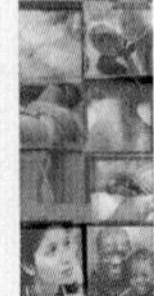

- Why is the dialogue effective when the nurse's question and response prompted Mrs. Randall to cry?
- How did the nurse respond to Mrs. Randall's crying? Provide rationale.
- In addition to assessing Mrs. Randall's breast lump, what other areas will the nurse assess?

Objective Data

Common and Specialty or Advanced Techniques

The **CBE** is an important part of a woman's health care. It provides an opportunity to identify breast disease, initiate early treatment, and demonstrate techniques for SBE. It is a good time to remind patients that mammography may not always detect breast cancer and that they should perform SBE monthly. Variations in clinician technique and experience affect actual findings. As with any examination, the more breast examinations you perform, the more likely it is that you will be to identify abnormalities or variations. Additionally, using a standardized and systematic approach to palpate the breasts increases the likelihood of detecting breast changes and abnormalities. The following sections review actual techniques.

The comprehensive head-to-toe assessment includes the most important and common assessment techniques. You may add focused or advanced techniques if you are concerned about a specific finding. Generally, the registered nurse (RN) does not examine the breasts of patients unless a condition exists in the breast, such as recent breast surgery. The advanced practice registered nurse (APRN) includes a breast assessment with the comprehensive assessment, such as an annual physical examination. Common and advanced practice techniques are summarized in the table.

Equipment

- Ruler marked in centimeters
- Small pillow
- Pamphlet or handout for SBE
- Gloves (if drainage is present)
- Adequate lighting

Technique	Purpose	Screening or Registered Nurse Assessment	Focused or Advance Practice Examination
Inspection of the breast	To assess lactation, healing, infection	X	
Complete breast examination	A yearly examination by a health care professional (medical doctor, nurse practitioner, physician's assistant) as an adjunct to mammography to detect and evaluate breast abnormalities at an early stage		X
Transillumination of breast mass	Using a strong light to differentiate between a fluid-filled or solid mass		X

Table title: **Basic Versus Focused/Specialty or Advanced Techniques Related to Breasts and Axillae Assessment**

Preparation

Keep in mind that hands-on palpation of the breasts may cause the patient to feel apprehensive and embarrassed. Adopting a professional, gentle, and reassuring approach is important. Before beginning, inform the patient that you will be examining the breasts. Provide as much privacy as possible and answer any questions the patients may have. This is an opportune time to ask a female patient whether she performs monthly SBE. If not, instructing her and watching return demonstration can provide an opportunity to verify technique and provide helpful correction as indicated.

The best time to examine the breasts is when they are least congested and smallest (in adult women, Days 4 to 7 of the menstrual cycle).

The breast examination involves inspection and palpation. Expose both breasts fully initially during inspection to assess for symmetry, but then cover or drape one breast while palpating the other. At the beginning of the exam, the patient should be sitting; ask the patient to move the arms into different positions (first at the sides, then over the head, then against the hips while leaning forward). For palpation, the patient should be supine.

Comprehensive Physical Assessment

Technique and Normal Findings	Abnormal Findings
Inspection Begin with the patient sitting with arms at the sides (Fig. 19.6). Inspect skin appearance for	
• **Color and texture**: Skin tone determines actual color. Pale, linear stretch marks (striae) may be evident after pregnancy or if a woman has gained then lost significant weight.	**Erythema (redness)** and heat can indicate infection or inflammation. **Hyperpigmentation** can signify cancer. A unilateral vascular appearance could indicate increased blood flow to a malignancy (produced by dilated superficial veins). **Peau d'orange** (i.e., orange peel) appearance is caused by breast edema from blocked lymph drainage and indicates advanced cancer (Fig. 19.7). Rash or ulceration may occur in **Paget disease** of the breast. See also Table 19.4 at the end of this chapter.

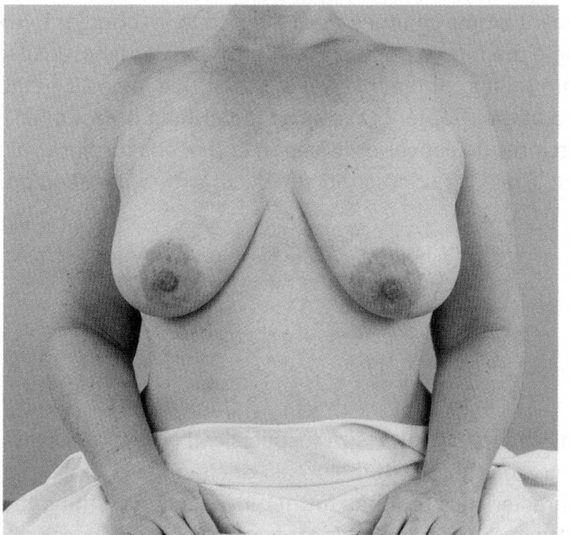

Figure 19.6 Patient sitting with arms at side as breast examination begins.

(table continues on page 542)

Technique and Normal Findings (continued)	Abnormal Findings (continued)
	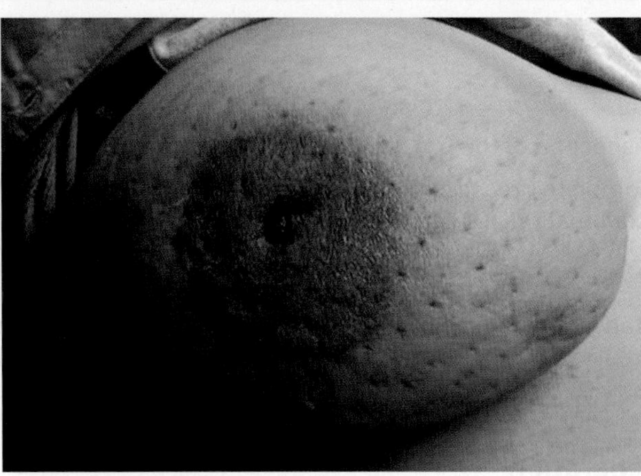 **Figure 19.7** Peau d'orange.
• **Size and shape**: Wide variation exists, from small to very large (pendulous).	If a patient has pendulous breasts, it is easier to visualize irregularities if she leans forward with her arms on her hips.
• **Symmetry**: The left breast is often slightly larger than the right breast.	Approximately 20% of women have one breast that is smaller compared to the other (Tenna et al., 2012).
• **Contour**: Should be uninterrupted.	Retractions or dimpling may occur with breast cancer (Fig. 19.8).

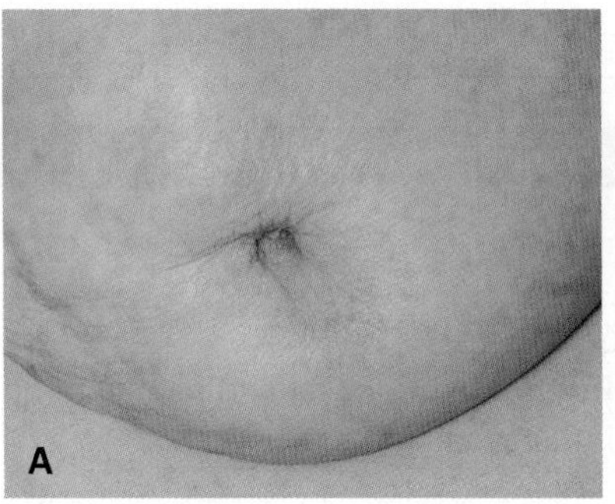

Figure 19.8 Retraction signs. **A.** Nipple retraction. **B.** Dimpling of skin.

Technique and Normal Findings (continued)	Abnormal Findings (continued)
• **Nipple and areola characteristics**: Areolae should be round or oval and pink to dark brown or black. Most nipples are everted, but it may be normal for one or both nipples to be inverted.	Recent nipple changes from everted to inverted or in the angle the nipple points may indicate malignancy (caused from pulling of the malignant tissue; see Table 19.4 at the end of the chapter.) Discharge (other than breast milk) can indicate cancer or infection and needs further evaluation. Cracking or crusting can occur with breastfeeding.
An extra nipple (supernumerary nipple) along the embryonic nipple line (from axilla to groin bilaterally) is a common variation. If present, it is most often found 5–6 cm (about 2 or 2½ in.) below the breast. On initial inspection, it looks like a mole, but on careful inspection, you will see a tiny nipple and areola.	
After inspecting with the arms at the side, reinspect with the patient lifting the arms over head (Fig. 19.9A), pressed firmly on the hips (Fig. 19.9B), standing and leaning forward from the waist (Fig. 19.9C), and then lying supine (Fig. 19.9D).	Any change in color, size (especially if unilateral), symmetry, or contour of the breast or change in nipple characteristics requires further investigation. Lifting the arms over the head adds tension to the suspensory ligaments and accentuates any dimpling or retraction. Leaning forward may reveal breast or nipple asymmetry.

(table continues on page 543)

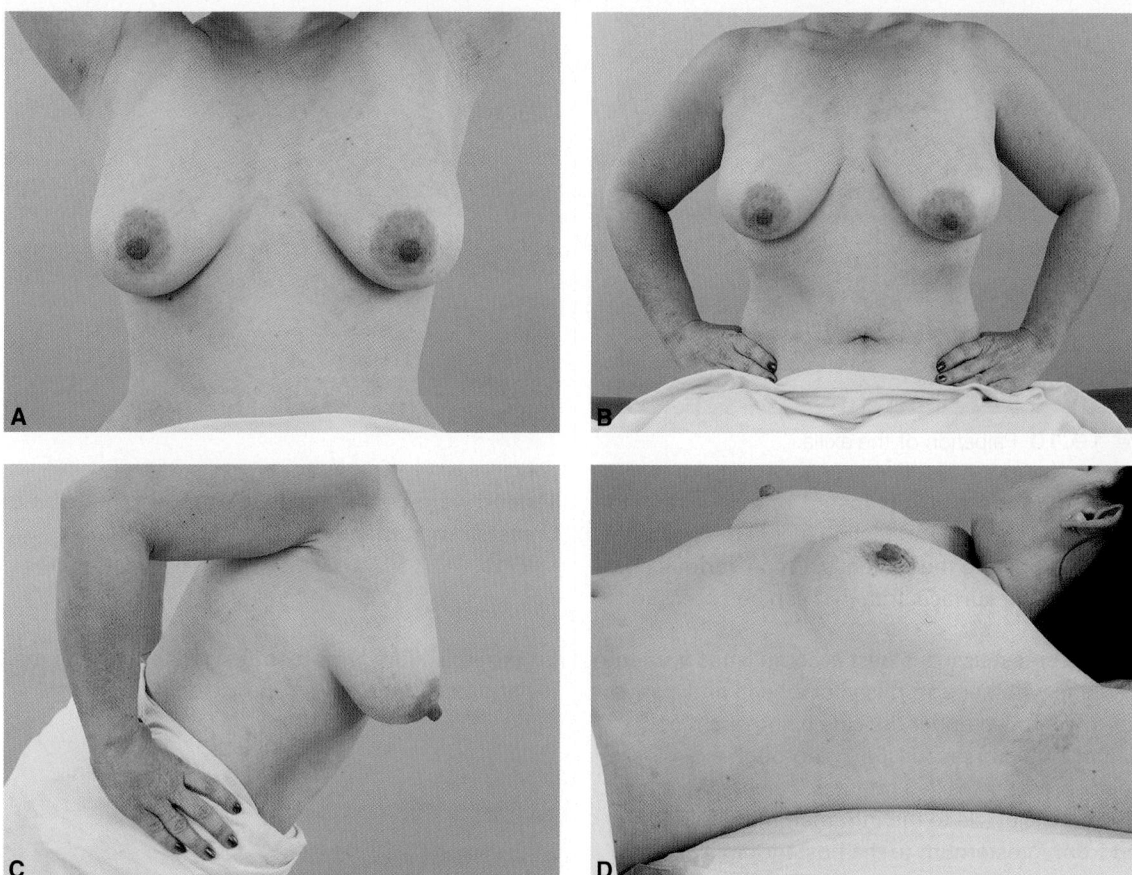

Figure 19.9 **A.** Arms over head. **B.** Arms pressed firmly on the hips. **C.** Leaning forward from the waist. **D.** Lying supine.

In addition, inspect the axillae while the patient is sitting, noting any rashes, infection, texture changes, or unusual pigmentation.

Breasts are symmetrical; skin is smooth and even without redness, bulging, or dimpling. No rash, edema, or lesion is found. Nipples are symmetrical and protuberant. Nipples and areolae are the same color and smooth or wrinkled in appearance. No discharge (unless the woman is pregnant or lactating), cracking, or crusting noted.

These signs suggest underlying cancer but may also be from benign lesions (e.g., fat necrosis, mammary duct ectasia). Rashes or infection may occur from laundry detergent or deodorant. Velvety axillary skin or deep pigmentation is associated with malignancy.

Palpation

Palpating the supraclavicular and intraclavicular areas and the axillae is best performed while the patient is sitting. Instruct the patient to gently raise the arm. Support the arm and wrist to aid in muscle relaxation. Use the right hand to palpate the left axilla and the left hand to palpate the right axilla (Fig. 19.10). Point your fingers toward the midclavicle, directly behind the pectoral muscles.

Feel for the central nodes, which are against the chest wall, because these are the most easily palpable. *One or more small, soft, nontender nodes are common findings.* Also assess the other axillary lymph nodes, but be aware that these are more difficult to palpate. Pectoral nodes are located inside the border of the pectoral muscle. Lateral nodes are located along the upper humerus, high in the axilla.

Firm, hard, enlarged nodes (greater than 1 cm [about ½ in.) that are fixed to underlying tissues or skin suggest malignancy.

(table continues on page 544)

Technique and Normal Findings (continued)	Abnormal Findings (continued)
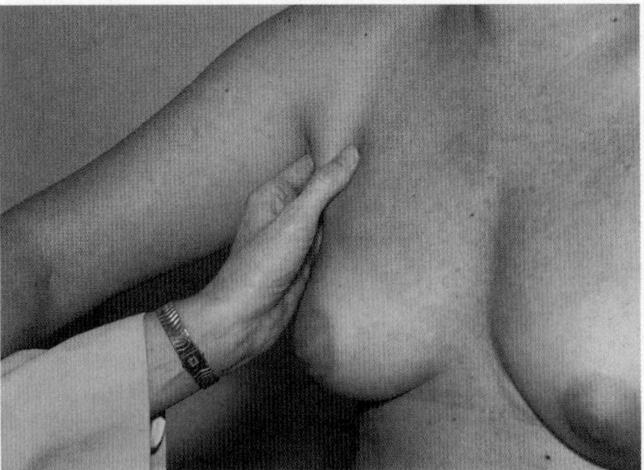 Figure 19.10 Palpation of the axilla.	
Subscapular nodes are best palpated with the examiner standing behind the patient, feeling inside the posterior axillary fold. Adjusting the patient's arm in various positions increases the surface area that can be assessed.	Tender, warm, enlarged nodes suggest infection of the breast, arm, or hand.
Palpating the breast tissue is best accomplished with the patient supine with her arm raised overhead and a small pillow or towel rolled under the side being examined. This will flatten the breast tissue. A thorough examination of each breast takes 2–3 minutes. Palpate the entire breast from the clavicle to the inframammary fold (bra line) and from midsternum to the posterior axillary line, making sure to examine the tail of Spence (Fig. 19.11).	Enlarged axillary lymph nodes are sometimes mistaken for nodules in the tail of Spence and vice versa.
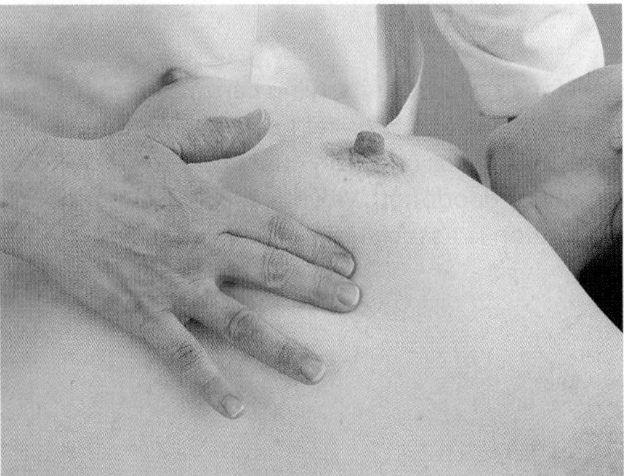 Figure 19.11 Palpation of the breasts with the patient supine.	
Various techniques for palpation can be performed. The ACS (2014) currently recommends using the **vertical pattern** (Fig. 19.12A) because some evidence supports that this is the most effective means of examining the entire breast. For this reason, this technique is described in detail in the following discussion. The **circular pattern** (Fig. 19.12B) and **wedge pattern** (Fig. 19.12C) patterns are also commonly used.	

(table continues on page 545)

Technique and Normal Findings (continued)	Abnormal Findings (continued)
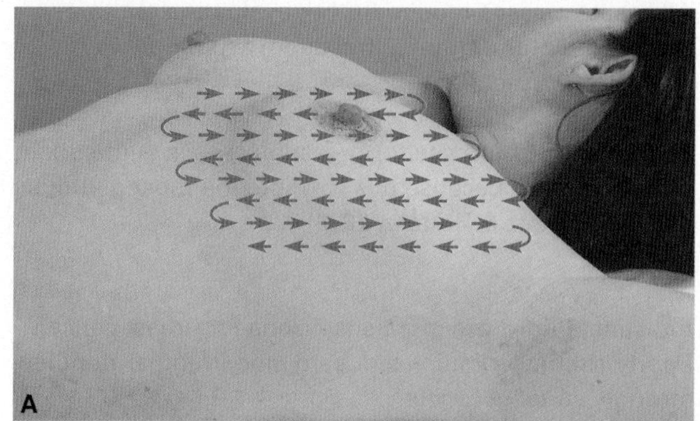 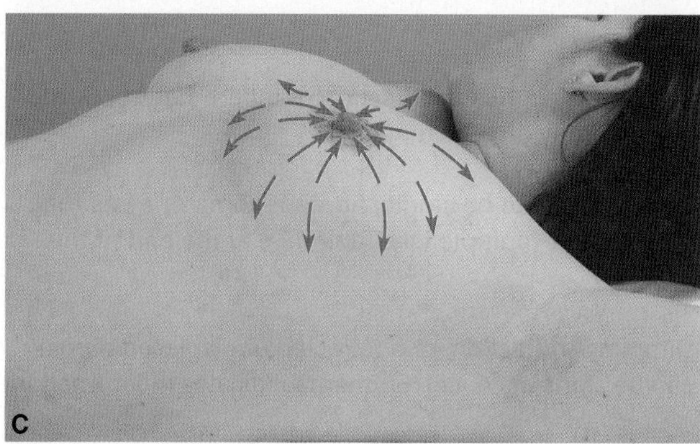	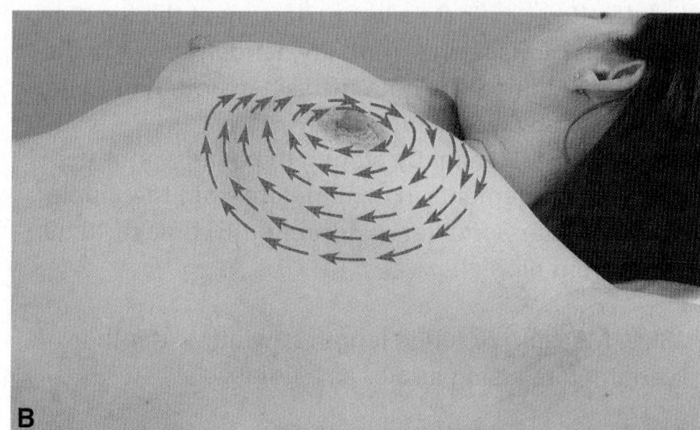 **Figure 19.12** **A.** Vertical strip pattern. **B.** Circular pattern. **C.** Wedge pattern.
Vertical Pattern. Using the finger pads of the first three fingers, palpate in small concentric circles beginning in the axilla and moving in a straight line down toward the bra line. Apply light, medium, and then deeper pressure at each examining point to reach the entire breast tissue. Continue in vertical overlapping lines until the sternal edge is met. Be systematic with the examination to ensure that you always assess the entire breast for consistency, tenderness, and nodules.	Sliding the fingers along the breast to palpate each section increases the likelihood of palpating the entire breast.
Consistency. Breast tissue shows wide variations. Nodular masses may be present before menses, disappearing after menses has occurred. *The breast of a nulliparous woman feels smooth, elastic, and firm. Before menstruation, breasts are often engorged secondary to increased progesterone. The patient may notice nodules, a slight enlargement, and tenderness during this time. Upon examination, the lobes may be more prominent with distinct margins. After pregnancy, breasts feel softer and have less tone.*	Mammary duct ectasia (dilated, painful mammary ducts) should be suspected when a lump or thickening is palpable. This benign condition may result from hormonal changes, smoking, or lack of vitamin A. Additionally, an inverted nipple may block the mammary ducts, which can cause inflammation and mammary duct ectasia.
When assessing a pendulous breast, the examiner may feel the **inframammary ridge**, which is a firm transverse ridge of breast tissue. This finding is expected.	Do not rush through the examination of a pendulous breast because lumps are harder to identify because of the increased size.
Tenderness. Breasts are often tender during the premenstrual period.	Tenderness or pain in the breast at other times may be from infection or trauma.

(table continues on page 546)

Technique and Normal Findings (continued)	Abnormal Findings (continued)
Nodules. If you palpate a lump, document the location, size, shape, consistency, mobility, tenderness, and distinctness. Additionally, note the skin over the lump, the nipple, and any lymphadenopathy.	All breast masses require further evaluation and may require a mammogram, ultrasound, aspiration, or biopsy (discussed later).
• **Location**: Document by stating the quadrant or use clock measurements in centimeters from the nipple (e.g., right upper outer quadrant or [R] breast, 10:00; 2 cm from nipple).	The most common site for breast masses is in the upper outer quadrant because this is where the most glandular tissue lies (Katz & Dotters, 2012).
• **Size**: Measure or judge length × width × depth in centimeters, using a ruler as a guide.	Indistinct lumps are more suspicious for breast cancer. Poorly circumscribed, fixed, hard, and irregular nodules strongly suggest cancer.
• **Shape**: Oval, round, lobular, nodular, or indistinct? • **Consistency**: Smooth, soft, firm, or hard? • **Mobility**: Movable or immobile? • **Tenderness**: Tender or not?	Tenderness indicates infection or inflammation. Some cancers may also be tender.
• **Distinctness**: One lump or multiple nodules?	Cancer tends to be single; fibroadenoma or cysts may be single or multiple (see Table 19.5 at the end of the chapter).
• **Skin**: Dimpled, retracted, erythematous?	Dimpling, retraction, or a retracted or displaced nipple can be signs of cancer. Erythema indicates inflammation.
• **Nipple**: Retracted or displaced?	
• **Lymphadenopathy**: Palpable lymph nodes? ■ Breast tissue is soft and homogeneous. No masses or tenderness. No lymphadenopathy.	Lymphadenopathy means swelling of the lymph nodes, which may occur postmastectomy, from blocked lymph nodes, or from infection.
Palpating the Nipple. Gently compress the nipple between your thumb and index finger to assess for discharge (Fig. 19.13). If discharge is evident, note the color, consistency, and amount. Massage around the areola if discharge is present to determine where it originates. ■ Nipple without discharge. 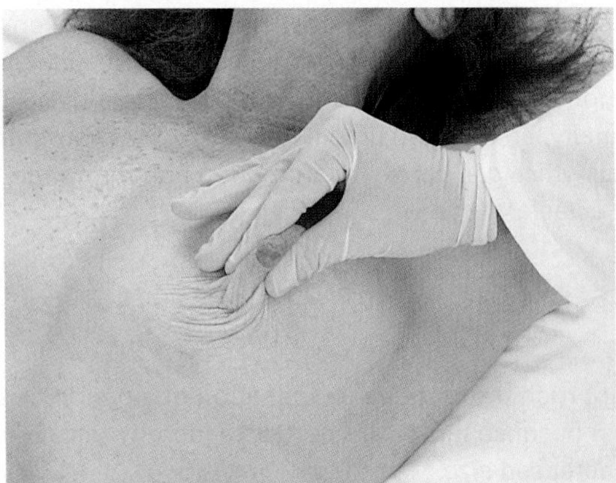 **Figure 19.13** Palpating the nipple.	If discharge is evident, it is important to obtain a cytological smear for examination.

(table continues on page 547)

Technique and Normal Findings (continued)	Abnormal Findings (continued)
Bimanual Technique. If a patient has pendulous breasts, the bimanual technique may be more efficient in palpating lumps. With this technique, the patient should sit upright, leaning slightly forward. Place one hand underneath the breast (on the inferior surface) while palpating the breast tissue with the other hand (Fig. 19.14). 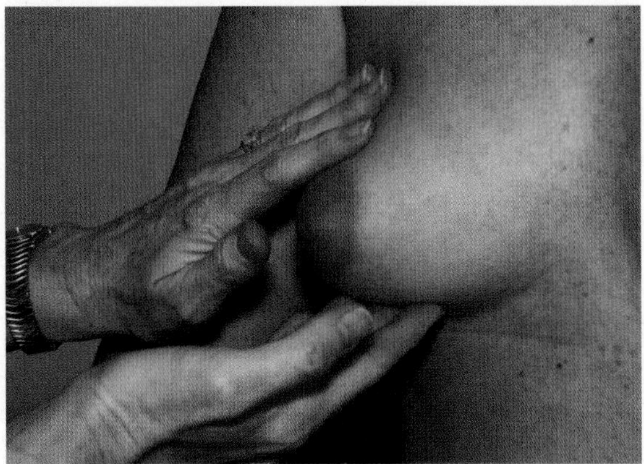 **Figure 19.14** Palpating the breasts using bimanual technique.	
Male Breasts Examining the male breast involves inspecting the nipple and areola for swelling, ulceration, or drainage. Additionally, palpate the areola and breast tissue for nodules or masses.	Firm, glandular tissue (**gynecomastia**) may occur when there is an imbalance of estrogen and androgen. An ulcer or hard, irregular mass suggests cancer. Obese men may have gynecomastia with increased fatty tissue. Gynecomastia also occurs with use of anabolic steroids, diseases, and as an adverse effect of some medications (see Table 19.4 at the end of the chapter).
Additional Techniques **Transillumination. Transillumination** of a breast mass may be performed in a darkened room to differentiate between a solid and fluid-filled mass. When a strong light is pressed up against a mass filled with fluid, the rays will pass through, but when pressed up against a solid mass, they will not. This technique is rarely used, having largely been replaced by mammography.	A solid mass is likely to be malignant, whereas a fluid-filled mass is more frequently a benign cyst (Katz & Dotters, 2012).
Examining a Patient Postmastectomy. A woman who had had a mastectomy may be more self-conscious about being examined than one who has not undergone this procedure. You must be empathetic and sensitive to her feelings. Malignancy can occur at the scar site or in other areas of the breast.	Masses, inflammation, color changes, and thickening may signify a recurrence of breast cancer.

(table continues on page 548)

Technique and Normal Findings (continued)	Abnormal Findings (continued)
Inspect the scar and axilla for signs of inflammation, rash, color changes, thickening, and irritation. Lymphedema may be evident in the axilla and arm secondary to impaired lymph drainage postmastectomy. Palpate the surgical scar and chest wall with the pads of two fingers in a circular motion (as previously described) to assess for breast changes (lumps, tenderness, thickening, swelling). Palpate the axillae and supraclavicular lymph nodes; assess for swelling and irritation. It is important to ask the patient to demonstrate SBE and to reiterate the importance of performing these monthly checks.	If the patient has undergone breast reconstruction, lumpectomy, augmentation, or reduction, perform the breast examination as described, paying close attention to the scar tissue.

Documenting Normal Findings

Inspection: (+) Symmetrical breasts, everted nipples. Palpation: (−) Palpable masses in breast or axilla, nipple discharge, rashes, or dimpling.

Teaching the Breast Self-Examination

After completion of CBE, it is appropriate to teach the patient how to perform a **SBE**. This practice is better than attempting to teach while performing the examination because it allows you to concentrate on the examination separately from concentrating on teaching. See Box 19.2.

Lifespan Considerations

Women Who Are Pregnant or Lactating

During pregnancy, breasts and nipples increase in size, which may cause mild discomfort. Linear stretch marks (**striae**) may be evident. Striae may disappear completely when breasts return to the prepregnant size. A blue vascular pattern may also be visible from increased blood flow. Nipples and areolae darken and widen. Montgomery glands become more prominent. Breasts may feel nodular, and nipples may expel yellow colostrum (milk precursor) after the first trimester.

If the woman is breastfeeding, milk production occurs most often by the third postpartum day. Breasts may become larger, reddened, warm, and engorged, especially at this time. Frequent breastfeeding will stimulate milk production, drain the breast sinuses, and resolve the symptoms. If these symptoms occur at other times during lactation, they could indicate **mastitis**, which usually requires antibiotic therapy as well as more frequent nursing to resolve. Nipples often become sore, but generally, this resolves spontaneously. If they become cracked and irritated, bleeding may occur.

After pregnancy and lactation, breasts return to their prepregnant state but often are less firm. The nipples and areolae usually remain darker than in the prepregnant state.

Newborns and Infants

As discussed previously, newborns may have enlarged breast tissue for the first few weeks of life from maternal estrogen. They also may secrete a clear white fluid from the nipples during this period. Should these findings occur, reassure parents or other caregivers that they are normal and will resolve spontaneously.

Children and Adolescents

On inspection, the symmetrical nipples of prepubescent children lie between the fourth and fifth ribs just lateral to the midclavicular line. The nipples and areolae are flat and darker than the rest of the breast tissue.

During puberty, girls begin to develop breasts (usually between 8½ and 10 years of age). As previously mentioned, breast tissue may be asymmetrical during growth. This temporary asymmetry may upset adolescents, who may need reassurance that this is expected and will resolve on its own. Breast tenderness may also occur. It is important to educate the adolescent girl about expected body changes that will occur during this time period. See Figure 19.5 for a review of Tanner staging.

Breast development before age 7 years in Caucasian girls or age 6 years in African American girls is termed precocious puberty and may be secondary to either dysfunction of the thyroid gland or a tumor of the ovaries or adrenal gland. Isolated breast development in the absence of other hormone-dependent changes (e.g., menses, pubic hair) in girls younger than age 8 years is termed **premature thelarche** (Diamantopoulos, 2007). Delayed development may occur in association with anorexia nervosa, malnutrition, or hormonal imbalance. Girls may be considered to have a developmental delay if

BOX 19.2 Breast Self-Examination Teaching Points

Begin teaching the SBE by assisting the patient to establish a regular SBE schedule. As previously stated, the best time for a SBE is when the breasts are least congested (the fourth to seventh day of the menstrual cycle, which coincides with the end of the menstrual period). In postmenopausal patients, the time of the month for the SBE is irrelevant because breast size remains stable. For these patients, a day of the month that they will remember (e.g., the first day of the month) may be a helpful suggestion.

Starting in their 20s, women may perform SBEs. Although most women will never get breast cancer, it is important for them to be aware of how their breasts feel and look so that they can immediately detect any changes. Emphasize to the patient that if she notices a significant change, such as dimpling or bulging of a section of the breast; a nipple that is inverted when it was previously outward; or a rash, soreness, swelling, or redness, then she should call her primary care provider for an appointment. Also inform the patient that many breast lumps are benign but that if a lump is cancerous, the survival rate is very high if it is detected and treated before it becomes invasive.

Women with breast implants should still perform monthly SBEs. Help these patients identify the edges of the implants so they can determine what is normal for them. Implants actually push breast tissue outward and may make abnormalities easier to feel.

Instruct the patient to begin SBE by disrobing and lying down with one arm under the head and a pillow under the side she is going to examine first. (If her right arm is under her head, she should place a pillow under her right side.) The patient should use the pads of the middle three fingers to feel the entire breast in an up-and-down pattern (Fig. A). The patient should make sure she checks the entire breast. Using a soft pressure allows the patient to feel the breast surface, a medium pressure gets a little deeper, and a firm pressure allows her to feel the tissue closest to the ribs and chest. Teach her to use all three levels of pressure during her SBE. She should repeat all the previous steps on her other breast.

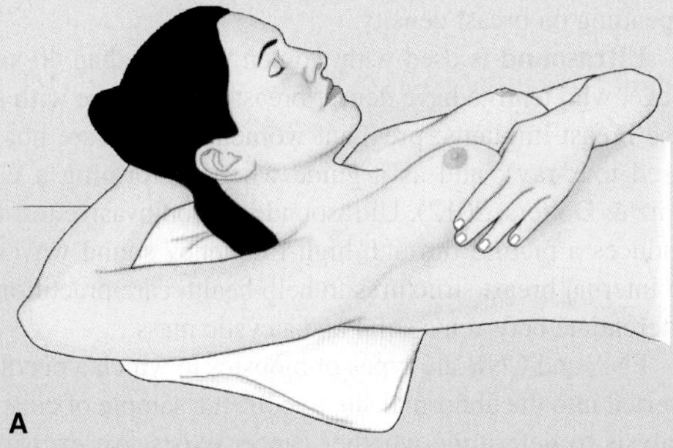

A

Next, she should look at her breasts in a mirror. Instruct her to keep her shoulders straight and her arms on her hips. Her breasts should be fairly equal in size, shape, and color (there may be some variation), without any swelling, discoloration, dimpling, or drainage from the nipple.

Instruct the patient to raise her arms over her head to look for equal movement of the breasts. Sometimes, raising the arms accentuates dimpling or the lagging behind of a breast if either is present (Fig. B).

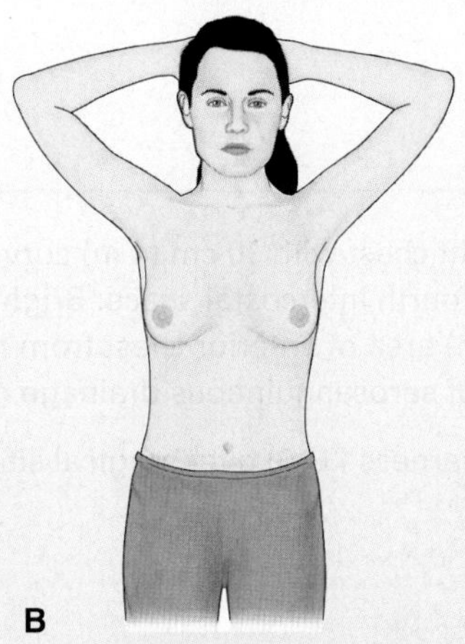

B

While the patient looks in the mirror, she should squeeze each nipple gently for any drainage. Generally, none is expressed (unless the woman is pregnant or breastfeeding, in which case there may be clear or milky white drainage).

From here, the patient should feel each breast in the same manner she did while supine (Fig. C). Often, women like to perform SBE while in the shower because the soap and water make the skin slippery.

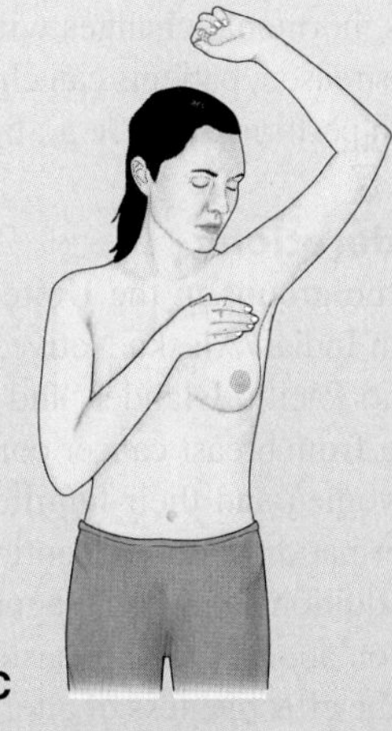

C

Instruct the patient to examine her underarm while she either stands or sits. It is easiest to feel the armpit with the arm only slightly raised because the skin is loose. The skin tightens when the arm is fully raised and makes it difficult to examine.

breast development has not occurred by age 13 years. Further evaluation is warranted if any of these conditions occur.

The breasts of an adolescent girl are uniform and firm. A mass at this age is most often benign (a cyst or fibroadenoma; see Table 19.4 at the end of the chapter). Adolescence is a good time to introduce patients to what their breasts normally feel like so that they will be more likely to perform SBE as they get older.

Older Adults

As a result of the relaxation of the suspensory ligaments and atrophy of the glandular tissue, the breasts of postmenopausal

Documenting Case Study Findings

Remember Mrs. Randall, who was seen by the visiting nurse for recent breast cancer surgery. She is concerned about her red and weepy skin. Think critically about the assessments that you will perform to evaluate Mrs. Randall for infection, inflammation and healing.

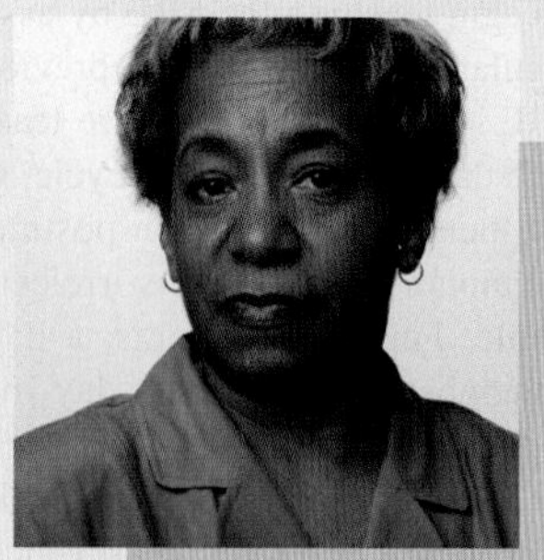

Inspection: Right chest with 10 cm (4 in) curved scar extending from axilla to right sternal border fourth intercostal space. Bright red erythema present over 15 by 20 cm (6 by 8 in) area of anterior chest from radiation treatment. Dermis is exposed, small amount of serosanguineous drainage noted.

Palpation: Tenderness (3/10) over surgical site.

women sag, flatten, and look more pendulous. On palpation, they may feel more granular. Nipples become flatter and smaller, and the inframammary ridge is more prominent from thickening. As women age, care providers should remind them to continue monthly SBEs and yearly CBEs because mature women are at increased risk for breast cancer. With the cessation of menses, hormonal changes will no longer affect their breasts. For this reason, patients can choose a convenient day of each month to perform SBEs (e.g., first day of month).

Cultural Considerations

The five major ethnic groups in the United States (African American, American Indian/Alaska Native, Asian American, Native Hawaiian and Pacific Islander, and Hispanic) have a greater risk of dying from breast cancer compared with Caucasians. Minority women and their families may not be receiving enough information about prevention, screening, and health promotion. Additionally, when diagnosed, they may be given less information about what the mastectomy procedure involves and about the effectiveness of alternative methods to make well-informed decisions about which breast cancer treatment option to choose—if they are indeed presented with a choice of options in the first place. Be aware of these issues and intervene considering these issues.

Critical Thinking

Laboratory and Diagnostic Testing

Mammography, ultrasound, MRI, and aspiration biopsy (fine-needle aspiration [FNA], core needle biopsy [CNB], or excisional biopsy) aid in accurately diagnosing breast cancer in 70% to 80% of cases (Esserman & Joe, 2014). A screening mammogram is suggested for patients at 40 years of age to detect nonpalpable breast masses (ACS, 2013; NCI, 2012).

Mammography consists of two x-rays (digital or conventional film). If a palpable mass has been detected, or if the woman has nipple discharge, magnification and additional views are necessary. A woman between 30 and 40 years of age may benefit from a mammogram if a mass is suspected, depending on breast density.

Ultrasound is used with women younger than 40 years of age, who tend to have denser breast tissue; those with silicone breast implants; pregnant women (so they are not exposed to x-ray); and as a guide when performing a CNB (Katz & Dotters, 2012). Ultrasound is a noninvasive test that produces a picture through high-frequency sound waves of the internal breast structures to help health care practitioners differentiate between a solid and a cystic mass.

FNA and CNB are types of biopsies in which a needle is inserted into the abnormal site to collect a sample of cells for analysis to determine whether cancer exists. An excisional biopsy is similar to a lumpectomy, in which the lump or suspicious area and a portion of the surrounding tissue are removed and examined. It is the standard procedure for lumps that are smaller than 1 in. in diameter and is performed on an outpatient basis.

MRI is a supplemental tool to mammography. This noninvasive painless test uses a magnetic field (not x-ray), radio waves, and a computer to detect and stage breast cancer and other breast abnormalities. It may be used for women with dense breast tissue (as in those younger than 40 years of age),

TABLE 19.2 Common Diagnostic Testing for Breasts	
Technique	**Purpose**
Mammography	Low-dose x-ray of the breasts to aid in the diagnosis of breast disease; should be performed as a screening tool annually beginning at age 40 years
Ultrasound	Noninvasive test using high-frequency sound waves; differentiates between a solid and cystic mass; is used as a guide in needle aspirations
MRI	Uses a magnetic field (not x-rays), radio waves, and a computer to detect and stage breast cancer and other breast abnormalities
Excisional biopsy	An excision (cut) made into the breast to remove a portion of a suspicious lump and the surrounding tissue to examine for cancerous cells
Microscopy	Viewing cells under a microscope to enhance cellular features
Ductogram	Examination of the breast ducts to determine cause of unilateral, single-pore nipple discharge
Cytological smear	Smearing and staining a cell sample (obtained from breast discharge) to determine cause
Thyroid-stimulating hormone	Blood test drawn to determine whether nipple discharge is secondary to a thyroid problem

with breast implants, or with scar tissue from previous breast surgery. It also may provide more detailed information to help determine treatment choices for a woman with breast cancer.

The clinical situation may indicate a need for additional tests (see Table 19.2).

Diagnostic Reasoning

You use assessment findings as the basis for ongoing care. An accurate and complete assessment provides a firm foundation for setting outcomes, providing individualized interventions, and evaluating progress.

Nursing Diagnoses, Outcomes, and Interventions

When formulating nursing diagnoses, it is important to use critical thinking to cluster data and identify patterns that fit together. You compare clusters of data with the defining characteristics (abnormal findings) for the diagnosis to ensure the most accurate labeling and appropriate interventions.

TABLE 19.3 Common Nursing Diagnoses Associated With Breast Cancer			
Nursing Diagnosis	**Point of Differentiation**	**Assessment Characteristics**	**Nursing Interventions**
Disturbed body image	Viewpoint or perspective of one's physical self that is significantly different from objective reality	Missing body part, avoiding looking at body part, behaviors of avoidance	Acknowledge feelings as normal when coping with change. Explore strengths. Encourage new clothes or wig in anticipation of changes.
Ineffective coping	Failure to address stressors; using methods to handle stressors that worsen or fail to solve the problems	Substance abuse, complaining without acting, lack of resolution of the problem, overeating, sleeping too much, isolating oneself	Observe causes of ineffective coping. Help identify resources. Discuss changes and previous successful coping strategies. Evaluate suicide risk.
Ineffective role performance	Behaviors that are out of the patient's usual context or character; failure to execute usual tasks	Inadequate resources to accomplish chores, change in normal responsibilities	Validate accomplishments. Locate community resources. Suggest physical accommodations.*
Grieving	Sadness related to loss of health, body part, function, or person	Sadness, crying, anger, depression, altered eating and sleep patterns, reliving past experiences	Encourage patient to express feelings and affirm that they are part of the grief process. Refer to spiritual counseling if indicated.

*Collaborative interventions.

A nursing diagnosis is a clinical judgment about responses to health problems or life processes. See Table 19.3 for a comparison of nursing diagnoses, abnormal findings, and interventions commonly related to the breast assessment in a patient with cancer (NANDA-International, 2012).

You use assessment information to identify patient outcomes. Some outcomes related to breast health include the following (Moorhead, Johnson, Maas, & Swanson, 2013):

- Patient looks at and touches changed or missing body part.
- Patient returns to previous social involvement.
- Patient verbalizes increased self-acceptance through positive self statements.
- Patient performs a SBE monthly.

After the outcomes have been established, you implement care to improve the status of the patient. You use critical thinking and evidence-based practice to develop the interventions. Some examples of nursing interventions for breast care are as follows (Bulechek, Butcher, Dochterman, & Wagner, 2013):

- Allow for privacy when examining breast tissue.
- Provide a mirror for the patient to visualize tissue and incisions.
- Teach SBE and encourage its monthly performance.

Progress Note: Analyzing Findings

The initial subjective and objective data collection is complete; the nurse has spent time reviewing the findings and other results. Mrs. Randall's skin is causing her discomfort. The radiation therapy is causing anorexia and fatigue. The following nursing note illustrates how subjective and objective data are collected and analyzed and nursing interventions are developed.

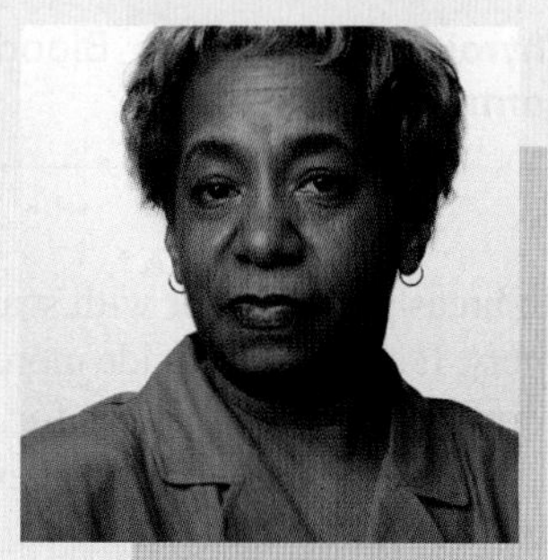

Subjective: "I'm tired, real tired. And I'm worried that my breast won't heal." She also states that she has no appetite and is fatigued.

Objective: Appears tired, crying intermittently. Skin color pale, moving slowly. Right chest with 10-cm (4-in.) curved scar extending from axilla to right sternal border 4th intercostal space. Bright red erythema present over 15 by 20 cm (6 by 8 in.) area of anterior chest from radiation treatment. Dermis is exposed, small amount of serosanguineous drainage noted. Tenderness (3/10) over surgical site with palpation.

Analysis: Fatigue related to recent cancer diagnosis, surgery, radiation treatments, and situational grieving. Impaired skin integrity related to radiation treatments.

Plan: Allow time to talk and express thoughts. Validate her concerns and appropriateness of her feelings. Assess support systems and who might be available to assist with home maintenance and meal preparation while she is fatigued. Evaluate the need for supplements to provide nutrition for wound healing. Observe her caring for erythematous skin. Keep skin clean, avoid skin irritation, and instruct on signs and symptoms of infection and when she should call physician.

Critical Thinking Challenge

- How will the nurse transition from collecting data about coping to collecting physical assessment data?
- What additional assessment data will be collected to evaluate adverse effects from the treatments?
- How do the coping, fatigue, treatment adverse effects, and ability to care for herself relate to each other?

Collaborating With the Interprofessional Team

Chore Services workers perform light household duties such as laundry, meal preparation, general housekeeping, and shopping. They direct services at maintaining patient households rather than providing hands-on assistance with personal care.

The following conversation illustrates how the nurse might organize data from Mrs. Randall and make recommendations about the patient's situation when making a referral to Chore Services.

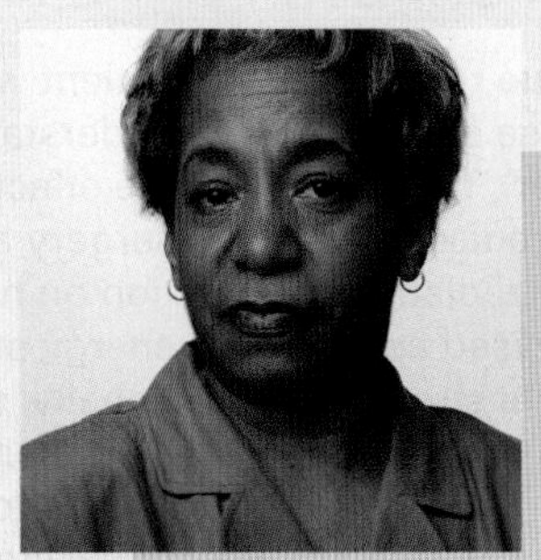

Situation: "Mrs. Randall is a 66-year-old woman who underwent a modified radical mastectomy for breast cancer 6 weeks ago and is currently receiving radiation therapy."

Background: "She has been experiencing severe fatigue and anorexia and is a good candidate for Chore Services to assist with shopping, cooking, and cleaning. She has a decreased appetite and cannot cook her meals or do her housework."

Assessment: "Increasing her food intake and rest will aid in healing, coping, and comfort. She seems very overwhelmed with all the changes she has had to deal with in the last 6 weeks."

Recommendations: "Please evaluate her mobility, strength, and home maintenance abilities. In particular, she may need an evaluation for housework and meals. Please let me know of your recommendations after your first visit. Your assessment in getting her some resources is greatly appreciated."

Critical Thinking Challenge

- What is the nurse's role in coordinating collaborative care with Chore Services?
- What family or community assessment information might be helpful?
- What other interventions might you recommend for Mrs. Randall?
- How will the nurse evaluate the effectiveness of the recommendations?

Pulling It All Together

The nurse uses assessment data to formulate a nursing care plan for Mrs. Randall based on a complete and accurate assessment. After completing these interventions, the nurse will reassess Mrs. Randall and document the findings in the chart to show critical thinking. The plan of care integrates separate parts of the nursing process. This thinking is illustrated in a care plan or case note similar to the following:

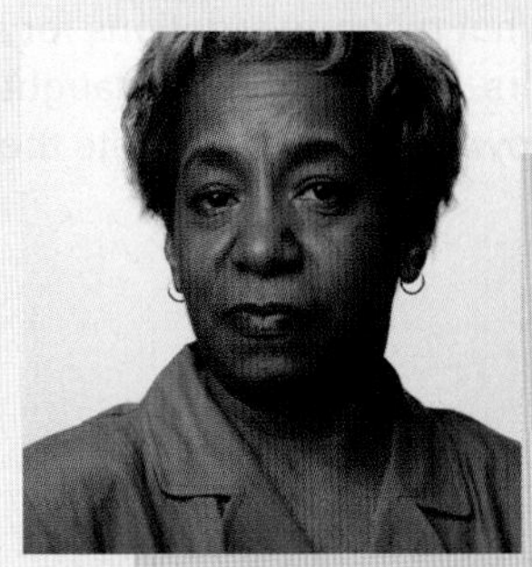

(case study continues on page 554)

Nursing Diagnosis	Patient Outcomes	Nursing Interventions	Rationale	Evaluation
Fatigue related to disease state (breast cancer), recent modified radical mastectomy, radiation, decreased appetite, and life stress	Patient will verbalize understanding of the effects of recent surgery and radiation on her overall energy state. Additionally, she will verbalize feelings related to her emotional state (stress from diagnosis and current treatments). She will also identify personal strengths and accept support within the next 2 weeks.	Educate the patient about radiation treatments and the expected course. Allow her time to ask questions. Offer emotional support. Allow time to talk and express thoughts. Validate her concerns and appropriateness of her feelings. Assess support systems and who might be available to assist with housework.	It is expected that a patient will experience fatigue at times with such recent surgery and while undergoing radiation. Confirming her feelings and assuring her that she will improve will aid in her recuperation. Effectiveness of coping is determined by the number, duration, and intensity of stressors. Her feelings are appropriate for the situation. Talking about her issues and finding support will help support her personal strengths during this difficult period.	Mrs. Randall is feeling less fatigued and more hopeful. She is looking forward to the end of her radiation treatments. Chore Services have recommended a worker for the next 6 weeks to come once a week to shop and do housecleaning. Mrs. Randall appreciates the support. Continue to follow patient regarding her ability to perform household chores.

Applying Your Knowledge

Using the previous steps of diagnostic reasoning, organizing, and prioritizing, consider all the case study findings woven throughout this chapter. When answering the following questions, begin drawing conclusions and see how the pieces of assessment must work together to create an environment for personalized, appropriate, and accurate care. Consider Mrs. Randall's case with her issues related to breast cancer, treatment, and side effects of treatment.

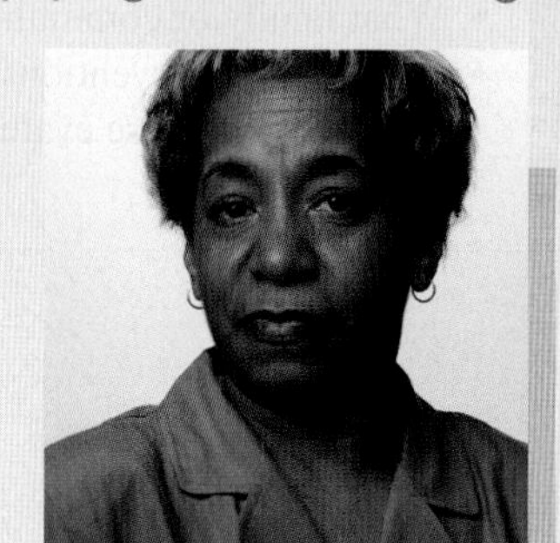

- What age group of women has the highest risk for breast cancer?
- Why is cancer in the upper outer quadrant of the breast at such high risk?
- Are Mrs. Randall's psychosocial or physical needs in this case more important?
- What lifestyle factors might be contributing to Mrs. Randall's risk for breast cancer?
- What recommendations for screening and follow-up would you suggest for Mrs. Randall and her daughters?
- How would you evaluate the success of interventions for Mrs. Randall?

Key Points

- To describe clinical findings, nurses should divide the breast into four quadrants by imagining lines that intersect at the nipple.
- The lymphatic spread of breast cancer may cause enlarged lymph nodes, most commonly in the tail of Spence.
- Women who are pregnant experience breast changes and enlargement beginning in the first 2 months of pregnancy.
- Breast enlargement may occur in newborns as a result of the influence of maternal hormones.
- Breast development in adolescent girls occurs over a 3-year period; the stage is identified by Tanner staging.
- Gynecomastia is common in approximately one third of adolescent boys; it usually resolves in 1 to 2 years.
- A new breast lump, change in existing lump, or bloody discharge from the nipple needs further investigation to rule out breast cancer.
- Nurses teach female patients how to perform a SBE as part of health-related patient teaching.
- Risk assessment for breast cancer includes seeking information about gender, race/ethnicity, menstrual history, combination oral contraceptive use, history of childbirth, breastfeeding, genetic risk factors (e.g., BRCA1 and/or BRCA2), alcohol abuse, tobacco use, combined and estrogen-alone menopausal hormone therapy (MHT), abnormal breast biopsy results, personal history of breast cancer, overweight or obesity (especially after menopause), physical inactivity, previous chest radiation, diethylstilbestrol (DES) exposure, and family history.
- Common signs and symptoms related to the breasts and axillae include breast pain, lumps, discharge, rash, swelling, and trauma.
- Palpation of the breasts may cause apprehension or embarrassment in patients; nurses provide reassurance and privacy.
- The best time to palpate the breasts is 4 to 7 days after the menstrual cycle begins.
- Size and shape of the breasts show wide variation.
- A supernumerary nipple is an expected variation.
- The sequence for inspecting the breasts is with the patient sitting with arms at the side, arms overhead, arms pressed on the hips, leaning forward at the waist, and lying supine.
- A vertical pattern of palpation is recommended.
- With pendulous breasts, a bimanual palpation technique is used.

Review Questions

1. When teaching the SBE, the nurse should inform the woman that it is best to perform the exam in which of the following times? Select all that apply.
   A. Just before the menstrual period
   B. Just after the menstrual period
   C. On the 4th to 7th days of the menstrual cycle
   D. On the 10th day of the menstrual cycle

2. A male patient presents to the clinic with a complaint of a hard, irregular, nontender mass on his chest under the areola. Upon examination, the nurse notes that the mass is immobile and suspects
   A. gynecomastia.
   B. benign lesion.
   C. Paget disease.
   D. carcinoma.

3. Gynecomastia may occur in an older male secondary to
   A. testosterone deficiency.
   B. lymphatic engorgement.
   C. trauma.
   D. decreased activity level.

4. When examining the breast of a 75-year-old woman, the nurse would expect to find which of the following?
   A. Enlarged axillary lymph nodes
   B. Multiple large firm lumps
   C. A granular feel to the breast tissue
   D. Pale areola

5. It is important to examine the upper outer quadrant of the breast because it is
   A. more prone to injury and calcifications.
   B. where most breast tumors develop.
   C. where most of the suspensory ligaments attach.
   D. the largest quadrant of the breast.

6. A 23-year-old nulliparous woman is concerned that her breasts seem to change in size all month long and they are very tender around the time she has her period. The nurse should explain to her that
   A. nonpregnant women usually do not have these breast changes and this is cause for concern.
   B. breasts often change in response to stress so it is important to assess her life stressors.
   C. cyclical breast changes are normal.
   D. breast changes normally occur during pregnancy and she should have a pregnancy test.

7. A patient with BBD is likely to
   A. develop breast cancer later in life.
   B. require hormone replacement therapy.
   C. be a teenager.
   D. resolve after menopause.

8. The nurse palpates a fine, round, mobile, nontender nodule and suspects that it is
   A. a fibroadenoma.
   B. a cyst.
   C. a fibrocystic breast change.
   D. breast cancer.

9. Peau d'orange appearance is highly suggestive of which of the following?
   A. Breast cancer
   B. Gynecomastia
   C. Papillomas
   D. Colostrum

10. The correct position in which to place the patient to palpate the breasts is
   A. left lateral position with arm over head.
   B. sitting forward with hands on hips.
   C. supine with arm over head.
   D. supine with arms at side.

The Jensen suite offers these additional resources to enhance learning and facilitate understanding of this chapter:

- thePoint online resource, http://thepoint.lww.com/Jensen2e
- *Laboratory Manual for Nursing Health Assessment: A Best Practice Approach*
- *Pocket Guide for Nursing Health Assessment: A Best Practice Approach*
- *Lippincott DocuCare,* an electronic health record simulation software, http://thepoint.lww.com/docucare
- *Adaptive Learning | Powered by PrepU*, http://thepoint.lww.com/prepu

References

American Cancer Society. (2012). Cancer screening in the United States: 2012. *CA: A Cancer Journal for Clinicians*, 62(2), 129.

American Cancer Society. (2013). *What are the risk factors for breast cancer?* Retrieved from http://www.cancer.org/cancer/breastcancer/detailedguide/breast-cancer-risk-factors

American Cancer Society. (2014). *Breast awareness and self-exam.* Retrieved from http://www.cancer.org/cancer/breastcancer/moreinformation/breastcancerearlydetection/breastcancer-early-detection-acs-recs-bse

American College of Obstetricians and Gynecologists. (2011). Breast cancer screening. *Obstetrics and Gynecology*, *118*(2, Pt. 1), 372

American College of Radiology & Society of Breast Imaging. (2010). Guideline on imaging screening for breast cancer. *Journal of American College of Radiology*, *7*(1), 18.

Bulechek, G. M., Butcher, H. K., Dochterman, J. M., & Wagner, C. M. (2013). *Nursing interventions classification (NIC)* (6th ed). St. Louis, MO: Mosby

Canadian Task Force on Preventive Health Care. (2011). Recommendations on screening for breast cancer in average risk women. *Canadian Medical Association Journal*, *183*(17), 1991.

Centers for Disease Control and Prevention. (2013). *Breast cancer statistics.* Retrieved from http://www.cdc.gov/cancer/breast/statistics/

Colvin, A. W., & Abdullatif, H. (2013). Anatomy of female puberty: The clinical relevance of developmental changes in the reproductive system. *Clinical Anatomy*, *26*, 115–129.

de Onis, M., Garza, C., Victora, C. G., Bhan, M. K., & Norum, K. R. (2004). The WHO Multicentre Growth Reference Study (MGRS): Rationale, planning and implementation. *Food and Nutrition Bulletin*, *25*(1, Suppl. 1), 1–89.

Diamantopoulos, S. (2007). Gynecomastia and premature thelarche: A guide for practitioners. *Pediatrics in Review*, *28*, e57–e67.

Esserman, L. J., & Joe, B. N. (2014). *Breast biopsy*. Retrieved from http://www.uptodate.com/contents/breast-biopsy

Ferrara, P., Giorgio, V., Vitelli, O., Gatto, A., Romano, V., Del Bufalo, F., & Nicoletti, A. (2009). Polythelia: Still a marker of urinary tract anomalies in children? *Scandinavian Journal of Urology and Nephrology*, *42*, 47–50.

Hassiotou, F., & Geddes, D. (2013). Anatomy of the human mammary gland: Current status of knowledge. *Clinical Anatomy*, *26*, 29–48.

Herman-Giddens, M. E. (2013). The enigmatic pursuit of puberty in girls. *Pediatrics*, *132*(6), 1125–1126.

Katz V. L., & Dotters D. (2012). Breast diseases: Diagnosis and treatment of benign and malignant disease. In G. M. Lentz, R. A. Lobo, D. M. Gershenson, & V. L. Katz (Eds.), *Comprehensive gynecology* (6th ed.). Philadelphia, PA: Elsevier Mosby.

Lemaine, V., & Simmons, P. S. (2013). The adolescent female: Breast and reproductive embryology and anatomy. *Clinical Anatomy*, *26*, 22–28.

Melmed, S., Polonsky, K. S., Larsen, P. R., & Kronenberg, H. M. (2011). *Williams textbook of endocrinology* (12th ed.). Philadelphia, PA: Saunders.

Moorhead, S., Johnson, M., Maas, M. L., & Swanson, E. (2013). *Nursing outcomes classification (NOC): Measurement of health outcomes* (5th ed.). St. Louis, MO: Elsevier

National Cancer Institute. (2012). *Mammograms.* Retrieved from http://www.cancer.gov/cancertopics/factsheet/detection/mammograms

National Cancer Institute. (2013). *Breast cancer risk in American women.* Retrieved from http://www.cancer.gov/cancertopics/factsheet/detection/probability-breast-cancer

NANDA-International. (2012). *Nursing diagnoses: Definitions and classification 2012–2014* (9th ed). Oxford, United Kingdom: Wiley-Blackwell.

Onstad, M., & Stuckey, A. (2013). Benign breast disorders. *Obstetrics & Gynecology Clinics of North America*, *40*, 459–473.

Rakel, R. E. (2011). *Textbook of family medicine* (8th ed.). Philadelphia, PA: Elsevier.

Scurr, J. C., White J. L., & Hedger, W. (2010). The effect of breast support on the kinematics of the breast during the running gait cycle. *Journal of Sports Sciences*, *28*(10), 1103–1109. doi:10.1080/02640414.2010.497542.

Tenna, S., Cogliandro, A., Cagli, B., Barone, M., Delle Femmine, P., & Persichetti, P. (2012). Breast hypertrophy and asymmetry: A retrospective study on a sample of 344 consecutive patients. *International Journal of Plastic Surgery*, *54*(1), 9–12.

U.S. Department of Health & Human Services. (2013). *2020 Topics & objectives – Objectives A-Z*. Retrieved from http://www.healthypeople.gov/2020/topicsobjectives2020/

U.S. Department of Health & Human Services, Office of Minority Health. (2013). *National breast and cervical cancer early detection program (NBCCEDP)*. Retrieved from http://www.cdc.gov/cancer/nbccedp/data/summaries/national_aggregate.htm#overview

U.S. Preventive Services Task Force. (2009). *Screening for breast cancer*. Retrieved from http://www.uspreventiveservices taskforce.org/uspstf/uspsbrca.htm

Tables of Abnormal Findings

TABLE 19.4 Breast Abnormalities

Carcinoma (skin, areola, and nipple retraction)

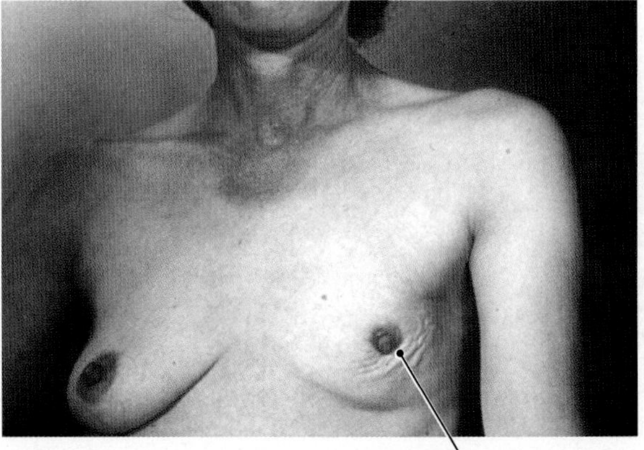

Carcinoma (bulging of breast and skin changes)

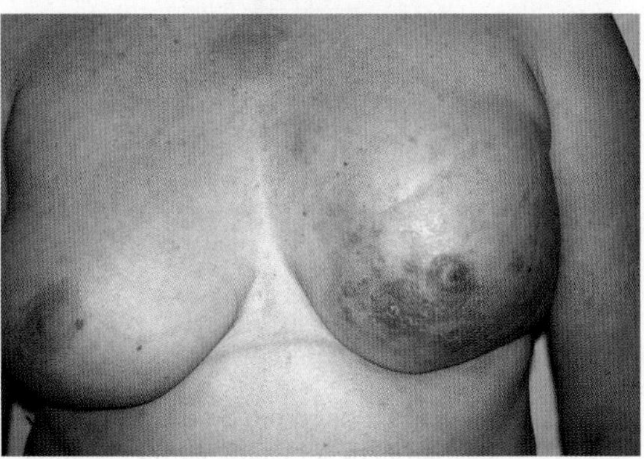

Paget disease (Follicular Keratosis)

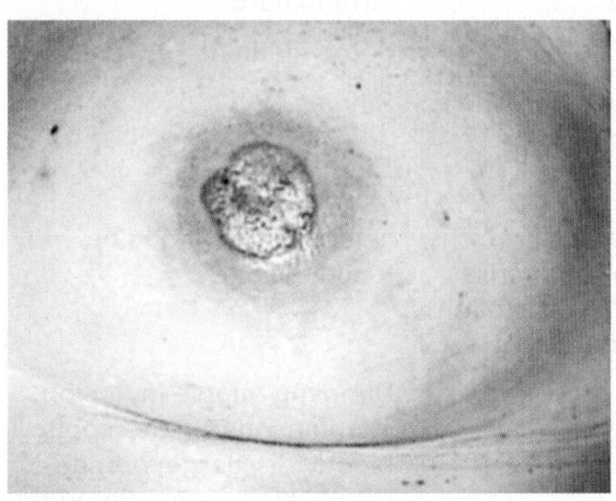

Mastitis

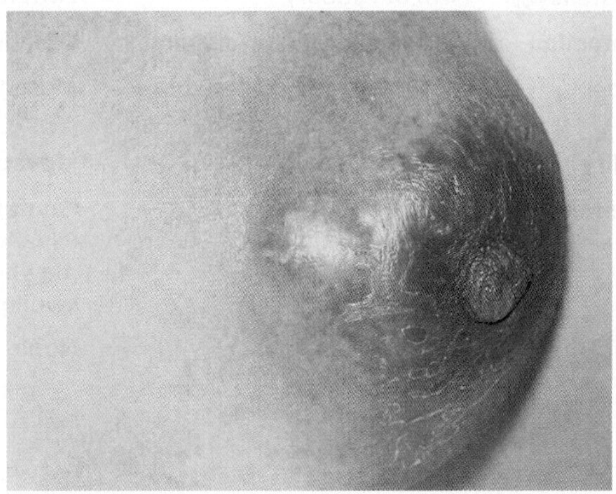

Mastectomy

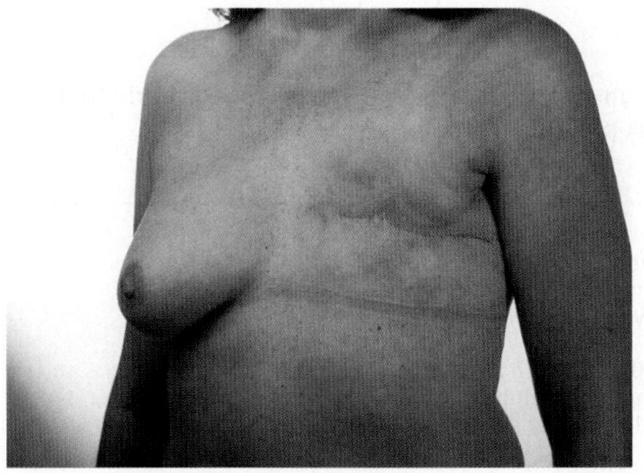

Gynecomastia

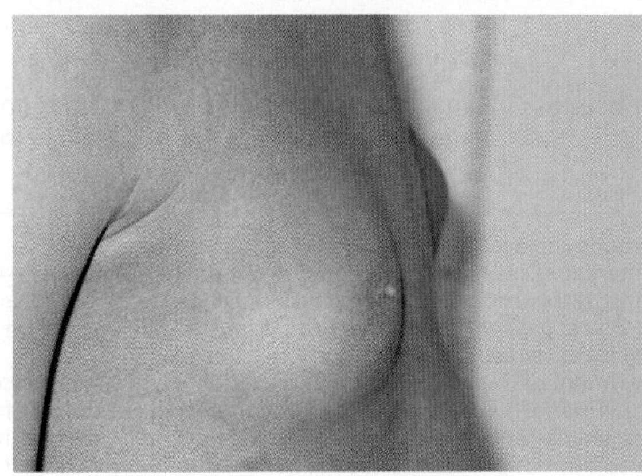

TABLE 19.5 Breast Lumps

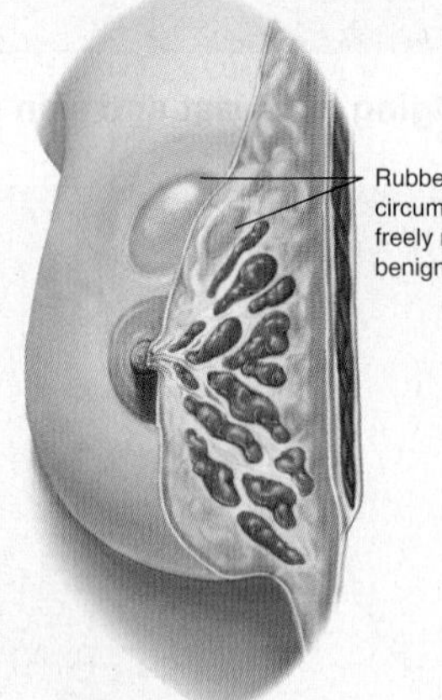

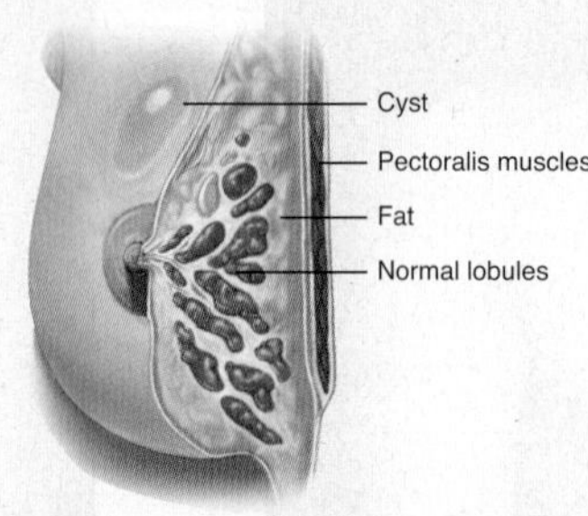

Characteristics	Fibroadenoma	Benign Breast Disease	Cancer
Likely age	Appears most often before 30 years (15–39 years; some up to 55 years)	30–50 years; incidence decreases after menopause	30–80 years; risk increases after 50 years
Shape/size	Oval, round, lobular, 1–5 cm	Round, lobular, variable size	Irregular, star-shaped, variable size
Consistency	Firm or rubbery	Firm to soft, rubbery	Firm to hard
Demarcation	Well demarcated, clear margins	Well demarcated	Poorly defined
Number	Most often single; may be multiple	Most often multiple; may be single	Single
Mobility	Freely movable	Movable	Fixed
Tenderness	Painless	Painful; breast tenderness, which usually increases before menses, may be noncyclical; breasts often swollen, usually bilateral	Nontender, but may be tender
Suspicious signs	None	None	Dimpling, nipple inversion, spontaneous single-nipple bloody discharge, orange-peel texture (peau d'orange), axillary lymphadenopathy
Pattern of growth	Rapid growing during pregnancy, with HRT, or if immunosuppressed; approximately 10% disappear spontaneously	Size may increase or decrease rapidly	Continually increases in size (at varying rates)
Risk to health	None; they are benign—must diagnose by biopsy	Benign, although general lumpiness may mask other cancerous lump	Serious, needs early treatment

HRT, Hormone replacement therapy.

From Centers for Disease Control and Prevention. (2013). *Breast cancer statistics*. Retrieved from http://www.cdc.gov/cancer/breast/statistics; Centers for Disease Control and Prevention. (2013). *Breast cancer rates by race and ethnicity*. Retrieved from http://www.cdc.gov/cancer/breast/statistics/race.htm;

U.S. Department of Health & Human Services, Office of Minority Health. (2007). *Health status of Asian American and Pacific Islander women*. Retrieved from http://minorityhealth.hhs.gov/templates/content.aspx?ID=3721; and National Cancer Institute. (2013). Breast cancer. Retrieved from http://www.cancer.gov/cancertopics/types/breast

20

Abdominal Assessment

Learning Objectives

1. Identify anatomical landmarks that guide assessment of the abdomen and documentation of findings.
2. Demonstrate knowledge of the anatomy and physiology of the body systems in the abdominal assessment.
3. Identify important topics for health promotion and risk reduction related to the anatomical systems found within the abdomen.
4. Collect subjective data related to the abdominal assessment.
5. Collect objective data related to the abdominal assessment using physical examination techniques.
6. Consider the condition, age, gender, and culture of the patient to individualize the abdominal assessment.
7. Identify expected and unexpected findings related to the systems in the abdominal assessment.
8. Analyze subjective and objective data from the abdominal assessment and consider initial interventions.
9. Document and communicate data from the abdominal assessment using appropriate medical terminology and principles of recording.
10. Identify nursing diagnoses and initiate a plan of care based on findings from the abdominal assessment.

Mr. Renaud, a 41-year-old Caucasian man, was admitted to the hospital with a gastrointestinal (GI) bleed. He has been on the acute care unit for 5 days following a 3-day stay in the intensive care unit (ICU). His temperature is 36.5°C (97.7°F) tympanic, pulse 102 beats/min, respirations 20 breaths/min, and blood pressure 148/92 mmHg. His current medications include a drug that blocks acid production and a liquid antacid. He is currently homeless and living in a shelter.

You will gain more information about Mr. Renaud as you progress through this chapter. As you study the content and features, consider Mr. Renaud's case and its relationship to what you are learning. Begin thinking about the following points:

- What techniques are used when assessing the anatomical systems within the abdomen?
- How will the nurse prioritize health promotion and teaching needs?
- How will the nurse organize the assessment during the shift?
- How does the nurse incorporate the different phases of the nursing process while performing the assessments?
- When Mr. Renaud's GI bleed is resolved, what recommendations do you expect the nurse, physician, and other members of the health care team to make as they continue to care for him?
- How will you evaluate whether your initial interventions are effective?

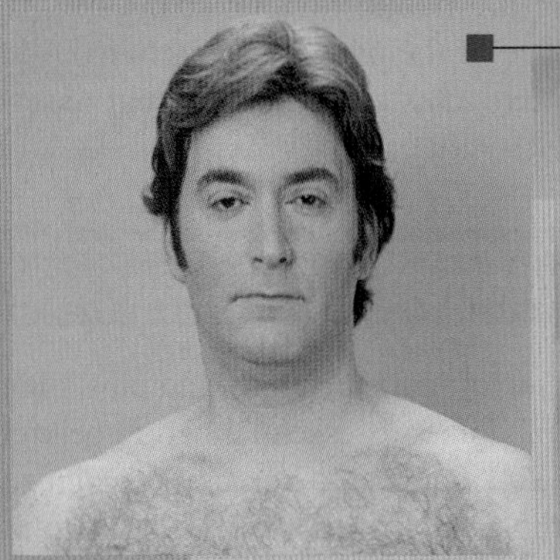

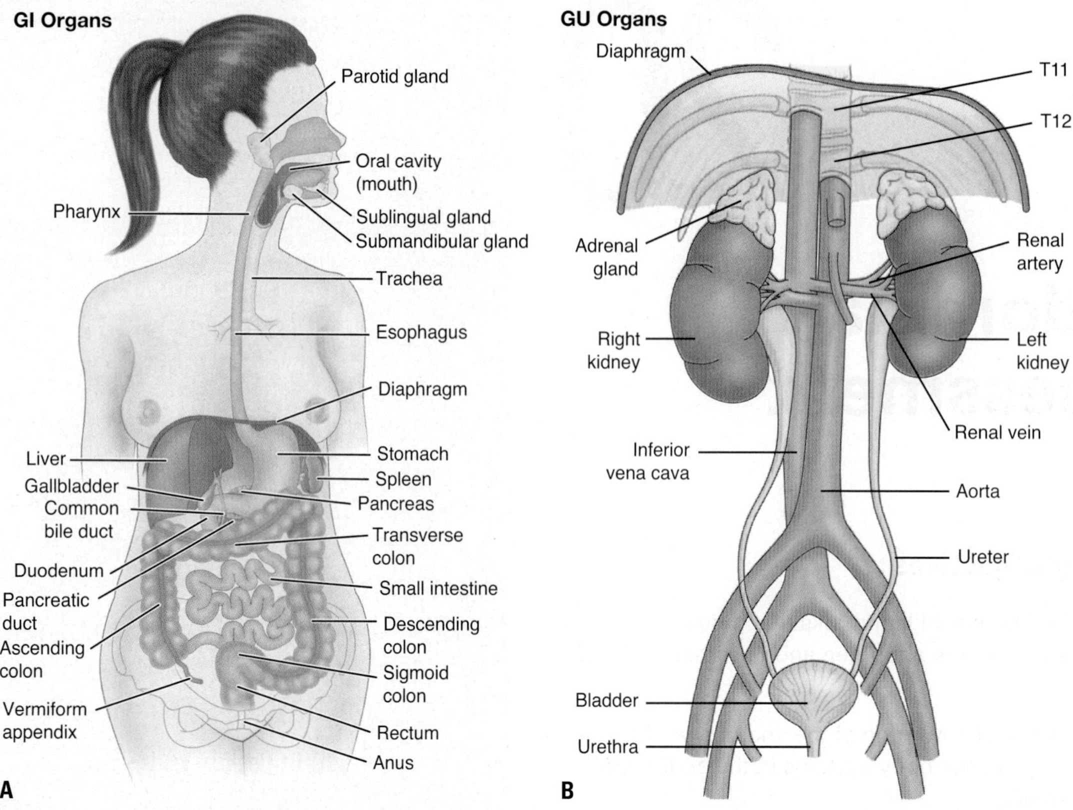

Figure 20.1 **A.** Overview of the gastrointestinal system. **B.** Overview of the genitourinary system.

It is not possible to perform an assessment of the abdomen without realizing that every system (except respiratory) is found within the abdominal cavity. Awareness of this fact will enable you to obtain valuable information about the functioning of the GI, cardiovascular, reproductive, neuromuscular, and genitourinary (GU) systems.

This chapter primarily addresses issues within the GI system. The GI system is responsible for the ingestion and digestion of food, absorption of nutrients, and elimination of solid waste products from the body. Parts of the GI system also reside in the head, neck, and thoracic regions (see Chapters 12 and 16). Findings need to be evaluated based on the organ systems found in those regions as well.

GI symptoms are common and send people of all ages in search of relief. Diagnosis of abdominal diseases depends heavily on accurate and thorough history taking. During the health history, it is essential to delineate the sequence of the patient's symptoms. Additionally, it is important to master the abdominal assessment to provide quality health care.

Structure and Function

Understanding the anatomy and physiology of the structures of the abdomen is essential before beginning an assessment (Figs. 20.1 and 20.2). You must recognize normal structures and their functions before identifying abnormalities. Understanding the physiology associated with each organ and its interactions will help you accurately interpret findings from the assessment (Boxes 20.1 and 20.2).

Anatomical Landmarks

The abdomen is a large cavity extending from the xiphoid process of the sternum down to the superior margin of the pubic bone. It is bordered in the back by the vertebral column and paravertebral muscles and at the sides and front by the

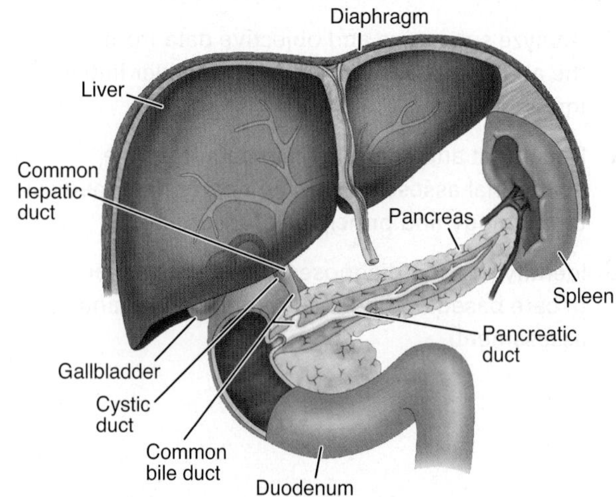

Figure 20.2 Overview of the accessory organs of the gastrointestinal system.

BOX 20.1 Major Organs of the Gastrointestinal/Genitourinary System and Their Functions

Esophagus
- Propels food into the stomach, controlled by the cardiac sphincter—a one-way valve at the distal end

Stomach
- Site for both mechanical and chemical digestion:
  - Churns food into small particles that become liquid when mixed with gastric juices
  - Stores food and slowly releases it into the small intestine
  - Secretes hydrochloric acid to aid in digestion; mucous cells secrete substances to coat the stomach lining; chief cells secrete pepsinogen, which is converted to pepsin to aid in digestion of protein; secretes gastrin, which stimulates secretion of acid and pepsinogen and increases gastric motility
  - Secretes intrinsic factor that protects vitamin B_{12} from stomach acid and facilitates its absorption by the parietal cells in the small intestine
  - Absorbs water, alcohol, and some medications
  - Destroys some food-borne bacteria
  - Allows emptying of stomach contents based on pressure gradient, a little at a time; gravity assists with emptying

Small intestine
- 5.5–6.1 m (18–20 ft) in adults
- Propels contents by wormlike movements known as peristalsis
- Primarily responsible for absorption of nutrients

Duodenum
- 25 cm (10 in.)
- Primary site for chemical digestion
- Enzymes, hormones, and bile from pancreas and liver enter and aid in absorption of nutrients:
  - Peptidases help break down proteins.
  - Enterokinase converts trypsinogen to active trypsin.
  - Maltase, lactase, and sucrase break down carbohydrates.
  - Cholecystokinin, secreted from duodenal wall, stimulates gallbladder to secrete bile.
  - Gastric inhibitory peptide inhibits gastric motility.
  - Secretin, secreted by duodenal wall, stimulates pancreatic secretions to neutralize gastric acid.

Jejunum and ileum
- Jejunum: 2.4 m (8 ft)
- Ileum: 3.7 m (12 ft)
- Absorb water, nutrients, and electrolytes for use in body

Large intestine
- Ascending and descending colon
- 1.5–1.8 m (5–6 ft)
- Absorbs salt and water and excretes waste products of digestive process from the rectum (defecation)
- Aids in synthesis of vitamin B_{12} and potassium

Kidneys
- Control blood pressure through the production of renin
- Stimulate red blood cell production by secreting erythropoietin
- Remove waste products filtered by the kidneys from the body

Bladder
- Aids in the removal of waste products from the body in the form of urine

Aorta
- Supplies oxygenated blood to the cells and organs of the lower half of the body

BOX 20.2 Accessory Organs of the Gastrointestinal System and Their Function

Liver (located in RUQ)
- Produces and secretes bile to emulsify fat
- Metabolizes protein, carbohydrates, and fats
- Converts glucose to glycogen and stores it
- Produces clotting factors, fibrinogen, and plasma proteins such as albumin
- Detoxifies drugs and alcohol
- Stores fat-soluble vitamins A, D, E, and K; vitamin B_{12}; and copper and iron
- Converts conjugated bilirubin from blood to unconjugated bilirubin

Gallbladder
- Located on back side of liver in RUQ
- Stores and concentrates bile

Pancreas
- Located in LUQ
- Endocrine functions:
  - Secretes insulin and regulates blood glucose levels
  - Secretes glucagons that store carbohydrates
  - Inhibits insulin and glucagon secretion
  - Secretes pancreatic polypeptide that regulates release of pancreatic enzymes
- Exocrine functions:
  - Secretes digestive enzymes. Amylase digests starches into maltose. Lipase breaks down lipids into fatty acids and glycerol.
  - Trypsinogen, chymotrypsinogen, and procarboxypeptidase are activated in the small intestine to break down proteins into amino acids.

lower rib cage and abdominal muscles. Four layers of large flat muscles form the ventral abdominal wall and are joined at the midline by a tendinous seam, the linea alba.

Reference Lines

For convenience in description, two methods are used to map the location of findings in the abdominal area. The most common is the *quadrant method*, which divides the abdominal wall into four quadrants by imaginary vertical and horizontal lines bisecting the umbilicus. The quadrants are the right upper quadrant (RUQ), left upper quadrant (LUQ), right lower quadrant (RLQ), and left lower quadrant (LLQ) (Fig. 20.3A). For most assessments and findings, this method is sufficient.

A more specific method is to divide the abdomen into nine regions by drawing two vertical lines at the midclavicular lines (MCLs) and two horizontal lines, one beginning at the lower edge of the costal margin and the other beginning at the anterosuperior iliac spine of the iliac bones. The regions are named from right to left and top to bottom: right hypochondriac, epigastric, left hypochondriac, right lumbar, umbilical, left lumbar, right inguinal, hypogastric, and left inguinal. Findings that require a more specific location can be mapped to these regions (Fig. 20.3B).

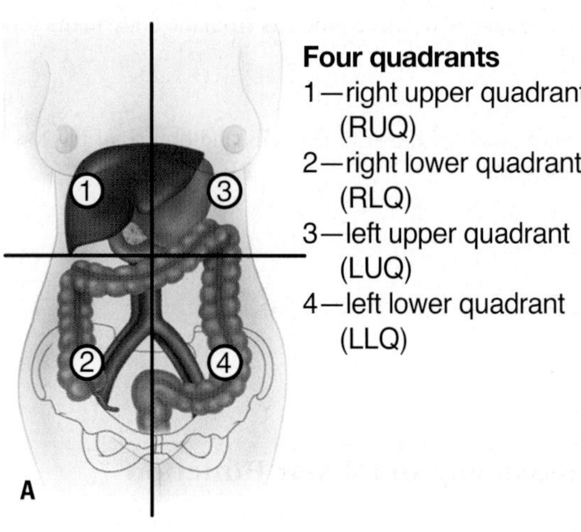

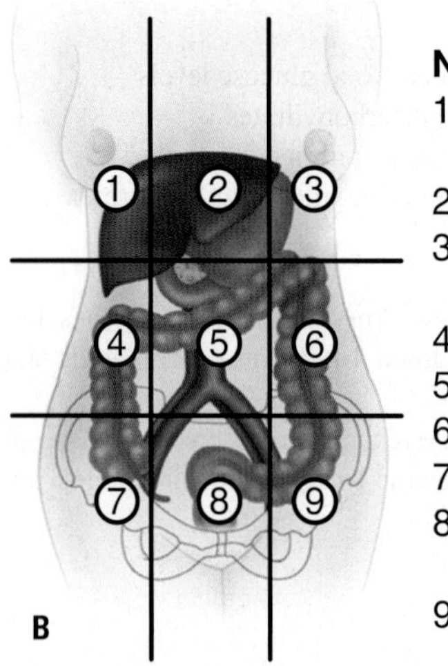

Figure 20.3 A. Division of the abdomen into four quadrants. **B.** Division of the abdomen into nine regions.

Abdominal Organs

Gastrointestinal Organs

The major GI organs found within the abdominal cavity include the stomach, small intestines, and colon. **Accessory organs** of the GI system within the abdomen include the liver, pancreas, and gallbladder.

Genitourinary Organs

The organs of the GU system found within the abdominal cavity include the kidneys, ureters, and bladder; the spermatic cord in males; and the uterus and ovaries in females. Disease processes in these organs can produce abdominal symptoms.

The kidneys control blood pressure through the production of renin, stimulate red blood cell production by secreting erythropoietin, and filter and remove waste products from the body. The ureters and bladder aid with removal of waste products in the form of urine. The volume in the bladder can be measured through a bladder scan; the probe is positioned so that it points toward the top of the full bladder (Fig. 20.4).

The spermatic cord protects the vas deferens, blood vessels, lymphatics, and nerves that run from scrotum to penis (see Chapter 23). The ovaries produce ova and secrete estrogen and progesterone. The uterus allows fertilization of the oocyte with sperm and, if conception occurs, provides an environment for fetal development (see Chapters 24 and 25).

Blood Vessels, Peritoneum, and Muscles

The aorta and branching arteries and veins are found within the abdominal cavity. They supply oxygenated blood to the cells and organs of the lower half of the body. The spleen also resides in the abdominal cavity; it stores red blood cells and platelets, produces new red blood cells and macrophages, and activates B and T lymphocytes.

The **peritoneum**, mesentery, and muscles are also part of the abdominal cavity. The peritoneum is a serous membrane that covers and holds the organs in place. It contains a parietal layer that lines the walls of the abdomen and a visceral layer that coats the outer surface of the organs. A small amount of fluid between these layers allows them to move

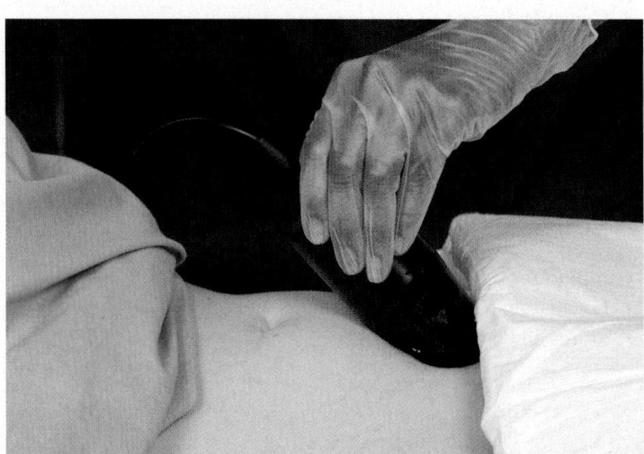

Figure 20.4 Bladder scan. The scan head is pressed above the pubic bone at a downward angle toward the bladder.

smoothly within the cavity. The fanlike mesentery receives its blood supply from the dorsal aorta and supplies blood vessels and nerves to the intestinal tract. The muscles protect and support the digestive system within the abdominal cavity. Muscles also assist with ingestion, mastication, and swallowing of food, and with the voluntary defecation of its by-products.

Ingestion and Digestion

The digestive process consists of mechanical and chemical digestion. Mechanical digestion is the breakdown of food through chewing, peristalsis, and churning. Chemical digestion is the breakdown of food through a series of metabolic reactions with hydrochloric acid, enzymes, and hormones.

The digestive process begins in the mouth where food is ingested and mastication (chewing) begins. During this process, saliva mixes with the food when a bolus of food forms. The bolus passes into the oropharynx and esophagus, which propel the bolus by means of slow peristaltic movements into the stomach. In the stomach, the bolus is mixed with digestive juices and hydrochloric acid and churned into a liquid called chyme.

Absorption of Nutrients

Absorption of nutrients takes place almost exclusively in the small intestine. In the first portion of the small intestine—the duodenum—pancreatic juices and bile are secreted into the chyme. This makes the nutrients in the chyme available for absorption by the many villi that line the walls of the remaining two portions of the small intestine: the jejunum and the ileum.

Elimination

Any food particles not absorbed by the small intestine pass into the large intestine, where a few electrolytes and water are further absorbed. Eventually, the remaining waste products are excreted as feces. On average, waste products of food ingested today are eliminated 48 hours later.

Lifespan Considerations: Older Adults

In older adults, production of saliva and stomach acid is reduced and gastric motility and peristalsis slow. These changes can lead to difficulties with swallowing, absorption, and digestion. Elderly people also have changes in dentition that may affect their ability to chew and may result in painful mastication. Chewing difficulties, accompanied by limited financial resources, can dramatically alter dietary choices (less protein, more carbohydrates). These factors, along with generally reduced muscle mass and tone, may contribute to constipation in older adults.

Fat accumulates in the lower abdomen in women and around the waist in men, making physical assessment more challenging. The liver decreases in size and liver function declines, making it harder for older adults to process medications. Renal function also declines, which decreases the ability to eliminate medications. The older adult also experiences a diminished sensation of thirst, which may result in a lower consumption of liquids, contributing to urinary tract infections (UTIs) and constipation.

Cultural Considerations

African Americans have higher rates of obesity, hypertension, diabetes mellitus, and metabolic syndrome than Caucasians (Liu et al., 2013). African American adults are twice as likely as Caucasians to be diagnosed with diabetes by a physician. American Indian/Alaska Native adults are more than twice as likely as Caucasians to be diagnosed with diabetes. In Hawaii, Native Hawaiians are more than 5.7 times as likely as Caucasians living in that state to die from complications of diabetes. Mexican American adults are 1.8 times more likely than Caucasians to be diagnosed with diabetes. Native Hawaiians/Pacific Islanders are 3 times more likely to be diagnosed with the disease (U.S. Department of Health & Human Services, Office of Minority Health, 2012).

Urgent Assessment

If a patient has an acute abdominal problem, the history and physical examination will be focused on that problem, so that much of the history taking discussed in the next section will be eliminated. Severe dehydration from nausea and vomiting, fever, and acute abdominal pain are potentially life-threatening symptoms that require prompt attention.

Subjective Data

A comprehensive history normally preceding the physical assessment involves asking the patient about his or her health status. It comprises a broad range of questions to discern possible difficulties associated with each organ and system within the abdomen. Approach the history from a head-to-toe direction and avoid skipping around with questioning. In many problems of the GI tract, a well-developed health history can point to a diagnosis in 80% to 90% of cases. If time is limited, a focused history on the abdomen will be sufficient.

Assessment of Risk Factors

The nurse assesses current problems first using symptom analysis. Next, the nurse assesses personal and family history to determine genetic risk factors. After this initial history, the nurse assesses other risk factors and teaches about those that may be modified so that assessment is linked to health promotion and teaching.

History and Risk Factors	Rationale
Personal History Are you having any abdominal difficulties now?	This question opens discussion with a general approach.
Have you had any unplanned changes in weight, either a loss or a gain?	Unexplained weight changes may indicate undiagnosed cancer, anorexia nervosa, bulimia nervosa, thyroid disorder, psychosocial issues, or socioeconomic concerns.
Do you have any special dietary needs or concerns, or cultural or religious beliefs, that affect your diet?	Special needs may indicate a nutrient imbalance or cause of symptoms. A 24-hour diet recall is helpful to determine what may be normal for the patient (see Chapter 7). If the patient has been sick for a prolonged period, ask what he or she "normally eats at each meal" rather than what was eaten in the previous 24 hours.
Have you had a fever or chills?	Fever may indicate an infection that could affect food or fluid intake.
Have you had any dizziness?	Dizziness may result from possible dehydration linked to inadequate fluid or caloric intake.
How old are you?	Risk of colorectal cancer increases with age (American Cancer Society [ACS], 2013a). Colorectal cancer is the second leading cause of U.S. cancer deaths. It is often asymptomatic, but if caught early, it is very curable.
Did you have a blood transfusion before the mid-1980s? Have you been vaccinated against hepatitis A or B?	Those who received blood transfusions prior to the mid-1980s (before the blood supply was tested for hepatitis B) may be at higher risk for the illness. Hepatitis B vaccine has been available to at-risk patients since the mid-1980s; since 1991, most U.S. born infants have been vaccinated. Question patients about whether they received all three doses.
Do you have a history of endometrial, ovarian, or breast cancer?	Personal history of endometrial, ovarian, or breast cancer also increases risk.
Have you ever had varicella (chickenpox)?	Varicella, which always precedes herpes zoster (shingles), may appear along a dermatome on one side of the abdomen and back.
General Gastrointestinal Questions. Have you had any previous treatments or hospitalizations for GI problems such as gastroesophageal reflux disease (GERD), peptic ulcer diseases (PUD), inflammatory bowel disease (IBD; either ulcerative colitis or Crohn disease), irritable bowel syndrome (IBS), anemia, thalassemia, or celiac disease?	The patient history may reveal an exacerbation of a previously diagnosed condition or a genetic predisposition or familial propensity for a particular disorder. Long-standing ulcerative colitis (more than 10 years) without remission increases the patient's risk for colorectal cancer. Crohn disease may contribute to malnutrition or multiple surgical resections of the bowel, resulting in short bowel syndrome.
Have you had any previous GI diagnostic tests such as stool for occult blood, coloscopy, upper GI series, barium enema, computed tomography (CT) scan, or magnetic resonance imaging (MRI)?	
Do you have a history of previous abdominal or pelvic surgeries?	Previous surgeries increase risk for adhesions, infections, obstructions, and malabsorption. Appendicitis must be ruled out as the cause of the current problem.
Have you had any recent insertions of GI tubes?	GI tubes can be a source of infection.
Have you had any recent trauma, such as motor vehicle accident, occupational injury, or sports injury?	A history of trauma can provide insight into a previous surgery or injury, which may be causing current symptoms.
Have you had any recent infection with mononucleosis?	Mononucleosis can cause hepatosplenomegaly.

(table continues on page 565)

History and Risk Factors	Rationale
Do you have a history of malabsorption disease?	This condition in self or family members may indicate lactose intolerance, food allergies, or celiac disease.
Do you have sickle cell anemia?	Abdominal pain is associated with sickle cell crisis.
Do you have history of eating disorders?	Eating disorders often begin in adolescence, with tendencies continuing into adulthood.
Have you ever had intestinal polyps?	History of intestinal polyps increases risk for colorectal cancer.
Chewing and Swallowing. Have you had any history of thyroid disease, neck masses, recent infection, vision changes, trouble swallowing, or sore throat?	Hypothyroidism and hyperthyroidism affects metabolism, weight, and elimination. Neck masses may indicate cancer or infection. Infections increase the caloric requirements. Visual changes may occur with nutritional imbalances. Difficulty swallowing may indicate an undiagnosed cancer or infection. Throat pain may impede swallowing (see also Chapter 15).
What is the date of your last dental exam?	Poor dentition affects the intake of major food groups and nutritional status.
Breathing. Do you have a history of breathing problems, shortness of breath, or chronic obstructive pulmonary disease (COPD)?	Respiratory problems diminish energy level and can decrease food intake. Some foods increase mucus in the throat. See also Chapter 16.
Weight Gain. Do you have a history of cardiovascular disease, high blood pressure, or congestive heart failure (CHF)?	Weight gain and increased sodium in the diet may exacerbate these problems.
Genitourinary Issues. What is the color of your urine? Do you have any urinary burning, frequency, or urgency?	Dark urine may indicate inadequate fluid intake or blockage in the biliary system.
Do you have a history of sexually transmitted infections?	They may cause lower abdominal pain.
Females: What is the date of your last menstrual period?	Unplanned pregnancy is often a cause of nausea and vomiting.
Do you have any vaginal discharge?	Discharge may indicate an infection.
Men: Do you have a history of prostate difficulties?	An enlarged prostate may be a source of urinary difficulty and result in decreased intake of fluids.
Do you have any penile discharge?	Penile discharge may indicate a sexually transmitted infection.
Joint Pain. Do you have a history of fractures, joint pain, or weakness?	Joint pain may result in long-term use of nonsteroidal antiinflammatory medications, which can cause GI bleeding. Joint issues may make food preparation difficult. Decreased mobility may result in constipation.
Neurological System. How many alcoholic drinks do you have each day?	Excessive alcohol intake is the number one cause of liver disease. Excessive drinking may lead to decreased caloric intake.
Have you had any numbness, back problems, or loss of bowel/bladder control?	Numbness and changes in the bowel or bladder are symptoms of significant spinal injury.
Metabolism. Do you have a history of diabetes or thyroid problems?	Diabetes may cause polyphagia, polydipsia prior to diagnosis, improper carbohydrate metabolism, insulin resistance, and obesity.
	These findings are associated with an abnormal metabolism and weight changes.

(table continues on page 566)

History and Risk Factors	Rationale
Skin. Have you had any changes in your skin, hair, or nails?	Inadequate nutrition or imbalances in electrolytes or hormones may be exhibited in the skin, hair, or nails.
Have you had any rashes, itching, or lesions?	Rashes and itching suggest liver disease or malnutrition.
Lymphatic and Hematological Systems. Have you had any food allergies or infections? Do you have sickle cell anemia?	Food allergies may cause belching, bloating, flatulence, diarrhea, or constipation. Sickle cell anemia may cause significant pain and anemia.
Alcohol or Substance Abuse. Use the CAGE questionnaire if the patient has (or signs and symptoms lead you to suspect he or she has) a significant history of either alcohol or substance abuse. See Chapter 9.	
Occupation. • What is your profession? • Where do you work? • Are you vigilant about using personal protective equipment at work?	Health care workers are at high risk for hepatitis C, for which no vaccine exists yet.
Foreign Travel. • Have you traveled to, or lived in, parts of the world where sanitation is less than optimal? • Have you eaten food prepared in places that are not sanitary? • Have you received the hepatitis A vaccine?	Hepatitis A is transmitted by the oral–fecal route, usually within 30 days of exposure. The disease is vaccine-preventable (Friedman, 2013).
Lifestyle. • Do you use, or have you abused, intravenous (IV) drugs? • How many sexual partners have you had? • Have you ever had sex with sex workers?	Hepatitis B is transmitted through contact with bodily secretions (i.e., blood, semen, saliva, vaginal fluids) of infected people. Patients may not be aware of previous infection because symptoms may have felt like flu. Transmission time for hepatitis B is 6 weeks to 6 months. Hepatitis C is the most commonly diagnosed form of hepatitis in the United States. It is transmitted through contact with the blood of infected people. IV drug users are at high risk for hepatitis C; 70% of patients with hepatitis C develop serious liver complications of cirrhosis or hepatoma.
Medications Have you been taking any over-the-counter (OTC) or prescribed medications?	Patients will frequently take antacids that may interact with other medications.
Family History Is there a family history of colorectal cancer in a first-degree relative?	Such a family history increases the patient's risk for this disease.
Do you have any family history of GERD, PUD, IBD, IBS	Many of these conditions run in families.

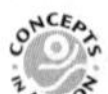

Risk Reduction and Health Promotion

It is important to provide nutritional counseling to patients with food allergies, poor nutrition, and obesity at least annually, if not at every visit. The health goals related to the abdomen include the following:

- Increase the proportion of adults who receive a colorectal cancer screening examination.
- Reduce the rate of new cases of end-stage renal disease (ESRD).
- Reduce cirrhosis deaths.

(U.S. Department of Health & Human Services, 2013)

Colorectal Cancer

Colorectal cancer is the third most commonly diagnosed cancer in the Unites States, and the second leading cause of U.S. cancer deaths (ACS, 2013a). In 2013, the estimated number of new cases of colorectal cancer was 142,820. Nonmodifiable risk factors include age, personal or family history of colorectal cancer, history of IBD (Barter & Dunne, 2011), and history of Type 2 diabetes. African Americans and Jews of Eastern European descent have the highest colorectal cancer mortality rates. Modifiable risk factors include sedentary lifestyle, dietary intake high in red and processed meats, obesity, smoking, and alcohol use (ACS, 2013b). The goal is to reduce mortality rates through early detection and treatment. Educating patients about their risk factors and ensuring that every patient older than 50 years is appropriately screened for colorectal cancer is the key to promoting health.

Food-Borne Illnesses

Food-borne illnesses affect the very young, elderly, and immunocompromised patients most seriously. Risk of food-borne illness increases with emerging pathogenic organisms, improper food storage or preparation, an increasingly global supply of foods, international travel, and inadequately treated water supplies. Severity of food-borne illness can range from annoying stomach upset to devastating dehydration; it is the leading cause of illness globally (LaRocque, Ryan, & Calderwood, 2012). Food allergies, especially those caused by peanuts, are on the rise. Estimates are that food allergies affect almost 4% of children younger than 6 years and 1% to 2% of adults (U.S. Department of Health & Human Services, 2013). Objectives for food-borne illnesses are to reduce infections by food-borne pathogens and to reduce deaths related to anaphylactic shock resulting from food allergies. Education about food handling in retail areas and at home, as well as food labeling, proper food preparation and storage, and hand washing are the methods identified to achieve these objectives.

Hepatitis

Hepatitis A, B, and C diseases are caused by viruses, some drugs, or toxic agents. The symptoms are similar regardless of the cause. Anorexia, nausea, vomiting, fever, and jaundice are typical symptoms. hepatitis A is transmitted via the oral–fecal route, affects adults more severely than children, and resolves within a year. Approximately 30% of persons in the United States test positive for previous hepatitis A infection. Since the availability of hepatitis A vaccine in 2006, the incidence of that disorder has greatly declined (Friedman, 2013).

Hepatitis B and C are transmitted via blood and body fluid exposure. They result in chronic disease. Chronic Hepatitis B infection afflicts 400 million people worldwide and 2.2 million people in the United States. Perinatal infection is the common mode of transmission of hepatitis B in infants. The infection rate among infants born to hepatitis B–positive mothers is 90% (Teo et al., 2009). Identifying at-risk mothers and vaccinating them and their infants would reduce this transmission. Complications of hepatitis B include cirrhosis and cancer. Risk factors include advanced age, alcohol use, cigarette smoking, and coinfection with hepatitis C. Hepatitis B is preventable with immunizations.

Hepatitis C afflicts 170 milllion people worldwide, and 1.8% of the United States population. Chronic hepatitis C develops in up to 85% of patients with acute hepatitis C. Those with chronic hepatitis C develop liver fibrosis, cirrhosis, and liver cancer (Friedman, 2013). Health care workers, men who have sex with men, and IV drug users are at a greater risk of contracting disease. There is no vaccination for hepatitis C. Reducing the incidence of hepatitis A, B, and C are objectives for improving population health through screening, education, and immunization programs (U.S. Department of Health & Human Services, 2013).

Hepatitis A and B immunizations are recommended for all infants; people whose work may expose them to blood, body fluids, or unsanitary conditions (i.e., health care, food services, sex workers); and those traveling to parts of the world where these illnesses are prevalent.

Screening and Patient Teaching

Risk of colorectal cancer increases with age. Initial screening for all people is recommended at 50 years, with serial fecal occult blood and colonoscopy for anyone whose results are positive. Follow-up screening is based on findings and risks, with colonoscopy repeated every 3 to 10 years.

Patient teaching concerning alcohol and substance abuse, and the possible effects on the organs in the abdomen, should be covered with all patients, especially those at high risk for abuse (see Chapter 9).

Common Symptoms

The focused health history should address common symptoms of the abdomen: indigestion, anorexia, nausea, vomiting, hematemesis, abdominal pain, **dysphagia** (difficulty swallowing), **odynophagia** (painful swallowing), changes in bowel function, constipation, diarrhea, and jaundice. It should also include questions about the possibility of GU disorders. Additional questions can include suprapubic pain, dysuria, urgency, frequency of urination, hesitancy, decreased urine stream in males, polyuria, nocturia, urinary incontinence, kidney or flank pain, ureteral colic, pelvic pain, and vaginal discharge in females. Some common symptoms should be assessed in all patients to screen for the presence of GI disease. Nurses can use any special concerns from patients about GI problems to identify focal areas. A thorough history of symptoms assists with identifying a current problem or diagnosis.

Common Abdominal Symptoms

- Indigestion
- Anorexia
- Nausea, vomiting, hematemesis
- Abdominal pain
- Dysphagia, odynophagia
- Change in bowel function:
  - Constipation
  - Diarrhea
- Jaundice/icterus
- Urinary/renal symptoms:
  - Urinary incontinence
  - Kidney or flank pain
  - Ureteral colic

Signs/Symptoms	Rationale/Abnormal Findings
Indigestion	
Have you had heartburn?	Heartburn suggests gastric acid reflux.
Do you have excessive gas, belching, or abdominal bloating or distention?	Increased intake of gas-forming foods, chewing gum, carbonated beverages, and motility problems can cause gas.
Have you noticed an unpleasant fullness after normal meals?	Gastric-emptying problems, outlet obstruction, and cancer can cause fullness.
Do you feel full shortly after starting to eat? Are you unable to eat a full meal?	Early satiety can result from diabetic gastroparesis, anticholinergic drugs, or hepatitis.
Anorexia	
How is your appetite?	**Anorexia** is loss of appetite and can be related to stress, difficulty with ingestion, socioeconomic issues, age-related issues, or dementia.
Do you deliberately eat small meals?	With anorexia nervosa, food intake is intentionally limited.
Have you ever vomited after eating?	Bulimia nervosa is a disease in which the patient deliberately vomits after eating.
Nausea, Vomiting, Hematemesis	
Do you have nausea or vomiting? Have you ever vomited blood?	Nausea and vomiting may result from infections, food poisoning, or stress. Hematemesis may indicate gastric ulcer, gastritis, or esophageal varices from alcoholic cirrhosis.
Abdominal Pain	
Do you have any pain or discomfort? • Where is the pain located? (Ask where the pain starts, and whether it radiates or moves.) • How intense is the pain? • How long does the pain last? • How would you describe your pain? (Note if gnawing or sharp. Note whether fever, chills, or pallor is present.) • What aggravates the pain? • What makes the pain go away? • What is your goal in relation to the pain? • What is your functional goal?	Discerning pain characteristics can greatly assist in diagnosis of the problem by pinpointing the type of assessment and diagnostic procedures required: • **Visceral pain** occurs when hollow organs are distended, stretched, or contract forcefully. It may be difficult to localize. The patient may describe it as gnawing, burning, cramping, or aching. If severe, it may be associated with sweating, pallor, nausea, vomiting, or restlessness. • **Parietal pain** results from inflammation of the peritoneum. It is usually severe and localized over the involved structure. Patients describe it as steady, aching, or sharp, especially with movement. • **Referred pain** occurs in more distant sites innervated at approximately the same spinal level as the disordered structure (see Chapter 6).
Dysphagia/Odynophagia	
• Do you have any difficulty swallowing or pain with swallowing? • Does it feel like food gets stuck in your throat or esophagus?	Dysphagia may result from stress, esophageal stricture, GERD, or tumor.
Change in Bowel Function	
What was your normal bowel pattern before symptoms developed?	The nurse needs to establish the patient's normal pattern, which may range from several times a day to once a week. This sets a basis for determining any current constipation or diarrhea.
Constipation. What is the change from your expected pattern? Are there any changes in your diet, medications, or physical activity?	Usually, functional **constipation** results from inadequate fiber and fluids in the diet. It also can result from medications such as anticholinergics or narcotics.

(table continues on page 569)

Signs/Symptoms	Rationale/Abnormal Findings
Diarrhea	**Diarrhea** can result from an infection such as with *Clostridium difficile*. It also can be associated with food intolerances, or it may be a medicinal adverse effect.
• What is the change from your expected pattern? • Is it associated with nausea or vomiting? • Do you get diarrhea with a change in your diet, or only when you eat certain foods? • Is pain relieved with moving your bowels?	
Jaundice/Icterus	
Have you noticed a change in • the color of your skin or the whites of your eyes?	Jaundice can result from obstruction of the common bile duct by gallstones or pancreatic cancer.
• the color of your urine or stool?	Dark urine is from impaired excretion of bilirubin into the GI tract. Gray or light stool is common in obstructive jaundice.
Have you recently traveled to, or had meals in, areas of poor sanitation?	Recent travel may indicate exposure to hepatitis A.
Have you had any recent exposure to blood or body fluids of an infected partner, use of shared needles for IV drugs, or blood transfusion?	Exposure to blood or body fluids may indicate infection with hepatitis B or C.
Urinary/Renal Symptoms	
Do you have	Many patients perceive these symptoms as abdominal in nature.
• Pain on urination or difficulty voiding (dysuria)?	Pain may be from infection or irritation of either the bladder or urethra. Women often report internal urethral discomfort; men typically feel a burning proximal to the glans penis.
• Urgency or frequency of urination?	Urgency may result from UTI or sexually transmitted infection.
• Suprapubic pain?	Suprapubic pain is usually from cystitis.
• (*in males*) Hesitancy or decreased urine stream?	Hesitancy may be from benign prostatic hypertrophy (BPH).
• Polyuria? (How frequent?)	Polyuria is a common symptom of diabetes.
• Nocturia? (How frequent?)	In males, nocturia is usually from BPH.
• Hematuria? (Painful or not painful?)	Painful hematuria is usually the result of bladder infection in younger patients or those with renal calculi. Painless hematuria is common in older adults with UTIs and in patients with bladder cancer.
Urinary Incontinence	
• Do you ever leak urine, especially when coughing or sneezing?	Patients need careful questioning on this topic because they often do not volunteer this information because of embarrassment.
• Have you had times where you could not make it to the bathroom fast enough?	Urinary incontinence may result from urinary sepsis, pelvic floor disorders, or multiparity.
• Have you ever lost urine before getting to the bathroom?	Types of urinary incontinence are as follows: • *Stress incontinence*: occurs with coughing, sneezing, or increasing intraabdominal pressure • *Urge incontinence*: sudden urge and loss of continence with little warning • *Total incontinence*: inability to retain urine (also ask patient about bowel incontinence)

(table continues on page 570)

Signs/Symptoms	Rationale/Abnormal Findings
Kidney or Flank Pain. Do you have pain? Is it dull, achy, and steady? Did you have any burning, urgency, or bladder pain prior to its development?	Renal calculi and pyelonephritis can cause flank pain.
Ureteral Colic. Do you have severe, colicky pain in your flank? Is it associated with nausea or vomiting?	Ureteral obstruction by blood clots or stones will cause a colicky cramping type of pain.

Documenting Normal Findings

Patient reports normal appetite, denies food intolerance, excessive belching, trouble swallowing, heartburn, or nausea. Bowel movements are daily, brown, soft; denies changes in bowel habits, pain with defecation, rectal bleeding, or black tarry stools. Denies hemorrhoids, passing of gas, constipation, or diarrhea. Denies abdominal pain. No jaundice, liver, or gallbladder problems, also no history of hepatitis.

Lifespan Considerations: Older Adults

Additional Questions	Rationale/Abnormal Findings
How do you get your groceries and prepare your meals?	Assess for risks for nutritional deficits: limited access to a grocery store, reduced income, compromised cooking facilities, physical disability (e.g., impaired vision, decreased mobility, decreased strength, neurological deficit).
Do you eat alone or share meals with others?	Risks for nutritional deficit include living alone, not bothering or remembering to prepare meals, social isolation, and depression.
Ask for a 24-hour diet recall, starting with breakfast (see Chapter 7). • Do you have any trouble swallowing these foods? • What do you do right after eating—walk, take a nap?	A 24-hour recall may not provide sufficient information, because daily patterns may vary. Attempt to get a week-long diary of food intake. Food consumption may vary based on income.
How often do you move your bowels? (Ask the patient to describe what is meant by constipation.) • How much liquid and what types do you drink daily? • How much bulk, fiber, and fresh fruits and vegetables are in your diet? • Do you take anything for constipation? How often do you use it?	Many older adults have concerns about their bowel function. As the GI system changes with age, appetite may decrease, and constipation may result.
What medications do you take daily?	Consider GI side effects (e.g., nausea, vomiting, anorexia, dry mouth) of all prescribed and OTC medications that the patient may take.

Cultural Considerations

Additional Questions	Rationale/Abnormal Findings
African Americans Do you or your parents have sickle cell disease or trait?	Sickle cell anemia has an autosomal recessive inheritance pattern. Most states screen for the disease at birth. Symptoms begin to emerge in the second 6 months of life and include jaundice and splenomegaly.

(table continues on page 571)

Additional Questions	Rationale/Abnormal Findings
Do you, or does anyone in your family, have glucose-6-phosphate dehydrogenase (G6PD) deficiency?	G6PD is a drug-induced anemia caused by a genetic lack of the G6PD enzyme in red blood cells. It is an X-linked recessive trait. Aspirin-containing medications, sulfonamides, antimalarials, and fava beans can trigger hemolysis.
Are you or is anyone in your family lactose intolerant?	Lactose intolerance tends to have a familial distribution and can develop at any age. Patients present with abdominal discomfort, bloating, belching, and diarrhea.
Asian Americans	
Do you have heartburn, upset stomach, loss of appetite, or weight loss? Any family history of gastric cancer?	Incidence of gastric and primary liver cancers is higher in Asian Americans. Heartburn and indigestion are often treated with OTC preparations, so that patients may not report that they use them. Such medications may cover symptoms, leading to a delay in diagnosis until metastasis has occurred (Phan, 2011).
Americans of Jewish Descent	
Do you have a personal or family history of ulcerative colitis or Crohn disease?	IBDs have a familial predisposition (Barter & Dunne, 2011).
Do you have a personal or family history of lactose intolerance?	Lactose intolerance may accompany the IBD and cloud the history (Stern, Cifu, & Altkorn, 2010).
Americans of Mediterranean Descent	
Do you or does anyone in your family have lactose intolerance?	There is a familial predisposition as mentioned above.
Do you or does anyone in your family have chronic anemia or thalassemia?	The thalassemias are a group of hereditary hypochromic anemias. They are often confused with iron-deficiency anemia and lead poisoning but they do not respond to iron supplementation. Minor pallor and splenomegaly may be present.
Native Americans	
• Do you drink alcohol? If so, how much and how often? • Have you ever had yellow skin or yellow eyes? • Have you had liver disease, gallbladder disease, or pancreatitis? • Do you have diabetes?	Alcoholism and diabetes are more prevalent in the Native American population.

Therapeutic Dialogue: Collecting Subjective Data

The nurse's role relative to subjective data collection is to gather information to improve the patient's health status and to help determine the cause of the patient's current symptoms. Remember Mr. Renaud, introduced at the beginning of this chapter. This 41-year-old man was admitted to the hospital with a GI bleed that is related to his ongoing alcohol intake. In addition to obtaining an abdominal assessment, the nurse will assess Mr. Renaud's needs to begin establishing a discharge plan.

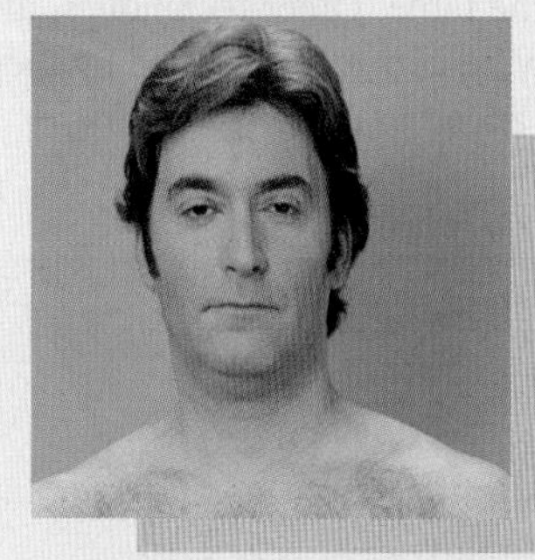

(case study continues on page 572)

Nurse: Hi, Mr. Renaud. We need to start thinking about where you're going after discharge. What are your thoughts?

Mr. Renaud: I don't want to go back to that dirty mission. I would rather be on the streets than in there.

Nurse: Tell me more about that (pause).

Mr. Renaud: The people are too rough and I always get bedbugs there.

Nurse: It sounds like you don't like the mission, but we want you to have a safe place to go (pause).

Mr. Renaud: I don't want to go there, but I've lost everything to alcohol—my wife, my kids, my house.

Nurse: Your drinking has created some problems for you. How are you feeling about quitting?

Mr. Renaud: I've tried before, but it doesn't work.

Nurse: It's hard making a change. If you think that you're ready to try again, I could talk with a social worker about finding a rehab placement for you.

Critical Thinking Challenge

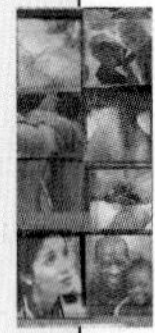

- Consider the question regarding alcohol use. What therapeutic communication skills did the nurse use?
- How might your life experiences influence your attitude toward Mr. Renaud?
- How does the nurse address the issue of homelessness?
- How might your values influence the patient assessment?

Objective Data

Common and Specialty or Advanced Techniques

The routine head-to-toe assessment includes the most important and common assessment techniques. Nurses may add specialty or advanced steps if concerns exist over a specific finding. The most common techniques, which are therefore essential to learn for use in clinical practice are summarized in the table. Other techniques, also summarized in the table, may be added if indicated by the clinical situation or used in advanced practice.

Equipment

- Stethoscope
- Measuring tape
- Pen or marker
- Reflex hammer or tongue blade to ascertain abdominal reflexes
- Pillow placed under the knees to relax the abdominal musculature

Preparation

Make sure the environment is warm and private. Adequate lighting is essential. Have the patient empty the bladder before the assessment. He or she should lie supine with the arms at the sides. Using a sheet for draping, expose only as much of the abdomen as necessary as you proceed through the assessment. Be sure to explain what you are doing and to perform the assessment systematically, slowly, and without quick movements. Throughout, observe the patient's face for signs of discomfort. Distract the patient with questions or conversation to avoid tensing of the abdominal musculature, which will make the assessment more difficult and the findings obscure.

Clinical Significance

The order of assessment of the abdomen is different from previous systems. Inspection is followed by auscultation for bowel sounds *before* percussion and palpation. Failure to adhere to this order may result in the alteration of bowel sounds from either percussion or palpation, leading to inaccurate findings.

Basic Versus Focused/Specialty or Advanced Techniques Related to Abdominal Assessment

Technique	Purpose	Screening or Registered Nurse Assessment	Focused or Advanced Practice Examination
Inspect abdomen.	To identify shape and contour	X	
Inspect urine.	To identify if cloudy, clear, or bloody and also to assess level of hydration	X	
Inspect emesis.	To assess bleeding, hydration, acid–base balance	X	
Inspect stool.	To assess for infection, presence of *C. difficile*, need for rectal drainage system	X	
Auscultate abdomen.	To assess for sounds from peristalsis	X	
Perform bladder scan.	To evaluate whether urine is present in the bladder	X	
Lightly palpate abdomen.	To assess overall impression	X	
Percuss abdomen.	To assess whether normal, gas, or fluid filled	X	
Percuss kidney.	To assess for tenderness		X UTI
Percuss liver.	To measure size		X Liver size
Percuss spleen.	To identify whether enlarged		X Splenomegaly
Percuss bladder.	To evaluate whether urine in the bladder		X Bladder distention
Deeply palpate abdomen.	To locate masses and organs		X Masses, tumors
Palpate liver.	To measure the size		X Liver size, texture
Palpate spleen.	To identify whether enlarged		X Splenomegaly
Palpate kidney.	To assess for tenderness and enlargement		X Suspect UTI
Test for fluid wave.	To evaluate whether gas or fluid is present		X Ascites
Test for shifting dullness.	To evaluate whether gas or fluid is present		X Ascites
Palpate abdominal aorta.	To identify whether enlarged		X Abdominal aneurysm
Palpate bladder.	To evaluate whether urine is present in the bladder		X Bladder distention
Palpate lymph nodes.	To assess for inflammation and drainage		X Suspect cancer
Assess abdominal reflex.	To assess central neurological symptoms		X Neurological deficit

Technique and Normal Findings	Rationale/Abnormal Findings
Inspection Inspect the abdomen. Look at the condition of the skin and umbilicus. Look at the abdomen for contour, peristaltic waves, and pulsations (Fig. 20.5). Inspect for size, shape, and symmetry. Note whether the umbilicus is inverted or everted and its position. Inspect from different angles to evaluate color, surface characteristics, contour, and surface movements. Note visible veins on the abdomen. Have the patient take a deep breath and bear down to determine any hernias or organomegaly. 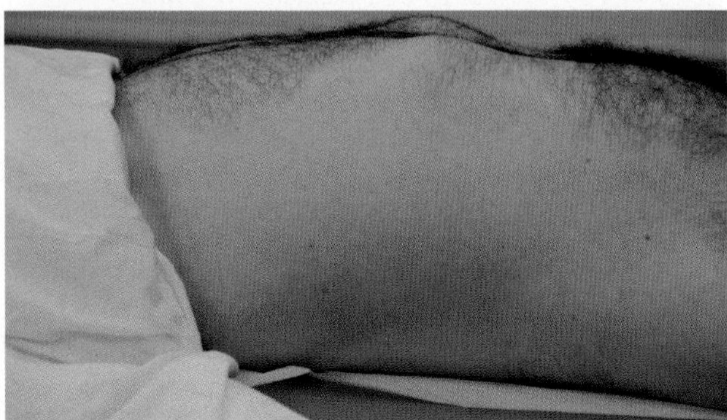 **Figure 20.5** Inspecting the abdomen.	Unexpected skin findings include scars, **striae** (stretch marks), and veins. The umbilicus may have a hernia or inflammation.
Assess for distention. If present, determine whether it is generalized or only in one area. Ask the patient if the abdomen looks or feels different from normal. Inspect for any visible aortic pulsations, peristalsis, and respiratory pattern. Evaluate for ascites.	Several simultaneous conditions can cause distention. Consider all possible contributory factors. Unexpected contours include bulging flanks, suprapubic bulge of full bladder, enlarged liver or spleen, or a tumor. A peristaltic wave may indicate GI obstruction, although in thin patients it may be a normal finding. Pulsation of the aorta may be increased and lateralized in an abdominal aortic aneurysm. **Ascites** is collection of fluid in the abdomen.
Bladder Scan. Scan the bladder according to the manufacturer's directions. Turn on the scanner and set the dial for male or female. Apply small amount of gel on the scanner head or above the pubic bone. Press the scan head above the pubic bone and at a downward angle (see Fig. 20.4). Press the button to display the volume; repeat three to four times to identify the largest volume. Remove gel and replace clothing.	Bladder scans identify the volume in the bladder and ability to void and empty the bladder. They are commonly used to identify the need for catheterization. After voiding, 50–100 ml (about 1¾ to 3½ oz) may be present in the bladder; more than 200 ml (about 6¾ oz) usually indicates incomplete emptying.
Urine. ■ Urine is clear and light yellow.	Cloudy urine may indicate a UTI. Sediment may indicate kidney disease. Blood in the urine can be caused by renal injury, renal disease, or trauma from a catheter. Dark urine may be due to dehydration. Cola-colored urine is the result of massive muscle breakdown and should be reported immediately.
Emesis. ■ There is no emesis.	Medications or diseases may cause emesis. Green emesis usually results from reduced peristalsis with irritation. Coffee-ground emesis is digested blood; bloody emesis is an active bleed with undigested blood.
Stool. ■ Stool is soft and light brown.	Foul-smelling stool may result from *C. difficile* infection. This bacterial infection leads to very liquid and light brown stool. Dark stool can be from iron supplements or digested blood. Melanotic stool is noted with partially digested blood from GI bleeding.

(table continues on page 575)

Technique and Normal Findings (continued)	Rationale/Abnormal Findings (continued)
Auscultation ***Bowel Sounds.*** Auscultate all four quadrants for bowel sounds. Begin by placing the warmed diaphragm of the stethoscope gently in one quadrant (Fig. 20.6). It is recommended to start at the point of the ileocecal valve, slightly right and below the umbilicus, and proceed clockwise. This is a very active area of bowel sounds. Bowel sounds are high-pitched gurgles or clicks that last from one to several seconds. There are 5–30 gurgles per minute or one sound every 5–15 seconds in the average adult. Sounds indicate bowel motility and peristalsis. If no sounds are audible, listen for up to 5 minutes.	Bowel sounds increase and decrease and indicate GI motility. They may be hyperactive at a point above a partial bowel obstruction and decreased or nonexistent below the point of obstruction. Increased bowel sounds, called **borborygmi**, occur with diarrhea and early intestinal obstruction. Decreased bowel sounds (hypoactive bowel) occur with adynamic ileus and peritonitis. High-pitched tinkling bowel sounds indicate intestinal fluid or air under tension in a dilated bowel. High-pitched rushing sounds indicate partial intestinal obstruction. Hyperactive sounds occur more than 30 gurgles per minute.
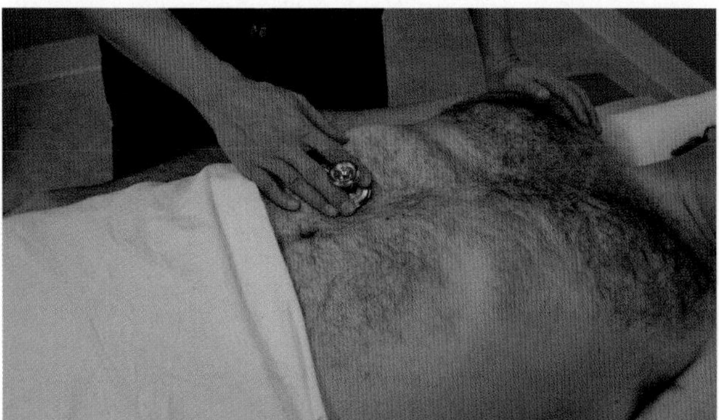 **Figure 20.6** Auscultating the abdomen.	
Vascular Sounds. Auscultate all four quadrants for vascular sounds. Best heard with the bell of the stethoscope, they include bruits, venous hums, and friction rubs.	
Listen for bruits over the aorta in the epigastric region and over the renal and iliac arteries (Fig. 20.7).	**Bruits** are swishing sounds that indicate turbulent blood flow resulting from constriction or dilation of a tortuous vessel. Bruits in the hepatic area indicate liver cancer or alcoholic hepatitis. Bruits over the aorta or renal arteries indicate partial obstruction of the aorta or renal artery.
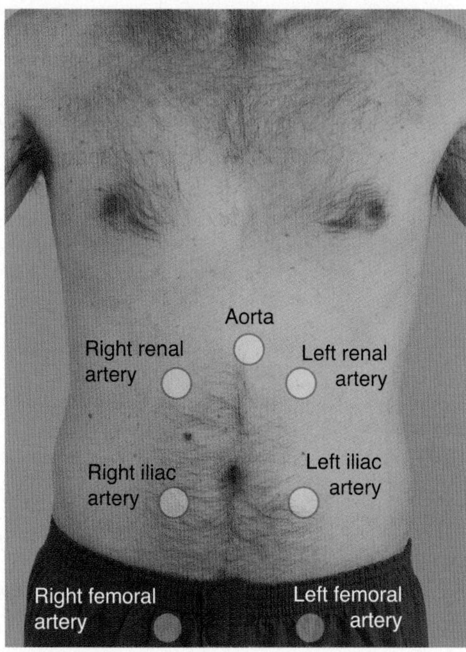 **Figure 20.7** Site for auscultating for bruits.	

(table continues on page 576)

Technique and Normal Findings (continued)	Rationale/Abnormal Findings (continued)
Venous hums are best heard in the epigastric region, near the liver and over the umbilicus (Fig. 20.8). 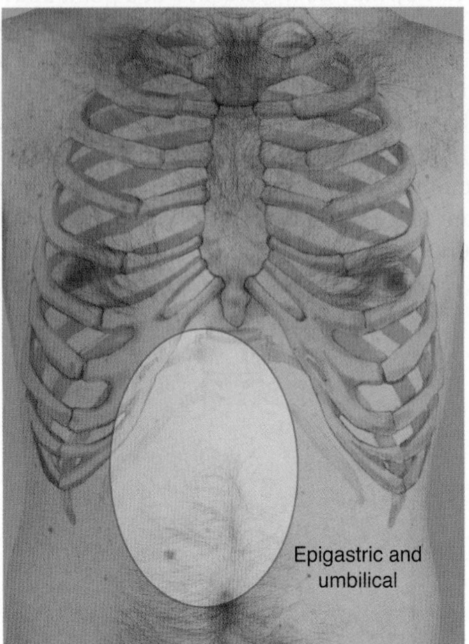 Figure 20.8 Site for auscultating for venous hums.	**Venous hums** are a soft-pitched humming noise with systolic and diastolic components. They indicate partial obstruction of an artery and reduced blood flow to the organ.
Finally, auscultate over the liver and spleen for friction rubs (Fig. 20.9). 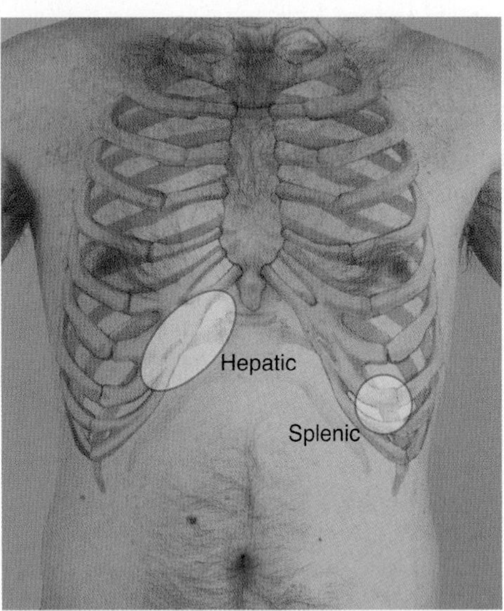 Figure 20.9 Site for auscultating for friction rubs.	**Friction rubs** are grating sounds that increase with inspiration. They may indicate a liver tumor, splenic infarction, or peritoneal inflammation.
Percussion Percussion is used to determine organ size and tenderness. It also detects any fluid, air, or masses in the abdominal cavity.	

(table continues on page 577)

Technique and Normal Findings (continued)	Rationale/Abnormal Findings (continued)
Percuss all four quadrants, listening carefully for tympany or dullness. Ask the patient whether abdominal pain is present. If an area is painful, percuss that area last. Ask the patient to point to the area of maximal tenderness and to suck in the abdomen. Place your hand 15 cm (about 6 in.) over the abdomen and ask the patient to push the stomach to your hand while coughing.	Pain indicates peritoneal inflammation and can indicate spontaneous infection in the area of the pain, appendicitis in RLQ, ruptured stomach ulcer or diverticulum in the LLQ, cholecystitis in the RUQ, or cystitis over the symphysis pubis.
All these maneuvers move peritoneal surfaces without contact. Normal percussion findings include dullness over the liver in the RUQ and hollow tympanic notes in the LUQ over the gastric bubble. Over most of the abdomen, tympanic sounds should be heard; they indicate the presence of gas.	Dullness may be heard over organs, masses, or fluid, such as ascites, GI obstruction, pregnancy, or an ovarian tumor.
Kidneys. Assessing kidney tenderness is accomplished by fist or blunt percussion at the costovertebral angle (CVA) posteriorly. (The CVA is where the rib cage meets the spine.) With the patient sitting, place the palm of your nondominant hand over the CVA and hit that hand with the fist of your dominant hand (Fig. 20.10). Repeat on the other side. Slight or no pain noted during fist percussion. 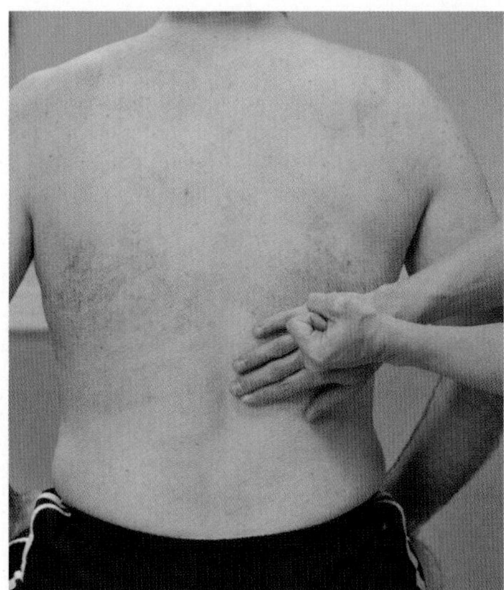 **Figure 20.10** Percussing for kidney tenderness at the costovertebral angle.	Significant pain upon blunt percussion at the CVA is a positive sign and can be indicative of a kidney infection (pyelonephritis) or kidney stones, which cause stretching or inflammation of capsules surrounding these organs.
Liver. A liver span test gives you an estimate of the size of the liver in the MCL. To assess the upper edge of the liver, start at the right MCL at the 3rd intercostal space (ICS) over lung tissue. Percuss down until you hear resonance change to dullness over the liver between the 5th and 7th ICSs (Fig. 20.11). Place a mark where the dullness begins. To determine the lower border of the liver, start at the right MCL at the level of the umbilicus and percuss upward until tympany turns to dullness, usually at the sternal border. Mark this area with a pen. Measure the distance between the two marks (Fig. 20.12). *Liver span is 6–12 cm (about 2½–5 in.).*	Abnormal findings include hepatomegaly and the firm hepatic edge indicating cirrhosis.

(table continues on page 578)

Technique and Normal Findings (continued)	Rationale/Abnormal Findings (continued)
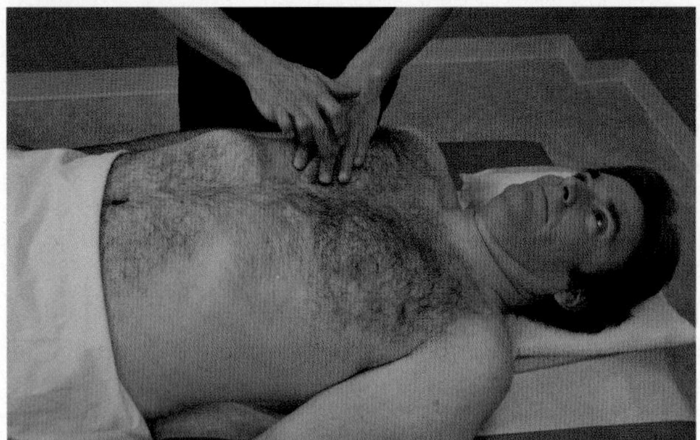 Figure 20.11 Percussing the liver. 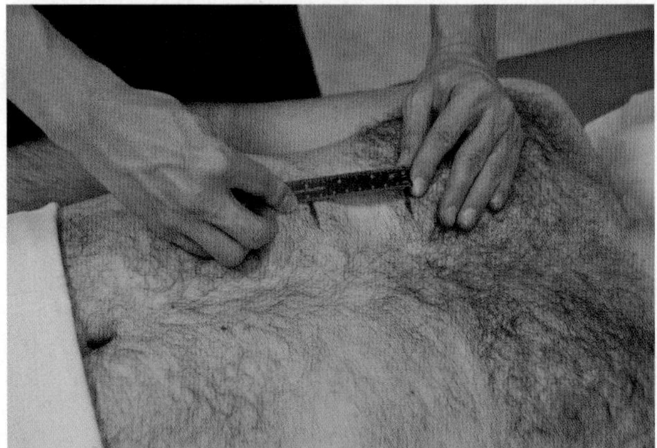 Figure 20.12 Measuring the liver border. If the liver span in the MCL is greater than 12 cm, measure it in the midsternal line. Normal midsternal liver span is 4–8 cm (about 1½–3 in.) (Fig. 20.13). 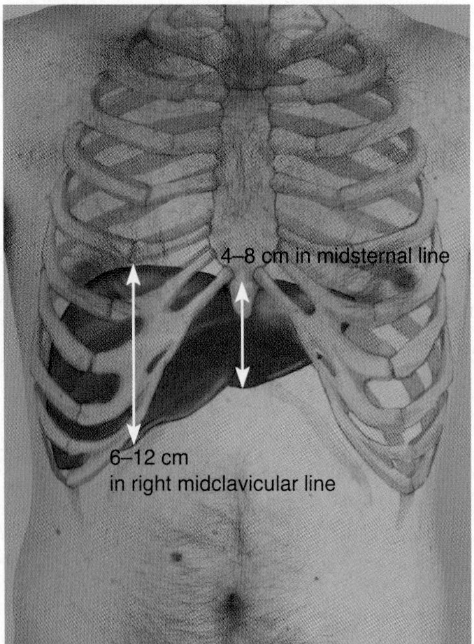 Figure 20.13 Normal liver span.	

(table continues on page 579)

Technique and Normal Findings (continued)	Rationale/Abnormal Findings (continued)

Spleen. Three methods are used to assess the approximate size of the spleen:

1. Percuss from the left MCL along the costal margin to the left midaxillary line (MAL). If you hear tympany, splenomegaly is unlikely.
2. Percuss at the lowest ICS at the left MAL. Ask the patient to take a deep breath and hold it; percuss again. Tympany is normal, but with splenomegaly, tympany turns to dullness on inspiration.
3. Percuss from the third to the fourth ICS slightly posterior to the left MAL, and percuss downward until dullness is heard. Dullness of the normal spleen is noted around the 9th–11th ribs.

Dullness at the MAL is indicative of splenomegaly (Fig. 20.14).

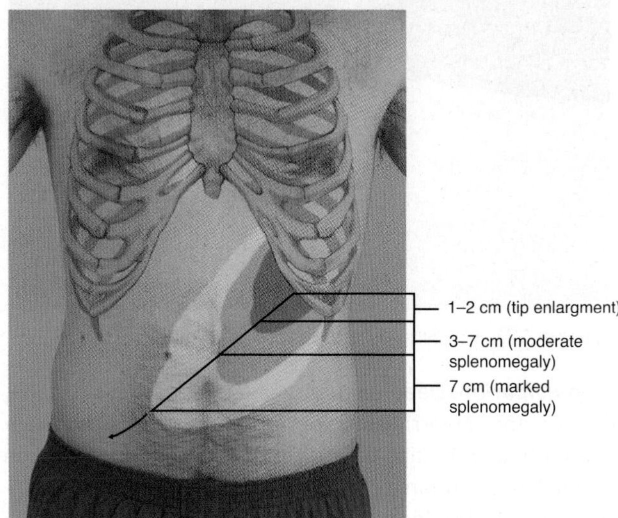

Figure 20.14 Indicators of splenomegaly.

Bladder. Assessing bladder size is achieved by percussing for bladder distension. Begin at the symphysis pubis and percuss upward toward the umbilicus, noting any dullness. *An empty bladder does not rise above the symphysis pubis.*

Tenderness over the symphysis pubis may indicate a UTI or pelvic inflammatory disease (PID).

Palpation

Light Palpation. Both light and deep palpations are used to assess the abdomen. Begin with light palpation in all four quadrants for a general survey of surface characteristics and to put the patient at ease. Press down 1–2 cm (about ½–1 in.) in a rotating motion, then lift your fingertips and move to the next location (Fig. 20.15). Observe for nonverbal signs of pain, such as grimacing and guarding. No tenderness should be noted. If guarding is present, place a pillow under the patient's knees and have him or her take a few deep breaths. While the patient is concentrating on breathing, lightly palpate the rectus abdominis muscles on expiration. The patient cannot voluntarily guard this muscle during expiration.

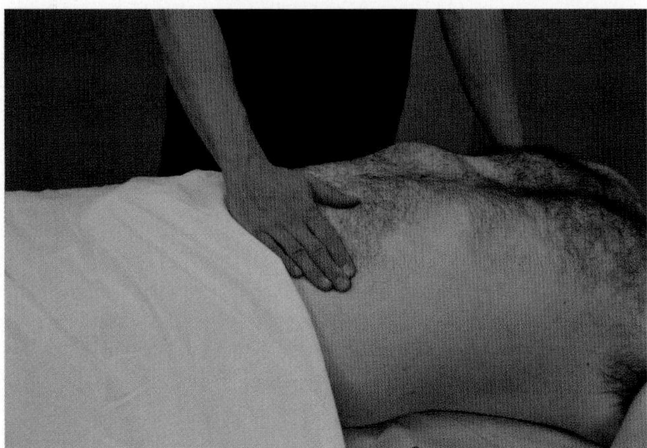

Figure 20.15 Lightly palpating the abdomen.

⚠ *SAFETY ALERT*

Do not palpate the abdomen of patients who have had an organ transplant or of a child with suspected Wilms tumor. Transplanted organs are often located in the anterior portion of the abdomen and are not as well protected as the original organ. In the case of Wilms tumor, palpating may cause the tumor to seed into the abdomen.

Involuntary guarding is a sign of possible peritoneal inflammation and should be carefully evaluated.

(table continues on page 580)

Technique and Normal Findings (continued)	Rationale/Abnormal Findings (continued)
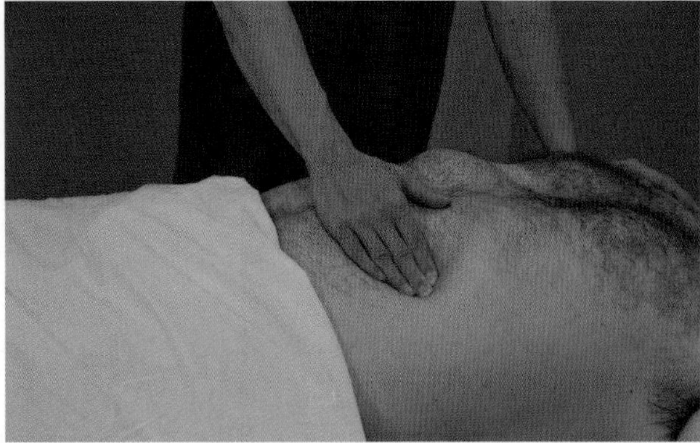 Figure 20.16 Single-handed deep palpation.	
Deep Palpation. Deep palpation is used to assess organs, masses, and tenderness. To perform single-handed deep palpation, use the tips of your fingers and depress 4–6 cm (about 1½–2½ in.) in a dipping motion in all four quadrants (Fig. 20.16). Tenderness may be noted in an adult near the xiphoid process, over the cecum, or over the sigmoid colon. Bimanual deep palpation is necessary when palpating a large abdomen. Place your nondominant hand on your dominant hand and depress your hands 4–6 cm (about 1½–2½ in.) (Fig. 20.17).	If you find a mass, note its location, size, shape, consistency, tenderness, pulsation, mobility, and movement with respiration. Refer to Figure 20.1 for the location of abdominal and accessory organs. Size and changes over time offer insight into pathology and the extent of involvement.
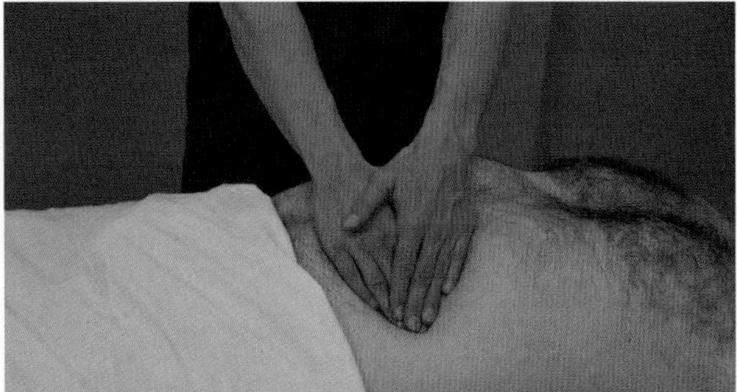 Figure 20.17 Bimanual deep palpation.	
Liver. To palpate the liver, place your right hand at the patient's right MCL under the costal margin. Place your left hand on the patient's back at the 11th and 12th ribs; press upward to elevate the liver toward the abdominal wall (Fig. 20.18). Have the patient take a deep breath.	An enlarged liver is palpable below the costal margin. Assess its size as described under "Percussion." An enlarged liver may indicate a tumor or cirrhosis.
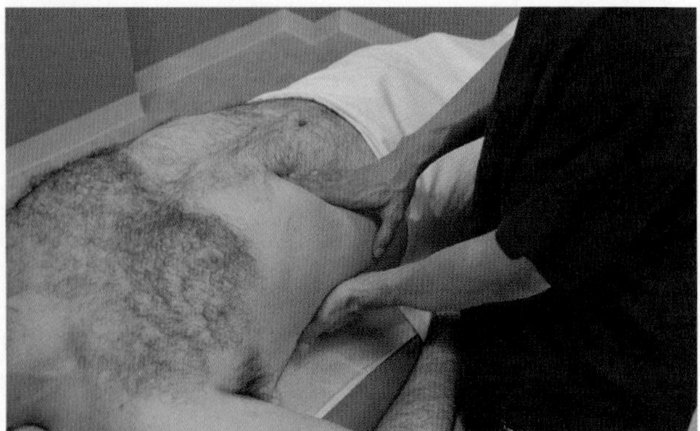 Figure 20.18 Pressing upward to elevate the liver.	

(table continues on page 581)

Technique and Normal Findings (continued)	Rationale/Abnormal Findings (continued)
Press your right hand gently but deeply in and up during inspiration. The liver edge is palpable against your right hand during inspiration.	
The hooking technique is another method to palpate the liver. Place your hands over the right costal margin and hook your fingers over the edge. Have the patient take a deep breath and feel for the liver's edge as it drops down on inspiration then rises up over your fingers on expiration (Fig. 20.19).	
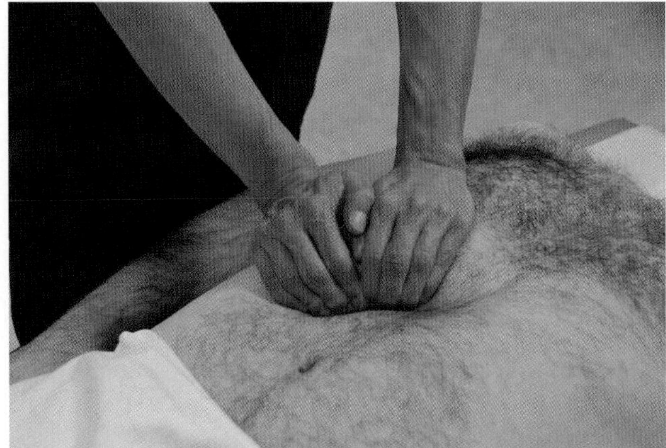 Figure 20.19 Using the hooking technique to assess the liver.	
Spleen. To palpate the spleen, stand on the patient's right side. Place your left hand under the patient's left CVA and pull upward to move the spleen anteriorly (Fig. 20.20). Place your right hand under the left costal margin. Have the patient take a deep breath; during exhalation, press inward along the left costal margin and try to palpate the spleen. An alternative approach is to have the patient turn onto the right side to move the spleen more forward (Fig. 20.21).	In an enlarged spleen, you can palpate the spleen tip. Enlarged spleen occurs with mononucleosis, HIV, cancers of the blood and lymphatic system, infectious hepatitis, and red blood cell abnormalities of spherocytosis, sickle cell anemia, and thalassemia.
A normal spleen is not palpable.	
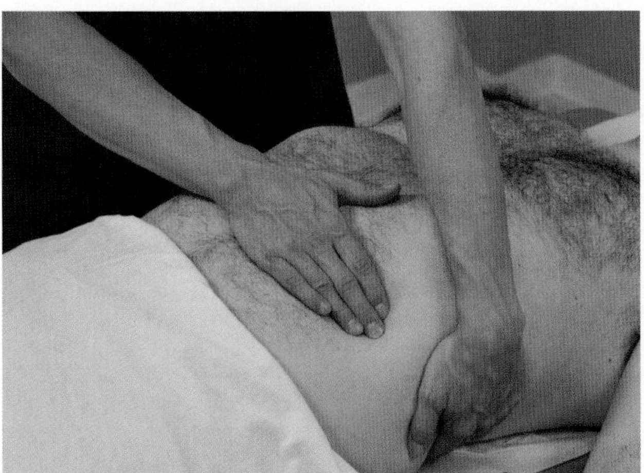 Figure 20.20 Placing the hand under the patient's left costovertebral angle to move the spleen.	

(table continues on page 582)

Technique and Normal Findings (continued)	Rationale/Abnormal Findings (continued)
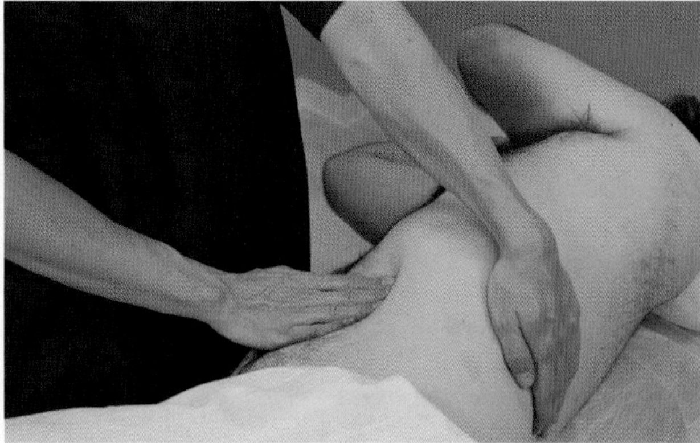 Figure 20.21 Palpating the spleen with the patient on the right side.	
Kidneys. To assess the left kidney, stand on the patient's right side and place your left hand in the left CVA. Place your right hand at the left anterior costal margin. Have the patient take a deep breath, then press your hands together to "capture" the kidney. As the patient exhales, lift your left hand and palpate the kidney with your right hand (Fig. 20.22).	Kidneys enlarged from hydronephrosis or tumors may be palpable.
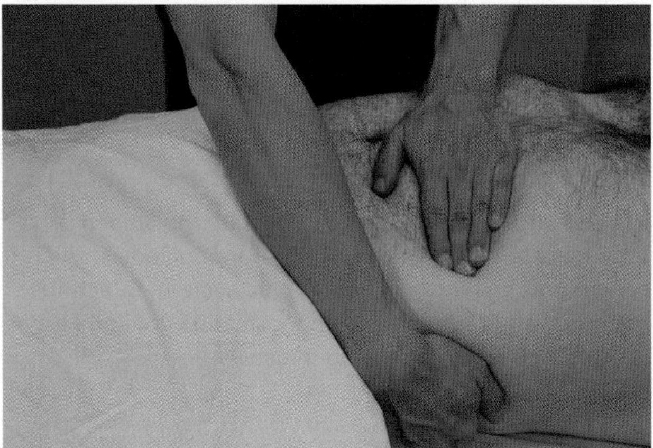 Figure 20.22 Palpating the left kidney.	
To assess the right kidney (only palpable if enlarged), remain on the patient's right side; place your right hand on the right CVA and your left hand on the right costal margin. When the patient exhales, palpate the right kidney (Fig. 20.23). *It is common to be unable to palpate the kidneys except in slender patients.*	
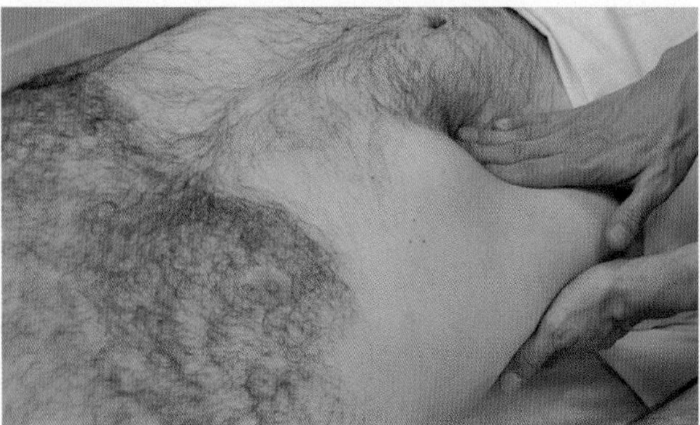 Figure 20.23 Palpating the right kidney.	(table continues on page 583)

Technique and Normal Findings (continued)	Rationale/Abnormal Findings (continued)
Abdominal Aorta. To palpate the abdominal aorta, place your fingers in the epigastric region, slightly toward the left of the MCL. Palpate for aortic pulsations on either side of the aorta (Fig. 20.24). You can assess the width of the aorta by placing one hand on either side of the aorta. Pulsations of the aorta are palpable; the aorta should measure 2 cm (about ¾ in.). 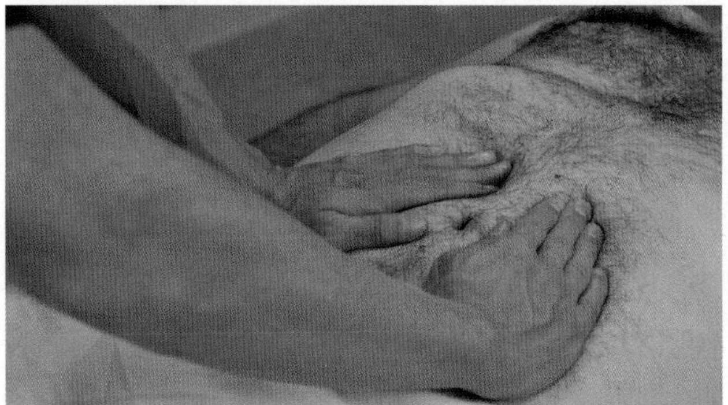 **Figure 20.24** Palpating for aortic pulsations.	An enlarged aorta (greater than 3 cm [about 1¼ in.]) or one with lateral pulsations that are palpable can indicate an abdominal aortic aneurysm.
Bladder. Palpate the bladder using deep palpation in the hypogastric area. The empty bladder is neither tender nor palpable.	A palpable bladder is either full or enlarged from an underlying mass arising in the bladder or pelvis. A tender bladder usually indicates a UTI.
Lymph Nodes. Inguinal lymph nodes lie deep in the lower abdomen. They can be palpated using the pads of your fingers just below the inguinal ligament for the superficial superior lymph nodes and along the inner aspect of the upper thigh for the superficial inferior nodes. They drain the exterior iliac, pelvic, and paraaortic areas. Inguinal lymph nodes are nontender and slightly palpable.	If lymph nodes are palpable, note size, shape, mobility, consistency, and tenderness. Enlarged lymph nodes indicate an infection in the regions drained, such as orchitis in males, an infection of the lower extremities, or metastatic disease involving the anus or vulva.
Eliciting the Abdominal Reflex The abdominal reflex is a superficial cutaneous reflex measured by stroking the abdomen lightly with a tongue blade or the handle of a reflex hammer. The abdomen is stroked in all four quadrants toward the umbilicus. The umbilicus moves toward the stimulus. This reflex may be masked and not determinable in obese patients.	The abdominal reflex is absent in patients with upper and lower motor neuron diseases. See Chapter 22.
Assessing for Ascites Assessing for ascites, which is detectable only after 500 ml (about 17 oz) of fluid has accumulated, is done in two ways: shifting dullness or fluid wave.	Ascites is found in patients with cirrhosis or primary or metastatic tumors of the liver.
Shifting Dullness. Shifting dullness can be detected by percussing dullness in the umbilical area when the patient is supine (Fig. 20.25) then having the patient lie on the right side and percussing again (Fig. 20.26). You can repeat this maneuver by having the patient turn to the left side.	Dullness will move to the most dependent area.

(table continues on page 584)

Technique and Normal Findings (continued)	Rationale/Abnormal Findings (continued)
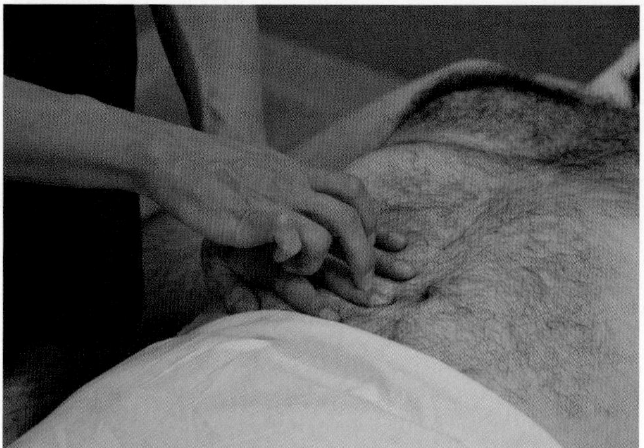 Figure 20.25 Percussing for dullness in the umbilical area with the patient supine.	
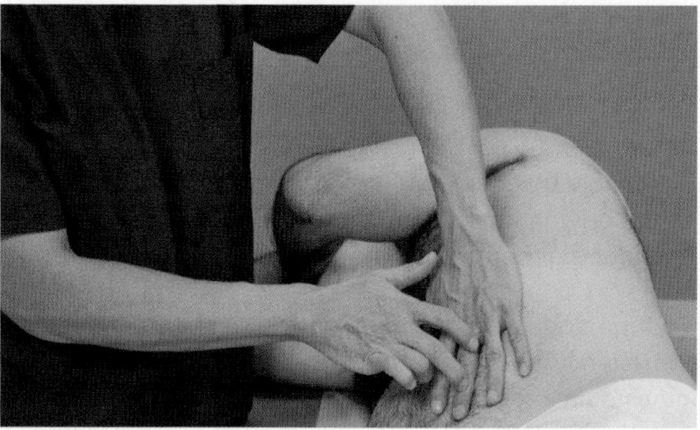 Figure 20.26 Percussing for dullness in the umbilical area with the patient turned to the side.	
Fluid Wave. Have the patient place his or her hand vertically in the middle of the abdomen. Place your hands on both sides of the patient's abdomen and tap one side while palpating the other (Fig. 20.27).	If ascites is present, the tap will cause a fluid wave through the abdomen and you will feel the fluid with the other hand.
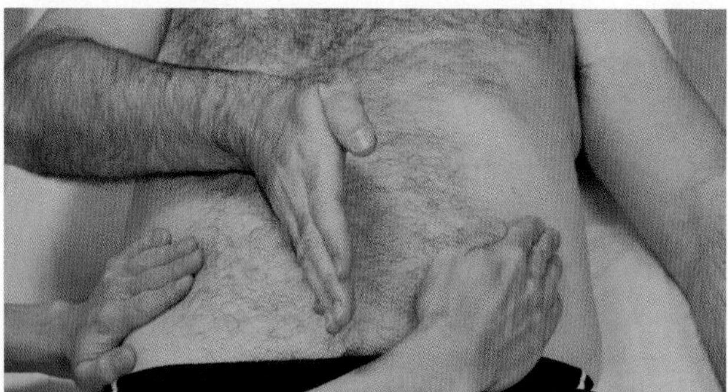 Figure 20.27 Assessing for a fluid wave to determine presence of ascites.	
Assessing for Peritoneal Irritation Assess for **Blumberg sign** or rebound tenderness to check for peritonitis. In a site away from the painful area, push down your hand at a 90-degree angle slowly and deeply, then lift up quickly. A negative and normal response is no pain when the pressure is released.	Pain when pressure is released indicates peritoneal irritation or **peritonitis**. It may indicate appendicitis or infection. A cough that causes abdominal tenderness in a specific area may also signal peritoneal irritation.

(table continues on page 585)

Technique and Normal Findings (continued)	Rationale/Abnormal Findings (continued)
Inflammation of the Gallbladder To check for inflammation of the gallbladder, assess for a **Murphy sign** or **inspiratory arrest**. Holding your fingers beneath the liver border, apply mild pressure, and ask the patient to breathe deeply. Normally, no pain occurs and the test result is negative.	Pain with breathing indicates inflammation of the gallbladder. The patient feels sharp pain when the liver pushes the inflamed gallbladder over the pressure and the patient abruptly stops breathing in, causing an inspiratory arrest.
Appendicitis The **iliopsoas muscle test** is performed when appendicitis is suspected. With the patient lying supine, lift the right leg straight up, keeping the knee straight. Push down over the lower part of the right thigh while the patient pushes up. No pain is normal and a negative test result.	Pain with contraction occurs when the iliopsoas muscle is inflamed, with an inflamed or perforated appendix. Pain is usually felt in the RLQ.

Documenting Normal Findings

No scars noted, old silver striae bilaterally. Flat, symmetrical, faint aortic pulsations LUQ. Approximately 20 clicks and gurgles a minute in RLQ, borborygmi upper quadrants, occasional clicks in LLQ. Tympanic to percussion, some scattered dullness all four quadrants. Relaxed, nontender, soft to palpation in all four quadrants. Liver span 8 cm (about 3 in.) R MCL, nontender, soft smooth edge 1 cm inferior to R costal margin. Gallbladder nonpalpable, nontender. Spleen tympanic on inspiration in lowest L anterior axillary interspace, nonpalpable. Kidney nonpalpable bilaterally, no CVA tenderness. Bladder percussed at symphysis pubis, nonpalpable. Aorta 2.5 cm (about 1 in.) wide with mild anterior pulsation. Appendix not identified, no tenderness.

Lifespan Considerations: Older Adults

Many elders are plagued with poor dentition, which may result in pain when chewing, dramatic changes in diet and weight, and long-term difficulties. Decreased production of saliva and stomach acid leads to changes in the digestive process. Motility and peristalsis decrease with age, which may result in more bloating, distention, and constipation. Other contributing factors are decreased muscle mass and tone. The liver shrinks and becomes less functional, resulting in less absorption of medications metabolized by the liver. Renal function decreases, resulting in a diminished ability to eliminate medications. Decreased liver and renal function in the elderly often results in lower than normal medication's therapeutic effects.

Inspection of the abdomen is more challenging in older adults and results are often less accurate. This is because of the fat that accumulates in the lower abdomen of women and around the waist of men as they age.

Cultural Considerations

Some health problems are more common in certain races and ethnic groups. African Americans more commonly present with sickle cell anemia, G6PD deficiency, and lactose intolerance (Stern et al., 2010). In those with sickle cell disease, you may find splenomegaly and jaundice on examination. In sickle cell crisis, patients may present with complaints of acute abdominal pain and vomiting. Lactose intolerance may cause abdominal cramping and diarrhea. **Obesity**, defined as weight greater than 120% of ideal weight, is generally higher in racial and ethnic minorities than in Caucasians. It is highest in non-Hispanic black women. See also Chapter 7.

GI cancers, especially stomach cancer, are more often seen in Asian Americans (Phan, 2011). Patients with these illnesses present with long-standing complaints of heartburn, indigestion, anorexia, and weight loss. Asian Americans have a higher incidence of infection with *Helicobacter pylori* (Atherton & Blaser, 2012).

Lactose intolerance and IBD are more prevalent in Americans of Jewish ancestry (Barter & Dunne, 2011). The most common presenting symptoms are abdominal cramping, diarrhea, and rectal bleeding. African Americans have the highest colorectal cancer incidence and mortality rates of all racial groups in the United States. Ashkenazi Jews have a greater risk of colon cancer than other ethnic group and are believed to carry a gene linked to the development of familial colorectal cancer (ACS, 2013b).

Americans of Greek and Italian descent more commonly present with lactose intolerance, thalassemia, and anemia (Stern et al., 2010). These illnesses cause abdominal cramping, diarrhea, jaundice, and splenomegaly.

Alcoholism, liver and gallbladder disease, pancreatitis, and diabetes are more common in Native Americans. GI symptoms in this group include jaundice, anorexia, ascites, abdominal pain, steatorrhea, weight loss, polyuria, polydipsia, polyphagia, and weakness.

Lactose intolerance is common among all cultural groups. In Europe and the United States, approximately, 7% to 20% of Caucasians are lactose intolerant. Approximately 80% to 95% of Native Americans, 65% to 75% of Africans and African Americans, and 50% of Hispanics are also lactose intolerant. In eastern Asia, 90% may be intolerant (Stern et al., 2010).

Documenting Case Study Findings

You have just finished conducting a physical assessment of Mr. Renaud, the 41-year-old Caucasian man admitted to the hospital with a GI bleed. Review the following important findings revealed in each step of objective data collection for this patient. Consider how these results compare with normal findings. Pay attention to how the nurse clusters data to provide a more complete and accurate understanding of the condition.

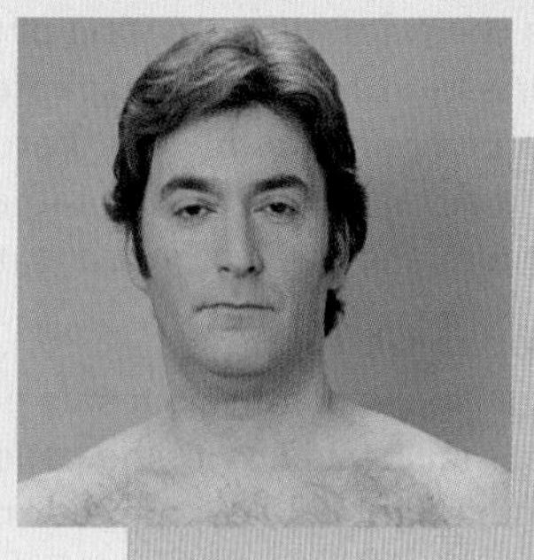

Inspection: Abdomen distended symmetrically. Umbilicus everted with significant ascites. Skin jaundiced with prominent venous network. Abdominal girth is 85 cm (about 33½ in.). Weight has decreased from 65 to 55 kg (about 143 to 121 lb). Height 1.78 m (about 5 ft 10 in.). Arms and legs lack muscle mass and tone.

Auscultation: Bowel sounds hyperactive in all four quadrants. No bruits present.

Palpation: Abdomen firm and slightly tender with muscle guarding. Lower border of the liver palpated 4 cm below (1½ in.) the sternal border at the right MCL. Fluid wave and shifting dullness are present. No masses present, liver smooth.

Percussion: Lower border of the liver percussed 4 cm (1½ in.) below the sternal border at the right MCL. Abdomen tympanic at the dome of the abdomen, flanks slightly dull.

Critical Thinking

Laboratory and Diagnostic Testing

Few specific laboratory tests focus on the abdomen and GI system. A complete blood count should be done to determine signs of anemia and infection. Iron-deficiency anemia in men, postmenopausal women, and elderly patients always warrants an endoscopy and colonoscopy to rule out GI cancer.

A basic metabolic panel (BMP) gives a good overview of various changes that can result from the malfunction of abdominal organs. Glucose level gives an indication of pancreatic endocrine function. The electrolytes sodium, potassium, chlorine, and carbon dioxide point to the state of the patient's hydration, which may be affected by vomiting or dehydration. The blood urea nitrogen (BUN) and creatinine levels are indicators of basic kidney function. Liver function tests (including alanine aminotransferase [ALT] and aspartate aminotransferase [AST] levels) indicate the health of the liver. Levels of these enzymes, which are necessary for digestion and absorption of nutrients, remain normal until liver compromise is significant. Amylase and lipase levels are also tested to determine the exocrine function of the pancreas. These studies would need to be added to the BMP.

If ulcer disease is suspected, a breath test for *H. pylori* is indicated. It is imperative that this test be done *before* any acid reducers (especially the proton pump inhibitors) are ordered to assist with pain relief (Atherton & Blaser, 2012). If a patient has been taking OTC proton pump inhibitors, he or she must stop the medication for 2 weeks before the breath test will be accurate.

Several specialized tests are performed to identify specific problems along the alimentary canal and its accessory organs. These tests are briefly discussed in the following sections.

Esophagogastroduodenoscopy

Esophagogastroduodenoscopy (EGD), also called endoscopy, determines the condition of the mucosa of the esophagus, stomach, and duodenum. The patient is usually given conscious sedation; the back of the throat is numbed with a spray anesthetic. The endoscope is passed and the entire upper GI tract is assessed through pictures taken and subsequent biopsies of any abnormalities. EGD is usually ordered and performed in patients with suspected gastric ulcer disease, active GI bleeding, or cancer of the esophagus or stomach.

Barium Enema

Barium enema is used in a radiological procedure in which the patient receives an enema of barium sulfate to outline the large intestine. This test helps determine whether the patient has IBD or cancer of the colon. It can be done as single contrast, with only the barium, or double contrast, in which the barium is removed after the initial part of the assessment, air is inserted, and a closer look at the walls of the colon is possible.

> ⚠ *SAFETY ALERT*
> *A barium enema should not be performed on a patient suspected of having an acute inflammatory condition, such as appendicitis, diverticulitis, or ulcerative colitis, or who has a perforated hollow organ. The barium enema can cause an inflamed area of the bowel to rupture. Death may result.*

Colonoscopy

Colonoscopy is done to determine the general condition of the colon and rectum and is used to identify polyps, ulcerations, and tumors. It is recommended as standard practice for patients older than 50 years to have screening for colorectal cancer. The patient is given conscious sedation, the colonoscope is passed, and the entire length of the colon is visualized. Pictures of the walls of the colon are taken; small polyps and tumors can be removed and biopsied as part of this test. This test requires preprocedure preparation of the bowel to remove all feces for the most accurate results.

Endoscopic Retrograde Cholangiopancreatography

Endoscopic retrograde cholangiopancreatography (ERCP) is performed to assess the ducts draining the liver and pancreas, to identify and remove gallstones in the common bile duct, and to diagnose pancreatic cancer. ERCP is similar to but more extensive than EGD; the patient receives conscious sedation and the endoscope is passed through the mouth into the stomach and duodenum to the area of the common bile ducts.

Computed Tomography Scan

CT scan is a radiological procedure performed with and without contrast to identify soft tissue problems that may arise in the abdominal cavity. Cysts, abscesses, infections, tumors, aneurysms, and enlarged organs such as the liver and gallbladder may be identified in this manner.

Magnetic Resonance Imaging

MRI is a radiological procedure performed with the patient lying within in a large magnetic tube. It is used to evaluate the condition of organs, ducts, and blood vessels. Patients with pacemakers, ventricular assist devices, and joint replacements cannot undergo MRI because the magnetic force can cause problems with the metal components of their embedded life-sustaining equipment.

Diagnostic Reasoning

Nursing Diagnoses, Outcomes, and Interventions

Table 20.1 provides a comparison of nursing diagnoses, abnormal findings, and interventions commonly related to the abdominal assessment (NANDA, 2012).

Nurses use assessment information to identify patient outcomes. Some outcomes that are related to system problems include the following:

- Diarrhea: Patient will defecate a formed soft stool every day to every third day.

TABLE 20.1 Common Nursing Diagnoses Associated With the Abdomen

Diagnosis	Point of Differentiation	Assessment Characteristics	Nursing Interventions
Imbalanced nutrition, less than body requirement	Dietary intake that is inadequate in quantity, quality, or both for metabolic needs	Body weight decreased, BMI less than normal	Provide nutritional supplements (e.g., milk shakes). Administer antiemetics as ordered*
Diarrhea	At least three liquid stools per day	Passage of loose unformed stools	Obtain stool specimens to determine infection (e.g., *Clostridium difficile* infection)
Constipation	Decrease in normal frequency of defecation with hard dry stool	Abdominal distention, pain, tenderness, firm abdomen, no stool for days	Obtain order for stool softener if patient is on opioids, increase intake of fiber, assist with ambulation, ensure adequate intake of fluids
Incontinence	Involuntary passage of urine occurring with sudden desire to urinate (urge)	Voiding more than every 2 hours while awake, awakening at night to urinate, voiding more than eight times in a 24-hour period	Review medications that may contribute to incontinence, perform bladder scan to evaluate if residual is present, teach principles of bladder training.

*Collaborative interventions.

- Constipation: Patient will maintain the passage of soft, formed stool every 1 to 2 days without straining.
- Patient will report relief from or decrease in the incidence and severity of incontinent episodes (Ackley & Ladwig, 2013).

After the outcomes have been established, nursing care is implemented to improve the status of the patient. The nurse uses critical thinking and evidence-based practice to develop the interventions. Some examples of nursing interventions for the GI system are as follows:

- Diarrhea: Consider inserting tube into rectum to drain stool and prevent skin breakdown.
- Constipation: Make sure to monitor last bowel movement and administer bulk stool softeners and laxatives as ordered.
- Incontinence: Teach patient to pace fluids and avoid fluids before bedtime (Ackley & Ladwig, 2013).

The nurse then evaluates care according to the patient outcomes that were developed, reassessing the patient and continuing or modifying interventions as appropriate.

An accurate and complete nursing assessment is an essential foundation for holistic nursing care. Even as a beginner, the nursing student can use the patient assessment to implement new interventions, evaluate the effectiveness of those interventions, and make a difference in the quality of patient care.

Progress Note: Analyzing Findings

Remember Mr. Renaud, whose difficulties have been outlined throughout this chapter. The initial subjective and objective data collection is complete, and the nurse has spent time reviewing the findings and other results. Unfortunately, Mr. Renaud vomits bright red blood, so it is necessary to reassess him and document the findings. The following nursing note illustrates how subjective and objective data are collected and analyzed and nursing interventions are developed.

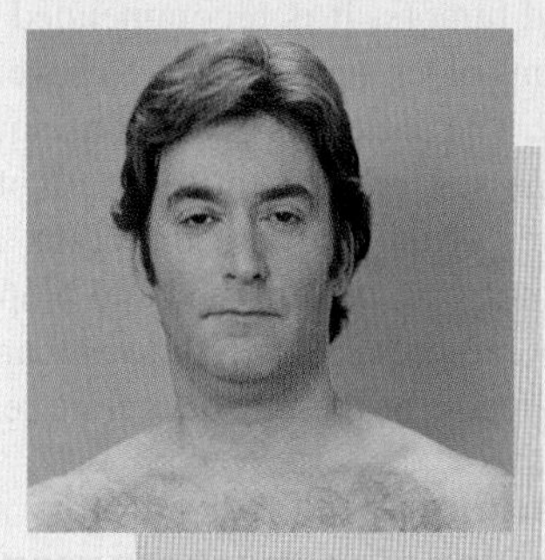

Subjective: I just felt it coming on fast. I knew I shouldn't have eaten that food. Am I going to have to go back to the ICU?

Objective: Vomited 250 ml (about 8 oz) of emesis with partially digested food and about 20% with bright red blood. Gastroccult tested positive for blood. T 37°C (98.6°F) tympanic, P 124 beats/min, R 24 breaths/min, BP 100/62 mmHg, oxygen saturation 93%. Sitting in bed with head of bed elevated. Abdomen slightly tender, firm, and distended with hyperactive bowel sounds. Tympany present over most of abdomen. Patient states feeling nauseous, fatigued, and anxious.

Analysis: Fluid volume deficit due to GI blood loss.

Plan: Saline lock intact. Notify primary care provider about emesis. Inform patient about plans and assure that the nurse will be readily available if needed. Provide oral hygiene and hold food or fluids until discussed with primary care provider. Administer medication for nausea according to physician's orders.

Critical Thinking Challenge

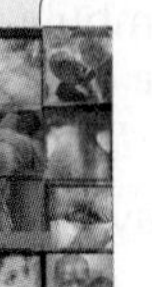

- Why is information on the vital signs included as part of the nursing note?
- How has the nurse altered the assessment focus from the earlier conversation about discharge planning?
- What additional information might be documented on patient flow sheets?

Collaborating With the Interprofessional Team

Mr. Renaud, admitted 5 days ago with a GI bleed, is having a new onset of bleeding. The new bleeding, drop in blood pressure, and increase in pulse need collaborative interventions, so the physician needs to be contacted.

The following conversation illustrates how the nurse might organize the data and make recommendations about the patient's situation to the physician.

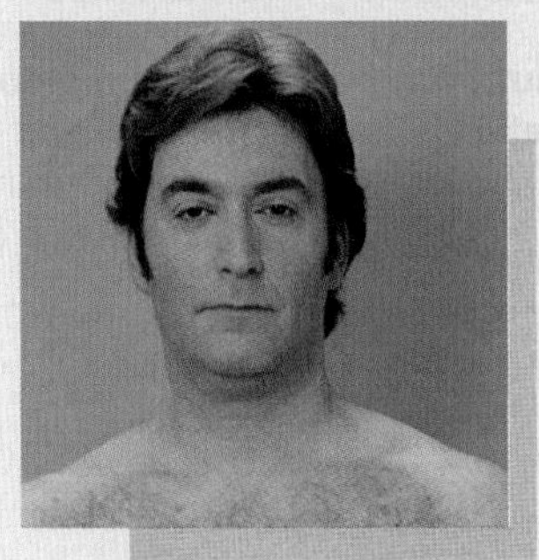

Situation: "Hi Dr. Plete. This is Kathy on 3 East. I'm taking care of Mr. Renaud, a 41-year-old patient on your team."

Background: "He was admitted 5 days ago with GI bleed and has been stable for the past few days."

Assessment: "He just vomited 250 ml (about 8 oz) of emesis with partially digested food and about 50 ml (about 2 oz) of blood; the Gastroccult was positive. His pulse is P 124 beats/min, R 24 breaths/min, BP 100/62 mmHg, and oxygen saturation is 93%. Usually, his pulse is around 100, and the blood pressure is about 150/90 mmHg. He has a saline lock in but no IV fluids, and I just gave him the as-needed antinausea medication."

Recommendations: "I'll see if that works in a half hour. For now, I've asked him to have nothing by mouth and was wondering if you wanted me to start IV fluids. I can also call the lab to have them order a stat hemoglobin and hematocrit. He has three units of packed red blood cells on hold if they are needed. What would you like to do?"

Critical Thinking Challenge

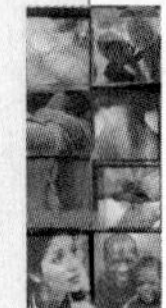

- Consider all the objective data that were collected. Why did the nurse omit some of the physical assessment findings previously documented in the SOAP note?
- Which of the assessments are within the nursing domain and which are within collaborative practice with the physician?
- What further assessments will you perform, and how frequently?

Putting It All Together

The nurse uses assessment data to formulate a nursing care plan for Mr. Renaud. After completing interventions, the nurse will reevaluate Mr. Renaud and document findings in the chart to show critical thinking. This is often in the form of a care plan or case note similar to the following:

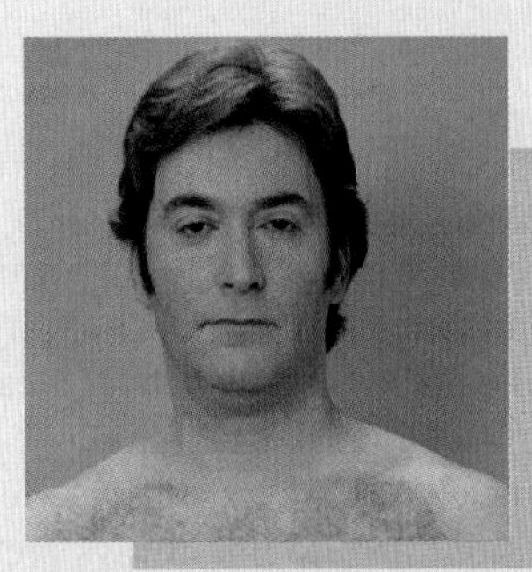

(case study continues on page 590)

Nursing Diagnosis	Patient Outcomes	Nursing Interventions	Rationale	Evaluation
Fluid volume deficit	Maintain blood pressure and pulse within normal limits	Monitor P and BP every 15 minutes until stable. Assess for signs of hypovolemia including postural hypotension, poor skin turgor, thirst, sunken eyeballs, and weakness. Also monitor intake and output and daily weights. Assess IV site for infection, inflammation, and infiltration.	Decreased intravascular volume results in decreased tissue oxygenation. Signs of hypovolemia may be noted with continued bleeding or insufficient replacement. The IV site may be a source of infection because the skin is broken.	IV fluids started with normal saline at 100 ml/h.* IV site without redness, tenderness, or swelling. Patient placed on nothing by mouth. No further episodes of vomiting, no stools. BP 122/66 mmHg, P 110 beats/min, skin turgor poor, eyeballs sunken, states feeling better.

*Collaborative interventions.

Applying Your Knowledge

Using the previous steps of diagnostic reasoning, organizing, and prioritizing, consider all the case study findings woven throughout this chapter. When answering the following questions, begin drawing conclusions and see how the pieces of assessment must work together to create an environment for personalized, appropriate, and accurate care.

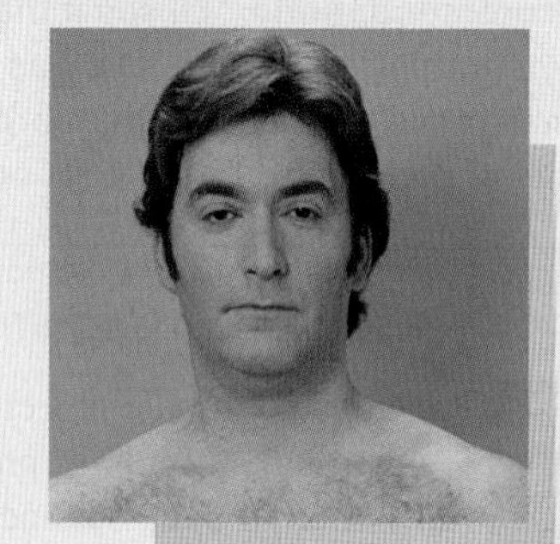

- What techniques are used when assessing the anatomical systems within the abdomen?
- How will the nurse prioritize health promotion and teaching needs?
- How will the nurse organize the assessment during the shift?
- How does the nurse incorporate the different phases of the nursing process while performing the assessments?
- When Mr. Renaud's GI bleed is resolved, what recommendations do you expect the nurse, physician, and other members of the health care team to make as they continue to care for him?
- How will you evaluate whether your initial interventions are effective?

Key Points

- Auscultation of the abdomen is always performed before percussion and palpation, which can alter bowel motility and diminish the nurse's ability to hear bowel sounds.
- The nurse assesses tender areas last to avoid referred pain and additional discomfort.
- The elderly are less likely to feel pain with abdominal conditions and do not always present with classic symptoms and laboratory findings. They are more likely to have vague diffuse pain and tend to have a less acute presentation.
- Patients who present with fever, chills, leukocytosis, and rebound tenderness warrant a rapid assessment and referral to an acute care facility.
- Abdominal pain lasting more than 6 hours or pain that wakes a patient from sleep requires evaluation and possible referral.
- Hypoactive bowel sounds are common in patients with constipation and paralytic ileus.
- Hyperactive bowel sounds are common in patients with gastroenteritis and diarrhea.
- The location of the bruit can determine its cause.

- Venous hums are continuous sounds found in the epigastric region and around the umbilicus and caused by portal hypertension.
- Eighty percent to 90% of GI diseases can be diagnosed by obtaining a thorough health history.
- Colorectal cancer is the second leading cause of U.S. cancer deaths.
- Food-borne illnesses affect the very young, the elderly, and immunocompromised patients more seriously.
- Hepatitis C is the most common blood-borne U.S. viral infection.

Review Questions

1. When performing an abdominal assessment, what is the correct sequence?
   A. Inspection, palpation, percussion, auscultation
   B. Palpation, percussion, inspection, auscultation
   C. Inspection, auscultation, percussion, palpation
   D. Auscultation, inspection, palpation, percussion

2. A patient reports a long history of changes in bowel pattern. Which is the *best* question to determine normal bowel habits?
   A. How often do you have a bowel movement?
   B. What was your bowel pattern before you noticed the change?
   C. Is there a family history of irritable bowel syndrome?
   D. Have any of your parents or siblings had cancer of the colon?

3. When palpating the abdomen, the nurse notices a mass at the anterior right costal margin in the MCL. Which organ is most likely involved?
   A. Liver
   B. Spleen
   C. Sigmoid colon
   D. Kidney

4. What percussion sound is heard over most of the abdomen?
   A. Resonance
   B. Hyperresonance
   C. Dullness
   D. Tympany

5. A patient with a history of kidney stones presents with complaints of pain, hematuria, and nausea with vomiting. What assessment technique will illicit kidney pain?
   A. Rovsing sign
   B. Psoas sign
   C. Percussion for CVA tenderness
   D. Blumberg sign

6. When auscultating the abdomen, the nurse hears a bruit to the right of the midline slightly below the umbilicus. The nurse documents this finding as a bruit of which of the following?
   A. Right renal artery
   B. Right femoral artery
   C. Right iliac artery
   D. Abdominal aorta

7. A patient with a history of cirrhosis tells the nurse that his abdomen seems to be getting larger and that he has gained 9.7 kg (20 lb) in the last 6 months. How will the nurse determine whether the abdominal enlargement is from accumulation of fluid or fat from the weight gain?
   A. By listening for a fluid wave
   B. By percussing the abdomen for shifting dullness
   C. By auscultating for lymph nodes
   D. By stroking the abdomen to elicit the abdominal reflex

8. A patient with a tympanic abdomen complains of pain in the RUQ. Which sign would the nurse expect to be positive?
   A. Murphy sign
   B. Psoas sign
   C. Rovsing sign
   D. Obturator sign

9. Which assessment technique would best confirm splenic enlargement?
   A. Deep palpation under the left costal margin
   B. Fist percussion of the spleen with the patient in a sitting position
   C. Deep palpation over the RUQ with the patient lying on the right side
   D. Percussion along the left MAL spleen and gentle palpation

10. When documenting a finding in the region over the stomach and centered above the umbilicus, the nurse most accurately identifies the region as
    A. epigastric.
    B. hypogastric.
    C. RUQ.
    D. LUQ.

The Jensen suite offers these additional resources to enhance learning and facilitate understanding of this chapter:

- thePoint online resource, http://thepoint.lww.com/Jensen2e
- *Laboratory Manual for Nursing Health Assessment: A Best Practice Approach*
- *Pocket Guide for Nursing Health Assessment: A Best Practice Approach*
- *Lippincott DocuCare,* an electronic health record simulation software, http://thepoint.lww.com/docucare
- *Adaptive Learning | Powered by PrepU*, http://thepoint.lww.com/prepu

References

Ackley, B., & Ladwig, G. (2013). *Nursing diagnosis handbook: An evidence-based guide to planning care* (10th ed.). St. Louis, MO: Mosby.

American Cancer Society, Inc. (2013a). *What are the key statistics about colorectal cancer?* Retrieved from http://www.cancer.org/cancer/colonandrectumcancer/detailedguide/colorectal-cancer-key-statistics

American Cancer Society, Inc. (2013b). *What are the risk factors for colorectal cancer?* Retrieved from http://www.cancer.org/cancer/colonandrectumcancer/detailedguide/colorectal-cancer-risk-factors

Atherton, J., & Blaser, M. (2012). *Helicobacter pylori* infections. In D. L. Longo, A. S. Fauci, D. L. Kasper, S. L. Hauser, J. L. Jameson, & J. Loscalzo (Eds.), *Harrison's principles of internal medicine* (18th ed.). New York, NY: McGraw-Hill.

Barter, C., and Dunne, L. (2011). Abdominal pain. In J. E. South-Paul, S. C. Matheny, & E. L. Lewis (Eds.), *Current diagnosis and treatment in family medicine* (3rd ed.). New York, NY: McGraw-Hill.

Centers for Disease Control and Prevention. (2013). *Hepatitis A FAQs for health professionals.* Retrieved from http://www.cdc.gov/hepatitis/hav/havfaq.htm#travel

Cunningham, F., Leveno, K., Bloom, S., Hauth, J., Rouse, D., & Spong, C. (2010). Maternal physiology. In F. G. Cunningham, K. J. Leveno, S. L. Bloom, J. C. Hauth, D. J. Rouse, & C. Y. Spong (Eds.), *Williams obstetrics* (23rd ed.). New York, NY: McGraw-Hill.

Friedman, L. (2013). Liver, biliary tract & pancreas disorders. In M. A. Papadakis, S. J. McPhee, & M. W. Rabow (Eds.), *Current medical diagnosis & treatment 2013.* New York, NY: McGraw-Hill.

LaRocque, R., Ryan, E., & Calderwood, S. (2012). Acute infectious diarrheal diseases and bacterial food poisoning. In D. L. Longo, A. S. Fauci, D. L. Kasper, S. L. Hauser, J. L. Jameson, & J. Loscalzo (Eds.), *Harrison's principles of internal medicine* (18th ed.). New York, NY: McGraw-Hill.

Liu, J., Hickson, D. A., Musani, S. K., Talegawkar, S. A., Carithers, T. C., Tucker, K. L., … & Taylor, H. A. (2013). Dietary patterns, abdominal visceral adipose tissue, and cardiometabolic risk factors in African Americans: The Jackson heart study. *Obesity (Silver Spring), 21*(3), 644–651. http://dx.doi.org/10.1002/oby.20265

NANDA International. (2012). *Nursing diagnoses: Definitions and classification 2012-2014* (9th ed). Oxford, United Kingdom: Wiley-Blackwell.

Phan, A. (2011). Gastric and esophageal cancer. In H. M. Kantarjian, R. A. Wolff, & C. A. Koller (Eds.), *The MD Anderson manual of medical oncology* (2nd ed.). New York, NY: McGraw-Hill.

Stern, S., Cifu, A., & Altkorn, D. (2010). I have a patient with acute diarrhea. How do I determine the cause? In S. C. Stern, A. S. Cifu, & D. Altkorn (Eds.), *Symptom to diagnosis: An evidence based guide* (2nd ed.). New York, NY: McGraw-Hill.

Stewart, M., & Schroeder, N. (2013). Dietary treatments for childhood constipation: Efficacy of dietary fiber & whole grains. *Nutrition Reviews, 7*(2), 98–109.

Teo, E. K., Lok, A. S. F. (2009). *Epidemiology, transmission and prevention of hepatitis B virus infection.* Retrieved from http://www.uptodate.com/home/index.html

U.S. Department of Health & Human Services. (2013). *2020 Topics & Objectives – Objectives A-Z.* Retrieved from http://www.healthypeople.gov/2020/topicsobjectives2020/

U.S. Department of Health & Human Services, Office of Minority Health. (2012). *Diabetes data/statistics.* Retrieved from http://minorityhealth.hhs.gov/templates/browse.aspx?lvl=3&lvlid=62

Tables of Abnormal Findings

TABLE 20.2 Abnormal Abdominal Findings

Finding	Description
Common Sites of Referred Pain	Abdominal pain may present with pain directly over the organ involved or the pain may be referred to a site where the organ was located in fetal development because the human brain has no felt image for internal organs. During fetal development, the organs migrate to their final location, but the nerves persist in the former location, and the patient feels the referring sensation. Pain in referred areas without representative history or other physical findings may not have an abdominal origin.

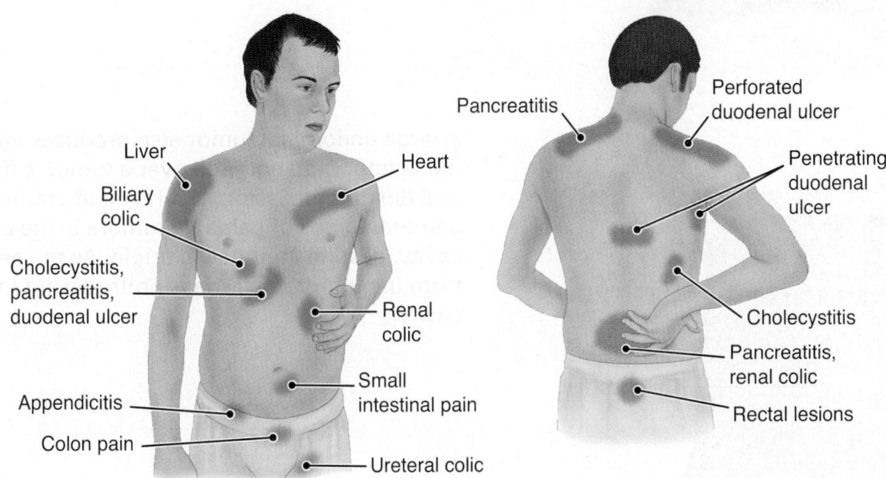

Finding	Description
Abdominal Distention	Abdominal distention occurs for a variety of reasons including obesity, gaseous distention, tumors, and ascites.
Obesity	Obesity causes protuberance of the abdomen resulting in a thickened abdominal wall and fat deposits in the mesentery and **omentum**. Percussion sounds over an obese abdomen present as normal tympanic sounds.

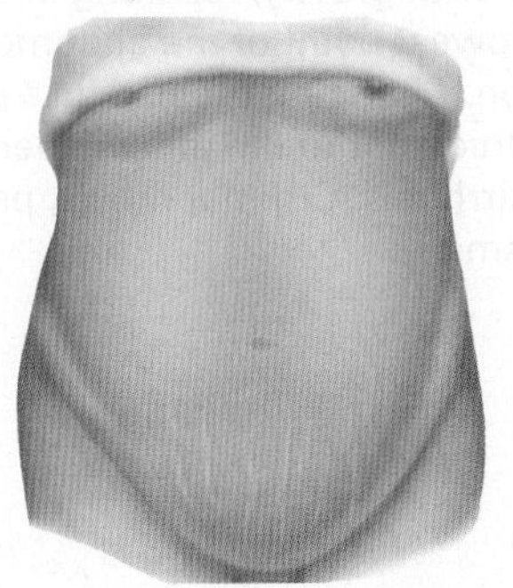

(table continues on page 594)

TABLE 20.2 Abnormal Abdominal Findings *(continued)*

Finding	Description
Gaseous Distention 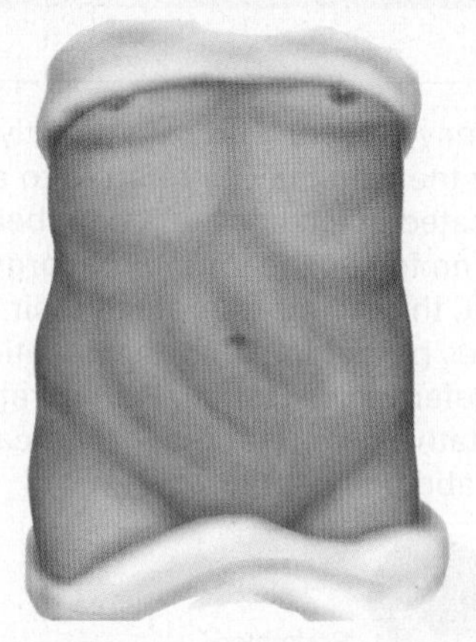	Gaseous distention is a result of increased production of gas in the intestines from the breakdown of certain foods and fluids. The average adult passes 500 ml of gas *per rectum* per day. It is also associated with altered peristalsis in which gas cannot move through the intestine. The altered peristalsis is seen in paralytic ileus and intestinal obstruction. Gaseous distention can be found in one area or generalized over the entire abdomen. Percussion sounds will be tympanic over the area of distention.
Abdominal Tumor 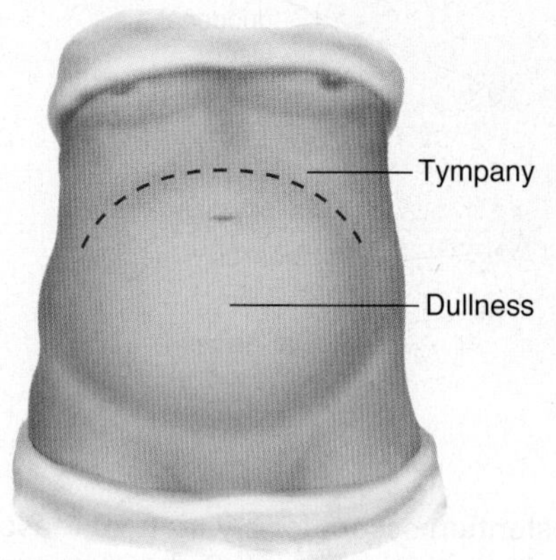	A large abdominal tumor also produces abdominal distention. The abdomen over a tumor is firm to palpation and dull to percussion. Ovarian and uterine tumors are common types of palpable tumors in the abdominal cavity, despite their pelvic origin. As the organs enlarge from the tumor, their mass protrudes into the abdominal cavity.
Ascites 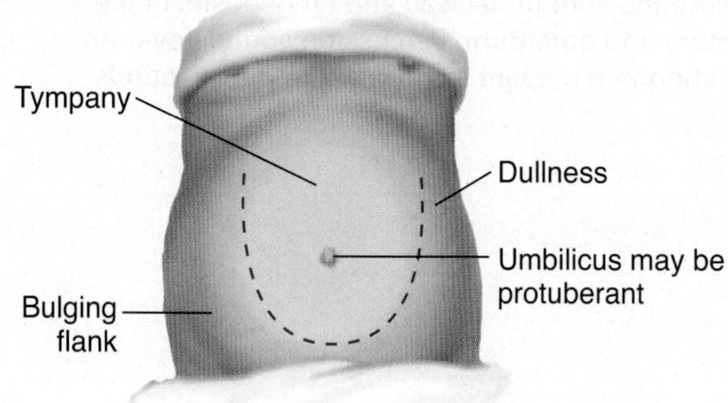	**Ascites** is the accumulation of fluid in the abdomen. The fluid descends with gravity, resulting in dullness to percussion in the lowest point of the abdomen based on patient's position. Changing the patient's position should move the fluid shift to the most dependent point. Ascites occurs in cirrhosis, CHF, nephrosis, peritonitis, and metastatic neoplasms.

(table continues on page 595)

TABLE 20.2 Abnormal Abdominal Findings *(continued)*

Finding	Description
Abnormal Bowel Sounds	Auscultation of the abdomen results in bowel, vascular, and rubbing sounds. Bowel sounds may be hyperactive or hypoactive and occur in any quadrant of the abdomen. Hyperactive sounds are common in gastroenteritis and diarrhea. Hypoactive sounds are common in constipation and paralytic ileus. High-pitched bowel sounds with cramping are commonly heard in intestinal obstruction.
Abnormal Vascular Sounds 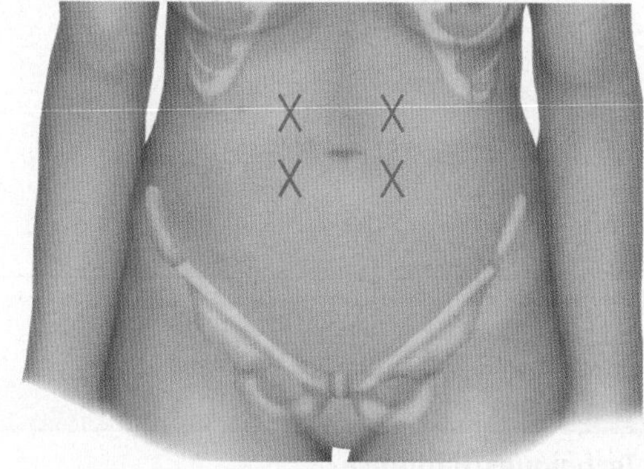	The most common abnormal vascular sound is a bruit. Its sound is blowing. Depending on location of the sound, the cause of the bruit can be determined. Bruits located in the midline below the xiphoid process are caused by aortic obstruction. Bruits located at the left and right costal borders at the MCL are caused by stenosis of the renal arteries. Other vascular sounds include venous hums and friction rubs.
Bruits 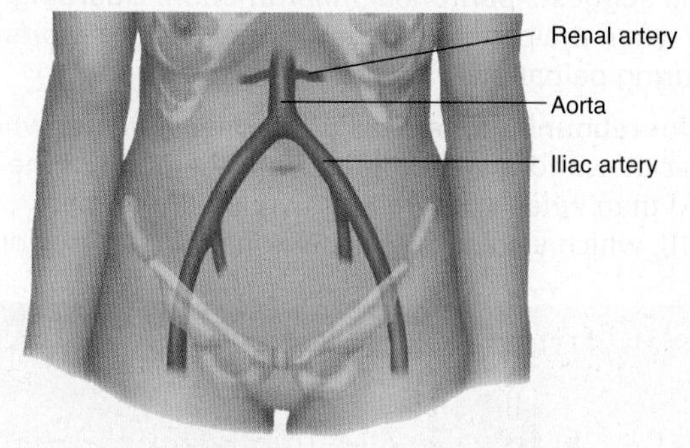	Bruits located at the left and right MCL between the umbilicus and the anterior iliac spine are caused by stenosis of the iliac arteries.
Venous Hums 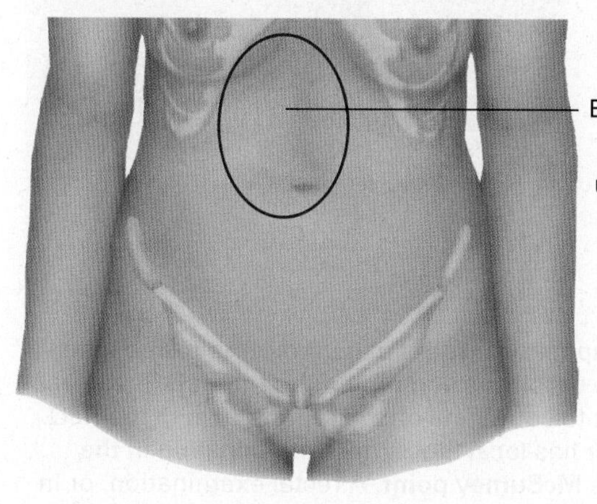	Venous hums are continuous sounds found in the epigastric region and around the umbilicus. They are caused by portal hypertension.

(table continues on page 596)

TABLE 20.2 **Abnormal Abdominal Findings** *(continued)*

Finding	Description
Friction Rubs 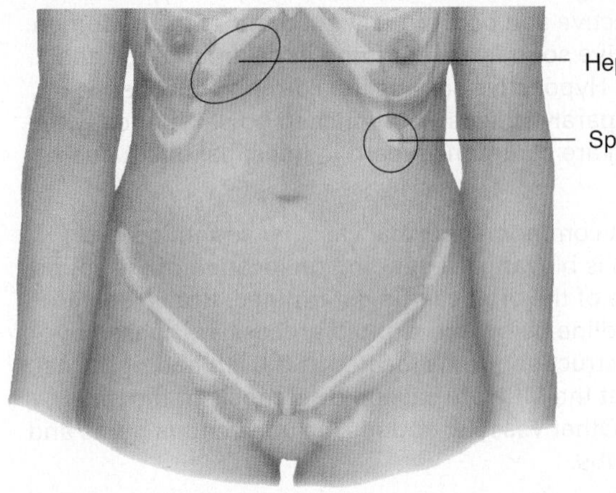	Friction rubs are harsh grating sounds found in the RUQ and LUQ, over the liver and spleen. They are caused by tumors or inflammation of the underlying organs.

TABLE 20.3 **Common Tests for Abdominal Problems**

Abdominal Problem	Special Techniques/Rationale
Acute Abdomen	Apply light and deep palpation. A firm boardlike abdominal wall suggests *peritoneal inflammation.* Guarding occurs when the patient flinches, grimaces, or reports pain during palpation. Check for **rebound tenderness** (tenderness greater when you quickly withdraw your hand from the point of the pain [A] than when you press slowly on the tender area [B]), which also suggests *peritoneal inflammation.*
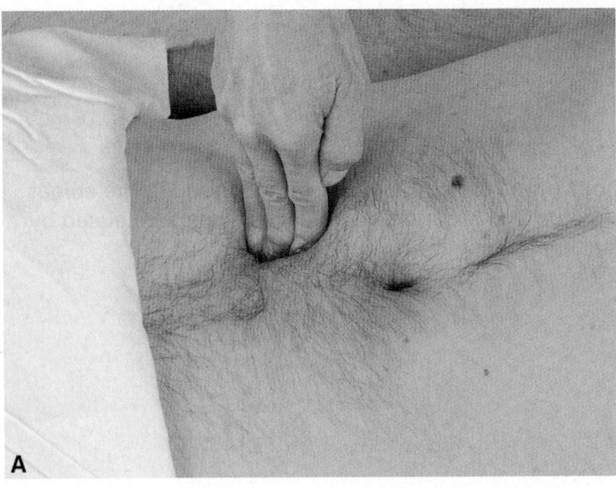 A	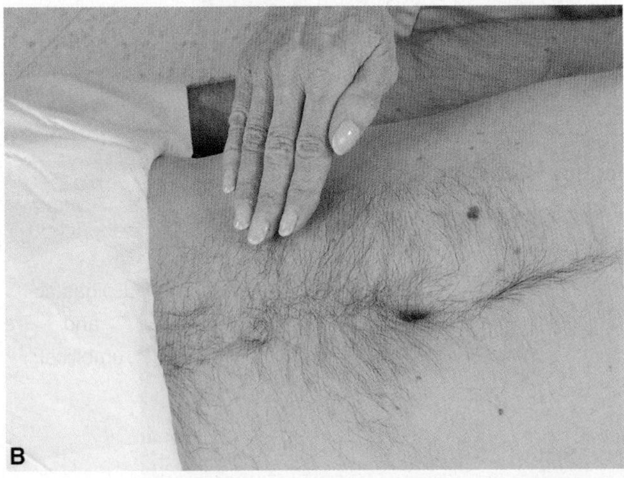 B
Appendicitis	In classic appendicitis, the patient reports pain beginning at the umbilicus and moving to the RLQ. If you ask the patient to cough, he or she reports pain in the RLQ. The patient has local tenderness on palpation in the RLQ, at the **McBurney point**. A rectal examination, or in women, a pelvic examination, will reveal local tenderness, especially if the appendix is retrocecal.

(table continues on page 597)

TABLE 20.3 Common Tests for Abdominal Problems *(continued)*

Abdominal Problem	Special Techniques/Rationale
	Other peritoneal findings include the following: **Rovsing sign (*shown at left*)**: press deeply and evenly in the LLQ and quickly withdraw your fingers. The patient reports pain in RLQ during LLQ pressure, suggesting appendicitis. **Psoas sign:** Place your hand just above the patient's right knee. Ask the patient to raise that thigh against your hand and turn to the left side. Extend the right leg at the hip to stretch to the **iliopsoas** muscle. A positive sign is pain in the RLQ with this maneuver, suggesting appendicitis or peritoneal inflammation.
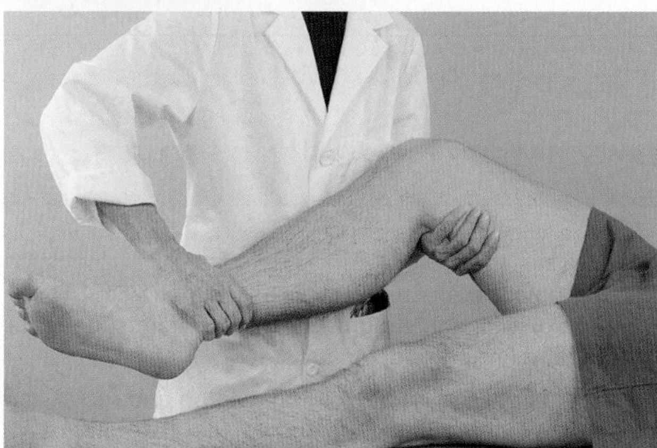	**Obturator sign (*shown at left*)**: Flex the patient's right thigh at the hip with the knee bent and rotate the leg internally at the hip, which stretches the internal obturator muscle. RLQ pain constitutes a positive obturator sign, suggesting an inflamed appendix or peritoneal inflammation.
Abdominal Aortic Aneurysm 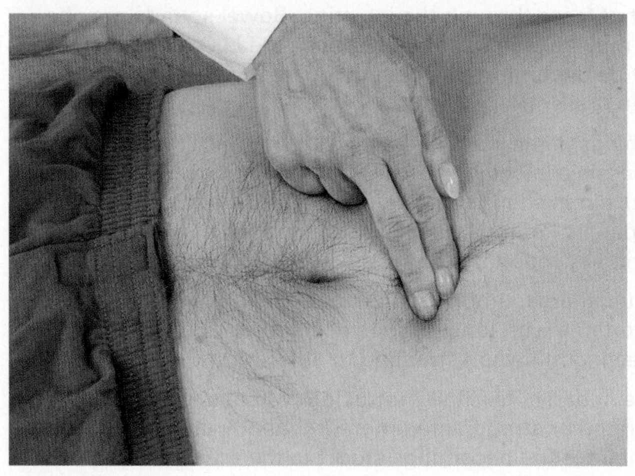	Patients complain of boring tearing pain and referred pain. Auscultation reveals bruits or exaggerated pulsations. A mass may be palpable over the aorta. Femoral pulses may be diminished or diffuse. Patients may seem in shock: hypotensive; tachycardic; tachypneic; pale, cool, clammy skin; cool extremities.

(table continues on page 598)

TABLE 20.3 Common Tests for Abdominal Problems *(continued)*

Abdominal Problem	Special Techniques/Rationale
Acute Cholecystitis 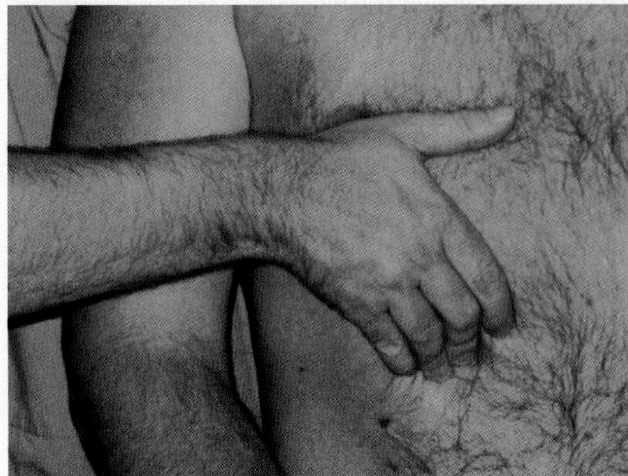	Auscultate, percuss, and palpate the abdomen for tenderness. Bowel sounds may be active or decreased. Tympany may increase with an ileus. There may be RUQ tenderness. Assess for the Murphy sign by hooking your thumb under the right costal margin at the edge of the rectus abdominis muscle (as shown to the left); ask the patient to take a deep breath. Sharp tenderness and a sudden stop in inspiratory effort constitutes a positive Murphy sign, suggesting cholecystitis.

TABLE 20.4 Gastrointestinal Diseases

Disease	Signs and Symptoms
Cancer of the stomach	This form of cancer, difficult to detect on physical examination, is associated with epigastric distress, abdominal fullness, anorexia, and weight loss. In late stages, patients may have ascites, a palpable liver mass, and lymph node enlargement.
Cancer of the colon	Colon cancer occurs most frequently in the descending and sigmoid colon and rectal areas. Patients report changes in bowel habits, blood in stool, and smaller diameter of bowel movement. Pain may accompany late stages of rectal cancer. A palpable mass may be found on rectal examination or on deep palpation of the LLQ.
Constipation	Results from delayed movement of feces through the intestine. Bowel sounds may be diminished on auscultation. You may be able to palpate feces in the LLQ with deep palpation. Palpation in general may be uncomfortable depending on the amount of feces and the length of time it has been present.
Diverticulitis	Diverticula are common outpouchings of the walls of the intestine in which feces may get trapped, causing inflammation, possible infection, abscess, and perforation. Patients present with severe pain (usually LLQ), diminished bowel sounds on auscultation, nausea, vomiting, and a long history of constipation. Peritoneal signs (see appendicitis) may be present if the bowel perforates. The patient may report that he or she had "left-sided appendicitis."
Hernias	Hernias may be found in the inguinal area, umbilical area, or along an old incision. Inguinal hernias are more uncomfortable with long periods of standing and diminish with rest. Patients may complain of feeling full when straining to defecate. Umbilical hernias usually resolve in early life. Their protrusion worsens with crying. Incisional hernias become incarcerated or strangulated more frequently than other types. Incarceration involves the loop of intestine becoming "stuck" in the scar tissue of the incision. Strangulation is compromise of the blood supply to the loop of bowel, resulting in death of the tissue involved. It constitutes a surgical emergency. A hiatal hernia causes the stomach to move through the esophageal opening and rise above the diaphragm. Symptoms include acid reflux, esophageal constriction, and subsequent esophageal damage.

(table continues on page 599)

TABLE 20.4 **Gastrointestinal Diseases** *(continued)*

Disease	Signs and Symptoms
IBD	This inflammatory condition involves all layers of the GI tract and can occur anywhere from mouth to anus. Problems of malnutrition and vitamin absorption are common. Abdominal pain is not relieved with defecation. Diarrhea and steatorrhea are common.
Crohn disease	Crohn involves the mucosal and submucosal layers of the colon. It increases the risk for colon cancer if not in remission after 10 years; it can also cause bowel perforation and toxic megacolon.
Ulcerative colitis	Colitis presents with cramping pain in the lower abdomen, relieved with defecation. Watery diarrhea with mucus in the stool and rectal bleeding are common. Surgery that removes the colon can cure the problem.
IBS	Also known as spastic colon, this condition has symptoms of diarrhea, constipation, or both. It usually presents as intermittent constipation, with hard compacted stools, and abdominal pain relieved by defecation. Many patients have a range of stools from pebbles to liquid over several days.
Liver failure	Liver failure can develop within 2–8 weeks of onset of jaundice. It results from the acute onset of massive necrosis of liver cells, leading to sudden and severe impairment of liver function. Causes include acetaminophen toxicity, *viral hepatitis*, drug reaction, toxins (mushroom poisoning), *ischemic hepatitis, autoimmune hepatitis*, and the fatty liver of pregnancy.
Pancreatitis	This inflammation of the pancreas alters the flow of digestive enzymes to the small intestine. Symptoms include nausea, vomiting, weight loss, severe boring pain in LUQ, and referred pain to the back or shoulder.
Paralytic ileus	Lack of peristalsis, usually in the small intestine, may follow surgery, peritonitis, or spinal cord injury. The presentation is intermittent colicky pain, with visible peristaltic waves on inspection and vomiting. Bowel sounds are absent. The abdomen is distended. Prompt attention is necessary to prevent bowel necrosis or perforation.
Peritonitis	This inflammation of the lining of the abdominal cavity presents with fever, nausea, and vomiting. Findings include abdominal pain of varying character, cutaneous hypersensitivity, abdominal rigidity, and guarding. Bowel sounds are diminished. Positive signs include psoas, obturator, Rovsing, and Murphy.
Pyelonephritis	Auscultate, percuss, and palpate the abdomen for tenderness. Bowel sounds may be active or decreased. Tympany may increase with an ileus; tenderness may be present anteriorly over the affected kidney on deep palpation. Check for CVA tenderness on the posterior thorax to be positive over the inflamed kidney.
Splenic rupture	This serious abdominal condition resulting in hemorrhage usually follows abdominal trauma but can accompany mononucleosis from an enlarged spleen, which is subsequently traumatized. Presentation is severe LUQ pain, radiating to the left shoulder. Hemorrhagic shock can develop.
Ulcer	Ulcers form when gastric mucosa becomes permeable, protective mucus is reduced as a result of inflammation, or exposure to bile or other irritating substances (e.g., medications, alcohol) is prolonged. *Gastric ulcers* present with gnawing pain, heartburn, anorexia, vomiting (possible hematemesis), eructations, and weight loss. *Duodenal ulcers* present with intermittent RUQ pain 2–3 hours after eating. Stools may be positive for occult blood.

21

Musculoskeletal Assessment

Learning Objectives

1 Demonstrate knowledge of the anatomy and physiology of the musculoskeletal system.

2 Identify important topics for health promotion and risk reduction related to the musculoskeletal system.

3 Collect subjective data related to the musculoskeletal system.

4 Collect objective data related to the musculoskeletal system using physical examination techniques.

5 Identify normal and abnormal findings related to the musculoskeletal system.

6 Analyze subjective and objective data from assessment of the musculoskeletal system and consider initial interventions.

7 Document and communicate data from musculoskeletal assessment using appropriate medical terminology and principles of recording.

8 Consider the condition, age, gender, and culture of the patient to individualize the musculoskeletal assessment.

9 Identify nursing diagnoses and initiate a plan of care based on findings from the musculoskeletal assessment.

Mrs. Gladys Runningbird is an 82-year-old Native American who recently fell and needed hospitalization. Twelve days ago, she was transferred from the hospital to a skilled nursing facility. Today, her temperature is 36.6°C (97.8°F) orally, pulse 82 beats/min, respirations 18 breaths/min, and blood pressure 122/64 mm Hg. Current medications include alendronate sodium (Fosamax) for osteoarthritis. Dietary supplements include a multivitamin, vitamin D, calcium, and magnesium.

You will gain more information about Mrs. Runningbird as you progress through this chapter. As you study the content and features, consider Mrs. Runningbird's case and its relationship to what you are learning. Begin thinking about the following points:

- How are physiological and psychological data connected?
- What nursing diagnoses might be activated on this patient's problem list? Provide rationale.
- What areas will the nurse assess as part of a comprehensive musculoskeletal assessment?
- What additional assessments should the nurse add?
- What are expected findings for Mrs. Runningbird based on her age versus findings based on her osteoarthritis?
- How will the nurse evaluate the effectiveness of the occupational therapy that Mrs. Runningbird is getting?

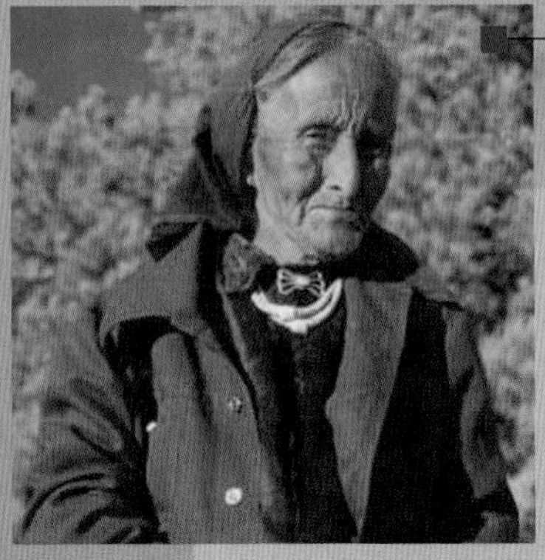

This chapter discusses the structure and function of the musculoskeletal system. It provides instructions for a comprehensive musculoskeletal assessment, including health history, physical examination (with specific procedures for joint difficulties), and related laboratory and diagnostic tests. A patient undergoes a complete musculoskeletal examination during the first visit to a health care provider or when a condition that involves all the joints is suspected. More commonly, a patient with a musculoskeletal complaint undergoes a focused assessment on a specific area with injury or pain, such as a shoulder, knee, or elbow.

Structure and Function

The musculoskeletal system is composed of skeletal muscle and five types of connective tissues: bone, cartilage, ligaments, tendons, and fascia. Muscles and bones facilitate movement through the joints, or articulations. Connective tissues are located all around the muscles, bones, and joints and serve protective functions. The more elastic the connective tissue found around a joint, the greater the range of motion (ROM) in that joint will be. The specialized forms of connective tissue in the musculoskeletal system are described in Table 21.1.

Bones

Bone is a living structure made up of a tough organic matrix strengthened by deposits of calcium phosphate. Two types of bones exist: compact bone, which forms the shaft and outer layer, and spongy or cancellous bone, which makes up the ends and center. Bones are classified by shape as short, flat, irregular, or long. Long bones are basically hollow tubes of compact bone with widened ends containing cancellous bone. Bones lengthen from the ends at areas called epiphyses.

Bones provide the framework for the body. They also protect vital tissues and are the primary site for storage and regulation of minerals, such as calcium and phosphate. Their marrow cavities serve as sites of hematopoiesis, or the manufacturing of blood cells.

Muscles

The 600 skeletal muscles in the body make up 40% to 50% of its weight. Muscles may be cardiac, smooth, or skeletal. This chapter discusses only skeletal, or voluntary, muscles. Skeletal muscles consist of fibers bound together in bundles and attached to bone by tendons. They contract and relax to move joints. Muscles give the body shape and produce heat during movement.

Joints

A joint, or articulation, is the area where two bones come together. The function of joints is to provide mobility to the skeleton. Joints may be classified by the type of cartilage involved:

- Fibrous (synarthrotic) joints are immovable, such as in the sutures in the cranium.
- Cartilaginous (amphiarthrotic) joints are slightly moveable, such as the costal cartilage between the sternum and ribs and the symphysis pubis.
- Synovial (diarthrotic) joints—the most common type—are freely movable and are named for their major type of movement: ball and socket (hip and shoulder), hinge (elbow and knee), pivot (atlas and axis), condyloid (wrist), saddle (thumb), and gliding (intravertebral).

TABLE 21.1 Connective Tissues

Type	Functions	Example
Cartilage	Allows bones to slide over one another, reduces friction, prevents damage, absorbs shock	Articular cartilage found on the ends of bones
Tendons	Connect muscles to bones	Biceps brachii tendon in the shoulder, which connects the biceps muscle over the head of the humerus to the glenoid fossa
Ligaments	Connect bone to bone to stabilize joints and limit movement	Anterior cruciate ligament (ACL) in the knee, which prevents lateral movement of the knee
Bursae	Fluid-filled sacs in areas of friction to cushion bones or ligaments that might rub against each other	Subacromial bursa in shoulder to reduce friction during adduction
Meniscus	Cartilage disc between bones to absorb shock and cushion joints	The medial and lateral menisci in the knee, which cushion the tibia and femur
Fascia	Flat sheets that line and protect muscle fibers, attach muscle to bone, and provide structure for nerves, blood vessels, and lymphatics	The outer layer of fascia, which tapers at each end to form tendons

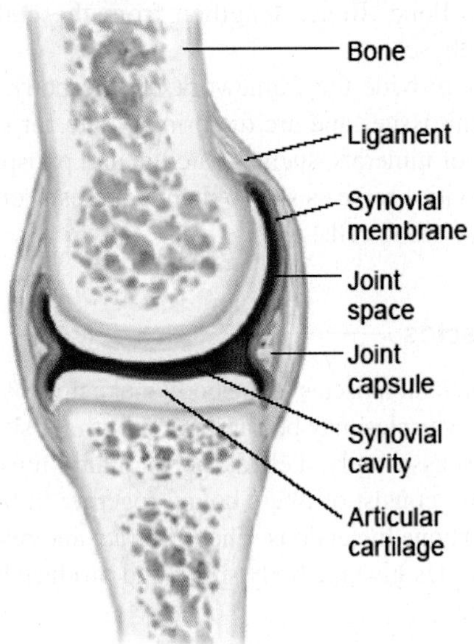

Figure 21.1 Example of a synovial joint.

Usually, one of the bone ends is stable and serves as an axis for the motion of the other. The joint shape and ligaments determine the movement the joint can make (Fig. 21.1).

Temporomandibular Joint

The temporomandibular joint (TMJ) is where the mandible and temporal bone articulate (Fig. 21.2). The TMJ is palpable below and slightly anterior to the tragus of each ear. It permits three movements of the jaw for chewing and speaking: opening and closing, **protrusion** and **retraction**, and gliding from side to side.

Shoulder

The shoulder joint is where the humerus articulates with the glenoid fossa of the scapula (Fig. 21.3). Because it is a ball-and-socket joint, the shoulder permits many types of movement (Tables 21.2 and 21.3). Four strong muscles and their tendons, collectively known as the rotator cuff, surround the shoulder to support and stabilize it. A large bursa protects the bones and ligaments of the shoulder during movement. The scapula and clavicle connect to form the shoulder girdle. The **acromion process** of the scapula is at the top of the shoulder. The greater tubercle of the humerus is downward and lateral to the acromion and the coracoid process of the scapula is a few centimeters medially.

Elbow

The elbow is the articulation of the humerus, radius, and ulna (Fig. 21.4). Its hinge action permits **flexion** and **extension**. A large **bursa** lies between the **olecranon process** and the skin. The olecranon process is centered between the medial and lateral epicondyles of the humerus. The sensitive ulnar nerve runs between the olecranon process and medial epicondyle. The radius and ulna articulate at two radioulnar joints, one at the elbow and the other at the wrist. These bones move together to permit **pronation** and **supination** of the hand and forearm.

Wrist and Hand

The wrist, or radiocarpal, joint is the articulation of the radius (on the "thumb side") and a row of carpal bones. Its condyloid action permits flexion, extension, and **deviation** (lateral movement of the hand). The midcarpal joint is the articulation between parallel rows of carpal bones. It allows flexion, extension, and some rotation. The metacarpophalangeal and intraphalangeal (proximal, medial, and distal) joints permit finger movement (see Table 21.2 and Fig. 21.5).

Hip

The hip joint is the articulation between the acetabulum and the head of the femur (Fig. 21.6). This ball-and-socket joint permits a wide ROM. Powerful muscles, strong ligaments, a fibrous capsule, and the insertion of the femur head into the acetabulum provide stability. Three bursae facilitate movement.

The iliac crest is palpable from the anterior superior iliac spine to the posterior. The ischial tuberosity is palpable when the hip is flexed. The greater trochanter of the femur is a depression on the upper lateral side of the thigh and is best palpated with the person standing.

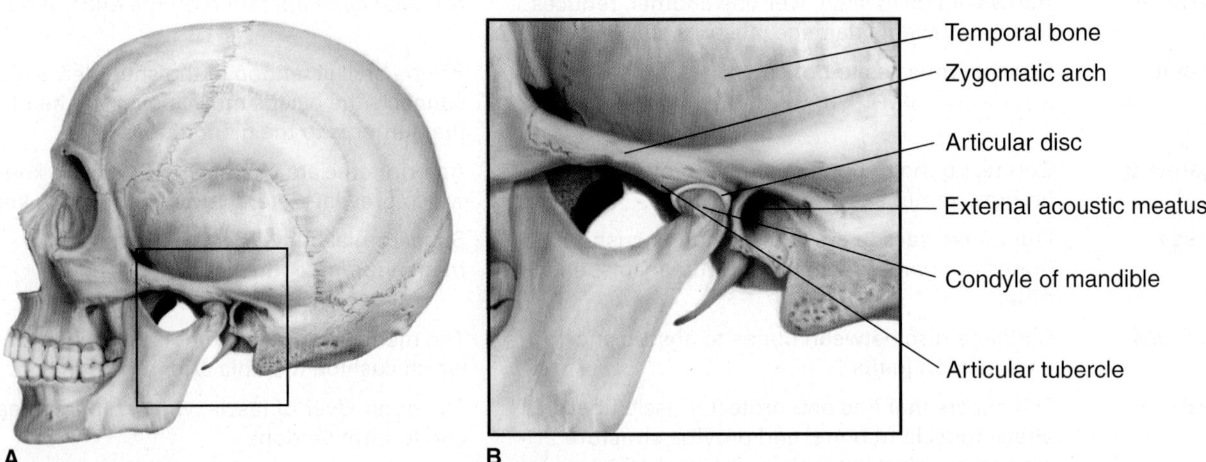

Figure 21.2 The temporomandibular joint (TMJ). **A.** Location of the TMJ within the skull. **B.** Close-up view of the TMJ.

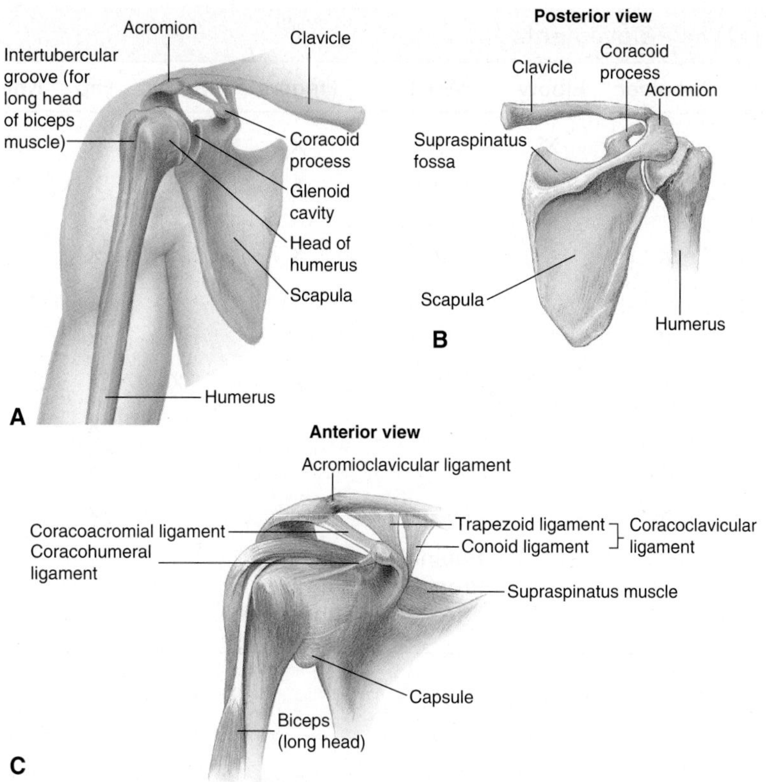

Figure 21.3 Shoulder. **A.** Anterior view. **B.** Posterior view. **C.** Ligaments.

TABLE 21.2 Terms for Joint Movement

Movement	Description
Flexion	Decreases the angle between bones or brings bones together • **Dorsiflexion:** Bending the ankle so that the toes move toward the head • **Plantar flexion:** Moving the foot so that the toes move away from the head
Extension	Increases the angle to a straight line or zero degrees
Hyperextension	Extension beyond the neutral position
Abduction	Movement of a part away from the center of the body
Adduction	Movement of a part toward the center of the body
Rotation	Turning of the joint around a longitudinal axis • **Internal rotation:** Rotating an extremity medially along its axis • **External rotation:** Rotating an extremity laterally along its axis • **Pronation:** Turning the forearm so the palm is down • **Supination:** Turning the forearm so the palm is up
Circumduction	A circular motion that combines flexion, extension, abduction, and adduction
Inversion	Turning the sole of the foot inward
Eversion	Turning the sole of the foot outward
Protraction	Moving a body part forward and parallel to the ground
Retraction	Moving a body part backward and parallel to the ground
Elevation	Moving a body part upward
Depression	Moving a body part downward
Opposition	Moving the thumb to touch the little finger

TABLE 21.3 Joints and Their Movements

Movements	Neck	Shoulder	Elbow	Wrist	Fingers	Spine	Hip	Knee	Ankle	Toes
Flexion	X	X	X	X	X	X	X	X	Dorsiflexion	X
Extension	X	X	X	X	X	X	X	X	Plantar flexion	X
Hyperextension	X	X		X	X	X	X			X
Rotation	X					X				
Circumduction		X					X			
Abduction	X	X			X	X	X			X
Adduction		X					X			
Internal rotation		X					X			
External rotation		X					X			
Other				Supinate Pronate	Finger–thumb opposition				Inversion Eversion	

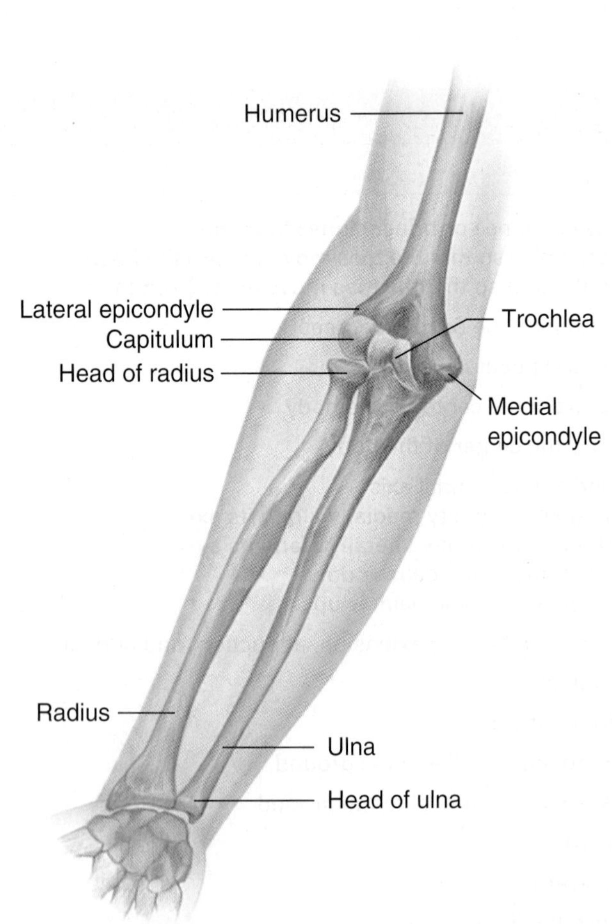

Figure 21.4 Bones of the elbow.

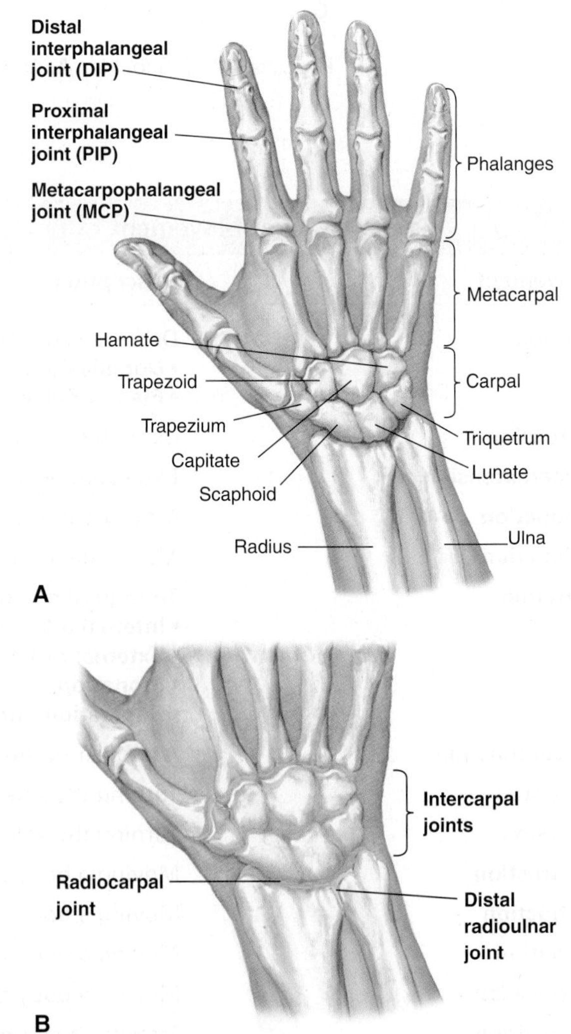

Figure 21.5 Bones of the **(A)** hand and **(B)** wrist.

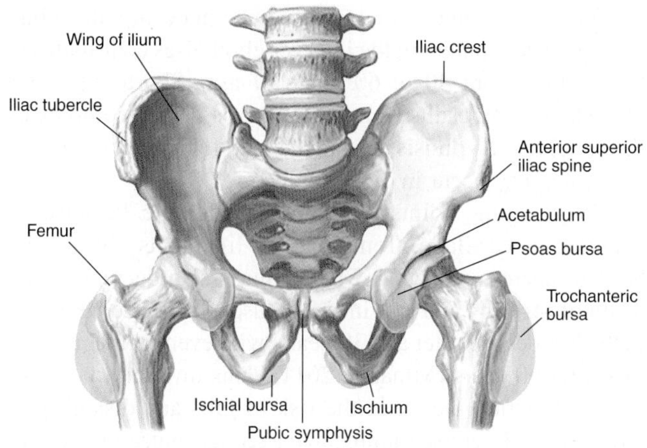

Figure 21.6 Anterior view of the hip joint.

Knee

The knee is the articulation involving the femur, tibia, and patella (Fig. 21.7). The medial and lateral menisci cushion the tibia and femur. The cruciate ligaments cross within the knee to provide anterior and posterior stability and to control rotation. The collateral ligaments felt in the depressions on both sides of the patella connect the joint at both sides to give medial and lateral stability and to prevent dislocation. Several **bursae** prevent friction. The tibial tuberosity is palpable on the midline of the tibia. The lateral and medial condyles of the tibia are to the sides and slightly above the tuberosity. The patella is above the condyles. The medial and lateral epicondyles of the femur can be felt above the patella.

Ankle and Foot

The ankle, or tibiotalar joint, is the articulation of the tibia, fibula, and talus (Fig. 21.8). It is a hinge joint limited to flexion and extension. The terms used to describe its movements are **dorsiflexion** and **plantar flexion**. The medial and lateral malleoli are palpable on either side of the ankle. Strong ligaments extend from each malleolus onto the foot to provide lateral stability of the ankle.

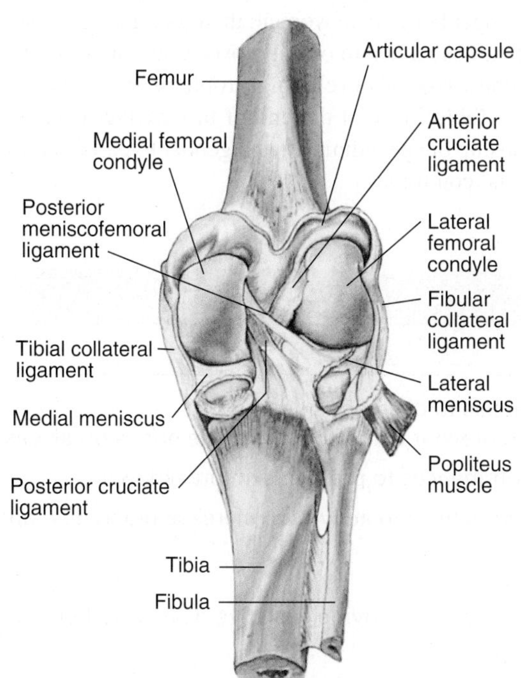

Figure 21.7 The right knee, posterior extended view.

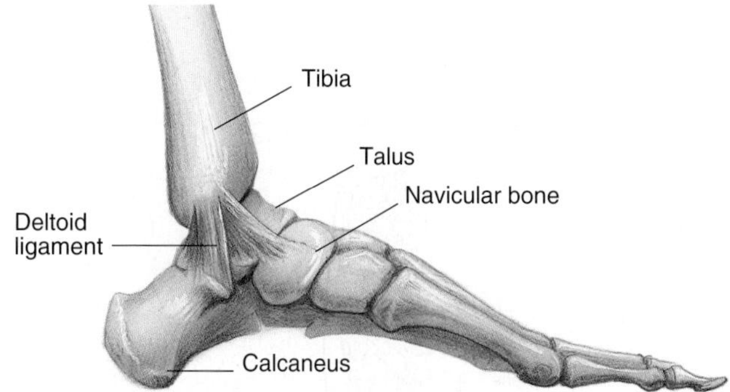

Figure 21.8 Bones of the ankle and foot.

The subtalar joint in the foot permits **inversion** and **eversion**. Weight bearing is distributed between the heads of the metatarsals and the calcaneus (i.e., the heel) by the longitudinal arch. The metatarsophalangeal and intraphalangeal joints permit flexion, extension, and abduction of the toes.

Spine

The spine is a column comprising 33 vertebrae: 7 cervical, 12 thoracic, 5 lumbar, 5 sacral, and 3 to 4 coccygeal (Fig. 21.9). Intervertebral discs separate and cushion the vertebrae. The vertebral spinous processes are palpable down the middle of the back, with paravertebral muscles on either side. The spinous processes of C7 and T1 are palpable at the back of the neck. The inferior border of the scapula normally is between T7 and T8, and a line drawn between the iliac crests crosses L4.

The vertebral column has four curves, best seen from the side. The cervical and lumbar curves are concave (inward), whereas the thoracic and sacrococcygeal curves are convex. These curves and the intervertebral discs allow the spine to absorb a considerable amount of shock. Abnormal postures include kyphosis, scoliosis, and **lordosis** (i.e., saddle back or swayback).

Lifespan Considerations: Older Adults

Aging affects all components of the musculoskeletal system (Table 21.4). Bone resorption occurs more rapidly than deposition. This loss of bone density is termed osteoporosis. Some degree of osteoporosis occurs in all people, but it is most evident in women with smaller bony frames. Women experience rapid loss of bone density for the first 5 to 7 years after menopause. After the initial rapid phase, bone loss continues but slows. Men also experience bone loss but at more advanced ages and much slower rates than women. Bone mass is related to race, heredity, hormonal factors, physical activity, and calcium intake. Smoking, calcium deficiency, high salt intake, alcohol intake, and physical inactivity increase bone loss. Resistance exercise and soy isoflavones decrease bone resorption (Ma, 2013).

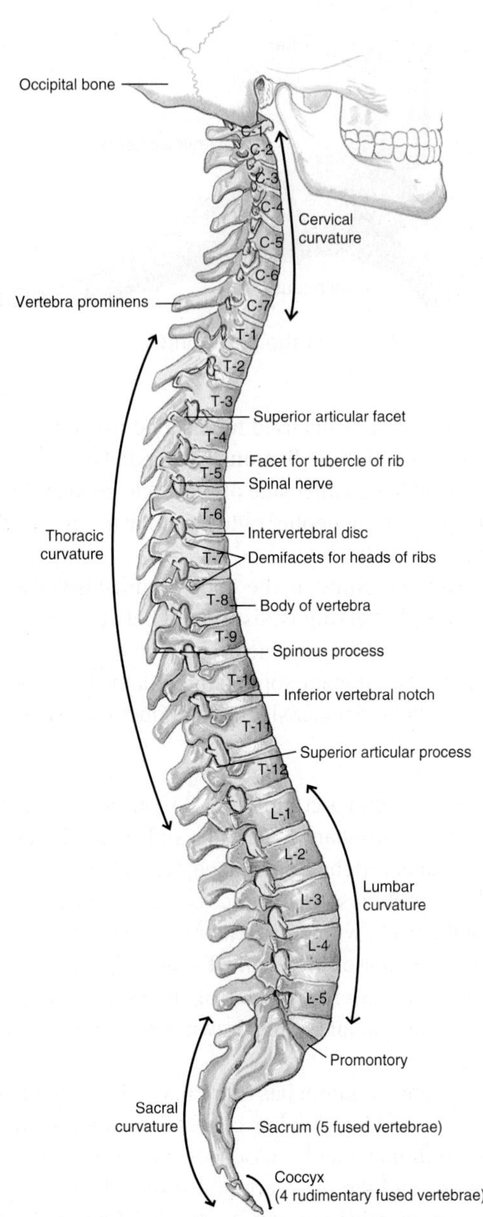

Figure 21.9 Sagittal view of the vertebral column (spine).

Postural changes and decreased height occur with aging. Loss of water content in the intervertebral discs contributes to height loss from 40 to 60 years of age. Shortening after 60 years of age results from osteoporosis, which compresses the vertebrae. **Kyphosis**, an exaggerated forward curvature of the spine, may occur in older adults.

With aging, joints become less flexible because of changes in cartilage. Tendons and ligaments shrink and harden, decreasing ROM. Muscle mass also decreases as a result of **atrophy** and loss in size. Muscle mass decreases 3% to 8% per decade after age 30 years, with even greater muscle loss after 60 years (Minaker, 2011). This involuntary loss of muscle function increases the risk of falls and disability in older adults. Exercise training and adequate nutrition are successful in improving muscle mass and strength.

Subcutaneous fat distribution changes with aging. Men and women usually gain weight after 40 years of age, predominantly in the abdomen and hips. After 80 years of age, subcutaneous fat continues to decrease, causing bony prominences to be more obvious.

Cultural Considerations

Many variations related to ethnicity are visible in the musculoskeletal system. Bone density is most likely related to body weight rather than a particular genetic background (Finkelstein et al., 2008). The curvature of long bones is related to both ethnicity and body weight. African Americans have straight femurs, whereas Native Americans have anteriorly curved femurs. The femoral curve in Caucasians is intermediate. Thin people of all cultures have less curvature than obese people. Caucasians, Mexican Americans, and African Americans have no difference in metabolism of vitamin D; however, conversion of active metabolites by sunlight is less efficient in African Americans (Frost, 2012).

Gender also affects the skeletal system. Men have larger and stronger bones than women; therefore, men are less prone to difficulties related to osteoporosis. Caucasian women have the highest risk of developing problems from loss of bone density. Table 21.10 at the end of this chapter describes the relationship of age, ethnicity, and gender to particular musculoskeletal conditions.

TABLE 21.4 **Musculoskeletal Changes With Aging**

Physiological Change	Nursing Implications
Decreased bone density	Encourage weight-bearing exercise to decrease bone loss. Teach patients about hazards to prevent falls because fragile bones break easily.
Increased bony prominences	Decrease pressure on bony prominences to prevent skin breakdown.
Cartilage degeneration	Encourage warm baths or showers prior to activity to increase blood flow and decrease joint stiffness.
Joint stiffness and lax ligaments	Encourage active ROM in all joints. Assess patient's ability to perform ADLs; provide assistive devices to help the patient perform self-care.
Muscle atrophy	Teach isometric exercises to maintain muscle strength.

Urgent Assessment

Assessment of patients reporting musculoskeletal difficulties focuses on identifying the specific problem, alleviating pain, and preventing complications. Look for alignment of limbs, joints, and the spine. Observe for symmetry of size, shape, position, and movement of extremities. If a joint is swollen and tender following an injury, a strain or sprain is likely. If a bone is not aligned, it may be fractured, whereas if a joint is not aligned, it may be dislocated.

> **SAFETY ALERT**
> *You should not attempt to correct malalignment because doing so can compound injury to muscle, nerves, or blood vessels. Instead, immobilize the extremity. Fractures require prompt care to prevent further injury or deformity. Focus your efforts on keeping the patient calm, quiet, still, and comfortable.*

Damage to soft tissue often occurs at the same time as bone fracture. If soft-tissue injury and bleeding are found, apply pressure to stop the bleeding and assess for swelling, pain, numbness, and guarding. Muscle contractions contribute to discomfort, so helping the patient to relax is essential. Nursing actions include taking vital signs, monitoring pulses, and assessing color, temperature, and capillary refill distal to the injury to evaluate tissue perfusion.

The GALS (*g*ait, *a*rms, *l*egs, *s*pine) locomotor screen (Doherty, Dacre, Dieppe, & Snaith, 1992) is a method of quickly inspecting gait, arms, legs, and spine. The patient performs eleven tasks while the examiner asks two questions: "Do you have any pain or stiffness anywhere?" and "Do you have any difficulty washing, dressing, or climbing stairs/steps?" Some educators and researchers have modified the first question to be more specific, that is, "Do you have any pain or stiffness in your muscles, joints, back, or neck?"

Subjective Data

Assessment of Risk Factors

Numerous factors affect the musculoskeletal system. Ask the patient about family history, personal history, medications and supplements, sports and hobbies, and working conditions. In addition, note the patient's age, gender, and ethnicity. Knowledge of risk factors helps identify topics for health-promotion teaching.

History and Risk Factors	Rationale
Personal History	
What is your age?	Table 21.10 at the end of the chapter reviews age-related musculoskeletal diseases. Osteoporosis affects 55% of people older than 50 years of age (National Osteoporosis Foundation [NOF], 2013). Failing eyesight and musculoskeletal changes increase older adults' risk for falls. Longer life expectancy has increased the number of people with disabilities. Young children are at risk for injury resulting from impulsive actions, such as running into the street after a ball. Adolescents are also at risk from impulsive actions, involvement in sports, and driving.
Note the patient's gender.	The incidence of many musculoskeletal diseases differs by gender (see Table 21.10 at the end of the chapter). Women are four times more likely than men to develop arthritis, and 50% of women will have an osteoporosis-related fracture in their lives (Agency for Healthcare Research and Quality [AHRQ], 2011).
What is your ethnic heritage or race?	Prevalence of some disorders varies by ethnicity. See Table 21.10 at the end of the chapter.
Have you ever had any musculoskeletal trauma or injury, or have you ever been diagnosed with a musculoskeletal difficulty? (Ask specifically about fractures, stroke, polio, infections of the bone or muscles, diabetes, cancer, and parathyroid problems.) • When did it occur? • How was it treated? • What was the outcome?	Following hip replacement, hip dislocation can occur with hip flexion greater than 90 degrees or adduction of the joint past the midline. A person who has had a stroke is at increased risk of **subluxation**, or partial dislocation, of the shoulder; this can occur from the weight of the arm and the lack of muscle tone to hold the joint together. A prior history of cancer is the only notworthy factor associated with an increased likelihood of cancer (Henschke et al., 2013).

(table continues on page 608)

History and Risk Factors	Rationale
How many servings of dairy products do you have per day?	Calcium is essential for bone growth and remodeling. Vitamin D is essential for calcium absorption.
Occupation, Lifestyle, and Behaviors What type of work do you do? • Does your work involve any repetitive motion? Lifting or twisting? • How do you protect yourself from injury while working?	Some occupations increase risk of musculoskeletal injury through repetitive movements, twisting, frequent or heavy lifting, vibration, exposure to cold, and pushing or pulling heavy objects. Ergonomics and safety equipment can protect workers against injury.
What hobbies and sports do you enjoy? • How do you protect yourself from injury while exercising or participating in sports? • Do you consistently use car seats, helmets, and protective gear?	Sports such as basketball, baseball, football, and soccer contribute to knee injuries. Skiing increases risks for lower extremity injuries, whereas skateboarding can lead to upper extremity injuries. Stretching and warming up before strenuous exercise decreases injury. Car seats, helmets, and protective gear decrease the severity of injury during accidents.
What is your weekly or monthly income? How many people live on that income?	Women of lower socioeconomic status are more likely to report limitations in activity and arthritis, obesity, and osteoporosis.
Have you ever smoked cigarettes or cigars? • If yes, how many cigarettes per day? • For how many years?	Smoking increases the risk of developing a vertebral fracture by 13% in women and 32% in men (Abate, Vanni, Pantalone, & Salini, 2013). Smoking is an independent dose-related risk factor. Smoking cessation may partially reverse the risk.
Have you ever consumed alcohol? • If yes, how many drinks per week? • What do you drink?	Alcohol use is associated with increased risk of osteoporosis. Alcohol raises parathyroid hormone levels, which causes calcium loss from bones. Regular consumption of 2–3 oz of alcohol every day interferes with absorption and use of calcium and vitamin D (NOF, 2013).
Medications What medications do you take? (Ask women about current and past birth control methods. Ask postmenopausal women about hormone replacement therapy [HRT].) • Do you take calcium and vitamin D supplements? • Do you take any pain or antiinflammatory medications? Muscle relaxants? • Do you take any steroids? • Do you use complementary or alternative therapies (e.g., chondroitin, glucosamine)?	Vitamin D deficiency has been linked to osteoporosis (van Schoor et al., 2008). Oral contraceptive use in young adults may contribute to risk of osteoporosis, whereas HRT may help prevent it (Dane, Dane, Cetin, & Erginbas, 2007; MacLean et al., 2008). Pain or antiinflammatory medications and muscle relaxants can mask symptoms. Steroids can affect calcium absorption. Glucosamine and chondroitin have been found to improve joint pain resulting from osteoarthritis.
Family History Do your parents or siblings have any muscle, joint, or bone difficulties? • Who had the difficulty? • When did it occur? • How was it treated? • What was the outcome?	Some musculoskeletal problems have a familial association. Examples include osteoporosis, bone cancer, and rheumatoid arthritis.
Psychosocial History In a patient with a musculoskeletal injury, ask questions related to how will it affect his or her ability to work, participate in hobbies, or perform routine activities of daily living (ADLs) independently.	Psychosocial assessment related to the musculoskeletal system is important because difficulties that limit or compromise movement and mobility can have wide-ranging effects and consequences.
If the patient lives alone, can he or she perform self-care safely? Does the patient have pain that interferes with every aspect of living? Will immobility add stress or contribute to isolation and sensory deprivation? Are deformities altering sense of self or body image?	If the patient does not have sick leave benefits and cannot work, the financial strain may be immense.

Risk Reduction and Health Promotion

Use the health history to gather information to discover areas requiring health teaching. The following *Healthy People 2020* goals relate to the musculoskeletal system and pertinent health teaching:

- Reduce the proportion of adults with chronic joint symptoms who experience limitation in activity due to arthritis.
- Increase the proportion of adults who have seen a health care provider to treat their chronic joint symptoms.
- Reduce the proportion of adults with osteoporosis and the number of adults who are hospitalized for vertebral fractures associated with osteoporosis.
- Reduce activity limitation due to chronic back conditions.
- Reduce hip fractures among older adults.
- Increase the proportion of adults who are at a healthy weight.
- Increase the proportion of persons aged 2 years and older who meet dietary recommendations for calcium.
- Reduce work-related injuries resulting in medical treatment, lost time from work, or restricted work activity.
- Reduce the rate of injury and illness cases involving days away from work due to overexertion or repetitive motion.
- Increase the proportion of adults who perform physical activities that enhance and maintain muscular strength and endurance.
- Increase smoking cessation attempts by adult smokers. (U.S. Department of Health and Human Services [USDHHS], 2013)

Ask whether the patient has any congenital bone, muscle, or joint difficulties. If the patient's response is positive, ask about the impact on the patient's life. Knowledge of congenital problems can guide you to alter assessment and to anticipate findings during the physical examination. Assess how the patient is adapting to the deformity.

Ask about previous injuries or illnesses of muscles, joints, or bones. Long-lasting effects may include muscle weakness, decreased ROM, and impaired mobility. Specifically ask about fractures, sprains, strains, and dislocations, and also about childhood polio or scoliosis. If the patient reports previous injuries, ask about continuing effects.

Ask about surgery to the musculoskeletal system. Have the patient describe the procedure, when it occurred, and the results. Knowledge of previous surgeries provides additional information, allows you to anticipate findings during the physical assessment, and enables you to alter assessment procedures as needed to protect the patient.

To determine the effects of previous or current difficulties in the musculoskeletal system, you can perform a functional assessment. An example of this type of assessment is the Short Musculoskeletal Function Assessment (Swiontkowski, Engelberg, Martin, & Agel, 1999).

Encourage people of all ages to maintain a healthy weight and perform weight-bearing exercise at least three times per week. To help prevent functional scoliosis, instruct patients to alternate the shoulder on which they carry their shoulder bag or purse or to use a backpack instead to distribute the weight more evenly. Encourage all patients to use good body mechanics when lifting and pushing, to use protective equipment during sports and work, and to wear seat belts. Inform patients that exercises to increase strength and flexibility and improve posture decrease the risk of falls. Advise older adults that exercise training and adequate nutrition will help improve muscle mass and strength.

Bone Density

Loss of bone density and muscle strength are major concerns of aging that lifestyle modification can help control. Calcium and vitamin D are important for people of all ages, as are weight-bearing exercises. Although osteoporosis can be treated, no cure has been found. Prevention is very important, especially for women. Current treatment includes bisphosphonates, calcitonin, estrogen and/or HRT, raloxifene, and parathyroid hormone (NOF, 2013). HRT with estrogen may prevent bone loss but this therapy increases the risk of breast cancer and heart attacks.

The NOF (2013) recommends a comprehensive approach to prevent osteoporosis:

1. Consume the daily recommended amount of calcium and vitamin D. Limit caffeine, which increases excretion of calcium.
2. Perform at least 30 minutes of weight-bearing exercise three times per week.
3. Avoid smoking and excessive alcohol consumption.
4. Discuss your risk for osteoporosis with your health care provider.
5. Have a bone density test and take medication when appropriate.

> **Clinical Significance**
>
> Because bone deposition begins to decrease after 30 years of age, women particularly need to consume adequate calcium and perform weight-bearing exercises in the preceding decades. Weight-bearing exercise is required for older adults to prevent bone loss and muscle wasting. Walking, the most helpful form of exercise, is less detrimental to joints than other forms.

Scoliosis Screening

Scoliosis is the lateral curvature of the spine, usually affecting both the thoracic and lumbar spine, with a deviation in one direction in the thoracic and in the other direction in the lumbar spine. Scoliosis may be structural, caused by a defect in the spine, or functional, caused by habits (e.g., consistently carrying a heavy backpack on one shoulder). If not corrected early, scoliosis can progressively worsen. Severe forms can interfere with breathing. The problem often develops in early adolescence, especially in girls. That is why school screening for scoliosis is so important.

To screen for scoliosis, inspect the patient's back. While the patient stands, look for symmetry of the hips, scapulae, shoulders, and any skin folds or creases (Fig. 21.10A and B).

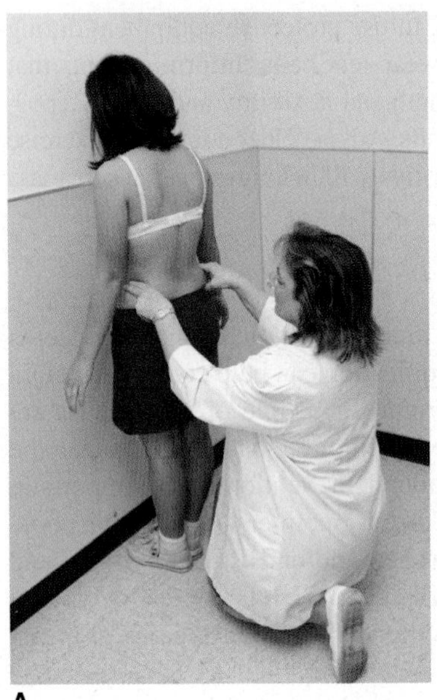
A

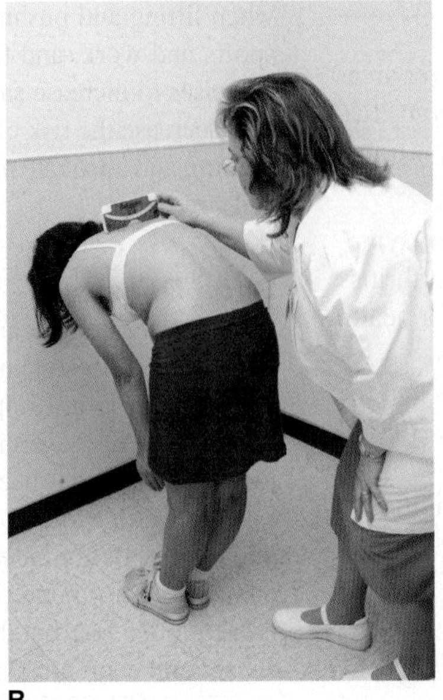
B

Figure 21.10 Screening for scoliosis. **A.** Standing behind the patient to assess symmetry of the hips, scapulae, shoulders, and any skin folds or creases. **B.** While the patient bends forward, look for any curves or protrusions on one side.

Ask the patient to bend forward with the arms hanging toward the floor. Look for any lateral curves or protrusions on one side. Next, ask the patient to slowly stand up while you continue inspecting the spine. You may use a **scoliometer** to obtain a measurement of the number of degrees that the spine is deviated. A deviation in the thoracic area usually has a corresponding deviation on the other side in the lumbar area. During palpation of the spine, palpate for any abnormal protrusions or deformities.

Today, scoliosis screening is regularly done in schools, but older people likely did not undergo such screening. Thus, you may discover cases in the older population. Severe cases can interfere with normal functioning of the organs within the chest.

Common Symptoms

Some common symptoms should be assessed in all patients to screen for the early presence of musculoskeletal disease. Any special patient concerns about joint difficulties will help identify focal areas for assessment. A thorough history of symptoms assists in identifying a current problem or diagnosis.

Common Musculoskeletal Symptoms

- Pain or discomfort
- Weakness
- Stiffness or limited movement
- Deformity
- Lack of balance and coordination

Signs/Symptoms	Rationale/Abnormal Findings
Pain or Discomfort Do you have any pain or discomfort in your muscles, bones, or joints?	Pain is subjective.
Where is the pain located? Is it only in that area, or does it radiate? Do you have pain in different areas at other times? If the pain is in more than one joint, is it symmetrical?	The location and timing of pain may help determine whether it originates in muscle (**myalgia**), bone, or joint (**arthralgia**). Pain limited to one joint is described as monoarticular; pain in several joints is polyarticular.
How badly does it hurt? Use a scale to measure the intensity (see Chapter 6).	
What does the pain feel like?	Patients may describe pain using many different terms. Burning pain may have a neurological cause. Bone pain may be aching, deep, and dull. Muscle pain is often cramping or sore. Patients often describe chronic pain as aching.

(table continues on page 611)

Signs/Symptoms	Rationale/Abnormal Findings
When do you feel pain? Is it constant, or does it come and go? Does it start suddenly or gradually?	Arthritic pain may get worse during cold damp weather. The joint pain of rheumatoid arthritis is often worse in the morning, whereas pain from osteoarthritis is usually worse at the end of the day.
Is there accompanying weakness, tingling, or numbness?	Weakness, tingling, and numbness indicate pressure on nerves.
What makes the pain worse? What helps relieve it?	Bone pain does not increase with movement, unless a fracture is present. Muscle and joint pain increases with movement.
For patients with chronic pain: What level of pain would you like to achieve?	Patients with chronic pain may never experience its absence. You and your patient need to determine what an acceptable level of pain is *together*.
Does the pain limit your activities?	Pain can limit ability to perform usual activities (e.g., walking, bathing, dressing, preparing food, working, sitting, changing positions, climbing stairs, lifting, pushing, pulling).
Weakness	
Do you have any muscle weakness?	Muscle weakness is associated with certain diseases.
Do all or just certain muscles feel weak?	Weakness may migrate from muscle to muscle or to groups of muscles. Knowing which muscles are involved helps determine the disease process. Distal weakness is usually of neurological origin, whereas proximal weakness is usually of muscular origin.
When does the weakness occur? How long does it last? What makes it worse? What helps the weakness? How bad is weakness on a scale of 1–10, with 10 being the worst?	Muscle weakness after prolonged activity may result from dehydration or electrolyte imbalances. Grading the degree of weakness can help patients see improvement or determine the time of day when they can perform better.
Does the weakness limit your activities?	
Stiffness or Limited Movement	
Do you have stiffness or limited movement in any part of your body?	Stiffness is one type of limited movement. It may result from pain in muscles or joints, swelling, or a disease process.
Is the stiffness in one or more joints?	Generalized body swelling from renal failure affects the entire body, whereas injury may involve only one joint.
Can you grade the stiffness on a scale of 0–10, with 10 being the inability to move?	
Is the stiffness constant or intermittent?	Early stages of rheumatoid arthritis may cause stiffness that is worse in the morning, whereas stiffness from osteoarthritis is usually worse at the end of the day.
Did the stiffness start after an injury or was onset gradual?	**Contracture** (shortening of tendons, **fascia**, or muscles) may result from injury or prolonged positioning. After a contracture develops, it is difficult for the patient to stretch and may require surgery.
What makes the stiffness worse? What helps the stiffness? Does the stiffness limit your activities?	

(table continues on page 612)

Signs/Symptoms	Rationale/Abnormal Findings
Deformity Do you have a deformity? Was it present at birth or did it develop later?	Disuse, including wearing a cast, leads to some wasting or shrinking of the muscle (atrophy).
Does it affect the entire body or is it localized?	Deformities may be general (decreased overall body size) or localized (disruption in limb length and alignment after a fracture).
Does it affect your ability to perform ADLs?	
Lack of Balance and Coordination Do you have any difficulties maintaining balance?	Unusual gait or inability to perform ADLs may result from a balance or coordination problem, which may indicate a neurological disorder.
Have you fallen recently?	
Have you noticed your movements are uncoordinated?	**Ataxia** (irregular uncoordinated movements) or loss of balance may be due to cerebellar disorders, Parkinson disease, multiple sclerosis, strokes, brain tumors, inner ear problems, or medications.

Documenting Normal Findings

Patient denies any discomfort, weakness, or stiffness in spine, bones, or joints. Patient reports no musculoskeletal difficulties with work, hobbies, or ADLs.

Lifespan Considerations: Older Adults

Additional Questions	Rationale/Abnormal Findings
Have you noticed any decrease in strength in the last year?	Decreased muscle strength is common as people age, especially in those with sedentary lifestyles.
Have you noticed an increase in stumbling or falling in the last year?	Older adults have an increased rate of falls because of postural changes. Loss of balance may also result from sensory or motor disorders, ear infections, adverse effects of some medicines, and other factors.
Do you use any aids to help you get around? Were you taught how to use the device?	Assistive aids help older adults walk but can cause falls if not used correctly.
Postmenopausal women: Do you take bisphosphonates, calcitonin, estrogens and/or hormone therapy, raloxifene, or parathyroid hormone?	Calcium supplementation, HRT, and weight-bearing exercise decrease the development of osteoporosis (Dane et al., 2007). Of the 10 million U.S. residents estimated to have osteoporosis, 8 million (80%) are women and 2 million (20%) are men (NOF, 2013).

Cultural Considerations

Additional Questions	Rationale/Abnormal Findings
What is your ethnicity? Where were you born?	Table 21.10 (at the end of the chapter) describes common musculoskeletal conditions based on ethnicity. Approximately 20% of Caucasian and Asian women aged 50 years or older are estimated to have osteoporosis as compared with 7% of men (NOF, 2013). Additionally, 52% of Caucasian and Asian American women aged 50 years or older have low bone mass, as compared with 35% of men (NOF, 2013). Low bone mass increases the risk of osteoporosis. It is estimated that 10% of Hispanic women aged 50 years or older have osteoporosis, with 49% having low bone mass (NOF, 2013). In African American women older than 50 years of age, 5% have osteoporosis, with an additional 35% having low bone mass (NOF, 2013).
	People of Asian American descent have lower fracture rates than Caucasians. Caucasian and Hispanic women have twice the risk for hip fracture as African Americans (AHRQ, 2011).
	Patients from countries with severe droughts or recent wars require assessment for signs of scurvy, including splinter hemorrhages in nails, ecchymosis, purpura, and hyperkeratotic papules on skin. These patients are also at risk for malnutrition, which increases the risk of osteoporosis.

Therapeutic Dialogue: Collecting Subjective Data

The nurse's role in subjective data collection is to gather information to improve the patient's health status and to help determine the cause of the patient's current symptoms. Remember Mrs. Runningbird, who was introduced at the beginning of this chapter. She is the 82-year-old Native American woman who has been in the skilled nursing facility for 12 days for rehabilitation. The nurse uses professional communication techniques to gather subjective data from Mrs. Runningbird.

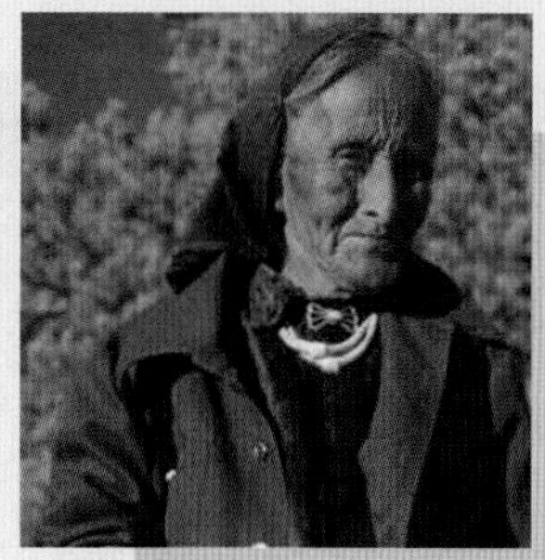

Nurse: Good morning, Mrs. Runningbird. How are you doing today? (pauses)

Mrs. Runningbird: Not so good.

Nurse: I'm sorry to hear that. Do you think that you're more stiff and cold than you were yesterday?

Mrs. Runningbird: No, I don't think so honey. Thank you for asking.

Nurse: I know that it's been hard for you being away from your home. You're doing a great job participating in your therapies.

Mrs. Runningbird: Oh, thank you. My legs and hands don't work the way that they used to.

Nurse: That must be difficult for you. I'm glad that you're here so that we can help you get better.

(case study continues on page 614)

Mrs. Runningbird: Yes, I'm really hoping that I can go home. I'll do whatever I can to get better.

Nurse: Let me help you get up and out of bed. I'll let you do what you can and help with the rest.

Critical Thinking Challenge

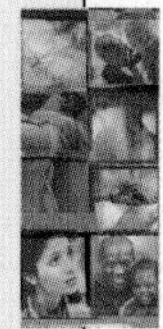

- What culturally appropriate behaviors did the nurse use?
- What other assessments might the nurse make regarding Mrs. Runningbird's coldness, stiffness, and loss of function?
- How might the nurse respond to Mrs. Runningbird? Support your response by drawing on what you understand about culturally competent care.
- What therapeutic communication techniques might be helpful to assess how Mrs. Runningbird is coping?

Objective Data

Common and Specialty or Advanced Techniques

Assessment involves inspection and palpation. Advanced practice health care providers may use percussion to assess for joint injury (see adjacent table for a list of standard and advanced techniques).

Inspection begins with the initial contact with the patient. Evaluate posture while the patient is sitting and standing. If the patient is ambulatory, evaluate his or her gait and coordination.

Equipment

- **Goniometer** (Fig. 21.11) for measuring the angle at which a joint can flex or extend
- Tape measure to assess circumference of extremities or length of bones

Basic Versus Focused/Specialty or Advanced Techniques Related to Musculoskeletal Assessment

Technique	Purpose	Screening or Registered Nurse Assessment	Focused or Advanced Practice Examination
Assess posture.	Assess for kyphosis, scoliosis, or lordosis.	X	
Observe gait, balance, and coordination.	Assess risk for falling and ease of movement.	X	
Inspect extremities.	Observe for deformities.	X	
Palpate extremities for swelling or tenderness.	Identify areas of inflammation.	X	
Observe joint ROM.	Conduct a general overview of functional ability.	X	
Assess muscle tone, strength, size, and symmetry.	Grade muscle bulk and function.	X	
Inspect the spine.	Observe for symmetry and pressure areas.	X	
Specifically inspect, palpate, and measure ROM in TMJ, cervical spine, shoulder, elbow, wrist, hand, hip, knee, ankle, foot, and thoracic and lumbar spine for injuries.	Perform if an area is specifically affected, such as assessment of an ankle following a sprain.		X Head-to-toe assessment for systemic disease

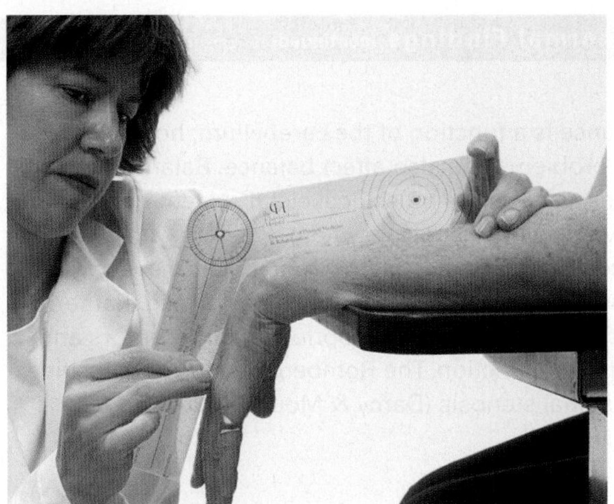

Figure 21.11 A goniometer is used to measure the angle at which a joint can extend or flex.

Preparation

Assemble needed supplies, as listed earlier. Make sure the room is warm and private. Wash and warm your hands. Help the patient to remove clothing so that the limbs and spine are visible. Drape the patient so that only the areas being currently observed are visible.

Weighing the patient is an important part of a comprehensive musculoskeletal examination. Obesity puts extra stress and strain on joints, increases the risk of degenerative joint disease, and decreases mobility.

> **Clinical Significance**
>
> Although nurses should compare each extremity to the other, they should examine last those areas that the patient has identified as tender or painful.

Initial Survey

Technique and Normal Findings	Abnormal Findings
Posture Observe the patient's posture while he or she stands with feet together. Observe the configuration of the head, trunk, pelvis, and extremities. Assess for symmetry in shoulder height, scapulae, and iliac crests. Also observe the patient's posture while sitting. Posture is erect with the head midline above the spine. Shoulders are equal in height.	Scoliosis or low back pain may cause the patient to lean forward or to the side when standing or sitting. Acromegaly may result in an enlarged skull and increased length to the hands, feet, and long bones. **SAFETY ALERT** *When assessing the musculoskeletal system, take measures to prevent patient falls. Ask about the patient's ability to transfer and to walk or stand. Encourage the patient to maintain balance by holding the examination table or wall when standing.*
Gait and Mobility Watch the patient walk across the room while observing from the side and from behind. Gait can predict a person's risk of falling. Gait assessment tools are useful tool for determining risk and can be found online. One example is The Gait Assessment Rating Scale (Ojai School of Massage). General categories include variability, guardedness, weaving, waddling, and staggering. Walking is normally smooth and rhythmic with the arms swinging in opposition to the legs. The patient rises from sitting with ease. **SAFETY ALERT** *Before assessing gait, ask whether the patient uses an assistive device, such as a cane or walker. Ensure that the patient has the equipment at the examination and knows how to correctly use it.*	Gait abnormalities include hesitancy, unsteadiness, staggering, reaching for external support, high stepping, foot scraping, inability to raise the foot completely off the floor, persistent toe or heel walking, excessive pointing of toes inward or outward, asymmetry of step height or length, limping, stooping, wavering, shuffling, waddling, excessive swinging of shoulders or pelvis, and slow or rapid speed. Table 21.11 at the end of this chapter describes some abnormal gait patterns. Gait abnormalities may result from muscle weakness, joint deterioration, malalignment of lower extremities, paralysis, poor coordination, poor balance, fatigue, or pain.

(table continues on page 616)

Technique and Normal Findings (continued)	Abnormal Findings (continued)
Balance Ask the patient to walk on tiptoes, heels, heel-to-toe fashion (tandem walking), and backward. Ask the patient to step to each side and to sit down and stand. Advanced assessment of balance includes the Romberg test, standing, and hopping on one foot. If the patient has a gait abnormality, you will not be able to assess balance. To perform the Romberg test, ask the patient to stand with feet together and eyes open; then have him or her close the eyes. If cerebral function is intact, the patient can do this without swaying (negative test). ■ Patient is balanced when standing and has a negative Romberg test result.	Balance is a function of the cerebellum; however, inner ear problems can also affect balance. Balance may be assessed with the musculoskeletal system but also involves the neurological system. Patients with cerebellar ataxia will generally be unable to balance even with the eyes open, so the test cannot be performed. Rather, the test is a function of the proprioception receptors and pathways function. The Romberg test is 90% sensitive for spinal stenosis (Darcy & Moughty, 2013).
Coordination Ask the patient to rapidly pat the table or his or her thigh, alternating between the palm and dorsum of the hand. To assess fine motor coordination of the hand, ask the patient to perform finger-to-thumb **opposition**. Assess gross motor coordination in the legs by having the patient run the heel of one foot up the opposite leg from ankle to knee. ■ Patient performs rapid alternating movements of the arms and finger–thumb opposition and runs the heel of one foot down the opposite shin.	The dominant side usually has slightly better coordination. Poor coordination may be due to pain, injury, deformity, or cerebellar disorders. Coordination is often tested during assessment of the musculoskeletal system, but it is actually an assessment of the neurological system.
Inspection of Extremities Look for any swelling, lacerations, lesions, deformity, length of long bones, size of muscles, and symmetry.	Asymmetry in bone length may be from injury. Asymmetry in muscle size may be from neurological damage (e.g., polio). Disuse, including while wearing a cast, leads to some wasting or shrinking of the muscle (atrophy).
Size and Shape of Extremities. Assess both extremities at the same time to evaluate symmetry. Assess bilaterally for muscle tone and strength for comparison. Note the size and shape of extremities and muscles, as well as alignment and any deformity or asymmetry. • Are the limbs of equal length?	Disuse, including while wearing a cast, will lead to some wasting or shrinking of the muscle (atrophy). Swelling or edema may be the result of trauma, inflammation, or lymph node resection.
Limb Measurements. Compare the circumference of the arms and legs. Compare the length of the radius by having the patient place the arms together from elbow to wrist. Observe the knee height with the patient sitting. Limb circumference may be measured on the forearms, upper arms, thighs, and calves. Measure circumference at the midpoint (measure the length first to determine the midpoint); the dominant side may be 1 cm (about half an inch) larger in circumference. Measure arm length from the acromion process to the tip of the middle finger. Measure true leg length from the anterior superior iliac crest to the medial malleolus (Fig. 21.12). Measure apparent leg length from the umbilicus to the medial malleolus.	Discrepancy in leg length of more than 1 cm (about half an inch) may cause gait difficulties, hip and back pain, and apparent scoliosis. Unequal apparent leg length, but equal true leg length, is seen with hip and pelvic abnormalities. Unequal arm length does not cause as many difficulties as unequal leg length. Unequal circumference may be result from disuse or neurological disorders.

(table continues on page 617)

Technique and Normal Findings (continued)	Abnormal Findings (continued)
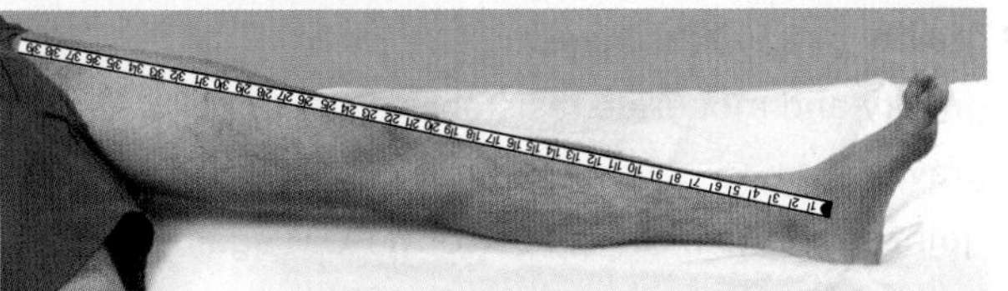 **Figure 21.12** True leg length is measured from the anterior superior iliac crest to the medial malleolus.	
Palpation Palpate joints for contour and size; palpate muscles for tone. Feel for any bumps, nodules, or deformity. Ask whether any tenderness is felt when being touched.	Asymmetry in muscle size and tone may be due to disuse or neurological disease. If the patient feels discomfort when touched, it may be due to inflammation or infection.
Joint Range of Motion. Assess both extremities at the same time to evaluate symmetry. Simultaneously observe and palpate each joint while the patient performs active ROM. If the patient cannot perform active ROM, carefully support the limb on either side of the joint and perform passive ROM. Ask the patient about any tenderness or discomfort. If ROM is limited, use a goniometer to measure the angle of the joint at its maximum flexion and extension (see Fig. 21.11). Listen to and feel the joint while the patient moves. *A healthy joint moves smoothly and quietly.*	Note limitation of movement, **crepitus** (cracking or popping), and nonverbal and verbal expressions of discomfort or pain. Ask the patient whether any tenderness or discomfort with movement is present. Do not apply force; be gentle, and stop if there is resistance or complaint of discomfort. Crepitus may be heard as a popping sound and may be felt as grating in the joint as it moves. *SAFETY ALERT* *When performing passive ROM, do not force the joint. Stop if resistance or reports of discomfort are present.*
Muscle Tone and Strength. When assessing muscle tone and strength, it is necessary to compare one side with the other. Upper and lower extremity muscle strength is 5/5 bilaterally.	Table 21.5 defines terms used when describing alterations in muscle tone. Table 21.6 describes the rating scale for muscle strength. Table 21.7 indicates what to say to the patient when assessing muscle strength.

Documenting Normal Findings

Patient denies any discomfort, weakness, or stiffness in spine, bones, or joints. Patient reports no musculoskeletal difficulties during work, hobbies, or ADLs.

TABLE 21.5 Terms for Describing Alterations in Muscle Tone

Atony	Lack of normal muscle tone or strength
Hypotonicity	Diminished tone of skeletal muscles
Spasticity	Hypertonic, so the muscles are stiff and movements awkward
Spasm	Sudden violent involuntary contraction of a muscle
Fasciculation	Involuntary twitching of muscle fibers
Tremors	Involuntary contraction of muscles

TABLE 21.6 Rating Scale for Muscle Strength		
5/5 (100%)	Normal	Complete ROM against gravity and full resistance
4/5 (75%)	Good	Complete ROM against gravity and moderate resistance
3/5 (50%)	Fair	Complete ROM against gravity
2/5 (25%)	Poor	Complete ROM with the joint supported; cannot perform ROM against gravity
1/5 (10%)	Trace	Muscle contraction detectable, but no movement of the joint
0/5 (0%)	Zero	No visible muscle contraction

Muscle strength can be described on a 0 to 5 scale, with 5 being the strongest, as percentage or by words.

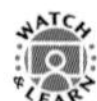

Comprehensive Physical Examination

Clinical Significance

Handle the extremities of patients with fragile bones gently to prevent fractures.

Advanced health care practitioners use special assessment procedures for the musculoskeletal system. These tests are described in Table 21.8.

TABLE 21.7 Instructions for Testing Muscle Strength

Muscle	Examiner Activity	Patient Instructions
Neck	Place hand on side of patient's head.	"Turn your head toward my hand."
Deltoid	Put hand on patient's upper arm and try to push arm down.	"Hold your arm straight out to the side. Try to prevent me from pushing down your arm."
Biceps	With elbow bent, place hand on patient's lower arm and have patient try to flex arm.	"Prevent me from straightening your arm."
Triceps	With elbow bent, place hand on patient's lower arm and have patient try to straighten arm.	"Prevent me from bending your arm."
Wrist	With wrist extended, place hand on dorsal surface of the patient's hand, and ask patient to try to flex the wrist. Place hand on palm and ask patient to push to hyperextend wrist.	"Prevent me from pushing your hand downward." "Push against my hand."
Fingers	Push on dorsal surface of patient's fingers. Hold patient's fingers together. With patient's fingers spread apart, prevent patient from bringing fingers together.	"Do not let me bend your fingers." "Do not let me straighten your fingers." "Spread your fingers apart." "Bring your fingers together."
Hip	With patient supine, push down on his or her leg above the knee.	"Keeping your leg straight, raise your leg (do a leg lift)."
Quadriceps	Push down on patient's leg above the knee. Place your hand on the front of the patient's lower leg and prevent extension of knee.	"While sitting, raise your leg. "Straighten your leg."
Hamstring	With patient's leg extended, place hand on back of the patient's lower leg and prevent flexion.	"Bend your knee."
Ankle	With patient's ankle flexed, push against sole of patient's foot. With patient's ankle flexed, push against dorsum of patient's foot.	"Bend your foot up." "Push against my hand."

TABLE 21.8 Advanced Musculoskeletal Assessment Techniques

HANDS

Phalen Test

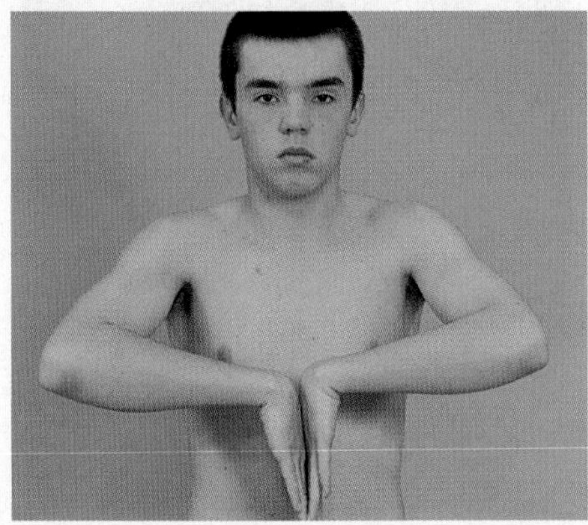

Evaluates for carpal tunnel syndrome. Ask the patient to flex the wrists 90 degrees and hold the backs of the hands to each other for 60 seconds. The expected response is denial of any discomfort. Positive signs include numbness, burning, or pain.

Carpal Compression

Evaluates for carpal tunnel syndrome. Perform direct compression over the carpal tunnel on the volar side of the wrist for up to 30 seconds. Pain, numbness, or tingling is a positive test result.

Tinel Sign/Test

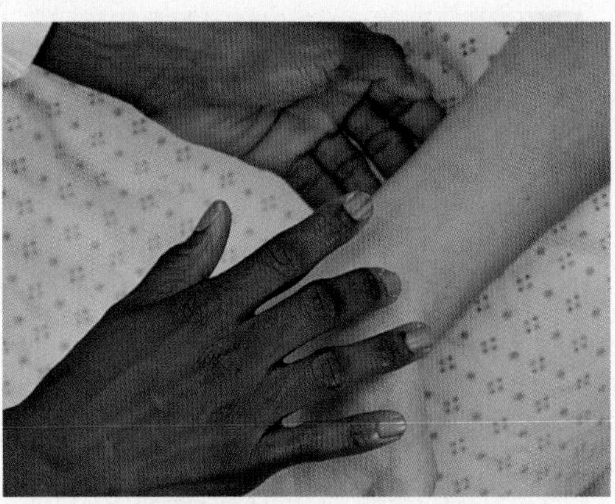

Evaluates for carpal tunnel syndrome. Percuss lightly over the median nerve located on the inner aspect of the wrist. Pain, numbness, or tingling is a positive (abnormal) finding.

ARM

Drop Arm Test

Assesses for rotator cuff injury. Ask the patient to abduct the arm to shoulder level or 90 degrees. If the patient cannot fully abduct and remain there, the drop arm test result is positive as the arm drops rapidly to the patient's side or the patient complains of severe shoulder pain.

Neer Impingement Test

Tests shoulder impingement. Stabilize the scapula and with the thumb pointing down, then passively flex the arm. Presence of pain is a positive test.

"Empty Can" Test

Tests supraspinatus impingement. Passively abduct the shoulder to 90 degrees, then flex to 30 degrees and point thumbs down. In this position, place resistance as the patient lifts upward. Pain or weakness suggests tendinopathy or tear.

Hawkins Impingement Test

Tests supraspinatus muscle impingement. Stabilize the scapula, then passively abduct the shoulder to 90 degrees, flex the shoulder to 30 degrees, flex the elbow to 90 degrees, and internally rotate the shoulder. Presence of pain is a positive test result.

(table continues on page 620)

KNEES

Bulge Test

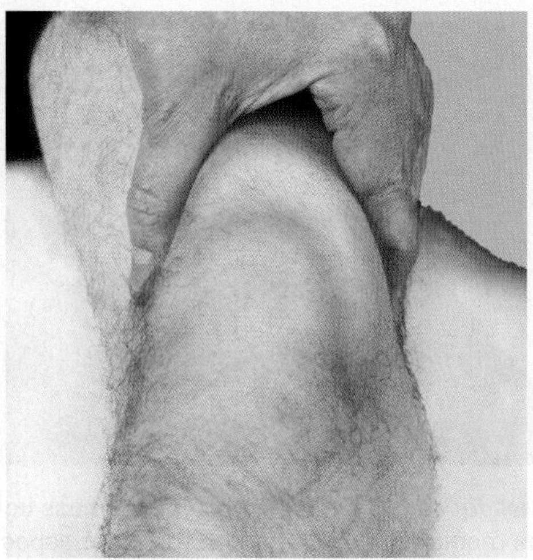

Differentiates soft tissue swelling from accumulation of excess fluid behind the patella. With the patient supine, milk upward along the medial aspect of the knee two, three, or four times. Then press on the lateral side of the knee and check for any bulging on the medial side. A bulge indicates mild joint effusion or liquid accumulation in the area, which is not a normal finding.

Loculation Test

Evaluates for loculated fluid. Attempt to hyperextend the knee by placing one hand superior to the patella and the other posterior to the heel. More than 2 or 3 cm (¾–1¼ in.) hyperextension is abnormal. With both hands, flex and extend the knee. Repeat while performing medial and lateral rotation. Determine whether any "locking" or "catching" is present.

Ballottement/Suprapatellar Pouch Effusion

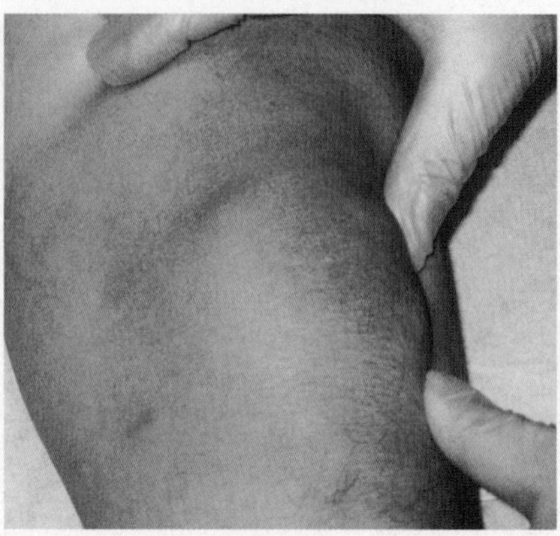

Evaluates presence of large accumulation of fluid behind the knee. With the patient supine and the knee extended, press on the quadriceps muscle just above the knee with one hand and keep that pressure there. This compresses the suprapatellar pouch. Palpate the patella with the other hand. If fluid is present, the patella will rebound or ballot against the fingers.

Drawer Sign

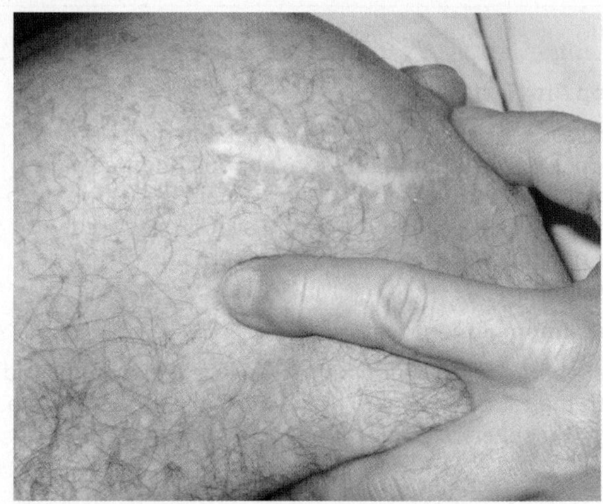

Checks for knee injury. Ask the supine patient to flex the knee to a right angle. While standing at the patient's feet, grasp the leg just below the knee and see whether you can move it toward and away from yourself.
A normal finding is that you cannot move the leg that way. A positive sign is the head of the tibia moves more than half an inch from the joint. This test may also be used for ankle injuries.

(table continues on page 621)

TABLE 21.8 Advanced Musculoskeletal Assessment Techniques *(continued)*

McMurray Test

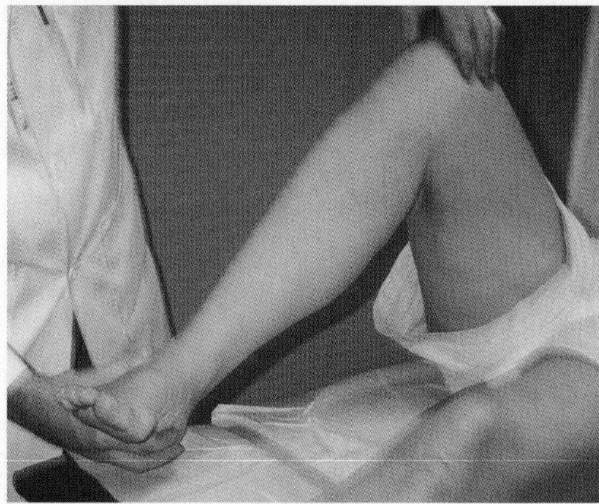

Checks for meniscus cartilage injury. Have the patient lie supine and flex the hip and knee. Support the knee with one hand and hold the foot with the other, rotating the foot laterally. Slowly extend the patient's knee while assessing for the positive findings of pain or clicking. Repeat the procedure, rotating the lower leg medially.

Lachman Test

Checks for knee laxity. Flex the knee only 20–30 degrees (rather than 90 degrees as in anterior drawer sign), then attempt to pull tibia anteriorly relative to the femur. An injured ACL will show an increase movement forward (positive sign). This test is thought to be more sensitive than the anterior drawer sign.

HIP

Thomas Test

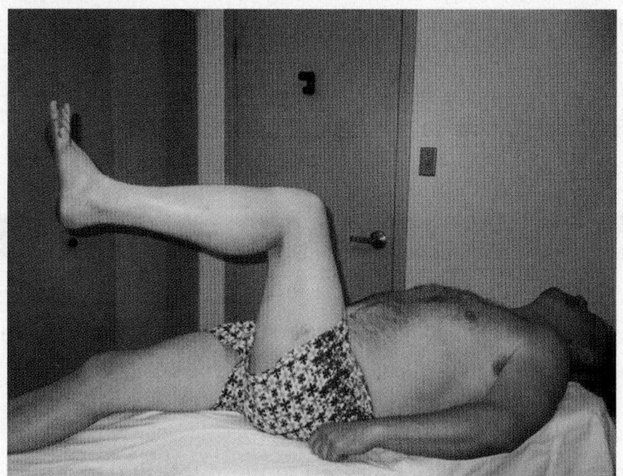

Assesses presence of a flexion contracture of the hip. Ask the supine patient to extend one leg and flex the hip and knee of the other leg, bringing the knee to the chest. A flexion contracture of the hip will cause the extended leg to rise up off the examination table.

Patrick or FABERE Test

Tests for sacroiliac or hip joint being source of the pain. Have the patient lie supine and place the foot of his or her involved side on his opposite knee. Inguinal pain is a general indication that there is pathology in the hip joint or surrounding muscles. Extend the ROM by placing one hand on the flexed knee joint and the other hand on the anterior superior iliac spine of the opposite side. Press down on each of these points. If the patient complains of increased pain posteriorly, this indicates injury in the sacroiliac joint. Anterior hip/groin pain indicates hip involvement.

(table continues on page 622)

TABLE 21.8 Advanced Musculoskeletal Assessment Techniques *(continued)*

Lasègue Test (Straight Leg Raising)

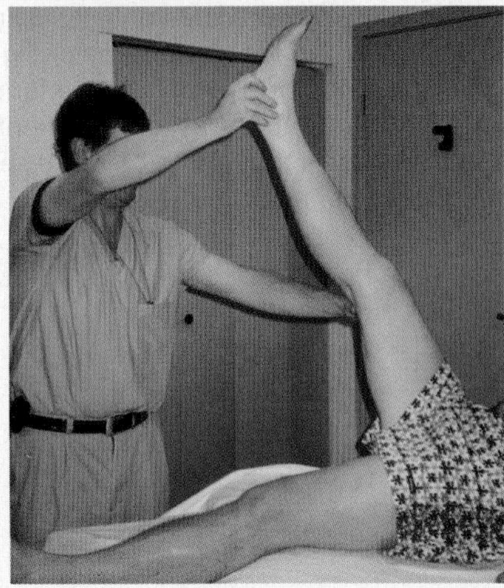

Checks for herniation of the lumbar disc and nerve irritation or pressure. With the patient supine and both legs extended, support and raise one leg. Report of pain is a positive response.

Trendelenburg Test

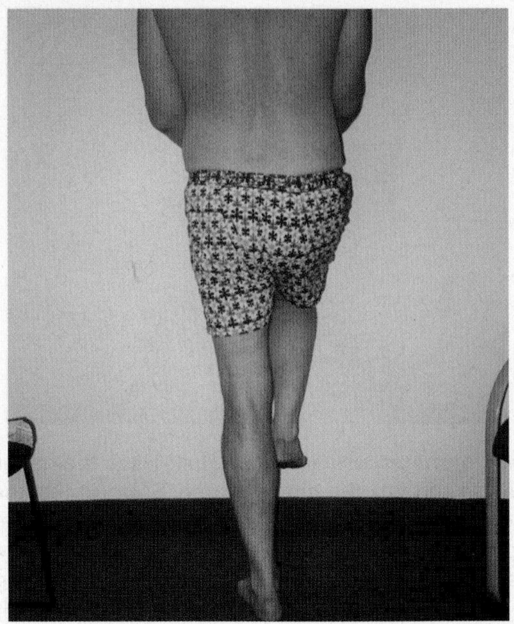

Assesses for hip disease with muscle weakness. Observe from behind the patient. Ask the patient to stand first on one foot, then the other. Normally, the pelvis remains level horizontally, which is a negative Trendelenburg sign. An abnormal or positive finding is that the other hip drops when the patient stands on the weak side.

ACL, anterior cruciate ligament; FABERE, *F*lexion, *A*bduction, *E*xternal *R*otation, *E*xtension.

Technique and Normal Findings	Abnormal Findings
Temporomandibular Joint	
Inspection. Inspect the TMJ for symmetry, swelling, and redness. The jaw is symmetrical bilaterally.	Asymmetrical facial or joint musculature may indicate previous or current facial fractures or surgery.
Palpation. Place your finger pads in front of the tragus of each of the patient's ears (Fig. 21.13). Ask the patient to open and close the jaw while you palpate the joints. You should feel a shallow depression; the mandible motion should be smooth and painless. The muscles are symmetrical, smooth, and nontender.	Discomfort, swelling, limited movement, and grating or crackling sounds are unexpected and require further evaluation for dental or neurological problems or TMJ syndrome. TMJ dysfunction may present as ear pain or headache. Swelling or tenderness suggests arthritis or myofascial pain syndrome (inflammation of the fascia surrounding the muscle).
Range of Motion. Ask the patient to open the jaw as wide as possible, push the lower jaw forward (protrusion), return the jaw to neutral position (retraction), and move the jaw from side to side 1 or 2 cm (about ½–¾ in.). The joint has an audible and palpable click when opened. The mouth opens with 3–6 cm (about 1¼–2½ in.) between the upper and lower teeth. The jaw moves with ease.	Difficulty opening the mouth may be due to injury or arthritic changes. Pain in the TMJ may indicate malalignment of the teeth or arthritic changes.

(table continues on page 623)

Technique and Normal Findings (continued)	Abnormal Findings (continued)
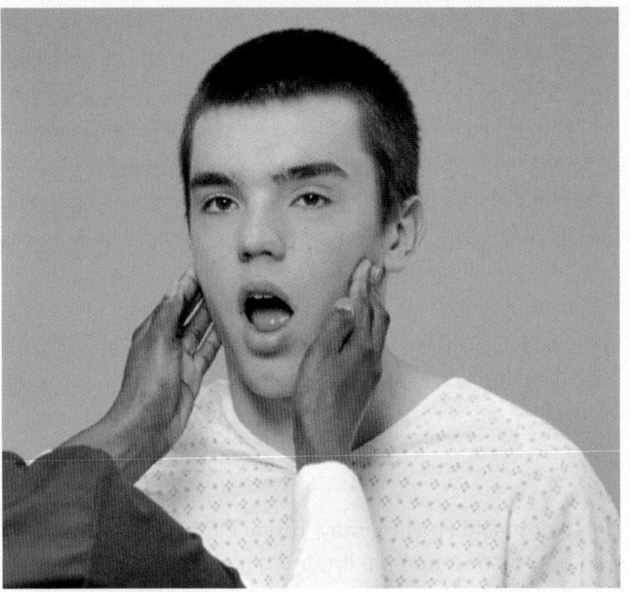 Figure 21.13 Palpating the temporomandibular joint.	
Muscle Strength. Ask the patient to repeat the above movements while you provide opposing force. This tests cranial nerve V (the trigeminal nerve). The strength of the muscles is equal on both sides of the jaw; the patient can perform the movements against resistance. Muscle strength is 5/5, with no pain, spasms, or contractions.	Decreased muscle strength may be because of muscle or joint disease.

Documenting Normal Findings

The TMJ is symmetrical bilaterally. The muscles are smooth with normal strength of 5/5. The joint moves smoothly through all ROM without pain. A slight popping sound is heard when the jaw is widely opened. The teeth align correctly.

Technique and Normal Findings	Abnormal Findings
Cervical Spine	
Inspection. With the patient standing, inspect the cervical spine from all sides. It should position the head above the trunk (Fig. 21.14). Observing from the side, check for the concave curve of the cervical spine. As viewed from behind, the patient holds the head erect and the cervical spine is in straight alignment. From the side, the neck has a concave curve.	Degenerative joint disease of the cervical vertebrae may cause lateral tilting of the head and neck. Lateral deviation of the neck (i.e., torticollis) may be due to acute muscle spasms, congenital difficulties, or abnormal head posture to correct vision problems. Weight lifting will cause hypertrophy of the neck muscles, resulting in a thickened appearance of the neck.
Palpation. Stand behind the patient to palpate the cervical spine and neck. C7 and T1 spinous processes should be prominent. The paravertebral, sternocleidomastoid, and trapezius muscles are fully developed, symmetrical, and nontender.	Osteoarthritis, neck injury, disc degeneration because of aging or occupational stress, and spondylosis can cause decreased ROM, pain, and tenderness on palpation. Pain on palpation may indicate inflammation of the muscles (**myositis**). Neck spasm may indicate nerve compression or psychological stress.

(table continues on page 624)

Technique and Normal Findings (continued)	Abnormal Findings (continued)
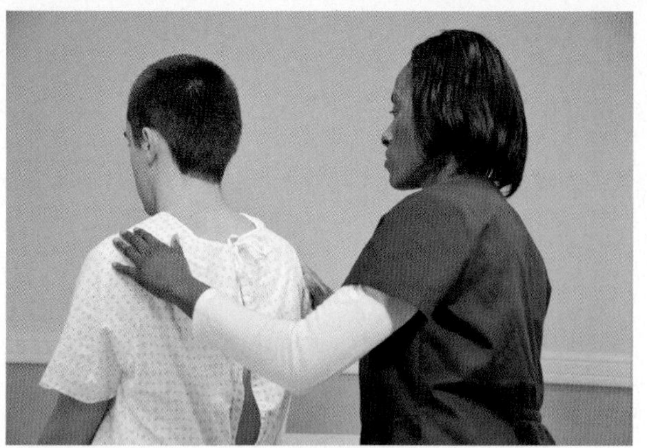 **Figure 21.14** Inspecting the cervical spine from behind the patient.	
Range of Motion. Ask the patient to touch the chin to the chest (flexion), look up toward the ceiling (**hyperextension**), attempt to touch each ear to the shoulder without elevating the shoulder (lateral flexion or bending), and turn the chin to the shoulder as far as possible (rotation) (Fig. 21.15). Neck ROM is normal: flexion 45 degrees, hyperextension 55 degrees, lateral flexion 40 degrees, and rotation 70 degrees to each side.	Pain or muscle spasms may impair ROM. Hyperextension and flexion may be limited because of cervical disc degeneration, spinal cord tumor, or osteoarthritic changes. Pain may radiate to the back, shoulder, or arms. Pain, numbness, or tingling may indicate compression of spinal root nerves.

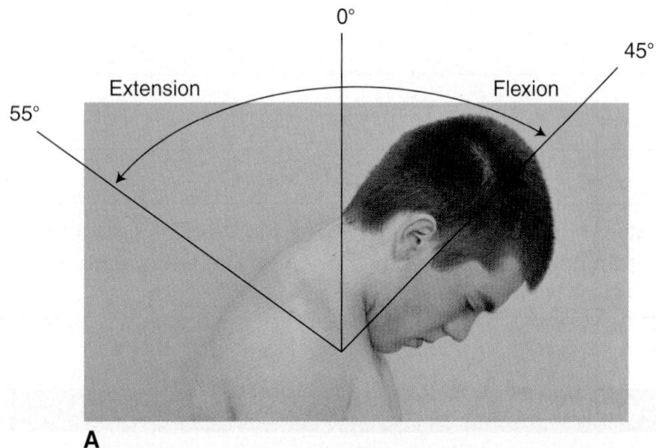

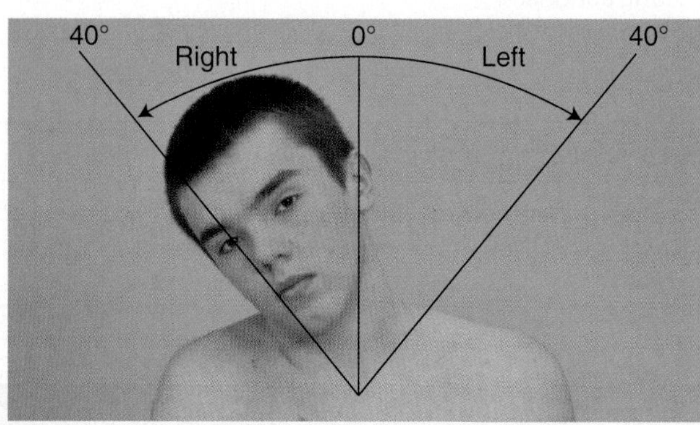

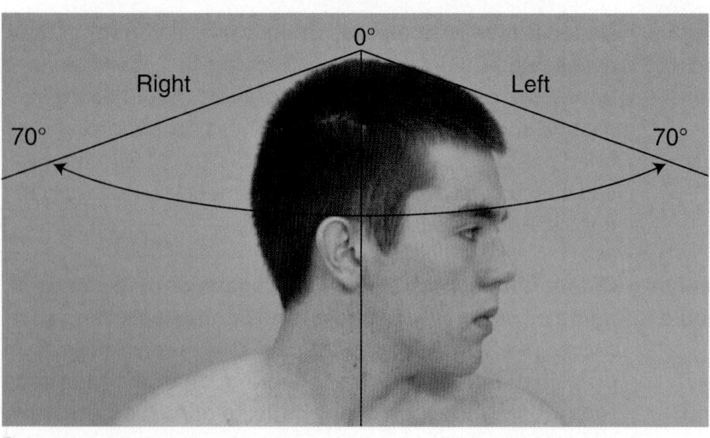

Figure 21.15 Assessing neck range of motion. **A.** Flexion. **B.** Testing lateral flexion or bending by moving the ear to shoulder left and right. **C.** Assessing rotation by moving the chin to shoulder left and right.

(table continues on page 625)

Technique and Normal Findings (continued)	Abnormal Findings (continued)
Muscle Strength. Ask the patient to rotate the neck to the right and left against the resistance of your hand. This tests cranial nerve XI (the spinal accessory nerve). Muscle strength is sufficient to overcome resistance.	Weakness or loss of sensation in arms may result from cervical cord compression.

Clinical Significance

After suffering any trauma, do not move patients with neck pain until the neck has been stabilized. Moving the patient could cause subluxation or dislocation of the cervical vertebrae and permanent injury to the spinal cord.

Documenting Normal Findings

Viewed from behind, the neck is straight and holds the head in alignment with the spine. Viewed from the side, the neck is slightly concave. Muscle size is symmetrical bilaterally. The neck has full ROM and moves smoothly and painlessly. Muscle strength is 5/5. The patient denies tenderness during palpation. C7 and T1 spinous processes are prominent and palpable. The muscles are fully developed. No nodules, swelling, crepitus, or muscle spasms are noted.

Technique and Normal Findings	Abnormal Findings
Shoulder	
Inspection. Compare both shoulders anteriorly and posteriorly for size and contour. Observe the anterior aspect of the joint capsule for abnormal swelling. No redness, swelling, deformity, or muscular atrophy is present. Shoulders are smooth and bilaterally symmetrical. Right and left shoulders are level. Each shoulder is at an equal distance from the vertebral column.	Shoulder joints may have some deformity because of arthritis, trauma, or scoliosis. Redness and swelling may indicate injury or inflammation. Unequal shoulder height may indicate scoliosis.
Palpation. Stand in front of the patient and palpate both shoulders, noting any muscular spasm, atrophy, swelling, heat, or tenderness. Start at the clavicle and methodically explore the acromioclavicular joint, scapula, greater tubercle of the humerus, area of the subacromial bursa, biceps groove, and anterior aspect of the glenohumeral joint. Muscles are fully developed and smooth.	Tenderness may be because of inflammation of the muscles, overuse of unconditioned muscles, or sports injuries. **SAFETY ALERT** *Suspect a cardiac origin for reports of shoulder pain without tenderness or inflammation. Assess for shortness of breath, nausea, and diaphoresis. If these symptoms are present, the patient needs to be sent to an emergency department for assessment of cardiac ischemia.*
Range of Motion. Ask the person to perform forward flexion, extension, hyperextension, abduction, adduction, and **internal** and **external rotation** (Fig. 21.16). Cup one hand over the patient's shoulder during ROM to detect any crepitus. Movement is fluid. ROM is normal: forward flexion 180 degrees, hyperextension 50 degrees, abduction 180 degrees, adduction 50 degrees, internal rotation 90 degrees, and external rotation 90 degrees.	Limited ROM, pain, crepitation, and asymmetry may result from arthritis, muscle or joint inflammation, trauma, or sports injury. Inability to externally rotate the shoulder suggests a rotator cuff injury.

(table continues on page 626)

Technique and Normal Findings (continued)	Abnormal Findings (continued)

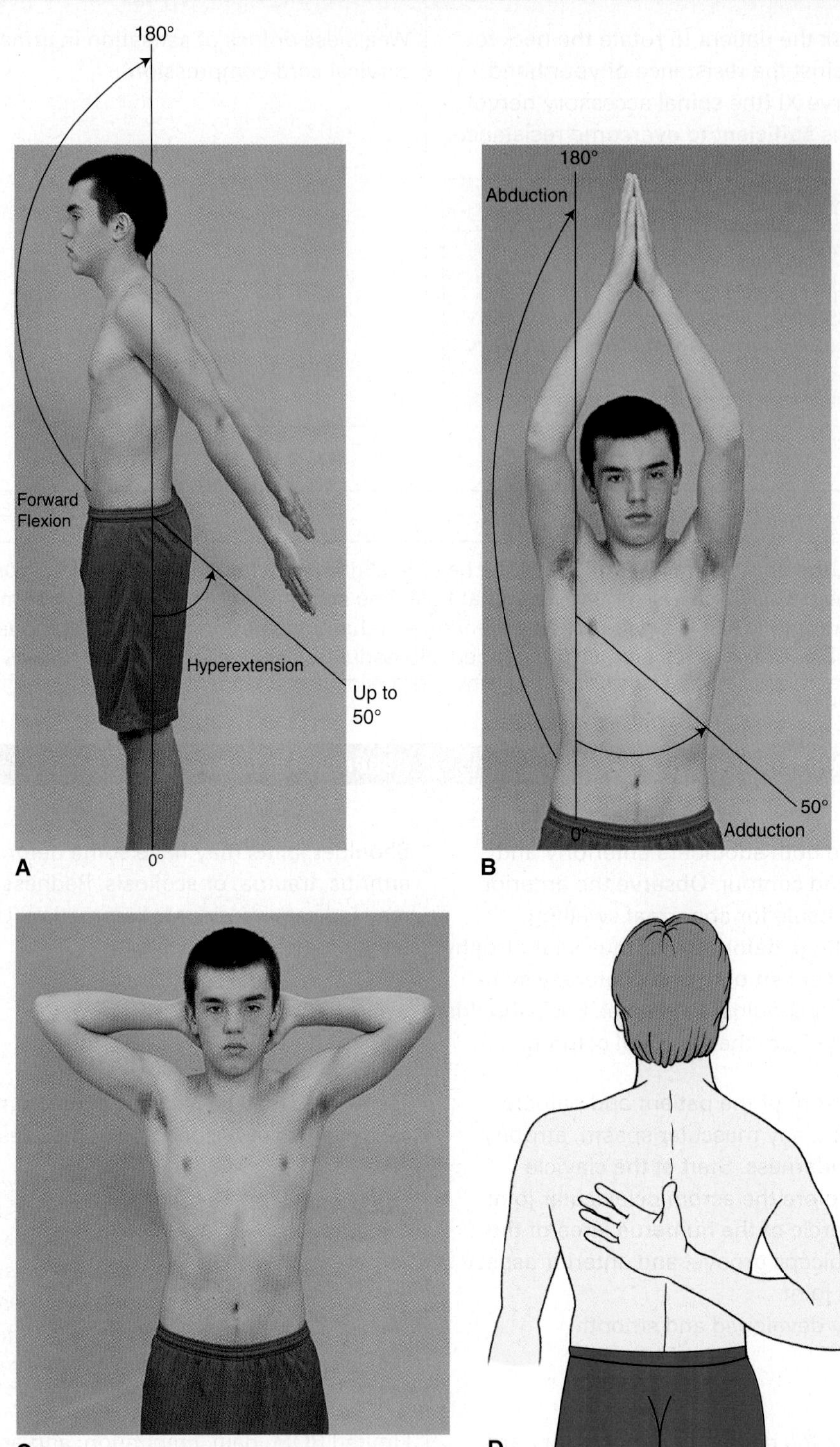

Figure 21.16 Assessing shoulder range of motion. **A.** Extension. **B.** Abduction/adduction. **C.** External rotation. **D.** Internal rotation.

Technique and Normal Findings	Abnormal Findings
Muscle Strength. Ask the patient to shrug both shoulders, flex forward and upward, and abduct against resistance. Shrugging the shoulders tests cranial nerve XI (spinal accessory nerve). Patient can perform full ROM against resistance.	Decreased ability to shrug the shoulders against resistance may indicate compressed spinal cord root nerve or spinal accessory nerve (CN XI).

Documenting Normal Findings

Shoulders are of equal height and equidistant from the spinal column. Muscle size is symmetrical bilaterally. Both shoulders have full ROM and move smoothly and painlessly. Muscle strength is 5/5. The patient denies tenderness during palpation. No nodules, swelling, crepitus, or muscle spasms are noted.

Technique and Normal Findings	Abnormal Findings
Elbow ***Inspection.*** Inspect the size and contour of the elbow in both the extended and flexed positions. Check the olecranon bursa for swelling. Elbows are symmetrical with no swelling.	Subluxation of the elbow shows the forearm dislocated posteriorly. This may occur when an adult tugs on a small child's forearm or swings the child holding onto the child's forearms. Swelling and redness of the olecranon bursa are easily observed because of the proximity to the skin. **Effusion** or synovial thickening is observed as a bulge on either side of the olecranon process and indicates gouty arthritis.
Palpation. Support the patient's forearm and passively flex the elbow to 70 degrees. Palpate the olecranon process and medial and lateral epicondyles of the humerus (Fig. 21.17). The tissues and fat pads should feel solid. Check for any synovial thickening, swelling, nodules, or tenderness. Elbows are smooth with no swelling or tenderness. 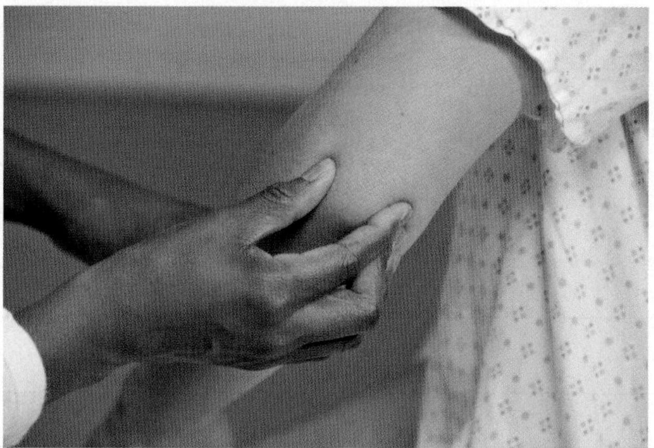 **Figure 21.17** Palpation of the elbow.	Epicondyles and tendons are common sites for inflammation and tenderness. Soft boggy swelling occurs with synovial thickening or effusion. Local heat or redness may indicate synovial inflammation. Subcutaneous nodules at pressure points on the olecranon process or ulnar surface may indicate rheumatoid arthritis.
Range of Motion. Ask the patient to bend and straighten the elbow. Then have the person pronate and supinate the forearm by laying the forearm and ulnar surface of the hand on a table. Have the patient touch the palm and then the hand dorsum to the table (Fig. 21.18). ROM is normal: flexion 150–160 degrees, extension 0 degrees, pronation and supination 90 degrees. Some people cannot extend the elbow fully (only to 5 to 10 degrees). Some people can hyperextend the elbow from –5 to –10 degrees.	Decreased ROM, pain, or crepitation may be from arthritis, muscle or joint inflammation, trauma, or sports injury. Redness, swelling, and tenderness of the olecranon process may be because of bursitis. Lateral epicondylitis (tennis elbow) is inflammation of the forearm extensor and supinator muscles and tendons, causing disabling pain at the lateral epicondyle of the humerus that radiates down the lateral side of the forearm. Medial epicondylitis (golf elbow) is the same as tennis elbow, except it affects the flexor and pronator muscles and tendons.

(table continues on page 628)

Technique and Normal Findings (continued)	Abnormal Findings (continued)
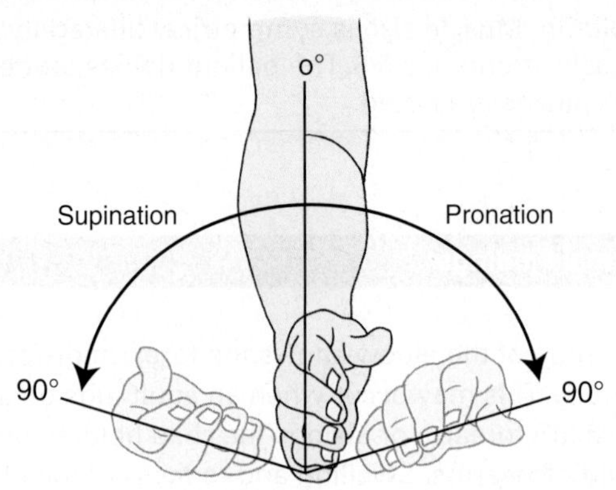 **Figure 21.18** Supination and pronation of the elbow.	
Muscle Strength. While supporting the patient's arm, apply resistance just proximal to the patient's wrist and ask the patient to flex and then extend both elbows (Fig. 21.19). Patient can perform full ROM against resistance. 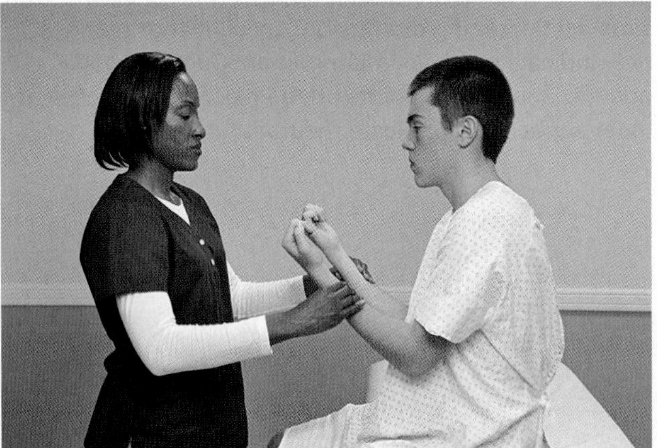 **Figure 21.19** Assessing biceps muscle strength.	Decreased strength may be from pain, nerve root compression, or arthritic deformity. People may compensate for weakened biceps or triceps muscles by using the shoulder muscles.

Documenting Normal Findings

Elbows are equal in size and shape. Muscle size is symmetrical bilaterally. Both elbows have full ROM and move smoothly and painlessly. Muscle strength is 5/5. The patient denies tenderness during palpation. No nodules, swelling, crepitus, or muscle spasms are noted.

Technique and Normal Findings	Abnormal Findings
Wrist and Hand ***Palpation.*** Hold the patient's hand in your hands. Use your thumbs to palpate each joint of the wrist and hand for tenderness (Fig. 21.20). Joint surfaces are smooth without nodules, edema, or tenderness.	Painful joints in the fingers are common in osteoarthritis. A firm mass over the dorsum of the wrist may be a ganglion. Rheumatoid arthritis may cause edema, redness, and tenderness of the finger and wrist joints.

(table continues on page 629)

Technique and Normal Findings (continued)	Abnormal Findings (continued)

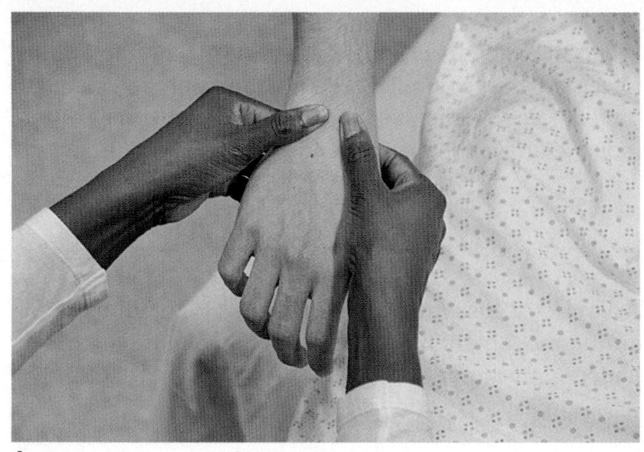

A

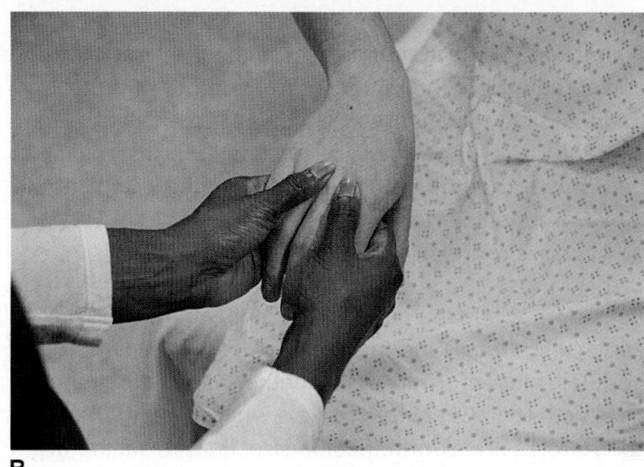

B

Figure 21.20 Palpating the joints of the **(A)** wrists and **(B)** hands.

Range of Motion. Observe wrist and hand ROM (Fig. 21.21).

Wrist motions are normal: flexion 90 degrees, extension return to 0 degrees, hyperextension 70 degrees, ulnar deviation 55 degrees, radial deviation 20 degrees. Metacarpophalangeal joints motion are normal: flexion 90 degrees, extension 0 degrees, hyperextension up to 30 degrees. Proximal and distal interphalangeal joints perform flexion (making a fist), extension, and abduction. The thumb performs **opposition** with each fingertip and the base of the little finger.

Joint or muscle inflammation may cause decreased or unequal ROM. Previous trauma may limit ROM.

70°
Extension
0°
Flexion
90°

Figure 21.21 Wrist and hand flexion and extension.

Muscle Strength. Perform each motion discussed above against resistance. Ask the patient to grasp your first two fingers tightly while you pull to remove your fingers.

Muscle strength is equal bilaterally and sufficient to overcome resistance.

Weak muscle strength may be due to arthritic changes or fractures of the metatarsals or phalanges.

(table continues on page 630)

Technique and Normal Findings (continued)	Abnormal Findings (continued)
Hip ***Inspection.*** While standing, assess the iliac crest, size and symmetry of the buttocks, and number of gluteal folds. Assist the patient to the supine position with legs straight. Look for any swelling, lacerations, lesions, deformity, size of the muscle, and symmetry. Look at the hips from the anterior and posterior views. Hips are rounded, even, and symmetrical.	When the patient is lying supine, external rotation of the lower leg and foot indicates a fractured femur. Unequal gluteal folds or unequal height of iliac crests may indicate uneven leg length or scoliosis.
Palpation. While the patient is supine, palpate the hip joints, iliac crests, and muscle tone. Feel for any bumps, nodules, and deformity. Ask whether there is any tenderness with touch. Feel for crepitus when moving the joint. Buttocks are symmetrical in size. Iliac crests are at the same height on both sides.	Asymmetry, discomfort when touched, or crepitus during movement may occur with hip inflammation or degenerative joint disease.
Range of Motion. Observe for full active ROM of each hip as follows (Fig. 21.22): • Flexion (lift straight leg to 90 degrees or draw knee to chest to 120 degrees) • Extension (standing position or lying on the examination table with the leg straight) • **Abduction** (lift, if standing, or slide, if lying, foot and straight leg to the side, away from body to 45 degrees) • **Adduction** (swing foot and straight leg in front and past the other leg to 30 degrees) • Internal and external ROM (with the hip and knee flexed, move the leg medially 40 degrees and then laterally 45 degrees). Have the patient stand or placed in a prone position to test hyperextension. Ask the patient to move the straight leg backward, away from the body (15 degrees). Have the patient, while standing or lying on one side, move the foot and leg in a circle beside the body (**circumduction**). Patient can perform full ROM without discomfort or crepitus.	Straight leg flexion that produces back and leg pain radiating down the leg may indicate a herniated disc. When the patient is lying down, one leg longer than the other or limited internal rotation may indicate a hip fracture or dislocation.

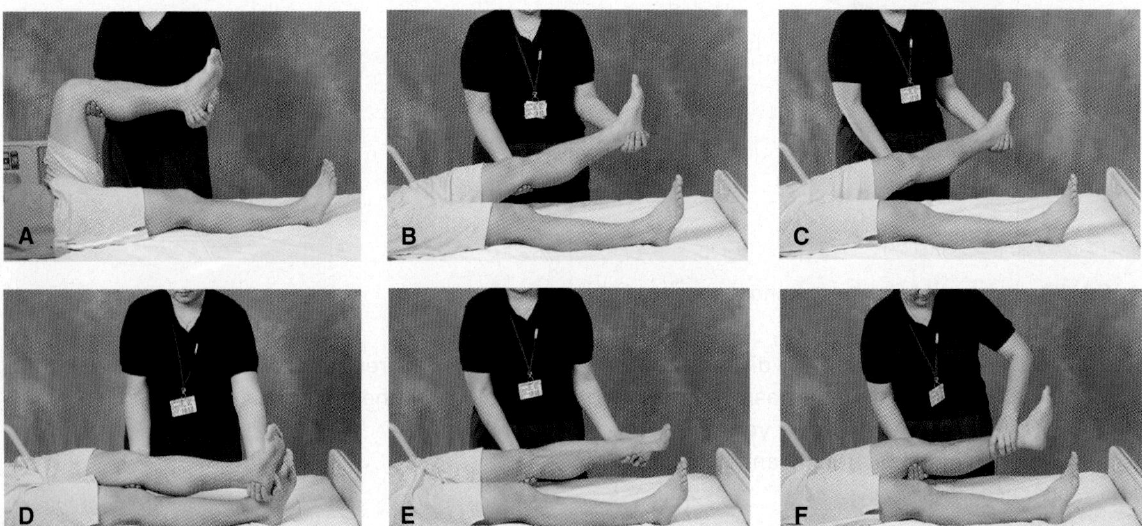

Figure 21.22 Hip range of motion. **A.** Flexion. **B.** Extension. **C.** Abduction. **D.** Adduction. **E.** Internal rotation. **F.** External rotation.

(table continues on page 631)

Technique and Normal Findings (continued)	Abnormal Findings (continued)
Muscle Strength. With the patient lying down, apply pressure to the top of the leg while the patient flexes the hip. Apply pressure to the side while the patient abducts the hip. ■ Patient can perform full ROM against resistance.	Asymmetry of strength may be due to pain or muscular or neurological disease. ⚠ *SAFETY ALERT* *Do not test adduction or flexion greater than 90 degrees in anyone with a hip replacement. Doing so may cause dislocation.*

Documenting Normal Findings

The muscles are well formed, firm to touch, and symmetrical. Hip joints have full active ROM through flexion, extension, hyperextension, abduction, adduction, circumduction, and internal and external rotation. Muscle strength is 5/5. Patient denies any discomfort while still or moving.

Technique and Normal Findings	Abnormal Findings
Knee	
Inspection. Inspect the knee with the patient both standing and sitting. Inspect contour and shape. Look for any swelling, lacerations, lesions, deformity, size of the muscle, and symmetry. Look for symmetry in the length of long bones: When the patient is standing, is one hip higher than the other? When seated, is one knee higher than the other? When seated, does one knee protrude further than the other? ■ Hollows on each side of the patella. Knees are symmetrical and aligned with thighs and ankles.	Swelling of the knee indicates inflammation, trauma, or arthritis. Muscle atrophy may accompany disuse or chronic disorders. A part of a limb twisted toward or out from the midline is labeled **varum** and **valgum,** respectively. For example, genu valgum is knock-kneed, whereas genu varum is bowlegged. Asymmetry in leg muscle size may be from disuse or nerve or muscle injury.
Palpation. With the knee flexed, palpate the quadriceps muscle for muscle tone. Palpate downward from approximately 10 cm (about 4 in.) above the patella; evaluate the patella and each side of the femur and tibia (Fig. 21.23). 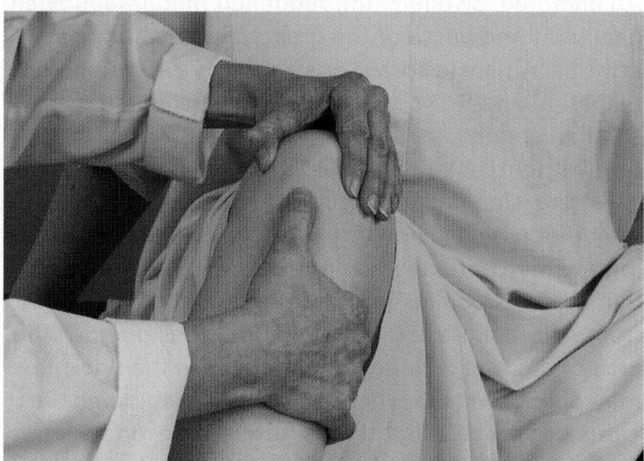 **Figure 21.23** Palpating the knee.	Pain, swelling, thickening, or heat may indicate synovial inflammation, arthritis, or torn **meniscus**. Painless swelling may occur with osteoarthritis. Bursitis causes swelling, heat, and redness.

(table continues on page 632)

Technique and Normal Findings (continued)	Abnormal Findings (continued)
Palpate the tibiofemoral joints with the leg flexed 90 degrees. Assess the tibial margins and the lateral collateral ligament. Palpate for any bumps, nodules, or deformity. Ask whether any tenderness occurs during touch. Feel for crepitus when moving the joint. Quadriceps muscle and surrounding tissue are firm and nontender. Suprapatellar bursa is not palpable. Joint is firm and nontender.	
Range of Motion. Observe for full active ROM of each knee with the patient seated. Flex the knee to 130 degrees and return to extended position. Knee can perform full ROM without discomfort or crepitus.	Inability to perform full ROM may be due to contractures, pain associated with trauma or inflammation, or neuromuscular disorders. *SAFETY ALERT* *Do not encourage the patient to hyperextend or rotate the knee. Attempting to do so may cause injury.*
Muscle Strength. With the patient seated, apply pressure to the anterior lower leg while the patient extends the leg. Also, with the leg bent, ask the patient to maintain that position while you pull the lower leg as if to straighten it. Muscle strength is equal bilaterally and able to overcome resistance.	Injury or deconditioning may lead to asymmetry of strength.

Documenting Normal Findings

The knees are aligned with the long axis of the leg. The muscles are well formed, firm to touch, and symmetrical. Joints have full active ROM through flexion and extension. No bulging or swelling is noted. Muscle strength is 5/5. Patient denies any discomfort while still or moving.

Technique and Normal Findings	Abnormal Findings
Ankle and Foot ***Inspection.*** Inspect the feet with the patient both standing and sitting. Look for any swelling, lacerations, lesions, deformity, size of the muscle, and symmetry. Look for toe alignment. Feet are the same color as the rest of the body. They are symmetrical, with toes aligned with the long axis of the leg. No swelling is present. When the patient stands, the weight falls on the middle of the foot. Advanced health care providers may perform the anterior drawer test to assess for ankle sprains or the Lachman or McMurray test. See Table 21.8.	An enlarged, swollen, hot, reddened metatarsophalangeal joint and bursa of the great toe indicates gouty arthritis. An ankle sprain or strain may cause pain on palpation and ROM. Crepitus may indicate a fracture. Often, a sprain cannot be differentiated from a fracture without an x-ray. With hallux valgus (bunion), the great toe is angled away from the midline, crowding the other toes. Flexion of the proximal interphalangeal joint with hyperextension of the distal joint indicates hammertoe. A callus or corn forms on the flexed joint from external pressure. With flatfoot (pes planus), the arch of the foot is flattened and touches the floor; this may only be visible when the person is standing. Pes varus describes a foot that is turned inward toward the midline. Pes valgus is a foot turned outward from the midline. Pes cavus is an exaggerated arch height.

(table continues on page 633)

Technique and Normal Findings (continued)	Abnormal Findings (continued)
	A corn is a conical area of thickened skin caused by pressure. Corns may be painful and do occur *between* toes. Callus is thickened skin from pressure and usually occurs on the sole of the foot. Calluses are usually not painful. Pain in the heel that occurs early in the morning or with prolonged sitting, standing, or walking may be due to plantar fasciitis, an inflammation of the plantar fascia where it attaches to the calcaneus. An inward turning foot is talipes equinovarus (clubfoot).
Palpation. Palpate for muscle tone. Feel for any bumps, nodules, or deformity. Holding the heel, palpate the anterior and posterior aspects of the ankle, the Achilles tendon (calcaneal tendon), and the metatarsophalangeal joints in the ball of the foot (Fig. 21.24). Palpate each interphalangeal joint, noting temperature, tenderness, and contour. Ask about tenderness during touch. Feel for crepitus when moving the joint. Ankle and foot joints are firm, stable, and nontender. 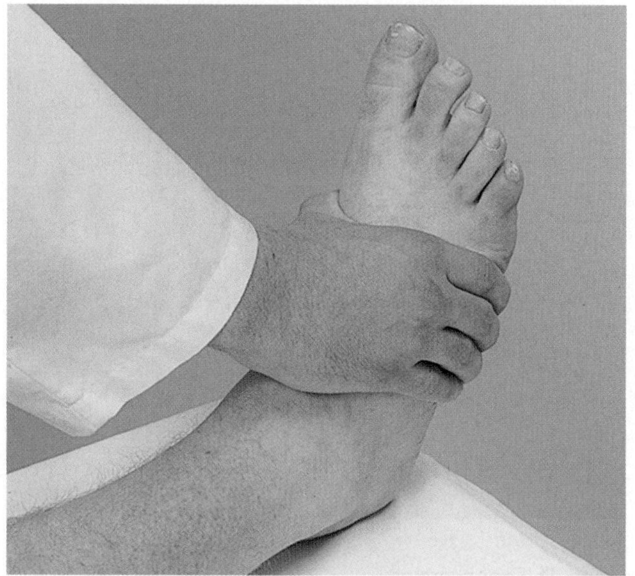 **Figure 21.24** Palpating the foot.	Pain or discomfort in the ankle or foot during palpation may indicate arthritis or inflammation. Pain and tenderness along the Achilles tendon may be due to bursitis or tendinitis. Small nodules on the tendon may occur with rheumatoid arthritis. Cooler temperature in the ankles and feet than in the rest of the body may be due to vascular insufficiency, which will lead to musculoskeletal dysfunction.
Range of Motion. Observe for full active ROM of the ankle. Assess dorsiflexion by asking the patient to raise the toes toward the knee. Plantar flexion requires the patient to point toes downward toward the ground. Inversion occurs when the sole of the foot is turned toward the opposite leg. Eversion is when the sole of the foot is turned away from the other leg (Fig. 21.25). Ask the patient to curl the toes and return them to straight position (flexion and extension). To assess hyperextension, ask the patient to keep the soles on the ground and raise the toes upward. For abduction, ask the patient to spread the toes wide open, as far apart from each other as possible.	Limited ankle or foot ROM without swelling indicates arthritis. Inflammation and swelling with limited ROM indicates trauma.

(table continues on page 634)

Technique and Normal Findings (continued)	Abnormal Findings (continued)
Adduction occurs when the toes return to their original position. Ankle ROM is normal: dorsiflexion 20 degrees, plantar flexion 45 degrees, inversion 30 degrees, and eversion 20 degrees. The toes can flex, extend, hyperextend, and abduct.	

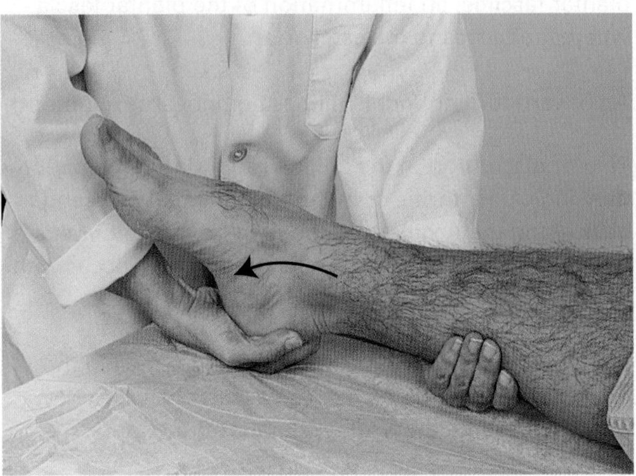
A

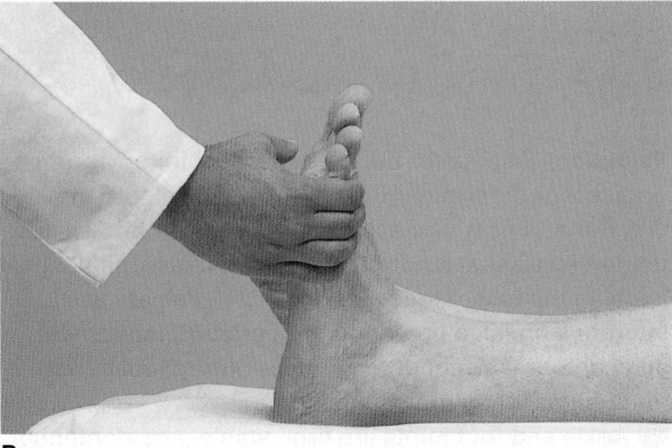
B

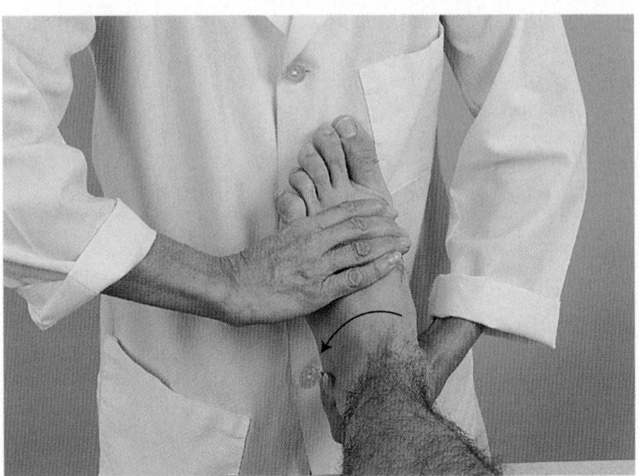
D

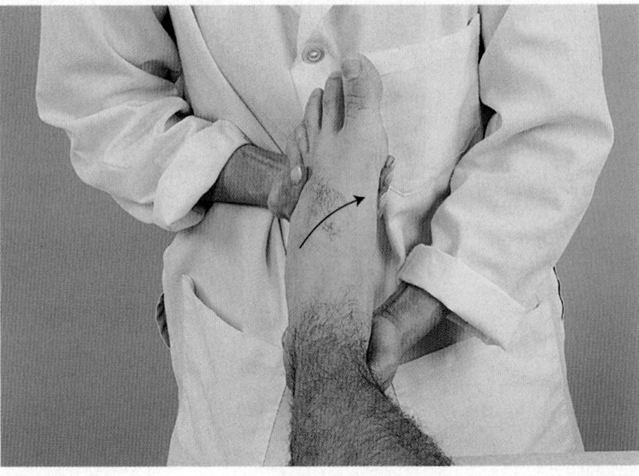
C

Figure 21.25 **A.** Plantar flexion. **B.** Dorsiflexion. **C.** Foot inversion. **D.** Foot eversion.

Technique and Normal Findings	Abnormal Findings
Muscle Strength. Ask the patient to perform dorsiflexion and plantar flexion against the resistance of your hand. Then ask the patient to flex and extend the toes against your resistance. Muscle strength is equal bilaterally and able to overcome resistance.	Asymmetry of strength may be due to pain, inflammation, deconditioning, or chronic disease.

Documenting Normal Findings

The ankles and feet are symmetrical and the same color as the rest of the body. The muscles are well formed, firm to touch, and symmetrical. The ankles have full active ROM through dorsiflexion, plantar flexion, inversion, and eversion. The toes abduct, flex, and extend. Muscle strength is 5/5. Patient denies any discomfort while sitting, standing, or walking.

Technique and Normal Findings	Abnormal Findings
Thoracic and Lumbar Spine ***Inspection.*** With the patient standing, look at the patient from the side for the normal S pattern (convex thoracic spine and concave lumbar spine) (Fig. 21.26). Observe the patient from behind, noting whether the spine is straight (Fig. 21.27). Observe if the scapulae, iliac crests, and gluteal folds are level and symmetrical. Ask the patient to bend forward and reassess that the vertebrae are in a straight line and the scapulae are equal in height. The spine is in alignment both standing and sitting.	Kyphosis, a forward bending of the upper thoracic spine, may accompany osteoporosis, ankylosing spondylosis, and Paget disease. Lordosis, and exaggerated curvature in the lumbar spine, is common in late pregnancy and obesity. A flattened lumbar curve may occur with lumbar muscle spasms. A list is a leaning of the spine to one side; this may occur with paravertebral muscle spasms or a herniated disc. **Scoliosis** is a lateral spinal curvature with a compensatory lumbar curve in the opposite direction.

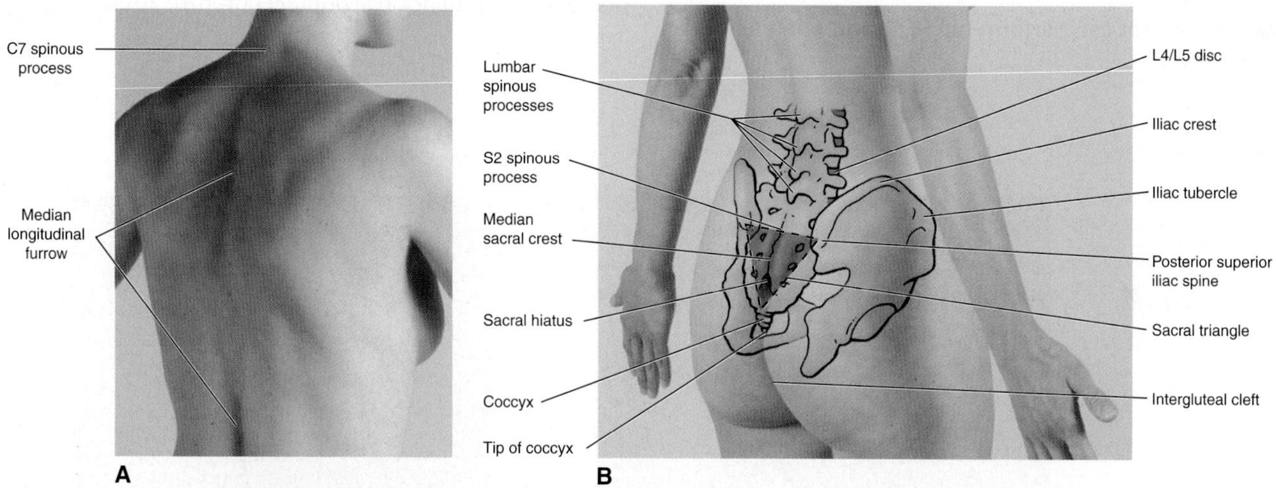

Figure 21.26 Assessing the spine and upper back. **A.** Upper portion. **B.** Lower portion.

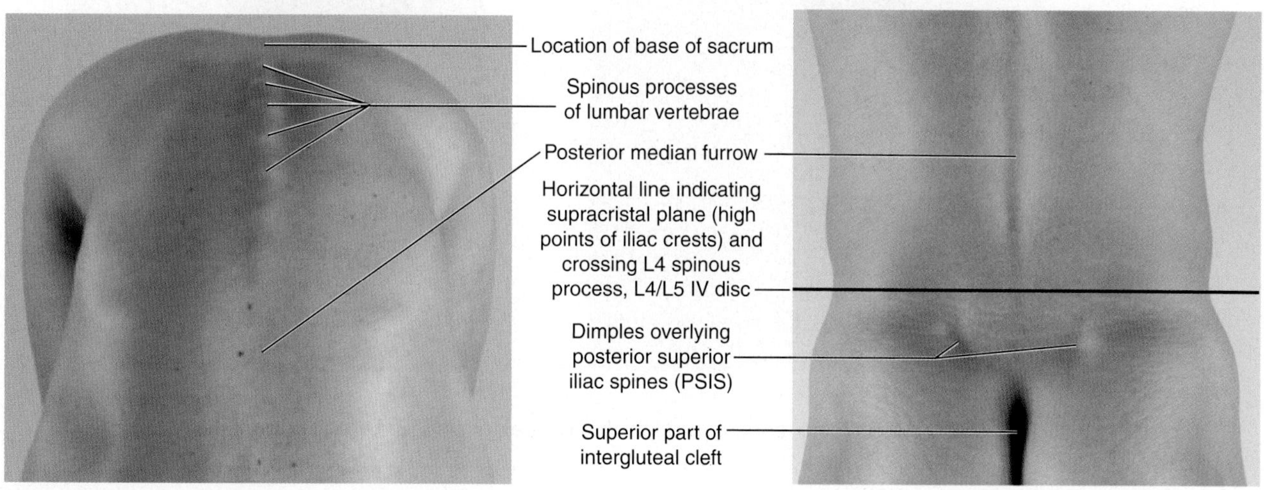

Figure 21.27 Lower back.

Technique and Normal Findings	Abnormal Findings
Palpation. Palpate the spinous processes. Feel for any bumps, nodules, or deformities. Ask about tenderness during touch. Feel for crepitus when the spine bends. The spinous processes are in a straight line. Patient denies tenderness. The paravertebral muscles are firm. There is no crepitus.	Pain on palpation may indicate inflammation, disc disease, or arthritis. Unequal spinous processes may indicate subluxation.

(table continues on page 636)

Technique and Normal Findings (continued)	Abnormal Findings (continued)
Range of Motion. Observe for full active ROM of the spine. Ask the patient to stand and bend forward to 75–90 degrees. Ask the patient to lean backward (hyperextend) to 30 degrees (Fig. 21.28). The spine assessment also includes lateral flexion (or abduction) to 35 degrees on either side. Ask the patient to slide a hand on one side down that thigh and bend away from the midline toward the side. Do this on both sides. To perform rotation of the spine, ask the patient to keep legs and hips forward facing while the shoulders move turn to the side (30 degrees). Repeat to the other side.	Pain, back injury, osteoarthritis, and ankylosing spondylitis may result in limited ROM.
The patient can perform full ROM without crepitus or discomfort.	**SAFETY ALERT** *Stand beside the patient and be ready to provide support while the patient performs spine ROM. Patients may lose balance and fall.*
	Noteworthy findings for cauda equina syndrome (which is a surgical emergency) include progressive motor or sensory deficit, saddle anesthesia, sciatica, and bowel or bladder incontinence (Dawodu & Lorenzo, 2014).

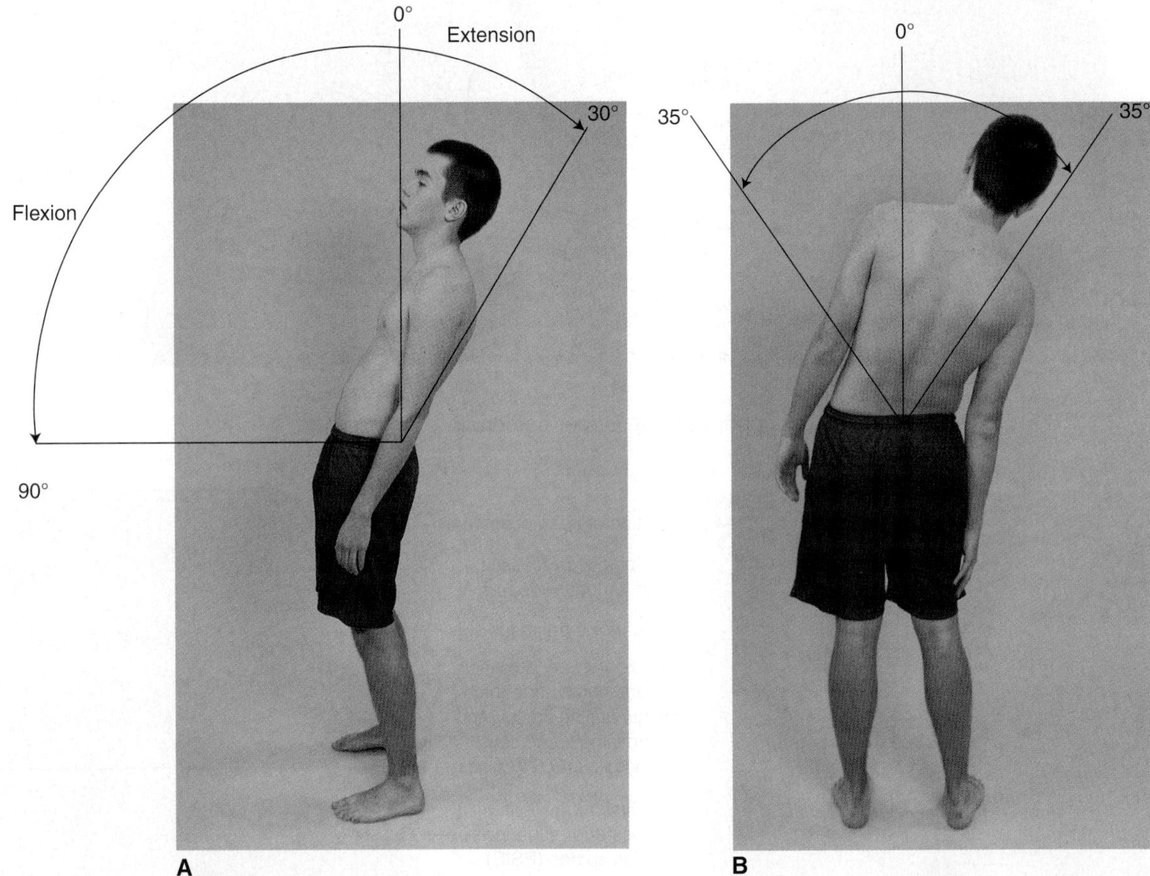

Figure 21.28 Spine range of motion. **A.** Hyperextension. **B.** Lateral flexion.

Documenting Normal Findings

The muscles are well formed, firm to touch, symmetrical. The spinous processes are straight and nontender. The thoracic and lumbar spines have full active ROM through flexion, extension, hyperextension, lateral flexion (or abduction), and rotation. Muscle strength is 5/5. Patient denies any discomfort while still or moving.

Risk for Falling

Several tools are available to assess whether a patient is at risk for falling. The most commonly used are the Morse Fall Scale (MFS) and the Hendrich II Fall Risk Model. A high score on either scale indicates a risk for falling and a need for preventive interventions, which may include frequent reminders, a bed alarm, and environmental cues. The Morse Fall Scale (Box 21.1) is more commonly used in hospitalized patients.

Lifespan Considerations: Older Adults

Allow extra time for older adults to complete each activity in the musculoskeletal assessment. You may want to divide the assessment into portions if an older patient appears fatigued.

Lifestyle affects the musculoskeletal system. Studies have found that improved gait speed indicates better and longer survival. Therefore, assessment of gait speed is recommended as a vital sign for older adults (Studenski et al., 2011).

Environmental Considerations

Some working conditions present potential risks to the musculoskeletal system. Workers required to lift heavy objects may strain and injure their backs. Jobs requiring substantial physical activity, such as construction work and fire fighting, increase the likelihood of sprains, strains, and fractures. Frequent repetitive movements may lead to misuse disorders such as carpal tunnel syndrome, pitcher's elbow, or vertebral degeneration. Musculoskeletal injuries may also occur when people sit for long periods at desks with poor ergonomic design.

BOX 21.1 Morse Fall Scale

Nursing fall risk assessment, diagnoses, and interventions are based on use of the Morse Fall Scale (MFS). The MFS is used widely in acute care settings, both in hospital and long-term care inpatient settings. The MFS requires systematic reliable assessment of a patient's fall risk factors upon admission, fall, change in status, and discharge or transfer to a new setting. MFS subscales include assessment of:

1. History of falling; immediate or within 3 months	No = 0 Yes = 25
2. Secondary diagnosis	No = 0 Yes = 15
3. Ambulatory aid	None, bed rest, wheel chair, nurse = 0 Crutches, cane, walker = 15 Furniture = 30
4. IV/heparin lock	No = 0 Yes = 20
5. Gait/transferring	Normal, bed rest, immobile = 0 Weak = 10 Impaired = 20
6. Mental status	Oriented to own ability = 0 Forgets limitations = 15

Risk Level	MFS Score	Action
No risk	0–24	None
Low risk	25–50	See standard fall prevention interventions
High risk	≥ 51	See high risk fall prevention interventions

From Morse, J. M. (2009). *Preventing patient falls* (2nd ed.). New York, NY: Springer.

Documenting Case Study Findings

The nurse has just finished conducting a physical examination of Mrs. Runningbird, the 82-year-old woman in the skilled nursing facility for rehabilitation following a fall at home. Unlike the samples of normal documentation previously charted, Mrs. Runningbird has abnormal findings. Review the following important findings that were revealed in each step of objective data collection for Mrs. Runningbird. Consider how these results compare with the normal findings presented in the samples of normal documentation. Begin to think about how the data cluster and which additional data the nurse might want to collect as he or she thinks critically about the situation and anticipates nursing interventions.

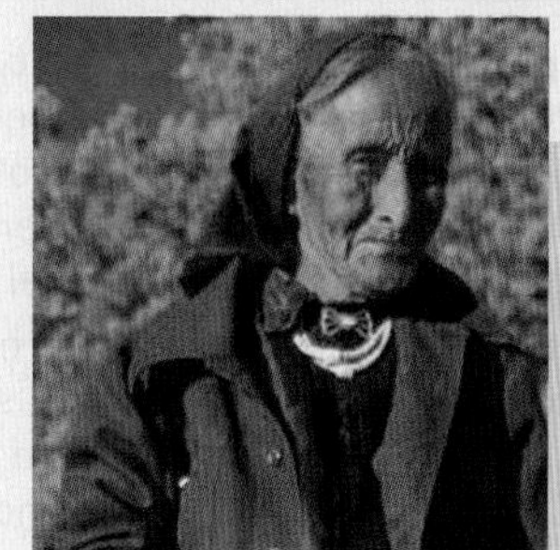

Inspection: Skin warm and pink. Mild kyphosis present. Heberden nodes present at the distal interphalangeal joint; Bouchard nodes present in the proximal interphalangeal joints in the hands. Diffuse swelling noted in all joints, most prominently in the hands. ROM approximately 50% of expected. Hip abduction and internal rotation are limited. Joints in knee and ankles are also swollen. Rheumatoid nodules are present. Gait slow but stable.

Palpation: Tenderness noted over joints in hands. Muscle strength 2/5 is decreased. Pulses 3/4. Capillary refill 2 seconds. Identifies sharp and dull touch accurately. Muscle strength in feet and legs is 3/4.

Critical Thinking

Laboratory and Diagnostic Testing

Laboratory tests can help identify specific musculoskeletal problems. Health care providers evaluate all test results within the context of other signs and symptoms.

Common laboratory tests for muscle injury include evaluations of lactate dehydrogenase (LDH), creatine kinase (CK), alanine aminotransferase (ALT), and aspartate aminotransferase (AST). Other tests can reveal responses to bone damage, such as evaluation of alkaline phosphatase. Uric acid levels are elevated in gouty arthritis. Inflammatory markers, such as erythrocyte sedimentation rate, C-reactive protein, and rheumatoid factor, are elevated with all inflammatory conditions, including rheumatoid arthritis and lupus.

Imaging tests are especially valuable in identifying musculoskeletal injuries and deformities. X-ray visualization shows bone fractures. Computed tomography (CT) and magnetic resonance imaging (MRI) can reveal soft tissue damage, including ligament and tendon injuries. Bone density scans can help identify patients with osteoporosis and those at risk for injury from falls.

Diagnostic Reasoning

When formulating a nursing diagnosis, it is important to use critical thinking to cluster data and identify patterns that fit together. Compare the clusters of data with the defining characteristics (abnormal findings) for the diagnosis to assure the most accurate labeling and appropriate interventions.

Nursing Diagnoses, Outcomes, and Interventions

Table 21.9 compares nursing diagnoses, abnormal findings, and interventions commonly related to the musculoskeletal system assessment (NANDA International, 2012).

You use assessment information to identify patient outcomes. Some outcomes that are related to system problems are as follows (Moorhead, Johnson, Maas, & Swanson, 2013):

- Patient does not fall.
- Patient dresses, grooms, and eats independently.
- Patient ambulates in hall three times daily.

Once you establish outcomes, you implement nursing care to improve the status of the patient. Use critical thinking and evidence-based practice to develop the interventions. Some examples of interventions are as follows (Bulechek, Butcher, Dochterman, & Wagner, 2013):

- Teach the patient to call for help before walking to bathroom.
- Open food packages and arrange the tray prior to encouraging the patient to eat independently.
- Communicate through documentation about the type of assistance needed.

You then evaluate the care according to the patient outcomes that you developed, reassessing the patient and continuing or modifying the interventions as appropriate. An accurate and complete nursing assessment is an essential foundation for holistic nursing care.

TABLE 21.9 Nursing Diagnoses Associated With the Musculoskeletal System

Diagnosis	Point of Differentiation	Assessment Characteristics	Nursing Interventions
Impaired physical mobility	Difficulty executing purposeful movements of the body or extremity without external supports	Limited ability to perform gross or fine motor skills, limited ROM, uncoordinated or jerky movements, difficulty with gait	Use footwear that facilitates walking and prevents injury. Use assistive devices. Screen for mobility skills (e.g., transitions to sitting or standing).
Activity intolerance	Lack of energy to initiate, sustain, or perform daily routines and behaviors	Report of fatigue or weakness, abnormal pulse or blood pressure, shortness of breath, dizziness, chest pain	Determine cause of intolerance. Promote reconditioning when the result of immobility. Gradually increase activity according to symptoms.
Self-care deficit (specify: bathing/hygiene, dressing/grooming, feeding, toileting)	Inability to perform activities of daily living for oneself	Grade ability to perform activity using a scale that includes being completely independent, requires use of equipment, requires help from another person, or completely dependent.	Observe patient's ability to perform skill. Ask for input on habits and preferences. Encourage patient to do as much independently as possible. Use adaptive devices such as Velcro or elastic in place of buttons or ties.
Impaired walking	Limitation of independent movement within the environment on foot	Cannot walk on even surfaces or uneven surfaces, climb stairs, or go required distances	Follow weight-bearing restrictions.* Use assistive devices such as a cane or walker. Obtain appropriate number of people to assist with walking the patient. Limit distractions during ambulation.

*Collaborative interventions.

Progress Note: Analyzing Findings

Remember Mrs. Runningbird, whose situation has been outlined throughout this chapter. The initial subjective and objective data collection is complete, and the nurse has spent time reviewing the findings and other results. The following nursing note illustrates how subjective and objective data are collected and analyzed and nursing interventions are developed.

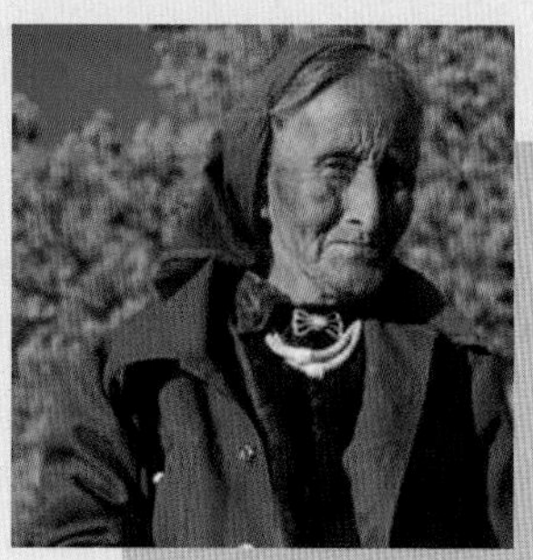

Subjective: "I feel stiff and cold. My legs and hands don't work the way that they used to."

Objective: Skin warm and pink. Diffuse swelling noted in all joints, most prominent in the hands. Rheumatoid nodules are present. ROM 50% in hands. Tenderness noted over joints in hands. Muscle strength 2/5 in hands and 3/5 in legs. Circulation + all four extremities. Identifies sharp and dull touch accurately. Hip abduction and internal rotation are limited. Gait slow but stable. Needs one-person assist and walker for ambulation to bathroom. Needs setup on fine motor skills for hygiene, dressing, and eating.

Analysis: Impaired physical mobility related to reduced strength and ROM

Plan: Allow patient to perform as much independently as possible. Provide encouragement for participation in physical and occupational therapies and positive reinforcement for small increments in improvement. Remind her to use walker and call for help before ambulating to bathroom.

Critical Thinking Challenge

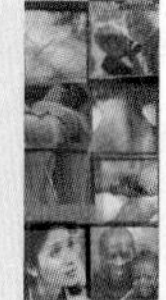

- What other assessments are important in addition to the musculoskeletal system?
- How will the nurse collect complete assessment information but avoid fatiguing Mrs. Runningbird?
- What functional patterns might the limited ROM and joint tenderness affect?
- Which is more of a concern for this patient—physiological or psychosocial assessment? Provide rationale.

Collaborating With the Interprofessional Team

Both occupational and physical therapists work with patients to increase mobility and functional abilities for rehabilitation. Generally, physical therapists focus on larger motor groups, whereas occupational therapists focus on fine motor skills and the upper body. Nurses may consult occupational therapists for patients with difficulties involving bathing, dressing, grooming, home and money management, assistive technology, or increasing ROM, tone, sensation, or coordination.

Mrs. Runningbird has been working with occupational therapy (OT) to increase function and to attain adaptive devices for her in the home. The following conversation illustrates how the nurse might communicate progress when OT comes.

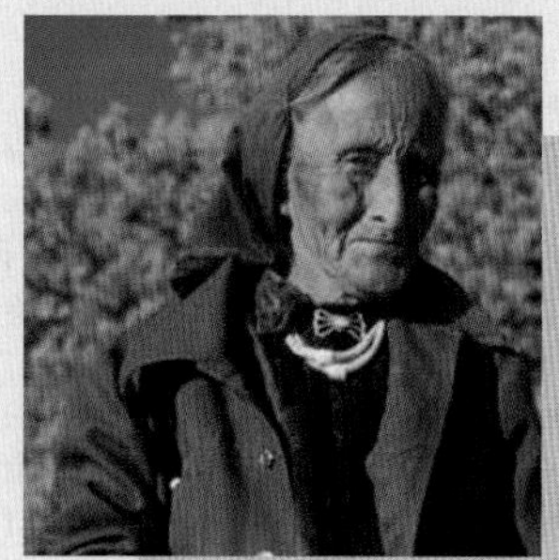

(case study continues on page 640)

Situation: "Hi Cheryl. I'm taking care of Mrs. Runningbird today. She said that you were going to work with her in the kitchen today." (Cheryl confirms)

Background: "She's a little discouraged because she doesn't feel like she's making progress."

Assessment: "I had a discussion with her about how she's coping with her decline in function. She feels frustrated that she's not making faster progress because she really wants to go home."

Recommendations: "I encouraged her and talked about how much improvement I've seen and she seemed encouraged by that. I think that if you also provided her with feedback on things that she is doing well, it will motivate her. We talked some about working with you today and seeing how she does in the kitchen because that's her biggest concern. She wants to be able to prepare her own meals but also is aware that a service that delivers meals might be an option. I told her how you would show her some tricks for cooking and also some ergonomic and lightweight cooking tools. Can you also work with her on opening jars? She's been having difficulty for a while and thinks that you might be able to help her."

Critical Thinking Challenge

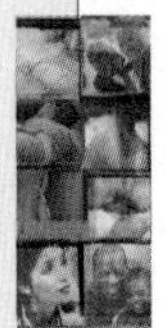

- Why didn't the nurse provide all the physical assessment data to the OT?
- What is the role of the nurse in providing the psychosocial information to the OT?
- What types of assessments will need to be completed prior to discharging the patient to home?

Pulling It All Together

The nurse uses assessment data to formulate a nursing care plan with patient outcomes and interventions for Mrs. Runningbird. Outcomes are specific to the patient, realistic to achieve, and measurable; they also have a time frame for completion. The interventions are actions that the nurse performs based on evidence and practice guidelines. After implementation of these interventions, the nurse reevaluates Mrs. Runningbird and documents the findings in the chart to show progress toward the patient outcome. The nurse uses critical thinking and judgment to continue or revise the diagnosis, outcomes, or interventions. This is often in the form of a care plan or case note similar to the one below.

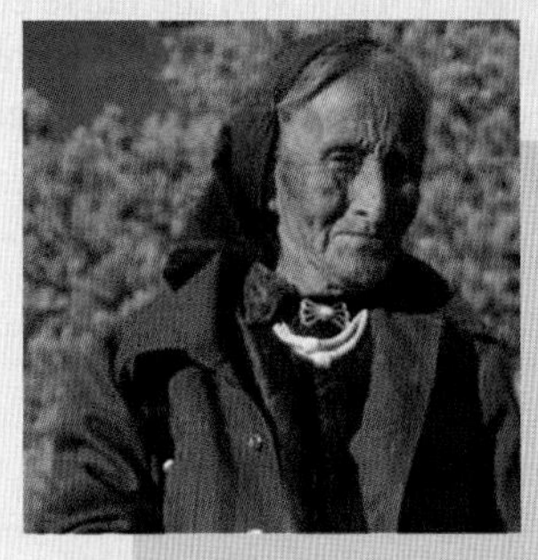

Nursing Diagnosis	Patient Outcomes	Nursing Interventions	Rationale	Evaluation
Impaired physical mobility related to joint swelling and tenderness as evidenced by limited ROM and reduced strength in hands	Demonstrates independent dressing, grooming, and toileting with assistive devices	Allow patient to do as much as possible. Provide positive feedback for progress each shift. Consult with OT on assistive devices. Collaborate on a plan for discharge and needed resources.	Independence provides increased control, functional ability, and a sense of accomplishment. OT can identify devices that might be helpful for discharge. A home care nurse may initially visit the patient to identify necessary resources.	Bathing and dressing with minimal assistance using elastic waist pants and Velcro shoes. Dressed the bottom half first and then the top. OT worked with patient today and identified assistive devices for the kitchen. Recommend home OT consult for at least one visit.

Applying Your Knowledge

Using the previous steps of diagnostic reasoning, organizing, and prioritizing, consider all the case study findings woven throughout this chapter. When answering the following questions, begin drawing conclusions and see how the pieces of assessment must work together to create an environment for personalized, appropriate, and accurate care.

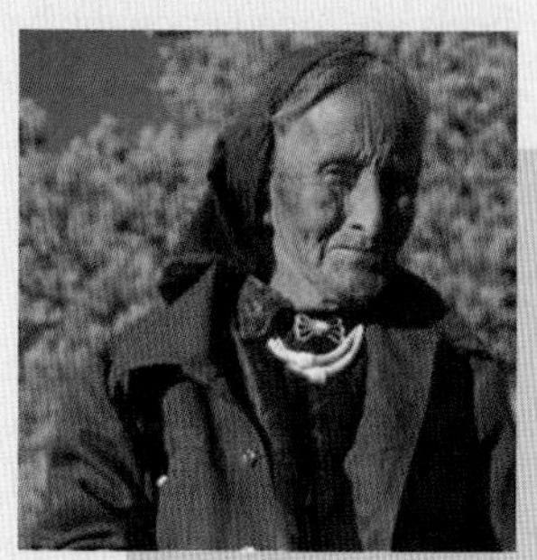

- How are physiological and psychological data connected?
- What nursing diagnoses might be activated on this patient's problem list? Provide rationale.
- What areas will the nurse assess as part of a comprehensive musculoskeletal assessment?
- What additional assessments should the nurse add?
- What are expected findings for Mrs. Runningbird based on her age versus findings based on her osteoarthritis?
- How will the nurse evaluate the effectiveness of the occupational therapy that Mrs. Runningbird is getting?

Key Points

- Functions of the musculoskeletal system include providing shape to the body and permitting movement.
- Identification of musculoskeletal risk factors is important for focused patient teaching aimed toward decreasing deformity or injury.
- Subjective data from the history and current condition guides performance of the physical assessment of the musculoskeletal system.
- The nurse should compare one side of the body with the other to determine whether symmetry is present.
- The nurse assesses each joint for ROM and muscle strength.
- Gait, coordination, and balance involve both the musculoskeletal and neurological systems.
- Nurses use inspection and palpation to assess the musculoskeletal system. Advance practice nurses may use percussion to assess injured joints.
- During passive ROM, examiners do not force joints beyond the development of resistance or the development of discomfort.
- Patients with fragile bones require gentle handling to prevent fracture.
- Nurses consider abnormal findings in ROM and muscle strength when developing nursing diagnoses and planning interventions.
- Nurses individualize assessment of the musculoskeletal system according to the patient's condition, age, gender, and ethnicity.

Review Questions

1. Mr. Brown was playing soccer and hurt his right knee. It appears swollen. What is the first assessment you should make?
   A. Palpate for crepitus in the knee.
   B. Compare the swollen knee with the other knee.
   C. Assess active ROM in the knee.
   D. Feel the knee for warmth.

2. Mrs. Johnson, a transcriptionist, reports pain and burning in her right hand. What assessment procedures should you perform next?
   A. Trendelenburg and drawer signs
   B. McMurray and Thomas tests
   C. Bulge test and ballottement
   D. Phalen and Tinel tests

3. Which of the following assessment tasks can you appropriately delegate to an unlicensed care provider?
   A. Height, weight, and vital signs
   B. Active and passive ROM
   C. History of current complaint
   D. Muscle strength

4. When doing an assessment of the spine of an older adult, you can expect to see which variation?
   A. Lordosis
   B. Torticollis
   C. Kyphosis
   D. Scoliosis

5. The patient's muscle tone is hypertonic so the muscles are stiff and the movements are awkward. The nurse documents these findings as
   A. atony.
   B. tremors.
   C. spasticity.
   D. fasciculation.

6. To correctly document that ROM in the fingers is full and active, you would write that the patient can
   A. perform rotation, lateral flexion, and hyperextension.
   B. make a fist, spread and close fingers, and do finger–thumb opposition.
   C. touch finger to own nose and to examiner's finger back and forth.
   D. perform supination, pronation, and lateral deviation.

7. When assessing a newborn, you note that one knee is lower than the other when the legs are flexed and the heels are together on the bed. You should correctly document this finding as positive
   A. ballottement.
   B. Thomas test.
   C. Allis sign.
   D. genu varum.

8. You are assessing a patient who has been diagnosed with a neuromuscular disorder. You note the patient cannot lift the right leg off the bed when you are applying resistance. You would document the muscle strength in the right leg as
   A. fair.
   B. 2/5.
   C. 50%.
   D. within normal limits.

9. You note that an adolescent has uneven shoulder height. To differentiate functional from structural scoliosis, you ask the patient to
   A. stand up straight while you check the height of the iliac crest.
   B. flex the elbow and pull against your resistance.
   C. shrug both shoulders while you provide resistance.
   D. bend forward at the waist while you palpate the spine.

10. A patient reports that a previous right hip replacement is suddenly painful. Which hip assessment technique should you omit?
   A. Adduction
   B. Hyperextension
   C. Extension
   D. Circumduction

11. A woman reports that her mother has osteoporosis and wants to know what she can do to prevent developing the disease herself. Which of the following responses is best?
   A. Engage in aerobic exercise at least three times per week.
   B. Eat at least one serving of dark green leafy vegetables daily.
   C. Consume three servings of dairy products per day.
   D. Perform muscle strengthening exercises every other day.

The Jensen suite offers these additional resources to enhance learning and facilitate understanding of this chapter:

- thePoint online resource, http://thepoint.lww.com/Jensen2e
- *Laboratory Manual for Nursing Health Assessment: A Best Practice Approach*
- *Pocket Guide for Nursing Health Assessment: A Best Practice Approach*
- *Lippincott DocuCare*, an electronic health record simulation software, http://thepoint.lww.com/docucare
- *Adaptive Learning | Powered by PrepU*, http://thepoint.lww.com/prepu

References

Abate, M., Vanni, D., Pantalone, A., & Salini, V. (2013). Cigarette smoking and musculoskeletal disorders. *Muscles, Ligaments and Tendons Journal, 3*(2), 63–69. doi:10.11138/mltj/2013.3.2.063

Agency for Healthcare Research and Quality. (2011). *Healthcare quality and disparities in women: Selected findings from the 2010 National Healthcare Quality and Disparities Reports. Fact Sheet* (AHRQ Publication No. 11-0005-1-EF). Rockville, MD: Author. Retrieved from http://www.ahrq.gov/qual/nhqrwomen/nhqrwomen.htm

Bulechek, G. M., Butcher, H. K., Dochterman, J. M., & Wagner, C. M. (2013). *Nursing interventions classification (NIC)* (6th ed.). St. Louis, MO: Mosby.

Dane, C., Dane, B., Cetin, A., & Erginbas, M. (2007). Comparison of the effects of raloxifene and low-dose hormone replacement therapy on bone mineral density and bone turnover in the treatment of postmenopausal osteoporosis. *Gynecological Endocrinology, 23*(7), 398–403.

Darcy, P., & Moughty, A. M. (2013). Images in clinical medicine. Pronator drift. *New England Journal of Medicine, 369*(16), e20. doi: 10.1056/NEJMicm1213343.

Doherty, M., Dacre, J., Dieppe, P., & Snaith, M. (1992). The "GALS" locomotor screen. *Annals of the Rheumatic Diseases, 51*(10), 1165–1169.

Dawodu, S. T., & Lorenzo, N. (2014). *Cauda equina and conus medullaris syndromes*. Retrieved from http://emedicine.medscape.com/article/1148690-overview

Finkelstein, J. S., Brockwell, S. E., Mehta, V., Greendale, G. A., Sowers, M. R., Ettinger, B., . . . Neer, R. M. (2008). Bone mineral density changes during the menopause transition in a multiethnic cohort of women. *Journal of Clinical Endocrinology and Metabolism, 93*(3), 861–868.

Frost, P. (2012). Vitamin D deficiency among northern Native Peoples: A real or apparent problem? *International Journal of Circumpolar Health, 71*, 18001. doi:10.3402/IJCH.v71i0.18001

Henschke, N., Maher, C. G., Ostelo, R. W., de Vet, H. C., Macaskill, P., & Irwig, L. (2013). Red flags to screen for malignancy in patients with low-back pain. *Cochrane Database of Systematic Reviews*, (28), CD0086868.

Ma, C. B. (2013). *Osteoporosis—Overview.* Retrieved from http://www.nlm.nih.gov/medlineplus/ency/article/000360.htm

MacLean, C., Newberry, S., Maglione, M., McMahon, M., Ranganath, V., Suttorp, M., . . . Grossman, J. (2008). Systematic review: Comparative effectiveness of treatments to prevent fractures in men and women with low bone density or osteoporosis. *Annals of Internal Medicine, 148*(3), 197–213.

Minaker, K. L. (2011). Common clinical sequelae of aging. In L. Goldman & A. I. Schafer (Eds.), *Cecil medicine* (24th ed.). Philadelphia, PA: Saunders Elsevier.

Moorhead, S., Johnson, M., Maas, M. L., & Swanson, E. (2013). *Nursing outcomes classification (NOC): Measurement of health outcomes* (5th ed.). St. Louis, MO: Elsevier.

Morse, J. M. (2009). *Preventing patient falls* (2nd ed.). New York, NY: Springer.

National Osteoporosis Foundation. (2013). *Are you at risk?* Retrieved from http://nof.org/articles/2

NANDA International (2012). *Nursing diagnoses: Definitions and classification 2012-2014* (9th ed.). Oxford, United Kingdom: Wiley-Blackwell.

Studenski, S., Perera, S., Patel, K., Rosano, C., Faulkner, K., Inzitari, M., . . . Guralnik, J. (2011). Gait speed and survival in older adults. *Journal of the American Medical Association*, 305(1), 50–58. doi:10.1001/jama.2010.1923

Swiontkowski, M. F., Engelberg, R., Martin, D. P., & Agel, J. (1999). Short musculoskeletal function assessment questionnaire: Validity, reliability, and responsiveness. *The Journal of Bone and Joint Surgery, 81-A*(9), 1245–1260.

U.S. Department of Health & Human Services. (2013). *2020 Topics & objectives - Objectives A-Z.* Retrieved on http://www.healthypeople.gov/2020/topicsobjectives2020/

van Schoor, N. M., Visser, M., Pluijm, S. M., Kuchuk, N., Smit, J. H., & Lips, P. (2008). Vitamin D deficiency as a risk factor for osteoporotic fractures. *Bone, 42*(2), 260–266.

Tables of Abnormal Findings

TABLE 21.10 Selected Musculoskeletal Problems: Onset, Gender, and Ethnicity

Problem	Age at Onset	Gender	Ethnicity
Amyotrophic lateral sclerosis (ALS)	Median age 55–66 years	More common in men	Most common in Caucasians
Ankylosing spondylitis	Women 17–35 years; men 20–30 years	Three times more common in men	Most common in Native Americans
Bursitis	Older than 40 years	Occurs in men and women, related to chronic stress or acute injury	Occurs in all ethnicities
Carpal tunnel syndrome	25–50 years	Three times more common in women; especially prevalent in pregnant women and in menopausal women	Most common in Caucasians
Dupuytren contracture	Older than 40 years	More common in men	Most common in Caucasians of northern European ancestry
Gout	Older than 70 years	Three times more common in men	Slightly more common in African Americans
Low back pain	30–50 years	More common in men	Affects all ethnicities
Multiple sclerosis	Average age 18–35 years but can occur at any age	Twice as common in women	Most common in Caucasians, but the more aggressive form occurs more frequently in African Americans
Multiple myeloma	Older than 50 years	More common in men	Two to four times more common in African Americans
Myasthenia gravis	Women 18–25 years; men older than 60 years	Twice as common in women	Occurs in all ethnicities
Osteoarthritis	Older than 50 years in women; 40–50 years in men	More common in women, although hip osteoarthritis is similar	Most common in Caucasians
Osteoporosis Types I and II	Postmenopausal women; 50–70 years in men	Type I more common in women	Type I most common in Caucasians
Osteosarcoma	Younger than 20 years and also 50–60 years	Slightly more common in men	Slightly more common in African Americans
Paget disease of bone	Older than 40 years	More common in men	Most common in Caucasians
Polymyalgia rheumatica	Older than 50 years	More common in women	Most common in Caucasians
Rheumatoid arthritis	20–40 years	Two to three times more common in women	Most common in Native Americans
Scleroderma	30–50 years	Two to eight times more common in women	Most common in Choctaw Indians followed by African, Hispanic, Caucasian, and then Japanese Americans
Scoliosis	10–15 years	Eight times more common in girls	Found in all ethnicities
Systemic lupus erythematosus (SLE)	20–30 years	Ten times more common in women	Most common in non-Caucasians

Adapted from: Firestein, G. S. (2012). *Kelly's textbook of rheumatology* (9th ed.). Philadelphia, PA: Elsevier; Canale, S. T., & Beaty, J. J. (2012). *Campbell's operative orthopedics* (12th ed.). Philadelphia, PA: Elsevier.

TABLE 21.11 Abnormal Gait Patterns

Gait	Pathological Condition	Description
Antalgic	Degenerative knee or hip disease	Patient walks with a limp to avoid pain. The gait is characterized by a very short stance phase.
Ataxic	Cerebellar lesion	Patient shows unsteady, uncoordinated walking with a wide base, feet thrown out, and a tendency to fall to one side.
Short leg	Discrepancy in length of one leg, flexion contracture of hip or knee, congenital hip dislocation	Patient limps with walking unless he or she wears adaptive shoes.
Footdrop or steppage	Peroneal or anterior tibial nerve injury, paralysis of dorsiflexor muscles, lower motor neuron damage, damage to spinal nerve roots L5 and S1	Patient lifts the advancing leg high so that the toes may clear the ground. He or she places the sole of the foot on the floor at one time, instead of placing the heel first. This problem may be unilateral or bilateral.
Apraxic	Frontal lobe tumors, Alzheimer disease	Patient has difficulty initiating walking. After starting to walk, the gait is slow and shuffling. Motor and sensory systems are intact.
Trendelenburg (compensated gluteus medius gait)	Developmental hip dysplasia, muscular dystrophy	The trunk lists toward the affected side when weight bearing is on that side. A waddling gait may develop if both hips are affected.

Other gait abnormalities are described in Chapter 22.

TABLE 21.12 Comparison of Musculoskeletal Conditions Affecting Multiple Joints

Assessment	Rheumatoid Arthritis	Osteoarthritis	Gouty Arthritis	Fibromyalgia
Risk factors	Physical and emotional stress	Obesity, aging	Family history, diet high in purine-rich foods, alcohol, stress	Family history Emotional stress
Pain	Upper extremities	Lower extremities	Base of big toe; may also affect feet, ankles, knees, elbows	Any joints, especially neck, back, shoulders, knees, hands
Onset	Young adulthood	50s–60s	Middle-aged men	Adult women, 22–55 years of age
Stiffness	Significant in mornings and after inactivity	Worse later in the day and after inactivity	None in acute cases, develops with chronic cases	Some stiffness, especially in the morning
Generalized complaints	Weakness, fatigue, low fever	None	Painful, monoarticular, nocturnal joints, later more joints, great toe most often	Sleep disturbance and morning fatigue
Physical examination—joints	Tender, swollen, may be warm	May be tender	Swollen, warm, tender, shiny, red	No swelling, tender to touch
Diagnostic tests	Elevated serum proteins in blood and synovial fluid—rheumatoid factor	X-ray, CT, MRI	Elevated uric acid in blood and urine Synovial fluid aspiration	Not definitive, rule out other diagnoses

TABLE 21.13 Comparing and Contrasting Assessment Findings in Common Conditions

Atrophy

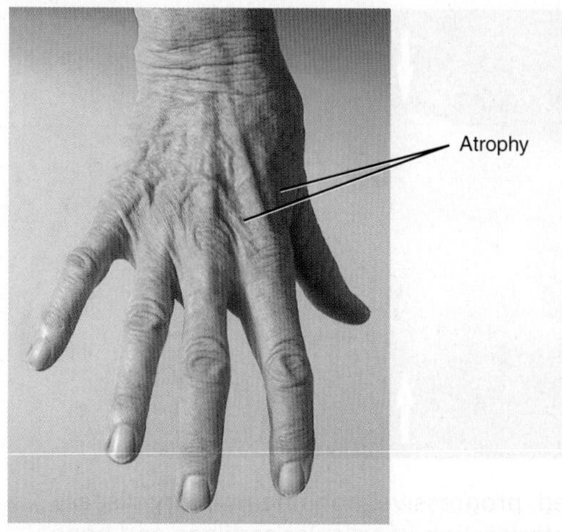

Hand of an 84-year-old woman

Decreased size can occur in any muscle. Causes include nerve damage, disuse, and nerve or muscle damage.

Joint Effusions

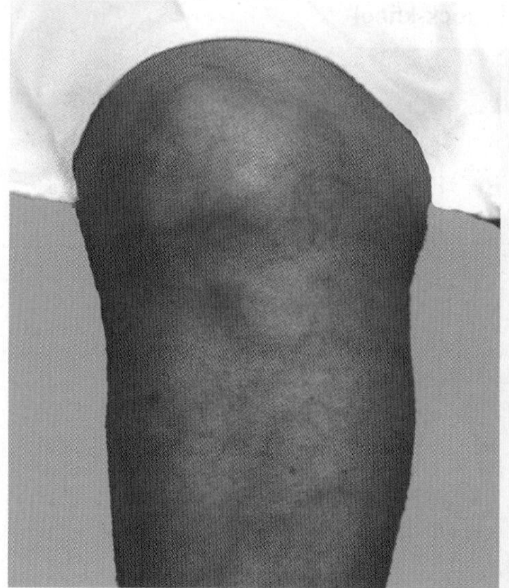

Inflammatory processes (commonly resulting from trauma, joint overuse, and rheumatoid arthritis) can cause synovial fluid to accumulate in a joint. When considerable fluid builds up, the joint appears swollen. The fluid is compressible (also called fluctuant). Treatment may involve rest, antiinflammatory agents, or surgical removal.

Joint Dislocation

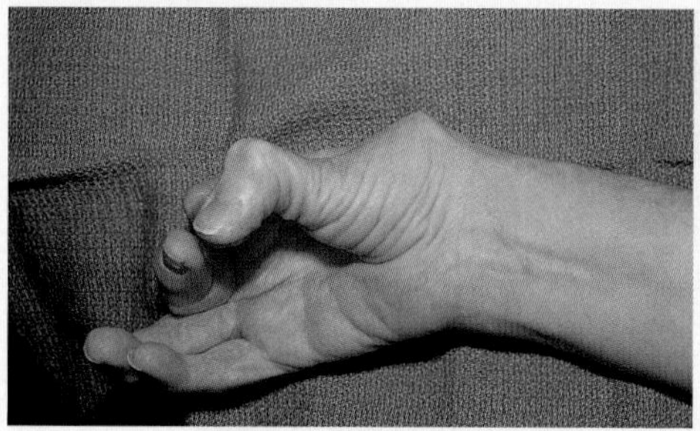

The ends of bones slip out of the usual position, usually from a sports-related injury, trauma, or a fall. Severe dislocation can cause tearing of the muscles, ligaments, and tendons that support the joint. Manifestations include swelling, pain, and immobility of the affected joint. Joints of the hand are most frequently dislocated, followed by shoulders. Hips, knees, and elbows are less commonly dislocated. Dislocations require medical intervention to prevent nerve damage.

Long-Standing Rheumatoid Arthritis

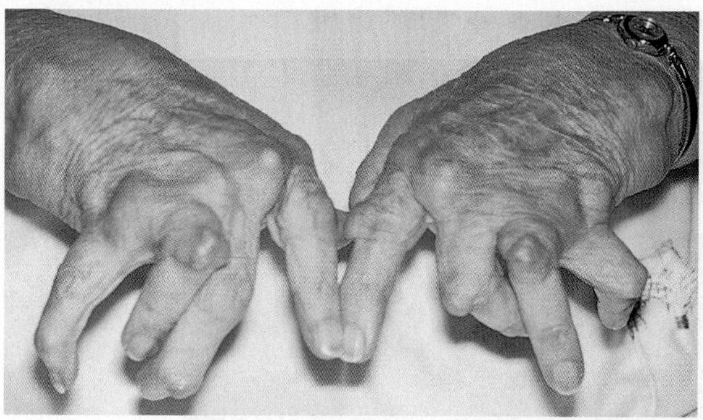

In this chronic, systemic, inflammatory disease of joints and connective tissue, inflammation causes thickening of synovial membrane. Fibrosis follows, with eventual bony ankylosis. The disorder is bilateral and symmetrical. Characteristics include heat, redness, swelling, and painful motion of affected joints. Associated symptoms include fatigue, weakness, anorexia, weight loss, low-grade fever, and lymphadenopathy.

(table continues on page 646)

TABLE 21.13 Comparing and Contrasting Assessment Findings in Common Conditions *(continued)*

Rotator Cuff Tear

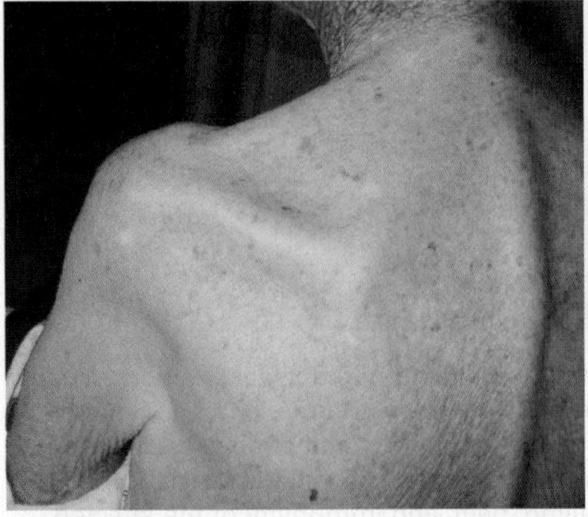

Manifestations include a hunched shoulder and limited arm abduction. A positive drop arm test result (arm is passively abducted, person cannot maintain position, and arm falls to side) is diagnostic. This condition may result from trauma while arm is abducted, falling on shoulder, throwing, or heavy lifting.

Osteoarthritis

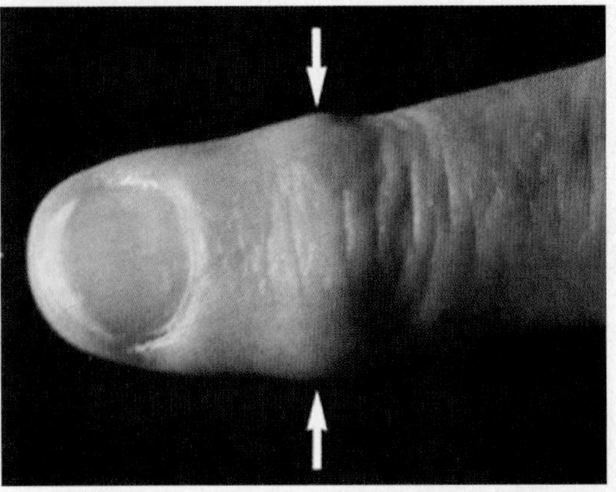

This localized, progressive, noninflammatory disease results in deterioration of articular cartilage and bone and deposition of new bone at joint surfaces. Incidence increases with age. Commonly affected joints include hands, knees, hips, and lumbar and cervical vertebrae. Manifestations include stiffness, swelling, hard bony protuberances, pain with motion, and limited motion.

Osteoporosis

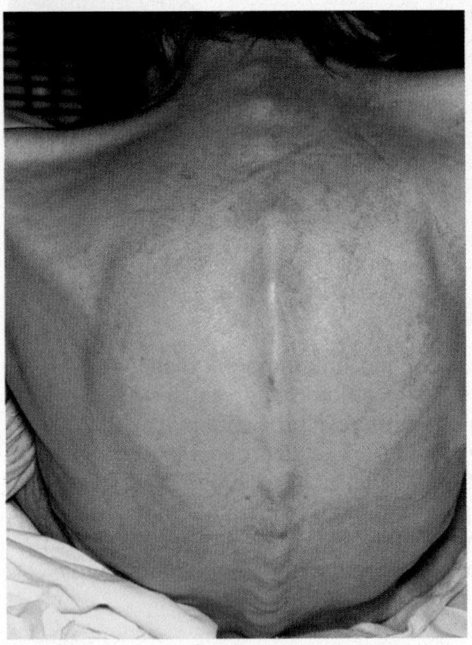

Osteoporosis occurs when bone resorption is faster than deposition. The weakened bone increases risk for fractures, especially in vertebrae, wrist, and hip. This occurs predominantly in postmenopausal Caucasian women. Risk factors include small bone frame, younger age at menopause, sedentary lifestyle, tobacco use, alcohol intake, and inadequate diet.

Genu Valgum (Knock-knee)

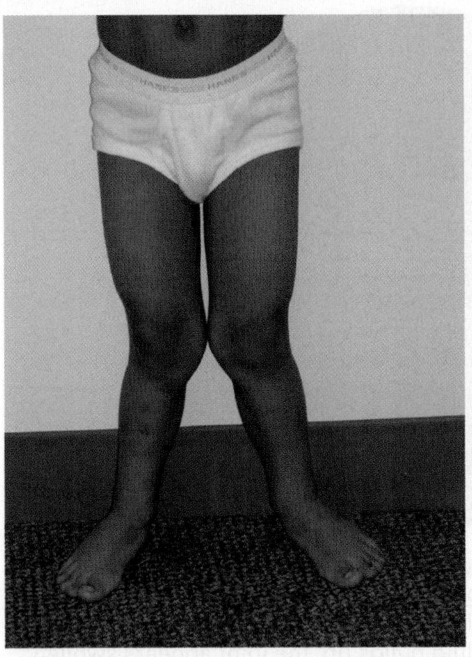

Many children have a temporary period of this condition, but persistent knock-knee may be genetic or the result of metabolic bone disease. The patient may need to swing each leg outward while walking to prevent striking the planted limb with the moving limb. The strain on the knee frequently causes anterior and medial knee pain. Physical therapy and surgical intervention may be required.

(table continues on page 647)

TABLE 21.13 Comparing and Contrasting Assessment Findings in Common Conditions *(continued)*

Ganglion Cyst

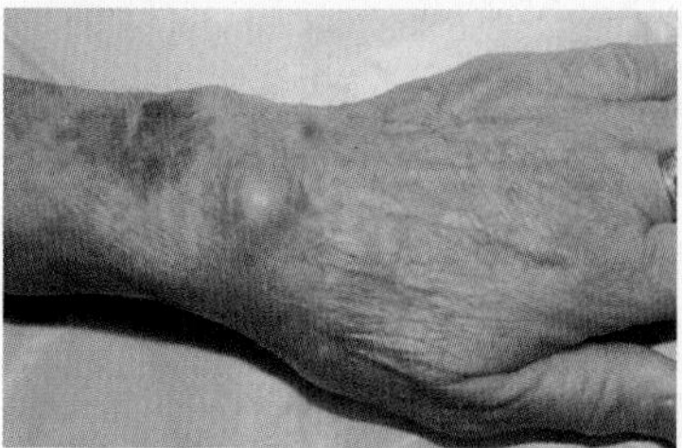

A soft, nontender, round nodule on the dorsum of the wrist that becomes more prominent during flexion. It is a benign tumor.

Epicondylitis

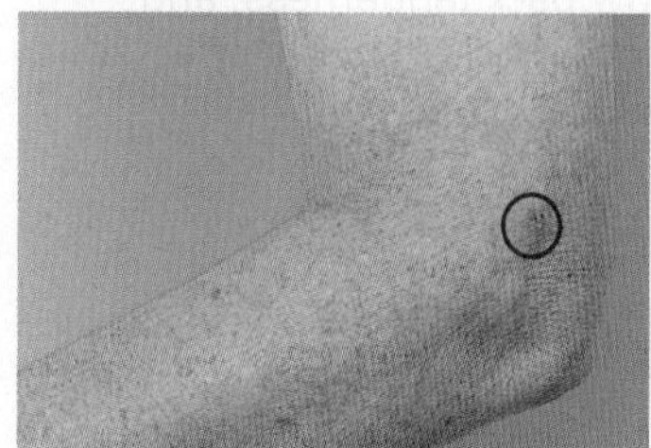

With this inflammation of the lateral epicondyle of the elbow, pain radiates down the extensor surface and increases with resisting extension of the hand. It results from activities combining excessive supination of forearm with an extended wrist. Inflammation of the medial epicondyle (golf elbow) is rarer and results from excessive wrist flexion and pronation.

Congenital Hip Dislocation

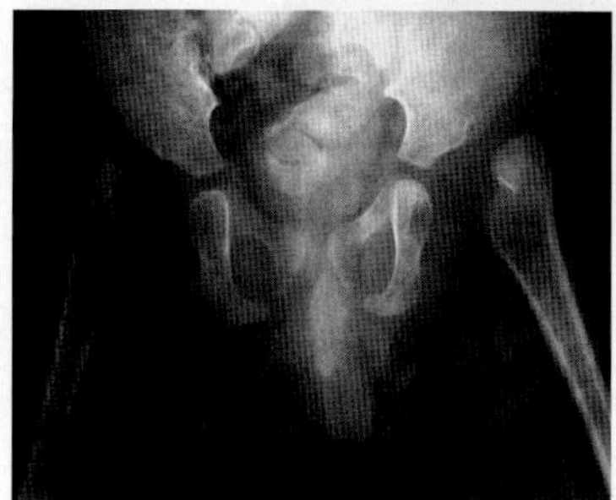

The head of the femur is displaced from the acetabulum. This condition is seven times more common in females. Signs include asymmetrical gluteal creases, uneven limb length, and limited abduction when the thighs are flexed. Diagnosis for newborns is a positive Barlow–Ortolani sign. Older children will have a positive Trendelenburg sign.

Bursitis (Olecranon Bursitis)

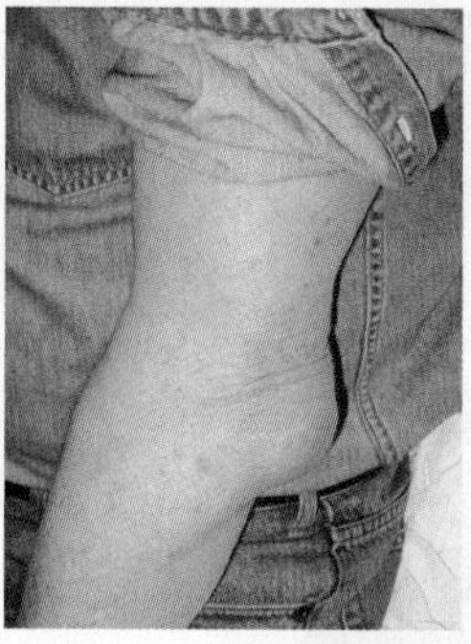

More than 150 bursae in the body cushion and lubricate joints, tendons, and ligaments. Bursitis is an inflammation of the bursa, which can follow injury, infection, or a rheumatic condition. Shoulders, elbows, and hips are common sites of bursitis; however, bursitis can occur in any joint, including knees, heels, and bases of big toes. Characteristics include swelling, tenderness, and pain that increases with movement.

Swan Neck and Boutonnière Deformity

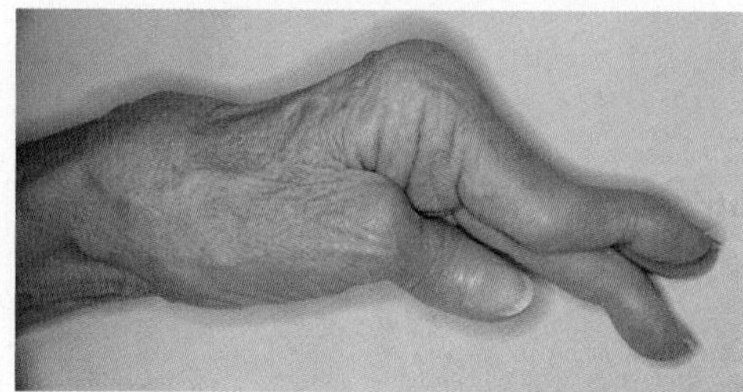

The fingers have a "swan-neck" appearance resulting from flexion contracture of the metacarpophalangeal joint with hyperextension of the distal joint. Boutonnière deformity causes flexion of the proximal interphalangeal joint with hyperextension of the distal joint. Both conditions occur with chronic rheumatoid arthritis and are often accompanied by ulnar deviation of the fingers.

Polydactyly

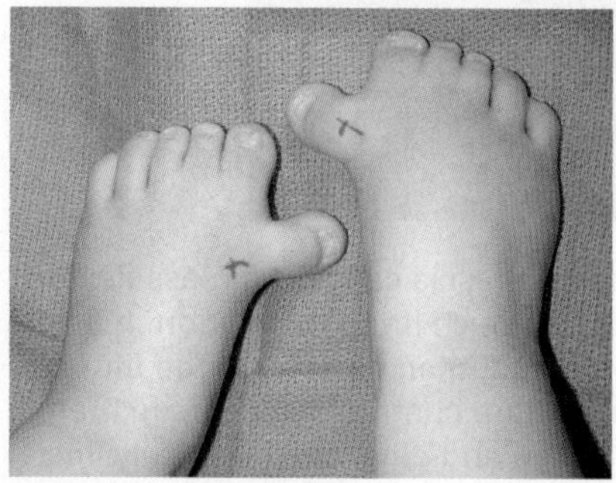

This congenital deformity results in extra fingers, usually at the thumb or fifth finger. Cosmetic removal is frequent, unless extra digit has full ROM and sensation.

(table continues on page 648)

TABLE 21.13 Comparing and Contrasting Assessment Findings in Common Conditions *(continued)*

Syndactyly

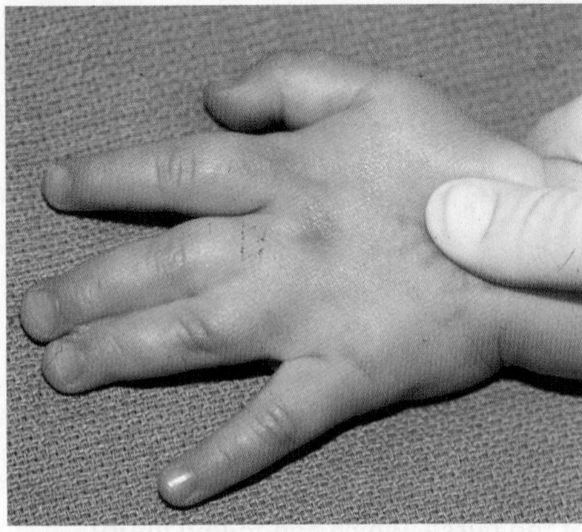

In this congenital deformity of webbed fingers, the metacarpals and phalanges of the webbed fingers are unequal in length and the joints do not align, which limits flexion and extension. Surgical separation is usual. Toes may also be webbed.

Dupuytren Contracture

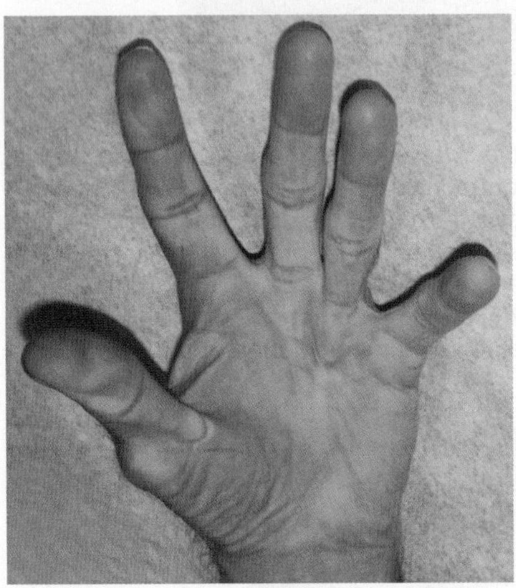

Hyperplasia of the palmar fascia causes painless flexion contracture of the digits, which impairs function. It usually starts in the fourth digit, then extends to the fifth and third. Dupuytren contracture commonly occurs in men older than 40 years of age and develops bilaterally. Incidence increases with diabetes, epilepsy, family history of Dupuytren contracture, and alcoholic liver disease.

Herniated Nucleus Pulposus

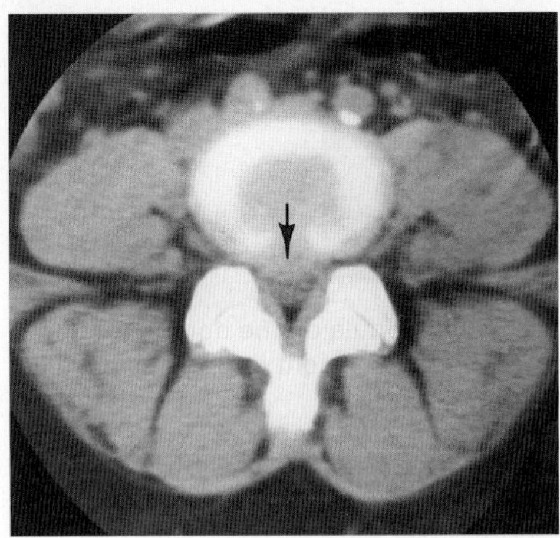

The intervertebral discs may slip out of position following trauma or strain. Rupture of the nucleus pulposus (soft inner portion) may put pressure on the spinal nerve root. Symptoms include sciatic pain radiating down the leg, numbness, paresthesia, listing from the affected side, decreased mobility, low back tenderness, and decreased motor and sensory function in the affected leg. Straight leg raises produce sciatic pain.

Talipes Equinovarus ("Club Foot")

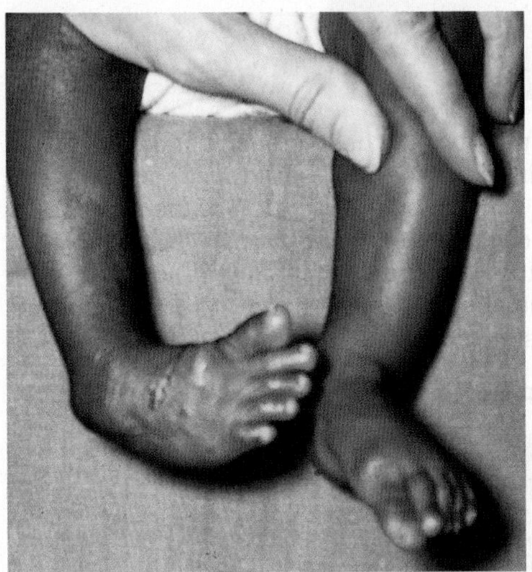

The foot is turned to the side, and the involved foot, calf, and leg are smaller and shorter than the normal side. One or both feet may be affected. This condition is not painful; however, if left untreated, significant discomfort and disability will develop. Treatment ranges from braces or casts to surgery.

(table continues on page 649)

TABLE 21.13 Comparing and Contrasting Assessment Findings in Common Conditions *(continued)*

Ulnar Deviation

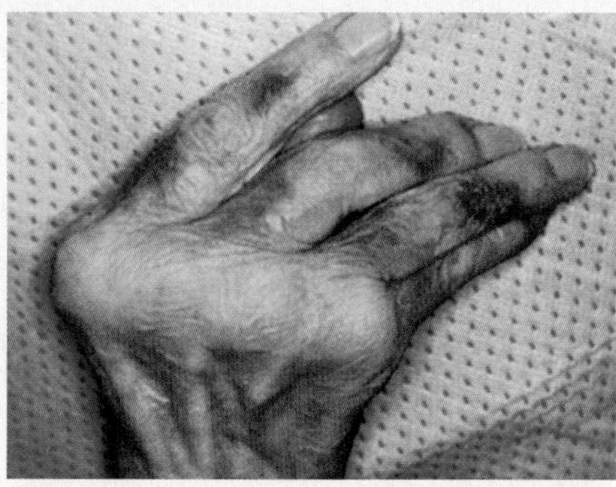

Stretching of the articular capsule and muscle imbalance in rheumatoid arthritis cause fingers to point in the ulnar direction.

Ankylosing Spondylitis

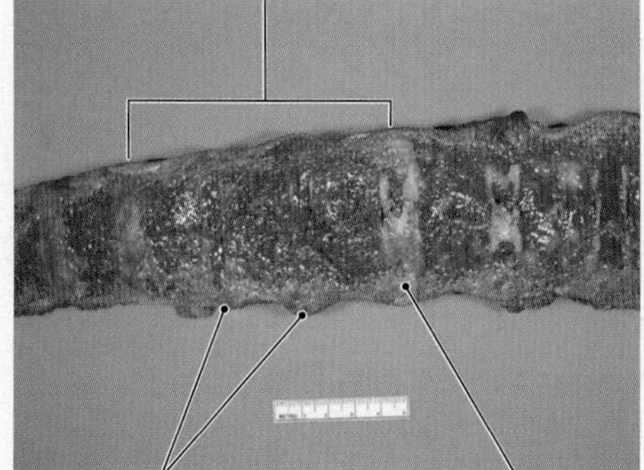

This chronic, progressive inflammation of the spine and sacroiliac and large joints in the extremities affects men 10 times more often than women. It is characterized by bony growths. Muscle spasms pull the spine forward and eliminate the cervical and lumbar curves. Flexion deformities can also occur in knees and hips.

Acute Rheumatoid Arthritis

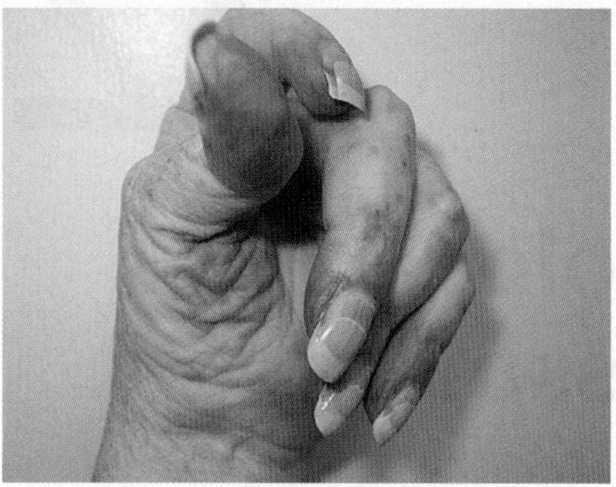

Inflammation results in painful, reddened, swollen joints and limited function. The condition is common in proximal interphalangeal joints.

Heberden and Bouchard Nodes

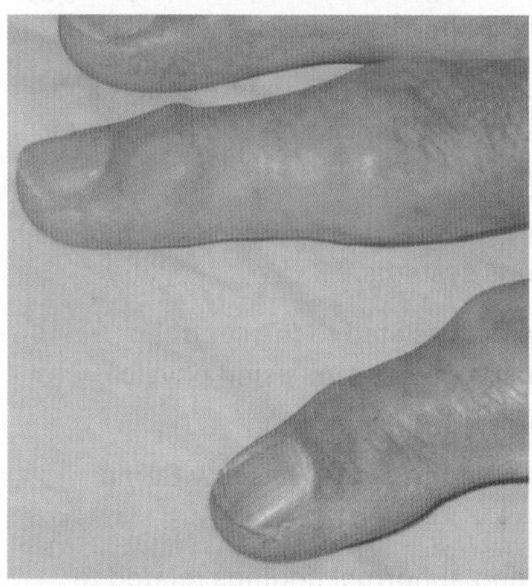

Hard, nontender bony growths on the distal (Heberden) and proximal (Bouchard) intraphalangeal joints. Frequently occurs with deviation of the fingers.

Carpal Tunnel Syndrome

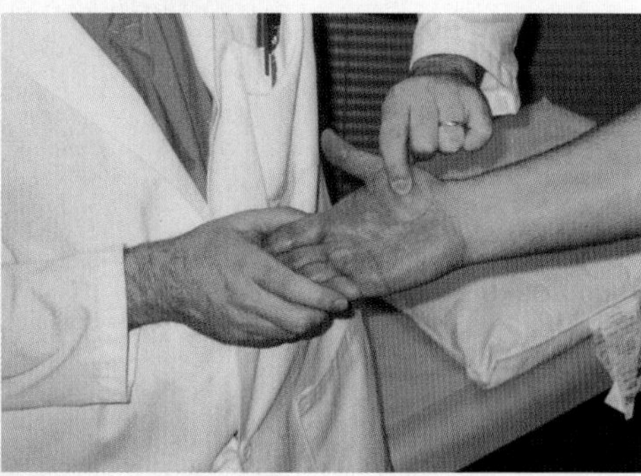

Carpal tunnel syndrome occurs from repetitive motion and develops in people aged 30–60 years. It occurs in women five times more frequently than men. Symptoms include burning, pain, and numbness from compression of the median nerve inside the carpal tunnel of the wrist. Atrophy of the thenar eminence at the base of the thumb is common. Diagnosis is made from a positive Phalen test or Tinel sign.

22

Neurological Assessment

Learning Objectives

1. Demonstrate knowledge of anatomy and physiology of the central and peripheral nervous systems.
2. Identify important topics for health promotion and risk reduction related to the central and peripheral nervous systems.
3. Collect subjective data related to the central and peripheral nervous systems.
4. Collect objective data related to the central and peripheral nervous systems using physical examination techniques.
5. Demonstrate knowledge of the Glasgow Coma Scale.
6. Identify normal and abnormal findings related to the central and peripheral nervous systems.
7. Analyze subjective and objective data from assessment of the central and peripheral nervous systems and consider initial interventions.
8. Document and communicate data from central and peripheral nervous assessment using appropriate medical terminology and principles of recording.
9. Consider the condition, age, gender, and culture of the patient to individualize the central and peripheral nervous assessment.
10. Identify nursing diagnoses and initiate a plan of care based on findings from the musculoskeletal assessment.

Mr. Gardner, a 56-year-old African American, has a history of atrial fibrillation, hyperlipidemia, hypertension, smoking, and mild vascular neurocognitive disorder. He was admitted to an acute care unit after being seen in the emergency department (ED) following a stroke. He lives alone, has poor hygiene, and is wearing multiple layers of mismatched clothing. He does not remember the last time he took his blood pressure medication. Vital signs are T 36.8°C (98.2°F) orally, P 88 beats/min, R 22 breaths/min, and BP 168/92 mm Hg. Mr. Gardner is alert, but he appears somewhat fearful and agitated. He asks for cigarettes and is oriented to name only. Speech is comprehensible but slurred.

You will gain more information about Mr. Gardner as you progress through the chapter. As you study the content and features, consider Mr. Gardner's case and its relationship to what you are learning. Begin thinking about the following points:

- What signs will the nurse assess to detect whether Mr. Gardner's situation is deteriorating?
- Is Mr. Gardner's condition at the end of the initial assessment stable, urgent, or an emergency?
- What ongoing health promotion and teaching needs are evident?
- How will the nurse individualize assessment to Mr. Gardner's specific needs, considering his condition, age, and culture?
- How will the nurse focus, organize, and prioritize ongoing objective data collection?
- How will the nurse evaluate the selection of the priority nursing diagnosis?

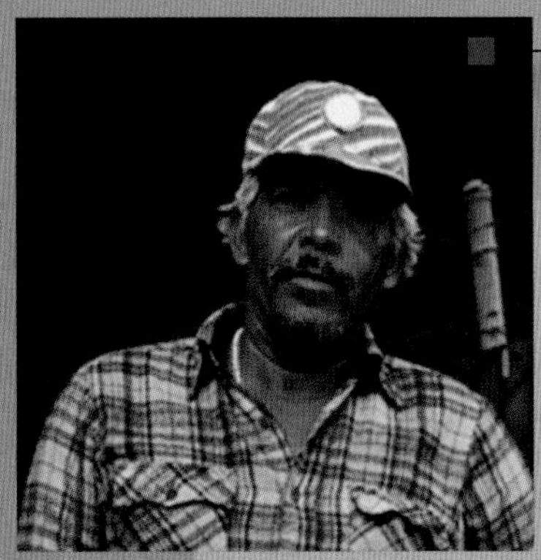

An intact appropriately functioning nervous system is critical for all human endeavors. It exerts unconscious control over basic body functions, such as respiration, temperature regulation, and movement coordination. The nervous system also enables very complex interactions with people and the environment. Assessment of neurological functioning serves multiple purposes. All those who perform neurological assessments use some of the same methods and, at times, share the same goals (e.g., detection of change in neurological status, particularly acute and life-threatening alterations). Generally, however, physicians and nurse practitioners assess neurological function primarily to identify pathology and to make a medical diagnosis. Nurses perform neurological assessment primarily to identify actual or potential health difficulties related to neurological dysfunction and the patient's response to those difficulties.

Common to all settings and types of neurological assessment is use of an organized approach to maximize the value of information derived from collected data. This approach consists of general patient observation, data gathering from the health history (often performed simultaneously), and a systematic neurological examination.

Structure and Function

The nervous system includes the central nervous system (CNS), consisting of the brain and spinal cord, and the peripheral nervous system (PNS), consisting of cranial, spinal, peripheral, and associated nerves.

The nervous system is classified according to function as either voluntary or involuntary (autonomic). In the voluntary division—also known as the somatic nervous system (SoNS)— PNS nerve fibers that connect the CNS to muscles and skin facilitate deliberate motor actions in response to stimuli. In the primarily unconscious autonomic division, PNS fibers connect the CNS with organs (including the heart and kidneys), smooth muscles, and glands.

Central Nervous System

Brain

The brain is a network of interconnecting neurons that control and integrate the body's activities (Fig. 22.1A). Each neuron contains a cell body, which serves as the control center; smaller receiving fibers called dendrites; and a connecting long fiber called an axon. Cell bodies are on the outside of the brain (gray matter or cerebral cortex), whereas axons that connect to other parts of the nervous system (white matter or brain tissue) are directed toward the center of the brain. (Axons are white because they are covered with a myelin sheath that speeds impulse conduction.) Neurons communicate with one another at synapses, small spaces between two neurons.

Important parts of the brain include the cerebrum, brainstem, and cerebellum (Fig. 22.1B).

Cerebrum. The cerebrum has two hemispheres, left and right, and comprises 83% of the total brain mass. In most people, the left hemisphere has more control over language and analytical abilities, which includes mathematics and logic, whereas the right hemisphere is more involved with visual–spatial skills, emotion, intuition, and musical and artistic abilities (Marieb & Hoehn, 2013). The cerebral cortex, which forms the outside of the cerebrum, contributes to motor and sensory function, intellect, and language.

Each hemisphere of the cerebral cortex has four lobes: frontal, temporal, parietal, and occipital (Fig. 22.2). The precentral gyrus in the frontal lobe controls motor function on the opposite side of the body; the left side of the brain controls the right side of the body, and the right side of the brain controls the left side of the body. The postcentral gyrus in the parietal lobe receives input on sensory function, including temperature, touch, pressure, and pain, also from the opposite side of the body. Motor and sensory function is organized from head to toe on both the left and right sides, similar to a person hanging upside down (Fig. 22.3).

> **Clinical Significance**
>
> A patient who has a cerebrovascular accident (stroke) in the right side of the brain will have motor and sensory deficits on the left side of the body. Conversely, a patient with a stroke in the left side of the brain will have right-sided motor and sensory deficits.

The cerebral cortex also is responsible for visual imaging, auditory processing, and language comprehension and expression. Each of the four lobes contributes to different functions (Fig. 22.4). The *frontal lobe* is responsible for complex cognition (orientation, memory, insight, judgment, arithmetic, and abstraction), language (verbal and written), and voluntary motor function. It integrates this cognitive function with emotional responses, personality, impulse control, and social behavior. The motor function area, previously discussed, is located at the foot of the frontal lobe. The *parietal lobe* recognizes the size, shape, and texture of objects and interprets touch, pressure, and pain. The sensory areas previously discussed are located at the front of the parietal lobe. Language is processed in the *Wernicke area* (located in the parietal lobe of the left hemisphere) and the *Broca area* (located in the frontal lobe). The **Wernicke** area integrates understanding of spoken and written words, whereas the **Broca** area regulates verbal expression and writing ability. The primary visual area is the *occipital lobe* at the back of the brain, with visual associative areas that interpret and integrate stimuli. The *temporal lobe* registers auditory input and is responsible for hearing, speech, behavior, and memory.

Additionally, some scientists identify a fifth lobe—the *limbic lobe*—which consists of the hippocampus and amygdaloid nucleus, a more primitive part of the brain (Gould, 2013). It is primarily concerned with self-preservation, including recall of pleasurable, unpleasant, or potentially dangerous events. It also recalls mood and emotional

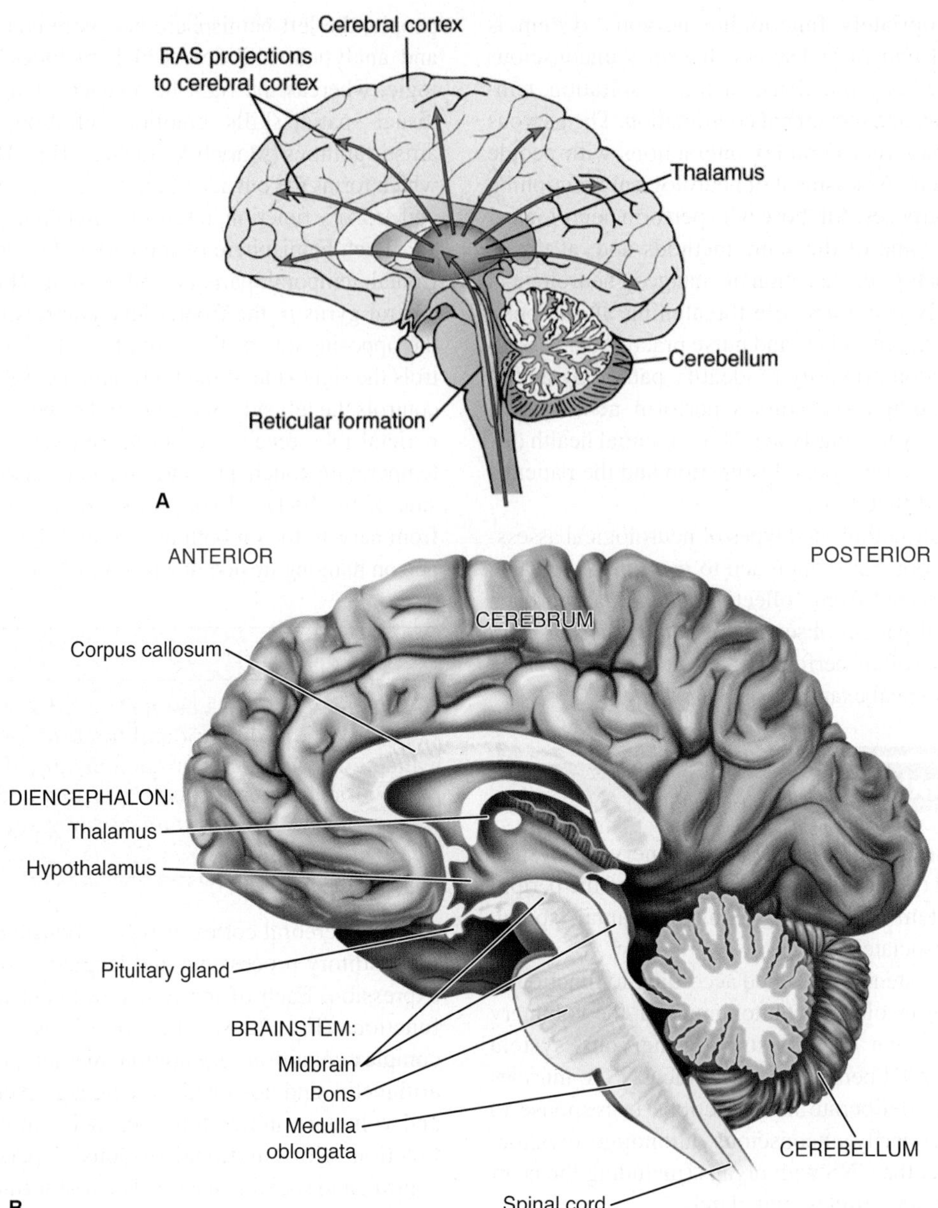

Figure 22.1 **A.** Interconnecting neurons that control and integrate the body's activities. **B.** The brain and its important divisions.

responses in relation to events, including aggression, interpretation of smell, feeding and sexual behaviors, and autonomic responses associated with emotion.

> **Clinical Significance**
>
> Because the areas that involve speech are in the brain's left hemisphere, patients who have a stroke there are more likely to have language deficits. Damage to the Wernicke area may lead to difficulty understanding verbal communication, called **receptive aphasia.** Damage to the Broca area causes problems with speaking or finding words; this is called **expressive aphasia**. **Global aphasia** is both expressive and receptive.

The cerebrum contains the basal ganglia, thalamus, hypothalamus, and limbic system (Gould, 2013). The *basal ganglia* are four paired tracts of gray matter on both sides of the thalamus deep within the brain tissue (Fig. 22.5A). They modulate automatic movements, receiving input from the cerebral cortex and sending output to the brainstem and thalamus to facilitate smooth motor function (e.g., fluid swinging of the arms while walking). The *thalamus*, directly above the brainstem, is the major relay station and gatekeeper for both motor and sensory stimuli to the cerebral cortex. The *hypothalamus* controls vital functions of temperature, heart rate, blood pressure, sleep, the anterior and posterior pituitary, the autonomic nervous system, and emotions. It maintains overall autonomic control. The *limbic system* is more primitive and mediates survival

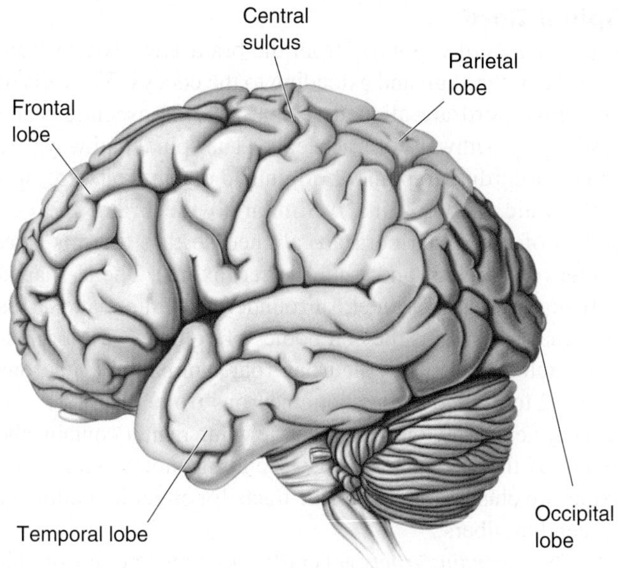

Figure 22.2 Lobes of the cerebral cortex.

behaviors such as fear, aggression, mating, and affection (Fig. 22.5B).

Brainstem. The brainstem is integral to intact neurological functioning. Both afferent and efferent fibers pass through it from the spinal cord to the cerebrum and cerebellum. Afferent (sensory) stimuli travel through the brainstem to the cerebral cortex; efferent (motor) fibers leave the cortex to pass through the brainstem and spinal cord.

The brainstem includes the medulla, midbrain, pons, and reticular formation. The cell bodies of cranial nerves (CNs) III to XII are in the *medulla*, which also contains the vital autonomic centers for respiratory, cardiac, and vasomotor function (Table 22.1). The medulla works with the pons to regulate smooth breathing rhythm. The medulla also controls involuntary functions such as sneezing, swallowing, vomiting, hiccoughing, and coughing. The *midbrain* contains many motor neurons; it relays information to and from the brain through ascending sensory tracts and descending motor pathways. The *pons* contains the ascending and descending neuron tracts and assists the midbrain to relay information. It contains two respiratory centers: one that controls the length of inspiration and expiration and the other that controls respiratory rate (Gould, 2013). The *reticular formation* relays sensory information, excitatory and inhibitory control of spinal motor neurons, and control of vasomotor and respiratory activity. It is responsible for increasing wakefulness, attention, and responsiveness of cortical neurons to sensory stimulation.

Cerebellum. The cerebellum is under the occipital lobe in the posterior part of the brain (see Fig. 22.1). It coordinates voluntary movement, posture, and muscle tone and maintains special orientation and equilibrium. It ensures adjustments in movement to maintain overall balance and coordination through connections to the motor cortex, brainstem, and neurological pathways. It integrates information from the cerebral cortex, inner ear, muscles, and joints. Alcohol intake can affect the cerebellum, causing the characteristic loss of balance and coordination. The cerebellum rests against the opening at the base of the skull known as the foramen magnum.

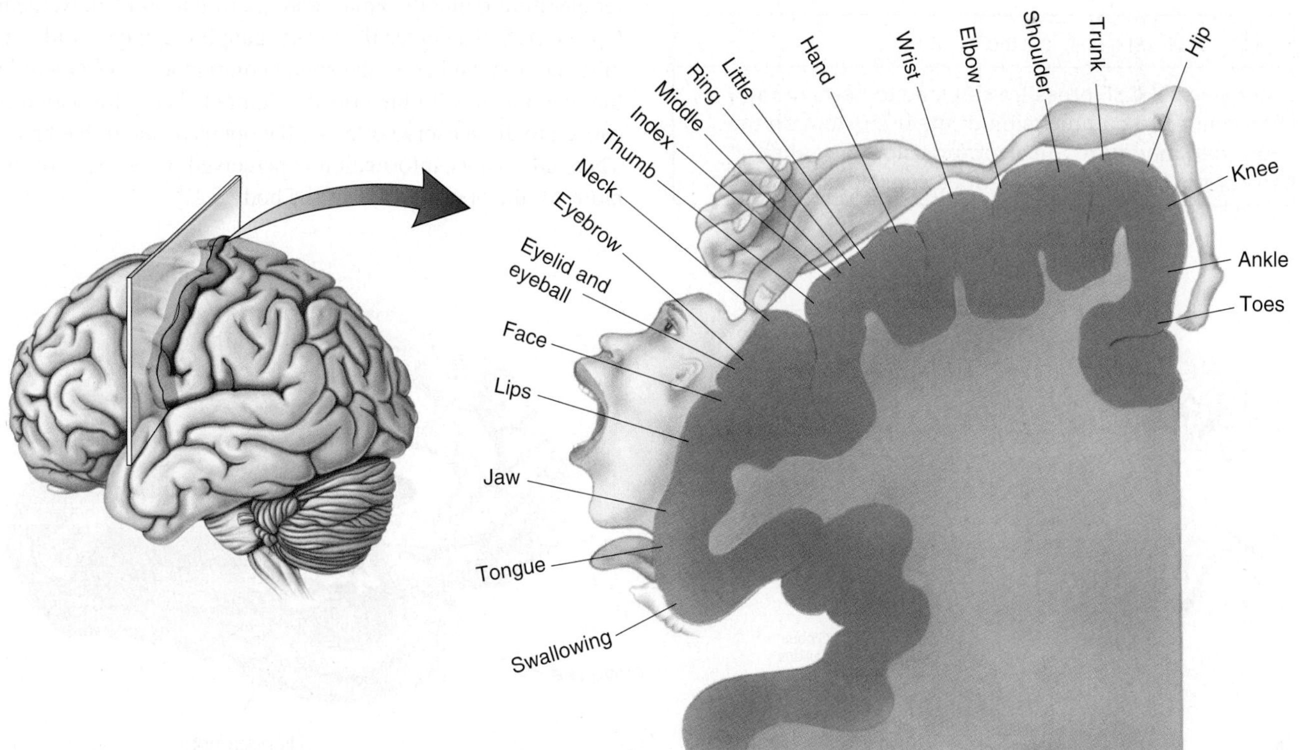

Figure 22.3 The homunculus, showing the organization of sensory function.

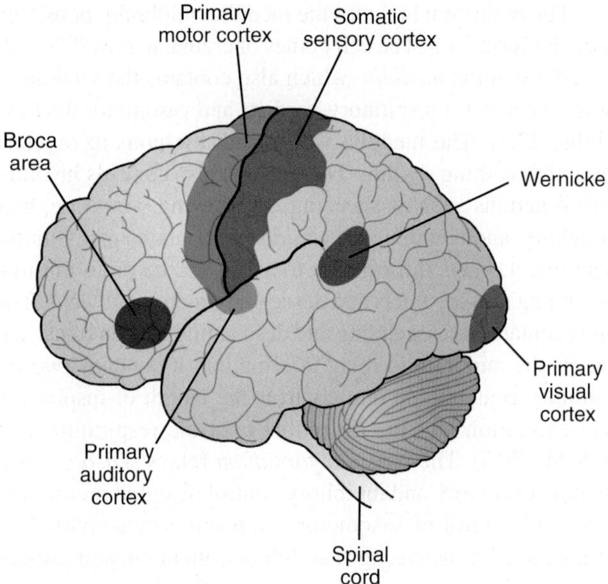

Figure 22.4 Four lobes of the brain contributing to different functions.

Protective Structures of the Central Nervous System

The meninges and skull cover and protect the brain. The ventricles of the brain are fluid-filled cavities that connect with the spinal cord. Cerebrospinal fluid (CSF) circulates within the space surrounding the brain, brainstem, and spinal cord. In addition to carrying nutrients, the CSF cushions and allows for shifts of fluid between the brain and spinal cord.

> **Clinical Significance**
>
> Increases in CSF pressure can lead to herniation of the brain and compression of the brainstem on the foramen magnum. Such compression may alter respiratory function and reduce consciousness.

Spinal Cord

The spinal cord continues from the brainstem, exiting from the base of the skull and extending to the coccyx. The cells of the spinal cord are aligned so that specific ascending and descending pathways or tracts exist. The spinal pathways are named according to point of origin and destination (e.g., spinothalamic, corticospinal). Similar to the brain, the cell bodies of the spinal cord are aligned so that there is gray matter (cell bodies) and white matter (axons). The H-shaped gray matter is at the center, surrounded by white matter. This gray matter contains the cell bodies of voluntary motor neurons, autonomic motor neurons (parasympathetic neurons from S2 to S4 and sympathetic neurons from T1 to L2), and sensory neurons (Gould, 2013). The white matter contains the axons of the ascending and descending motor fibers. The axons are clustered into specific tracts for either ascending or descending fibers.

The *ascending tracts* generally carry specific sensory information from the periphery to higher levels of the CNS (Fig. 22.6). Input from sensory receptors in the skin, organs, and muscles travels through the peripheral nerves to the dorsal root of the spinal nerve and into the spinal cord. These *dorsal columns* (also called posterior columns) carry information about localized touch (stereognosis), deep pressure, vibration, position sense (proprioception), and movement (kinesthesia) (Gould, 2013). They travel up the same side of the spinal cord to the brainstem. At the medulla, they synapse, cross to the opposite side of the body, and travel to the sensory cortex. Because of the crossing of the fibers in the medulla, right-sided sensations are perceived on the left side of the brain, and left-sided sensations are perceived on the right side of the brain. Additionally, specialized ascending tracts for pain and temperature (spinothalamic) and coordination of movement (spinocerebellar) enter the dorsal ganglia, synapse with another neuron, and cross the spinal column here (instead of in the medulla as with the dorsal columns). The information is carried to the sensory cortex on the opposite site of the brain. Thus, all sensory information is perceived on one side of the brain for the opposite side of the body.

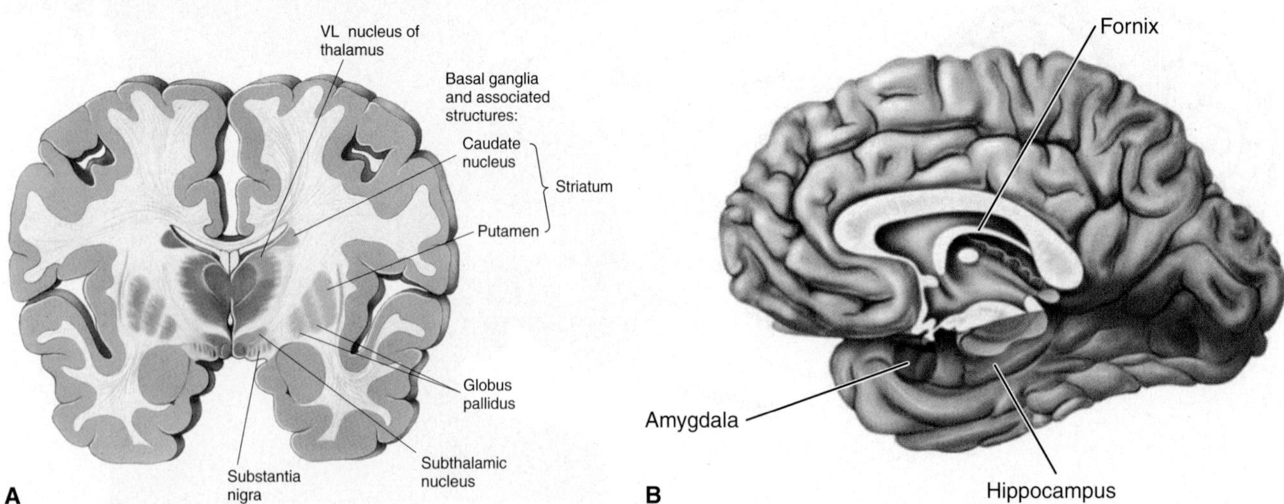

Figure 22.5 **A.** The basal ganglia. **B.** The primitive limbic system.

TABLE 22.1 **Cranial Nerves**		
Cranial Nerve	**Anatomy**	**Physiology**
I. Olfactory (sensory)	Originates in the nasal mucosa; ends in the temporal lobe	Smell and smell interpretation, including peristalsis, salivation, and sexual stimulation
II. Optic (sensory)	Originates in the retinal cells in the optic disc; travels over the optic nerve to end in the occipital lobe	Vision, including visual acuity and peripheral vision
III. Oculomotor (motor)	Originates in the midbrain and supplies motor fibers to the eye, eyelid, ciliary muscles, and iris	Extraocular movements (EOMs): • Upward • Medial • Downward • Up and in Eyelid raising and pupil constriction
IV. Trochlear (motor)	Originates in the midbrain and supplies motor fibers to the superior oblique muscle of the eye	EOMs: down and in
V. Trigeminal (sensory and motor)	Originates in the pons; has three branches: *ophthalmic* (sensory), *maxillary* (sensory), and *mandibular* (sensory and motor)	*Ophthalmic branch*: sensation to the cornea, conjunctiva, nasal mucosa, forehead, and nose *Maxillary branch*: sensation to the skin of the cheek and nose, lower eyelid, upper jaw, teeth, oral mucosa *Mandibular branch*: sensation to the lower jaw and motor function to muscles of mastication
VI. Abducens (motor)	Originates in the pons and supplies motor fibers to the lateral rectus muscle	EOMs: lateral
VII. Facial (sensory and motor)	Originates in the pons and supplies sensory fibers to the anterior two thirds of the tongue and soft palate and motor fibers to the muscles of the face	Taste and sensation for the anterior two thirds of the tongue and soft palate; serves as the primary motor nerve for facial expression
VIII. Acoustic (sensory)	Cochlear sensory fibers originate in the cochlea and transmit auditory sensation to the ear, pons, and temporal lobe. Vestibular sensory fibers originate in the semicircular canals of the ear and vestibular ganglion and end in the pons	Hearing Equilibrium
IX. Glossopharyngeal (sensory and motor)	Sensory divisions from the external ear, tympanic membrane, upper pharynx, and posterior one third of the tongue end in the medulla; motor divisions supply the pharyngeal muscle and parotid gland	Pharyngeal muscle elevation for swallowing and speech; parotid gland secretion; general sensory (pain, touch, temperature) function
X. Vagus (sensory and motor)	Major parasympathetic nerve of the body; originates in the medulla; sensory from larynx, esophagus, trachea, carotid bodies, thoracic and abdominal viscera, and stretch and chemoreceptors from the aorta; motor supplies the pharynx, larynx, thoracic, and abdominal viscera	Provides most parasympathetic innervation to a large region; effects include digestion, defecation, slowed heart rate, and reduced contraction strength
XI. Spinal accessory (motor)	Originates in medulla with two branches; cranial root innervates muscles of the larynx and pharynx; spinal root innervates trapezius and sternocleidomastoid muscles	Swallowing and speaking; innervates the muscles that turn the head and elevates the shoulders (shoulder shrug)
XII. Hypoglossal (motor)	Originates in the medulla and ends at the tongue	Tongue movement

Information from Standring, S. (2008). *Gray's anatomy: The anatomical basis for clinical practice* (40th ed.). London, United Kingdom: Elsevier Churchill Livingstone; Kandel, E. R., Schwartz, J. H., Jessell, T. M., Siegelbaum, S. A., & Hudspeth, A. J. (Eds.). (2012). *Principles of neural science* (5th ed.). Philadelphia, PA: Elsevier.

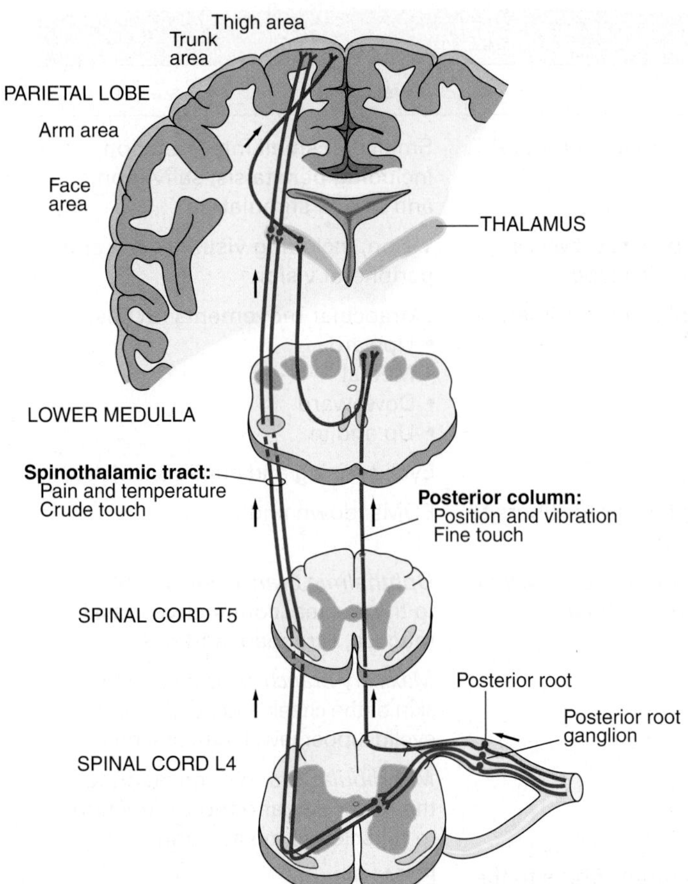

Figure 22.6 Ascending tracts of the brain carry sensory information from peripheral nerves to the central nervous system.

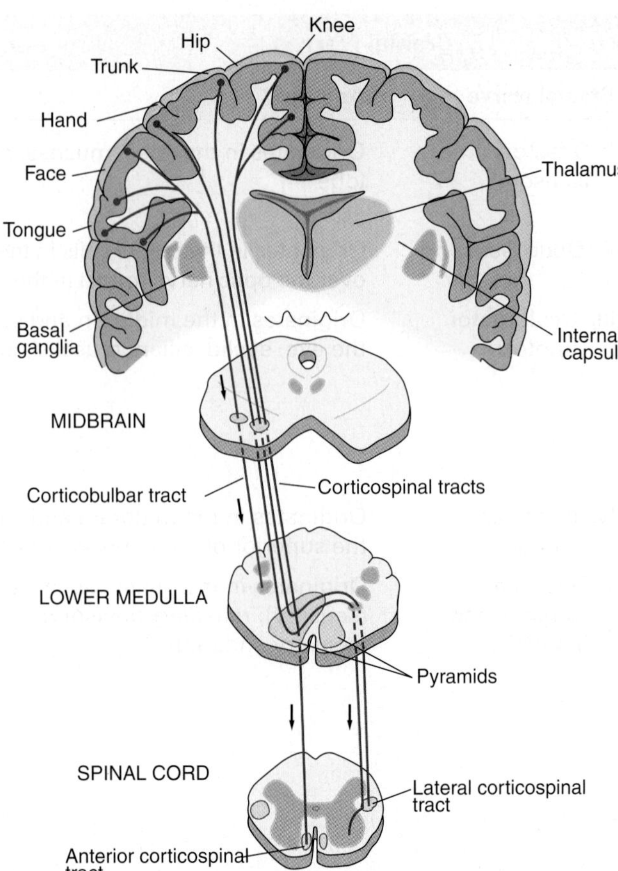

Figure 22.7 Descending tracts carry motor and muscle information from the cortex to the cranial and peripheral nerves.

> **Clinical Significance**
>
> When half of the spinal cord is severed (e.g., by a gunshot wound), the patient may experience **Brown-Séquard syndrome** sensory loss. Manifestations include loss of pain and temperature sensation on the opposite side of the injury because these fibers cross in the spinal cord. Localized touch, deep pressure, vibration, position sense, and movement remain on the same side of the body because these fibers cross in the medulla.

The *descending tracts* carry information related to motor function and muscle movement (Fig. 22.7). They control voluntary movement, carrying impulses from the cortex to the cranial (corticobulbar tract) and peripheral (corticospinal tract) nerves (Gould, 2013). The corticobulbar and corticospinal tracts are referred to as the *pyramidal tract.* Axons originate in the motor cortex, travel to the brainstem, and cross at the medulla. Similar to the sensory tracts, the motor tracts on the left side of the brain control the right side; those on the right side of the brain control the left. The neurons exit the spinal cord at the ventral root of the spinal nerve, and impulses are carried to the peripheral motor nerves.

Another group of fibers in the descending tract carries information involving all motor systems except those of the pyramidal tract. This *extrapyramidal tract* originates in the reticular formation and is modulated by the brainstem, basal ganglia, and cerebellum. It travels down and synapses in the ventral root of the spinal cord; however, it does not directly innervate the peripheral motor system. This tract controls gross automatic movements such as reflexes, walking, complex movements, and postural control.

> **Clinical Significance**
>
> Some medications prescribed to patients with psychiatric illnesses have extrapyramidal adverse effects. Such patients need ongoing assessment for involuntary and irregular muscle movements, restlessness, and spasms of the neck, tongue, or jaw. Patients with Parkinson disease may have poor skeletal muscle tone, drooling, tremor, and shuffling gait related to loss of neurons in the extrapyramidal tract. Involuntary writhing movements related to damage to this tract also may accompany cerebral palsy.

Peripheral Nervous System

The peripheral motor system includes neurons outside the CNS. The CNs, spinal nerves, and autonomic nervous system all belong to the **peripheral motor system**.

Cranial Nerves

The 12 paired CNs exit from the brain rather than the spinal cord (Fig. 22.8). Some CNs have only a sensory component, some have only a motor component, and others have both. Many CNs originate in the midbrain, pons, or medulla and innervate the eyes, ears, nose, mouth, and throat. An exception is the vagus nerve, which provides motor and sensory function to the heart and abdomen. See Table 22.1 for a complete description of the CNs.

Spinal Nerves

The spinal nerves arise from the spinal cord and innervate the rest of the body. They are described by their location in relation to the vertebrae, such as the 6th cervical (C6) or 4th thoracic (T4). Unlike the CNs, the spinal nerves each have afferent sensory fibers (located in the dorsal root) and efferent motor fibers (located in the ventral root). The combination of motor and sensory fibers is referred to as the spinal nerve. The 31 pairs of spinal nerves include 8 cervical, 12 thoracic, 5 lumbar, 5 sacral, and 1 coccygeal nerve (Fig. 22.9). Each level innervates a specific body part from head to toe on the right and left sides. This is visualized by evaluating the area of skin innervated by the afferent sensory fibers in the dorsal root of a spinal nerve called a **dermatome**.

Although the dermatomes provide a general idea of the innervation by each nerve, some overlap exists (Fig 22.10):

- C1–3 control movement in and above the neck.
- C4–6 are at the level of the shoulder and diaphragm for breathing independently.
- C7–8 are at the level of the fingers and hand grasp to perform self-care and transfers with arms.
- T1–6 provide trunk stability for balance when sitting.
- T6–12 are for the thoracic muscles and upper back for respiratory and transfer strength (Gould, 2013).
- L1–2 are at the level of legs and pelvis.
- L3–4 are hamstrings and ankles.

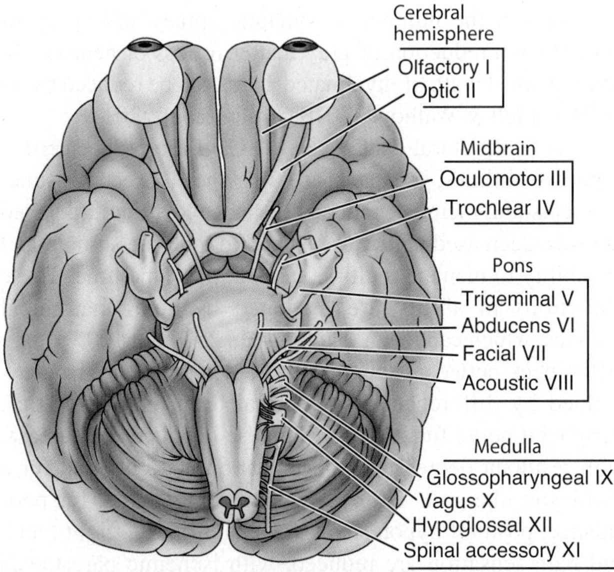

Figure 22.8 The 12 paired cranial nerves.

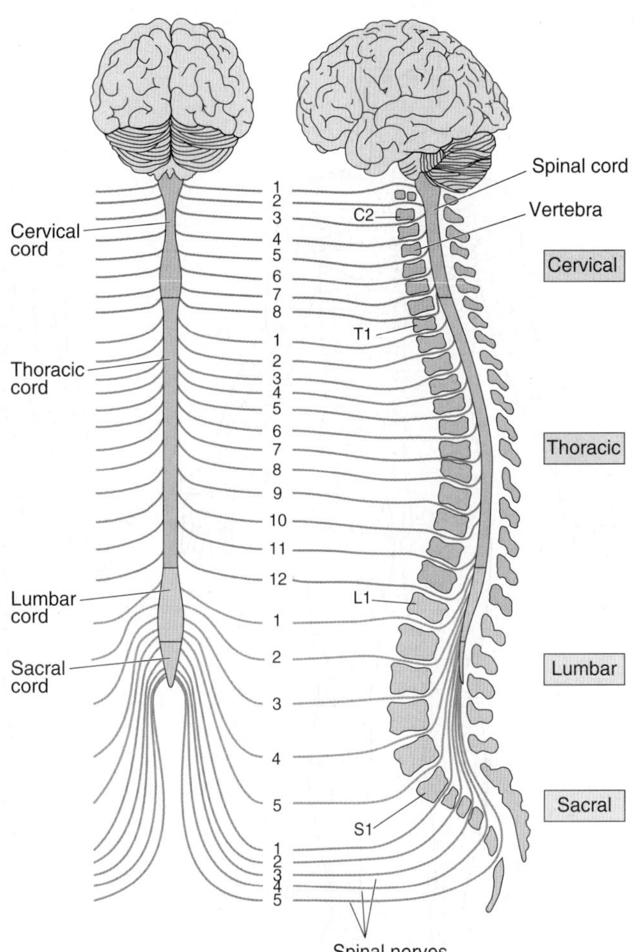

Figure 22.9 The spinal nerves.

Level of injury to the spinal cord affects function at and below the site of trauma. Thus, a patient with an injury at T6 would have arm movement and sensation but no leg movement or sensation. The patient with a lesion or spinal cord injury at L1–2 has varying control of the legs and pelvis. One with difficulties at L3–4 has weakened hamstrings and ankles, which may permit ambulation with braces and a cane.

Autonomic Nervous System

The **autonomic nervous system** maintains involuntary functions of cardiac and smooth muscle and glands. It has two components: *sympathetic* (fight or flight) and *parasympathetic* (rest and digest). These two systems balance the body and maintain homeostasis (Gould, 2013). The sympathetic ganglia are located in the spine from T1 to L2. The major neurotransmitter is epinephrine (also known as adrenaline). The cell bodies of the parasympathetic nervous system are located in the brainstem and spinal segments S2–4. The ganglia are located near the structures that they innervate; the neurotransmitter is acetylcholine.

The autonomic nervous system can both sense changes and make changes based on input. To regulate heart rate and blood pressure, it receives input from chemoreceptors and baroreceptors. Based on such input, the sympathetic system secretes epinephrine to increase blood pressure, heart rate, and contractility; the parasympathetic system secretes acetylcholine to reduce heart rate and force of contraction. Many

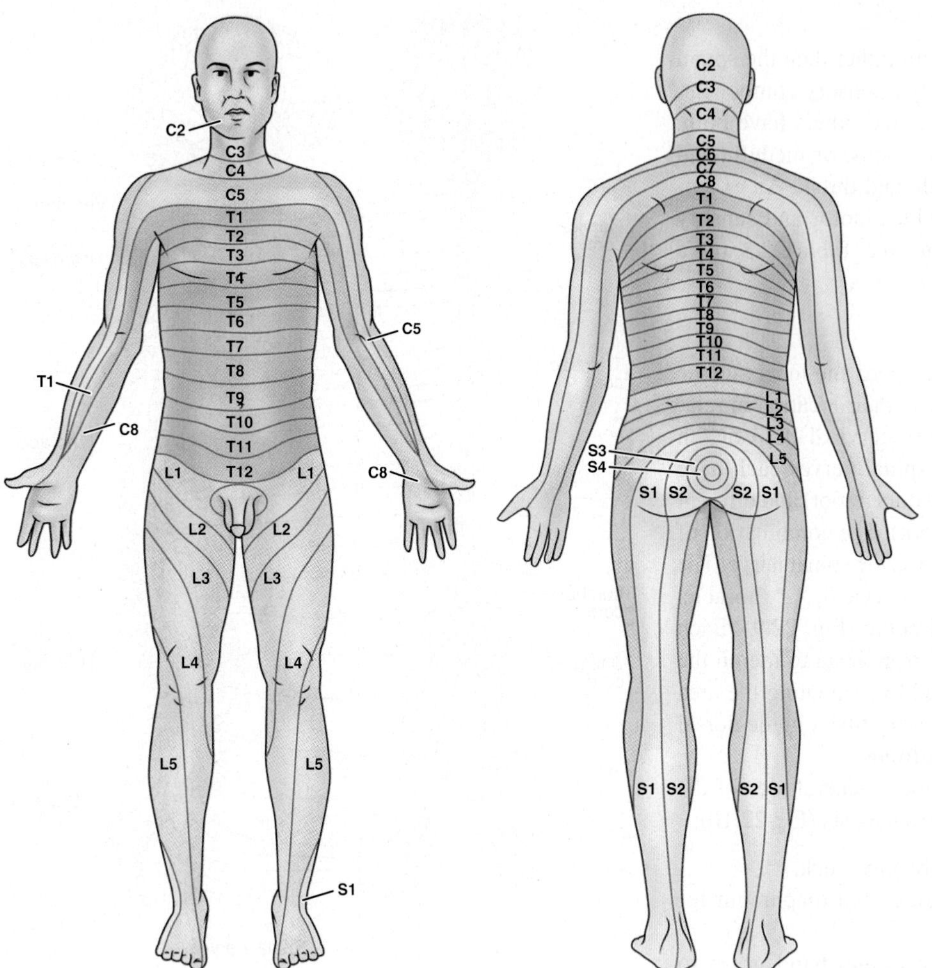

Figure 22.10 Dermatomes.

times, the two systems work in opposite ways to provide balance to the body's overall function.

Reflexes are involuntary responses to stimuli. They maintain balance and tone. Reflexes also provide quick responses in potentially harmful situations, such as withdrawing the foot when stepping on a sharp object. The simplest type of **reflex arc** involves a receptor-sensing organ, afferent sensory neuron, efferent motor neuron, and effector motor organ (Fig. 22.11). A commonly tested reflex is the "knee-jerk" reaction when the knee is tapped; this is a deep tendon reflex (DTR) when the patellar tendon is stimulated. The patellar tendon is the sensing organ, which travels through the sensory neuron to the dorsal root ganglion. It synapses in the spinal cord and travels out through the motor neuron to the quadriceps muscle, where this motor organ contracts and causes the knee to jerk. The muscle must also be strong enough to cause the reflex. Other reflexes include the superficial (e.g., corneal, abdominal), visceral (pupillary response to light), and neonatal (rooting, grasp, Babinski).

Lifespan Considerations: Older Adults

The structure of the CNS continuously changes from birth throughout the lifespan. Thus, normal aging, even when free from dementia, is associated with structural brain changes. There are decreases in the brain volume and the ventricles holding the cerebral spinal fluid expand in healthy aging. The major changes have been noted in the frontal and temporal cortexes as well as in the putamen, thalamus, and nucleus accumbens. The reduction in brain volume that occurs in healthy aging is most likely related to the shrinkage of neurons and reduction in the number of synaptic spines and synapses rather than a reduction of gray matter or loss of neurons. In addition, the length of myelinated axons can be reduced by up to 50% (Fjell & Walhovd, 2010; Touhy & Jett, 2012).

These structural changes in the CNS can reduce certain cognitive abilities, such as processing speed, executive function, episodic memory, reduced response to stimuli, delayed reflexes, decreased ability to respond to multiple stimuli, and the ability to manage multiple tasks at the same time. These reductions in ability are mediated by neuroanatomical changes, which can mean that between 25% and 100% of the differences between younger and older people can be explained by differences in structural brain characteristics. Peripheral nerve function and impulse conduction decrease, with resultant decreased proprioception and potential for a Parkinson-like gait. Thus, older adults are at risk for poor balance, postural hypotension, falls, and injury. Light touch and pain sensation are reduced, with ischemic paresthesia common in the extremities. Overall cognitive function with

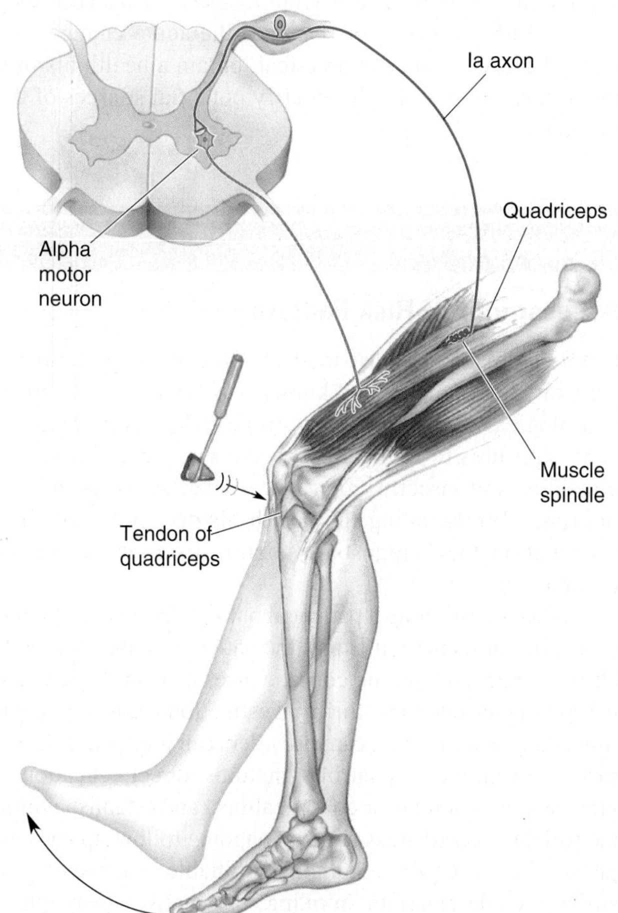

Figure 22.11 A commonly cited reflex arc is the "knee-jerk" reaction, which is a deep tendon reflex that results with stimulation of the patellar tendon.

aging varies greatly depending on overall lifestyle choices and heredity (Fjell & Walhovd, 2010; Touhy & Jett, 2012).

Cultural Considerations

African American adults are 1.6 times as likely as Caucasians to have a stroke. In general, American Indian/Alaska Native adults are 2.4 times more likely to have a stroke than Caucasians. Normally, Asian American adults are less likely than Caucasian adults to have suffered a stroke; they are less likely to die from a stroke. Hispanic women are 20% more likely to have a stroke than Caucasian women (U.S. Department of Health & Human Services, Office of Minority Health [USDHHS OMH], 2012)

Urgent Assessment

After baseline information has been gathered, it is often neither practical nor necessary to perform a complete neurological examination. Choice of which elements to assess in a given setting depends on many variables. Recognition of situations requiring acute assessment and rapid communication of findings is critical to preventing or limiting negative outcomes for patients (Box 22.1).

When situations such as those in Box 22.1 are identified, rapidly assessing key areas included in the neurological examination is the first step in determining the nature of the problem and possible urgent interventions. This abbreviated acute assessment includes the following (details of each element are described more completely later):

- Rapidly assess level of consciousness (LOC) using the Glasgow Coma Scale (GCS), which scores verbal response,

BOX 22.1 Indicators of Significant Changes in Neurological Status

- Acute change in mental status: increasing restlessness, agitation, or confusion
- Changes in consciousness not explained by known causes (e.g., sedatives). These range from patterns of increasing difficulty in arousing the patient to complete lack of responsiveness to any stimulus.
- Seizure activity
- Onset of flexor or extensor posturing, either spontaneously or in response to noxious stimuli
- Flexor posturing = adduction of arm with flexion at elbow and wrist, extension and internal rotation of leg with plantar flexion of foot
- Extensor posturing = adduction, internal rotation, and extension of arm; extension and internal rotation of leg with plantar flexion of foot
- Change in size and decreased reactivity to light in one or both pupils
- Onset of conjugate or dysconjugate eye deviation
- Progressing weakness (paresis) or paralysis of an extremity or one side of the body; observe for facial weakness on the same side
- Changes in ability to identify sensation
- Significant changes in vital signs (beyond parameters established by physician)
- Changes in blood pressure may threaten tissue oxygenation or result in direct injury from hemorrhage. For example, a patient with cerebrovascular insufficiency who is usually hypertensive may suffer a cerebral infarction if blood pressure drops too low. In a patient with an untreated ruptured cerebral aneurysm or intracerebral hemorrhage, hypertension may trigger additional hemorrhage.
- Change in heart rate or rhythm may threaten adequate perfusion or indicate potential etiology (e.g., atrial fibrillation with emboli, causing stroke).
- Fever may indicate infection or dysfunction of the autonomic nervous system and is associated with worsened outcome after traumatic brain injury and acute stroke.
- Significant or progressively rising blood pressure may lead to widening pulse pressure, decreasing pulse, and decreasing respirations, the classic signs of increased intracranial pressure (ICP) (**Cushing response**); these are late signs of lower brainstem compression.
- Irregular breathing patterns may indicate progressing brainstem compression.

BOX 22.2 Glasgow Coma Scale

The GCS is a tool for assessing a patient's response to stimuli. Scores range from 3 (deep coma) to 15 (normal).

Eye opening response	Spontaneous	4
	To voice	3
	To pain	2
	None	1
Best verbal response	Oriented	5
	Confused	4
	Inappropriate words	3
	Incomprehensible sounds	2
	None	1
Best motor response	Obeys command	6
	Localizes pain	5
	Withdraws	4
	Flexion	3
	Extension	2
	None	1
Total		3–15

From Teasdale, G., & Jennett, B. (1974). Assessment of coma and impaired consciousness. A practical scale. *Lancet*, *304*, 81–84.

eye opening, and motor function (Box 22.2). If the patient can respond verbally, assess basic orientation. This also allows a basic speech/language assessment (comprehension and production of spoken language and speech quality, such as garbled or slurred).

- Assess **pupillary reaction**: assess size (before and after light stimulus) and speed of response to light.
- Perform gross assessment of extremity strength. If the patient can follow commands, ask him or her to lift each extremity off the bed, noting whether the patient can maintain limb elevation against gravity and then against resistance from you. Also note any facial asymmetry (either at rest or during facial movement).
- Perform gross assessment of **sensation** (only possible if the patient can communicate) by examining ability to identify presence and location of light touch on all extremities and both sides of the face.
- If consciousness is impaired, assessing selected other CNs may help differentiate neurological from metabolic causes, particularly **extraocular movements** (EOMs), **gag reflex**, and **corneal reflex**.

Vital signs are part of this acute assessment because they may be either a cause or result of the acute change (see Box 22.1). As soon as is practical, obtain a health history; this information will help identify potential sources of the problem.

Subjective Data

Assessment of Risk Factors

Obtain a history of past medical diagnoses, particularly head or spinal trauma, and known risk factors for common neurological conditions (e.g., stroke). Note chronic or recent exposures to toxins; any recent viral infections; vaccinations; and insect, spider, tick, snake, or scorpion bites or stings. While taking the health history, you may elicit information that suggests a seizure disorder, stroke, or traumatic injury.

When questioning a patient about risk factors, the goal is to identify how likely it is that the patient will develop, or is already experiencing, the consequences of neurological and neurovascular diseases. Such investigation creates an environment in which health care providers can implement necessary interventions to control symptoms, direct education to prevent new problems or complications, and establish within the patient's record areas needing ongoing follow-up and emphasis. For example, common modifiable risk factors for stroke include cigarette smoking, obstructive sleep apnea, cardiovascular disease, overweight, physical inactivity, high blood pressure, high cholesterol, diabetes mellitus, heavy or binge drinking, use of certain birth control pills or hormone therapies that include estrogen, and use of cocaine and methamphetamines (American Heart Association [AHA], 2012b). Other risk factors include personal and family history of stroke, myocardial infarction, or transient ischemic attack; being older than the age of 55 years; ethnicity (African Americans have a higher risk of stroke than people of other races); and gender (men have a higher risk of stroke than women). Women are usually older when they have strokes and are more likely to die of strokes than men. After assessment, nurses identify focused teaching areas and evaluate in ongoing visits the patient's progress toward change.

The following screening questions are important in establishing the patient's risk for neurological disease.

History and Risk Factors	Rationale
Biographical Information From the chart, obtain the following: • Age • Heredity • Gender • Date and result of last blood pressure reading • Date and result of last measurement of cholesterol level	Increased age and male gender increase risk for stroke. Another risk factor is stroke in a parent, grandparent, or sibling. African Americans have a higher risk of death from stroke than Caucasians, partly because African Americans have higher risks of elevated blood pressure, diabetes mellitus, and obesity (AHA, 2012).

(table continues on page 661)

History and Risk Factors	Rationale
Past Medical History Have you ever been diagnosed with a neurological problem, such as a seizure? • When did you have it? How often? • Tell me about your seizure history: associated warning signs (aura), motor activity, loss of consciousness, incontinence, sleepiness after the seizure (postictal phase), and precipitating factors. • How was the seizure treated? • Was the treatment effective?	Various scales have been developed to identify seizure severity. Criteria include seizure frequency, seizure type, seizure duration, postictal events, postictal duration, automatisms, seizure clusters, known patterns, warnings, tongue biting, incontinence, injuries, and functional impairment.
Have you ever had a head injury? • When? • How was it treated? • What were the outcomes?	A head injury is suspected if there is a • Witnessed loss of consciousness of longer than 5 minutes • History of amnesia of longer than 5 minutes • Abnormal drowsiness • Three or more episodes of vomiting within 4 hours of injury • Dangerous mechanism of injury • Seizure in a patient with no history of epilepsy (Bethel, 2012).
Have you ever had a stroke? • When did you have it? • How was it treated? • What were the outcomes?	An exact time of onset, definite focal symptoms, neurological signs, and ability to lateralize the signs to the left or right side of the brain suggest a stroke (Runchey & McGee, 2010).
Have you ever had any infectious or degenerative diseases, such as meningitis or multiple sclerosis?	Symptoms of meningitis include high fever, stiff neck, drowsiness, and photosensitivity. Symptoms of degenerative disease include weakness, tingling or numbness, difficulty seeing, and elimination control difficulties.
Have you had any changes in your emotional state or coping strategies related to your health? • Personality change • Alterations in level of independence • Loss of role function related to altered ability to carry out responsibilities, interact with others • Depression, apathy, or irritability • Change in ability to tolerate stress • Issues related to chronic conditions, progressive deterioration in function, or hospitalization	Information regarding past and current emotional state and coping strategies is obtained through attention to functional health patterns. Family relationships and socioeconomic background provide valuable clues to the patient's support system and capacity to manage the social and financial effects of disabilities frequently associated with neurological conditions.
Do you have a history of high blood pressure? • When was it diagnosed? • How is it being treated?	Epidemiological studies have demonstrated that elevated blood pressure is the most important determinant of the risk of stroke. Systolic blood pressure greater than 140 mm Hg, diastolic blood pressure greater than 90 mm Hg, or both is a risk factor for stroke (Lackland, 2013)
Risk Factors Do you have any of the following conditions that place you at risk for neurovascular disease? • Diabetes mellitus • Carotid artery disease • Atrial fibrillation • Sickle cell disease	Atrial fibrillation increases risk for stroke because quivering atria can lead blood to stagnate and then form small clots. A clot that breaks off can circulate to the brain and block the artery, causing an embolic stroke. In sickle cell disease, blood cells tend to be stickier, causing clots to form more easily in narrowed arteries.

(table continues on page 662)

History and Risk Factors	Rationale
Do you have any of the following lifestyle choices that place you at risk for neurovascular disease? • Smoking • High-fat diet • Obesity • Physical inactivity	Many risk factors for stroke are the same as for cardiovascular disease (see Chapter 17).
What environmental or occupational hazards might you have that increases the risk of neurological trauma? • Lack of seat belt use • No helmet worn when biking, snowboarding, engaging in other high-risk sports • Incorrect use of car seats for children • Use of drugs or alcohol while driving • Falls (lack of window guards, pull bars, safety gates) • Ignorance of firearm safety	Men are almost twice as likely as women to sustain traumatic brain or spinal cord injuries, partly because they engage in riskier activities (National Center for Injury Prevention and Control [NCIPC], 2013a).
Medications Are you taking any medications for central or peripheral neurological difficulties?	
Family History Does anyone in your family have a history of stroke, neuromuscular disease, or other neurological condition?	

Risk Reduction and Health Promotion

An important purpose of the health history is to gather information to promote health and provide health teaching. Health promotion activities for the nervous system focus on preventing disease, identifying difficulties early, and reducing complications of existing or established diagnoses. The most important focus areas for the neurological system involve prevention of stroke and unintentional injury. The health goals include the following:

- Reduce stroke deaths.
- Increase the proportion of adults with high blood pressure who are taking action (e.g., losing weight, increasing physical activity, and reducing sodium intake) to help control their blood pressure.
- Increase the proportion of adults who are at a healthy weight and reduce the proportion of adults who are obese.
- Reduce the proportion of adults who engage in no leisure time physical activity and increase the proportion of adults who engage regularly, preferably daily, in moderate physical activity for at least 30 minutes.
- Reduce tobacco use by adults.

(USDHHS, 2013)

Stroke Prevention

Risk factors for stroke are similar to those for cardiovascular disease; thus, stroke prevention involves modification of unhealthy lifestyle choices. The majority of known risk factors—cigarette smoking, dyslipidemia, hypertension, diabetes mellitus, abdominal obesity, and psychosocial factors—are modifiable by preventive measures and adjunctive drug therapies.

Patients should control blood pressure by maintaining a healthy diet and using antihypertensive medications as prescribed. At every visit, ask patients about smoking and, for those with a positive response, about the desire for cessation. Provide all patients with information about a diet low in saturated fat and high in fruits and vegetables. Ask overweight and obese patients about their willingness to reduce calories. Additionally, advise all patients to exercise aerobically three to seven times a week for 20 to 60 minutes per session.

Injury Prevention

When investigating risk for traumatic injury, also provide information about prevention. Recommend use of protective helmets and gear to patients who engage in sports involving physical contact. During assessment of driving habits, advise patients about the importance of using seat belts and discourage use of alcohol and drugs while driving. Provide patient with teaching materials to reinforce concepts, especially for adolescents and young adults who are at highest risk of brain and spinal cord injury.

Common Symptoms

When recording the history of the present illness or problem, provide a detailed account of each symptom, its nature (location, quality, and severity), date of onset, precipitating factors, and duration (constant, intermittent, or worse at any particular time of day). Also note what, if anything, makes the symptoms worse or better, and what has been the general pattern of progression (e.g., rapid, static, progressively worse, remitting, exacerbating).

During assessment of the neurological system, ask all patients about common neurological symptoms to screen for the early presence of disease. If a patient is concerned about specific neurological problems, assess these focused areas with follow-up questions. A thorough history of symptoms assists with identifying the current problem or diagnosis. Direct your questions toward a history of problems with headaches, weakness or paralysis, loss of sensation, and involuntary movements or sensations.

Common Neurological Symptoms

- Headache or other pain (see Chapter 12)
- Weakness of single limb or one side of body
- Generalized weakness
- Involuntary movements or tremors
- Difficulty with balance, coordination, or gait
- Dizziness or vertigo
- Difficulty swallowing
- Change in intellectual abilities
- Difficulties with expression or comprehension of speech/language
- Alteration in touch, taste, or smell
- Loss or blurring of vision in one or both eyes, diplopia (double vision)
- Hearing loss or tinnitus (ringing in the ears)

Signs/Symptoms	Rationale/Abnormal Findings
Headache or Other Pain Do you have a headache or other pain (see Chapter 12).	
Limb or Unilateral Weakness Do you have any weakness on one side or in one limb? • How long does it last? • Is there any associated speech difficulty?	The three most predictive findings for the diagnosis for acute stroke are facial paresis, arm drift/weakness, and disturbed speech. Report patients with positive findings to a physician for diagnosis and treatment.
Generalized Weakness Do you have generalized weakness? • Does it occur mostly in the hands and feet or core muscles? • Do any repetitive actions lead to such weakness? • Are there any associated symptoms such as rash or joint inflammation?	Causes may be infectious, neurological, endocrine, inflammatory, rheumatic, genetic, metabolic, electrolyte-induced, or drug-induced. Neuropathy primarily occurs in distal muscles. A rash is a sign of systemic lupus erythematosus. Repetitive actions exacerbate myasthenia gravis. Common neurological causes include demyelinating disorders, amyotrophic lateral sclerosis, Guillain-Barré syndrome, multiple sclerosis, myasthenia gravis, and degenerative disc disease.
Involuntary Movements or Tremors Have you noted any shaking or tremors? • Do they occur at rest? With movement? While maintaining a fixed position?	Resting tremors worsen at rest and decrease with activity; they are usually a symptom of Parkinson disease. Gradual onset of positional tremors suggests essential tremor; acute onset suggests a toxic or metabolic disorder. Intention tremors are worst with movement toward an object; they may result from multiple sclerosis (Touhy & Jett, 2012).
Balance/Coordination Difficulties Do you have any difficulty with balance, coordination, or walking?	Multiple sclerosis, Parkinson disease, stroke, and cerebral palsy are neurological causes of impaired gait. Refer to Chapter 21 for further information.
Dizziness or Vertigo Have you had any periods of dizziness? • Can you describe what it feels like without using the word "dizziness"? • Is it associated with nausea and vomiting? • Does changing positions make it better or worse?	Common causes include multiple sclerosis, Parkinson disease, cerebellar ischemia or infarction, benign or malignant neoplasms, and arteriovenous malformation of blood vessels in the brain. Positional changes usually worsen dizziness associated with the inner ear.

(table continues on page 664)

Signs/Symptoms	Rationale/Abnormal Findings
Difficulty Swallowing Have you had any difficulty swallowing? • Are any foods or liquids particularly difficult to consume?	**Dysphagia**, associated with CNS dysfunction, is a common symptom of stroke or neuromuscular disease. Generally, soft foods are more easily tolerated than chewy foods or liquids.
Intellectual Changes Have you noticed intellectual changes or difficulty with concentration, memory, or attention? (You also may ask family members or friends of patients about this.)	Common causes of memory loss include Alzheimer disease, dementia, depression, stroke, some medications, and metabolic imbalances. Refer to Chapter 28 for more information.
Speech/Language Difficulties Do you notice any difficulties with expression or comprehension of speech/language? • Any difficulty understanding speech? • Any difficulty forming words? • Any difficulty finding words and putting sentences together?	**Aphasia** is a common symptom of stroke, especially when it affects the speech centers in the left hemisphere (Touhey & Jett, 2012). Neuromuscular disease also affects the speech center, such as in Alzheimer disease or other forms of dementia.
Changes in Senses of Taste, Touch, or Smell Have you noticed alterations in touch, taste, or smell? • Any numbness, tingling, or hypersensitivity? • Where do you feel it?	**Paresthesia**, abnormal prickly or tingly sensations, is most common in the hands, arms, legs, and feet but can occur over other body parts. Causes include neurological disease or traumatic nerve damage such as carpal tunnel syndrome or cervical stenosis.
Lost or Blurred Vision Have you had a loss or blurring of vision in one or both eyes, or double vision? • When do you notice it? • Are there associated symptoms such as weakness or impaired speech? • Does this create any safety issues? Can you drive?	Central causes of **diplopia** (double vision) include stroke, vascular malformation, tumor, mass, trauma, meningitis, hemorrhage, and muscular sclerosis.
Hearing Loss or Tinnitus Have you noticed any hearing loss or tinnitus (ringing in the ears)? • Do you have a history of hearing loss? • Was it a sudden or slow onset? • Is it in one or both ears?	Common causes of sensorineural hearing loss include noise, autoimmune disorders, Ménière disease, ototoxic medications, and head trauma (Touhy & Jett, 2012). Refer to Chapter 14 for more information.

Documenting Normal Findings

Patient without headache, weakness, tremors; no difficulty with balance, coordination, or gait. Denies dizziness or vertigo; dysphagia; change in intellectual abilities; difficulty with concentration, memory, attention span, expression or comprehension of speech/language; alteration in sense of touch, taste, or smell. No loss or blurring of vision or diplopia; no hearing loss, tinnitus, altered sensation, numbness, or paresthesia.

Lifespan Considerations: Older Adults

Additional Questions	Rationale/Abnormal findings
Do you have a history of Alzheimer disease, dementia, stroke, Parkinson disease, or epilepsy?	These conditions are found more frequently in the elderly. Hypertension, atrial fibrillation, diabetes, congestive heart failure, chronic renal disease, female gender, previous cerebrovascular disease, and ischemic stroke increase risk of neurovascular disease (Touhy & Jett, 2012).
Have you fallen or had a head injury? *To the patient or caregiver*: Have you noticed any cognitive impairment; language difficulties (slow, slurred, and difficult or impossible to understand speech); hearing, taste, smell, or vision losses; and balance or emotional difficulties?	Those 75 years or older have the highest rate of traumatic brain injury–related hospitalization and death (NCIPC, 2013b). Falls are the most common cause, followed by car accidents.

Cultural Considerations

Additional Questions	Rationale/Abnormal Findings
From the chart, note ethnicity, gender, and area of residence.	These variables are relevant in some disorders (e.g., incidence of multiple sclerosis is higher in temperate climates; stroke occurs more often in African Americans than in Caucasian Americans).
Is there any history of head injury?	Hospitalization rates for traumatic brain injury are highest among African Americans and American Indians/Alaska Natives (NCIPC, 2013b). African Americans have the highest death rate from traumatic brain injury (NCIPC, 2013b). Certain military duties (e.g., paratrooper) increase risk for brain injury (NCIPC, 2013b).
Are you exposed to pesticides at work or home?	Maternal exposure to pesticides is linked to increased incidence of menstrual disorders, infertility, spontaneous abortion, stillbirth or infant death, low birth weight, and congenital abnormalities. Living in areas of pesticide use also increases risks. Implications for farm workers, especially migrant workers, are of particular concern (Kelley, Flocks, Economos, & McCauley, 2013). Folic acid deficiency also is linked to neural tube defects. Incidence of neural tube defects is highest among Hispanic women, partially as a result of exposure to pesticides (Brender, Felkner, Suarez, Canfield, & Henry, 2010; Tinker et al., 2013).
How old is your home? Do you know if the paint has lead in it?	Old lead-based paint continues to be the most significance source of lead exposure in the United States. The most common cause of lead exposure is dust and chips from deteriorating paint that included lead (manufactured before 1978). Exposure is higher in those living in old homes in poor repair (U.S. Environmental Protection Agency [EPA], 2013). Exposure to lead paint also is of concern for children; lead has been found in toys (EPA, 2013). Severe lead exposure can lead to damage to the brain and nervous system and death; mild exposure can lead to developmental delays and contribute to hyperactivity (EPA, 2013). Lead also can cause pregnancy difficulties and reproductive problems in both men and women (EPA, 2013).

Therapeutic Dialogue: Collecting Subjective Data

Remember Mr. Gardner, introduced at the beginning of this chapter, who was seen in the ED for acute stroke. He is confused, and health care providers are finding it challenging to communicate with him. The nurse needs to accurately assess the patient's neurological status; later, the nurse will interview Mr. Gardner to gather details about the lifestyle practices that have led to him having a stroke at a young age.

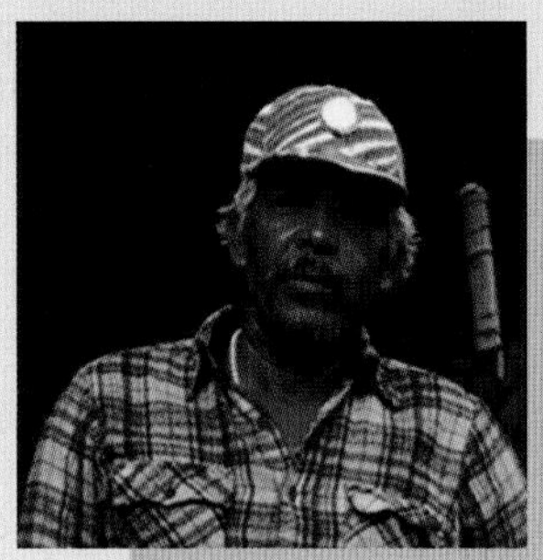

Nurse: Mr. Gardner, I would like to ask you a few questions to find out more about your stroke. Is that all right?

Mr. Gardner: (Nods head yes). (Speaks slowly) Can I have a cigarette?

Nurse: Your cigarettes are put away. I would like to ask you a few questions. Tell me where you are now.

Mr. Gardner: I'm at home. Who are you?

Nurse: I'm your nurse. My name is Trevor. You're in the hospital because you had a stroke. You're at Mountain View Hospital. Tell me what day it is today.

Mr. Gardner: Is it Wednesday? (correct answer is Monday)

Nurse: Today is Monday, July 10th, 2014. Tell me what your name is.

Mr. Gardner: Bill Gardner (smiles)

Critical Thinking Challenge

- Why did the nurse provide information on the correct day, date, and place? Provide rationale.
- Considering this patient's speech deficits, should the nurse ask open- or closed-ended questions for orientation? Provide rationale.
- How would you respond to the patient's request for a cigarette? Provide rationale.

Objective Data

Common and Specialty or Advanced Techniques

The routine head-to-toe assessment includes the most important and common techniques of neurological assessment. Examiners add specialty or advanced steps if concerns exist over a specific finding, as the clinical situation demands, or as a regular part of advanced practice (refer to the adjacent table.)

Equipment

- Penlight or flashlight
- Tongue blade
- Cotton swab
- Optional: tuning fork, reflex hammer, supplies for CNS testing

Preparation

You should anticipate that patients may attempt to minimize or to hide neurological deficits. For example, when you ask, "What year were you born?" the patient might say, "Well, if I told you that, then you'd know how old I was (and laughs)." You can return to this question later to evaluate long-term memory or change the question slightly to get a different response.

With healthy people, you can integrate the neurological examination with history taking. For example, you can evaluate function of the CNs during conversation and while observing the patient's facial expressions. You perform neurological screening for patients at high risk for problems, such as following a motor vehicle collision, or for patients with a documented history of previous neurological illness. You add techniques according to the specific injury or disease process as part of a focused neurological examination.

Basic Versus Focused/Specialty or Advanced Techniques Related to Neurological Assessment			
Technique	**Purpose**	**Screening or Registered Nurse Assessment**	**Focused or Advanced Practice Examination**
Assess LOC.	Alertness	X	
Assess attention.	Cognitive functions and processing	X	
Assess communication/speech.	Aphasia or dysarthria	X	
Inspect pupillary responses.	CN II function and ICP	X	
Check for abnormal posturing.	Severity of deficits	X	
Test function of CNs III–VII.	Basic evaluation	X	
Evaluate muscle tone and strength.	Upper and lower motor function	X	
Check gait and balance.	Basic cerebellar function	X	
Evaluate complex cognitive function.	Orientation, cognition, memory		X
Check function of CNs I–XII.	Comprehensive evaluation		X
Check coordination.	Advanced cerebellar function		X
Assess deep tendon and superficial reflexes.	Intact reflex arc		X

Comprehensive Physical Assessment

Physical examination of the nervous system provides information about its functional integrity. Because of how the nervous system is organized, a deficit or group of deficits often provides the information needed to localize the area of pathology. This information, combined with the history and diagnostic testing, allows determination of the nature (e.g., traumatic, neoplastic, vascular, infectious, degenerative) of the pathological process.

Nurses mainly use inspection and palpation in neurological examination. Clinicians use percussion when testing DTRs; they limit auscultation of the nervous system to evaluation of vascular sufficiency.

Begin the comprehensive neurological assessment with general observation of how the patient relates to the environment. Observe the patient during initial contact, before the formal process of history taking begins, and also during the entire encounter with the patient. When observing for level of alertness and responsiveness, focus on attention span, mood, and affect. Behavioral and emotional status can be described as calm, cooperative, restless, combative, confused, agitated, or not testable. Assessment of general appearance includes grooming, cleanliness and arrangement of clothing, use of prosthetic devices (e.g., eyeglasses, hearing aids), and any visible evidence of trauma or other surface abnormalities (e.g., birthmarks; skin tumors; asymmetry of face, gaze, or extremities).

Often, this initial interaction allows you to assess speech and language, general movement, and gait and balance. These are discussed in depth in Chapter 9. The initial interaction with the patient often provides data that directs further focused assessment of individual functions during the physical examination.

Technique and Normal Findings	Abnormal Findings
Level of Consciousness Begin by assessing LOC. The initial outcome determines the extent and method of the rest of the examination. People visibly express LOC through degree of response to stimulus, with the highest level being spontaneous alertness. Be sure to apply stimulus in the correct order (see Table 22.2), moving to a more intense stimulus only when the previous attempt is unsuccessful. First arouse the patient by speech, then by touch, and then by pressure to the nail beds (Fig. 22.12) or by pinching a large muscle mass on an extremity.	The GCS (see Box 22.2) can facilitate the assessment of patients with impaired consciousness. Primarily, the GCS determines the degree of conscious impairment by evaluating behavioral responses in three areas: motor responses, verbal responses, and eye opening. The examiner lists, for each category, the patient's best response. The GCS weights each response numerically to quantify overall response. The minimum score is 3; the maximum is 15.

(table continues on page 668)

TABLE 22.2 **Assessment of Consciousness: Applying Stimulation**

Order of Stimulation	Example
Spontaneous	Enter room and observe arousal.
Normal voice	State patient's name; ask him or her to open eyes.
Loud voice	Use loud voice if no response to normal voice.
Tactile (touch)	Touch patient's shoulder or arm lightly.
Noxious stimulation (pain)	Apply nail bed pressure to elicit pain response, telling patient that you will be applying pressure.

Technique and Normal Findings (continued)

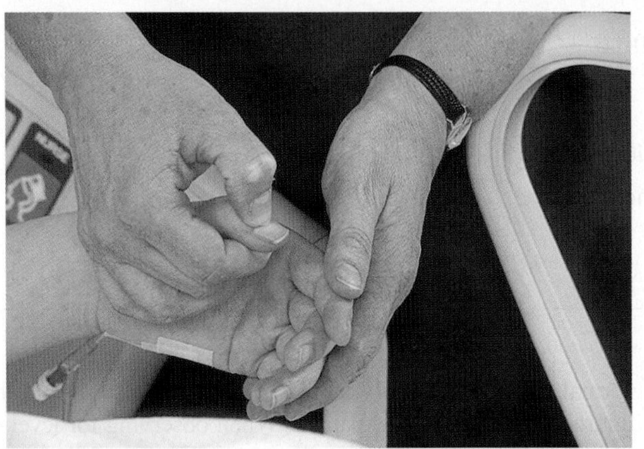

Figure 22.12 The nurse is applying pressure to the nail beds to arouse a patient who has not responded to speech or touch.

⚠ *SAFETY ALERT*

Do not pinch a small fold of skin, which may cause soft tissue trauma.

Pressure to the nail beds also can be useful in determining gross motor function when the patient's LOC makes formal strength testing impossible.

Objective description of the patient's response is critical to evaluating changes in LOC over time. A wide range of terms has been used to describe LOC (Table 22.3). Despite careful definition within a particular institution, these terms are by nature subjective and must be used carefully to allow accurate comparisons of serial assessments by different practitioners. Description of specific response to stimulus provides the best chance of identifying change that may initially be subtle.

Patient alert, opens eyes spontaneously.

Cognitive Function

If results of LOC assessment show that the patient can interact, evaluate cognitive function. (Many components of cognitive evaluation may have been completed during history taking). Remember to conduct specific cognitive tests so that patients do not feel that their intelligence is being challenged.

Abnormal Findings (continued)

- Motor response is scored according to the most functional response from either upper extremity (e.g., if a patient follows commands with the right hand but not the left, the motor score indicates ability to follow commands).
- Verbal response includes orientation, conversation, speech, sounds, and no response as an indicator of cognitive function.
- Eye opening is in response to activity in the environment, verbal cues, nonnoxious stimuli, or noxious stimuli pressure as an indicator of LOC.

Although accepted as a relatively objective assessment of consciousness, the GCS itself is also vulnerable to differences in scoring of the same patient situation, especially in eye opening, verbal responses and the motor area (Adeleye, Owolabi, Rablu, & Orimadegun, 2012). Consistency in training staff to use the GCS, with periodic review, may be needed to produce reliable results. GCS is predictive of outcome from a traumatic brain injury when combined with the patient's age and pupillary response.

(table continues on page 669)

TABLE 22.3 **Levels of Consciousness**	
Term	**Definition**
Alert wakefulness	Patient appreciates the environment and responds quickly to stimuli.
Confusion	Patient is disoriented to time, place, or person; has shortened attention span; shows poor memory; or has difficulty following commands.
Drowsiness	Patient responds to stimuli appropriately but with delay and slowness; may respond to some but not all (also described as **lethargy** or **obtunded** state).
Stupor	Patient is unresponsive and can be aroused only briefly by vigorous, repeated stimulation.
Coma	Patient is unresponsive and generally cannot be aroused.

From Hickey, J. V. (2009). The neurological physical examination and neurological assessment. In J. V. Hickey (Ed.), *The clinical practice of neurological and neurosurgical nursing* (6th ed.). Philadelphia, PA: Lippincott Williams & Wilkins.

Technique and Normal Findings (continued)

Cognitive function includes basic orientation, concentration, and attention span as well as more complex functions such as memory, calculation ability, abstract thinking, reasoning, and judgment. Complex cognitive function can be tested informally whenever you interact with the patient, especially when teaching, establishing goals and priorities, and planning for home care. Doing so provides information about the patient's ability to learn, to reason, and to make judgments. See Chapter 9 for discussions of assessment of attention, concentration, memory, calculation, and abstract thinking.

Abnormal Findings (continued)

The Mini-Mental State Examination (MMSE) is a tool commonly used to assess dementia. The features are presented in Box 22.3 (Folstein, Folstein, & McHugh, 1975). See Chapter 9 for the Mini-Cog tool. Many of these tools are copyrighted and have specific directions for use.

BOX 22.3 Categories of Questions for the MiniMental Status Examination

Category	Description
Orientation to time	From date of birth to current time, day, date. Orientation to time has been correlated with future decline.
Orientation to place	Ask, where are you? This is sometimes narrowed down to address, or to floor or room number.
Registration	Have the patient repeat named prompts (e.g., pony or table) right away
Attention and calculation	Calculate serial sevens, or spell the word "world" backwards. It has been suggested that serial sevens may be more appropriate in a population where English is not the first language.
Recall	State the items from registration, about 1 or 2 minutes later
Language	Identify a pencil and a watch
Repetition	Speak back a phrase
Complex commands	May include three-step directions. May involve drawing figure shown.

Patients may also be asked about items related to functional ability, such as telling the time using a clock face. In general, when a patient complains of memory problems, a brief screening test is needed to establish whether there is a cause for concern that would prompt further investigation or referral (Gill et al., 2013).

(table continues on page 670)

Technique and Normal Findings (continued)	Abnormal Findings (continued)
Orientation. Assess orientation by directly questioning the patient about person, place, and time. Display sensitivity to the patient's environment and communication ability. Asking "What month (year, season) is it?" may be more reasonable than "What day is it?" if the patient has been hospitalized for several days with few cues about day of the week. For patients with **aphasia** (impaired ability to interpret or use the symbols of language), you may need to ask about place through "yes" or "no" questions rather than "Where are you?" Ask the patient to identify himself or herself and also to identify visitors or family pictures. Also ask the patient about his or her age (National Institutes of Health [NIH], 2013). The patient is "oriented."	
Communication (Speech/Language) Communication is another function to assess continuously throughout the interaction. Observe clarity and fluency of speech through basic conversation. Ask the patient to repeat words or phrases with multiple combinations of consonants and vowels (e.g., "aggravating conversation") to test speech articulation. Formal testing includes assessment of comprehension, repetition, naming, reading, and writing (see Chapter 9). Speech is clear and articulate.	Deficits in articulation are referred to as **dysarthria.** In some cases, distinguishing speech/language deficits from confusion is difficult. Typically, those patients with speech/language deficits behave appropriately to situation and environment, especially to visual cues. This is less likely in confused patients. Consultation with a speech pathologist for formal assessment of communication and cognitive function will clarify the type of deficit. Patients with a language deficit might be unable to express needs but usually can follow simple commands (e.g., "Open and close your eyes," "Squeeze your hand"; NIH, 2013). Confused states can be described as acute (delirium) or chronic (dementia, with multiple causes).
Pupillary Response Basic assessment of pupils includes size, shape, and reactivity to light (see Chapter 13). Darken the room and instruct the patient to gaze into the distance to dilate the pupils. Ask him or her to keep looking straight ahead. Hold a light on the side (avoid pointing it into the eye). Observe for nystagmus in one or both eyes. Bringing the light in quickly from the side, observe the reaction of the same and then the other pupil for the consensual light reflex. Use a preprinted guide or scale on a penlight to identify the size. Record both the initial size and response size as R 6 → 4, L6 → 4. Pupils are round, equal, and constrict briskly (within 1 second) in response to light, both directly and consensually (when one pupil constricts to light, the other does, too). This is also recorded as PERRL (*p*upils *e*qual, *r*ound, *r*eactive to *l*ight). Test accommodation by having the person shift the gaze from a distant to near object. *Accommodation includes constriction of the pupils and convergence of the eyes bilaterally.* When documented with the pupils, it is charted as PERRLA (A is for accommodation).	Describe the reaction as brisk, sluggish, fixed, pinpoint or blown. **Nystagmus** is a jerking movement of the eye that can be quick and fluttering or slow and rolling, similar to a tremor. Causes include medications (e.g., antiseizure medications), cerebellar disease, weakness in the extraocular muscles, and damage to CN III (oculomotor). See also Chapter 13 and Table 22.7 at the end of this chapter.

(table continues on page 671)

Technique and Normal Findings (continued)	Abnormal Findings (continued)
Also assess the gaze for eye contact and drifting. If the eyes deviate, assess whether it is conjugate (move together) or dysconjugate (move separately). ■ Gaze is purposeful and conjugate.	
Abnormal Movements Observation of abnormal movements is an additional element of inspection. They include abnormal reflex posturing (spontaneous or in response to painful stimuli) and involuntary movements caused by various neurological disorders affecting the extrapyramidal motor system. ■ Movements are smooth and symmetric.	Abnormal posturing includes flexion abnormal, extension abnormal, hemiplegia, quadriplegia, and paralysis (see Table 22.8 at the end of this chapter). Abnormal movements include tic, myoclonus, fasciculation, dystonia, tremor, chorea, and athetosis (see Table 22.9 at the end of this chapter).
Cranial Nerve Testing There are 12 pairs of CNs. Each member of the pair innervates structures on the same side from which it arises (the ipsilateral side). A lesion of the CN or its nucleus results in an ipsilateral peripheral nerve deficit. A lesion in the cerebral cortex in the area that supplies the CN nucleus, or the tracts traveling from the cerebral cortex to the CN nucleus, results in a contralateral CNS deficit. Example: Facial weakness caused by a lesion in the right frontal motor control center occurs on the left side of the face. A lesion affecting the right facial nerve itself produces weakness on the entire right side of the face. Aside from a thorough screening assessment for a suspected problem, it is rarely necessary to assess complete CN function (see Table 22.4). Examples of selected testing include the following: • Observe functional near and far vision; assess pupil constriction and EOMs; assess corneal reflexes (included earlier under acute assessment) if LOC is acutely impaired. • Observe facial expression, test facial strength and sensation, observe uvula rise with "ah," test gag reflex, and observe tongue movement when assessing potential for dysphagia (difficulty swallowing). Alertness and attention span are also relevant for this purpose. ■ PERRLA, EOMs intact. Positive gag and corneal reflexes. Facial strength 41 with intact sensation bilaterally.	Use of the gag reflex as part of assessment varies widely. Many practitioners continue to use absence of gag reflex as an indicator for risk of aspiration; however, they may overestimate risk when absence of gag reflex is the only deficit found. Conversely, they may miss other risks if gag reflex is the only function tested and found intact (Leder, 1997). Refer to Table 22.4 for a description of unexpected findings.
Motor Function Examination of the motor system focuses on assessment of symmetry of muscle bulk, tone, and strength.	Distinct patterns of abnormality are found with CNS motor pathway (upper motor neuron [UMN]) lesions compared with peripheral motor nerve pathway (lower motor neuron [LMN]) lesions. See Table 22.10 at the end of this chapter for a description of UMN and LMN deficits.

(table continues on page 674)

TABLE 22.4 **Summary of Cranial Nerve Assessment**

Cranial Nerve	Technique	Abnormal Findings
I. Olfactory (sensory)	Usually deferred, CN I is tested when symptoms involve smell or abnormal findings warrant evaluation. First assess patency by closing off one nostril and asking the patient to inhale; perform the same technique on the opposite side. Occlude one nostril. Tell the patient to close the eyes, place a familiar scent near the open nostril, and ask the patient to inhale and identify the scent. Repeat on the opposite side. Commonly used fragrances include orange, peppermint, cinnamon, and coffee.	Only a few neurological conditions are linked with olfactory deficits. It is important to test for patency of the naris, which can influence ability to smell. Other influences include allergies, mucosal inflammation, increased age, and excessive tobacco smoking. An olfactory tract lesion may compromise ability to discriminate odors (anosmia).
II. Optic (sensory)	Monitor while working with the patient. Ask him or her to identify how many fingers you are holding up. Use the Snellen chart to evaluate far vision and near vision with small print. Test visual fields using confrontation. See Chapter 13 for tests of visual acuity and visual fields.	Visual acuity less than 20/20 is abnormal. Inability to read small print is common in older adults as a result of age-related loss of accommodation.
III. Oculomotor (motor), IV. trochlear (motor), and VI. abducens (motor)	Assess pupils for size, shape, and equality. Assess the six cardinal positions of gaze. Observe for nystagmus in one or both eyes	Nystagmus may manifest as quick and jerky movements or slow pendulous movements, where the eye moves back and forth in the socket. Note whether the movement is fine or coarse and constant or intermittent. Check if the plane of movement is either up and down or back and forth. Nystagmus is associated with disease of the vestibular system, cerebellum, or brainstem.
V. Trigeminal (sensory and motor), includes corneal	Evaluate sensory function by touch and motor function with movement. To evaluate the sensory component, ask the patient to close the eyes. Using a cotton swab and broken tongue blade or swab, ask the patient to identify sharp or dull sensations when he or she feels them. Be sure to evaluate all three divisions of the nerve at the scalp (ophthalmic), cheek (maxillary), and chin (mandibular) areas on each side. Evaluate motor function by observing the face for atrophy, deviation, and fasciculations. Ask the patient to tightly clench the teeth; palpate over the jaw for masseter muscle symmetry. Ask the patient to open the jaw against resistance; normal movement is symmetrical. The corneal reflex is not normally tested unless motor or sensory abnormalities are noted. Have the patient remove any contact lenses. Instruct him or her to look up. Inform the patient that you will touch the eye with a cotton swab wisp. Bring the swab in from the side and lightly touch the cornea, not the conjunctiva. Normally the patient blinks bilaterally as stimulation is applied.	Decreased or dulled sensation, weakness, or assymetrical movements are unexpected findings associated with CN V. A weak blink from facial weakness may result from paralysis of CN V or VII. A depressed or absent corneal response is common in contact lens wearers.

(table continues on page 673

TABLE 22.4 Summary of Cranial Nerve Assessment *(continued)*

Cranial Nerve	Technique	Abnormal Findings
VII. Facial (sensory and motor)	Assess by evaluating taste. Place sweet, sour, salty, and bitter solutions on the anterior two thirds of the tongue on both sides; also test the posterior one third of the tongue for CN IX. The patient should properly identify the taste. Evaluate motor function by observing facial movements during conversation. Additionally, the patient completes facial movements and symmetry is observed. Ask the patient to raise the eyebrows, squeeze the eyes shut, wrinkle the forehead, frown, smile, show teeth, purse lips, and puff out the cheeks. Normal movements are strong and symmetrical.	Fasciculations or tremors are abnormal. Asymmetric movements may be noted with the lower eyelid sagging, loss of the nasolabial fold, or mouth drooping. These findings are common following a stroke or with Bell palsy.
VIII. Acoustic (sensory)	Evaluate hearing during normal conversation using a simple whisper test or with an audiometer. Refer to Chapter 14 for more information.	Inability to hear conversation is abnormal; note the presence of a hearing aid.
IX. Glossopharyngeal (sensory and motor)	Evaluate sensory function with CN VII. Evaluate motor function with CN X upon swallowing.	Impaired taste or swallowing is common following a stroke.
X. Vagus (sensory and motor), includes gag reflex	Evaluate the motor component by asking the patient to open the mouth and stick out the tongue, which should be symmetrical. Place a tongue blade on the middle of the tongue and have the patient say "ah"; observe the uvula and soft palate for symmetry. Evaluate the sensory component by stimulating the gag reflex, which is tested only when a problem is suspected. Inform the patient that you will be touching the posterior pharyngeal wall and it may cause gagging. Observe for upward movement of the palate and contraction of the pharyngeal muscles with the gag reflex.	Injury to the vagus or glossopharyngeal nerve causes the uvula to deviate from midline. Asymmetry of the soft palate or tonsillar pillars is also abnormal. An impaired gag reflex, coughing during oral feeding, and changes in voice after swallowing are all associated with aspiration. Closely evaluate patients with any of these symptoms.
XI. Spinal accessory (motor)	Evaluate the sternomastoid and trapezius muscles for bulk, tone, strength, and symmetry. Ask the patient to press against resistance on the opposite side of the chin. Also ask the patient to shrug the shoulders against resistance. The movements should be strong and symmetrical.	Weakness or asymmetry in movement accompanies neurological and musculoskeletal problems.
XII. Hypoglossal (motor)	Evaluate this function with CN X. First, inspect the tongue; next, ask the patient to stick out the tongue and observe for symmetry. Ask the patient to say, "light, tight, dynamite" and note that the letters l, t, d, and n are clear and distinct.	Fasciculations, asymmetry, atrophy, or deviation from midline may occur with general neuromuscular conditions or lesions of the hypoglossal nerve.

Technique and Normal Findings (continued)	Abnormal Findings (continued)
Muscle Bulk and Tone. Inspect muscle bulk by observing and palpating muscle groups to check for any wasting (atrophy). This inspection provides some information about muscle tone as well. The relaxed muscle shows some muscular tension. To further assess tone, determine degree of resistance of muscle groups to passive stretch. Instruct the patient to relax totally and to let the examiner move his or her limbs. Commonly tested groups include deltoids, biceps, triceps, hamstrings, and quadriceps. ■ Good muscle bulk and tone.	If there is absolutely no resistance to movement, the muscles are said to be **flaccid** or **atonic.** If the tone seems to be only decreased or "flabby," note the finding as **hypotonia.** Increased resistance of the muscles to passive stretch is called **hypertonia. Spasticity** also can occur with UMN disorders. It is characterized by increased resistance to rapid passive stretch, especially in flexor muscle groups in the upper extremities, resulting from hyperexcitability of the stretch reflex. In certain conditions, this resistance is strongest on initiation of the movement and "gives way" as the examiner slowly continues the movement. This characteristic has prompted the use of the term **clasp-knife spasticity**; it describes the type of hypertonicity noted in patients with Parkinson disease. **Rigidity** is characterized by a steady persistent resistance to passive stretch in both flexor and extensor muscle groups. This phenomenon has led to the descriptive phrases **"lead-pipe" rigidity** or "plastic" rigidity. **Cogwheel rigidity** is seen in patients with Parkinson disease and is manifested by a ratchet-like jerking noted in the extremity on passive movement.
Muscle Strength. Assess muscle strength (pyramidal motor system) by asking the patient to move extremities or selected muscle groups both independently and against the examiner's resistance. In addition to the muscle groups mentioned earlier, evaluate strength by hand grasp, pronator drift, dorsiflexion, and plantar flexion. Grade strength of movement on a scale of 0–5+: 0—No muscle contraction 1—Barely detectable, flicker 2—Active movement with gravity eliminated 3—Active movement against gravity 4—Active movement against some resistance 5—Active movement against full resistance *Strength is 4–5+.*	Motor strength of 0–3+ indicates weakness. Also can describe strength as the following: Moves well upon request Weak movement upon request Moves well when stimulated Weak movement when stimulated No movement
During conversation, observe for ptosis or facial palsy (NIH, 2013). An early or mild upper extremity weakness can be detected by observing for **pronator drift.** Ask the patient to close the eyes and outstretch the arms straight ahead with palms upward (supinated) for 10 seconds (Fig. 22.13). ■ The patient extends the hands for 10 seconds without drifting. 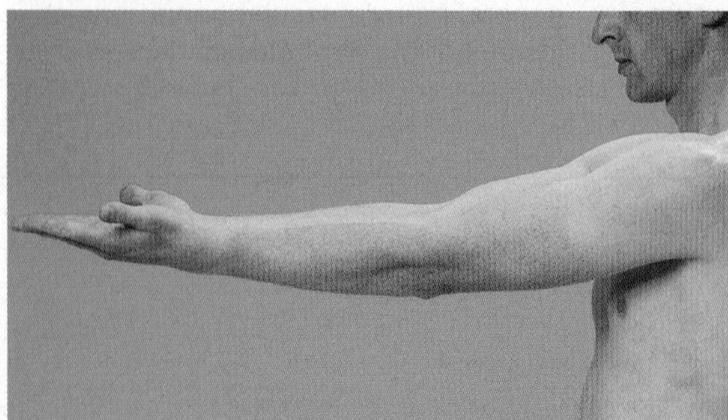 **Figure 22.13** Assessing for pronator drift.	Pronation of the hands and downward drift of the arm indicate weakness. Pronator drift is indication of a subtle UMN disorder.

(table continues on page 675)

Technique and Normal Findings (continued)	Abnormal Findings (continued)
Also ask the patient to press the feet against resistance to assess strength or extend the leg at 30 degrees; drift is present if the leg falls before 5 seconds (NIH, 2013). Refer to Chapter 21 for a complete description of strength testing.	
Gait and posture combine functions of the pyramidal and extrapyramidal motor systems, other cerebellar function, and sensory systems. If possible, ask the patient to walk down a corridor. Points to observe include smoothness of gait, position of feet (narrow vs. wide base), height and length of step, and symmetry of arm and leg movement. Also ask the patient to walk on heels and toes, then tandem-walk (i.e., heel-to-toe in a straight line) (Fig. 22.14). The patient walks smoothly without swaying. 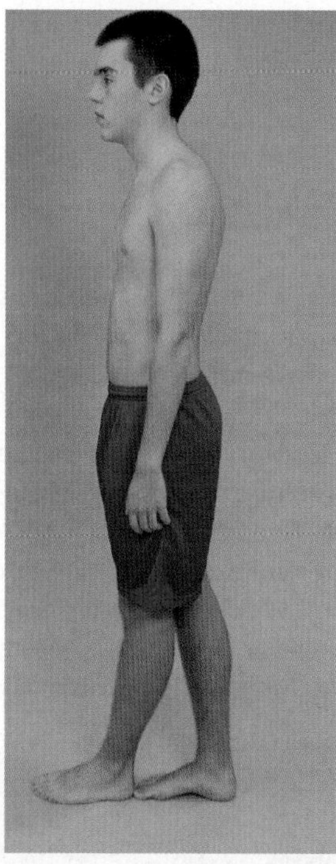 **Figure 22.14** Assessing the tandem walk to evaluate gait and posture.	Abnormal gaits include spastic hemiparesis, scissors, parkinsonian, cerebellar ataxia, sensory ataxia, waddling, dystonia, and athetoid (see Table 22.11 at the end of this chapter).
In the **Romberg test**, ask the patient to stand with feet together and arms at sides (Fig. 22.15). Note any swaying (stand close enough to prevent the patient from falling). Ask the patient to close the eyes during the Romberg test for additional assessment. Slight swaying may be normal because visual cues help humans maintain balance. The patient can maintain position without opening the eyes.	Moderate swaying with eyes open and closed indicates vestibulocerebellar dysfunction. Pronounced increase in swaying (sometimes ending with a fall) with the eyes closed usually indicates a lesion in the posterior columns of the spinal cord.

(table continues on page 676)

Technique and Normal Findings (continued)	Abnormal Findings (continued)

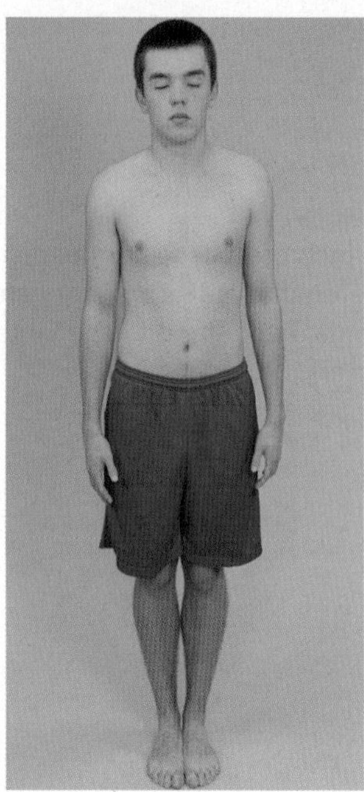

Figure 22.15 Positioning for the Romberg test.

Cerebellar Function

Assessment of finger-to-nose coordination or rapid alternating movements tests upper extremity cerebellar function. Ask the patient to touch the tip of your finger with the tip of his or her forefinger (test each hand separately) and then to touch his or her own nose and to repeat this maneuver several times while you move your finger (Fig. 22.16). To assess rapid alternating movements, instruct the patient to slap his or her thigh with first the palm of the hand and then the back as fast as possible (Fig. 22.17). It is not uncommon for people to perform better with their dominant hand.

Ataxia is unsteady, wavering movement with inability to touch the target. During rapid alternating movements, lack of coordination is **adiadochokinesia**. Deficits in any of these maneuvers indicate an ipsilateral cerebellar lesion. Note any tremor. Other signs of cerebellar dysfunction can include hypotonia, nystagmus, and dysarthric speech. Dysarthric speech noted with cerebellar lesions may exhibit a peculiar quality called "scanning speech," which is characterized by alternating patterns of slowness and explosiveness as each syllable is spoken. Refer to Table 22.11 at the end of the chapter.

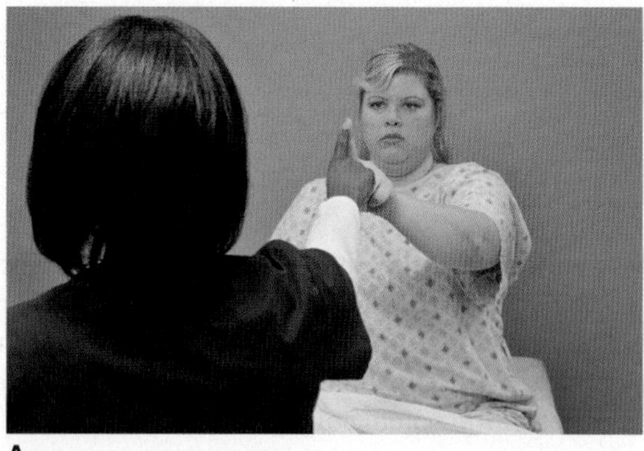

A B

Figure 22.16 Assessing coordination function. **A.** The patient touches the examiner's finger with her forefinger. **B.** The patient touches her own nose.

Assess lower extremities by the heel-to-shin test. With the patient seated or supine, ask him or her to take the heel of one foot and, without deviation, move it steadily down the shin of the other leg.

Well coordinated movements.

(table continues on page 677)

Technique and Normal Findings (continued)	Abnormal Findings (continued)
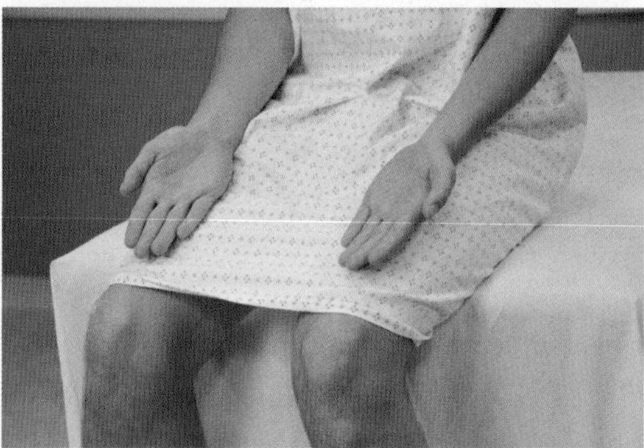 Figure 22.17 Assessing rapid alternating movements.	
Sensory Function When assessing sensation, it is important that the patient's eyes remain closed to avoid visual cues from influencing responses. Have the patient identify where he or she feels the sensation, but avoid cueing the patient by asking, "Do you feel this?" Allow 2 seconds between each stimulus to avoid summation (in which the patient perceives frequent small stimulations as one long stimulation). Begin with light stimulation and proceed with increased pressure until the patient reports a sensation. Stronger stimulation is needed over the central torso and back than on areas that are more sensitive. Observe areas of sensory decrease or loss. Compare findings between sides. Screening may be performed by testing the most distal areas and proceeding centrally if deficits are noted. Testing involves the arms (not hands), legs, trunk, and face (NIH, 2013). Complete testing of all nerves is rare. Clinically, patterns of sensory loss are assessed depending on the problem or area of injury.	When interpreting sensory deficits, keep in mind that this testing includes the peripheral nerves, sensory tracts, and cortical perception. Consider the patient's clinical situation and whether the problem is generalized or specific, such as trauma to a nerve. Spinal cord injury generally follows the pattern of the dermatome, whereas sensory loss in diabetic neuropathy is distal. See also Table 22.12 at the end of this chapter.
Light Touch. Pull at the end of a cotton swab so that it becomes wispy. Ask the patient to close the eyes and apply light touch to the skin with the swab (Fig. 22.18). Ask the patient to state where he or she feels the sensation. Patient correctly identifies light touch.	Hyperesthesia refers to increased touch sensation. Anesthesia refers to absent touch sensation. Reduced touch sensation is hypesthesia.
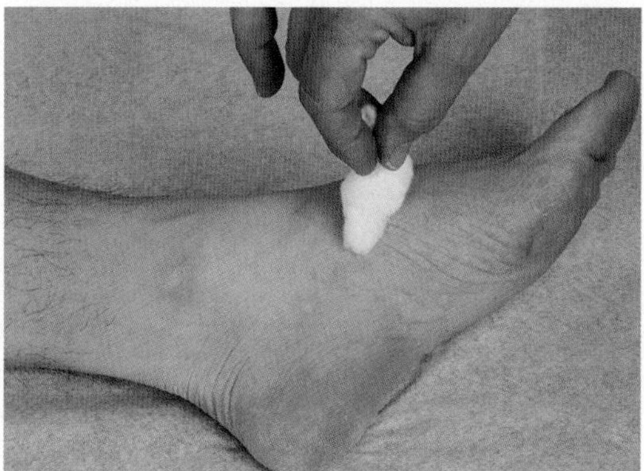 Figure 22.18 Applying a cotton swab to assess light touch sensation.	

(table continues on page 678)

Technique and Normal Findings (continued)	Abnormal Findings (continued)
Superficial Pain Sensation. Break a tongue blade or cotton swab so that the end is sharp. Ask the patient to close the eyes; lightly touch the patient's skin with the sharp end. Ask the patient to state where he or she feels the sensation. Pain sensation is intact.	Hyperalgesia refers to increased pain sensation. Analgesia refers to absent pain sensation. Reduced pain sensation is hypalgesia. **SAFETY ALERT** *Patients with neuropathy need to be taught to visually inspect their feet because they may have injuries that go unnoticed.*
Temperature Sensation. (This test is not usually performed.) Test temperature sense only if pain or touch sensation is abnormal. Use one prong of a tuning fork that has been warmed with the hands or use test tubes containing warm and cold water. Ask the patient to close the eyes. Touch the skin with warm or cold objects. Have the patient identify when he or she feels warm or cold. Temperature sensation is intact.	Abnormal temperature sensation is common in neuropathies. **SAFETY ALERT** *Patients with neuropathy need to learn to use a body part with good sensation to determine the temperature of hot surfaces. Getting into a bath that is too hot can cause inadvertent burns to the feet. Similarly, a patient with neuropathy can be easily burned by a heating pad that is too hot.*
Point Localization. Ask the patient to close the eyes. Using a finger, gently touch the patient on the hands, lower arms, abdomen, lower legs, and feet. Have the patient identify where he or she feels the sensation but avoid cueing the patient by asking, "Do you feel this?" Observe areas of sensory loss. Compare side to side. Point localization is intact.	Observe the pattern of sensory loss by mapping it out during testing. "Stocking-glove" distribution suggests peripheral nerves; dermatomal distribution suggests isolated nerves or nerve roots; reduced sensation below a certain level is associated with the spinal cord. A crossed face–body pattern suggests the brainstem, and hemisensory loss suggests a lesion or stroke (Weiner, Goetz, Shin, & Lewis, 2010).
Vibration Sensation. (This test is not usually done.) Strike a low-pitched tuning fork on the side or heel of the hand to produce vibrations. Ask the patient to close the eyes. Holding the fork at the base, place it over body prominences, beginning at the most distal location. The toes, ankle, shin, finger joints, wrist, elbow, shoulder, and sternum may all be tested (Fig. 22.19). If the sensation is felt at the most distal point, no further testing is necessary. Ask the patient to state where the sensation is felt and when it disappears. To stop the sensation, dampen the tuning fork by pressing on the tongs. Vibration sense is intact. 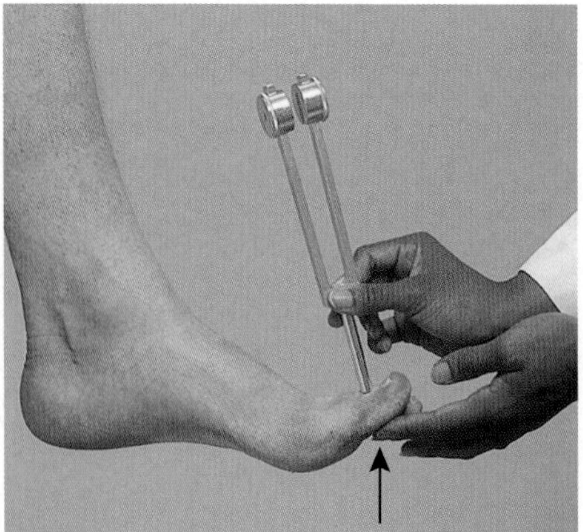 **Figure 22.19** Testing vibration sensation.	Peripheral neuropathy is more severe distally and improves centrally. It is a common consequence of peripheral vascular disease and diabetic neuropathy. Often, vibration sense is the first lost. With damage to a specific dermatome, the line of sensory loss is usually marked and specific.

(table continues on page 679)

Technique and Normal Findings (continued)	Abnormal Findings (continued)
Motion and Position Sense. This is only done if other findings are abnormal. Ask the patient to close the eyes. Move the distal joints of the patient's fingers and then the toes up or down. If the patient cannot identify these movements, test the next most proximal joints (e.g., wrist if finger movement is not sensed). Motion and position sense are intact.	Involuntary, writhing, snakelike movements of a limb (athetosis) result from loss of position sense. The brain cannot sense where the limb is in space so the limb moves on its own; the patient must use vision to consciously control the limb's movements.
Stereognosis. This test evaluates cortical sensory function and is not usually done. Ask the patient to close the eyes and identify a familiar object (e.g., coin, key) placed in the palm (Fig. 22.20). The patient correctly identifies the object. 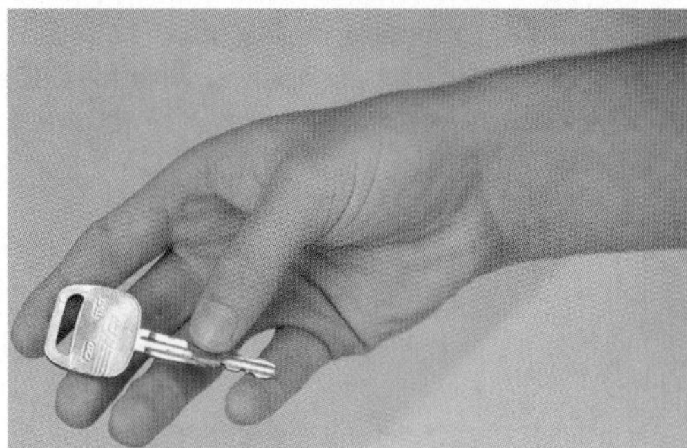 **Figure 22.20** Testing stereognosis.	Inability to identify objects correctly (**astereognosis**) may result from damage to the sensory cortex caused by stroke.
Graphesthesia. This test also evaluates cortical sensory function and is not usually done. Use a blunt object to trace a number (e.g., "8") on the patient's palm. Ask the patient to identify which number has been traced (graphesthesia) (Fig. 22.21). The patient correctly identifies the number. 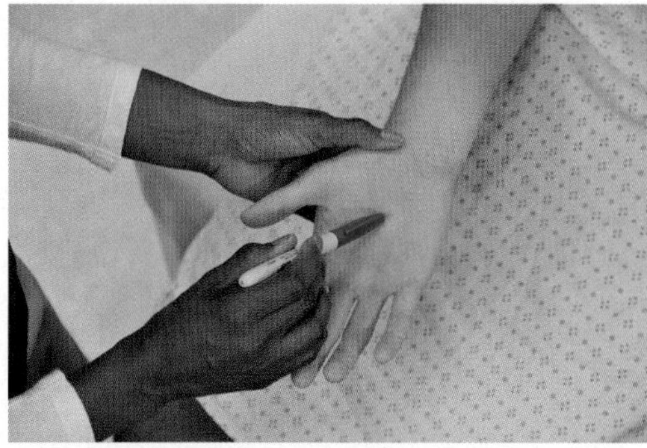 **Figure 22.21** Assessing graphesthesia.	Cortical sensory function may be compromised following a stroke.
Two-Point Discrimination. This test is only done if other findings are abnormal. Ask the patient to close the eyes. Hold the blunt end of two cotton swabs approximately 5 cm (2 in.) apart and move them together until the patient feels them as one point (the ends of an opened paperclip may also be used). The fingertips are most sensitive, with a minimal distance of 3–8 mm (about ¼ in.), whereas the upper arms and thighs are least sensitive, with a minimal distance of 75 mm (about 3 in.). Generally, there is more discrimination distally than centrally.	Cortical sensory function may be lost with a stroke. *(table continues on page 680)*

Technique and Normal Findings (continued)	Abnormal Findings (continued)
Extinction. This test is only done if other findings are abnormal. Ask the patient to close the eyes. At the same time, touch a body area on both sides. Ask the patient to state where he or she perceives the touch. ■ Sensations are felt on both sides.	Cortical sensory function may be lost after a stroke. The stimulus on the opposite side of the damaged cortex may be lost or reduced.
Reflex Testing Reflex testing includes muscle stretch reflexes (DTRs) and superficial (cutaneous) reflexes. Pathological reflexes may or may not be elicited.	
DTRs. Advanced practice nurses and physicians generally test DTRs. Nevertheless, direct care nurses should understand how to test them to better incorporate the findings of other practitioners into identifying patterns of neurological deficit.	**Clonus** is characterized by alternating flexion/extension movements (jerking) in response to a continuous muscle stretch. In unconscious patients, DTRs may be tested in the usual manner; however, depth of coma alters the response. Deep coma is associated with loss of all reflexes as well as loss of muscle stretch and tone.
DTRs tested include biceps, triceps, brachioradialis, patellar, and Achilles (Table 22.5). These reflexes are observed for symmetry when tested bilaterally and for briskness of reflex movement. DTRs are graded on a scale of 0–4, with 0 representing absent reflexes and 4 corresponding to significantly hyperactive responses. • 4+—Very brisk, hyperactive with clonus • 3+—Brisker than average • 2+—Average, normal • 1+—Diminished; low normal • 0—No response	
The reflex response depends on the force of the stimulus, accurate location of the striking area over the tendon, and patient's relaxation level. Refer to Chapter 3 for use of the reflex hammer and technique. To ensure accurate location, have the patient flex the muscle to find the tendon and then relax it for testing. Pathological reflexes are primitive responses that indicate loss of cortical inhibition (see Table 22.13 at the end of this chapter). ■ DTRs are 2+ bilaterally without clonus.	
Superficial Reflexes. Superficial reflexes are elicited by stimulation of the skin. These are done only when other findings are abnormal. Record the response to stimulation as present, absent, or equivocal (i.e., present or difficult to determine).	
Plantar Response. Test by stroking the sole of the foot with a blunt instrument such as the edge of a tongue blade or the handle of a reflex hammer. Apply the stimulus firmly but gently to the lateral aspect, beginning at the heel and stopping short of the base of the toes. The toes flex (a flexor–plantar response).	Pathological reflexes include **abnormal plantar reflexes** and the **triple flexion response**. With abnormal plantar reflexes, the great toe extends upward and the other toes fan out (an extensor–plantar response, or Babinski sign; Fig. 22.22). Triple flexion describes reflex withdrawal of the lower extremity to plantar stimulus through flexion of ankle, knee, and hip.

(table continues on page 682)

TABLE 22.5 **Deep Tendon Reflexes**

Deep Tendon Reflex: Level Tested	Technique
Biceps: C5 and C6 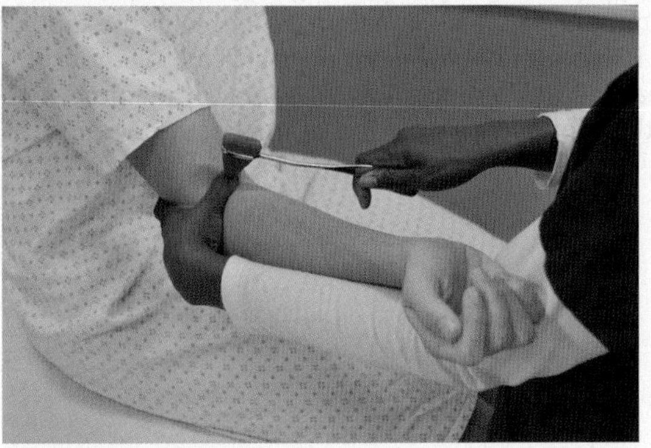	Have the patient partially flex the elbow and place the palm down. To assist with relaxation, the patient may rest the arm against the nurse's. Place one finger or thumb on the biceps tendon. Strike the finger or thumb with the reflex hammer briskly so that the impact is delivered through the digit to the biceps tendon. Observe for flexion at the elbow and contraction of the biceps muscle. If the patient's reflexes are symmetrically diminished or absent, ask the patient to clench the teeth or squeeze one hand tight with the opposite hand to aid in detection (reinforcement).
Triceps: C6–8 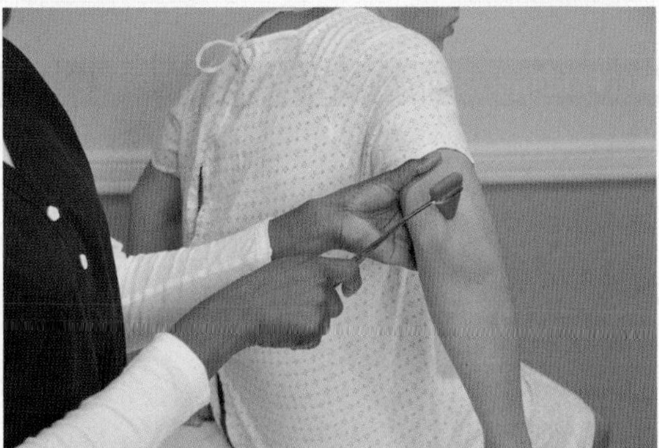	Have the patient flex the arm at the elbow and turn the palm toward the body if supine. If the patient is seated, it may be easiest for the nurse to hold the patient's arm in a relaxed dangling position. Palpate the triceps muscle and strike it directly just above the elbow. Observe for extension of the elbow and contraction of the triceps muscle.
Brachioradialis: C5 and C6 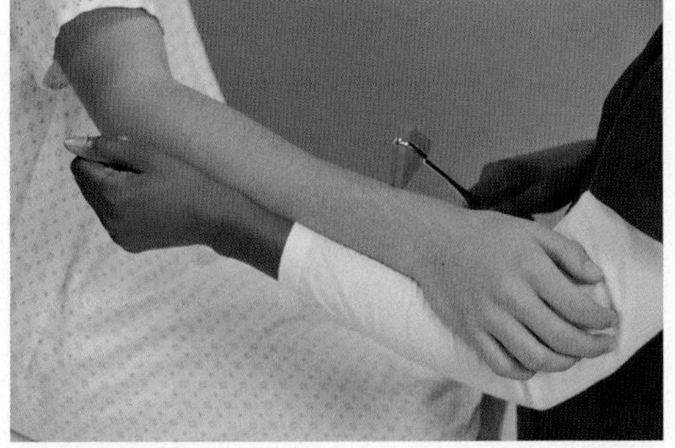	Have the patient flex the arm (up to 45 degrees) and rest the forearm on the nurse's arm with the hand slightly pronated. Palpate the brachioradial tendon approximately 5 cm (1–2 in.) above the wrist and strike it directly with the reflex hammer. Observe for pronation of the forearm, flexion of the elbow, and contraction of the muscle.
Patellar: L2–4 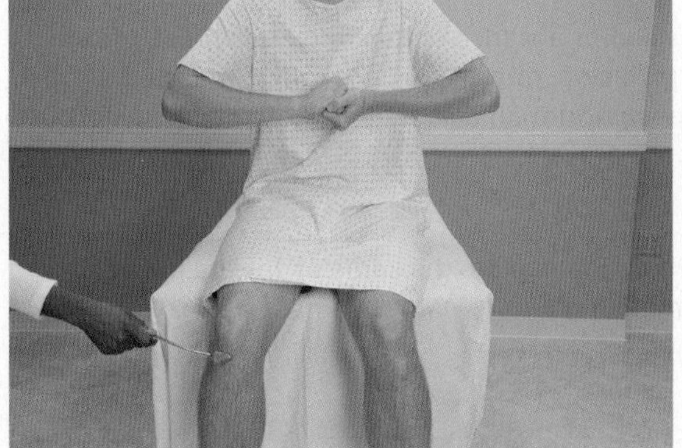	Have the patient flex the knee at 90 degrees, allowing the lower leg to dangle. Support the upper leg with the hand. Palpate the patellar tendon directly below the patella. Observe for extension of the lower leg and contraction of the quadriceps muscle. If the patient's reflexes are symmetrically diminished or absent, ask the patient to lock the fingers in front of the chest and pull one hand against the other (reinforcement).

(table continues on page 682

TABLE 22.5 Deep Tendon Reflexes *(continued)*

DTR: Level Tested	Technique
Achilles: S1 and S2 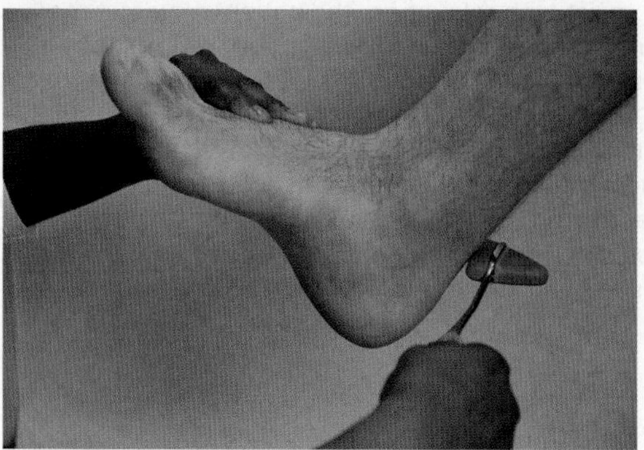	With the patient sitting and legs dangling, hold the patient's foot. (The patient may also kneel on a stool with the feet dangling.) Palpate the Achilles tendon; strike the tendon directly near the ankle malleolus. Observe for plantar flexion of the foot and contraction of the gastrocnemius muscle.

Technique and Normal Findings (continued)	Abnormal Findings (continued)
	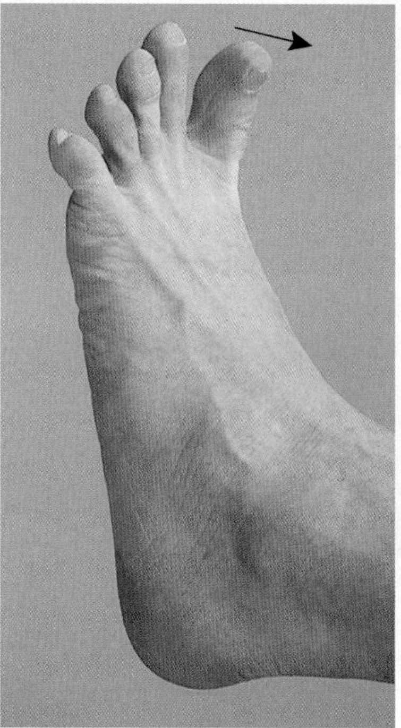 **Figure 22.22** Babinski sign.
Upper Abdominal. This test is to identify the integrity of T8–10. Stroke the upper quadrants of the abdomen with a tongue blade or reflex hammer. The umbilicus moves toward each area of stimulation symmetrically.	Depression or absence of this reflex may result from a central lesion, obesity, or lax skeletal muscles (e.g., postpartum). It also may be noted with spinal cord injury.
Lower Abdominal. This test is to identify the integrity of T10–12. Stroke the upper quadrants of the abdomen with a tongue blade or reflex hammer. The umbilicus moves toward each area of stimulation symmetrically.	Abnormal findings are the same as for the upper abdominal region.

(table continues on page 683)

Technique and Normal Findings (continued)	Abnormal Findings (continued)
Cremasteric (Male). This test helps identify the integrity of L1–2 in male patients. Stroke the inner thigh of the male patient. The testicle and scrotum rise on the stroked side.	Response is diminished or absent.
Bulbocavernous (Male). This test helps identify the integrity of S3–4 in male patients. Apply direct pressure over the bulbocavernous muscle behind the scrotum. The muscle should contract and elevate the scrotum.	Response is diminished or absent.
Perianal. This test helps identify the integrity of S3–5. Scratch the tissue at the side of the anus with a blunt instrument. The anus puckers. **Clinical Significance** The anal reflex also can be tested when administering rectal medications.	Response is diminished or absent.
Carotid Arteries Auscultation over the carotid artery may elicit a bruit that indicates stenosis and turbulent flow in the artery. Refer to Chapter 17 for technique. No bruit is heard.	Carotid stenosis is associated with an increased risk of stroke (Jayasooriya, Thaper, Shalhoub, & Davies, 2011).

Documenting Normal Findings

Neurological and Face: Well-groomed and relaxed with good eye contact. Alert and oriented with good attention span and judgment. Speech clear and appropriate. Immediate and recent memory intact. CNs II–XII grossly intact. PERRLA with L5 → 3 and R5 → 3, EOMs intact without ptosis or nystagmus. Can correctly identify light touch on face in all three areas.

Upper Extremities: Slight muscle tone tension felt during passive stretch. Muscle strength 5/5 in hands, wrists, elbows, and shoulders bilaterally. Performs rapid alternating movements smoothly and equally. Point-to-point testing smooth and accurate with eyes open and closed bilaterally. Sensation of pain and light touch intact bilaterally over dermatomes C4–T1. Vibration and position sense intact at fingers equally. Extinction, stereognosis, and graphesthesia intact bilaterally. Biceps reflex 2+, triceps and brachioradialis reflexes 1+ bilaterally. Abdominal reflexes brisk bilaterally.

Lower Extremities: Slight muscle tension noted during passive stretch for tone. Muscle strength 5/5 over feet, ankles, knees, and hips. Rapid alternating movement at toes moderately smooth. Point-to point testing smooth, accurate with eyes open and eyes closed. All movements equal bilaterally. Pain and light touch intact over dermatomes L2–S1 bilaterally. Vibration sense at great toes and position sense at random toes intact bilaterally. Patellar and ankle reflexes 2+ without reinforcement bilaterally. Babinski sign negative.

Gait and Balance: Posture upright, gait coordinated. Romberg with steady posture with eyes open and slight sway with eyes closed. Tandem walking smooth and coordinated. Coordinated walking on heels and toes, strength and coordinated movement with shallow knee bend and hop on one foot bilaterally.

Lifespan Considerations: Older Adults

As discussed earlier, aging is accompanied by expected changes in neurological function. Examples include lost nerve cell mass, atrophy in the CNS, decreased brain weight, and fewer nerve cells and dendrites. Such changes lead to slower thought and memory; however, plasticity enables the lengthening and production of dendrites to accommodate for this loss. Demyelination of nerve fibers leads to delayed impulse transmission. An increased latency period (period before next stimulation) causes slowed reflexes, which may produce mobility and safety issues. Fewer cells are in the spinal cord, although this does not appear to reduce function. Peripheral nerve conduction slows; therefore, assessment techniques, interpretation of findings, and linked interventions may require adjustments as appropriate.

Cultural Considerations

African Americans are more likely to have functional limitations as a result of a stroke. The nurse needs to carefully assess for these factors. These include being able to

- Walk up 10 steps without resting.
- Sit for about 2 hours.
- Reach up over your head.
- Use your fingers to grasp or handle small objects.
- Lift or carry something as heavy as 4 kg (about10 lb) (e.g., grocery bag).
- Go out to do things like shopping, movies, or sporting events.
- Participate in social activities like visiting friends.

(USDHHS OMH, 2014).

BOX 22.4 Neurological Screening Examination in a Healthy Patient

- Vital signs (temperature, pulse, respiration, blood pressure, pulse oximetry)
- LOC
- Communication/speech
- Orientation
- Motor (strength, pronator drift, balance, and coordination)
- Sensory (gross assessment of limbs and face)
- Pupillary reaction

National Clearinghouse Guidelines. (2012). *Diagnosis and initial treatment of ischemic stroke.* Retrieved from http://www.guideline.gov/content.aspx?id=38254&search=ischemic+stroke

Neurological Assessment in Selected Situations

Screening Examination of a Healthy Patient

Experienced nurses may complete a thorough screening assessment of a healthy patient in 10 to 15 minutes or less. Following a history and general observations, the nurse notes vital signs, including right and left radial pulses; right and left brachial blood pressures; and lying and standing blood pressure (immediate and after 3 minutes). See Box 22.4 for the components of a screening examination in a healthy patient.

Serial Neurological Assessment and Documentation

Although some neurological changes are evident instantaneously, most progress over time. Consistently accurate serial

Documenting Case Study Findings

Mr. Gardner, the 56-year-old man admitted with a stroke, has some abnormal findings. Compare these results with the expected findings presented in the samples of normal documentation. Begin to think about how the data cluster and what additional data might be needed to anticipate appropriate nursing interventions.

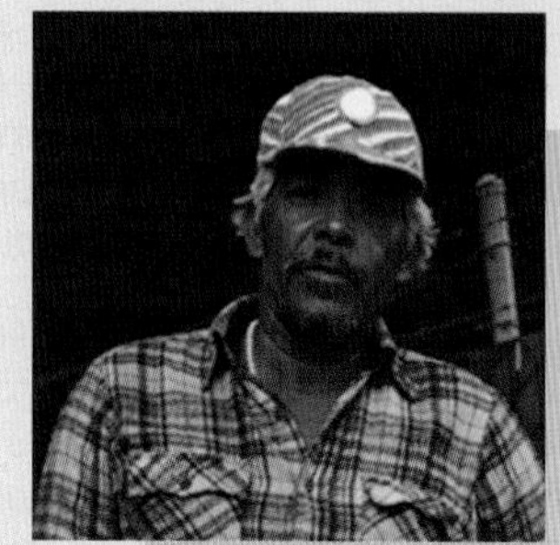

Inspection: A 56-year-old African American man with a history of hypertension, smoking, and mild baseline dementia. Lives alone, with poor hygiene and multiple layers of mismatched clothes. Does not remember the last time he took "high pressure pills." Is alert, appears somewhat fearful and agitated, asking for cigarettes, oriented to name only. Speech is comprehensible but slurred. Patient can follow one-step commands only—is easily distracted. Impaired short-term memory—remembers zero of three objects after 1 minute. Pupils equal, round, briskly reactive. Appears to have left visual field loss, EOMs intact. Left lower facial weakness, left tongue deviation.

Palpation: Muscle bulk symmetrical, tone slightly increased on left arm/leg. Strength 5/5 right arm/leg, 2/5 left arm, 3/5 left leg, left Babinski. Right arm/leg coordination grossly intact, left arm/leg not tested because of weakness, gait not tested (on bed rest). Diminished attention to objects/people on left side of bed, difficult to assess sensation because of varying patient attention. Remains hypertensive—see flow sheet for vital signs.

assessment is critical for timely identification and intervention. Orders for "neuro checks" usually mean to look for signs that, if present, would signify a critical or potentially life-threatening event. These signs typically include the patient's LOC (GCS score), pupillary size, equality and light responses, motor ability, and, when appropriate, additional elements linked to location of pathology or existing deficits (e.g., other selected CNs or sensory function). When intracranial pathology is not present (e.g., postoperative laminectomy), it is sufficient to observe for motor and sensory changes only and not use the GCS.

The patient's specific risk for acute neurological deterioration dictates the frequency of assessment. Even mild neurological decline should trigger increased frequency of assessment to observe for development of a pattern of deficits that may indicate urgent or emergency intervention.

Communication of findings is critical. Documentation of the neurological examination may be handwritten or entered electronically. Nurses typically use a flow sheet to track assessment changes over time, supported by a narrative note to detail assessments not addressed by the limitations of a flow sheet. A written note should be succinct but clearly describe relevant findings. Repetition of information recorded on a flow sheet is unnecessary.

Assessment of Meningeal Signs

A stiff neck (nuchal rigidity) is associated with meningitis and intracranial hemorrhage from irritation of the meninges. Ask the patient to relax and lie down. With the patient supine, slide your hand under and raise the patient's head gently, flexing the neck. Pain and resistance to movement are associated with **nuchal rigidity**. If neck stiffness is present, the **Brudzinski sign** may be present. The sign is positive if there is resistance or pain in the neck and flexion in the hips or knees. Evaluate for **Kernig sign** by flexing the leg at the hip. With the patient supine, raise the leg straight up (or flex the thigh on the abdomen) and extend the knee. The sign is present if there is resistance to straightening or pain radiating down the posterior leg. These are three classic signs of bacterial meningitis and when taken together have a sensitivity of 64% and specificity of 54% (Mehndiratta, Nayak, Garg, Kumar, & Pandey, 2012).

Assessing the Unconscious Patient

Assessment of unconscious patients deserves special consideration for the following reasons:

- Patients who present with acute unconsciousness require urgent evaluation to determine the cause of the impairment and, when appropriate, to implement prompt intervention.
- Unconscious patients are at risk for life-threatening complications secondary to loss of protective reflexes; these deficits may be noted during examination.
- They require special assessment techniques because they cannot participate in the examination.

You should quickly review the patient's history for possible causes of impaired consciousness. Review recent medications and laboratory values, which may reveal potential causes. Rapidly evaluate the patient's general cardiovascular and respiratory status so that any existing compromise can be treated promptly. Inspect the patient thoroughly for any visible clues, such as trauma, that might be the cause of the loss of consciousness.

Physical examination includes the following:

- LOC assessment using the GCS
- Pupillary assessment
- Brainstem assessment—gaze, facial symmetry, corneal reflex, gag reflex, cough, oculocephalic reflex (doll's eye maneuver) (Fig. 22.23) if cervical spine injury has been ruled out
- Motor function in addition to motor component of GCS (although formal strength testing cannot be done with an unresponsive patient, observe for hemiparesis/hemiplegia by comparing right and left extremity response to pain or noting frequency and location of any spontaneous movement.)
- Patterns of dysfunction associated with progressing herniation

If LOC assessment progresses to application of painful stimulus (included in eye opening in the GCS), you must employ a method to elicit the desired response without causing harm. Perform peripheral stimulation first by assessing nail bed pressure. Central stimulus, which is more reliable in evaluating patients with impaired LOC, may be applied by pinching the trapezius or pectoralis muscle. Applying pressure to the supraorbital notch can also be effective but is contraindicated when a facial fracture is suspected. Application of a "sternal rub" (knuckles applied to the skin over the sternum) also works, but it can easily bruise the skin if pressure is prolonged.

Use the oculocephalic reflex (doll's eye maneuver) to assess brainstem function in comatose patients. Ensure that the spinal cord is clear and intact before performing this test. Hold the patient's eyes open and turn the head first to one side quickly and then to the other. In a patient with an intact brainstem, the eyes move toward the opposite side. If brainstem or midbrain function is lost, the eyes move with the head, still pointing forward (similar to a doll with the eyes painted on).

Brain Herniation Syndromes

Patterns of neurological change occur when increasing intracranial pressure (ICP) causes tissue shifts between compartments within the brain. Mass effect from space-occupying lesions, such as brain edema, hematoma, hydrocephalus, or tumor, may occur bilaterally or unilaterally. If either process continues unchecked, the cerebellum down through the foramen magnum can herniate.

Altered mentation and decreasing LOC are usually the first signs of neurological deterioration. You should be alert to even subtle changes in the patient's behavior and level of responsiveness. With unilateral herniation, an ipsilateral (same-sided) dilating pupil, at first sluggishly reactive, may signify neurological worsening. As herniation progresses, which it may do rapidly, response only to pain, contralateral

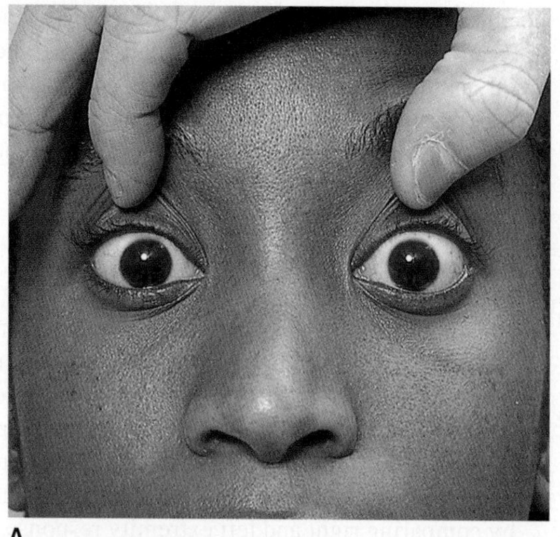

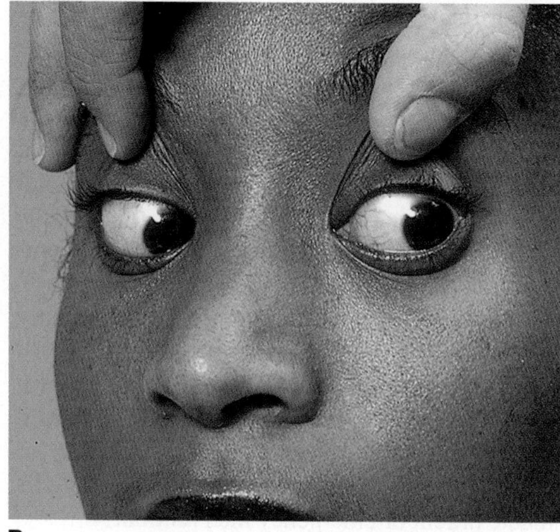

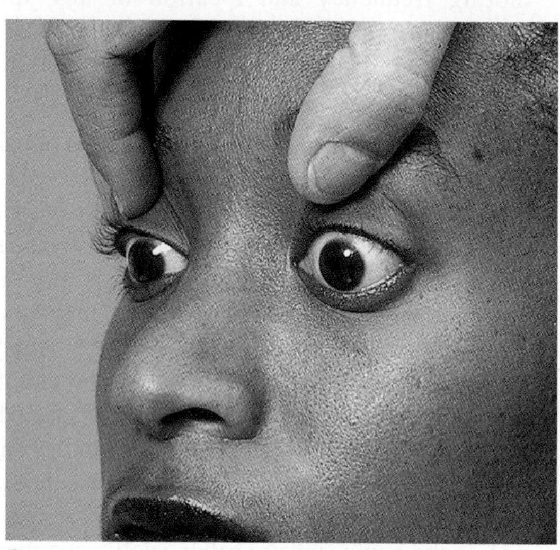

Figure 22.23 The oculocephalic reflex involves the doll's eye maneuver. **A.** The nurse holds the patient's upper eyelids open. The nurse then quickly turns the patient's head. **B.** If the eyes can move in the opposite direction of the head, this indicates that the brainstem is intact. **C.** In a comatose patient, the ability to move both eyes to one side is lost.

(opposite-sided) posturing of extremities, and brainstem abnormalities may be noticeable. With bilateral herniation, pupil change and reflex posturing are on both sides.

With cerebellar herniation, the patient has fixed pupils (size depends on site of original lesion), flaccid muscles, and no response to pain. The patient may rapidly experience **brain death** as well as respiratory and cardiovascular changes. Certain respiratory patterns may be seen with progressive neurological deterioration related to increased ICP or focal lesions of the brainstem (see Table 22.14 at the end of the chapter).

Critical Thinking

Laboratory and Diagnostic Testing

Diagnostic tests serve to further define the precise location and often the nature and extent of a lesion. Many diagnostic tests also provide information about the integrity of surrounding areas. A wide variety of diagnostic tests can aid in the identification of nervous system disease. Technological advances have made new equipment and techniques possible; such progress continues rapidly. Significant developments in genetic testing have allowed molecular diagnosis of infectious, congenital, and inherited neurological diseases, among multiple other applications. Although neurodiagnostic testing can be categorized in many ways, this review sorts tests as anatomical imaging, electrical conduction testing, and CSF/spinal procedures.

Anatomical Imaging

Computed tomography (CT) continues to be the staple of neurodiagnostic imaging. It consists of passage of multiple x-ray beams through tissue in sequential planes, displayed in shades of gray. Intravenous injection of a radiopaque medium ("contrast") provides bright enhancement of vascular structures and areas of blood–brain barrier breakdown. CT detects potential causes of increased ICP and multiple other intracranial pathologies.

The MRI is a noninvasive, nonradiological test that delivers highly detailed images of neuroanatomy and associated pathology. Duration of the procedure is usually significantly longer than CT. This, plus the effects of the strong magnetic field on most critical care monitors and equipment such as infusion pumps, makes MRI more problematic for critically ill patients. The procedure is noninvasive (barring intravenous infusion of contrast material for certain sequences), but patients may experience discomfort from the duration of the procedure, loud sounds, and possible feelings of claustrophobia. Patient movement disrupts the adequacy of images (as with CT), so sedation may also be indicated.

SAFETY ALERT

Preprocedure considerations include removal of metallic objects from hair, wrists, fingers, and piercings. Providers also must screen the environment for metal that could possibly become a missile if exposed to the strong magnetic field in the immediate area of the MRI scanner. Objects such as oxygen tanks, scissors, forceps, and stethoscopes have been implicated in potential or actual patient injury.

Angiography, an invasive procedure, involves intraarterial injection of contrast material to visualize the lumen of intracranial and extracranial vessels. It is the standard criterion for identification of aneurysms, arteriovenous malformations, and vasospasm following subarachnoid hemorrhage (Li, Lv, Yao, Li, & Xie, 2013). Disadvantages of cerebral angiography are associated with risk for complications after arterial access of vessels that typically already contain pathology.

SAFETY ALERT

Preprocedure nursing considerations include screening for allergy to shellfish or iodine or for presence of renal disease. (Premedication to lower risk of anaphylaxis will be considered; an alternative contrast material can reduce risk of renal failure.) The postprocedure focus is on observation and prevention of complications. Frequent serial assessment of the arterial puncture site, distal pulses, and limb color and temperature targets risk for bleeding, hematoma, or occlusion of the cannulated vessel.

Electrical Conduction Testing

The largely noninvasive electroencephalogram (EEG) records spontaneous electrical impulses from scalp electrodes positioned over the brain surface area. EEG detects abnormal electrical activity, such as seizures or alterations caused by neuronal damage from trauma, stroke, encephalopathies, or other cerebral pathology (Stefan & Lopes da Silva, 2013). Electromyography records electrical activity in muscles at rest, during voluntary contraction, and with electrical stimulation using inserted small needle electrodes. Nerve conduction studies record speed of conduction in motor and sensory fibers of peripheral nerves using surface electrodes. They are used to evaluate for neuromuscular disorders such as myasthenia gravis, neuropathy, or other peripheral nerve dysfunction.

Cerebrospinal Fluid/Spinal Procedures

Lumbar puncture involves insertion of a hollow needle into the spinal subarachnoid space to examine and measure the pressure of CSF. Placement is between L4 and L5 or L3 and L4 vertebrae to avoid the spinal cord, which typically ends at L1. Lumbar puncture is usually performed at the bedside (or in a clinic if done as an outpatient procedure), under strict asepsis.

SAFETY ALERT

After lumbar puncture, patients typically must remain flat in bed for 6 to 8 hours. If headache develops or becomes severe when a patient first gets up, bed rest may continue for up to 24 hours. Headache typically results from loss of the cushioning effect of CSF or from leakage of CSF from the puncture site into surrounding tissue. If the ICP is significantly elevated, lumbar drainage of CSF could potentially precipitate downward herniation of the brain into the foramen magnum. Thus, patients need frequent assessment for headache and LOC following a lumbar puncture.

Diagnostic Reasoning

Nursing Diagnoses, Outcomes, and Interventions

When formulating a nursing diagnosis, you use critical thinking to cluster data and identify related patterns. You compare clusters with defining characteristics (abnormal findings) for the diagnosis to ensure the most accurate labeling and appropriate interventions (Table 22.6) (NANDA International, 2012). Note how the potential interventions often include assessments. This illustrates how the nursing process is interwoven, with assessment a continuous part of nursing care.

You use assessment information to identify patient outcomes. Some outcomes related to neurological problems include the following (Moorhead, Johnson, Maas, & Swanson, 2013):

- Patient cares for both sides of the body and keeps affected side safe.
- Patient does not aspirate or fall and maintains a safe environment.
- Patient improves motor function and becomes independent with activities of daily living (ADLs).

After outcomes have been established, nursing care can be implemented. Use critical thinking and evidence-based practice to develop interventions. Some examples of nursing interventions for neurological care are as follows (Bulechek, Butcher, Dochterman, & Wagner, 2013):

- Use cues and anchors to promote attention to the affected side.
- Assess neurological and mental status frequently; inform physician of changes.
- Orient patient to time, place, and person frequently.

TABLE 22.6 Common Nursing Diagnoses Associated With the Neurological System

Diagnosis	Point of Differentiation	Assessment Characteristics	Nursing Interventions
Impaired verbal communication	Compromised ability to use speech (whether receiving, transmitting, or both)	Difficulty forming words or sentences, difficulty expressing thoughts verbally, inappropriate verbalization	Observe behavioral cues for needs. Maintain eye contact. Ask yes and no questions. Anticipate patient's needs. Use touch as appropriate.
Acute confusion	Abrupt onset of global transient changes and disturbances in attention, cognition, and consciousness	Fluctuation in cognition, increased agitation or restlessness, lack of follow-through in behavior	Perform mental status examination. Provide environmental cues (e.g., large clock, calendar). Orient to time, place, and person frequently.
Impaired memory	Problems with recollecting or remembering information from levels ranging from short-term memory to basic behaviors	Inability to recall facts, remember recent or past events, or learn new information	Encourage patient to use a calendar, keep reminder lists, set alarm watches, and make signs for room number or bathroom.
Unilateral neglect	Lack of awareness and attention to one side of the body	Inattention to one side, inadequate positioning, leaves food on plate on affected side	Provide safe, well-lit, and clutter-free environment. Set up environment so that most activity is on unaffected side. Encourage patient to compensate for neglect.
Risk for aspiration	Risk for oropharyngeal secretions, food, or fluid entering into the tracheobronchial passages	Reduced LOC, facial droop, depressed cough and gag reflexes, drooling, choking, and coughing on food	Auscultate lungs before and after feeding. Request swallowing evaluation by speech therapy. Elevate head of bed when eating.
Risk for intracranial adaptive capacity	Increased ICP in response to stimuli	Increases in ICP of more than 10 mm Hg for more than 5 minutes, resulting from brain injuries	Keep head and neck in midline. Avoid suctioning. Reduce environmental stimuli. Adjust sedation. Provide adequate oxygen.*
Ineffective brain tissue perfusion	Decrease in oxygen or blood supply resulting in failure to nourish brain	Abnormal pupils, weakness or paralysis, changes in motor response, altered mental status	Monitor neurological status using neurological flow sheet. Notify physician about changes in condition. Prevent injury.

*Collaborative interventions.

Progress Note: Analyzing Findings

The difficulties of Mr. Gardner have been outlined throughout this chapter. Initial subjective and objective data collection is complete. The nurse is reviewing the findings and other results.

Mr. Gardner is reassessed on the acute care unit following his admission from the ED. The following nursing note illustrates the collection and analysis of subjective and objective data and the development of preliminary nursing interventions.

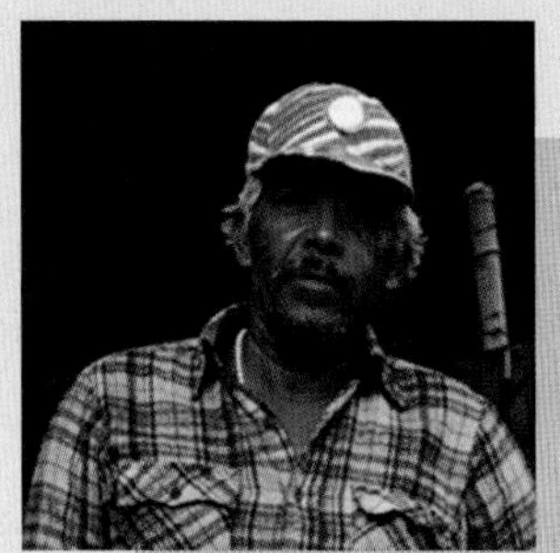

Subjective: A 56-year-old African American man with a history of hypertension, smoking, and mild baseline dementia. Lives alone, poor hygiene, wearing multiple layers of mismatched clothes. Does not remember last time he took "high pressure pills." Is alert, appears somewhat fearful and agitated, asking for cigarettes, oriented to name only. Speech is comprehensible but slurred.

Objective: Patient can follow one-step commands only—is easily distractible. Impaired short-term memory—remembers zero of three objects after 1 minute. PERRLA. Appears to have left visual field loss, EOMs intact. Left lower facial weakness, left tongue deviation. Muscle bulk symmetrical, tone slightly increased on left arm/leg. Strength 5/5 right

(case study continues on page 689)

arm/leg, 2/5 left arm, 3/5 left leg, left Babinski. Right arm/leg coordination grossly intact, left arm/leg not tested because of weakness, gait not tested (on bed rest). Diminished attention to objects and people on left side of bed, difficult to assess sensation because of varying patient attention. Remains hypertensive—see flow sheet for vital signs.

Analysis: Findings consistent with right hemisphere stroke, complicated by baseline impaired cognitive function. Potential for further impaired cerebral perfusion. Probable left unilateral neglect, high risk of falling, dysphagia, and aspiration risk.

Plan: Frequent neurological assessment to monitor for stroke progression. Monitor BP—currently untreated per stroke guidelines. Consult social work for support system and financial assessment—patient may be unable to return to independent living. Evaluate safe ADL performance with physical and occupational therapists. Implement fall prevention plan; discuss speech pathology consult for swallowing evaluation prior to starting diet.

Collaborating With the Interprofessional Team

Mr. Gardner may be at risk for aspiration because of his facial droop and tongue deviation. The nurse contacts speech therapy to evaluate the patient's ability to swallow without choking or aspirating. Nurses consult speech therapy when patient needs are associated with the following:

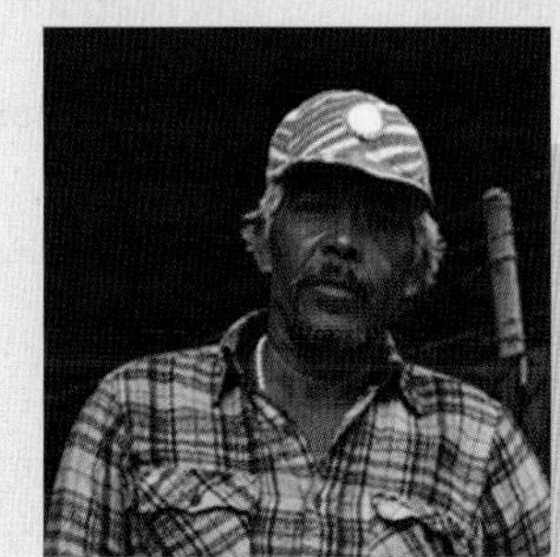

- Swallowing evaluation/management and diet recommendations
- Cognitive communication and language evaluations
- Difficulty with communication
- Oral or facial trauma
- Aphasia

The nurse is contacting speech therapy at this time for the risk of aspiration, a safety issue. Speech therapy also may be involved during this patient's rehabilitation for issues related to communication. The following conversation illustrates how the nurse might organize data and make recommendations to speech therapy.

Situation: "Hello, I'm E. J. Howick, Mr. Gardner's nurse on 5 East."

Background: "Mr. Gardner was admitted yesterday with a right-sided stroke. He hasn't started a diet yet. He has some left lower facial weakness and left tongue deviation that might interfere with ability to chew and swallow. He wants to eat, but he still has an order for nothing by mouth."

Assessment: "I'm worried that he's at risk for aspiration. I would like you to evaluate his swallowing before we start feeding him."

Recommendations: "For now, I'm going to keep him on nothing by mouth. After you see him, let me know what your evaluation is. We may have the physician change his diet order if he's safe to eat."

Critical Thinking Challenge

- Consider all the collected subjective data. Review the above report. Should the nurse communicate any other data to speech therapy?
- Critique the objective data. Is the organization logical? Would it be clearer to add to or take out any of the information?
- Critique the analysis and recommendations. What is the nurse's role in coordinating collaborative care with speech therapy?

Pulling It All Together

The nurse uses assessment data to formulate a nursing care plan with patient outcomes and interventions for Mr. Gardner. Outcomes are specific to the patient, realistic to achieve, measurable, and have a time frame. After interventions have been completed, the nurse will reevaluate Mr. Gardner and document the findings to show progress toward outcomes. The nurse uses critical thinking and judgment to continue or revise the diagnosis, outcomes, or interventions. This is often in the form of a care plan or case note similar to the one below.

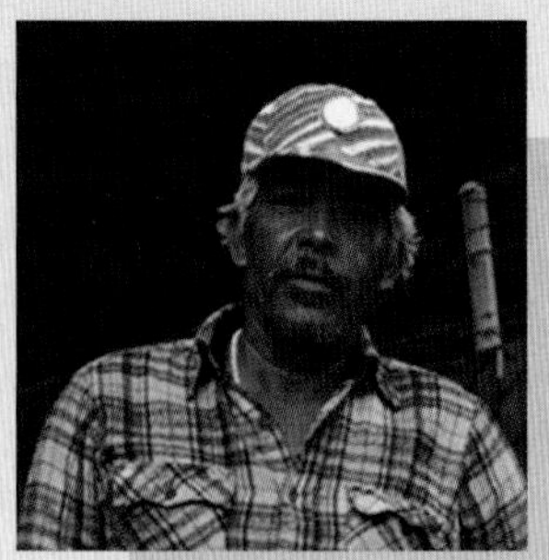

Nursing Diagnosis	Patient Outcomes	Nursing Interventions	Rationale	Evaluation
Unilateral neglect related to hemianopsia, left-sided weakness	Demonstrates measures to care for left side of body and keep it free from injury within 1 week	Assess neurological function every shift including muscle strength. Assist with dressing and grooming until strength returns. Place call bell on right side of bed.	The initial priority is patient safety and injury prevention. Assess function to determine improvements or decline. Assist patient with ADLs until he can care for himself.	Motor strength 2+ on left arm and leg; 4+ on right. Facial droop and tongue deviation persist. Needs assistance in two-handed tasks, such as bathing. Needs one-person assist with transfers. Continue to monitor; obtain physical therapy consult to assess for readiness for rehabilitation.

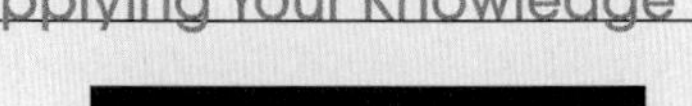

Applying Your Knowledge

Using the previous steps of diagnostic reasoning, organizing, and prioritizing, consider all the case study findings woven throughout this chapter. When answering the following questions, begin drawing conclusions and see how the pieces of assessment must work together to create an environment for personalized, appropriate, and accurate care. Note how assessment forms the foundation for accurate, individualized, and holistic nursing care.

- What signs will the nurse assess to detect whether Mr. Gardner's situation is deteriorating?
- Is Mr. Gardner's condition at the end of the initial assessment stable, urgent, or an emergency?
- What ongoing health promotion and teaching needs are evident?
- How will the nurse individualize assessment to Mr. Gardner's specific needs, considering his condition, age, and culture?
- How will the nurse focus, organize, and prioritize ongoing objective data collection?
- How will the nurse evaluate the selection of the priority nursing diagnosis?

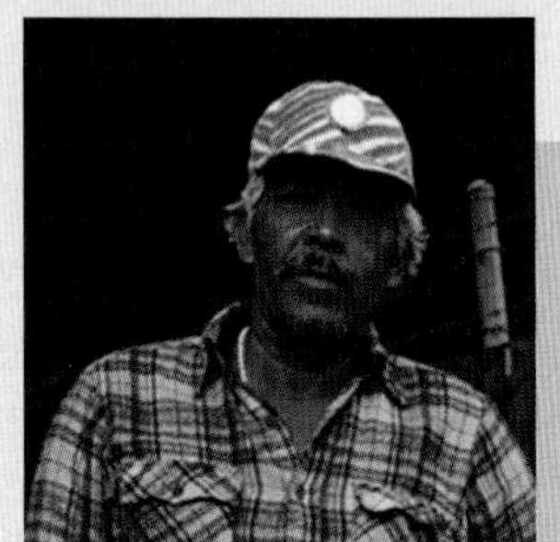

Key Points

- Nurses use experience, knowledge of anatomy and physiology, and the patient's acuity, current deficits, and risk for deterioration to select elements of the neurological examination most appropriate for the situation.
- Although some neurological changes are evident instantaneously, most progress over time. Consistent, accurate, and clearly communicated serial assessments are critical for timely identification and intervention.
- Early recognition of events requiring urgent intervention maximizes the patient's chance of optimal outcome.
- Common areas of health promotion include reducing the risk of neurovascular disease and injury prevention.
- Common symptoms associated with the neurological system include headache, weakness, blurred vision, impaired motor function, and impaired speech.

- When collecting a headache history, characteristics such as pain worse in the morning on awakening and pain precipitated or made worse by straining or sneezing may indicate potentially elevated ICP.
- Clinical situations that require urgent communication of neurological assessment findings include a change in LOC, pupillary reaction, and verbal or motor response.
- Consciousness and cognition are assessed early in the neurological examination because these functions direct the method used to elicit further information.
- Use of the GCS helps to provide relatively objective information about LOC but is most reliable after staff training.
- Assessment of the function of CNS is performed at the bedside through observation of vision, pupils, EOMs, facial expression and strength, and uvula and tongue movement.
- Spinal and peripheral nerve function may be assessed by testing for motor strength and sensation at different levels of the spinal cord according to the dermatomes.
- Abnormal reflexes include hyperactive or diminished DTR, decreased superficial reflexes, and abnormal reflexes such as a positive Babinski sign.
- Abnormal posturing occurs in late stages of injury, including abnormal flexion and abnormal extension responses.
- Abnormal motor function includes disorders of movement such as tremor and abnormal gait.
- Common nursing diagnoses are impaired verbal communication, acute confusion, impaired memory, unilateral neglect, risk for aspiration, risk for intracranial adaptive capacity, and ineffective brain tissue perfusion.
- Although neurological assessment findings can highlight location and acuity of neuropathology, diagnostic testing provides the critical next step in assessing type and etiology of the condition. Knowledgeable pre- and postprocedure care aids in maximizing information obtained and reducing patient stress and complications.

Review Questions

1. Use of the GCS provides relatively objective assessment of LOC. The three functions assessed are
   A. pupil reaction, orientation, and sensation.
   B. verbal response, eye opening, and motor response.
   C. eye opening, motor response, and sensation.
   D. verbal response, pupil reaction, and motor response.

2. The patient with a head injury and increasing ICP is likely to have which assessment findings?
   A. Decreased LOC and sluggish pupil
   B. Left-sided weakness and facial droop
   C. Right ptosis and right-sided loss of vision
   D. Dilated left pupil and receptive aphasia

3. The chart states that a 62-year-old woman has had a stroke in the right parietal area of the brain. The nurse expects to note which of the following?
   A. Tremors on the left side of the face
   B. Tremors on the right side of the face
   C. Weakness in the right arm
   D. Weakness in the left arm

4. The nurse performs blood pressure screening at the local community center. As part of the health promotion intervention, the nurse also discusses the following risk factors for stroke.
   A. Low blood pressure, lack of exercise, and diet high in fat
   B. High blood pressure, diet high in fat, and smoking
   C. Diet high in fat, smoking, and walking five times weekly
   D. Obesity, swimming five times weekly, high blood pressure

5. If the great toe extends upward and the other toes fan out in response to stroking the lateral aspect of the sole of the foot, this is documented as which of the following?
   A. Hyporeflexia
   B. Normal plantar reflex
   C. Cushing response
   D. Babinski sign

6. A 26-year-old man was in a motor vehicle accident and suffered a complete spinal cord injury to L3. The nurse assesses the patient for loss of motor function in the
   A. legs.
   B. abdomen.
   C. chest.
   D. arms.

7. A patient in a nursing home was admitted with a diagnosis of dementia. He started a fire because he was cooking at home and forgot that he left a pan on the stove. The nursing diagnosis that is highest priority is
   A. ineffective brain tissue perfusion.
   B. risk for injury.
   C. acute confusion.
   D. impaired memory.

8. While the nurse performs formal patient assessment, assistive personnel often observe changes when obtaining vital signs or assisting patients with ADLs. When discussing care for a patient with back pain, the nurse should particularly alert the assistant to watch for
   A. dizziness.
   B. bowel/bladder incontinence.
   C. difficulty swallowing.
   D. arm weakness.

9. When collecting a health history for the patient complaining of headache, the patient reports having as many as four episodes per day of severe right orbital pain lasting about 30 minutes with lacrimation and nasal congestion on the right. This is most consistent with
   A. cluster headache.
   B. migraine with aura.
   C. tension headache.
   D. migraine without aura.

10. Of the following changes, which is the earliest sign of progressing brain herniation that originates in the cerebral hemispheres?
   A. An enlarging pupil that is sluggishly reactive to light
   B. Altered mentation
   C. Widening pulse pressure with bradycardia
   D. Reflex posturing of extremities

The Jensen suite offers these additional resources to enhance learning and facilitate understanding of this chapter:

- thePoint online resource, http://thepoint.lww.com/Jensen2e
- *Laboratory Manual for Nursing Health Assessment: A Best Practice Approach*
- *Pocket Guide for Nursing Health Assessment: A Best Practice Approach*
- *Lippincott DocuCare*, an electronic health record simulation software, http://thepoint.lww.com/docucare
- *Adaptive Learning | Powered by PrepU*, http://thepoint.lww.com/prepu

References

Adeleye, A. O., Owolabi, M. O., Rablu, T. B., & Orimadegun, A. E. (2012). Physician's knowledge of the Glasgow Coma Scale in a Nigerian University Hospital: Is the simple GCS still too complex? *Frontiers in Neurology, 3*(28), 1–6.

American Heart Association. (2012a). Physical activity and exercise recommendations for stroke survivors: An American Heart Association scientific statement from the Council on Clinical Cardiology, Subcommittee on Exercise, Cardiac Rehabilitation, and Prevention; the Council on Cardiovascular Nursing; the Council on Nutrition, Physical Activity, and Metabolism; and the Stroke Council. *Circulation, 109*(16), 2031–2041.

American Heart Association. (2012b). *Stroke risk factors*. Retrieved from http://www.strokeassociation.org/STROKEORG/AboutStroke/UnderstandingRisk/Understanding-Stroke-Risk_UCM_308539_SubHomePage.jsp

American Nurses Association (ANA) and the John A. Hartford Foundation Institute. Normal changes in aging. (2007). Retrieved August 13, 2007, from http://consultgerirn.org/topics/age_related_changes/want_to_know_more/

American Psychiatric Association. (2013). *Diagnostic and statistical manual of mental disorders* (5th ed.). Arlington, VA: American Psychiatric Publishing.

Bethel, J. (2012). Emergency care of children and adults with head injury. *Nursing Standard, 26*(43), 49–56.

Brender, J. D., Felkner, M., Suarez, I., Canfield, M. S., & Henry, J. P. (2010). Maternal pesticide exposure and neural tube defects in Mexican Americans. *Annals of Epidemiology, 20*(1), 18–22.

Bulechek, G. M., Butcher, H. K., Dochterman, J. M., & Wagner, C. M. (2013). *Nursing interventions classification (NIC)* (6th ed.). St. Louis, MO: Mosby.

Fjell, A. M., & Walhovd, K. B. (2010). Structural brain changes in aging: courses, causes and cognitive consequences. *Review of Neuroscience, 21*(3), 187–221.

Folstein, M. F., Folstein, S. E., & McHugh, P. R. (1975). "Mini-mental state." A practical method for grading the cognitive state of patients for the clinician". *Journal of Psychiatric Research, 12*(3), 189–98. doi:10.1016/0022-3956(75)90026-6

Gill, D. P., Hubbard, R. A., Koepsell, T. D., Borrie, M. J., Petrella, R.J., Knopman, D. S., & Kukull, W. A. (2013). Differences in the rate of functional decline across three dementia types. *Alzheimer's & Dementia, 9*(5), 563–571.

Gould, D. J. (2013). *Lippincott's pocket neuroanatomy.* Philadelphia, PA: Lippincott Williams & Wilkins.

Jayasooriya, G., Thaper, A., Shalhoub, J., & Davies, A. H. (2011). Silent cerebral events in asymptomatic carotid stenosis. *Journal of Vascular Surgery, 54*(1), 227–36.

Kandel, E. R., Schwartz, J. H., Jessell, T. M., Siegelbaum, S. A., & Hudspeth, A. J. (Eds.). (2012). *Principles of neural science* (5th ed.). Philadelphia, PA: Elsevier.

Kelley, M. A., Flocks, J. D., Economos, J., & McCauley, L. A. (2013). Female farmworkers' health during pregnancy: health care providers' perspectives. *Workplace Health & Safety, 61*(7), 308–313.

Lackland, D. (2013). Hypertension: Joint National committee on detection,, evaluation and treatment of high blood pressure guidelines. *Current Opinion in Neurology, 26*(1), 8–12.

Leder, S. B. (1997). Videofluoroscopic evaluation of aspiration with visual examination of the gag reflex and velar movement. *Dysphagia, 12*(1), 21–23.

Li, Q., Lv, F., Yao, G., Li, Y., & Xie, P. (2013). 64-section multidetector CT angiography for evaluation of intracranial aneurysms: comparison with 3D rotational angiography. *Acta Radiologica*. Advance online publication.

Marieb, E. N., & Hoehn, K. (2013). *Human anatomy & physiology* (9th ed.). Boston, MA: Pearson.

Mehndiratta, T. A. B., Nayak, R., Garg, H., Kumar, M., & Pandey, S. (2012). Improved sensitivity of Kernig's and Brudzinski's sign in diagnosing meningitis in children. *Annals of Indian Academy of Neurology, 15*(4), 287–288.

Moorhead, S., Johnson, M., Maas, M. L., & Swanson, E. (2013). *Nursing outcomes classification (NOC): Measurement of health outcomes* (5th ed.). St. Louis, MO: Elsevier.

NANDA International. (2012). *Nursing diagnoses: Definitions and classification 2012–2014* (9th ed). Oxford, United Kingdom: Wiley-Blackwell.

National Center for Injury Prevention and Control. (2013a). *Spinal cord injury (SCI): Fact sheet*. Retrieved from http://www.cdc.gov/traumaticbraininjury/scifacts.html

National Center for Injury Prevention and Control. (2013b). *Traumatic brain injury in the United States: Fact sheet*. Retrieved from http://www.cdc.gov/traumaticbraininjury/get_the_facts.html

National Clearinghouse Guidelines. (2012). *Diagnosis and initial treatment of ischemic stroke*. Retrieved from http://www.guideline.gov/content.aspx?id=38254&search=ischemic+stroke

National Institutes of Health. (2013). *NIH stroke scales and clinical assessment tools*. Retrieved from http://www.ninds.nih.gov/doctors/NIH_Stroke_Scale.pdf

Runchey, S., & McGee, S. (2010). Does this patient have a hemorrhagic stroke? Clinical findings distinguishing hemorrhagic stroke from ischemic stroke. *The Journal of the American Medical Association, 303*(22), 2280–2286.

Standring, S. (2008). *Gray's anatomy: The anatomical basis for clinical practice* (40th ed.). London, United Kingdom: Elsevier Churchill Livingstone.

Stefan, H., & Lopes da Silva, F. H. (2013). Epileptic neuronal networks: methods of identification and clinical relevance. *Frontiers in Neurology, 4*(8), 1–15.

Tinker, S. C., Devine, O., Mai, C., Hamner, H. C., Reefnuis, J., Gilboa, S. M., . . . Honein, M. A. (2013). Estimate of the potential impact of folic acid fortification of corn masa flour on the prevention of neural tube defects. *Birth Defects Research: Part A, Clinical and Molecular Tetralogy, 97*(10), 649–657.

Touhy, T. A., & Jett, K. (2012). *Toward healthy aging* (8th ed.). St. Louis, MO: Elsevier.

U.S. Department of Health & Human Services. (2013). *2020 Topics & objectives - Objectives A-Z*. Retrieved from http://www.healthypeople.gov/2020/topicsobjectives2020/

U.S. Department of Health & Human Services, Office of Minority Health. (2012). *Stroke data/statistics*. Retrieved from http://minorityhealth.hhs.gov/templates/browse.aspx?lvl=3&lvlid=86#sthash.y5OfkIIu.dpuf

U.S. Department of Health & Human Services, Office of Minority Health. (2014). *Stroke and African Americans*. Retrieved from http://minorityhealth.hhs.gov/templates/content.aspx?ID=3022

U.S. Environmental Protection Agency. (2013). *Lead in dust, paint and soil*. Retrieved from http://www2.epa.gov/lead/hazardstandards-lead-paint-dust-and-soil-tsca-section-403

Weiner, W. J., Goetz, C. G., Shin, R. K., & Lewis, S. L. (2010). *Neurology for the non-neurologist* (6th ed.). Philadelphia, PA: Lippincott Williams & Wilkins.

Tables of Abnormal Findings

TABLE 22.7 Pupils in Comatose Patients

	Pathological Indication	Description
Unequal pupil size, physiological	Physiological anisocoria, not associated with any disease	May be congenital in 20% of the population
Unequal pupils size, pathophysiological	Anisocoria related to compression of the optic nerve	One pupil is 0.1 mm different from the other.
Constricted and fixed pupils (pinpoint)	Miosis related to hemorrhage in the pons or opiate narcotics	Pinpoint pupils (smaller than 0.1 mm) or small pupils (1–2.5 mm) suggest damage to the sympathetic pathways or metabolic encephalopathy.
Dilated and fixed pupils	Anoxia, sympathetic neural effects, atropine, tricyclics, amphetamines, or pilocarpine drops for glaucoma treatment; when associated with a head injury, prognosis is poor.	Pupils are greater than 6 mm bilaterally.
Horner syndrome	Preganglionic, central, or postganglionic lesion	Miosis (small pupil), ptosis (lid droop), anhidrosis (lack of sweat), and apparent enophthalmos (affected eye appears to be sunken)
Adie pupil	Denervation of the nerve supply resulting from diabetic neuropathy or alcoholism	Both the pupillary response and accommodation are sluggish or impaired in one eye.
Argyll Robertson pupil	Neurosyphilis, meningitis	Virtually no response to light but brisk response to accommodation bilaterally. Pupils are small and frequently irregular in shape.
Third nerve palsy	Third nerve palsy	Sudden ptosis, diplopia, and pain are some of the symptoms. Pupil is fixed and dilated, and extraocular motility is restricted.

From Kipioti, T. (2013). *Demystifying abnormal pupils.* Retrieved from http://www.optometry.co.uk/uploads/exams/articles/cet_22_february_2013_kipioti.pdf; for more on abnormal pupils, see Chapter 13.

TABLE 22.8 Abnormal Postures

	Pathological Indication	Description
Abnormal Extension 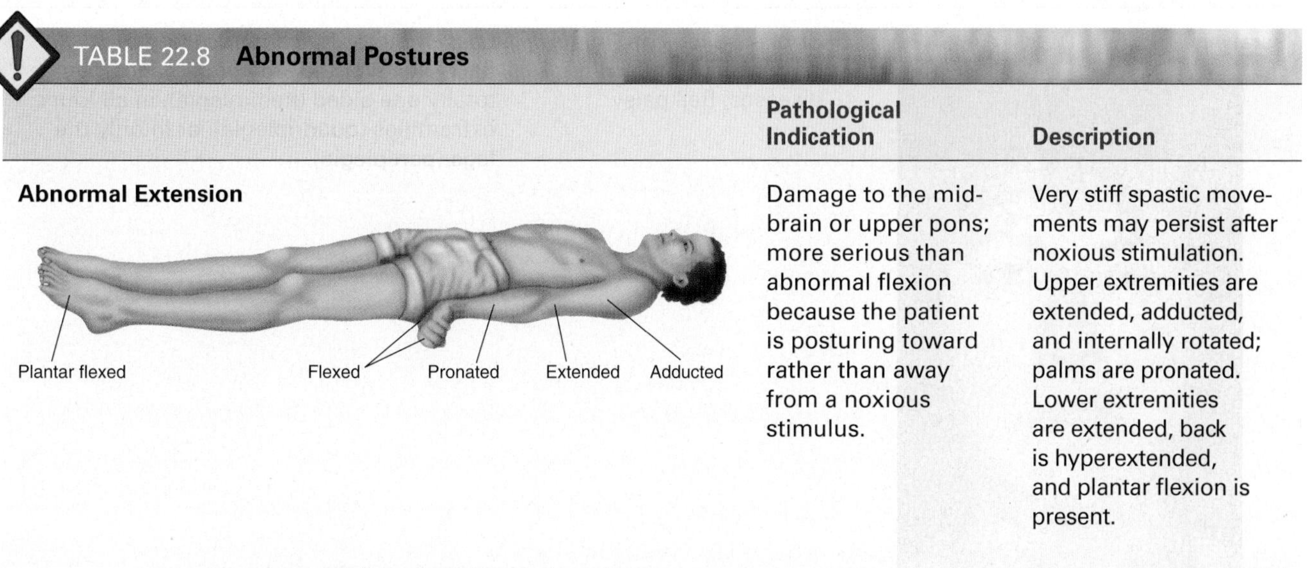	Damage to the midbrain or upper pons; more serious than abnormal flexion because the patient is posturing toward rather than away from a noxious stimulus.	Very stiff spastic movements may persist after noxious stimulation. Upper extremities are extended, adducted, and internally rotated; palms are pronated. Lower extremities are extended, back is hyperextended, and plantar flexion is present.

(table continues on page 694)

TABLE 22.8 Abnormal Postures *(continued)*

	Pathological Indication	Description
Abnormal Flexion Flexed Plantar flexed Internally rotated Flexed Adducted	Damage to the cerebral cortex	Very stiff spastic movements may persist after noxious stimulation. Upper extremities are flexed and arms are adducted. Lower extremities are extended, internally rotated with plantar flexion.
Hemiplegia Externally rotated Flaccid	Stroke	Sensation and motor strength are lost unilaterally.
Flexion Withdrawal	CNS depression or injury	Gross movements of all body parts are away from the noxious stimulus. Rather than localizing pain to one side, the patient may withdraw both arms when nail bed pressure is applied.
Flaccid Quadriplegia	Nonfunctional brainstem	Sensation and muscle tone are completely lost.

TABLE 22.9 Abnormalities of Movements

	Common Associations	Description
Paralysis	Stroke, spinal cord injury, chronic neuromuscular diseases, Bell palsy	Loss of motor function resulting in flaccidity over the area of damage; may be totally one-sided (hemiplegia), in all four extremities (quadriplegia), or in only the legs (paraplegia)

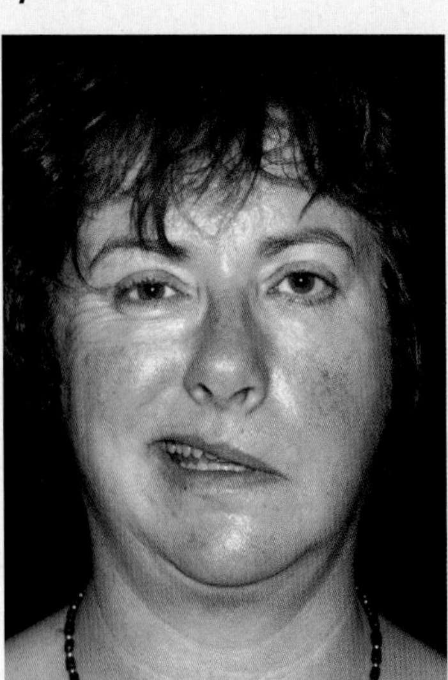

(table continues on page 695)

TABLE 22.9 **Abnormalities of Movements** *(continued)*

	Common Associations	Description
Resting Tremor 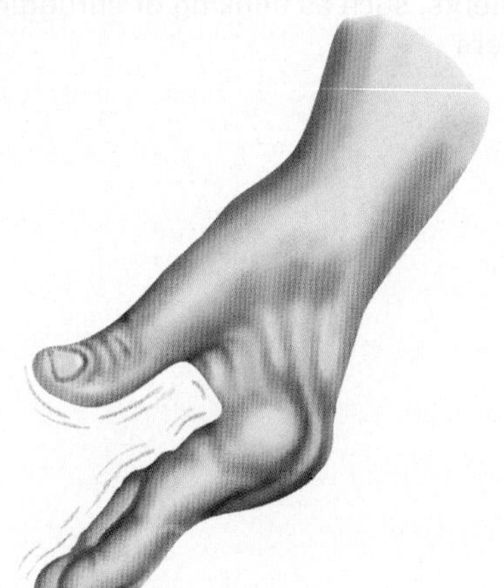	Parkinson disease	Prominent at rest; may decrease or disappear with voluntary movement
Intention Tremor 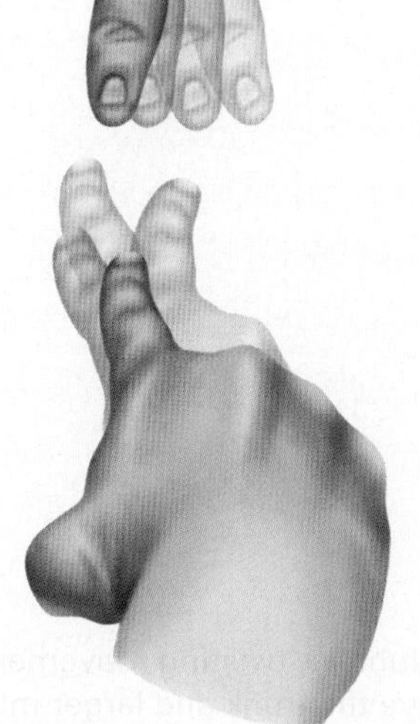	Multiple sclerosis with damage to the cerebellar pathways, or essential tremor	Absent at rest, increase with movement; may worsen as movement progresses
Fasciculation 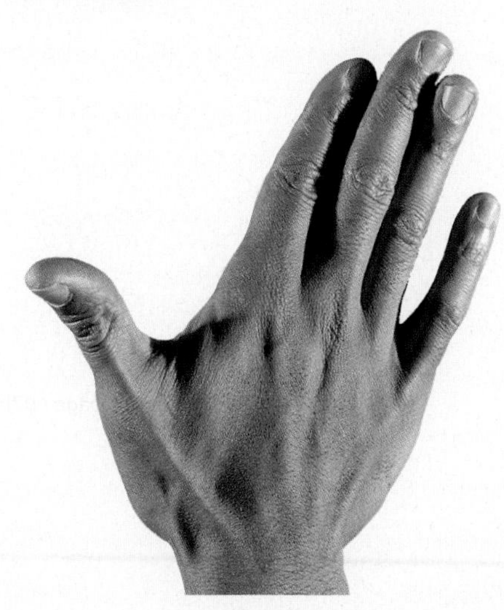	Deterioration of the anterior horn cells	Fine, flickering, irregular movements in small muscle groups seen under the skin; may not cause movement at the joint. Because fasciculations occur under the skin, it is difficult to see them clearly.

(table continues on page 696)

TABLE 22.9 Abnormalities of Movements *(continued)*

	Common Associations	Description
Tic 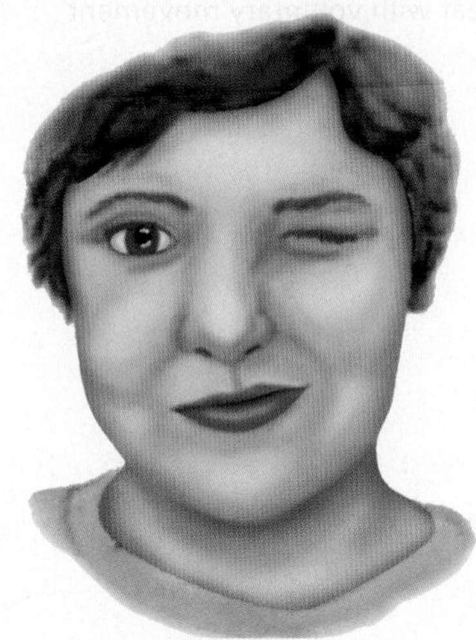	Tourette syndrome, use of psychiatric medications, and use of amphetamines (e.g., methamphetamine)	Brief, repetitive, similar but irregular movements, such as blinking or shrugging shoulders
Clonus/Myoclonus 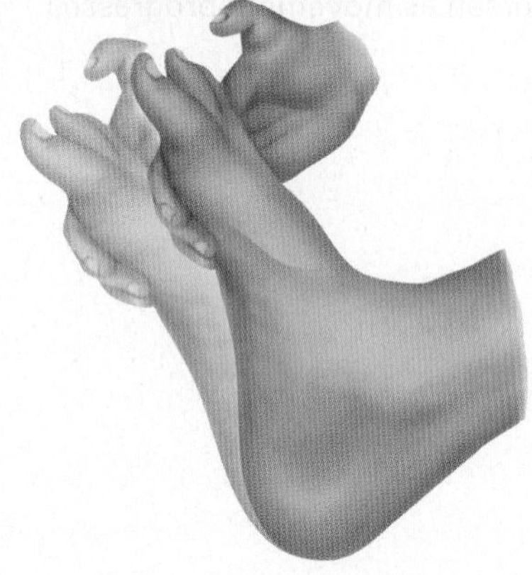	Seizures, hiccups, or just prior to falling asleep	Rapid, sudden, clonic spasm of a muscle that may occur regularly or intermittently
Dystonia 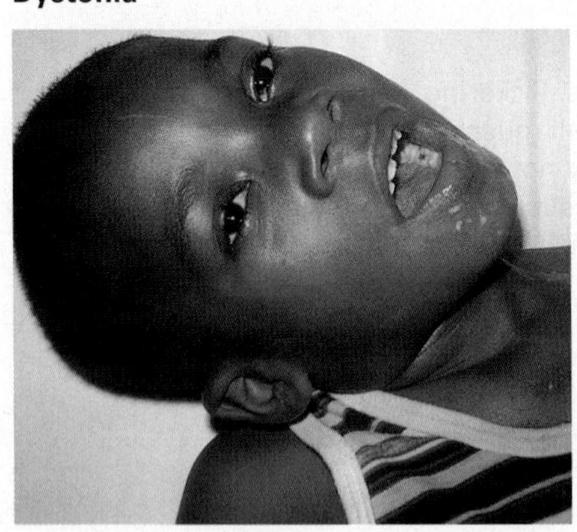	Use of psychiatric medications	Slow, involuntary, twisting movements that often involve the trunk and larger muscles; may be accompanied by twisted postures

(table continues on page 697)

TABLE 22.9 Abnormalities of Movements *(continued)*

	Common Associations	Description
Choreiform Movements	Huntington disease	Brief, rapid, jerky movements that are irregular and unpredictable; commonly affect the face, head, lower arms, and hands
Athetoid Movements	Cerebral palsy	Slow, involuntary, wormlike twisting movements that involve the extremities, neck, facial muscles, and tongue; may be associated with drooling and dysarthria

TABLE 22.10 Differential Diagnosis of Upper Motor Neuron Versus Lower Motor Neuron Lesions

Signs	Upper Motor Neuron Lesions	Lower Motor Neuron Lesions
Strength	Spastic paresis or paralysis (may be flaccid in acute phase)	Flaccid paresis or paralysis
Muscle tone	Increased (spasticity)	Decreased or absent (flaccidity)
Muscle stretch reflexes	Increased; presence of Babinski sign	Decreased or absent
Muscle atrophy	Absent (although disuse atrophy may occur with prolonged deficit)	Present
Muscle fasciculation	Absent	Present

UMN lesions involve motor areas of cerebral cortex and white matter tracts connecting to motor nerve nuclei in brain or spinal cord.
LMN lesions involve brainstem or spinal cord motor nuclei, nerve roots, or nerves.

TABLE 22.11 Abnormal Gaits

Picture	Pathologic Indication	Description
Spastic Hemiparesis 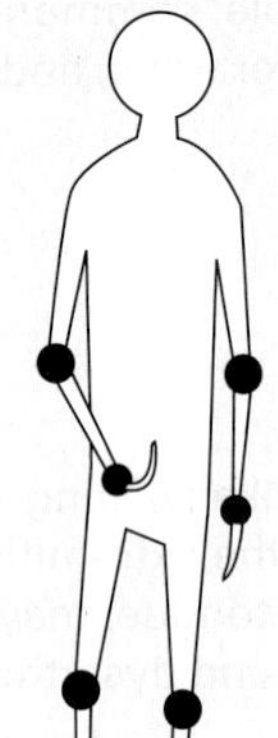	Stroke	One side of the body is normal. The other side is flexed from spasticity. The elbow, wrist, and fingers are flexed; the arm is close to the side. The affected leg is extended with plantar flexion of the foot. When ambulating, the foot is dragged, scraping the toe, or it is circled stiffly outward and forward.
Scissors 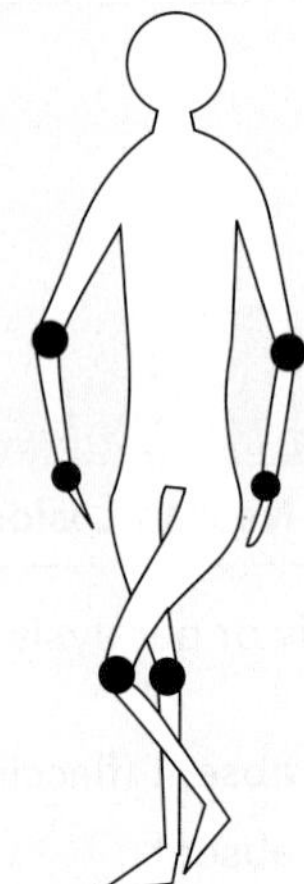	Spastic diplegia associated with bilateral spasticity of the legs	Moves the trunk to accommodate for the leg movements. Legs are extended and knees are flexed. Leg cross over each other at each step, similar to walking in water.
Parkinsonian 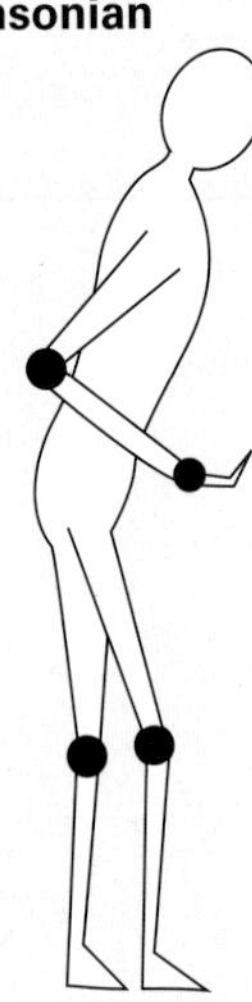	Parkinson disease	Stooped posture, head and neck forward and hips and knees flexed. Arms are also flexed and held at waist. There is difficulty in initiating gait, often rocking to start. Once in motion, steps are quick and shuffling. Has difficulty stopping once started.

(table continues on page 699)

TABLE 22.11 **Abnormal Gaits** *(continued)*

Picture	Pathologic Indication	Description
Cerebellar Ataxia 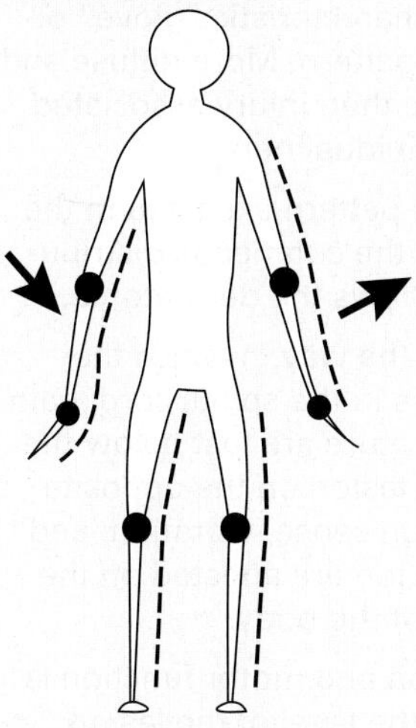	Cerebral palsy and alcohol intake	Wide-based gait. Staggers and lurches from side to side. Cannot perform Romberg because of swaying of the trunk.
Sensory Ataxia 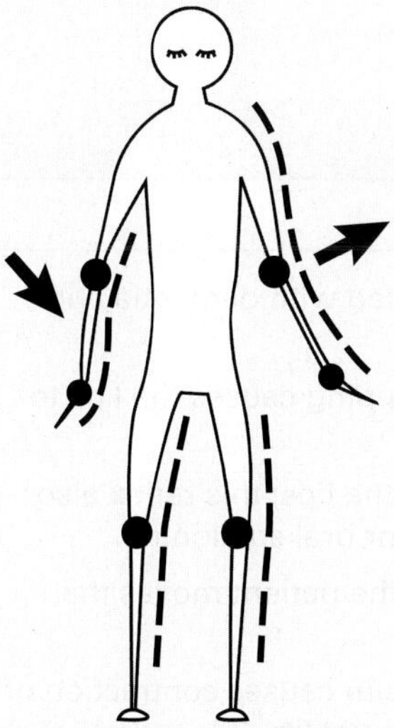	Cerebral palsy	Wide-based gait. Feet are loosely thrown forward, landing first on the heels and then on the toes. Patient watches the ground to help guide the feet. Positive Romberg sign from loss of position sense.
Dystrophic (Waddling)	Weak hip abductors	Wide gait. Weight is shifted from side to side with stiff trunk movement. Abdomen protrudes and lordosis is common.

TABLE 22.12 Abnormalities of Sensory Function

Abnormality	Pathological Indication	Description
Peripheral neuropathy	Diabetes mellitus or peripheral vascular disease	Sensory loss is distributed peripherally in a characteristic "glove" or "stocking" pattern. More diffuse and less specific than injury associated with an individual nerve.
Individual nerves	Trauma or injury	Follows the pattern expected in the nerve, with the cutaneous distribution that follows the dermatome.
Spinal cord hemisection	Brown-Séquard syndrome from spinal cord injury, tumor, or mass	Because of the way in which the nerves cross in the spinal cord, pain and temperature are lost below the level of the lesion on the opposite side. Position sense, vibration, and motor function are affected on the same side of the body.
Complete transection of the spinal cord	Spinal cord injury, tumor, or mass	All sensation and motor function is lost below the level of the lesion.

TABLE 22.13 Pathological (Primitive) Reflexes

Procedure	Abnormal Findings in Adults
Grasp reflex. Apply palmar stimulation.	A grasping response is associated with dementia and diffuse brain impairment.
Snout reflex. Elicit by tapping a tongue blade across the lips.	The snout reflex is present if tapping causes the lips to purse.
Sucking reflex. Touch or stroke the lips, tongue, or palate.	Observe sucking movement of the lips; this reflex also may be noted during oral care or oral suctioning.
Rooting reflex. Stroke the lateral upper lip.	The rooting reflex is present if the patient moves the mouth toward the stimulus.
Palmomental reflex. Stroke the palm of the hand.	It is present if stroking of the palm causes contraction of the same-sided muscle of the lower lip.
Hoffman sign. Tap the nail on the third or fourth finger.	A positive Hoffman sign is if tapping elicits involuntary flexion of the distal joint of the thumb and index finger.
Glabellar reflex. Tap the forehead to cause the patient to blink.	Normally, the first five taps cause a single blink, and then the reflex diminishes. Blinking continues in patients with diffuse cerebral dysfunction.

From Hickey, J. V. (2009). The neurological physical examination and neurological assessment. In J. V. Hickey (Ed.), *The clinical practice of neurological and neurosurgical nursing* (6th ed.). Philadelphia, PA: Lippincott Williams & Wilkins.

TABLE 22.14 **Abnormal Respiratory Patterns Associated With Intracranial Conditions**

Pattern and Description	Effect
Cheyne-Stokes Respiration (Spindle Pattern) Breathing pattern with period of apnea (10–60 seconds) followed by gradually increasing depth and frequency of respiration, gradually decreasing in depth and frequency until period of apnea	Poor brainstem perfusion
Central Neurogenic Hyperventilation Rapid and deep respirations, sometimes greater than 40 breaths/min	Medulla or pons malfunction
Apneustic Breathing Sustained inspiratory effort, usually less than 12 breaths/min	Medulla or pons damage
Gasping Rapid, quick, difficult breaths; irregular respirations with varying rate and tidal volume	Extensive pons damage, severe hypoxia
Biot Breathing (Cluster Pattern) Several short breaths followed by long irregular periods of apnea	Pons malfunction, increased ICP
Apnea Absence of breathing	High cervical cord or extensive medulla damage, brain death

From Webber, C. L. (2007). *Neural control of breathing*. Retrieved from http://www.meddean.luc.edu/lumen/meded/medicine/pulmonar/physio/pf11.htm; for more on abnormal breathing patterns, see Chapter 16.

23

Male Genitalia and Rectal Assessment

Learning Objectives

1 Demonstrate knowledge of the anatomy and physiology of the male genitalia and rectum.

2 Identify important topics for health promotion and risk reduction related to male genitalia and rectal assessment.

3 Collect subjective and objective data on the male genitalia, rectum, and prostate.

4 Identify expected and abnormal findings in the inspection and palpation of the male genitalia, prostate, and rectum.

5 Analyze subjective and objective findings from the assessment of the male genitalia and rectum and consider initial interventions.

6 Document and communicate data from the male genitalia and rectal assessment using appropriate medical terminology and principles of recording.

7 Consider the condition, age, gender, and culture of the patient to individualize the assessment of the male genitalia and rectum.

8 Identify differential diagnoses and initiate a plan of care based on findings from the male genitalia and rectal assessment.

Mr. Gardner, a 50-year-old Caucasian man, was diagnosed with benign prostatic hyperplasia (BPH) 3 years ago. He is visiting the clinic today because he is having increased difficulty with urination. Mr. Gardner has been married to his second wife for 3 months. Mr. Gardner states he is in a monogamous relationship and that he had a vasectomy about 15 years ago. He denies having erectile dysfunction, difficulty with ejaculation, or any discharge from or lesions on his penis. He has two children from his first marriage and two stepchildren. Mr. Gardner's temperature is 37.0°C (98.6 °F), pulse 84 beats/min, respirations 16 breaths/min, and blood pressure 122/68 mm Hg. His current medications include tamsulosin (Flomax) for BPH and lovastatin for his elevated lipid levels. His dietary supplements include a multivitamin and fish oil tablets that he takes to prevent cardiovascular disease. The nurse understands the importance of using evidence-based tools for assessing the impact of BPH on Mr.2Gardner. After obtaining the initial information, the nurse asks Mr. Gardner to fill out an American Urological Association Symptom Index form for BPH.

This questionnaire was designed to identify the degree of symptomatology in each patient. There are seven items on the questionnaire that determine the severity of symptoms including obstruction or irritation. Total symptoms scores may range from 0 to 35.

You will gain more information about Mr. Gardner as you progress through this chapter. As you study the content and features, consider Mr. Gardner's case and its relationship to what you are learning. Begin thinking about the following points:

- Is Mr. Gardner's condition stable, urgent, or an emergency?
- What are potential causes for difficulties with urination?
- How will the nurse incorporate an evidence-based standardized questionnaire to determine the degree of symptomatology?
- How will the nurse help Mr. Gardner to relax during inspection and palpation of his genitalia and rectum?
- What factors contribute to the patient's concerns?
- How will the nurse work with Mr. Gardner to promote health and reduce risk for illness?
- How will the nurse evaluate whether the assessment has been complete and accurate?

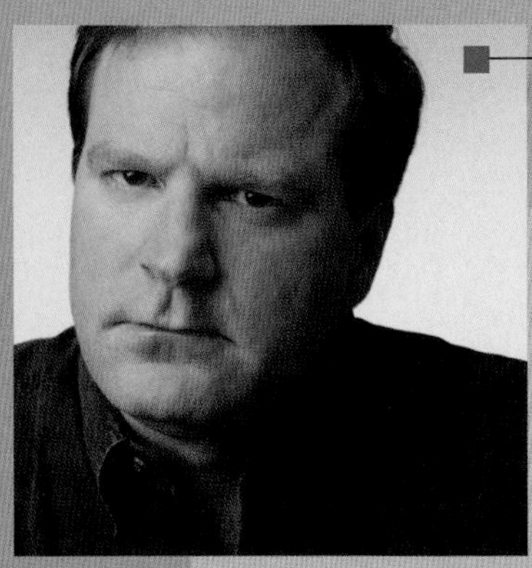

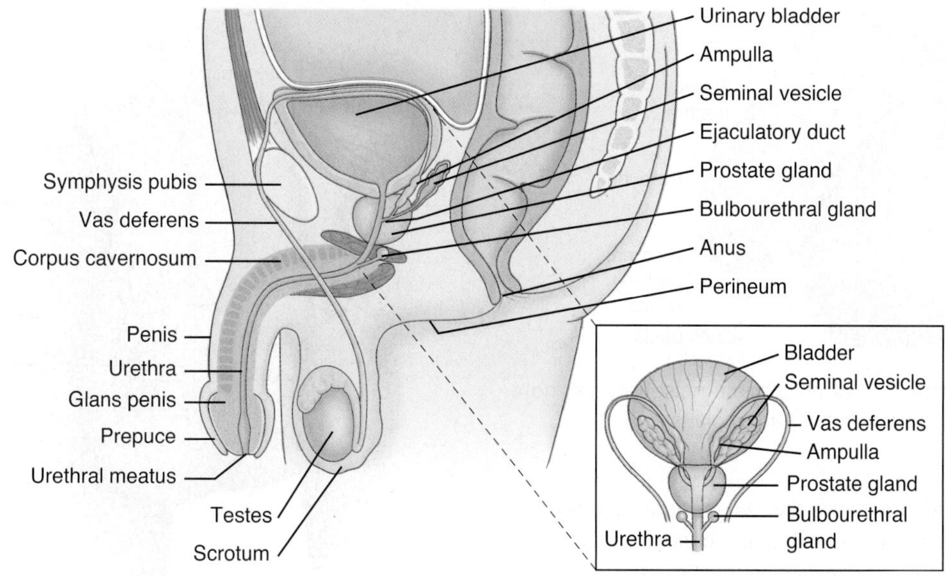

Figure 23.1 Overview of the male genitalia.

This chapter provides an overview of normal anatomy and focused physical assessment of the male genitalia, which includes the seminal vesicles, scrotum, penis, testicles, prostate gland, and epididymides (Fig. 23.1). Although the rectum and anus are terminal structures of the gastrointestinal tract (see Chapter 20), you will frequently integrate a holistic nursing assessment of these organs into the physical examination of the male genitalia. A basic understanding of pertinent anatomy helps you perform informed assessments with confidence.

During such a very intimate assessment, it is important to provide privacy for the patient. Ask open-ended questions; the patient's answers will help you guide the direction of the dialogue. The patient has the right for a chaperone to be present during the examination. In language the patient will understand, remember to explain each step of the assessment.

Educational opportunities often arise during assessment; you can teach health promotion and risk reduction while collecting subjective and objective data. All findings should be documented according to the protocols of your institution.

This chapter is designed to provide a foundation for you to conduct individualized health assessments in which you fully consider each patient's age, sexual orientation, and culture. Incorporated throughout are examples of evidence-based critical thinking, points of clinical significance, and key abnormal findings. A sensitive tactful approach to examination paves the way to providing excellent health care.

Structure and Function

External Genitalia

The penis has two functions: (1) it is the final excretory organ of urination, and (2) with sexual excitement, it becomes firm or erect to allow penetration for intercourse.

The penis can be subdivided into the root, shaft (or body), and glans penis (Fig. 23.2). The root of the penis lies deep within the perineum. The shaft has hairless thin skin that adheres loosely, allowing for expansion of the erect penis. The glans (head of the penis) is lighter in pigmentation than the rest of the organ.

The penis contains three distensible structures: two corpora cavernosa, which form the dorsum and sides of the penis, and a single corpus spongiosum, which forms the bulb. The urethra is located in the middle of the corpus spongiosum, which ends in the cone-shaped glans with its expanded base or corona. The small slit in the distal tip of the glans is the urethral meatus. The ridge of the corona separates the glans from the shaft.

When engorged with blood, the smooth spongy tissue of the penis becomes erect. An erection is a complex neurovascular reflex that ensues when a decreased venous outflow and an

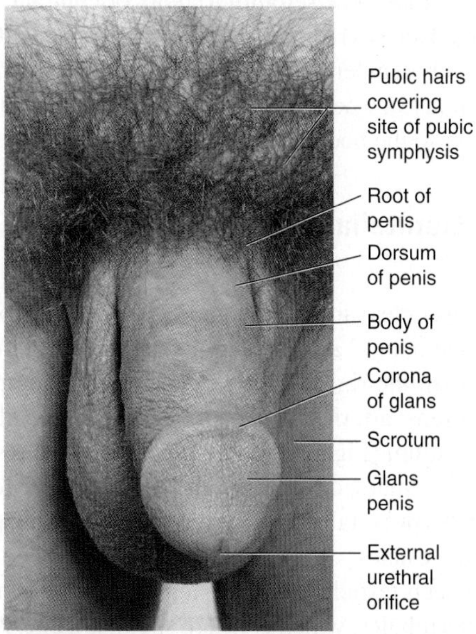

Figure 23.2 Surface anatomy of the penis.

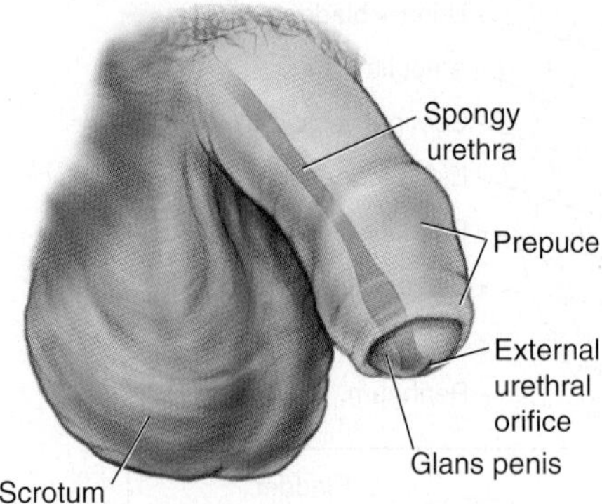

Figure 23.3 Depiction of an uncircumcised penis; note how the prepuce or foreskin covers the glans.

increased arterial dilation cause the two corpora cavernosa to fill with blood. This reflex is under the control of the autonomic nervous system and depends on local synthesis of nitric oxide. Psychogenic and local mechanisms can induce an erection. Any type of sensory input, including auditory, tactile, visual, or imaginative can cause a psychogenic erection. Tactile stimuli initiate the local reflex mechanisms.

Ejaculation occurs with emission of semen from the epididymides, vas deferens, prostate, and seminal vesicles. Ejaculation follows constriction of the arterial vessels supplying blood to the corpora cavernosa. After ejaculation, the penis returns to its normally flaccid condition.

In uncircumcised males, loose, hoodlike skin called the **prepuce** or foreskin covers the glans (Fig. 23.3). Pulling back the foreskin or prepuce exposes the **glans**. Sloughed epithelial cells and mucus collect between glans and foreskin, forming a white, cheeselike substance called **smegma**. Circumcision involves removal of the prepuce or foreskin.

The scrotum is a pouch covered with darkly pigmented, loose, rugous (wrinkled) skin. A septum divides the scrotum into two sacs, each of which contains a testis, epididymis, spermatic cord, and muscle layer known as the cremaster muscle. This allows the scrotum to relax or contract.

Spermatogenesis requires a temperature 3.5°F (2°C) lower than core body temperature. When the temperature rises, the scrotal sac relaxes; when temperature decreases, the scrotal sac moves closer to the body.

Internal Genitalia

Testes

The testes (testicles) are smooth and ovoid and approximately 3.5 to 5 cm about (1 ½ to 2 in.) long. Usually, the left testicle lies lower than the right. The spermatic cords (composed of the vas deferens, arteries, veins, and nerves) suspend the testes in the scrotum (Fig. 23.4). The function of the testicles is to produce spermatozoa (sperm) and testosterone. Testosterone stimulates pubertal growth of the male genitalia, prostate, and seminal vesicles.

Inside each testicle is a series of coiled ducts known as seminiferous tubules, which is where spermatogenesis occurs. Mature sperm are generated approximately every 90 days.

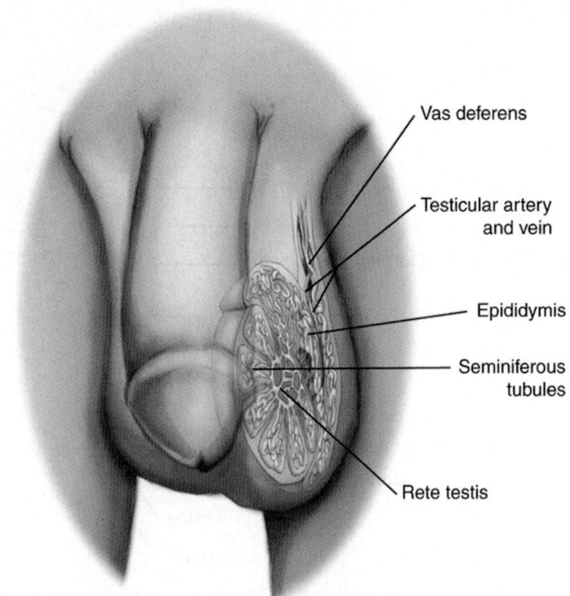

Figure 23.4 Anatomy of the testis.

As sperm are produced, they move toward the center of the testicle, traveling into the efferent tubules adjacent to the ductus epididymis.

Ducts

Ducts are responsible for moving sperm. The journey begins in the epididymides and continues to the vas deferens, ejaculatory duct, and urethra. The soft comma-shaped epididymis is on the posterolateral and upper aspect of the testicles. This structure provides for storage, maturation, and transit of sperm. The vas deferens (also called the ductus deferens) transports sperm from the epididymis to the ejaculatory duct. The vas deferens, arteries, veins, and nerves make up the spermatic cord, which ascends through the external inguinal ring and into the inguinal canal. Inside the canal, and just before the entrance into the prostate gland, the vas deferens unites with the seminal vesicle to form the ejaculatory duct.

After sperm enter the ejaculatory duct, they are transported downward through the prostate gland and into the posterior portion of the urethra. The urethra is approximately 18 to 20 cm (7 to 8 in.) long, extending from urinary bladder to meatus. The urethra can be divided into three sections: (1) posterior, (2) membranous, and (3) cavernous or anterior. It extends from the base of the bladder, traveling through the prostate gland down the shaft of the penis. The urethral opening is a small slit at the tip of the penis; it is the terminal route for both sperm and urine.

Glands

The seminal vesicles, prostate gland, and bulbourethral gland are the three structures that produce and secrete an ejaculation fluid known as semen. Semen provides an alkaline medium needed for motility and survival of the sperm. The seminal vesicles are small pouches located between the rectum and posterior bladder wall; the vesicles join the ejaculatory duct at the base of the prostate.

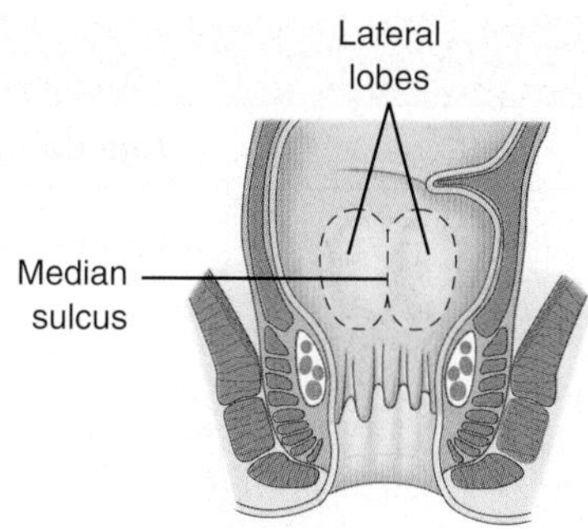

Figure 23.5 The prostate gland.

The prostate gland contains muscular and glandular tissue (Fig. 23.5). It has five lobes and is approximately 3.5 × 3.0 cm (about 1½ × 1¼ in.). The prostate gland surrounds the urethra at the bladder neck; its shape resembles that of a large chestnut. The physiological function of the prostate and its secretion is not fully understood; however, it produces the greatest volume of ejaculatory fluid. The right and left lobes of the prostate are divided by a slight groove known as the median sulcus. These two lobes are in close contact with the anterior rectal wall and are palpable during digital rectal examination (DRE). The median lobe is anterior of the urethra and cannot be palpated on a rectal examination. Prostatic cancer is known to have a tendency to locate in the gland's posterior and apical peripheral zone (and is thus palpable through the rectal wall), whereas BPH tends to affect the transition zone that surrounds the urethra.

> **Clinical Significance**
>
> **Benign prostatic hyperplasia** is another name for nodular hyperplasia of the prostate. It is one of the most common conditions affecting men older than 40 years of age. The middle and lateral lobes, which are usually located above the ejaculatory ducts, are typically involved in BPH. The exact cause of BPH is unknown, but the condition is believed to be associated with age-related hormonal changes. As men age, the fibromuscular structures of the prostate gland atrophy and collagen gradually replaces the muscular element of the prostate.

The bulbourethral glands are located on either side of the urethra immediately below the prostate gland.

Rectum and Anus

The rectum and anus constitute the terminal sections of the gastrointestinal (GI) tract and are included in the posterior portion of the male perineum examination.

Rectum

The rectum is approximately 12 cm long (about 4-3/4 in) and is located above the anus. The proximal end of the rectum is continuous with the sigmoid colon. The distal end, commonly referred to as the anorectal junction, is identifiable during a colonoscopy as having a sawtooth-like edge. Located above the anorectal junction, the rectum dilates and turns posteriorly into the hollow area of the coccyx and sacrum; this forms the rectal ampulla, which stores flatus and feces. Three semilunar transverse folds, known as rectal valves, are located in the rectum. The valves extend across half the diameter of the rectum with the inferior valve palpable on digital examination. The exact functions of these valves remain unknown; however, the valves may impede defecation while flatus is being expelled.

Anal Canal and Anus

The male's anal canal is approximately 2.5 to 4.0 cm (about 1 to 1½ in.) long and extends from the anorectal junction to the anus. It is lined with mucous membrane arranged in longitudinal folds called rectal columns, which contain a complex system of veins and arteries commonly referred to as the internal hemorrhoidal plexus. Between each column is a recessed area called the anal crypt. The perineal glands empty into the anal crypt. Around the anal canal are two concentric rings of muscles, the internal and external sphincters. The internal sphincter contains smooth muscle and is under involuntary control. The sensation to defecate comes when the rectum fills with stool, which causes reflexive stimulation that relaxes the internal sphincter. The striated external sphincter consists of skeletal muscles and is under voluntary control of defecation.

The anal canal perceives pain differently; the autonomic nervous system controls the upper portion, which is relatively insensitive to stimuli. Conversely, the lower portion, which is controlled by somatic sensory nerves, is sensitive to stimulation.

The anus is the terminal portion of the rectum. Its moist mucosal tissue is pink and surrounded by hyperpigmented perianal skin; hair may be present in an adult. Normally, the anus is closed except during defecation.

Lifespan Considerations

Children and Adolescents

Tanner's stages of maturation are used in the assessment of preadolescent and adolescent males. Stages of development of the males external primary and secondary sex characteristics are shown in Table 23.1.

Older Adults

In older men, degeneration of afferent neurons in the rectal wall can lessen the feeling of rectal distention and interfere with relaxation of the rectal sphincter, resulting in retention of stool. With this loss of tone of the autonomically controlled internal sphincter, the external sphincter cannot by itself control the bowels, and incontinence may result. With aging, pubic hair becomes finer, turns gray, and falls out as a result of alopecia. Testosterone levels decline with aging, which may affect both libido and sexual function. Erection becomes more dependent on tactile stimulation and less responsive to erotic cues. The penis may shrink; the testes drop lower in the scrotum. As the male ages, the fibromuscular structures of the prostate gland atrophy. Benign hyperplasia of the glandular tissue often obscures the atrophy of aging.

Aging affects sexual functioning: over 25% of men older than 65 years of age have **erectile dysfunction (ED)**. ED,

TABLE 23.1 **Tanner Staging: Male Development**

Stage	Male Development	Age Range (years)
1	There is no pubic hair. Testes and penis are small (prepubertal).	younger than 10
2	Sparse thin hair is at base of the penis. Testes enlarge. Scrotal skin becomes coarser and redder.	10–13
3	Scrotum and testes continue to grow. Penis lengthens, with diameter increasing slowly. Pubic hair increases, becoming darker, coarse, curly, and extending laterally.	12–14
4	Penis and testes continue to grow. Pubic hair extends across pubis but spares the medial thighs.	13–15
5	Penis is at its full size. Pubic hair is diamond shaped in appearance with adult color; texture extends to surface of medial thighs.	14–17

The Tanner stages present a scale of physical development for children, adolescents, and adults. The maturation process is based on external primary and secondary sex characteristics. Each person passes through each stage at different rates.
From Tanner, J. (1962). *Growth at adolescence*. Oxford, United Kingdom: Blackwell.

sometimes referred to as impotence, is the failure to consistently maintain a sufficiently ridged erect penis to allow for sexual intercourse. ED can also present as a lack of desire or inability to ejaculate. ED can have many causes, including neurological, vascular, physiological, psychological, and endocrinal. Episodes of impotence occur in about half of all adult men at one time or another in their lives and are not always pathological.

Cultural Considerations

When a patient becomes ill, his recognition of and reaction to illness are rooted in cultural beliefs, values, and social and family structures. Illness is more than just physical symptoms and pain. The concept of illness includes perceived difficulties with emotional, physical, and spiritual states. Appreciating the patient's perception of manhood, cultural beliefs, and sexual orientation will help you understand how the patient perceives health, illness, and disease. Establishing an open and trusting relationship with a patient requires a nonjudgmental attitude. As a dedicated nurse, you can develop an awareness of cultural beliefs and values through education, listening, and self-awareness.

Genital Piercing. For thousands of years, and in numerous societies, piercings have occurred in various forms and fashions. In the last 10 years, genital piercing has increased in popularity. Nevertheless, genital piercing can be an abnormal finding during assessment of the male genitalia. It is important to talk to the patient about the care of the piercing in a professional nonjudgmental manner. Because this site is highly prone to infection, discussion should involve how the patient cleans the piercing and ways to avoid infection. Inquire how the site feels to the patient, as it is possible for him to lose sensation in the area of the piercing. It may also damage strategic nerves, thus leading to an inability to achieve an orgasm (WebMD, 2013).

Investigate where the piercing was done; health risks such as hepatitis, tetanus, and tuberculosis, among other diseases, are possible when procedures are performed in an unsterile environment. U.S. laws concerning piercing vary in each state.

Urgent Assessment

⚠ *SAFETY ALERT*

Six conditions can result in an acute scrotum: ischemia, trauma, infection, inflammation, herniation, and emergency situations accompanying a chronic condition (e.g., testicular tumor with rupture). Although the differential diagnosis is broad, an accurate physical assessment and history can often accurately determine the condition. Imaging studies can correlate with the clinical assessment and expedite therapeutic decisions.

The signs and symptoms of the acutely ill genitourinary patient can range from subtle to obvious. An example of subtle signs is a patient complaining of fatigue or shortness of breath after exertion (possibly due to anemia from rectal bleeding). More obvious behaviors are a patient who complains of sudden and severe testicular pain (possibly testicular torsion) or urinary retention. All acute conditions need immediate evaluation. Patients presenting with an acute problem are anxious and tense; staying calm will help the patient relax and promote clear thinking.

It is important to compare two acute scrotal conditions: testicular torsion and epididymitis (Table 23.2). **Epididymitis** is inflammation of the epididymis; although painful, it is not usually an emergency. **Testicular torsion** is the twisting or rotation of the testes, resulting in acute ischemia. Because testicular torsion is a urological emergency, it is imperative for health care providers to understand the difference (Dunphy, Winland-Brown, Porter, & Thomas, 2011). Both diagnoses may present with the same chief concern of scrotal pain.

The Centers for Disease Control and Prevention (CDC) estimates that 1 of every 10 to 20 patients hospitalized in the United States develops a health care–associated infection (HAI) (also called a nosocomial infection) (CDC, 2013b). Urinary tract infection (UTI), a type of HAI, accounts for more than 30% of infections reported by acute care hospitals in the United States. Virtually all hospital-associated UTIs are caused by instrumentation of the urinary tract, mainly from indwelling urinary catheters. Prevention of a **catheter-acquired urinary tract infection (CAUTI)** is a key component of an acute-care hospital's patient safety and quality improvement program.

Anorectal difficulties can cause significant discomfort and concern. Because of the sensitive nature of this subject, patients often delay treatment. Colorectal cancer is common in adults and may be present with a benign condition. All complaints need thorough investigation. Early detection has been clearly shown to lower the mortality rate for colorectal cancer. The patient with rectal bleeding needs rapid assessment. Bleeding associated with anorectal difficulties can resolve spontaneously or with local pressure. The patient undergoing anticoagulation therapy, however, may need hospitalization. Inquire about medications and bleeding disorders.

A newborn with dark tarry stools or who is vomiting blood may have a vitamin K deficiency. An infant presenting with rectal bleeding could have necrotizing enterocolitis, a life-threatening disease that needs immediate action.

Subjective Data

Subjective data collection includes a focused health history related to common symptoms, assessments for prostate and testicular cancer, and assessment of risk factors. It is important to assess risk for sexually transmitted infections (STIs). While collecting information from the patient, opportunities for health promotion and health-related patient teaching will present themselves.

Assessment of Risk Factors

Numerous factors affect the male genitalia, rectum, and anus. Ask the patient about current problems, family history, personal history (including age, gender, and ethnicity), medications and supplements, and risk factors for infections or cancer. Knowledge of risk factors helps identify topics for health promotion teaching.

TABLE 23.2 Testicular Torsion Versus Epididymitis

Testicular Torsion	Epididymitis
Pain is acute.	Pain is gradual.
Nausea and vomiting occur in 50% of patients.	Nausea and vomiting are rare findings.
Fever is rare.	Fever occurs in 50% of patients.
Voiding symptoms, urethral irritation, and urethral discharge are rare.	Voiding symptoms, urethral irritation, and urethral discharge occur in 50% of patients.
0%–30% of patients have abnormal results in urinalysis.	Urinalysis will be diagnostic in 20%–95% of those with epididymitis.
Elevation of affected testicle does not lessen pain.	Elevation of affected testicle usually lessens pain.
Surgical intervention is immediately required.	Antibiotic therapy is indicated.

History and Risk Factors	Rationale
Personal History	
Do you have any current or chronic illnesses such as diabetes mellitus, hypertension, neurological impairment, respiratory problems (asthma, chronic obstructive pulmonary disease [COPD], chronic bronchitis), or cardiovascular disease?	Men with these illnesses are at increased risk for ED.
Medical and Surgical History	
• Was surgery ever performed on your penis, scrotum, or rectum? • What type of procedure was performed? What was the year and date? • How has this procedure affected you?	Surgery is used to treat enlarged prostate, testicular cancer, hydrocele, varicocele, and undescended testicle. Some men choose permanent sterilization through vasectomy. Rectal or anal conditions requiring surgery include hemorrhoids, anorectal fissures, and carcinoma of the rectum and anus.
• Have you ever been treated for an STI? • Where and when did you receive this treatment? • What type of STI was diagnosed? • How was it treated? • Did you have a test of cure following the procedure?	More than 50 different STIs have been identified. This is an important but sensitive topic for discussion. Tactful direct questioning is an essential part of the assessment. See Box 23.1 for STI risk factors.
• Have you ever had an injury to, or difficulties with, your scrotum, penis, or testes? If yes, please explain.	Examples include testicular torsion, hydrocele, spermatocele, and varicocele.
• Have you had a condition affecting the prostate gland, such as BPH or prostatitis?	Identification of previous difficulties may help when documenting current health concerns.
• Do you have a history of cancer? • When was the diagnosis? • What treatment did you have?	See Box 23.2 for risk factors for testicular, prostate, and penile cancers (common cancers found in men). Even with removal of a cancerous testicle, cancer can recur in the other testicle.
Sexual History	
• How old were you the first time you had sexual intercourse? • Was this by choice? • Do you prefer sexual relationships with men, women, or both? • In what type of sex do you engage (penile–vaginal, penile–rectal, recipient rectal, oral)? • How frequently do you have intercourse? • Do you have sex with multiple partners? • How many partners have you had in the last 6 months? • Do you or your partner frequently use drugs or alcohol before sexual intercourse? • Are you satisfied with your sexual relationship? • Do you use contraceptives? Do you use protective barriers every time you have intercourse? • Have you ever gotten someone pregnant? • What was the outcome of this situation? • Have you ever been pushed, slapped, or had something thrown at you? • Have you ever been kicked, bitten, or hit with a hand or object?	Often, nurses hesitate to initiate conversation about sexual history. Nevertheless, this information is important to help identify high-risk sexual practices, establish patient norms, and provide education. Sexual dysfunction can present as anxiety, anger, or depression. In addition, physical difficulties can lead to sexual difficulties. You must be careful not to impose your personal standards on the patient. **SAFETY ALERT** *Men as well as women can be victims of abuse, so it is important to ask these questions. Often, it is difficult for men to admit that they are being victimized. See Chapter 9.* *(table continues on page 709)*

BOX 23.1 Risk Factors for Sexually Transmitted Infections

- Engaging in sexual relations with a new partner or with multiple partners*
- Personal history of STIs or engaging in sexual activity with a partner with a history of STIs*
- Engaging in a relationship with a partner who has several partners*
- Failure to practice safe sex*

STIs can be transmitted through vaginal, rectal, or oral sex between homosexual or heterosexual partners. STIs are on the rise. In response to that increase, the CDC (2010) have published guidelines for sexually transmitted diseases, which include information on prevention, diagnosis, and treatment for all known STDs and is available online at 2010 STD Treatment Guidelines (http://www.cdc.gov/std/treatment/2010/).

*The risk factor is modifiable.

BOX 23.2 Risk Factors for Testicular, Prostate, and Penile Cancer

Testicular Cancer

- Age: highest incidence in young men ages 20–34 years
- Ethnicity and culture: highest incidence among Caucasian men in the United Kingdom and United States
- Cryptorchidism (undescended testicle at birth)
- History of testicular cancer in other testicle
- Family history: increased risk if brother has had testicular cancer

Prostate Cancer

- Second leading cause of cancer death in men
- Family history of prostate cancer
- Age: highest incidence is in older men; 75% of new cases occur in men older than 65 years of age
- Ethnicity: African American men have highest incidence of prostate cancer—two times higher than white men. Worldwide, highest prevalence is in North America and northwestern Europe.

Penile Cancer

- Phimosis (the foreskin of the penis cannot be pulled back over the glans)*
- Age 60 years or older
- Poor personal hygiene*
- Sexual promiscuity*
- Using tobacco products*
- Possible link with HPV*

*This risk factor is modifiable.

Data from American Cancer Society (ACS). (2013). *What are the key statistics about testicular cancer?* Retrieved from http://www.cancer.org/cancer/testicularcancer/detailedguide/testicular-cancer-key-statistics; National Cancer Institute at the National Institute of Health; American Urology Association; National Cancer Institute. (n.d.). *NCI Fact sheets.* Retrieved from http://www.cancer.gov/cancertopics/factsheet

History and Risk Factors	Rationale
Do you wear protective gear during contact sports?	Lack of protection can lead to injury of sensitive genitalia. This question can provide a good teaching opportunity to encourage the use of protective equipment.
Have you received a hepatitis A or B vaccine or screening for Hepatitis C?	**SAFETY ALERT** *The CDC (2012) recommend the hepatitis A vaccine for unimmunized men who have sex with men. The CDC recommends the hepatitis B vaccine for all unimmunized people at risk for STIs.* Hepatitis C is a liver disease caused by the hepatitis C virus (HCV). HCV infection sometimes results in an acute illness, but most often becomes a chronic condition that can lead to cirrhosis and liver cancer.
Do you perform self-genital examination?	This question serves as an excellent teaching opportunity. Stress to the patient the importance of the self-examination.
Do you have regular clinical examinations by a health professional?	Primary prevention helps patients maintain health. Age-appropriate health screenings should be discussed during the appointment.
Medications What medications do you currently take, including herbal supplements, recreational drugs, and over-the-counter (OTC) drugs?	Many medications and supplements can affect the genitourinary tract and its function.
Family History Is there a family history of testicular cancer?	Risk for testicular cancer is greater in men whose brother or father had the disease (American Cancer Society [ACS], 2013). See Box 23.2.
Is there a family history of prostate cancer?	Prostate cancer in a first-degree relative increases the patient's risk. African American men have the highest incidence of prostate cancer—two to three times higher than Caucasian men. Prevalence is highest in North America and Europe (ACS, 2013). See Box 23.2.

(table continues on page 710)

History and Risk Factors	Rationale
Is there a history of penile cancer in your family?	Although rare in the United States, some studies suggest an association between penile cancer and human papillomavirus (HPV) (CDC, 2013a). See Box 23.2.
Are any of your siblings infertile?	Encourage the patient to review his family tree for signs of infertility, especially if he is having difficulties impregnating his partner.
Is there a history of hernia in your family?	Congenital weakness may predispose the patient to developing a hernia.

Risk Reduction and Health Promotion

It is important for men to screen themselves for testicular cancer by performing self-examination. Screening for prostate cancer is through laboratory blood testing and physical examination.

Health Goals

The overarching goals of health promotion are to attain high-quality, longer lives free from preventable disease, disability, injury, and premature death; achieve health equity, eliminate disparities, and improve the health of all groups; create social and physical environments that promote good health for all; and promote quality of life, healthy development, and healthy behaviors across all life stages. Male health promotion is very important because many problems are preventable. Additionally, both testicular and prostate cancers have better outcomes if detected early. The following goals relate to prostate cancer, family planning, and STIs (U.S. Department of Health and Human Services; Healthy People 2020, 2013):

- Reduce the prostate cancer death rate.
- Increase male involvement in pregnancy prevention and family planning efforts.
- Reduce the number of new AIDS cases among adolescent and adult men who have sex with men.
- Reduce the proportion of adults with *Chlamydia trachomatis*, gonorrhea, syphilis, and genital herpes infections.

Testicular Self-Examination

The purpose of performing self-examination is not necessarily to find something currently wrong. By performing monthly self-examinations, men and adolescents older than 14 years of age become familiar with what is normal for them. After this "normal" has been established, changes are easier to identify. Thus, testicular cancer can be detected at an early (and most often curable) stage.

Testicular self-examination (TSE) is best performed after a warm shower or bath. Heat relaxes the scrotum, which makes the TSE easier. Steps for TSE are as follows:

1. Examine each testicle with both hands. Place the index and middle fingers under the testicle and the thumbs on top. Roll the testicle gently from side to side. You should not feel pain. Remember that one testicle may be larger; this finding is normal (Fig. 23.6).

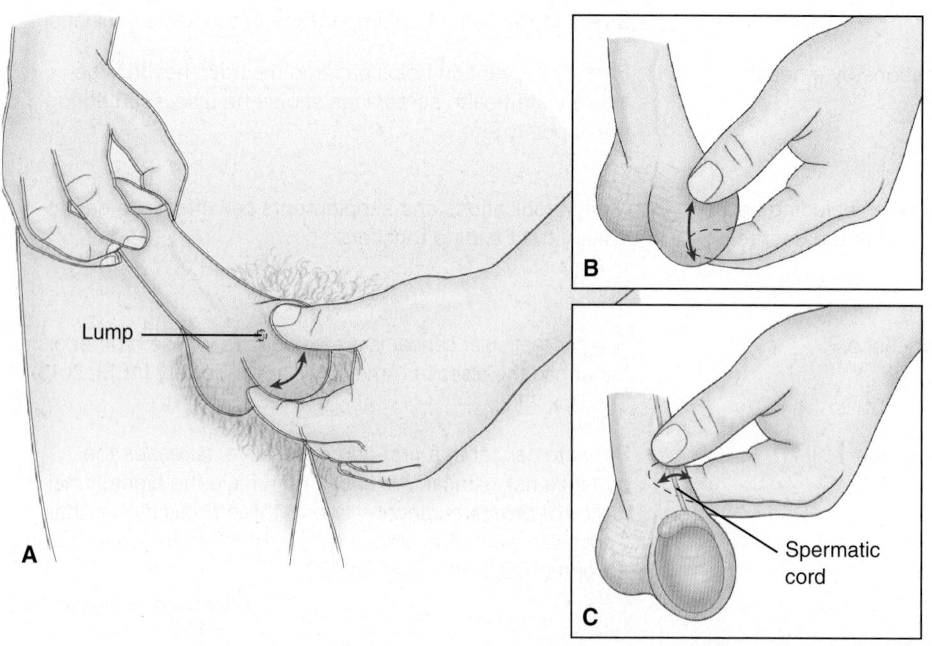

Figure 23.6 The testicular self-examination (TSE). **A.** The patient holds the penis in one hand away from the testicles while using the other hand to palpate one testicle at a time. The patient should roll the area side to side to feel for any lumps. **B.** He also should maneuver his fingers up and down. **C.** The patient should also run his fingers along the surface length of the spermatic cord to become familiar with how it feels, so that he does not mistake this for a lump.

2. Cancerous lumps usually are on the sides of the testicle, but can show up on the front. Become familiar with the location of the epididymis; this soft, tubelike structure behind the testes collects and carries sperm. If you become familiar with this structure, you won't mistake it for a lump.
3. Make an appointment with a physician, preferably a urologist, as soon as possible if you find a lump or any of the following warning signs: enlargement of the testes, pain or discomfort, heaviness in the scrotum, a dull ache in the groin, significant loss of size of one testicle, or a sudden collection of fluid in the scrotum (The Testicular Cancer Resource Center, 2012).

Screening for Prostate Cancer

In 2013, a long-awaited update from the U.S. Preventive Services Task Force (USPSTF) recommended against screening men for prostate cancer with the prostate-specific antigen (PSA) test. The task force's recommendation advised only against screening men aged 75 years and older; the update has extended that guidance to include all men. As per the USPSTF and the National Cancer Institute, evidence is insufficient to conclude whether screening for prostate cancer with prostate-specific antigen (PSA) or DRE reduces mortality resulting from prostate cancer. Based on an analysis of several studies, the USPSTF concluded that no more than 1 death would be avoided for every 1,000 men aged 55 to 69 years screened every 1 to 4 years for a decade (USPSTF, 2012).

Common Symptoms

Common Symptoms of the Male Genitalia, Prostate, and Rectum

- Pain
- Problems with urination
- ED
- Penile lesions, penile discharge
- Scrotal enlargement

Signs/Symptoms	Rationale/Abnormal Findings
Pain	
Please point to the painful area. • Do you feel the pain anywhere else? • When did it begin? How long have you had this pain? Have you ever experienced this pain before? • Can you rate your pain on a scale of 0–10, with 10 being the worst pain you have ever had? • What does the pain feel like? • Is the pain associated with nausea, vomiting, fever, abdominal distention, and burning on urination? Is your urine a different color? • What makes the pain worse or what better? What have you done to help alleviate the pain, if anything? How well did this intervention help? • What is your pain goal?	Various problems can lead to pain in the lower abdominal, pelvic, or rectal areas. Sudden distention of the ureter, renal pelvis, or bladder may cause flank pain. Pain around the costovertebral angle may be from distention of the renal capsule. Kidney stone pain may radiate down the spermatic cord and present as testicular pain. Pain in the groin or scrotum may result from a hernia or problems in the spermatic cord, testicles, or prostate. Testicular pain can occur secondary to any problem of the testes such as epididymitis, orchitis, hydrocele, spermatic cord torsion, and tumors. Understanding what interventions the patient uses to relieve the pain assists with developing a treatment plan. Always ask about use of OTC medications, current prescriptions, and herbal remedies.
Have you ever had a prolonged painful erection?	A long and painful erection is called **priapism**. It can occur in patients with leukemia or hemoglobinopathies (e.g., sickle cell anemia). This is not from sexual excitation—the prolonged erection results from vein thrombosis in the corpora cavernosa.
Are you experiencing rectal or anal pain?	Perianal abscess, rectal fissure, and hemorrhoids are among the most painful problems of the anus and rectum.
Difficulties with Urination	
• Do you have trouble starting a stream of urine? • Is there a change in the flow of urine? • Do you have sudden urges to urinate? • Can you estimate how much urine is passed with each void or urination? • Do you need to urinate at night? • Are you straining to urinate? • Have you been drinking more fluids than usual? • Do you involuntarily lose small amounts of urine?	Urgency and frequency may be from UTIs, prostatitis, STIs, or low-grade bladder cancer. Prostate enlargement is common in older men; because of the location of the gland, it can affect urine flow. The following are signs of partial prostate obstruction: recurrent acute UTIs, the sensation of residual urine, decreased caliber of the urine stream, hesitancy, straining, and terminal dribbling.

(table continues on page 712)

Signs/Symptoms	Rationale/Abnormal Findings
• What color is your urine? Do you ever notice red urine?	Blood in the urine can be associated with a benign disease, a clinically insignificant issue (e.g., eating red foods), or a life-threatening malignancy. It is therefore one of the most common and important signs for the nurse to investigate.
• Do you have persistent erections unrelated to sexual stimulation? • With an erection, do you have a curvature of the penis in any direction? • Do you have difficulty achieving erection? Is there pain associated with the erection? • When you have sexual stimulation or intercourse, how often do you ejaculate? What is the color, consistency, and amount of the ejaculate? • How strong is your sex drive? Over the last month, how would you rate your confidence in achieving and maintaining an erection? • If you were to spend the rest of your life with your sexual function just the way it is now, how would you feel about that?	The main types of sexual dysfunction include premature ejaculation, ED (difficulty achieving or maintaining erection), low libido (low sexual interest), delayed orgasm, and physical abnormalities of the penis. ED cannot be seen or palpated during an assessment; thus, this issue is important to discuss with the patient. Many men welcome the opportunity to discuss ED, but nurses are often reluctant to bring up the subject. Presenting the topic in a nonthreatening, nonjudgmental manner encourages the patient to talk about ED. An example of an opening statement for a patient whose hypertension is controlled with medication is, "High blood pressure medications often cause erectile dysfunction. Have you experienced any problems?"
Penile Lesions, Discharge, or Rash • When did you first note the lesion? Is there more than one? • Is pain, itching, burning, or stinging associated with the lesion? • Is there a discharge? When did the discharge begin? Is there an odor or color associated with it? • If you are sexually active, does your partner have the same symptoms? Has there been a change in sexual partners?	Direct tactful questioning about a history of exposure to STIs is important. A lesion should alert you to the possibility of an STI. Ask whether the patient has had genital warts, syphilis, gonorrhea, trichomoniasis, or other STIs. Ask whether any discharge is continuous or intermittent. Bloody penile discharge is associated with urethritis and neoplasm. Tactfully explore whether the patient has been with a new partner recently or if there has been a change in sexual habits.
Scrotal Enlargement • When did you first notice the enlargement? • Is there pain associated with it? Is the pain intermittent or constant. Is it associated with lifting or straining? • Has there been any recent trauma to your groin? • Have you ever had a hernia? Do you use a truss or any treatment? • Have you had any difficulties with fertility?	Although rarely fatal, scrotal enlargement and pain carry a risk of morbidity from testicular atrophy, infarction, or necrosis. Any patient with scrotal pain should be presumed to have testicular torsion until another diagnosis can be proven. Accurate history and assessing skills contribute to an accurate diagnosis. Assess the patient for varicoceles, which are often linked with infertility.

Documenting Normal Findings

Patient denies pain or discomfort. No difficulty with urination. States that he has no premature ejaculation, ED, low libido, delayed orgasm, or physical abnormalities of the penis. States no lesions, discharge, or scrotal enlargement.

Lifespan Considerations: Older Adults

Additional Questions	Rationale/Abnormal Findings
Are you noticing urinary dribbling, urgency, or frequency? Do you feel that your bladder does not completely empty?	Disorders of the prostate, including hyperplasia and cancer, are more common in older adults.
Often, older adults may notice a change in their sexual function as they age. Have you noticed any such changes?	Older adults may notice that it may take longer to obtain an erection or ejaculate. Also consider coexisting illnesses and medications that may affect sexual function.

Cultural Considerations

Additional Questions	Rationale/Abnormal Findings
Based on your age, ethnicity, and sexual preference, what do you perceive as your risk for developing HIV or other STIs?	In young men who have sex with men, black men have 1.6 times as many new HIV infections as white men, and 2.3 times as many as Hispanic men (Quinn, Bartlett, & McGovern, 2009). Men who have sex with men are also at higher risk for genital herpes. These men should be offered STI screening at the annual visit.

Therapeutic Dialogue: Collecting Subjective Data

Remember Mr. Gardner, who was introduced at the beginning of this chapter. He is a 50-year-old man with a history of BPH and increasing symptoms. The nurse uses professional communication techniques to gather subjective data from Mr. Gardner.

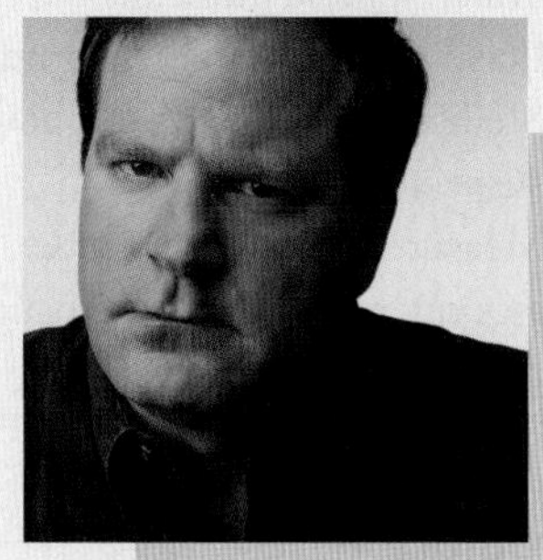

Nurse: Hi, Mr. Gardner. It looks like you're here because of difficulty urinating. I see that you have BPH.

Mr. Gardner: Yes, I've had it for 3 years.

Nurse: Can you tell me more about your symptoms?

Mr. Gardner: Well, I am having more trouble with urination.

Nurse: So is that difficulty with starting your urine stream?

Mr. Gardner: Yes, and when I go, it seems like it starts and stops.

Nurse: And sometimes, men also have some dribbling . . .

Mr. Gardner: Yes, I've had that too, and it's embarrassing. It also seems like my bladder never completely empties. I go and then I have to go back an hour or two later.

Nurse: That must be very uncomfortable.

Mr. Gardner: Yes, it is. I am newly married and I'm worried that this might affect my relationship if I have to have surgery.

Critical Thinking Challenge

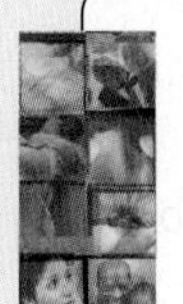

- How might the nurse be better prepared for the interview? What is your comfort level in discussing issues related to sexuality, reproduction, and male genitalia?
- What techniques will the nurse use to discuss concerns regarding these intimate issues?
- How will the nurse address Mr. Gardner's embarrassment?
- What concerns might Mr. Gardner have that could be further assessed? To what extent might you want to involve others in the dialogue?

Objective Data

Common and Specialty or Advanced Techniques

The most important and common assessment techniques used in the comprehensive male genital and rectal assessment are summarized in the table. Additional specialty techniques may be added if indicated by the clinical situation, or in advanced practice for diagnosis. Note that the function of the registered nurse is primarily inspection. Advanced education is required for the more invasive genital examination.

Equipment

- Latex gloves (check patient for allergies)
- Water-soluble lubricant
- Flashlight or penlight (for transillumination)
- Stethoscope (to listen for bowel sounds if hernia is suspected)
- Measurements of your index finger, which can be used as a ruler to measure the patient's penis, testes, and prostate gland

Preparation

It is important to maintain a confident, professional, matter-of-fact attitude throughout the examination. Upon entering the examination room, introduce yourself and include your title. Greet the patient by his full name and ask what he prefers to be called. Before beginning the genital examination, ask permission to perform it; this step is especially important if you are a woman. Asking permission allows the patient to gracefully ask for a male nurse for this part of the examination if he so prefers.

If performing a complete history and physical assessment, conduct the genital examination last. Doing so allows the patient to become more comfortable with the overall interaction. A parent should always be present for a child's genital examination. An adolescent should have a choice as to whether he prefers a parent or guardian present. An adult man accompanied by a companion should be given the option of having his companion present during the assessment.

Examine the patient in the supine position, on his side, and then standing. While the patient is standing, you should be seated in front of him.

Clinical Significance

If the patient has an erection during the physical examination, reassure him that this is a normal physiological response to touch that he could not have prevented. Do not stop the examination—doing so could cause further embarrassment.

Basic Versus Focused/Specialty or Advanced Techniques Related to Male Genital and Rectal Assessment

Technique	Purpose	Screening or Registered Nurse Assessment	Focused or Advanced Practice Examination
Inspect the genital hair, penis, and scrotum.	Inspect skin, assess gross deformities	X	
Inspect the inguinal region and the femoral area.	Inspect gross deformities	X	
Inspect the sacrococcygeal areas, perianal area, and anus.	Inspect gross deformities	X	
Palpate the genital hair, penis, and scrotum.	Masses, texture		X Genital examination
Palpate the scrotum, testes, epididymides, and vas deferens.	Masses, texture		X Genital examination
Transilluminate the scrotum.	Mass or fluid		X Mass or fluid
Palpate the inguinal canal.	Hernias		X Hernias
Palpate the sacrococcygeal areas, perianal area, and anus.	Hemorrhoids, fissures, stool		X Hemorrhoids, fissures, stool
Palpate the anal canal and the prostate.	Rectal tone and enlarged prostate		X Rectal tone and enlarged prostate
Examine stool.	Consistency, color		X Test for blood

Comprehensive Physical Assessment

Technique and Normal Findings	Abnormal Findings
Groin With the patient supine, inspect the groin. Observe genital hair distribution. ■ Skin is clear, intact, and smooth. Hair is diamond shaped or in an escutcheon pattern. Hair appears coarser than at the scalp and has no parasites.	Unexpected genital hair findings are no hair, patchy growth, or distribution in a female or triangular pattern with the base over the pubis. Observe for any infestations such as pediculosis, scabies, or other parasites. Look for inflammation, lesions, or dermatitis. Candidiasis infections cause crusty, multiple, red, round erosions and pustules; this infection is associated with immunological deficiencies. Tinea cruris (commonly referred to as "jock itch") is a fungal infection on the patient's groin and upper thighs. It appears with large, red, scaly patches that are extremely itchy. Tinea cruris rarely involves the scrotum. See Table 23.7 at the end of the chapter for a list and descriptions of potential infections.
Penis Observe the penis for surface characteristics, color, lesions, and discharge. Be sure to inspect the posterior side. ■ The dorsal vein is apparent on the dorsal surface of the penis. The penis has no edema, lesions, discharge, or nodules.	Unexpected conditions include piercings, phimosis (foreskin cannot retract), paraphimosis (foreskin is retracted and fixed), and balanitis (related to diabetes mellitus). See Table 23.8 at the end of this chapter for photos and descriptions of abnormal conditions.
In the patient with an uncircumcised penis, the prepuce covers the glans. Ask the patient to retract the prepuce. ■ The prepuce retracts easily. **Smegma** (a thin, white, cheesy substance) may be normally present around the corona. In the patient with a circumcised penis, the glans and corona are visible, lighter in color than the shaft, and free of smegma. Circumcised penises have varying lengths of foreskin: some have folds of skin, whereas others have no extra foreskin (see Fig. 23.1).	
Glans. Inspect the glans. ■ Glans is glistening pink, smooth in texture, and bulbous.	
Shaft. Inspect and palpate the shaft. ■ Shaft feels smooth without lesions or pain. Expected variations include ectopic sebaceous glands on the shaft that appear as tiny whitish-yellow papules.	Abnormal conditions of the glans include **hypospadias** (urethral meatus on underside) and **epispadias** (urethral meatus on upper side). See Table 23.8 at the end of the chapter.
External Urethral Meatus. Inspect and palpate the external urethral meatus (Fig. 23.7). ■ Meatus is located centrally on the glans. The orifice is slitlike and millimeters from the tip of the penis. The external urethral meatus has no discharge, stenosis, or warts. The glans can be opened by pressing it between the thumb and forefinger; the patient can be instructed to do this. Next, strip or milk the penis from the base toward the glans or head. Note color, consistency, or odor of any discharge. ■ The glans is smooth and pink with no discharge.	Discharge may be yellow, milky-white, or greenish and may have a foul odor. It needs immediate attention. See Table 23.7 at the end of the chapter.

(table continues on page 716)

Technique and Normal Findings (continued)	Abnormal Findings (continued)
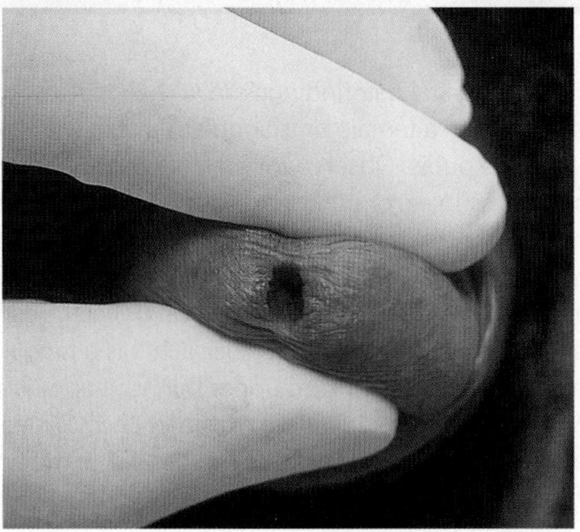 Figure 23.7 Inspecting and palpating the external urinary meatus.	
Scrotum Ask the patient to hold the penis out of the way. Inspect the scrotal septum. Inspect the anterior and posterior scrotum for any sores or rashes. *Scrotum is divided into two sacs. The scrotum could hang asymmetrically, with the left side lower than the right. Sebaceous cysts or sebaceous glands may be normally noted on the scrotal sac. The anterior and posterior scrotal skin appears darker in pigmentation with a rugous or wrinkled surface.*	Scrotal lesions, edema, and redness are unexpected. When examining the scrotum, certain diseases (e.g., diabetic neuropathy, syphilis) may render the testes totally insensitive to pain. Renal, cardiac, and hepatic illness may result in scrotal edema. If inconsistencies in size or texture are present, be alert for possible infection, tumor, or cyst. Abnormal scrotal conditions include testicular torsion, epididymitis, varicocele, hydrocele, and spermatocele. See Table 23.7 at the end of the chapter.
Sacrococcygeal Areas Inspect the sacrococcygeal areas for surface characteristics and tenderness. Skin is clear and smooth with no palpable masses or dimpling.	A dimple with an inflamed tuft of hair or a tender palpable cyst in the sacrococcygeal area suggests a **pilonidal cyst** or sinus. Generally, the patient is asymptomatic unless the area becomes infected. After infection, redness, tenderness, and a palpable cyst are present. When ruptured, the cyst drains purulent mucoid secretions. Often, the affected patient is febrile.
Perineal Area With the patient on his side, spread the buttocks and inspect the perineal area. Skin surrounding the anus is coarse with darker pigmentation. The anal sphincter is closed.	A penlight assists in inspecting for warts, loose sphincter, lesions, hemorrhoids, fissures, fistulas, or polyps. Infestations from pinworms or fungal infections make this area appear irritated and erythremic. See Table 23.9 at the end of this chapter.
Inguinal Region and Femoral Areas Instruct the patient to stand. Ask him to bear down. While he does so, inspect the inguinal canal area and femoral area for bulges or masses.	Bulges or masses suggest a **hernia**. If a bulge is noted, the inguinal canal needs to be palpated. See Table 23.10 at the end of the chapter.

Documenting Normal Findings

Penis free from skin lesions and indurations. Scant amount smegma present. Glans smooth. Urethral meatus at distal end of glans. No lateral curvature or flexion. Prepuce retracts easily. Urethral meatus opens readily and is free from discharge, no tenderness. Scrotum wrinkled, loose, no lesions. Spermatic cord palpable, smooth bilaterally. Left testes lower than right. Testes firm, smooth, slightly rubbery on palpation. Free from nodules, tenderness. Epididymis palpable and nontender on posterior surface bilaterally. Inguinal area symmetrical and no inguinal or femoral bulges. Nonpalpable lymph nodes bilaterally. Spermatic cord palpable into inguinal canal bilaterally. Sacrococcygeal and perianal areas with skin intact, coarse, color of surrounding skin. Anal opening darkly pigmented, hairless, moist, closed; external sphincter tone intact. Smooth, nontender rectal walls. Smooth, rubbery heart-shaped and walnut-sized prostate gland; slightly moveable and nontender; defined median sulcus.

Special Circumstances and Advanced Techniques

Technique and Normal Findings	Abnormal Findings
Testicles After inspection of the scrotal sac, palpate each testicle separately. Each testicle has a smooth, rubbery consistency; no nodules are palpable.	Irregularities in texture or size may indicate an infection, tumor, or cyst.
The epididymis is located discretely on the posterolateral surface of each testicle. The epididymis feels smooth and nontender.	Note the place of any concerns with the epididymis and whether the condition resolves itself when the patient is supine.
Vas Deferens Next, palpate the vas deferens, which is located in the spermatic cord and has accompanying arteries and veins (Fig. 23.8). It may be difficult to palpate; however, it should feel like a smooth, cordlike structure. Upon palpating from the testicle to the inguinal ring, no nodules or lesions are palpable. 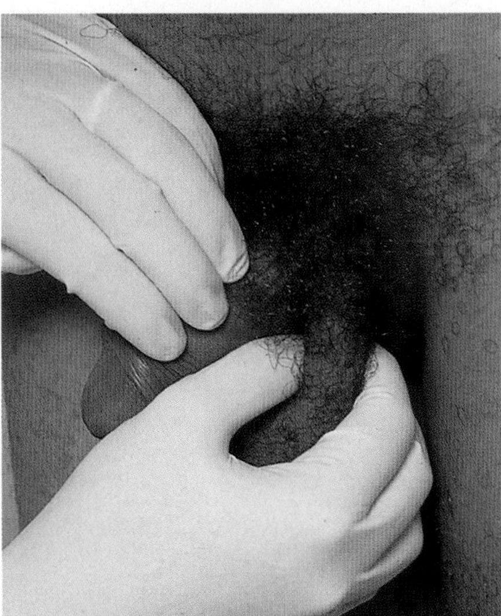 **Figure 23.8** Palpating the vas deferens.	An unexpected finding is tenderness, tortuosity, thickening, or a masslike structure. See Table 23.11 at the end of the chapter.
Transillumination of the Scrotum Transillumination of the scrotum is done to assess for evidence of a mass or fluid. The testes and epididymides do not transilluminate.	Note any masses proximal or distal to the testes. Assess for any pain or tenderness. **Hydroceles** and **spermatoceles** contain fluid and can be revealed during transillumination. Tumors, epididymitis, and hernias do not (see Table 23.11 at the end of the chapter).

(table continues on page 718)

Technique and Normal Findings (continued)	Abnormal Findings (continued)
After palpating the scrotum for a mass or fluid, transilluminate each pouch. Use a bright penlight or transilluminator and press the light against the scrotal sac. The sac does not contain additional fluids or contents.	
Hernias Palpate the inguinal canal for hernia. With the patient relaxed, insert your finger into the scrotal sac and follow it upward along the vas deferens into the inguinal canal. Which finger you use depends on the age of the patient; for an adult, use the middle finger. Palpate the oval external ring. If a hernia is present, you should feel the sudden presence of a viscus against your finger (Fig. 23.9).	**Hernia** occurs when a loop of intestine prolapses through the inguinal wall or canal or abdominal musculature. The patient reports pain on exertion or lifting. On examination, pain increases when maneuvers or positioning increases intraabdominal pressure. The only way to stop a hernia from worsening is to repair the defect surgically. Three of the more common hernias are direct inguinal, indirect inguinal, and femoral. See Table 23.10 at the end of the chapter.

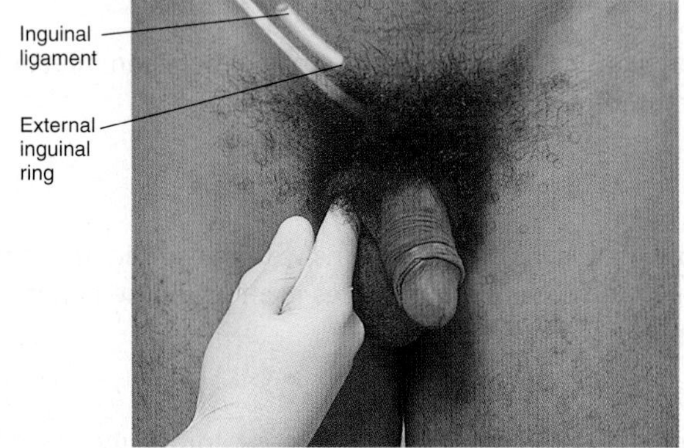

Figure 23.9 Palpating for a hernia.

Perianal and Rectal Examination

A standing position is preferred for rectal examination because it allows for visualization of the anus and palpation of the rectum. Have the standing patient place both feet together, slightly flex both knees, and bend forward over the examination table.

If the patient cannot stand, the rectal examination can be performed with the patient on his left side with the right leg flexed and the left leg semiextended (the Sims position; Fig. 23.10).

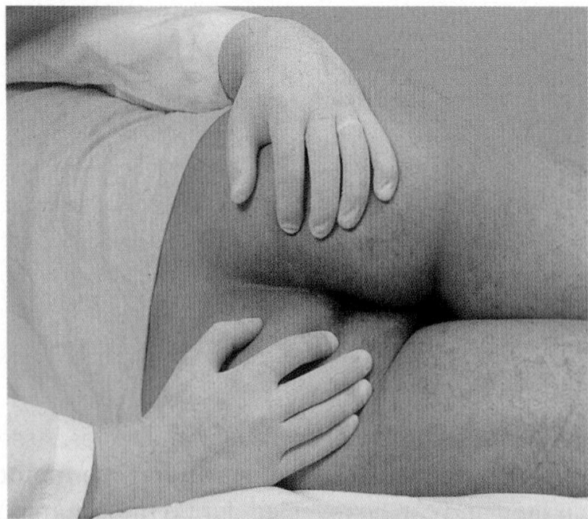

Figure 23.10 Sims positioning for rectal examination.

(table continues on page 719)

Technique and Normal Findings (continued)	Abnormal Findings (continued)
Anus. Spread the buttocks apart and inspect the anus. A penlight helps with visualization. Next, have the patient bear down. Observe the anus for lesions, warts, tags, hemorrhoids, fissures, and fistulas. It is helpful to use a clock for reference, 12-o'clock position being ventral midline and 6-o'clock position being dorsal midline.	
Apply a lubricant to the index finger of the gloved hand. Explain to the patient the lubricant is used for his comfort and might feel cool. Further explain that, initially, he may feel like he is going to have a bowel movement; however, this will not happen. Have the patient take a deep breath while you insert your finger into the rectum. Rectal tone can be assessed at this time. Full closure around the finger is palpable.	Look for thrombosed hemorrhoids, rectal fissures, or hard stool. Hemorrhoids can be classified as external or internal. **Hemorrhoids** are usually caused by constant or excessive straining upon defecation.
Rotate your index finger around the anal ring. The anal ring feels smooth without nodules, masses, or irregularities.	
Continue to advance your index finger into the anal canal. The lateral and posterior rectal walls feel smooth and uninterrupted. Internal hemorrhoids are not palpable.	A hypotonic or lax anal sphincter could be due to rectal surgery, neurological deficit, or trauma (often associated with anal sex). Hypertonic or tight sphincter may be associated with inflammation, scarring, or anxiety about the examination.
Note any nodules, masses, irregularities, or polyps. Pay attention to any discomfort felt by the patient. Rotate your index finger to palpate the anterior rectal wall, repeating the above process. There are no nodules, masses, irregularities, or polyps.	Patients complain of pain when anal fissures or fistulas are present. Local anesthesia may be necessary to complete the examination. Extreme rectal pain is associated with local disease. Because the anterior rectal wall is in contact with peritoneum, you may be able to detect the tenderness of peritoneal inflammation and nodularity of peritoneal metastases. Abnormalities may be related to BPH, prostatitis, and prostate cancer.
Prostate. At this point of the examination, the posterior surface of the prostate gland can be felt (Fig. 23.11). Explain to the patient that it may feel like he is going to urinate, but he will not. Note the prostate gland for its size, contour, consistency, and mobility. The normal prostate gland has the consistency of a rubber ball. The prostate is nontender, firm, smooth, and slightly movable. It is about 4 cm, heart-shaped and walnut-sized; less than 1 cm protrudes into the rectum. The lateral lobes should feel symmetrical and divided by the median sulcus. The sulcus may be obliterated when the lobes are neoplastic or hypertrophied. The DRE of the prostate allows palpation of the posterior surface, which is the area where cancer often starts.	Prostate enlargement is classified by the amount of projection into the rectum (see Table 23.3). If the prostate feels hard, this may indicate carcinoma, prostatic calculi, or chronic fibrosis. A rubbery or boggy glandular consistency may indicate BPH, a common finding in men older than 60 years of age. The gland may feel soft, tender, and boggy from infection. According to the National Institutes of Health, BPH is a condition of aging: 50% of men older than 60 years of age have BPH, as do 90% of men older than 70 years of age. Signs and symptoms of BPH are urine retention, hesitancy, urgency, dribbling, nocturia, and straining to void. If the problem becomes chronic, the patient can develop overflow incontinence from increased intra-abdominal pressure. See Table 23.4 for the American Urological Association's Symptoms Score Index for BPH. *SAFETY ALERT* *Acute urine retention needs immediate intervention.*

(table continues on page 720)

Technique and Normal Findings (continued)

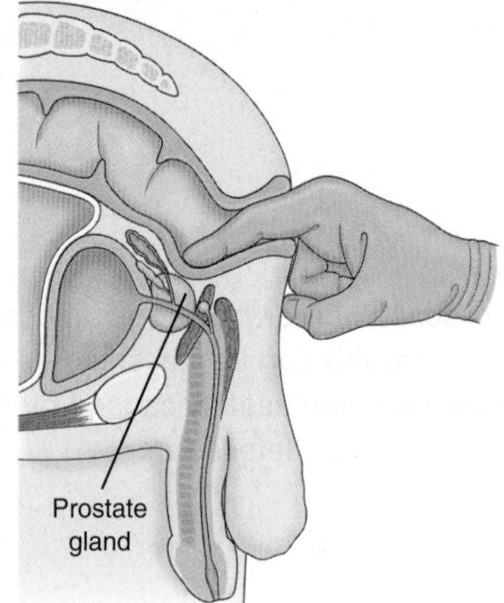

Figure 23.11 Palpating the prostate.

Abnormal Findings (continued)

TABLE 23.3 Classification of Prostate Enlargement

Grade	Protrusion Into Rectum
I	1–2 cm or 3/8–3/4 in.
II	2–3 cm or 3/4–1 1/8 in.
III	3–4 cm or 1 1/8–1 3/4 in.
IV	Greater than 4 cm or 1 3/4 in.

The seminal vesicles are not palpable unless they are inflamed. Prostatitis is an inflammation or infection of the prostate gland.

⚠ SAFETY ALERT

Do not massage the prostate if acute prostatitis is suspected because of the possibility of releasing bacteria and producing septicemia.

(table continues on page 721)

TABLE 23.4 American Urological Association Symptoms Score Index

Also known as the International Prostatic Symptom Score

	Not at all	Less Than 1 Time in 5	Less Than Half the Time	About Half the Time	More Than Half the Time	Almost Always
1. Over the past month, how often have you had a sensation of not emptying your bladder completely after you finished urinating?	0	1	2	3	4	5
2. Over the past month, how often have you had to urinate again less than 2 hours after you finished urinating?	0	1	2	3	4	5
3. Over the past month, how often have you found you stopped and started again several times when you urinated?	0	1	2	3	4	5
4. Over the past month, how often have you found it difficult to postpone urination?	0	1	2	3	4	5
5. Over the past month, how often have you had a weak urinary stream?	0	1	2	3	4	5
6. Over the past month, how often have you had to push or strain to begin urination?	0	1	2	3	4	5
	None	**1 Time**	**2 Times**	**3 Times**	**4 Times**	**5 or More Times**
7. Over the past month, how many times did you most typically get up to urinate from the time you went to bed at night until the time you got up in the morning?	0	1	2	3	4	5
Total symptom score						

Score: 0–7 Mild; 8–19 Moderate; 20–35 Severe.

Data from WebMD. (2012). *American Urological Association symptom index—Topic overview.* Retrieved from http://www.webmd.com/urinary-incontinence-oab/tc/american-urological-association-symptom-index-topic-overview

Technique and Normal Findings (continued)	Abnormal Findings (continued)
Stool. Upon removing your finger from examining the rectum, inspect the gloved finger for consistency and color of the stool. *The stool is brown and soft.*	Abnormal findings include stools with an unusual color, blood, purulent drainage, or mucus. Black tarry stool raises suspicion of upper GI bleeding. Very light tan or gray stool could indicate obstructive jaundice. A subtle loss of blood may not change the color of the stool; however, it may yield a positive guaiac test result, which is used to evaluate occult blood in the stool. A positive guaiac test result may indicate occult blood in the stool.
For 3 days prior to the examination, the patient should have refrained from eating red meat and ingesting vitamin C supplements. Use a guaiac test to evaluate for occult blood. See Box 23.3 instructions for testing.	
Upon completion of the examination of the rectum, explain to the patient that you are going to remove your finger. Offer the patient a cleansing wipe and a private few minutes to dress.	

BOX 23.3 Instructions for Testing Stool for Blood (Guaiac)

The guaiac slide test is a qualitative test. Instructions are:

- Obtain guaiac developer and slide.
- Open the flap of the cardboard guaiac slide.
- Dab the stool on the paper in the boxes of the slide (Fig. A).

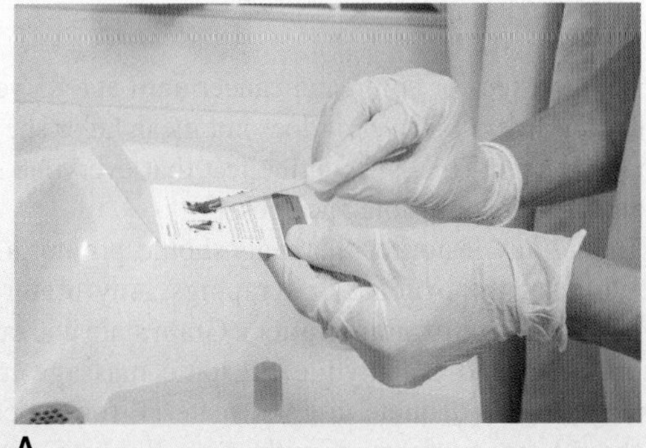

A

- Close the flap and remove your gloves.
- With clean gloves on, reverse the slide and open the flap.
- Apply two drops of developing solution to each box of guaiac paper (Fig. B).

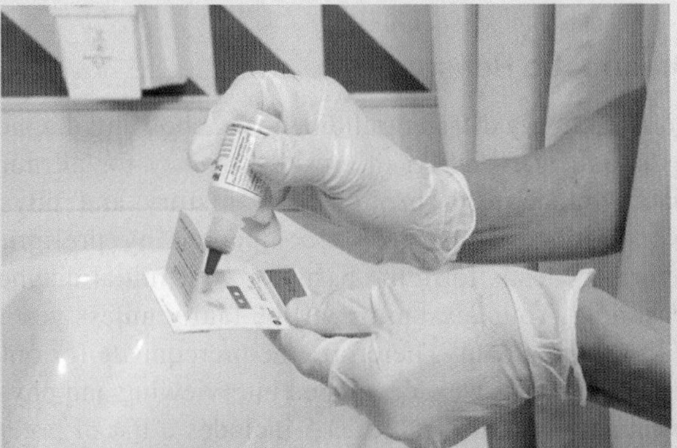

B

- Wait 30–60 seconds and note color of the paper (Fig. C). A bluish discoloration indicates a positive result that occult blood is present. This is a warning sign that a patient may have colorectal disease, including colon cancer. However, false-positive guaiac results may occur from a diet of red or rare meats, dietary peroxidases, or both. Intake of vitamin C (ascorbic acid) may cause false-negative results.

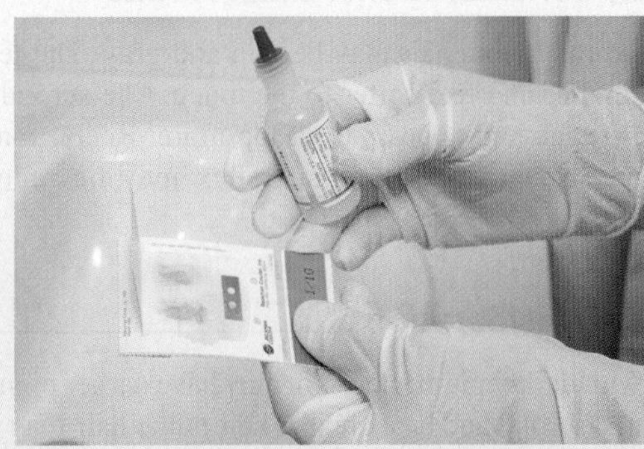

C

Documenting Case Study Findings

The APRN is assessing Mr. Gardner, the 50-year-old man with BPH. Unlike the samples of normal documentation charted previously, Mr. Gardner has unexpected findings. Consider how Mr. Gardner's symptoms are increasing. Consider what other data the nurse will collect while thinking critically and anticipating nursing interventions. Pay attention to how the nurse clusters data to provide a more complete and accurate understanding of the condition.

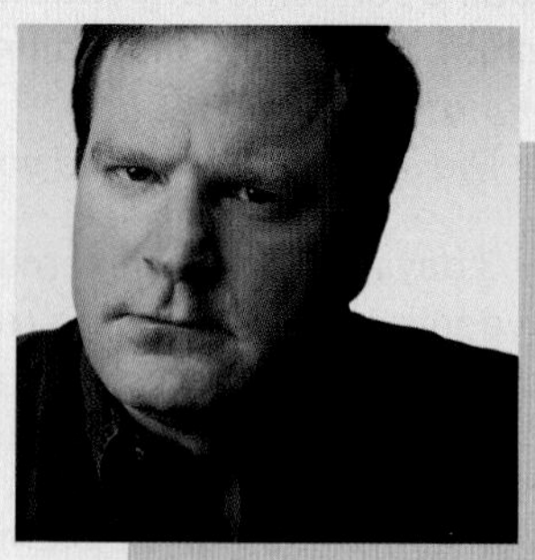

Inspection: Genital hair intact and appropriate to age. No odor. Glans and corona are visible, darker in color than the shaft of the penis with no smegma. Glans is slightly reddened around the **meatus.** The shaft of the penis is smooth without lesions or pain. Scrotum without swelling or inflammation. No masses or lesions in the inguinal or femoral area. Anal, sacrococcygeal area, perianal area, and anus are without redness, lesions, or masses. Skin is smooth and pink.

Palpation: The prostate is enlarged, symmetrical, firm, and smooth.

Lifespan Considerations: Older Adults

In older adults, pubic hair may be thin and gray. The testes may be smaller and feel softer to the touch. The scrotal sac has fewer rugae and appears to droop more. Rectal tone is intact, but strength of the rectal reflex may be reduced slightly.

Cultural Considerations

Patients with darkly pigmented skin may have darker pigmentation in the scrotal and anal areas. Their pubic hair may also be darker and coarser.

Critical Thinking

You will use assessment findings as the basis for ongoing care. An accurate and complete assessment provides a firm foundation for setting outcomes, providing individualized interventions, and evaluating progress.

Laboratory and Diagnostic Testing

Adult men should have their weight and blood pressure checked regularly. Men aged 35 years and older should have their cholesterol levels checked regularly. Beginning at age 50 years and continuing until age 75 years, men should be tested for colorectal cancer. Certain people may need to continue being tested for colorectal cancer until age 85 years. If your doctor orders this test, it does not mean he or she thinks you have cancer. This is a routine test that everyone should have along with applicable vaccines.

Finding any lesion of the penis should prompt a smear and culture of the exudate or scrapings. Any urethral discharge must also be examined after a Gram stain and cultured for gonococci and chlamydia. Prostatic massage may be necessary to get adequate urethral material for the culture; this should be performed with care because vigorous manipulation of the prostate may result in septicemia. Next, a urinalysis is done and culture with a colony count. If the diagnosis is still uncertain, it is wise to consult a urologist before proceeding with expensive testing.

Diagnostic Reasoning

Constructing a differential diagnosis, choosing diagnostic tests, and interpreting the results are key for all nurses. Data you acquire through your history and physical examination, sometimes accompanied by preliminary laboratory tests, form the basis for your initial diagnostic reasoning. Your reasoning will be faulty unless you start with accurate data. Therefore, the prerequisite for obtaining valid data is well-developed interviewing and physical examination skills. Table 23.5 includes a list of potential medical diagnoses, clinical clues, and important tests to consider.

TABLE 23.5 Differential Diagnosis, Symptoms, and Testing in Male Genital Assessment		
Differential Diagnosis	**Signs/Symptoms**	**Diagnostic Tests**
BPH	Unable to empty bladder, frequent urination, weak stream, dribbling after urination, nocturia	DRE, urinalysis, PSA urine cytology, IVP, postresidual volume of urine. (The American Urological Association no longer recommends measuring serum creatine on the initial evaluation.) Follow with referral to urologist if initial treatment does not eliminate symptoms.
	Active Alternatives: Most Common	
Bladder calculi **Bladder neck contracture** **Urethral stricture** **Urethritis**	Unable to empty bladder fully, weak stream, pain, hematuria, urgency, and frequency	Urinalysis, PSA, complete blood count, blood urea nitrogen, creatine; consider IVP, which can identify a postresidual volume of urine; DRE. Follow with referral to urologist if initial treatment does not eliminate symptoms.
	Active Alternative: Must not Miss	
Cancer of the prostate	Patient complaints include bladder outlet symptoms or acute urinary retention with very large or locally extensive tumors; nocturia. New onset ED, hematuria, and hematospermia are less common presentations of prostate cancer.	If positive findings on DRE and PSA, patient should be referred to urologist for a definitive diagnosis (involving biopsy) and staging.

IVP, intravenous pyelogram.

Nursing Diagnosis, Outcomes, and Interventions

When formulating a nursing diagnosis, it is important to use critical thinking to cluster data and identify patterns that fit together. You will compare these clusters with the defining characteristics (abnormal findings) for the diagnosis to ensure the most accurate labeling and appropriate interventions. Table 23.6 reviews nursing diagnoses, abnormal findings, and interventions commonly related to the male assessment (NANDA International, 2012).

Use assessment information to identify patient outcomes. Some outcomes that are related to male genital difficulties include the following:

- Patient will describe alternative safe sexual practices.
- Patient will remain free of infection.
- Patient will be continent of urine (Moorhead, Johnson, Maas, & Swanson, 2013).

After you have established the outcomes, you will implement nursing care to improve the status of the patient, using critical thinking and evidence-based practices to develop the interventions. Some examples of nursing interventions for male genital system care are as follows:

- Assess the patient's knowledge and understanding of safe sexual practices.
- Teach care for the infection-prone site.
- Teach the patient exercises to strengthen the pelvic floor (Bulechek, Butcher, Dochterman, & Wagner, 2013).

You then evaluate the care according to the patient outcomes that were developed, reassessing the patient and continuing or modifying the interventions as appropriate. Even as a beginner, you can use the patient assessment to implement new interventions, evaluate the effectiveness of those interventions, and make a difference in the quality of patient care.

TABLE 23.6 Common Nursing Diagnoses Associated With the Male Genital System

Diagnosis	Point of Differentiation	Assessment Characteristics	Nursing Interventions
Ineffective sexuality pattern	Concern, dissatisfaction, or verbalized difficulties with sex life	Alteration in relationship with significant other, changes or limitations in sexual activities and behaviors	After establishing a relationship with the patient, give the patient permission to discuss issues by asking, "Are you concerned about sexual function because of changes in your health?"
Risk for infection	Potential for invasion by pathogens	Inadequate knowledge, urinary reflux, recent trauma, or urinary catheter placement	Teach safe sex practices. Teach warning signs of genital tract infections. Remove urinary catheters as early as possible.
Urinary retention	Inability to completely empty the bladder	Increased urinary residual volume, slow stream, hesitant urination, dribbling	Obtain a postvoid bladder ultrasound. Teach double voiding and to avoid taking OTC cold medications that include a decongestant.
Risk for urge incontinence	Involuntary passage of urine with a sudden desire to urinate	Voiding more than once every 2 hours, awakening at night to urinate	Assess the patient for functional barriers to continence; teach spacing of fluids in consistent quantities over the day. Avoid consuming fluids late in the evening.

*Collaborative interventions.

Progress Note: Analyzing Findings

Remember Mr. Gardner, whose difficulties have been outlined throughout this chapter. Initial subjective and objective data collection is complete and the nurse has spent time reviewing the findings and other results. Unfortunately, Mr. Gardner has urinary retention, so it is necessary to reassess him and document the findings. The following nursing note illustrates how subjective and objective data are collected and analyzed and nursing interventions are developed.

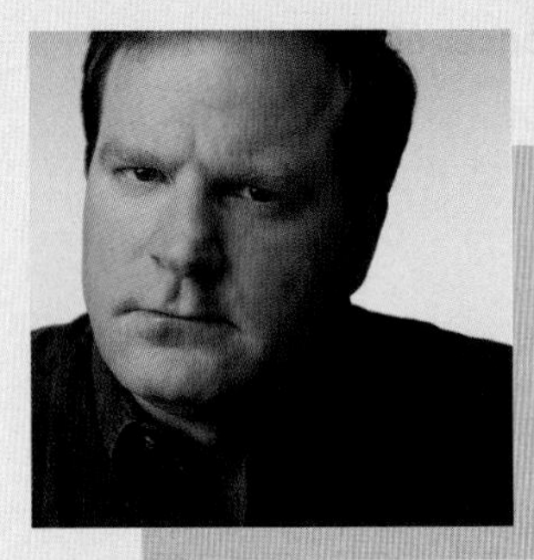

Subjective: "I can't urinate and it feels like my bladder is full."

Objective: Urinary residual volume 250 ml (8 oz), slow stream, hesitant urinary voiding, dribbling.

Analysis: Urinary retention related to partial obstruction

Plan: Inform urologist about residual volume. Teach the patient to avoid caffeine and alcohol because of the diuretic effects. Teach the patient to avoid pseudoephedrine and phenylephrine found in OTC cold medications. Teach double voiding. Teach to urinate every 2 or 3 hours and when first feeling the urge. Avoid rapid intake of fluids that may overdistend the bladder. Repeat bladder scan to ensure that residual volume is not increasing.

Critical Thinking Challenge

- What can Mr. Gardner do to improve his health?
- How can Mr. Gardner talk with his wife about his symptoms?
- At what point will the nurse contact the urologist regarding an acute assessment?

Collaborating With the Interprofessional Team

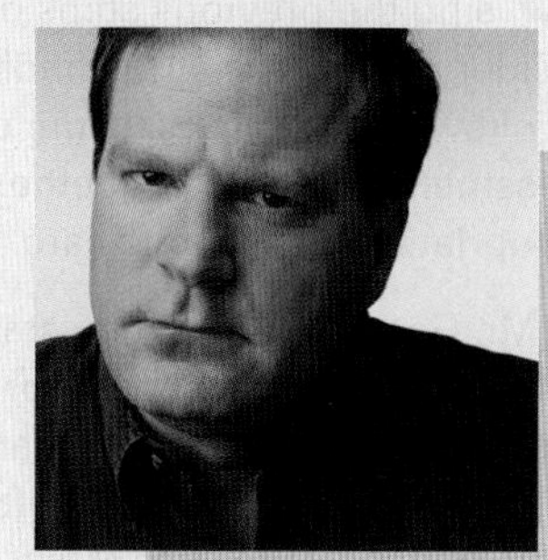

In this case, Mr. Gardner will need insertion of a urinary catheter if he cannot urinate. The nurse will need to talk with the urologist to obtain an order for a urinary catheter. Results that might trigger a consult with a urologist include urinary retention, incontinence, blood in the urine, prostate disease, kidney stones, infections of the urinary tract, infertility, and sexual dysfunction.

Mr. Gardner has been experiencing urinary retention; therefore, a urology consult is indicated. The following conversation illustrates how the nurse might organize the data and make recommendations about the patient's situation.

Situation: "Hi, I'm Denise, a nurse in the primary care clinic. Mr. Gardner is a 50-year-old man who has had BPH for the past 3 years."

Background: "He came in today with symptoms of incomplete bladder emptying and he had a bladder scan that showed a residual volume of 250 ml (8 oz). He is also having a slow stream, hesitant urinary voiding, and dribbling."

Assessment: "I am concerned that Mr. Gardner is experiencing urinary retention and will be at risk for reflux and an infection."

Recommendations: "He might be developing severe enough symptoms that he needs to have a urinary catheter inserted. When would you be able to evaluate him?"

Critical Thinking Challenge

- When will the nurse intervene with health promotion activities?
- At what point will the nurse talk with the patient's wife about his symptoms?
- What symptoms will prompt the nurse to call the urologist?

Pulling it All Together

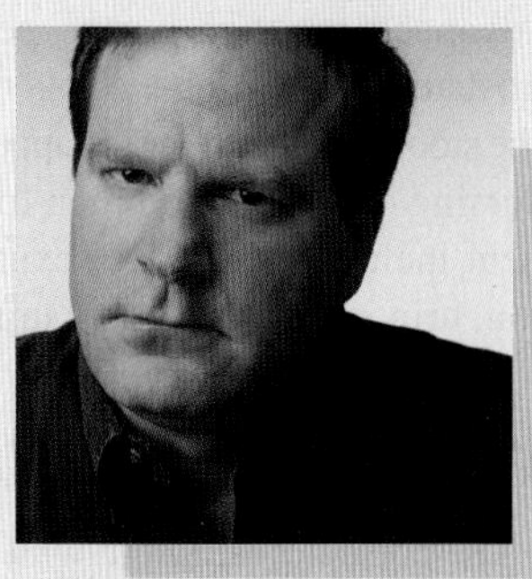

The nurse uses assessment data to formulate a nursing care plan with patient outcomes and interventions for Mr. Gardner. Outcomes are specific to the patient, realistic to achieve, measurable, and have a time frame for meeting the outcome. The interventions are actions that the nurse performs based on evidence and practice guidelines. After these interventions are completed, the nurse reevaluates Mr. Gardner and documents the findings in the chart to show progress toward the patient outcome. The nurse uses critical thinking and judgment to continue or revise the diagnosis, outcomes, or interventions. This is often in the form of a care plan or case note similar to the one below.

Nursing Diagnosis	Patient Outcomes	Nursing Interventions	Rationale	Evaluation
Urinary retention related to obstruction	Patient will be free from urinary tract distress.	Teach the patient to double void by urinating, resting for 3–5 minutes, and then trying again to urinate.	Double voiding promotes more efficient bladder emptying by allowing the muscles to contract, rest, and then contract again.	Patient states that he has tried double voiding but he has discomfort and dribbling. Urologist contacted for evaluation of symptoms and possible surgery for retention.

Applying Your Knowledge

Using the previous steps of diagnostic reasoning, organizing, and prioritizing, consider all the case study findings woven throughout this chapter. When answering the following questions, begin drawing conclusions and see how the pieces of assessment must work together to create an environment for personalized, appropriate, and accurate care.

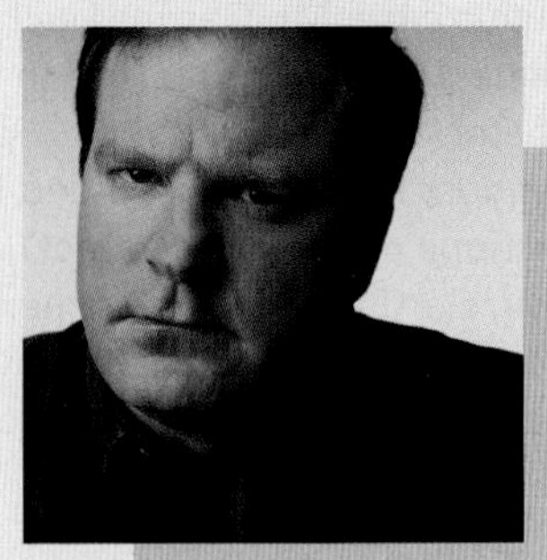

- Is Mr. Gardner's condition stable, urgent, or an emergency?
- What are potential causes for difficulties with urination?
- How will the nurse incorporate an evidence-based standardized questionnaire to uncover the degree of symptomatology?
- How will the nurse assist Mr. Gardner to relax during inspection and palpation of his genitalia and rectum?
- What factors contribute to the patient's concerns?
- How will the nurse work with Mr. Gardner to promote health and reduce risk for illness?
- How will the nurse evaluate whether the assessment has been complete and accurate?

Key Points

- The anatomy of normal male genitalia includes external and internal structures.
- Goals related to the male genital system include prevention of prostate cancer, appropriate family planning, and prevention of STIs.
- TSE and screening for prostate cancer are important health promotion activities.
- Common symptoms of male genital problems include pain, difficulties with urination, ED, penile lesions or discharge, and scrotal enlargement.
- During the intimate male genital assessment, it is important to provide the patient with privacy.
- The role of the registered nurse during a male genital examination primarily involves inspection.
- Acute scrotum pain may be caused by ischemia, trauma, infections, inflammation, herniation, and chronic conditions with an acute exacerbation; it needs immediate attention.
- Advanced practice nurses perform perianal, rectal, and prostate examinations.
- The stool is assessed for the appearance and presence of blood.
- Nursing diagnoses common following male genital assessment include ineffective sexuality patterns, risk for infection, urinary retention, and urge incontinence.

Review Questions

1. The correct position in which to place a healthy adult male client to examine the rectum and prostate is
   A. the left lateral Sims position with right knee flexed and left leg extended.
   B. the supine position with hips and legs flexed and feet positioned on the examining table.
   C. the modified knee–chest position with the patient prone and knees flexed under hips.
   D. leaning over the examination table with chest and shoulders resting on the table.

2. During a physical assessment, using the handle of the reflex hammer, you gently stroke the inner left thigh of the patient, which causes the ipsilateral testicle to rise. What superficial reflex is demonstrated?
   A. Abdominal reflex
   B. Babinski reflex
   C. Brachioradialis reflex
   D. Cremasteric reflex

3. A 20-year-old Caucasian man complains of a mass in his left testicle. In addition to his age and race, what else is a risk factor for testicular cancer?
   A. Colon cancer in his mother
   B. Personal history of cryptorchidism
   C. Urinary tract infection last month
   D. Congenital hydrocele

4. A 20-year-old male patient presents with scrotal pain. A suspected diagnosis that requires immediate referral is
   A. testicular torsion.
   B. hydrocele.
   C. epididymitis.
   D. inguinal hernia.

5. Which of the following would you recognize as an unexpected finding while examining the male genitalia?
   A. Smegma is present on the uncircumcised patient.
   B. Testes are palpable and firm within the scrotal sac.
   C. You note an impulse at the tip of your finger during hernia examination.
   D. The urethral meatus has a slitlike opening central to the distal tip of the glans.

6. When examining the scrotum of an adult Hispanic male, a normal finding is
   A. symmetrical scrotal sac with two movable testes.
   B. smooth, rubbery, saclike surface that is sensitive to gentle compression.
   C. asymmetrical sac with left side lower than right side.
   D. reddish colored skin that is darker than general body skin and has sebaceous cysts.

7. A young male presents for a sports physical examination. In addition to examining for hernias, it would be appropriate for you to do which of the following?
   A. Teach testicular self-examination.
   B. Evaluate for urinary retention.
   C. Examine for prostate cancer.
   D. Draw blood to measure prostatic surface antigen.

8. A patient complains of a soft, irregular mass on the left side of the scrotum he noticed while walking. The nurse palpates a mass that feels like "a bag of worms." These findings are consistent with which condition?
   A. Hydrocele
   B. Varicocele
   C. Spermatocele
   D. Epididymitis

9. A 70-year-old man presents with the following symptoms: straining to void, nocturia, dribbling, and hesitancy when voiding. These signs are consistent with what condition?
   A. Benign prostatic hypertrophy (BPH)
   B. Prostatitis
   C. Testicular cancer
   D. Phimosis

10. You are inspecting the groin of an older adult man who lives in a long-term care facility. Which of the following is an expected finding that you will document?
   A. Pediculosis in hair distribution
   B. Hypospadias on the glans
   C. Yellow discharge from the meatus
   D. Smegma under the foreskin

11. Which sexually transmitted infection presents with painful red superficial vesicles along the penis or on the glans?
   A. Gonorrhea
   B. Chlamydia
   C. Syphilis
   D. Herpes simplex virus 2 (HSV-2)

The Jensen suite offers these additional resources to enhance learning and facilitate understanding of this chapter:

- thePoint online resources, http://thepoint.lww.com/Jensen2e
- *Laboratory Manual for Nursing Health Assessment: A Best Practice Approach*
- *Pocket Guide for Nursing Health Assessment: A Best Practice Approach*
- *Lippincott DocuCare,* an electronic health record simulation software, http://thepoint.lww.com/docucare
- *Adaptive Learning | Powered by PrepU,* http://thepoint.lww.com/prepu

References

American Cancer Society (ACS). (2013). *What are the key statistics for cancer?* Retrieved from http://seer.cancer.gov/statfacts/html/prost.html

American Urological Association (AUA). (2013). *An AUA best practice policy and ASRM practice committee report.* Retrieved from http://www.auanet.org

Bulechek, G. M., Butcher, H. K., Dochterman, J. M., & Wagner, C. M. (2013). *Nursing interventions classification (NIC)* (6th ed.). St. Louis, MO: Mosby.

Centers for Disease Control and Prevention (CDC). (2010). *Sexually transmitted disease treatment guidelines, 2010.* Retrieved from http://www.cdc.gov/mmwr/preview/mmwrhtml/rr5912a1.htm

Centers for Disease Control and Prevention (CDC). (2012). *Viral hepatitis and men who have sex with men.* Retrieved from http://www.cdc.gov/hepatitis/Populations/msm.htm

Centers for Disease Control and Prevention (CDC). (2013a). *Human papillomavirus (HPV)-associated cancers.* Retrieved from http://www.cdc.gov/cancer/hpv/

Centers for Disease Control and Prevention (CDC). (2013b). *Surveillance for urinary tract infections.* Retrieved from http://www.cdc.gov/nhsn/acute-care-hospital/CAUTI/

Dunphy, L. M., Winland-Brown, J.E., Porter, B., & Thomas, D. (2011). *Primary care: The art and science of advance practice nursing* (3rd ed.). Philadelphia: F.A. Davis.

NANDA International (2012). *Nursing diagnoses: Definitions and classification 2012–2014* (9th ed.). Oxford, United Kingdom: Wiley-Blackwell.

Moorhead, S., Johnson, M., Maas, M. L., & Swanson, E. (2013). *Nursing outcomes classification (NOC): Measurement of health outcomes* (5th ed.). St. Louis, MO: Elsevier.

Quinn, T. C., Bartlett, J. A., & McGovern, B. H. (2009). *The global human immunodeficiency virus pandemic.* Retrieved from http://www.Uptodate.com

The Testicular Cancer Resource Center (TCRC). (2012). *How to do a testicular self-examination.* Retrieved from http://tcrc.acor.org/tcexam.html

U.S. Department of Health and Human Services; Healthy People 2020. (2013). *Topics & objectives: Objectives A–Z.* Retrieved from http://www.healthypeople.gov/2020/topicsobjectives2020/

U.S. Preventive Services Task Force. (2012). *Screening for Prostate Cancer.* Retrieved from http://www.uspreventiveservicestaskforce.org/prostatecancerscreening/prostatefinalrs.htm

WebMD. (2013). *Are there risks associated with genital piercings?* Retrieved from http://www.webmd.com/sex/genital-piercings?page=2.

TABLE 23.7 Sexually Transmitted Infections

STI	Findings and Clinical Implications
Scabies infection 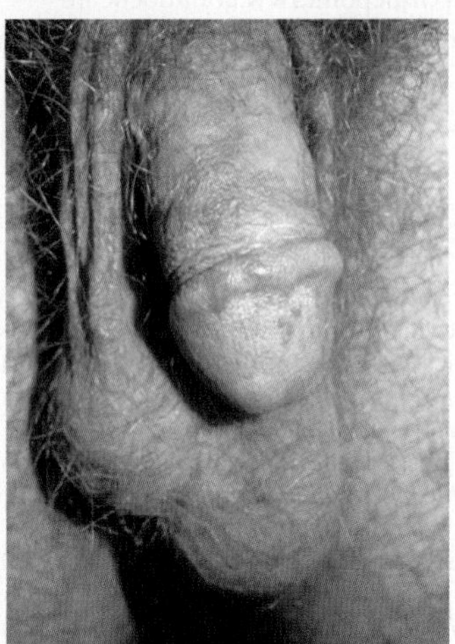	Scabies is a highly communicable skin condition caused by an arachnid (*Sarcoptes scabiei*), commonly known as the itch mite. It is transmitted by direct skin contact. The females live in burrows that appear as slightly darkened lines. Associated papules, vesicles, pustules, and intense itching are the usual findings.
Chlamydia 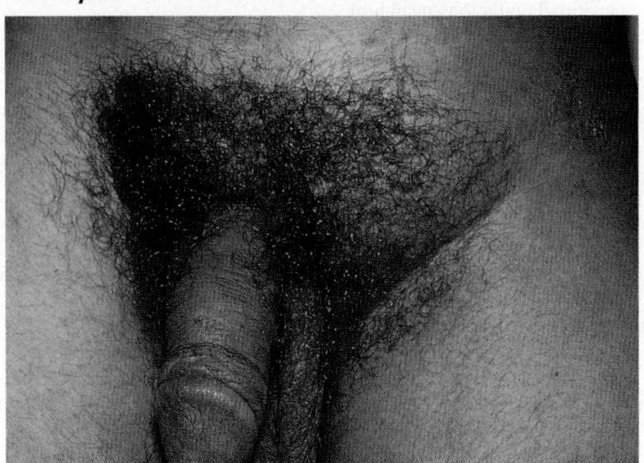	*Chlamydia trachomatis* is a bacterium with a variable incubation period, usually within 1 week of exposure. The most frequently reported bacterial STI in the United States, **this disease is reportable in every state**. In men, the urethra has a mucopurulent discharge. Urination is accompanied by a burning sensation. Chlamydia commonly presents asymptomatically. A chlamydia infection can cause nongonococcal urethritis and acute epididymitis. If urethral discharge is present, obtain specimen for diagnostic testing.
Gonorrhea 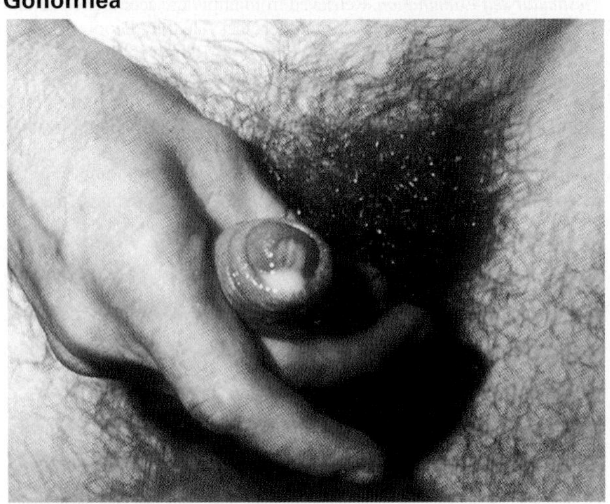	*Gonorrhoeae* organisms are gram-negative diplococci present in exudates and secretions of infected mucous surfaces. Transmission results from intimate contact; incubation period is 2–7 days. **This disease is reportable in every state**. Men may present with dysuria, urethral discharge, or rectal pain. Common sites include the urethra, epididymis, prostate, rectum, and pharynx. If urethral discharge is present, obtain specimen for diagnostic testing.

(table continues on page 729)

STI	Findings and Clinical Implications
Syphilis 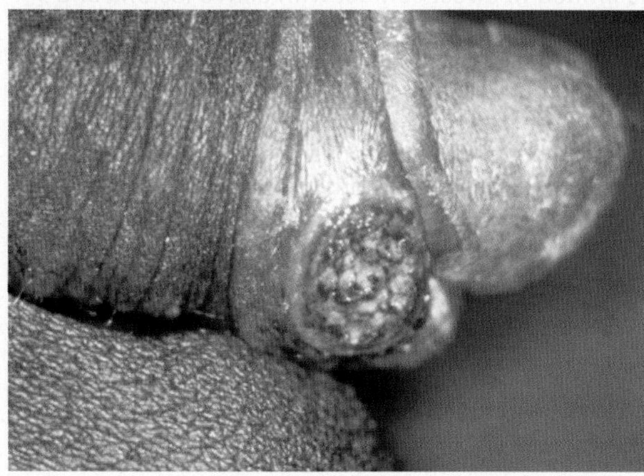	Syphilis is caused by *Treponema pallidum,* a thin fragile organism that penetrates intact skin or mucous membrane during sexual contact, multiplies, and rapidly spreads to regional lymph nodes. Primary incubation period for acquired syphilis is about 3 weeks, but it can occur 10–90 days after exposure. Secondary syphilis develops 6–8 weeks later. Latent and tertiary syphilis can occur years later. **Report all cases of syphilis to the appropriate public health department.** The five stages of syphilis are as follows: 1. ***Primary syphilis.*** Genital lesions are usually indurated and painless. Regional lymphadenopathy is usually present. Chancre persists for 1–5 weeks and heals spontaneously. 2. ***Secondary syphilis.*** Occurs 6–8 weeks later and is characterized by flulike symptoms. A macular, papular, anular, or follicular rash is present, often involving the palms and soles. The rash spontaneously heals in 2–6 weeks. Secondary syphilis is the most contagious stage. 3. ***Latent stage.*** Occurs after the second stage. It can last from 2 to 20 years. 4. ***Tertiary syphilis.*** This stage has the most devastating effects on the cardiovascular, neurological, musculoskeletal, and ophthalmic systems of the body. 5. ***Congenital syphilis.*** Occurs during mother-to-child transmission, usually when the mother has primary or secondary syphilis. Signs and symptoms in the infant include retinal inflammation, glaucoma, destructive bone and skin lesions, and central nervous system disorders.
Human papillomavirus (HPV) 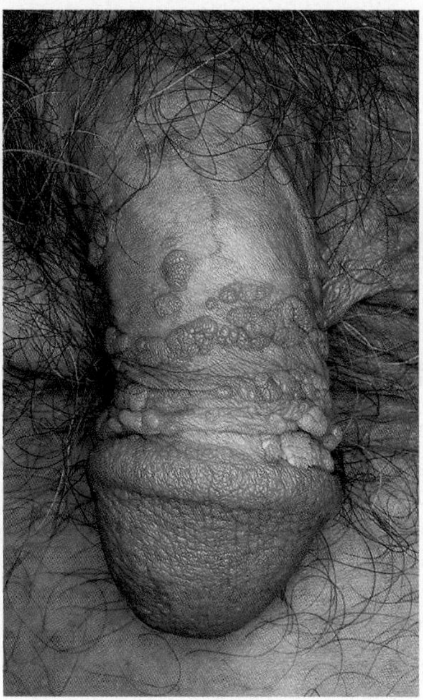	HPV produces epithelial tumors of the skin and mucous membranes. Many types of sexually transmitted HPV can infect the genital tract, rectum, and oral mucous membranes. The incubation period is uncertain, but it can range from 3 months to several years. Some strains of the virus can progress to genital warts, although most men with HPV never develop genital warts. Although rare, a complication is penile or anal cancer. Visible genital warts usually result from HPV type 6 or 11. These lesions can appear on the scrotum, perineum, perianal skin, and penis. Individual warts may become confluent and appear as a single, large, fleshy lesion. Recent studies indicate that men do not clear the virus as quickly as women. On October 25, 2011, the Advisory Committee on Immunization Practices recommended routine use of quadrivalent HPV vaccine in boys age 11–26 years (CDC, 2013a).

(table continues on page 730)

TABLE 23.7 Sexually Transmitted Infections *(continued)*

STI	Findings and Clinical Implications
Herpes simplex virus (HSV) types 1 and 2 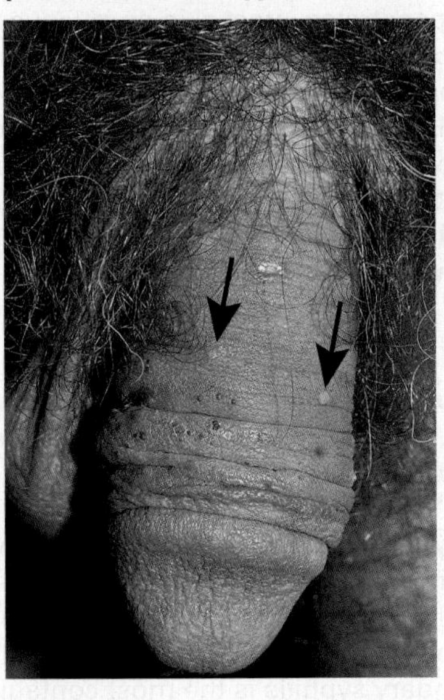	HSV-1 and HSV-2 are epidermotropic viruses. Transmission is limited to direct contact with active lesions or a virus-containing fluid such as saliva. Incubation period is 2–14 days. HSV-1 is associated with infection of the lips, face, buccal mucosa, and throat. HSV-2 is associated with genitalia. There may be an overlap in site of infection; type 1 strains can be recovered from the genital tract, and type 2 strains can be recovered from the pharynx following oral–genital activity. The usual sequence is painful papules followed by vesicles, ulceration, crusting, and healing.

Note: There are more than 50 different STIs. Six common STIs are presented in the table.
Information obtained from National Institute of Allergy and Infectious Diseases. (2013). *Sexually transmitted diseases*. Retrieved from http://www.niaid.nih.gov/topics/std/Pages/default.aspx; Centers for Disease Control and Prevention. (2012). *2011 sexually transmitted diseases surveillance: Table of contents*. Retrieved from http://www.cdc.gov/std/stats11/toc.htm

TABLE 23.8 Abnormal Conditions of the Penis

Genital Piercing

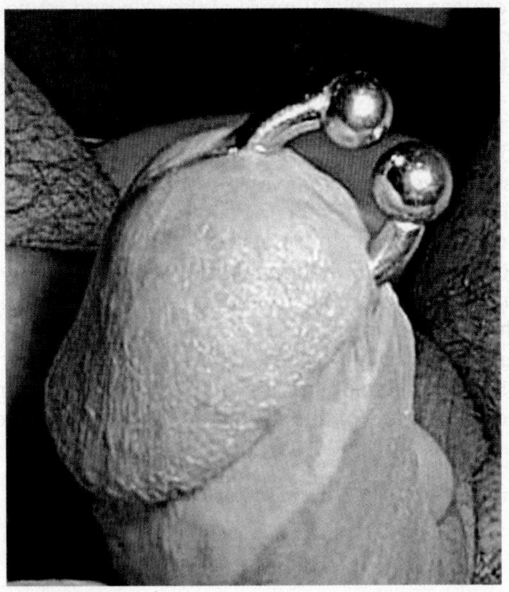

The "Prince Albert" is a common type of male genital piercing in which a ring is inserted through the urethra and out the bottom of the glans. The most common issue associated with piercing is infection. Other complications include bleeding and difficulty urinating.

Phimosis

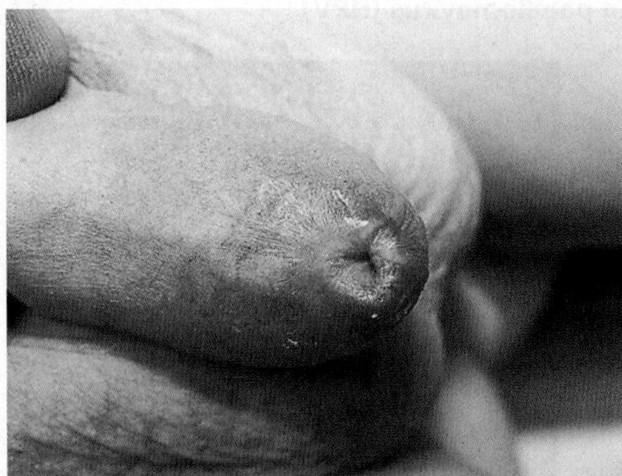

The prepuce cannot be retracted over the glans. It can occur during the first 6 years of life. It may be congenital or follow recurrent infections or *balanoposthitis* (inflammation of the prepuce and glans). Occasionally, the narrowed foreskin obstructs urinary flow, resulting in a dribbling stream or ballooning of the foreskin. Severe phimosis is treated by circumcision.

(table continues on page 731)

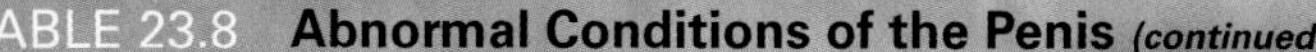

TABLE 23.8 Abnormal Conditions of the Penis *(continued)*

Paraphimosis

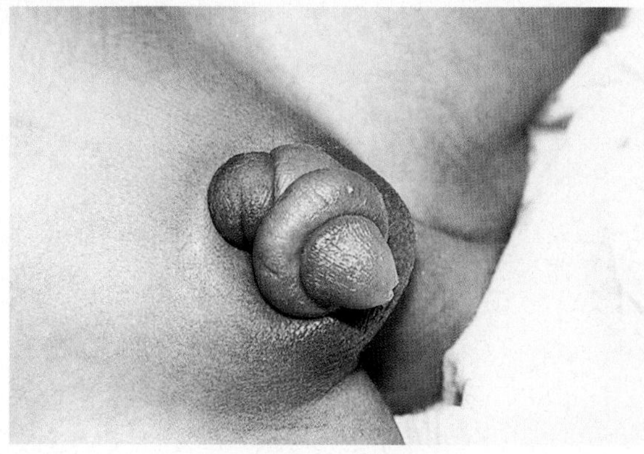

The retracted prepuce cannot be placed back over the glans. Paraphimosis may be severe enough to restrict circulation to the glans. In an uncircumcised male, the foreskin would always be pulled toward the urethral opening.

Hypospadias

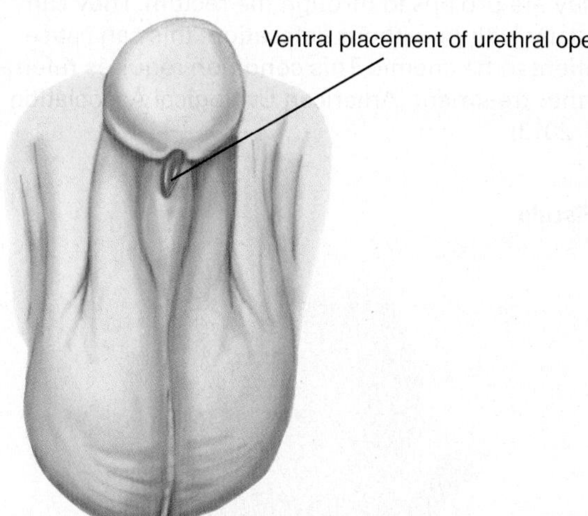

The urethral meatus opens on the ventral side of the penis. Hypospadias may be associated with underlying congenital anomalies in genital urinary development. The deviation of the meatus makes it difficult to urinate when standing. The physical appearance of the penis is altered, sometimes causing body image disturbances.

Balanitis or balanoposthitis

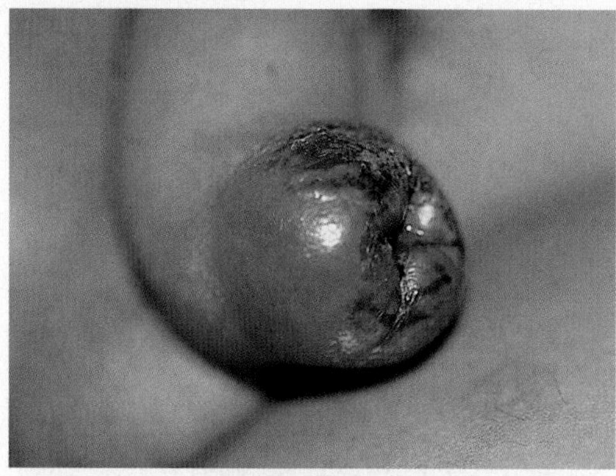

Inflammation of the glans and prepuce occurs in uncircumcised men. Many men with this condition have poorly controlled diabetes. Scars and narrowing of the urethral opening may cause inflammation, infections, and foul discharge. The scarring may make it difficult to clean under the foreskin.

Epispadias

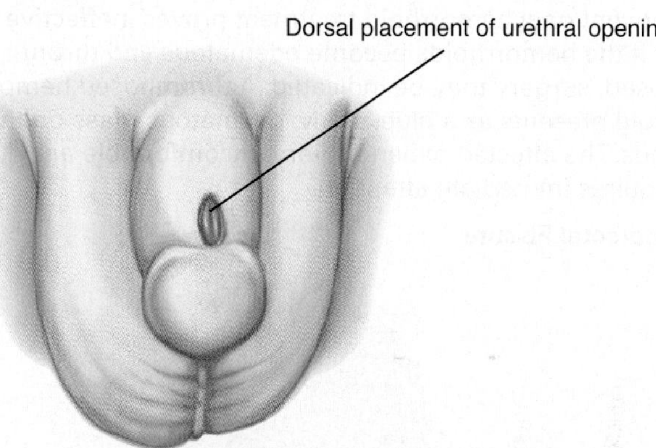

The urethral meatus opens on the dorsal surface of the penis. Epispadias may be associated with underlying congenital anomalies in genital urinary development. The deviation of the meatus makes it difficult to urinate when standing. The physical appearance of the penis is altered, sometimes causing body image disturbances. The lower urinary tract may be exposed in severe cases.

TABLE 23.9 Conditions of the Anus, Rectum, and Prostate

External Hemorrhoids

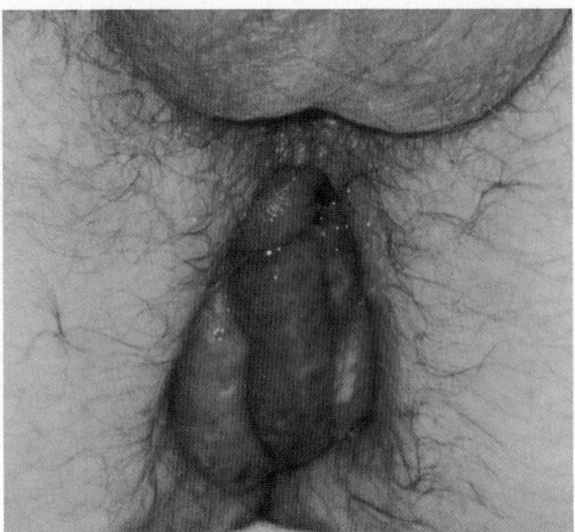

External hemorrhoids are varicose veins that originate below the pectinate line and are covered by anal skin. Patients complain of rectal itching, pain, or burning. External hemorrhoids are usually not visible at rest but become visible when standing or during defecation. If conventional hemorrhoid treatment proves ineffective or if the hemorrhoids become edematous and thrombosed, surgery may be indicated. A thrombosed hemorrhoid presents as a blue, shiny, edematous mass on the anus. The affected patient is very uncomfortable and requires immediate attention.

Internal Hemorrhoids

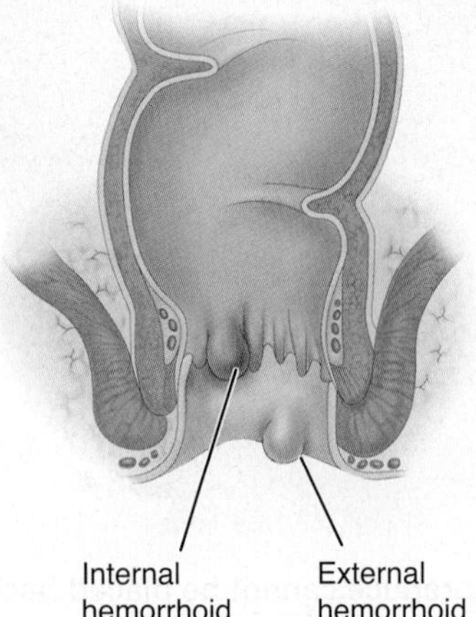

Internal hemorrhoids can be painless unless they are thrombosed, infected, or prolapsed. They occur above the pectinate line and are covered by the mucosa of the anal canal. Internal hemorrhoids create soft swelling and are difficult to palpate on a digital examination unless they are prolapsed through the rectum. They can bleed daily with or without defecation; this can cause the patient to be anemic. This condition requires referral for further treatment (American Urological Association [AUA], 2013).

Anorectal Fissure

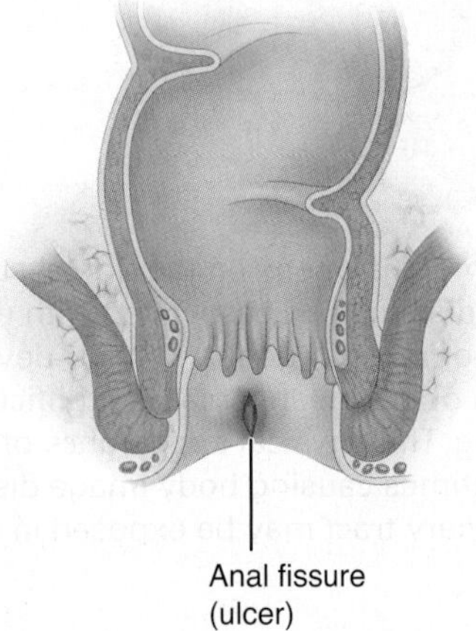

Anorectal fissure is a rip in the anal mucosa; it can occur midline or posterior or anterior to the anus. Usually, a fissure is caused by the passage of large hard stool. On observation, a sentinel skin tag may be seen at the lower end of the fissure. Ulcerations may appear at the site. The patient has bleeding, pain, and itching. Because the internal sphincter is spastic, anesthesia of the site is necessary for examination.

Anal Fistula

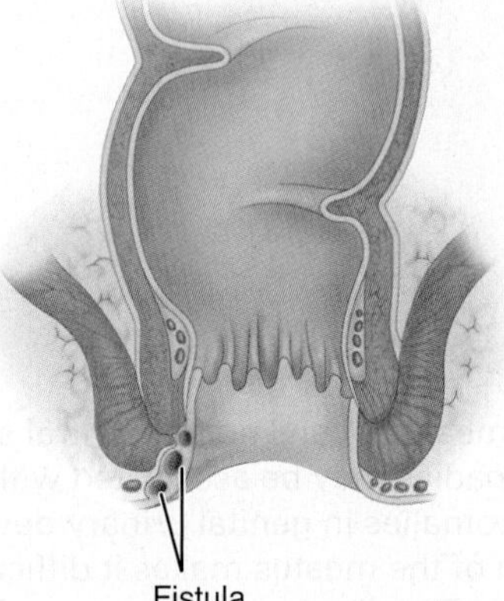

Anal fistula is an inflammatory tract or tube that opens at one end in the anus or rectum and at the other end onto the skin surface. It originates in the anal crypts. The fissure can occur spontaneously or from perirectal abscess. On compression, serosanguineous or purulent drainage may appear. Externally, the area appears raised, red, and granular. This condition requires referral for further treatment (AUA, 2013).

(table continues on page 733)

TABLE 23.9 Conditions of the Anus, Rectum, and Prostate *(continued)*

Rectal Polyp

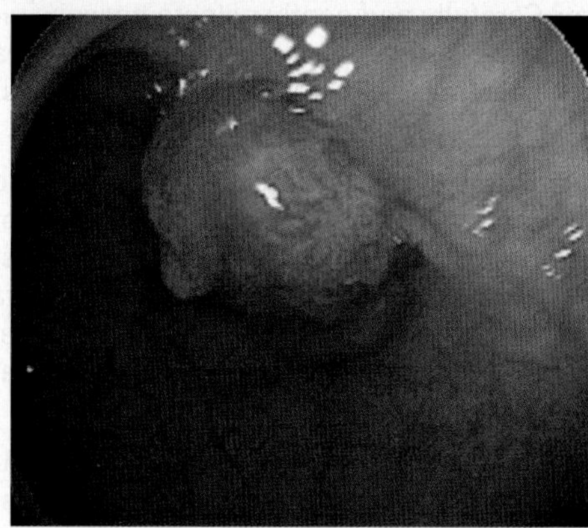

Polyps, which are common, can occur anywhere in the intestinal tract. They can be adenomatous or inflammatory in origin, occurring singly or in clusters. They can cause rectal bleeding and be seen protruding through the rectum on examination. On DRE, polyps can be palpated as soft nodules; they can be either pedunculated or sessile. You cannot, however, *always* palpate polyps. Colonoscopy is needed to differentiate between a polyp and carcinoma. Older adults are more prone to rectal polyps and are at higher risk for carcinoma, making a rectal examination particularly important in this population.

Carcinoma of the Rectum and Anus

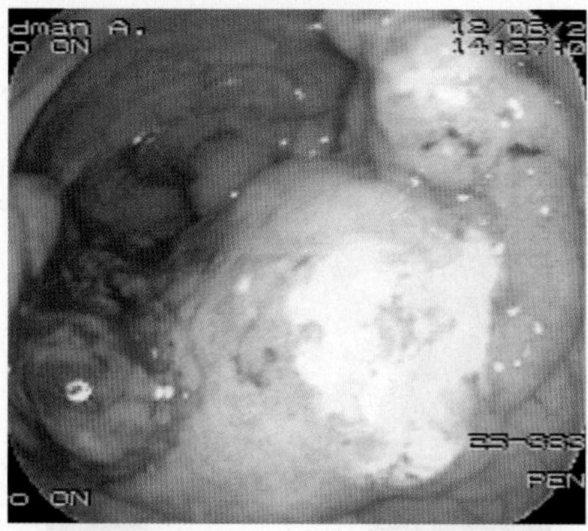

Although rare, cancers of the rectum and anus are becoming more common. The most common causes are anal intercourse, especially if associated with chronic irritation, such as with HPV. Symptoms of rectal and anal cancer include constant discharge, change in bowel habits, blood in the stool, and weight loss. On examination, a stony, irregular, sessile polypoid mass is palpated. It is nodular with areas of ulceration. The cancer initially is asymptomatic, so routine clinical rectal examination and regular screening are key to early detection.

Rectal Prolapse

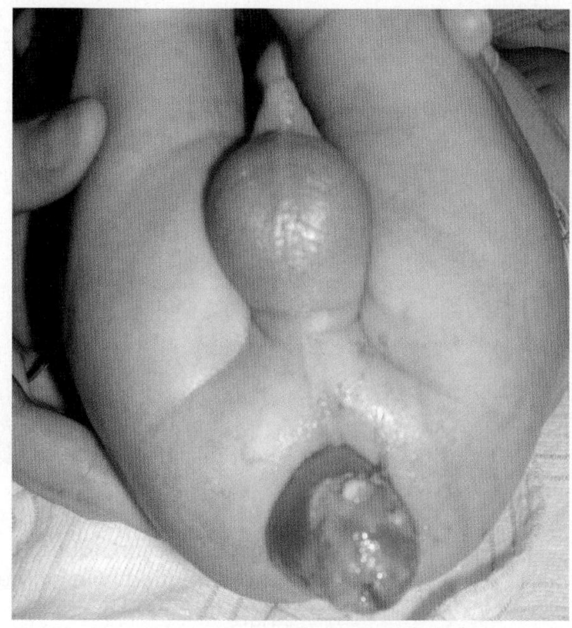

Rectal prolapse usually occurs during defecation; the rectal mucosa, with or without a muscular wall, prolapses through the anal ring. On examination, a prolapse may present in a doughnut shape. A complete prolapse includes the muscular wall and is larger than an incomplete prolapse, with circular folds. Children with cystic fibrosis may present with rectal prolapse.

Prostatitis

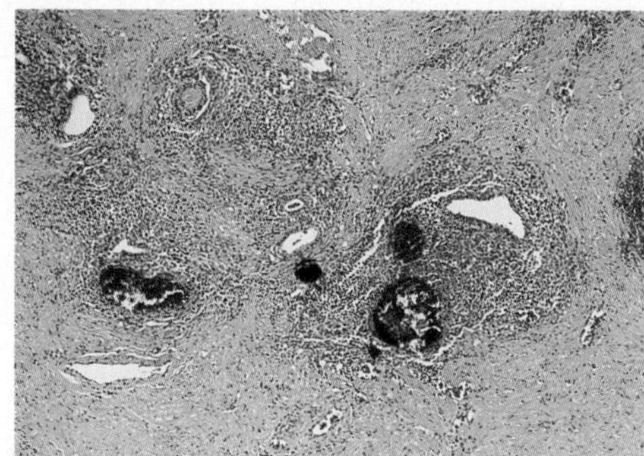

Inflammation or infection of the prostate gland can be acute or chronic. Acute **bacterial prostatitis** may result from ascending urethral infection, reflux of infected urine, extension of a rectal infection, or hematogenous spread. **Chronic prostatitis** results from autoimmune, allergic, neuromuscular, or psychological disorders of the bladder; detrusor hyperreflexia; or pelvic floor tension myalgia.

Signs and symptoms of acute and chronic prostatitis are similar; they include fever, chills, malaise, dysuria, frequency, inhibited urinary voiding, low back pain, suprapubic discomfort, and perineal pain. Many patients also complain of painful sexual intercourse, pain when defecating, and hematuria. Acute prostatitis usually presents with more severe symptoms than chronic prostatitis.

(table continues on page 734)

TABLE 23.9 Conditions of the Anus, Rectum, and Prostate *(continued)*

On examination, the prostate is tender, warm, swollen, and boggy. Carefully and gently palpate because vigorous massage can disseminate bacteria in the bloodstream, resulting in bacteriemia. The patient with prostatitis is seriously ill and needs immediate intervention.

Prostate Cancer

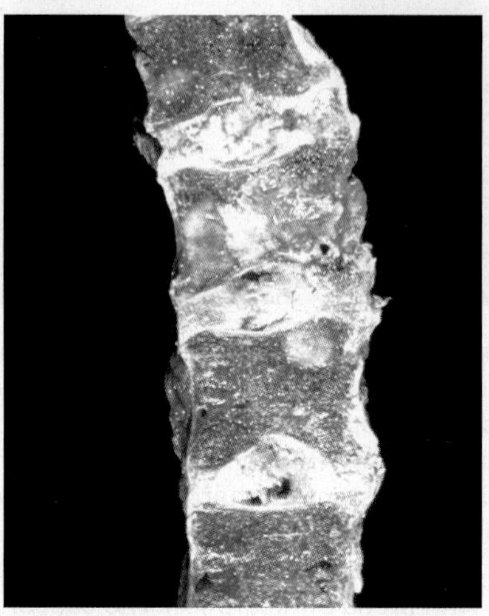

Prostate cancer is the most common cancer found in American men and ranks second in the number of cancer deaths. (Lung cancer is number one.) Prostate cancer is usually a very slow-growing cancer. In fact, more than 40% of men older than 50 years of age have been found to have prostate cancer on autopsy, and the prevalence increases with age.

Men are usually asymptomatic early in the disease. Latent symptoms include bone pain, weight loss, anemia, shortness of breath, lymphedema, and lymphadenopathy. Patient complaints also include bladder outlet symptoms or acute urinary retention with very large or locally extensive tumors but are most often due to BPH (Dunphy et al., 2011).

Prostate cancer is usually asymptomatic in its early stages. As the prostate enlarges, the patient may develop hesitancy, dribbling, frequency, urgency, nocturia, retention, slow stream, or feeling of bladder fullness. Diagnosis is made with a PSA blood test and rectal examination.

TABLE 23.10 Types of Hernias

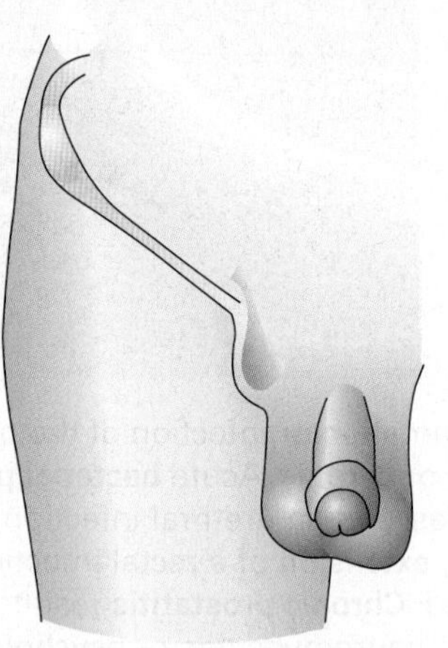

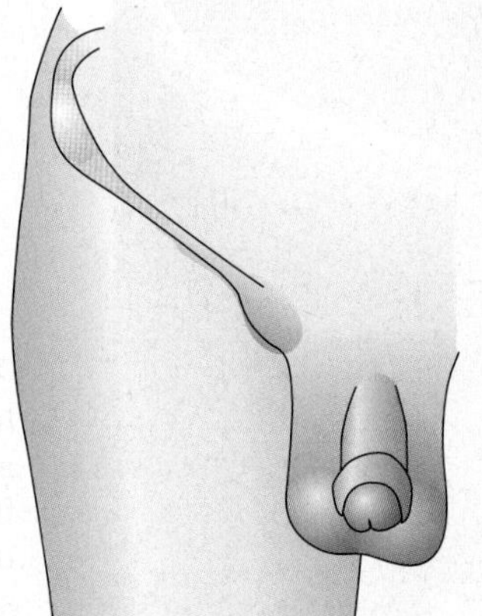

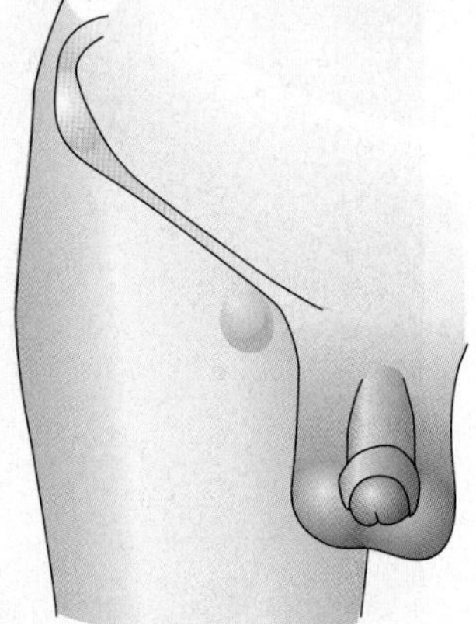

	Direct Inguinal	Indirect Inguinal	Femoral
Affected population	Middle-aged and elderly men	All ages	Least common; found more frequently in women
Bilaterality	55%	30%	Rare
Origin of swelling	Above inguinal ligament; directly behind and through external ring	Above inguinal ligament; hernial sac enters inguinal canal at internal ring and exits at external ring	Below inguinal ligament
Scrotal involvement	Rare	Common	Never
Impulse location	At side of examiner's finger in inguinal canal	At tip of examiner's finger in inguinal canal	Not palpable by examiner's finger in inguinal canal; mass below canal

TABLE 23.11 Scrotum and Testes Abnormalities

Abnormal Finding	Description
Testicular Torsion 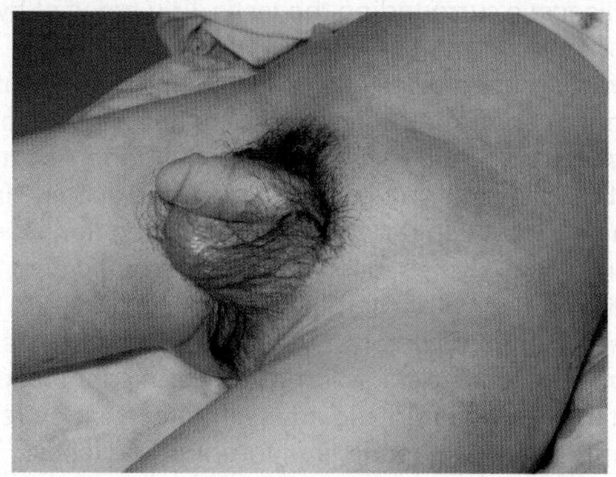	This sudden twisting of the spermatic cord typically occurs on the left side because the left cord is longer. Most common in late childhood or early adolescence, it is rare after 20 years of age. Testicular torsion results from faulty anchoring of the testis on the scrotal wall, which enables rotation. The anterior part of the testes rotates medially toward the other testes. Blood supply is impaired, resulting in ischemia and venous engorgement. Because the testis can become gangrenous within a few hours, *testicular torsion is considered a surgical emergency.*
Epididymitis 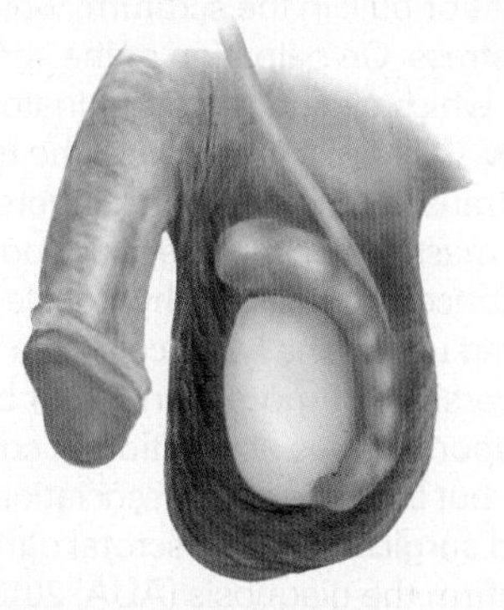	This acute infection of the epididymis is commonly caused by chlamydia, gonorrhea, or other bacterial infection (e.g., *Escherichia coli*). In men younger than 35 years old, the most common cause is an STI. Epididymitis is often linked to prostatitis, especially after surgical intervention or urethral instrumentation. Uncommon causes include tuberculosis, trauma, systemic fungal infections, and use of the drug amiodarone. Pain in the scrotum is severe, accompanied by swelling and fever. The scrotum can become greatly enlarged, inflamed, and painful to touch. Treatment with antibiotics is often needed.
Varicocele 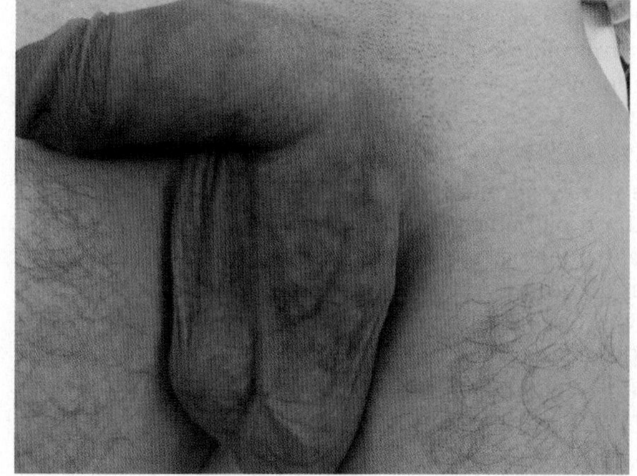	This dilated, tortuous, varicose vein most often occurs in the left spermatic cord, which is longer and inserts at a right angle into the left renal vein. Varicoceles are common in young males (5% of teens and 15% of adults) but rare before 10 years of age. In boys younger than 10 years of age, varicocele may correlate with malignancy. It is important to screen for varicocele in early adolescence because this condition is *the most common cause of infertility*. Correction of testicular atrophy in early adolescence results in improved sperm count. Increased fertility has been noted in 80%–90% of those who undergo surgical correction. No visual abnormality may appear on the scrotum, but a bluish tinge may be seen in light-skinned patients. When the patient is upright, you can palpate a soft irregular mass that feels distinctly like a "bag of worms" posterior and superior to the testis. The varicocele collapses when the patient is supine but enlarges when the patient bears down or does the Valsalva maneuver. Testes on the affected side may be smaller because of impaired circulation, so you will need to compare both testes (length, width, and depth). In advanced practice, orchidometers are often used to measure testicular volume in milliliters: • Grade 3: bag of worms more than 2 cm (3/4 in.) in diameter and easily visualized • Grade 2: 1–2 cm (3/8–3/4 in.) in diameter and easily palpable • Grade 1: (most common) very small, difficult to palpate; Valsalva maneuver may help Asymptomatic Grade 1 varicoceles with normal testicular volumes usually do not require intervention in adolescents, but ultrasound is recommended every 6 months to evaluate size.

(table continues on page 736)

TABLE 23.11 **Scrotum and Testes Abnormalities** ***(continued)***

Abnormal Finding	Description
Hydrocele 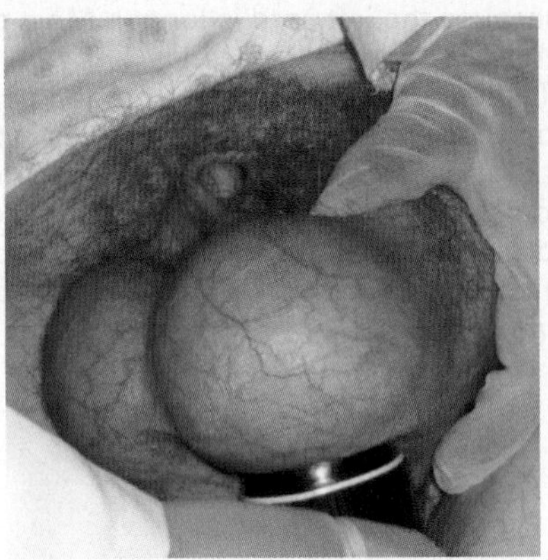	This circumscribed collection of serous fluid develops in the tunica vaginalis testis surrounding the testis. Two types of hydroceles occur: noncommunicating and communicating. In *noncommunicating hydrocele*, fluid collects only in the scrotum but is persistent. A communicating hydrocele has a patent process vaginalis testis, so fluid can move from the abdomen to the scrotum. Edema is intermittent; the scrotum is usually flat in the morning and swollen during the day or when the patient cries or performs the Valsalva maneuver. A *communicating hydrocele* is associated with a hernia. Incidence is 0.5%–2% of males. It primarily appears before 1 year of age; if it persists beyond 1 year of age, you should assume it to be in conjunction with a hernia. In older children and adults, hydrocele may result from epididymitis, trauma, hernia, and tumor of the testis. The patient will present with unilateral edema but no pain. He may complain of weight or bulk in the scrotum, which does not cause any apparent distress. On palpation of the scrotum, you will note a large mass, which can be transilluminated and will have a pink or red glow. If a hernia is involved, the hydrocele will not be evident during transillumination. Your fingers should be able to get around the mass; however, this is not possible if a hernia is present. If a noncommunicating hydrocele is present, no treatment is indicated unless the hydrocele is so large that it causes discomfort or persists for more than 1 year because, by then, there should be spontaneous absorption. A communicating hydrocele can resolve, but because of its association with hernia, this condition will need surgical repair. A scrotal ultrasound may be ordered to help confirm the diagnosis (AUA, 2013).
Spermatocele 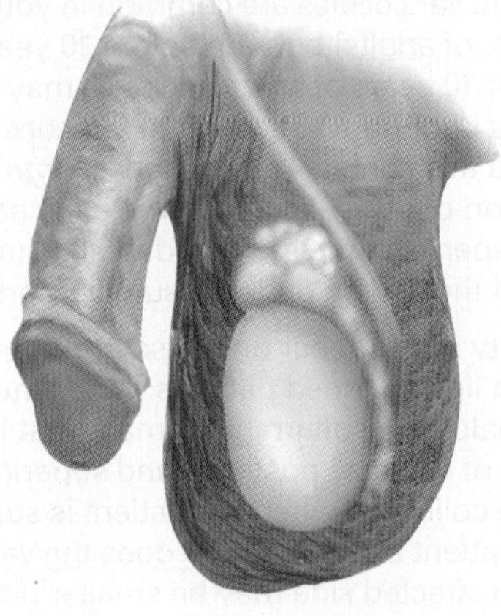	This benign scrotal mass or cyst, which contains sperm, develops on the head of the epididymis or testicular adnexa. An uncommon finding, it occurs in less than 1% of all males from the neonatal period to a peak at 14 years of age. For the nurse, it is virtually impossible to differentiate this from a simple epididymal cyst that does not contain sperm. The patient may complain of a lump in the scrotal sac or edema. Upon palpation, you will find a mobile cystic nodule, usually less than 1 cm (3/8 in.) in size, superior and posterior to the testis. The mass will be evident during transillumination and will have a pink or red glow. The spermatocele will not change in size when the patient performs the Valsalva maneuver. The advanced practice nurse orders a scrotal ultrasound for diagnostic purposes.

24

Female Genitalia and Rectal Assessment

Learning Objectives

1 Demonstrate knowledge of anatomy and physiology of the female genitalia and rectum.

2 Identify important topics for health promotion and risk reduction of the female genitalia and rectum.

3 Collect subjective data related to the female genitalia and rectum.

4 Collect objective data related to the female genitalia and rectum using physical examination techniques.

5 Identify expected and unexpected findings related to the female genitalia and rectum.

6 Analyze subjective and objective data from assessment of the female genitalia and rectum and consider initial interventions.

7 Document and communicate data from the assessment of the female genitalia and rectum using appropriate medical terminology and principles of recording.

8 Individualize health assessment of the female genitalia and rectum considering age, ethnicity, and culture of the patient.

9 Identify nursing diagnoses and initiate a plan of care based on findings from the assessment of the female genitalia and rectum.

Teresa Nguyen, a 28-year-old Vietnamese American woman, is being seen in the clinic for the first time with clear vaginal secretions and pelvic pain. Her temperature is 36.8°C (98.2°F) orally, pulse 82 beats/min, respirations 16 breaths/min, and blood pressure 102/66 mm Hg. She is taking no medications.

You will gain more information about Ms. Nguyen as you progress through this chapter. As you study the content and features, consider Teresa Nguyen's case and its relationship to what you are learning. Begin thinking about the following points:

- What are some causes of vaginal discharge?
- What are the implications of Teresa's presenting condition for her boyfriend?
- What cultural considerations should the nurse incorporate into the care provided for Teresa?
- What lifestyle factors might be contributing to Teresa's present condition?
- What recommendations for screening and follow-up would the nurse suggest for Teresa?
- How will the nurse evaluate if the assessment has been accurate and complete?

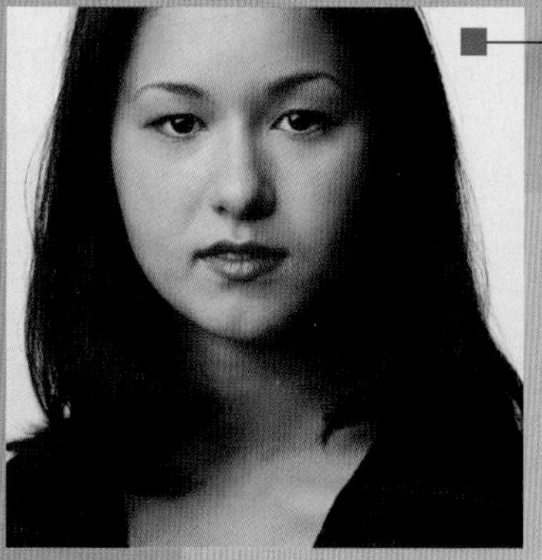

This chapter focuses on genital and rectal assessment of the female patient across the lifespan. By identifying key factors in the process of this assessment, you can explore opportunities for positive communication and accurate information regarding women's health. You can guide female patients in risk reduction and health promotion from the onset of puberty to the menopausal years and beyond.

Structure and Function

The female genitalia can be subdivided into external and internal parts. External genitalia include the mons pubis, labia majora, labia minora, prepuce, and clitoris. The internal genitalia are the vagina, fornix, uterus, cervix, fundus, fallopian tubes, ovaries, and supporting tissues.

External Genitalia

The collective external genitalia are also called the vulva (Fig. 24.1). The mons pubis is the most anterior structure; it is composed of subcutaneous fatty tissue covered by pubic hair. The mons pubis lies directly over the pubic bone and creates a cushion that protects the bone during intercourse. The labia majora consist of two folds that extend from the mons pubis downward to the perineum. The clitoris, the female equivalent of the penis, responds in an erectile fashion when stimulated. It consists of the glans that lies posterior to two crura (erectile tissue structures). Nerve fibers in the clitoris respond to touch and produce pleasurable feelings for the female. The ventral surface of the glans is known as the frenulum and it is where the labia minora, two small folds that extend from clitoral hood to the posterior fourchette of the vagina, fuse. The vestibule lies between the labia minora and is bound anteriorly by the clitoris and posteriorly by the perineum. Within the vestibule lie the urethra at the upper middle area, with bilateral paraurethral Skene glands at the 7-o'clock and 5-o'clock positions, respectively. The Skene glands produce clear fluid that aids in lubrication during intercourse. The vaginal introitus lies posterior to the urethra. The Bartholin glands, located at the base of the vestibule, secrete clear mucus into the vaginal introitus during intercourse. They are positioned at 7-o'clock and 5-o'clock positions of the posterior vestibule.

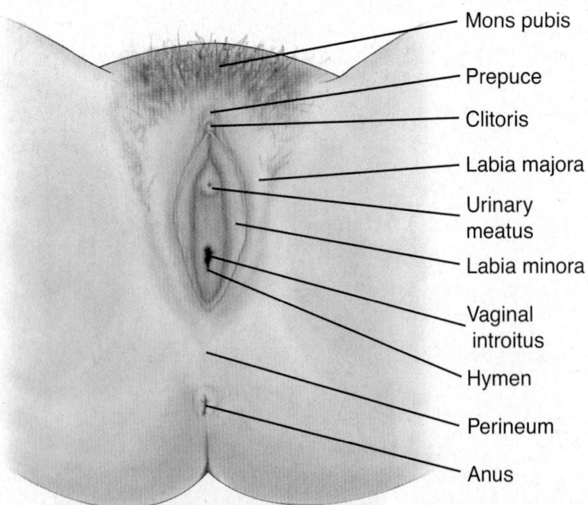

Figure 24.1 Anatomy of the external genitalia.

> **Clinical Significance**
>
> The perineum is the area between the vaginal introitus and rectum. This is the anatomic location where an episiotomy is sometimes done to facilitate difficult childbirth.

Internal Genitalia

Vagina

The vagina is a tube of muscular tissue that extends from vaginal introitus to uterus. The three-layer vaginal muscle wall is extremely flexible, especially during childbirth. It is lined with a glandular mucous membrane, within which are folds called rugae. These rugae become less prominent in advanced years. The vagina is approximately parallel to the lower portion of the sacrum. This position is the reason the anterior wall of the vagina measures 7 cm (about 2¾ in.) while the posterior wall is about 9 cm (about 3½ in.). The vesicovaginal septum separates the anterior wall of the vagina from the urethra and bladder. The rectovaginal septum separates the posterior wall of the vagina from the rectum.

Uterus

The hollow uterus, often referred to as the "womb," is the organ that holds the endometrial lining and is prepared to accept an implanted ovum (Fig. 24.2). It lies between the bladder and rectum and is approximately 7 to 8 cm long (about 2¾ to 3¼ in.) and 4 to 5 cm (1½ to 2 in.) at its widest part. The uterine walls consist of an outer layer called the peritoneum, a muscular layer called the myometrium, and an inner layer called the endometrium.

The uterus has two parts separated by a narrow isthmus: the corpus (body) and the cervix. If implantation occurs, the uterus accommodates the growing fetus for the remaining 9 months. If no fertilization occurs, the endometrial lining sheds and the patient will have a menstrual period. The freely mobile uterus is supported bilaterally by the round, cardinal, uterosacral, and broad ligaments.

Cervix

The cervix is the posterior portion of the uterus that protrudes into the vagina. The cervix is smooth, rounded, and has a midline opening called the os. In a woman who has never given birth (nulliparous), the os resembles a donut with a small hole in the middle. In a woman who has had one or more pregnancies and deliveries (parous), the opening resembles a horizontal slit.

Fallopian Tubes

The fallopian tubes transport ova from the ovary to the uterus. They are approximately 12 cm (4¾ in.) long and 1 mm in

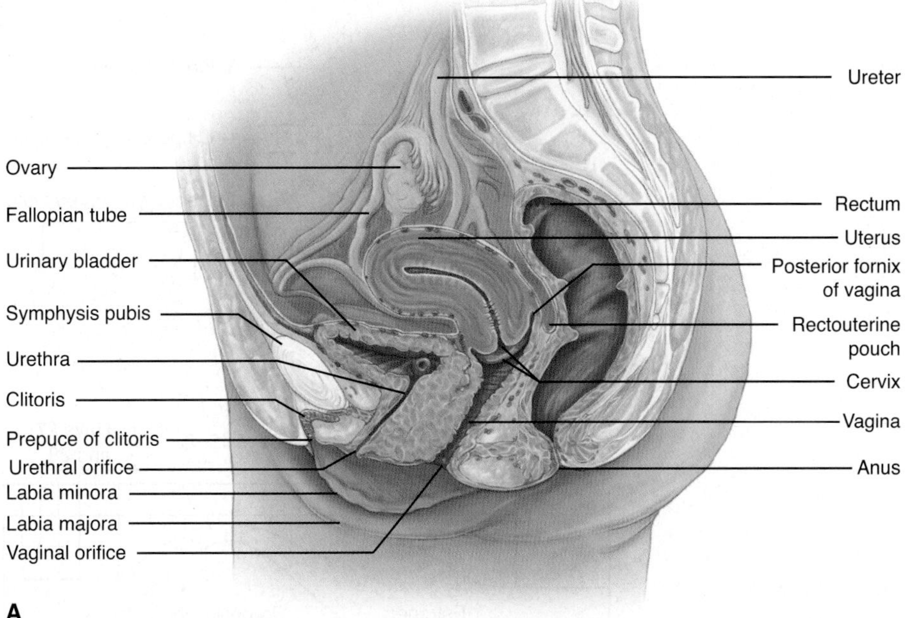

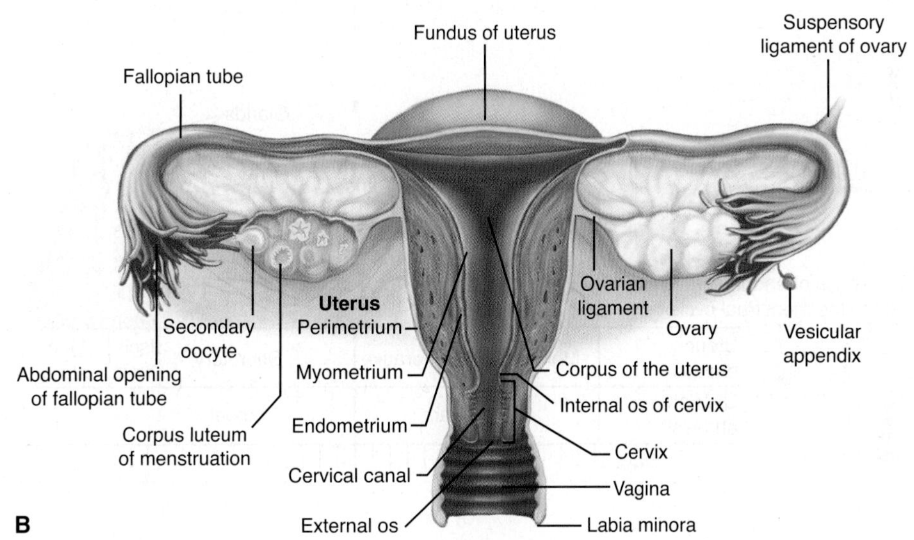

Figure 24.2 Internal female genitalia. **A.** Side view. **B.** Frontal view.

diameter. The tubes are composed of four layers of tissues: peritoneal (serous), subserous (adventitial), muscular, and mucous. These layers are responsible for the blood and nerve supply as well as providing the peristaltic condition necessary to move the ovum toward the uterus. The fallopian tubes are divided into three parts: isthmus, ampulla, and fimbriae. Fertilization most often occurs in the ampullary portion of the fallopian tubes.

Ovaries

The ovaries are two almond-shaped structures measuring approximately 3 cm × 2 cm (about 1¼ in by ¾ in.). They develop after puberty and shrink (atrophy) after menopause. The ovaries are held in place by the infundibulopelvic and ovarian ligaments. The ovaries provide ova to be fertilized by sperm and secrete two hormones: estrogen and progesterone (discussed later).

Rectum, Anal Canal, and Anus

Anatomy and physiology of the rectum, anal canal, and anus are covered in detail in Chapter 23.

Hormone Regulation

Many hormones regulate the female reproductive system. The main sources of these hormones are (1) the anterior pituitary gland, (2) the hypothalamus, and (3) the ovaries.

The anterior pituitary gland secretes follicle-stimulating hormone (FSH) and luteinizing hormone (LH). The function of FSH is to stimulate the growth and maturation of the ovarian follicle and the production of testosterone, which maintains spermatogenesis in the male. LH functions to luteinize the follicle, which increases production of progesterone by

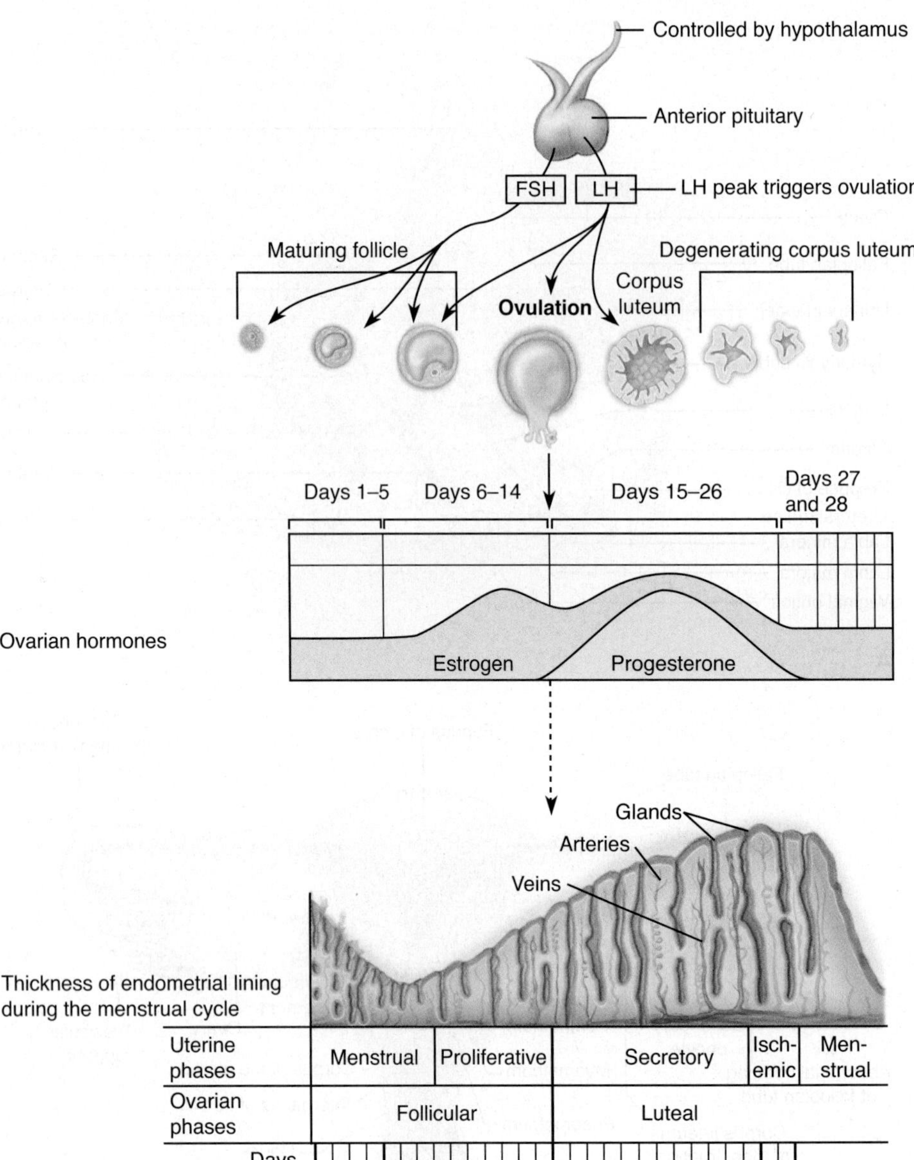

Figure 24.3 Relationship between hormonal levels **(center)**, follicular development **(top)**, and the menstrual cycle **(bottom)**.

the granulose cells (Fritz & Speroff, 2012). The luteinizing process ultimately produces the corpus luteum.

The hypothalamus is responsible for the release of FSH and LH by way of the gonadotropin-releasing hormones (GnRH) and luteinizing-releasing hormones (LnRH). The hypothalamus acts as an inhibitor of prolactin release via the secretion of prolactin inhibiting factor. These cyclic hormones drive the function of menstruation, reproduction, sexuality, and physical as well as emotional health (Fritz & Speroff, 2012). The pelvic organs are the recipients of the hormones (Fig. 24.3).

The ovaries, as already noted, produce estrogen and progesterone. Estrogen regulates the development of secondary sex characteristics; contributes to the growth of the vagina, fallopian tubes, and uterus; contributes to the proliferation of the endometrial lining; and plays a role in maturation of ovarian follicles. Progesterone develops the corpus luteum and is necessary for the successful implantation of the embryo. If no implantation happens, a menstrual cycle occurs.

Lifespan Considerations

Women Who Are Pregnant

The cervix of the pregnant woman is very different than that of the nonpregnant woman. Assessment of a pregnant woman is discussed in detail in Chapter 25.

Infants, Children, and Adolescents

On assessment of the newborn girl, it is not uncommon to see some pink discharge at the opening of the vagina. This is most often a result of maternal estrogen. In a girl, the genitalia continue growing, except for the clitoris (Fig. 24.4).

Genital assessment of the adolescent is not required unless there has been initiation of sexual activity or genital tract difficulties arise. The opportunity for patient education is greatest at this time, however. The adolescent is experiencing body changes, self-identity exploration, and relationship questions. You should be direct and honest with the teen. Establishment of a trusting and confidential nurse–patient relationship is vital. Sexually active adolescent females should have an annual examination.

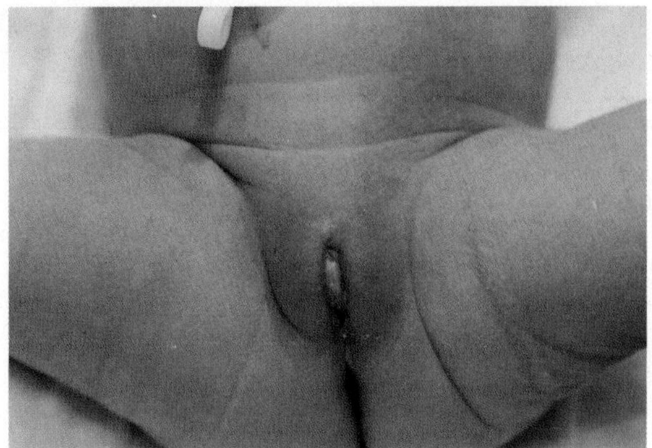

Figure 24.4 Surface anatomy of the female infant genitalia.

> **Clinical Significance**
>
> **Ambiguous genitalia** are a congenital anomaly found in some newborns. Hyperplasia of the adrenal glands causes excessive androgen production. The clitoris may resemble a penis, and the fusion of the labia resembles a scrotal sac. This potentially serious condition requires referral for diagnostic evaluation (Fritz & Speroff, 2012).

Older Adults

Women older than 65 years of age represent more than 15% of the female population (U.S. Census Bureau, 2014). As women age, they experience many changes in the genitourinary tract. Most of these are related to limited or absent estrogen in the system.

Menopause is defined as 12 consecutive months without menses (Fritz & Speroff, 2012). As estrogen levels decrease, the uterus becomes smaller, the ovaries shrink, the normal vaginal rugae flatten, and the epithelium atrophies. These normal changes may lead to difficulties such as vaginal infections, urinary tract infections (UTIs), dyspareunia, and diminished libido. Older women are at increased risk for endometrial cancers and need education regarding unexpected signs and symptoms. You have an opportunity to provide counseling and education about intimacy difficulties and physiological changes and to answer the patient's questions.

Cultural Considerations

Age of onset of puberty in girls has continued to decline, according to the American Congress of Obstetricians and Gynecologist Committee on Adolescent Health Care. The U.S. median age at menarche is 12.4 years. African American girls may begin puberty before 8 years of age. Onset of menses correlates with estrogen release by the hypothalamic-pituitary-ovarian axis (Fritz & Speroff, 2012). Budding of the breasts occurs first followed by development of pubic hair (see Chapter 19). Onset of menses follows breast budding by approximately 2 to 3 years. The **Tanner stages of maturation** are used to assess preadolescent and adolescent females (Marshall & Tanner, 1969). Female pubic hair stages are reviewed in Table 24.1.

Urgent Assessment

If the patient is experiencing severe pain or excessive vaginal bleeding, the assessment needs to be truncated to involve only questions pertinent to the immediate condition and necessary for current care. Severe pain may be related to an acute infection (e.g., pelvic inflammatory disease [PID]), UTI, gastrointestinal illness (e. g., appendicitis, pancreatitis, cholecystitis, strangulated hernia), or musculoskeletal trauma (ruptured bladder, spleen, or liver). It is important to perform a thorough symptom analysis to evaluate these problems. A ruptured ovarian cyst may be present, which needs to be assessed quickly. An ectopic pregnancy is also an urgent situation; suspect this condition if a normally menstruating female has had amenorrhea for a period of 5 to 6 weeks.

Subjective Data

The assessment of the female genital system is very invasive and can be uncomfortable for both the patient and the nurse. During initiation of the health history, allow the patient to become comfortable with you; as you acquire important data about the patient, you will feel more confident. It is important to project a respectful, nonjudgmental demeanor.

The room should be private and comfortable. You should be seated at eye level or lower than the patient. Reassure the patient that all information is kept confidential. It is best to obtain the history while the patient is dressed; this reduces potential patient embarrassment and vulnerability. If this is not possible, make sure the patient is completely covered, warm, and comfortable. Make eye contact but be careful of nonverbal communication. Often, minor cues give the greatest amount of information. Begin the interview with less personal basic biographical data.

Talking about sex with patients has a direct impact on unintended pregnancies and sexually transmitted infections (STIs). In cultures that have greater sexual fluency and candidness about sexuality, there are improved sexual experience, increased contraceptive use, fewer STIs, and fewer unintended pregnancies. Women want practitioners who know the way they feel about sex matters. Many women, however, are too embarrassed to bring up the topic, although most will discuss sexual concerns if their provider introduces the topic. The sexual history includes gathering data on the "5 Ps": *partners*, *pregnancy prevention*, *protection against STIs*, sexual *practices*, and *past history of STIs*.

Avoid making assumptions when talking with patients about sexual matters. Some common misconceptions are the following:

- Sexually experienced people know how to use safer sex techniques.
- People with good jobs and families do not experiment sexually.
- Single people have lots of partners and risky safer sex practices.
- Older people have fewer partners and infrequent sex.
- Married people are heterosexual and do not have sex with partners of the same gender.

With practice, you will become more fluent and comfortable talking about the female reproductive system, STIs, contraception, and sexuality.

TABLE 24.1 **Tanner Staging: Female Pubic Hair**

Stage	Description
Stage 1: Preadolescent 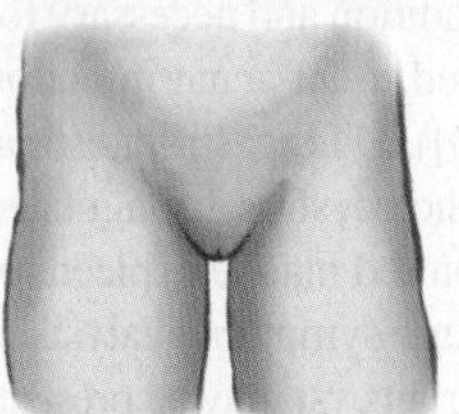	The vellus over the pubes is not further developed than that over the anterior abdominal wall (i.e., no pubic hair).
Stage 2 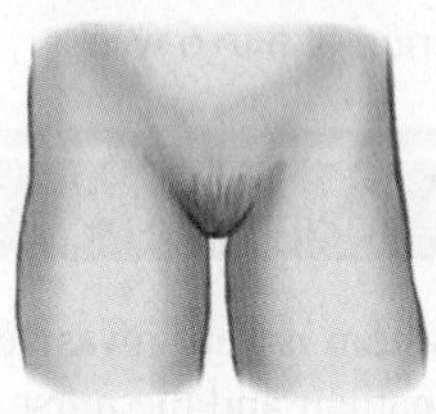	Long, slightly pigmented, downy hair that is straight or only slightly curled appears chiefly along the labia.
Stage 3 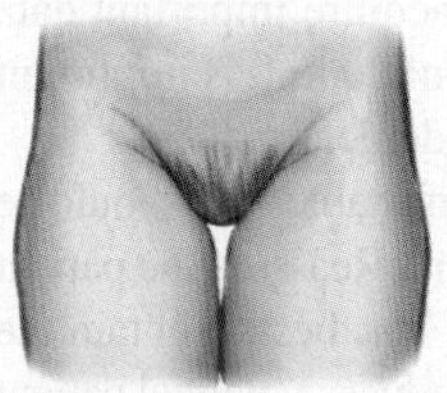	Hair is considerably darker, coarser, and more tightly curled. It spreads sparsely over the junction of the mons pubis.
Stage 4 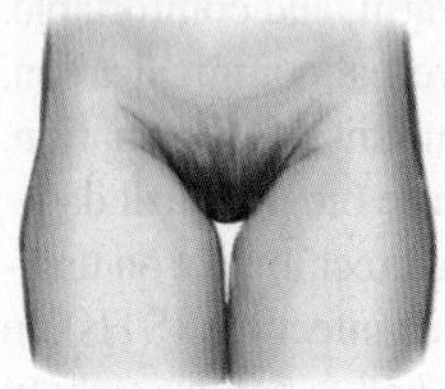	Hair is now adult in type, but the area covered by it is still considerably smaller than in most adults. No spread to the medial surface of the thighs observed.
Stage 5 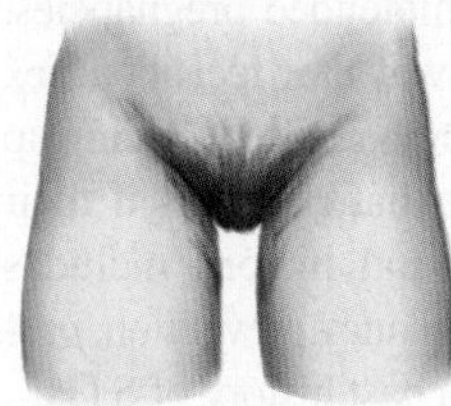	Hair is adult in quantity and type, distributed as an inverse triangle of the classically feminine pattern. Spread is to the medial surface of the thighs but not up the linea alba or elsewhere above the base of the inverse triangle.

Assessment of Risk Factors

History and Risk Factors	Rationale
Personal History	
Menstrual History. Ask about menstrual history first. • How old were you when you got your first menstrual period? • What was the first day of the last menstrual period? • What is the character or consistency of your flow? • Do you use tampons? • How many days do you experience flow during your cycle? • How many pads or tampons do you use per day? How many days is there heavy flow, moderate flow, or light spotting?	Menarche usually begins around 12 years of age. If a patient has not had menarche by age 16 years, an endocrine evaluation is recommended. The menstrual cycle is calculated from the first day of the last menstrual period to the first day of the next menstrual period. The usual cycle is 28–32 days, but cycles can be as short as 20 days or as long as 40 days without clinical intervention becoming necessary. Flow is approximately 25–60 ml (about ¾–2 oz) per menstrual period. Normal length is 2–8 days.
Obstetrical History • Have you ever been pregnant? • If so, how many times? • How many living children do you have? • Did you give birth vaginally or through cesarean operation? • Were there any complications before, during, or after your pregnancy? • Have you ever had a miscarriage? • Have you ever had an abortion? If yes, was it an elective termination, spontaneous miscarriage, or incomplete miscarriage?	**Gravida:** The number of pregnancies a woman has had, including any current pregnancy. **Para:** The number of births a woman has had after 20 weeks even if the fetus died at birth. **Term:** Infant born after 37 weeks' gestation. **Preterm:** Infant born after 20 weeks but before 37 weeks. **Abortion:** Number of pregnancies that were ended spontaneously or for therapeutic reasons. **Living:** Number of living children either delivered or adopted. A woman could be a gravida 1 (one pregnancy), and have two children (para 2). This occurs with twins.
Menopause • Have you stopped having menstrual periods? • Are your menstrual cycles irregular? • Do you experience any symptoms of irregularity or absence of menses?	**Menopause** is the cessation of menstrual periods for 12 months or more. **Perimenopause** is irregularity of menstrual cycles and accompanying symptoms (hot flashes, night sweating, mood swings, vaginal dryness, decreased sexual drive or **libido**) between 40 and 55 years of age and before actual cessation of menses (Panay, Hamoda, Arya, & Savvas, 2013).
Gynecological History • Have you ever had a Pap smear? If so, when was it done? • Have your Pap smear results always been normal? • If not, did you receive any treatment for it? When? • Have you had any previous procedures or surgeries?	A **Papanicolaou smear** (Pap smear) is a cytological evaluation of the cells of the cervix to screen for precancerous cervical lesions. It does ***not*** screen for STIs or any cancers other than cervical cancer. You need to provide the patient with the most up-to-date evidence-based information. By educating the patient regarding the importance of follow-up and collaborating with health care providers to ensure compliance, you play a part in the reduction of cervical cancers.
• Have you ever been treated for any vaginal infections? • Do you have frequent vaginal infections?	Risk factors for a vaginal yeast infection include treatment with antibiotics, hormone contraceptives, contraceptive devices, weakened immune system, pregnancy, diabetes mellitus, and sexual activity (Sobel, 2013).
• Do you use over-the-counter vaginal medication? • Have you ever had any pelvic infections?	Frequent use of over-the-counter (OTC) vaginal creams or suppositories can potentially mask other more serious infections.

(table continues on page 744)

History and Risk Factors	Rationale
• Do you use scented vaginal products such as sprays or scented tampons or pads?	Use of scented products may result in a contact dermatitis of the vulva or vagina.
• Do you douche? How often do you douche?	Educate the patient about problems that can arise from douching, such as vaginal infections, imbalance of normal vaginal flora (i.e., altered pH), and the possibility of transferring a vaginal infection into the uterus. The consequence can be PID.
Immunizations. Have you received the vaccine against the **human papillomavirus (HPV)**? • When did you receive it? • Did you receive all three doses?	Recommended routine vaccination of girls aged 11–12 years with three doses of quadrivalent human papillomavirus vaccine. The vaccination series can be started as young as 9 years of age with the second dose 2 months after the first and the third dose 6 months after the first (Centers for Disease Control and Prevention [CDC], 2013). Vaccination also is recommended for girls and women aged 13–26 years who have not been previously vaccinated or who have not completed the full series.
Sexual History	
Sexual health is important to overall health, so I always like to ask patients about it. Is it OK to ask you a few questions about sexual matters? • Have you ever been sexually involved? Are you having sexual relations now? • What type (vaginal, oral, anal)?	Frank discussion opens opportunities for inquiry otherwise not brought up by the patient. You may be one of many persons to ask, but the first whom she is comfortable telling. Current statistics show that adolescents may not engage in vaginal intercourse but may have anal or oral sex (Guttmacher Institute, 2014).
• Approximately how many sexual partners have you had? Male, female, or both? Do you masturbate? • Are you currently in a sexual relationship? Is it monogamous?	Ascertaining a patient's experience is important to determine risks. It is important to provide accurate and health promoting information to homosexual, bisexual, and heterosexual females.
• Many patients have been sexually coerced or abused. Have you ever have sex when you didn't want to?	It is important to "normalize" and feel comfortable discussing sexual abuse; you will feel more comfortable with practice. Obtaining a history of sexual abuse not only opens discussion about it and the patient's current feelings but also allows you to proceed to the examination giving the emotional support necessary.
• Do you experience any pain or bleeding with or after intercourse?	Bleeding during intercourse may indicate an infection or possibly a cervical polyp.
• Do you experience urinary burning or infections related to intercourse?	**Dysuria** (burning with urination) or frequent UTIs may be related to bladder trauma resulting from intercourse. Educate the patient to empty her bladder before and after intercourse to reduce trauma and avoid introduction of bacteria into the urethra.
Sexual behavior	
• Has any illness, pregnancy, or surgery interfered with your ability to enjoy sex? • Is sex pleasurable for you? Do you have any issues with lubrication? Arousal? • Do you have any sexual concerns?	At first glance, sexual behavior may be seen as a biological or physical activity. However, sexuality is interwoven with social and cultural contexts, beliefs, attitudes, and values (Chandra, Mosher, Copen, & Sionean, 2011).
Contraception	
• Do you use condoms or other barrier methods during sexual intercourse? Sometimes or always? • Do you use any methods to prevent pregnancy? If so, what do you currently use? • Have you used anything different in the past to prevent pregnancy? • Have you had any difficulties with any contraceptive forms? Has it detracted or improved sexual pleasure? • Is your contraceptive method meeting your needs?	Evaluate whether intercourse "just happens" versus planning for sex. Condoms provide some but not complete protection against STIs; they provide protection only if used consistently. It is equally important for homosexual females to use barrier methods to prevent transmission of particular infections. Contraceptive use is different than practicing "safer sex." Contraceptives protect against pregnancies, not STIs. Only sexual abstinence provides 100% safety against pregnancy and STIs.

(table continues on page 745)

History and Risk Factors	Rationale
Sexually Transmitted Infections • Do you engage in unprotected sex? • Do you have multiple sexual partners? How many partners in the past month? 6 months? • Are you between 15 and 24 years old? • Are you experiencing any pain within or discharge from the pelvic region? • Have you any recent travel where you may have been at risk? Barrier methods? • Past history of STI? • Lesions on skin? Warts? Herpes? Lesions? • Voiding or burning with urination? Pain?	Screening, treating, and counseling of and about chlamydia and gonorrhea are currently recommended for all sexually active adolescents. *Chlamydia trachomatis* is currently the most common and frequently reported bacterial STI in the developed world (Hocking et al., 2013). Because of the asymptomatic nature of this infection, risk for infection is high. Long-term infection can cause PID and subsequent potential infertility. Pharyngitis may result from chlamydia infection.
Additional Health Risks for Women ***Obesity.*** Obesity is considered an independent risk factor for coronary heart disease. Central obesity (apple shape) increases this risk. Women with pear-shaped bodies are thought to be at less risk.	A body mass index (BMI) of 18.5–24.9 is considered normal, a BMI of 25–29 is overweight, and greater than 30 is considered obese (see Chapter 7). Women who exercise decrease cardiovascular risk. Additionally, the most active women have a 25% lower risk of breast cancer as compared with the least active (Hildebrand, 2013).
Osteoporosis. Osteoporosis is a bone disorder characterized by decreased bone mass, which leads to fragility and potential fracture, especially in females.	Bone mineral density screening is a simple and cost-efficient test recommended for all women age 65 years or older. Those at risk for osteoporosis (Caucasian or Asian women with a family history of osteoporosis, thin frame, tobacco use, glucocorticoid use, or any fracture after age 45 years) should be screened as well (National Osteoporosis Foundation [NOF], n.d.).
Hormonal Contraceptive and Tobacco Use • Do you smoke? • Are you using hormonal contraceptives? • How old are you?	Tobacco is contraindicated for any patient age 40 years or older who uses hormonal contraceptives. The combination of tobacco and hormonal contraceptives increases risk for vascular problems (e.g., deep vein thrombosis, pulmonary emboli) as well as risk for cardiovascular incident. Even light or "social" smoking doubles a female patient's risk of cardiovascular mortality (National Heart, Lung, and Blood Institute, 2011).
Medications and Supplements • Are you currently taking any prescribed medications? • Are you taking any OTC medications? • Have you recently been on any antibiotics? • Do you use any herbal therapeutics? • Do you currently take any vitamins?	Certain medications, including oral contraceptives, antidepressants, and antihypertensive agents, can cause changes in menstrual cycles, appetite, and libido. Certain antibiotics can strip the vagina of its normal flora and create an environment that promotes yeast infections. Antibiotics can interfere with the absorption of oral contraceptives; a backup method of contraception or abstinence is advised during the treatment period. Use of any herbal therapy requires caution. Although some positive effects with herbal preparations have been reported, herb-drug interactions have been reported. Often, herbal products affect other medications being taken; patients taking anticoagulants, digoxin, oral contraceptives, statins, and HIV medications should exercise caution. All herbal products should be reviewed for safety during pregnancy.

(table continues on page 746)

History and Risk Factors	Rationale
Family History Tell me about your family history of the following, including two generations: • Diabetes • Heart disease • Cancer • Thyroid problems • Gynecological conditions • Hypertension • Asthma • Allergies • Diethylstilbestrol use by mother • Multiple pregnancies • Congenital anomalies	Current studies show that the major factors in breast and ovarian cancer are the ***BRCA1*** and ***BRCA2* genes.** These genes may be transmitted from the father's side as well as the mother's side (National Cancer Institute [NCI], 2014). **Diethylstilbestrol (DES)** was a hormone given to pregnant women to prevent miscarriages from 1940 to 1970. Maternal DES use is associated with higher risks of cancers in children. Ongoing studies continue regarding DES exposure (Troisi et al., 2013).

SAFETY ALERT

Any patient taking isotretinoin (Accutane) for treatment of acne MUST have two negative pregnancy tests before starting therapy and continue with monthly pregnancy tests until treatment is discontinued. Because of the severe teratogenic effects of this medication, any woman of childbearing age must either abstain or use at least two forms of birth control 1 month before, after, and during treatment. Patients must register in the iPLEDGE program (FDA 2010) before starting isotretinoin therapy.

Risk Reduction and Health Promotion

An estimated 15 million new cases of **STIs** are reported each year. Of these, nearly 4 million occur in adolescents (CDC, 2013). Complications of STIs include cervical cancer, pelvic infections, infertility, and pelvic pain. Education is the most powerful tool you can offer regarding prevention of STIs. Maintain confidentiality during the sexual behavior portion of the history to elicit information from the patient, and offer the most current, evidence-based information to ensure greater understanding on the part of the patient.

Healthy People 2020 goals for health of the female reproductive system include the following:

- Increase the proportion of adolescents who abstain from sexual intercourse or use condoms if currently sexually active.
- Increase the proportion of sexually active persons who use condoms.
- Reduce the proportion of adolescents and young adults with *C. trachomatis* infections, gonorrhea, syphilis, HPV, and genital herpes.
- Increase those women age 18 years and older who have had a Pap smear (U.S. Department of Health and Human Services [USDHHS], 2013).

Topics for health promotion include menopause changes, prevention of HPV and cancer, prevention of STIs, genital self-examination, and female genital mutilation. Risk factors can be reduced through the provision of accurate evidence-based information. Give women throughout the lifespan an opportunity to ask questions and allow for open and nonjudgmental discussion about sexuality. Screen all adults who are at increased risk (multiple partners, intravenous (IV) drug use) for chlamydia, gonorrhea, HIV, hepatitis B, and syphilis.

Women with a history of multiple partners have the highest risk of contracting HPV and cervical cancer. It is important to discuss this statistic and to recommend monogamy, abstinence, or consistent use of condoms with each act of intercourse. Women currently using oral contraceptives are less likely to use any barrier methods such as condoms or diaphragms. When counseling women on oral contraceptive use, it is important to stress that the contraceptives used do not protect against STIs.

Incidence of cervical cancer has decreased in the past decades because of widespread use of Pap screening. The greatest risk factor for cervical cancer is infection with HPV. More than 100 types of HPV cause genital warts, some of which can lead to cancer of the cervix. Having unprotected sex increases the chance of contracting HPV. Not everyone infected with HPV develops cancer of the cervix. Other risk factors influence the likelihood of cervical cancer, such as tobacco use, infection with chlamydia or HIV, poor diet, low income, and family history of cancer. HPV testing can be done at the same time as the Pap smear; a simple swabbing of the external and endocervical areas is tested for the types of HPV (16, 18, 31, 33, 35, 45, 51, 52, and 56) that cause high-grade cervical lesions that lead to cancer. Women aged 21 to 65 years should receive cervical cancer screening every 3 years with cytology. Routine screening for ovarian cancer is not recommended.

SAFETY ALERT

HPV vaccines target HPV types 16 and 18, which cause 70% of cervical cancer cases. The only cervical cancer symptoms are precancerous changes in the cervix, which can be detected during regular pelvic examinations (Boardman, 2014). HPV testing along with cytological testing is significantly more sensitive than cytology testing alone.

The **HPV vaccine** consists of three separate doses and is recommended for females 9 through 26 years of age. Patients (and, in the case of minors, their parents) should be counseled to complete the series. The CDC and the United States Preventive Services Task Force (USPSTF) still recommend annual screening even if the patient has received the vaccine (USPSTF: http://www.uspreventiveservicestaskforce.org/uspstf/uspscerv.htm and CDC: http://www.cdc.gov/cancer/cervical/basic_info/screening.htm).

Common Symptoms

When assessing the patient who presents with a specific complaint, you perform a focused assessment. Ask questions systematically relating to the primary reason for seeking care. Begin with asking about the onset of the symptom. It is best to get specifics such as the number of hours, days, or weeks that the patient has been experiencing the symptoms. If bleeding is the problem, inquire about the number of pads or tampons used per hour or day. Ask about the location; many patients are not comfortable with anatomical descriptions and just say "down there." Use appropriate terminology in a matter-of-fact manner. Ask if pain involves the abdomen, bladder, vagina, urethra, uterus, or rectum. If possible, have the patient point to the area of concern. Inquire about the duration of the difficulty. Again, specifics help: How long does the symptom last? Is it ongoing? Ask about the character of the pain, bleeding, itching, discharge, or lesion.

You can provide the patient with a laundry list of descriptions such as dull, sharp, burning, stinging, color and consistency of blood, presence of clots, thick or thin discharge, and odor. Find out whether any associative factors exist, such as nausea, vomiting, fever, malaise, fainting, or change in urinary or bowel habits. Inquire about activities, products, or conditions (e.g., intercourse, menses, physical activity, hygiene products, self-treatment) that might aggravate symptoms. If the patient has experienced any relief, ask what has made it better. Has the symptom been experienced before and when? What was done for it? Finally, ask about the severity of the symptom. How bad is the pain, itching, or bleeding on a scale of 0 to 10, with 10 being the worst?

Common Female Genital or Rectal Symptoms

- Pelvic pain
- Vaginal discharge, burning, or itching
- Menstrual disorders
- Discomfort related to structural problems
- Sexual dysfunction
- Hemorrhoids

Signs/Symptoms	Rationale/Abnormal Findings
Pelvic Pain Do you have any pain or discomfort? • Location • Intensity • Duration • Description • Aggravating factors • Alleviating factors • Functional impairment • Pain goal	Measurable pain identification allows you to address symptoms individually. Ask the patient to rate the pain or discomfort from 0–10 with 10 being the worst pain ever. Differences between acute and chronic pain may alter the course of intervention and goals set. Always ask the patient to point to the area of pain or discomfort to gather more accurate and reliable data. Many gynecological problems differ in their pain characteristics. The description of burning versus dull and gnawing can help you and the primary care provider identify the problem sooner. Conditions involving the pelvic region increase in pain and intensity with activities such as exercise, intercourse, or prolonged standing. Relief may be in the form of OTC medications or remedies, such as warm baths or a heating pad. If the current difficulty is impairing functional ability, you need to address this as a priority as much as if you yourself had the pain or discomfort. The goal is to assist in expediting the relief of the presenting symptom and to contribute to the return of functionality in the patient.
Vaginal Burning, Discharge, Itching • Have you ever been treated for an STI? • If you were treated, were your partner(s) treated? • Did you have a follow-up examination to confirm efficacy of treatment? • Are you aware of the different types of STIs? • Do you currently have any vaginal discharge? If so, describe its color, odor, or consistency? • Do you have any itching or burning sensation involving your pubic hair, vulva, or vagina?	An STI survey allows you to educate the patient on all possible infections. Vaginal discharge is a common symptom of STIs; however, a patient with an STI may have few or no symptoms. Differentiate between external and internal itching. External itching can have any number of sources; examples include pediculosis pubis (commonly called "crabs"), contact dermatitis, herpes simplex virus, condyloma acuminatum (external genital warts), and atrophic vulvitis.

(table continues on page 748)

Signs/Symptoms	Rationale/Abnormal Findings
Menstrual Disorders	
• Have you ever experienced irregular menstrual cycles or skipped a cycle? • Do you experience cramps during your menses? • Do you take any medication for menstrual cramps? If so, how much and how often? Does it help? • Do you experience preflow bloating, mood swings, headaches, or breast tenderness? Does it go away once your flow begins?	**Amenorrhea** is the absence of menstrual periods. The most common causes of secondary amenorrhea are pregnancy and anovulation. **Dysmenorrhea** is pain with menses. Nonsteroidal antiinflammatory drugs have been shown effective for dysmenorrhea. Premenstrual syndrome is the emotional and physical symptoms that occur at the same time before menses each month.
• Are there any times other than your menstrual period that you experience bleeding or spotting?	Intermenstrual bleeding or spotting or bleeding could be normal or could indicate an ongoing infection.
• Do you experience any bleeding or spotting following intercourse? • Do any menstrual conditions cause you to miss work, school, or social functions?	Postintercourse bleeding or spotting could indicate an STI or possibly a cervical polyp.
Structural Difficulties	
• Have you ever been treated for any cancer of the reproductive organs? • Have you ever been treated for any gynecological conditions such as endometriosis, uterine fibroids, ovarian cyst, or unexpected bleeding? • Have you noticed any change in the amount of hair you have on the vulva, abdomen, or around the nipples? • Have you gained weight especially in the midabdomen in the past 6 months? • Have you noticed changes in your skin?	Patients with a history of endometriosis have increased risk of infertility (National Institute for Health and Clinical Excellence [NICE], 2013). Frequent ovarian cysts along with menstrual irregularities warrant evaluation for **polycystic ovarian syndrome**. In this condition, the patient presents with obesity, acne, **hirsutism** (increased hair along the abdomen and around the nipples), and **acanthosis nigricans** (areas of hyperpigmentation around the back of the neck and under arms). Vaginal ultrasound reveals multicystic ovaries. The patient may have variations in hormone levels, including increased free testosterone (Lucidi, 2013).
Sexual Dysfunction	
• Is sex pleasurable? • Do you get moist or have orgasm? • Do you have problems with lubrication?	Even though there is more sexual autonomy and satisfaction than in the past, there remains a gender difference in the perception of the right to have pleasurable sex. A woman needs to feel at ease in saying if sex doesn't feel right and communicate what feels good during sex.
Hemorrhoids	
Do you have hemorrhoids?	Hemorrhoids are very common, especially following childbirth. Hemorrhoids may be either external or internal.

Lifespan Considerations

Additional Questions	Rationale/Abnormal Findings
Women Who Are Pregnant	
Have you had any bleeding or cramping since you became pregnant?	Any bleeding or spotting following confirmation of pregnancy must be investigated further by a specialist.
Have you had any abnormal Pap smear results in the past?	Patients who have had abnormal results may have a recurrence during pregnancy. Those who have had surgery to remove abnormal cells may have scar tissue, which needs to be released during labor to permit a vaginal delivery.
Have you had any STIs in the past?	Verify that any STIs were treated per protocol. Assess risk of reexposure because many STIs can harm the fetus.

(table continues on page 749)

Additional Questions	Rationale/Abnormal Findings
What type(s) of contraception have you used? When was the last time you used it?	If the patient was using hormonal contraceptives within three cycles prior to conception, it is difficult to assess when ovulation occurred. A patient taking such contraceptives does not have true menses but rather has "withdrawal bleeds" when she is not taking progesterone for 7 days. Even if pregnant, if she continues taking her birth control pills, she may have withdrawal bleeds at the usual time. If her conception date is not clear, ultrasound dating in the first trimester can be offered.
Have you had any difficulties with infertility?	If the response is positive, fully document the patient's history, including any medication taken and type of assisted reproduction. In vitro pregnancies have a somewhat increased risk of multiple gestation and fetal loss.
Do you have any common symptoms of pregnancy? (See also Chapter 25.)	Morning sickness, growing pains, increased vaginal discharge or urination, breast tenderness/discharge, periumbilical pain, fetal hiccups, or Braxton-Hicks contractions may be uncomfortable.
Newborns, Infants, and Children	
Do you use bubble baths for your child?	Just as with women, contact with perfumed bath products or lotions may cause a contact dermatitis. For young girls, it is best to avoid bubble bath and fragrance-containing products.
Does your child have frequent pain with urination? Does your child (older than 2½ years of age) have control over the bladder?	Difficulties with bladder control may require a specialist. Sudden regression in bladder or bowel control may signal **sexual harm**.
Do you notice your child scratching his or her genitals?	Itching or scratching in the genitals could indicate infection, pinworm, sexual abuse, or may be hygiene related.
Have you noticed any vaginal discharge on the underwear? Do you notice any odor in the genital area?	Young children, especially toddlers, sometimes insert foreign objects in orifices including the vagina.
Older Adults	
Have you noticed any bleeding since your menses stopped?	Any bleeding that occurs after the patient has had 1 year without menses should be investigated.
Have you noticed any vaginal problems such as dryness, itching, or vaginal secretions?	Loss of estrogen in the vagina along with loss of normal rugae can lead to irritation and possible spotting from the vagina.
Are you currently having sexual relations? Have you experienced any pain with intercourse? Do you have a satisfactory sexual relationship with your partner?	Regular sexual activity is normal in older women and should be encouraged unless it causes pain. Recommendation of vaginal lubricants will help provide relief from vaginal dryness. The practitioner may prescribe local estrogen to help with dryness.
Have you noticed any vaginal pressure or loss of urine if you cough or sneeze? Have you noticed any rectal pressure or experienced difficulty with bowel movements or incontinence of feces?	Vaginal pressure may indicate uterine prolapse. With accompanying bladder symptoms, there may be bladder support (**cystocele**) problems. Rectal pressure may indicate a **rectocele**, prolapsed rectum, or mass and should be evaluated.

Cultural Considerations

Additional Questions	Rationale/Abnormal Findings
Have you ever had a pelvic examination? Would you prefer a female practitioner?	Some cultures and religions have rules about who can see women unclothed and when pelvic examinations are allowed. In many cultures, girls are socialized to protect and preserve their virginity and "private parts."

Therapeutic Dialogue: Collecting Subjective Data

Remember Teresa Nguyen, the woman who was introduced at the beginning of this chapter: a 28-year-old woman with vaginal discharge, pelvic pain, and fever. The following conversation shows how the nurse might approach this sensitive subject with the patient. Cultural, gender, and age considerations are incorporated into the interview style.

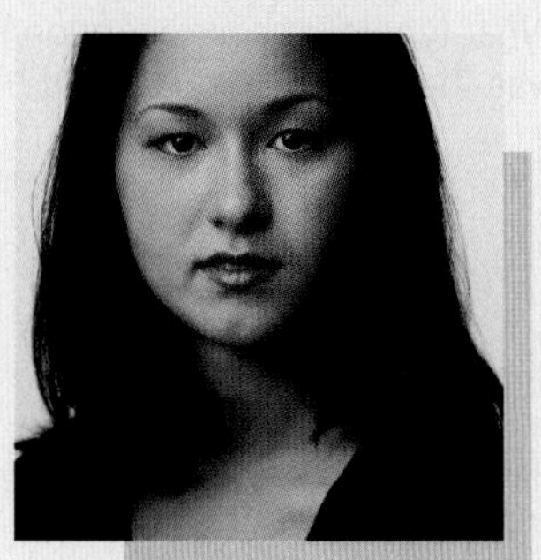

Nurse: Good morning, how are you today?

Teresa: Good, thank you.

Nurse: What name would you like me to call you?

Teresa: You can call me Teresa.

Nurse: Good, and you can call me Shelly. Let me look over your chart (looks at chart). It looks like you've been having some pelvic pain and vaginal discharge.

Teresa: Yes.

Nurse: Tell me a little more about those symptoms.

Teresa: Well, I really notice that the pain is bad when my boyfriend has sex with me.

Nurse: (Listens)

Teresa: I'm really afraid that I have an STI. My friends really don't like my boyfriend and they said that he cheated on me.

Nurse: You sound very concerned.

Teresa: I just don't want my parents to know. They are very traditional.

Nurse: You are protected by privacy laws, but we may need to notify the health department if an illness needs to be reported.

Critical Thinking Challenge

- How should the nurse proceed with questioning about privacy?
- What questions should the nurse ask regarding sexual activity and sexual practices? Give specific examples.
- What are your thoughts about Teresa's relationships with her parents? How might those affect the care?

Objective Data

Common and Specialty or Advanced Techniques

The routine head-to-toe assessment includes the most important and common assessment techniques. The examiner may add specialty or advanced steps if he or she is concerned about a specific finding. This table summarizes the most common techniques used in the comprehensive registered nurse (RN) assessment; these are essential to learn for clinical practice. The RN assessment includes inspecting the external genitalia. This is important because yeast infections are common during antibiotic treatment or with incontinence where skin irritation may occur. Inspection of the vagina, obtaining a Pap smear, and a bimanual examination are within the scope of practice of the nurse practitioner. These examinations require additional training and skills.

Basic Versus Focused/Specialty or Advanced Techniques Related to Female Genitalia and Rectal Assessment			
Technique	**Purpose**	**Screening or Registered Nurse Assessment**	**Focused or Advanced Practice Examination**
Inspect external genitalia	To observe for deformities, drainage, rashes, or lesions	X	
Palpate internal genitalia	To palpate vaginal wall for weakness, masses, or tumors		X Weakness, masses, tumors
Perform speculum examination	To increase visibility of vaginal walls and cervix		X Vaginal walls and cervix
Inspect cervix and os	To observe for redness, lesions, or drainage		X Cervix and os
Perform Pap smear and cultures	To detect atypical cells and cancer (Pap smear) and infections (culture)		X Cancer screening
Inspect vaginal wall	To inspect for lesions, irritation, drainage		X Vagina
Perform bimanual examination	To palpate for masses, tumors, pain, organs		X Masses, tumors, pain, organs
Perform rectovaginal examination	To palpate vaginal wall for rectocele		X
Perform rectal examination	To palpate for masses, tumors, pain		X Masses, tumors, pain

Equipment

- Examination gown
- Sheet or drape
- Nonsterile examination gloves (both latex and nonlatex)
- Water-soluble vaginal lubricant
- Lamp with either goose neck or speculum attachment
- Wooden/plastic spatula
- Cervical brush (broom)
- Endocervical brush
- Glass slide
- Slide fixative
- Liquid Pap base
- Culture tubes (DNA) for chlamydia and gonorrhea
- Sterile cotton swabs
- Large cotton swabs
- Small bottles with tops, one containing saline solution, one containing potassium hydroxide (KOH), and one containing acetic acid solution (white vinegar)
- Speculum (preferably warmed via heat source in examination drawer)
  - Pederson: narrow blades
  - Graves: wider blades
  - Pediatric: smaller Pederson with narrow blades and shorter length
  - Can be either metal or plastic

See Figure 24.5.

A

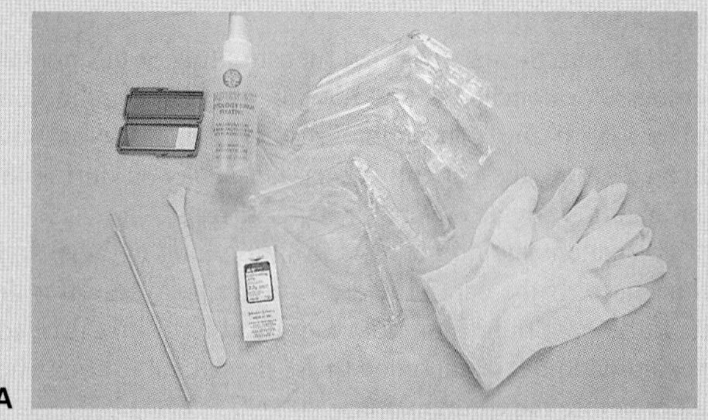

B

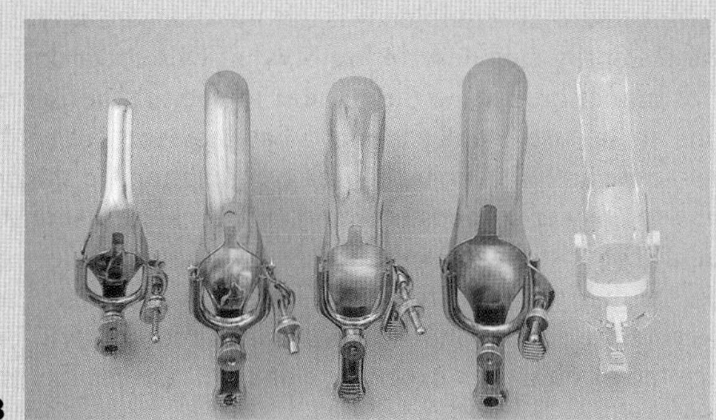

Figure 24.5 **A.** Materials used in the examination of the female genitalia. **B.** Types of specula.

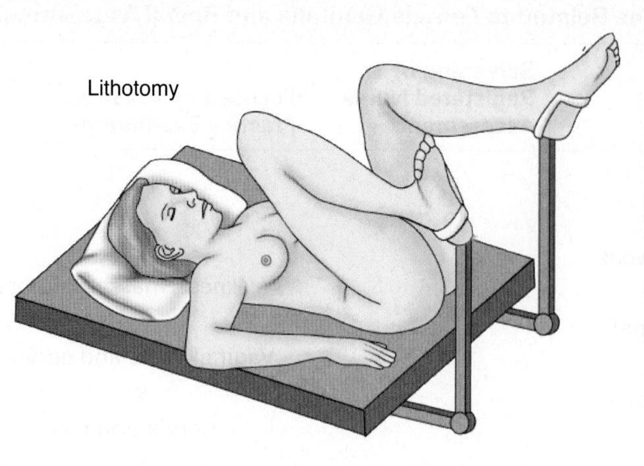

A

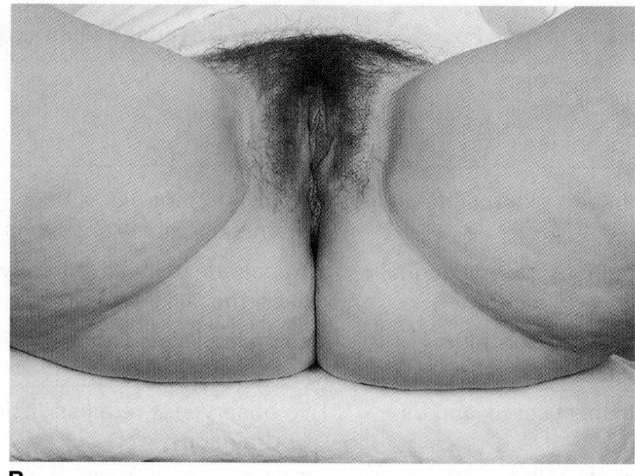

B

Figure 24.6 Lithotomy positioning for the examination of the female genitalia. **A.** Illustration showing the positioning of the lower extremities and buttocks. **B.** Frontal view of surface anatomy.

Preparation

It is important to provide a comfortable environment and to display confidence while staying in tune with the patient's feelings of fear or embarrassment. A room containing information pamphlets and three-dimensional models encourages inquiry and lessens anxiety. Ensure privacy throughout the examination. The table should be facing away from the door and instructions given to the staff so that you and the patient will not be disturbed during the examination.

Make sure the patient is not menstruating or has not had intercourse or douched before the Pap test. These conditions interfere with the cytological results. Unless otherwise indicated, allow the patient to keep her socks on during the examination. Provide covers for table stirrups.

The patient should not have to sit too long in the examination room. If the care provider is being delayed, offer the patient the opportunity to remain dressed until it is time for her examination. It is important to ask the patient to empty her bladder before the examination.

Make sure all equipment is set up and within reach. Offer a step-by-step description of what will occur during the examination. Allow the patient to see all the instruments to be used and explain what they are for. Take time—especially if this is the first examination for the patient—to answer all questions and concerns. Reassure the patient that if she is uncomfortable at any time to let you know so that you can stop or alter the examination. Empowering the patient and allowing patient control will enhance the examination experience and will ensure that the patient returns in the future.

Assist the patient into a semilithotomy position; help her to move down just before the examination (Fig. 24.6) and assist her in placing her feet into the stirrups. It is a good idea to make sure she is comfortable after her feet are placed. Elevating the patient's head and shoulders allows her to view the examination. It is also helpful to provide a mirror so that she might see the examination better (Fig. 24.7). Take time to encourage the patient to ask questions during the examination. When draping the patient, keep the genitals visualized without completely exposing the legs and knees. In addition, keep in mind the importance of making sure the patient can see your face and you hers. At this point, you can position the examination chair in front of the examination table.

Wash your hands and put gloves on both hands. Have the patient slowly move toward the end of the table. It is a good idea to reassure her that you will not let her fall. Holding your gloved hands out to the side of each knee, instruct the patient to allow her knees to drop into your hands, or allow her legs to go limp. It is important never to force her legs apart with your hands or arms. Talk through each step and let the patient know what you are going to do next.

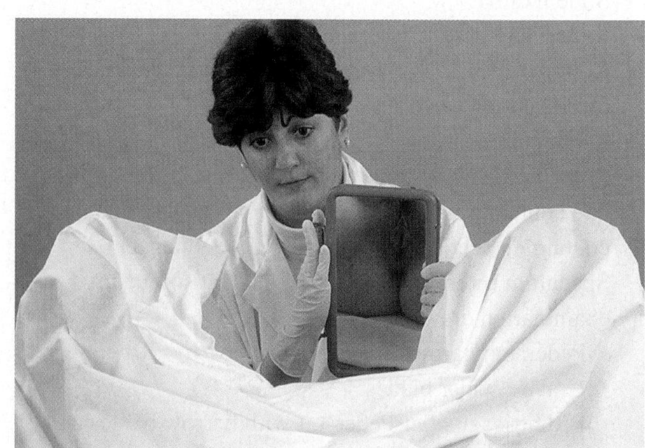

Figure 24.7 The nurse or health care practitioner may offer to the patient a mirror during the examination so she can watch what is happening.

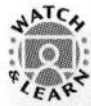

Comprehensive Physical Assessment

Technique and Normal Findings	Abnormal Findings
External Genitalia Begin the inspection with the mons pubis. Inspect the pubic hair for amount and distribution. The pubic hair of the older woman becomes thinner with age. Look at the hair and skin for lice or nits. Hair is evenly distributed and growing in a downward direction. No lice or nits are seen.	Pediculosis pubis (crab lice) commonly presents with itching (see Table 24.4 at the end of the chapter).
Inspect the skin for any redness, breakdown, papules, or vesicles. Observe the inguinal area bilaterally for erythema, fissures, or enlarged inguinal lymph nodes. Inspect the clitoris, noting size and shape. The clitoris is 1–1.5 cm (about ½–¾ in.) long.	Symptoms of **herpes simplex virus** 2 include vulvar or vaginal pain, flulike symptoms such as chills or fever, sores on the vulva or genital region, scattered vesicles along the labia, matching vesicles on the labia reflecting "kissing" lesions, surface ulcerations or crusted healing lesions, and inguinal lymphadenopathy (see Table 24.3 at the end of the chapter).
Inspect the labia majora for size and symmetry. Look for any swelling or redness. Because both labia majora and minora are composed of sebaceous and apocrine glands, they are prone to form small inclusion cysts. These are common and may come and go without notice.	Symptoms of condyloma acuminatum (warts) include vulvar or vaginal itching, vaginal secretions, and growths along the vagina or rectum. Examination may reveal fleshy pink or grey papilloma or wartlike projections at the vulva, vagina, or anus (see Table 24.3 at the end of the chapter).
Inspect the vaginal opening for swelling or redness (Fig. 24.8). No protrusions are seen from the vagina. 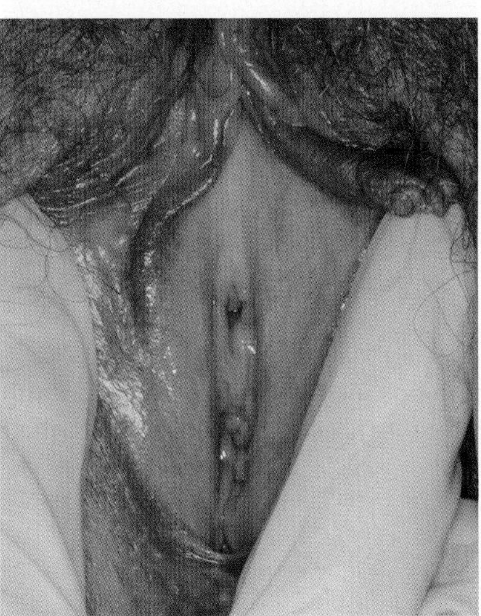 **Figure 24.8** Inspecting the vaginal opening (introitus).	Cancer of the vulva is usually asymptomatic until the lesion becomes large enough that itching, burning, pain, and bleeding or watery discharge from the lesion may be present. Any discharge or mucus is considered abnormal and requires a culture.
Inspect the vestibule for color, redness, swelling, odor, or discharge. Inspect the urethra for position and patency. There is no discharge or redness. Observe the Skene glands at the 1-o'clock and 11-o'clock positions lateral to the urethra. Skene glands are small, noninflamed, and occasionally not seen.	Candidiasis is associated with vulvovaginal and possibly rectal pruritus and dyspareunia. Examination may reveal vulvovaginal edema, erythema, excoriation, and thick white secretions, sometimes only along the inner vaginal walls (see Table 24.3 at the end of the chapter).

(table continues on page 754)

Technique and Normal Findings (continued)	Abnormal Findings (continued)
Inspection is completed with the perineum. The area between the introitus and anus is smooth with no lesions or tears. Scars from any episiotomies are healed. The anus is intact with no swelling, lacerations, or protrusions.	Look for abnormalities such as contact dermatitis (see Table 24.4 at the end of the chapter) and chancres of syphilis.
Internal Genitalia Using the thumb and middle finger of your gloved hand, separate the inner portion of the labia minora, insert your index finger approximately 1 cm (about ½ in.), and rotate the finger so that it is facing upward. Gently press your index finger forward to assess the urethra and Skene glands (Fig. 24.9). Do not do this very long because it will irritate the urethra and cause the patient discomfort. 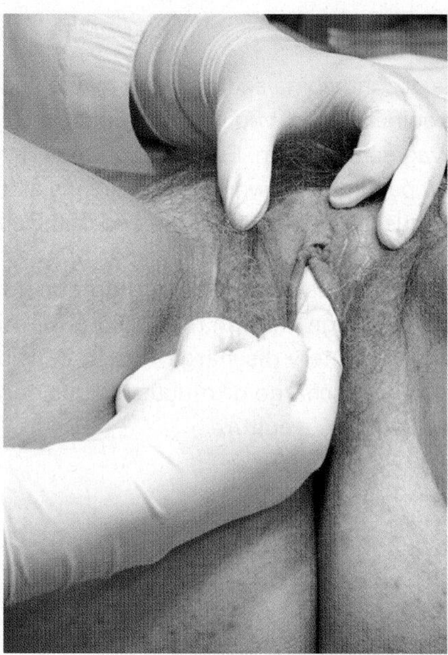 **Figure 24.9** Palpating the Skene glands and urethra.	
With your index finger still inserted approximately 1 cm (about ½ in.) into the vagina, rotate the finger downward again and palpate the Bartholin glands on each side with the index finger and the thumb (Fig. 24.10). The Bartholin glands are located bilaterally in the lower labial areas at approximately 8-o'clock and 4-o'clock positions. No swelling or tenderness is noted on either side.	Abnormal findings include an abscess of a Bartholin gland or urethral caruncle (see Table 24.4 at the end of the chapter).
While your finger is inserted, advance it to locate the cervix. (This will help avoid inaccurate placement of the speculum around the cervix.) Explain to the patient what you are doing. While your index finger is still in place, ask the patient to squeeze the vaginal muscles around your finger to check vaginal tone. Ask the patient to then bear down slightly to assess for pelvic organ prolapse.	Assessment of vaginal tone is important, especially if the patient has complaints of pelvic relaxation or urinary incontinence. **Pelvic organ prolapse** is not limited to older women; many times, obesity and gravity are factors (Rogers & Fashokun, 2014).

(table continues on page 755)

Technique and Normal Findings (continued)	Abnormal Findings (continued)
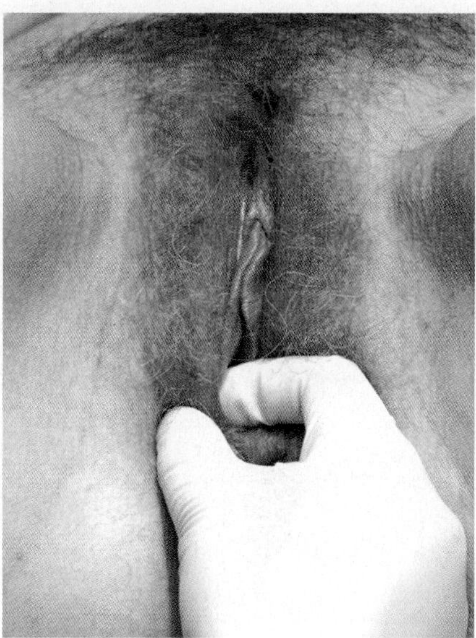 **Figure 24.10** Palpating the Bartholin glands.	
Speculum Examination Choose the speculum based on the patient's history, not weight or outward appearance. Warm the speculum in the examination table drawer if possible; if not, run the speculum under warm water. Hold the speculum between the index and middle finger of your dominant hand. Make sure the blades are pushed together and stay together during insertion to ensure comfort and to avoid pinching any part of the labia or vaginal walls between them. Place the thumb under the thumbscrew on the metal or the lever on the plastic type of speculum. With the opposite hand, insert the index finger as in the initial vaginal examination and place slight pressure downward.	⚠ *SAFETY ALERT* *Do not use a lubricant on the speculum because it can interfere with the cytological and culture results.*
Insert the speculum in an oblique position along the top of your finger (Fig. 24.11A). A constant downward insertion prevents the anterior blade of the speculum from hitting the urethra or bladder and causing discomfort or pain. As the speculum moves in and downward, slowly remove your index finger. Have the patient exhale slowly as the speculum is inserted; this helps relax the pubococcygeal muscles. Slowly rotate the speculum so that it is in a horizontal position (Fig. 24.11B) while continuing to press the bottom blade in a downward position at 45 degrees. After the blade has been completely inserted, slowly open the speculum blades while continually keeping a posterior pressure on the lower blade.	⚠ *SAFETY ALERT* *Do not try to force the complete blade in if it causes the patient discomfort or pain.*

(table continues on page 756)

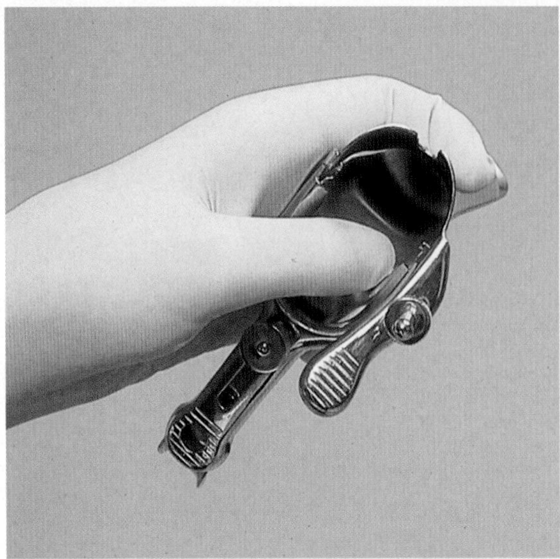

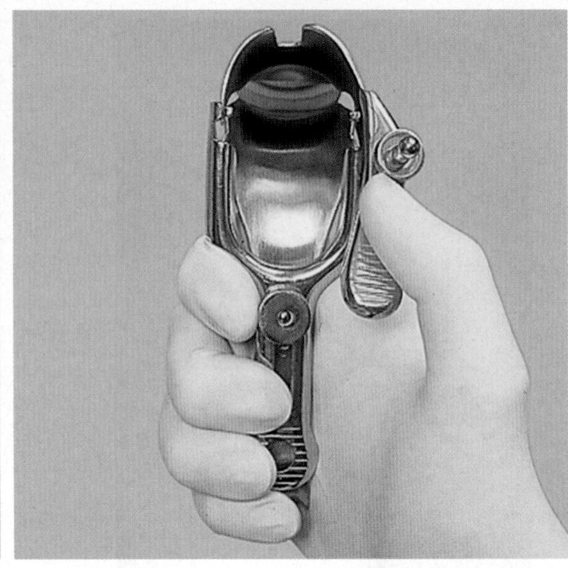

Figure 24.11 The speculum. **A.** Angle at entry. **B.** Angle at full insertion.

For most women, the speculum most often used is the Pederson. The length of this speculum is approximately 6 cm (2 ½ in.), which is the usual length of the vagina. After the speculum has been fully inserted, open the blades slowly by pressing on the thumb piece until the cervix comes into view at the end of the blades. As the cervix comes into view, lock the speculum into place by tightening the screw on the thumb piece. Check with the patient at all steps to make sure she is comfortable (Fig. 24.12).

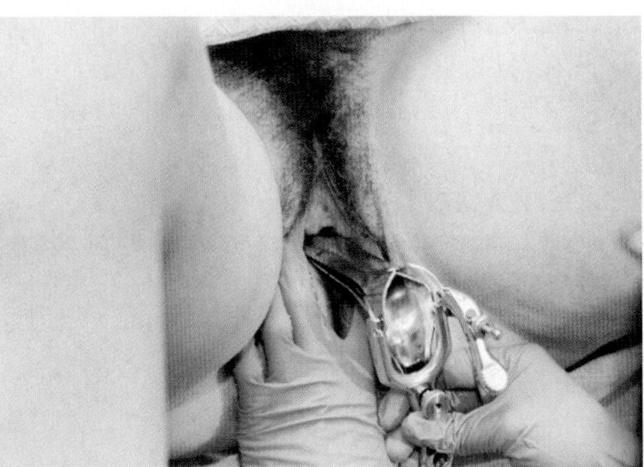

Figure 24.12 Inserting the speculum.

Cervix and Os. Inspect the cervix and vaginal walls (Fig. 24.13).

The cervix is smooth and pink and positioned midline in the vagina.

If the cervix is not visualized, the speculum may be too high. Repositioning with the blades pressed posterior may be necessary.

(table continues on page 757)

Technique and Normal Findings (continued)	Abnormal Findings (continued)

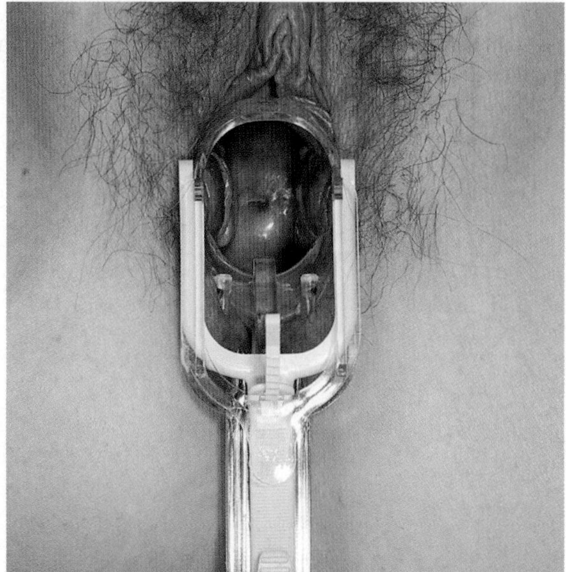

Figure 24.13 View of the normal cervix through the speculum.

The position is based on the angle of the uterus and may tilt anteriorly or posteriorly. The cervix of a nulliparous woman has a small round os, whereas that of the parous woman has a horizontal or fish-mouth appearance. Inspect the cervix and surrounding area for increased discharge. Clear secretions are present normally and may be more or less productive based on the woman's cycle or menstrual history. It is best not to remove too much of this secretion because doing so may compromise cervical cells needed for the Pap smear. If the woman has an intrauterine device, this is the time to check for the two clear strings.

If the patient has experienced any birth traumas, a tear of the cervix may result in an irregular slit. It is common in women who have had vaginal births to have one or several **Nabothian cysts.** These small benign nodules resemble yellow pustules. These are not treated but are documented as findings. A small polyp may be present at the opening or the os; it may be removed in the office and sent to the pathology department for testing (Fig. 24.14). Additional abnormal findings include cervical polyps, DES syndrome, cervical dysplasia, carcinoma in situ, and cervical cancer (see Table 24.6 at the end of the chapter).

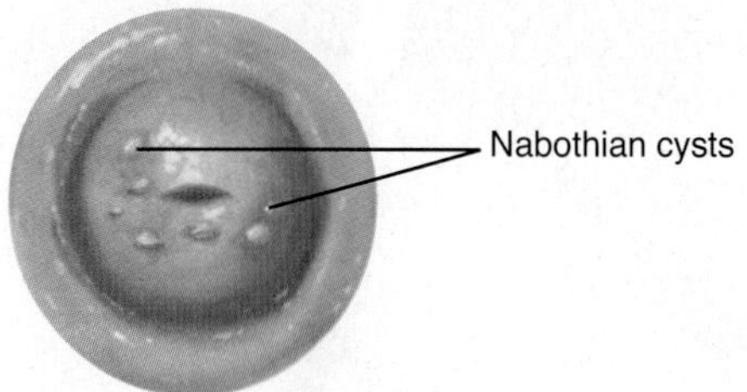

Figure 24.14 Nabothian cysts.

Pap Smear and Cultures. The Pap smear (named after Dr. George Papanicolaou), is a screening tool for cervical neoplasia. An Ayers spatula (either wood or plastic) is used in conjunction with an endocervical brush for glass-slide examinations. A plastic cytology broom is used to obtain both exocervical and endocervical cells for a liquid Pap examination.

Insert the longer portion of the spatula into the cervical os and rotate 360 degrees as you press it against the cervix to gently scrape the cells from the squamocolumnar junction of the cervix (Fig. 24.15). (This is also called the transformation zone and includes the outer and inner areas of the endocervix; it is the area with highest neoplastic involvement.) Spread the secretions obtained from the spatula on a clear glass slide and apply a fixative spray.

The Pap smear is used to evaluate cells from the cervix for precancerous or cancerous status. Newer technologies and techniques for obtaining the cervical cells have helped to improve screening and early detection. Currently, several types of cytological testing exist. The conventional Pap testing consists of acquisition of cervical cells by a wooden or plastic spatula and an endocervical brush, with the cells then "smeared" onto a slide with fixative applied. The conventional smear-to-slide method has a 20% false negative rate. (American Congress of Obstetricians and Gynecologists [ACOG], 2012). Liquid-based cytology (Thin-Prep) uses a similar technique except the practitioner uses a plastic spatula or broom and the cells removed are placed into a liquid solution.

(table continues on page 758)

Technique and Normal Findings (continued)	Abnormal Findings (continued)
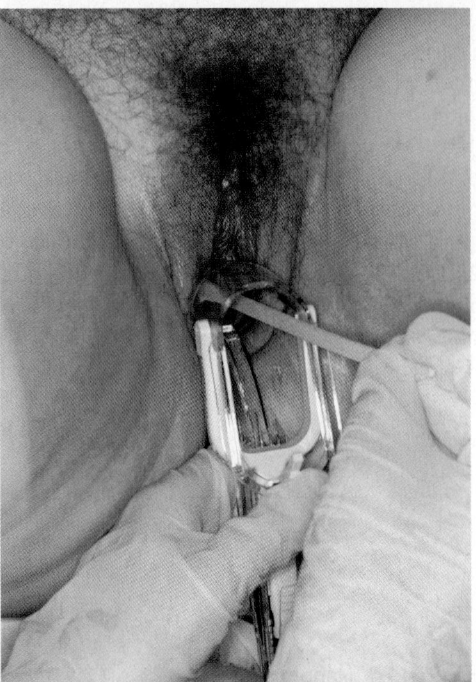 Figure 24.15 Using the spatula to retrieve ectocervical cells.	Collection of cells from the endocervix or cervix may cause some spotting or bleeding; this can occur with a Pap or with an STI screening.
Next, insert the endocervical brush into the endocervix and rotate 720 degrees to ensure an adequate cell sample (Fig. 24.16). Then gently roll out the endocervical brush on a clean glass slide, avoiding cell destruction. Apply a spray fixative and label the slide for cytology. 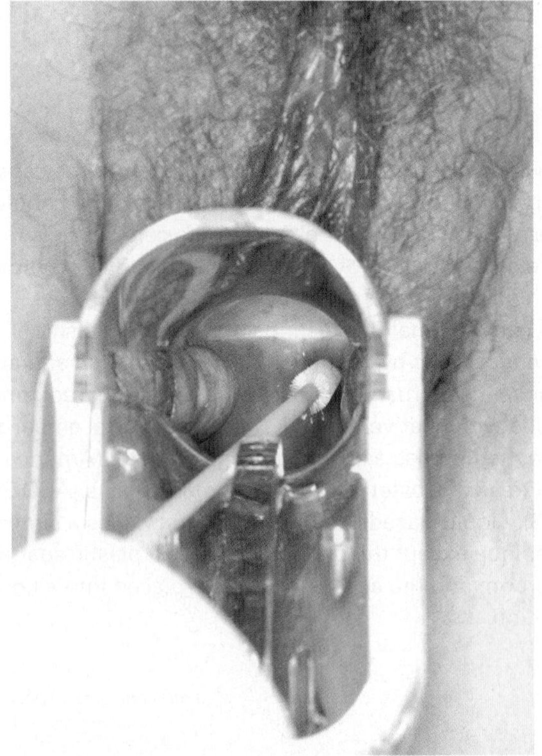 Figure 24.16 Using the endocervical brush.	⚠ SAFETY ALERT *It is important to do the Pap smear first so that bleeding is minimal on the cytology specimen. The cultures for chlamydia (CT) and gonorrhea (GC) are done after the Pap smear.*

(table continues on page 759)

Technique and Normal Findings (continued)	Abnormal Findings (continued)
If a liquid base Pap is to be taken, use the plastic broom; insert the tip of the broom into the endocervix and rotate it 720 degrees. Remove the tip of the broom and place it into the liquid solution (Fig. 24.17). 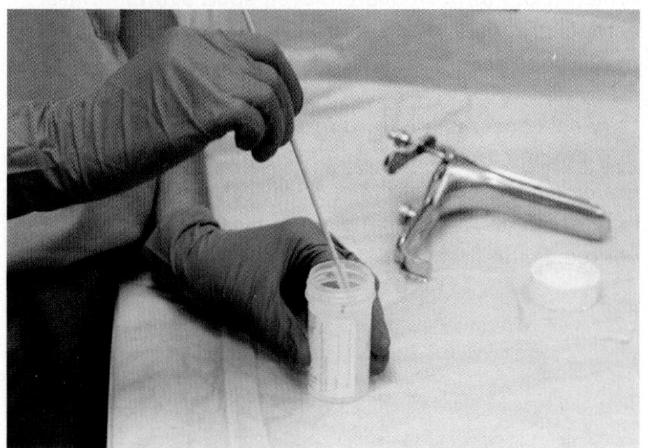 **Figure 24.17** Collecting cells in the solution during liquid-based Pap testing.	
For cultures, insert the Dacron probe into the endocervical canal and keep it there for 30 seconds to 1 minute. Remove the probe, avoiding contact with vaginal secretions, and place the specimen into the culture tube.	Most commonly, a DNA-based probe is used, which cultures both CT and GC at the same time.
Vaginal Wall. During insertion and removal of the speculum, inspect the vaginal wall. Inspect the lateral and anteroposterior walls for lesions, bleeding, erythema, and edema. In the older patient, it is not uncommon to see atrophic changes to the lining of the vagina from lack of estrogen; you will notice a lack or thinning of the vaginal rugae. This is very tender and uncomfortable, so you should proceed gently. Remove the speculum in the reverse order of insertion, giving careful attention to keeping the blades open until the blades are slid away from the cervix. Keep your thumb on the lever and slowly release it. As you rotate the speculum to an oblique position, slowly close the blades; avoid pinching the vaginal walls or labia, and avoid pulling the pubic hair.	Any secretion abnormal in amount, color, or odor is sampled for infection (see Table 24.5 at the end of the chapter). **Trichomoniasis** often presents with vaginal impurities, thin or thick secretions, a foul vaginal odor, purulent, yellow-to-green, frothy discharge, pain on pelvic examination, cervical redness (strawberry appearance), contact bleeding, pH higher than 4.5, and occasional dysuria. **Gonorrhea** is indicated by yellow vaginal secretions, pain with urination (dysuria), and dyspareunia. In addition, findings include purulent discharge from the cervix and tenderness or pain with the pelvic examination. Associated pharyngeal or anorectal infections may be present. **Bacterial vaginosis** presents with vaginal secretions that have a strongly "fishy" odor and vaginal itching or burning. Examination may reveal a creamy white-to-gray secretion that coats the vaginal walls. **Chlamydia** is often asymptomatic. Occasional clear or white secretion may be evident; bleeding may occur after intercourse. **Dyspareunia** (pain with intercourse) may be present. Examination shows changes in the cervix, which may be reddened or bleed easily. The pelvic examination may become painful.

(table continues on page 760)

Technique and Normal Findings (continued)	Abnormal Findings (continued)
Bimanual Examination Inform the patient that this part of the examination is to assess the organs by manually palpating from both inside and outside the size, shape, and position of the uterus and ovaries as well as assessing general support of the organs.	Cystocele, rectocele, and uterine prolapse are abnormal pelvic findings (see Table 24.5 at the end of the chapter). Additional abnormalities include endometriosis, leiomyoma (fibroid tumor), ovarian cyst, solid ovarian mass, ectopic pregnancy, and acute salpingitis. These may or may not be accompanied by pain.
At this time, remove the gloves and place a new glove on the hand that will be doing the internal examination. Insert the index and second fingers into the vagina in a downward fashion and slowly turn the fingers upward after they reach the cervix. Keep the thumb upward or tucked in during this time to keep it from pressing on the clitoris. Rest the fingers internally at the posterior area of the cervix. Palpate the cervix for size, shape, and movement. Place the nonexamining hand midway between the symphysis pubis and the umbilicus (Fig. 24.18). 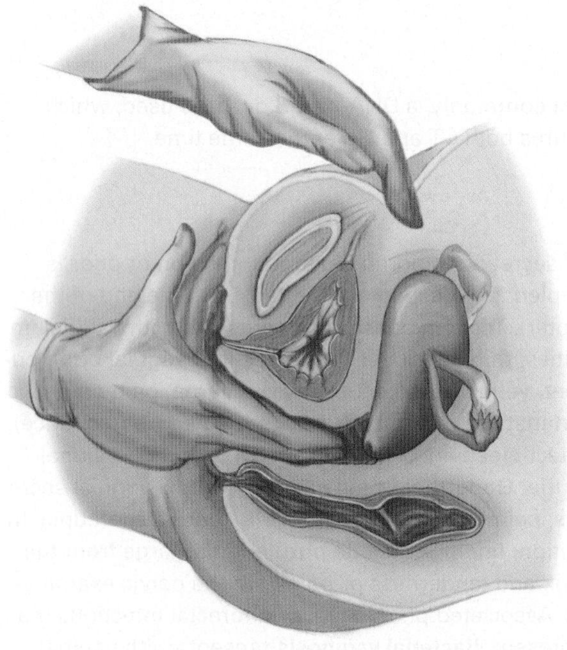 **Figure 24.18** Positioning of the hands in bimanual palpation of the cervix.	Cervical cancer is the third most common reproductive cancer (American Cancer Society [ACS], 2014). Preinvasive cancer of the cervix is often asymptomatic. In later stages, abnormal bleeding, especially after intercourse, is the first sign.
Next, palpate the uterus between the pads of the fingertips. Move the uterus upward so that your examining fingers can palpate between the top and back of the uterus (Fig. 24.19). This position allows for evaluation of the size and shape of the uterus as well as its ability to move without tenderness or resistance. *Normal size is approximately 7 cm × 4 cm (2¾ x 1½ in.) (size is occasionally larger in multigravid women).* ■ The uterus feels pear shaped and smooth and is freely mobile.	Leiomyomas can cause abnormal uterine bleeding and blockage, abdominal pressure, constipation, incontinence, and dysmenorrhea if large. Endometrial cancer is the most common malignancy of the reproductive system (ACS, 2014) and is associated with abnormal uterine bleeding, uterine enlargement, or mass.

(table continues on page 761)

Technique and Normal Findings (continued)	Abnormal Findings (continued)

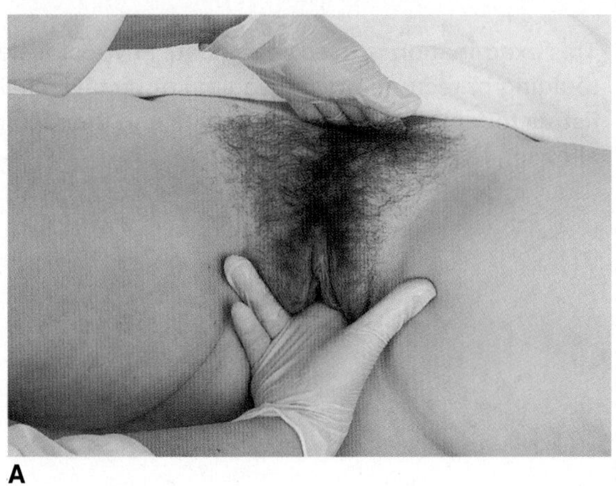

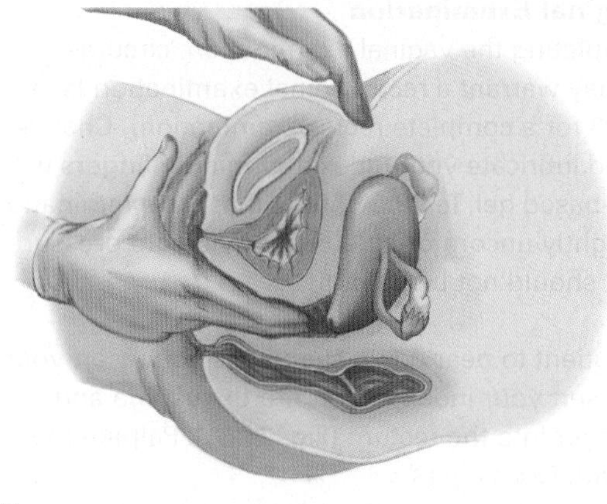

A B

Figure 24.19 Bimanual palpation of the uterus. **A.** External view. **B.** Internal position of the hands.

After you have assessed the uterus, let the patient know that you are now going to check her ovaries. With your two fingers still deep in the vagina and facing upward, move to the lateral side of the uterus. If you are using your right hand, move the fingers first to the patient's right and place the hand on the abdomen medial to the anterior superior iliac spine. Bring your two hands together as close as possible. With a slow sweeping motion, move the fingers down toward the introitus while allowing the adnexa to be palpated between them (Fig. 24.20). Repeat this procedure on the patient's left side. Perform the palpation quickly and gently. As stated above, this part of the examination should be brief because the ovaries are similar to gonads in their sensitivity. *The ovary is often not felt, especially in older menopausal women. If palpated, it feels like a small almond.*

With an ovarian cyst, findings may include pain, tenderness over the ovary, irregular menses, and intraperitoneal bleeding if it ruptures. A solid ovarian mass raises the possibility of ovarian cancer, which is the second most frequent reproductive cancer (ACS, 2014).

> ⚠ *SAFETY ALERT*
> *In an ectopic pregnancy, the most common symptoms are lower quadrant pain, nausea, and referred pain in the neck or shoulder from blood beneath the diaphragm. If severe hemorrhage occurs, the patient is at risk for shock.*

Salpingitis is also referred to as PID. Infection spreads throughout the uterus and up into the tubes. See Table 24.7 at the end of the chapter.

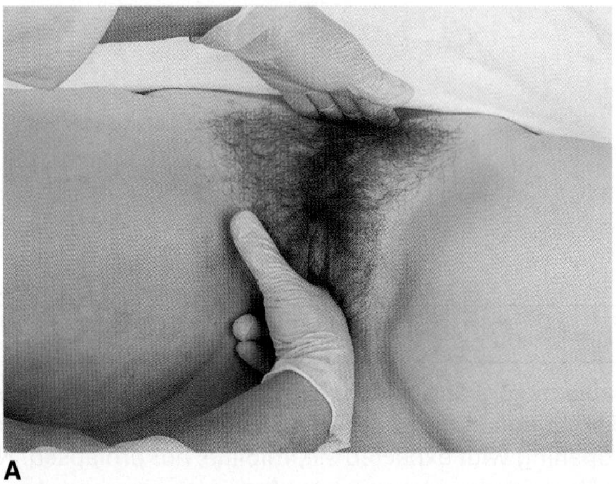

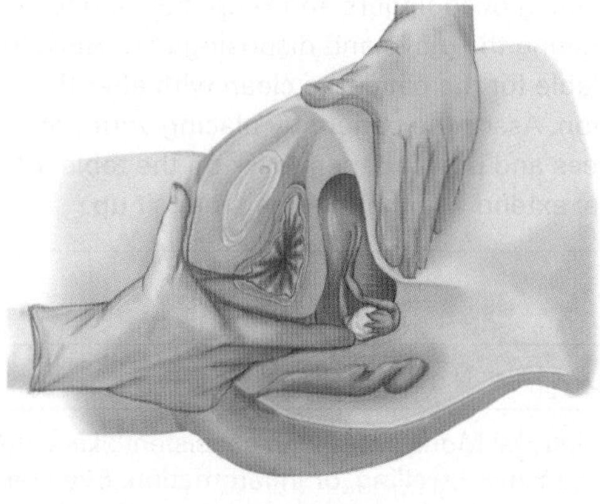

A B

Figure 24.20 Bimanual palpation of the ovaries. **A.** External view. **B.** Internal position of the hands.

(table continues on page 762)

Technique and Normal Findings (continued)	Abnormal Findings (continued)
Rectovaginal Examination After completing the vaginal examination, circumstances may warrant a rectovaginal examination (see Chapter 23 for a complete rectal examination). Change gloves and lubricate your index and middle fingers with the water-based gel. Tell the patient that the examination will be slightly uncomfortable and may create pressure, but that it should not be painful. Ask the patient to bear down slightly as you insert your fingers. Insert your index finger into the vagina and your middle finger into the rectum (Fig. 24.21). Palpate the septum with two fingers. The septum feels smooth and intact. The posterior portion of the uterus is smooth. 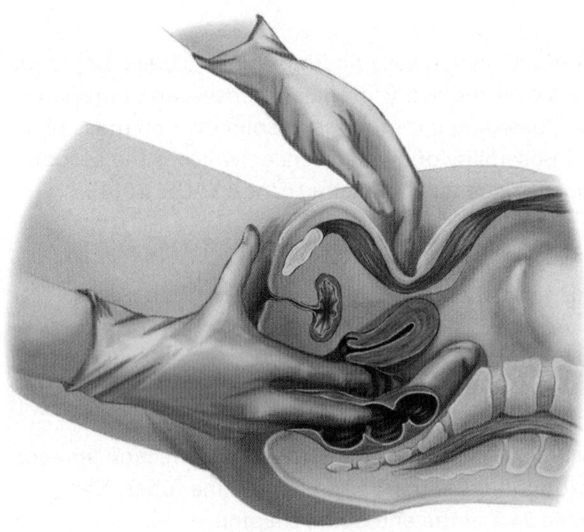 **Figure 24.21** Rectovaginal examination. Withdraw the gloved fingers and keep the hand lower while removing the glove and disposing of it. Have tissues available for the patient to clean with after the examination. Assist the patient by placing your hands on her knees and pushing them back on the table. At the same time, extend your hand to help her sit up.	This examination is used to evaluate any rectocele (bulging of rectum into the vagina) or **rectovaginal fistula** (opening between the vagina and the rectum allowing feces to enter the vagina).

Documenting Normal Findings

External genitalia: Mons pubis with consistent skin color; labia majora and minora symmetrical. No ecchymosis, excoriation, rashes, swelling, or inflammation. Even hair distribution in the shape of an inverted triangle. No tenderness on light or deep palpation. Clitoris not engorged. Urethral opening with expected slit, midline, not prolapsed. No odor or discharge. Vaginal opening with no discharge or lesions. No evidence of mutilation. Anal area pigmented and clear.

Internal genitalia: Cervix midline, smooth, evenly pink. Projects 3 cm (1¼ in.) into the vagina. Vaginal wall pink, moist, smooth, and rugated. No laceration of ulcers. Vaginal walls strong without bulging of walls. Vaginal muscle strong, tone intake.

Bimanual examination: Cervix smooth, firm. No pain when cervix is moved from side to side; no tenderness. Uterus not enlarged and moves freely, fundus round and firm. No tenderness or nodules.

Lifespan Considerations

Women Who Are Pregnant

The physical examination of the pregnant woman is discussed in Chapter 25. To review quickly, you first assess whether the membranes are ruptured. This can be done by inspection, in the case of gross rupture; using Nitrazine (either paper or swab) to test the pH of the discharge; or through a sterile speculum examination if you have received special training. Defer vaginal examination when the membranes are ruptured, especially if the patient does not appear to be in active labor.

Even with ruptured membranes, you would perform a vaginal examination if requested to do so by the primary health care provider, or if you suspect that birth might be imminent. Document cervical dilation (in centimeters), effacement (in centimeters), station (degree of descent into the pelvis of the presenting part), consistency of the cervix (firm, medium, soft), and position (posterior, mid position, anterior). Together, these values can be used to calculate the Bishop score. A Bishop score above 9 suggests that vaginal birth is very likely, even if induction or augmentation is necessary.

Children

Allow the parent to hold the child. Have the child place her feet together positioned "like a frog." Allow the child to take part in the examination. Have the parent let the child know it is okay to allow this examination by a practitioner, especially if she has been taught not to allow anyone to touch her genitals.

Adolescents

Ask the patient if she would like her mother or a friend to be present during the examination. Provide a mirror so that she may observe the examination and have opportunities to ask questions.

Place the examining finger just at the posterior fourchette and gently press downward; this will allow the pubococcygeal muscle to gradually relax, allowing the insertion of the finger. The patient can identify the muscles to relax when you are inserting the speculum. Do a one-finger vaginal examination before inserting the speculum; this allows you to estimate the vaginal capacity as well as the position of the cervix; it ensures a more comfortable examination. Inform the patient that the speculum you will use will be no larger than your index finger, which she just felt. Avoid using words such as "pain"; instead, use words such as "mild pressure."

Older Adults

Menopause usually occurs between 48 and 51 years of age, although variability is wide. The ovaries stop producing estrogen and progesterone, causing the uterus to droop and the cervix to shrink. Associated findings include thinning of the genital hair, thinning and loss of elasticity of vaginal mucosa, and diminished vaginal secretions as a result of lower estrogen levels. The fat pads atrophy and the labia and clitoris decrease in size.

Cultural Considerations

Latina women have the highest rates of cervical cancer of all groups of women. They also are more likely to die from cervical cancer than Caucasian women. African American women develop cervical cancer more often than Caucasian women and are more than twice as likely to die from it. Screening is very important to help reduce this disparity. In fact, 6 in 10 cervical cancers occur in women who have never received a Pap test or have not been tested in the past 5 years (Office on Women's Health, 2014).

Documenting Case Study Findings

The nurse has just finished a physical examination of Teresa Nguyen, the 28-year-old being seen with vaginal drainage and pelvic pain. Unlike the samples of expected documentation previously charted, Ms. Nguyen has unexpected findings. Review the following important findings revealed in each of the steps of objective data collection for Ms. Nguyen. Consider how these results compare with the expected findings presented in the samples of expected documentation. Begin to think about how the data cluster and what additional data the nurse might want to collect as the nurse thinks critically about Ms. Nguyen's problems and anticipates nursing interventions. This note is documented by the nurse practitioner who will work collaboratively with the RN.

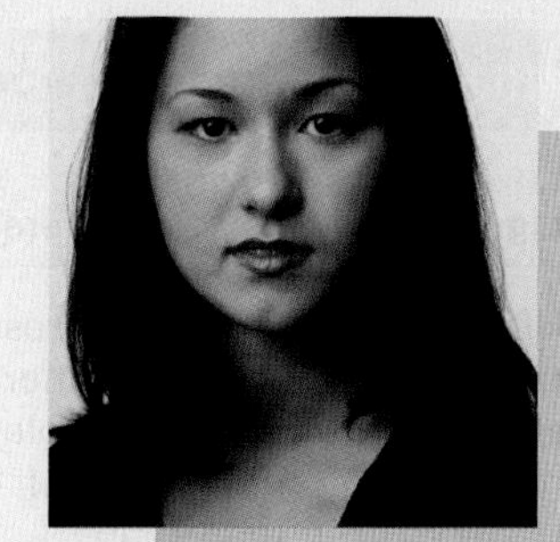

Inspection: External genitalia has even hair distribution, no lesions present. Bartholin's glands, urethra, Skene's gland (BUS) with no erythema, edema, or discharge. Vaginal introitus and walls pink, moist with normal rugae, good anterior and posterior wall support, moderate clear discharge present.

Palpation: Cervix smooth round and red, some tenderness on movement. Clear drainage present. Uterus normal size, shape, mid position, and freely mobile. Adnexa with no palpable masses but positive tenderness during examination. Perineum smooth. Anal area pink, with no hemorrhoids, fissures, or bleeding present. Nonspecific tenderness present over lower half of abdomen during bimanual examination.

Critical Thinking

The RN and advanced practice registered nurse (APRN) work collaboratively to provide care for patients with issues related to the female genital system. After collecting data, the RN and APRN identify unexpected findings and areas for health promotion. They cluster data to reveal significant patterns and make clinical judgments about outcomes and potential interventions.

Laboratory and Diagnostic Testing

The annual gynecological visit by the female patient is often the only physical examination she has. For this reason, complete laboratory work is typically done, including tests for anemia, cholesterol, thyroid, and diabetes. A white blood cell (WBC) count may be done to rule out infections. A urinalysis is commonly done at each visit. If the patient has signs or symptoms of urinary tract problems, a clean catch urinalysis and culture and sensitivity are done. If the patient is having any bleeding or lack of menses, a serum human chorionic gonadotropin is drawn to rule out pregnancy.

The **wet mount** analysis of vaginal secretions is done to identify which, if any, vaginal infections are present. A slide is made with the vaginal secretions and a single drop of KOH or saline or both. The examination findings are then matched with the signs and symptoms and the wet mount findings. Blood tests, such as measuring LH, FSH, and GnRH, are done if endocrinal irregularities are present or suspected.

Vaginal and abdominal ultrasounds are the standard diagnostic tests for abnormalities of the fallopian tubes, ovaries, uterus, and the endometrial lining. More in-depth testing is done if the woman has infertility difficulties.

The American Cancer Society's current Pap smear screening recommendations are as follows: For initial screening, women should undergo a Pap test within 3 years of onset of sexual activity or at age 21 years (whichever comes first). Women aged 21 years and older who have no sexual activity should still be screened. Women younger than 30 years of age should have a Pap test annually. Women older than 30 years of age who have had three normal Pap tests in a row have two options. They may receive a liquid-based Pap every 2 to 3 years; however, patients with a history of DES exposure or HIV or any previous cervical cancer diagnosis, should continue annual Pap testing. The second option is screening with a liquid-based Pap test and an HPV DNA hybrid capture (HC2) test. This hybrid capture is a culture specifically for the HPV virus. If the results of both tests are normal, the patient can go 3 years without screening. The American Cancer Society recommends discontinuation of Pap testing after 70 years of age. Women who have had total hysterectomy (for noncancerous reason) do not require Pap testing (ACS, 2014).

Nursing Diagnosis, Outcomes, and Interventions

The formation of the nursing diagnosis is based on all the information given. Many times, it is considered a presumptive diagnosis, especially if the patient has multiple problems. Validation of the data is needed to analyze the findings and the subsequent management of the patient's symptoms. Your role as a nurse is to see not only the condition of the patient but also the possibilities for education and long-term benefits to the patient. Table 24.2 provides a comparison of nursing diagnoses, abnormal findings, and interventions commonly related to assessment of the female genitalia (NANDA International, 2012).

TABLE 24.2 Nursing Diagnoses Associated With the Female Genital System

Diagnosis	Point of Differentiation	Assessment Characteristics	Nursing Interventions
Ineffective sexuality patterns	Limitations resulting from disease or therapy, alteration in sex role, change in interest of self or others	Altered body function, recent childbirth, reproductive surgery, medications, abuse	Gather sexual history. Determine patient and partner's knowledge. Observe for stress, loss, or depression. Explore physical causes of chronic disease.
Risk for infection	Potential for invasion by pathogens	Chronic illness, unsafe practices, rupture of amniotic membranes, recent surgery	Consider risk for methicillin-resistant *Staphylococcus aureus* (MRSA). Observe and report signs of infection. Use appropriate hand hygiene and follow standard precautions. Avoid use of indwelling catheters when possible. Administer medications as prescribed.*
Ineffective health maintenance	Lack of adaptation to changes, lack of knowledge, lack of interest in improving health behaviors	Inability to make appropriate judgments, ineffective family coping, unachieved developmental tasks	Assess the patient's feelings about not following safe practices. Assess family patterns. Assist the patient to community groups. Assess access to health care.

*Collaborative interventions.

You use assessment information to identify patient outcomes. Outcomes related to female genital problems include the following:

- Expresses ability to perform sexually despite physical imperfections
- States the risk factors for, causes of, and ways to prevent STIs
- States disease process, treatment effects, and side effects (Moorhead, Johnson, Maas, & Swanson 2013).

After the outcomes have been established, nursing care is implemented to improve the status of the patient. Some examples of nursing interventions for the female genitalia are as follows:

- Normalize the experience of difficulties related to sensitive sexual topics and allow time for patient to express concerns.
- Offer a variety of options for safe sex practices to provide choices and promote respect for differences.
- Teach about disease process, treatment effects, adverse effects, and expected outcomes (Bulechek, Butcher, Dochterman, & Wagner 2013).

You evaluate nursing care according to the patient outcomes that you developed by reassessing the patient and continuing or modifying the interventions as appropriate.

Genital and rectal assessment can be a sensitive and embarrassing experience for many patients and nurses. For this reason, it is important that you include the psychosocial dimension in this assessment and become comfortable talking about the sexual topics. You can modify the assessment process to the individual patient so that outcomes can be positive for all involved.

Progress Note: Analyzing Findings

Remember Teresa Nguyen, whose difficulties have been outlined throughout this chapter. The initial subjective and objective data collection is complete and the nurse practitioner has spent time reviewing the findings and other results. Unfortunately, Ms. Nguyen has a chlamydia infection, so it is necessary for the nurse practitioner to treat her with antibiotics. The following nursing note illustrates how data are collected and treatment is prescribed by the nurse.

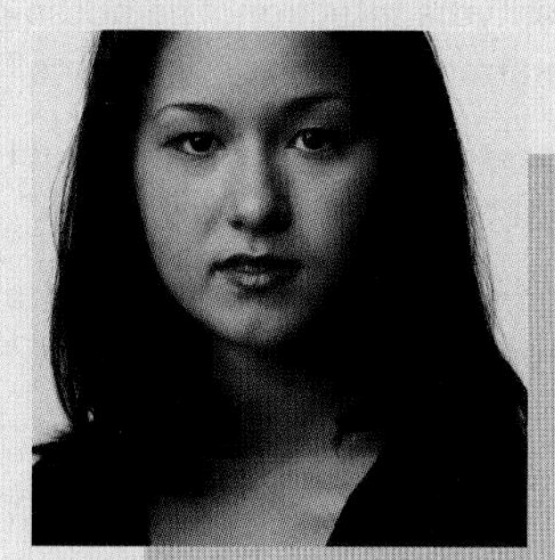

Subjective: States has pelvic pain and vaginal discharge. Increased during intercourse. Is present in the lower half of the abdomen, increases with palpation. States is 3/10 at rest, 8/10 with intercourse. Has had pain for 2 weeks, increasing in intensity. Pain has limited intercourse over the past 1½ weeks. Taking acetaminophen for pain with minimal effect. States that discharge is clear and increasing in amount.

Objective: Temperature 38.8°C (101.8°F) orally, appears flushed. Culture is positive for *C. trachomatis.* White blood cell count and erythrocyte sedimentation rate elevated.

Analysis: Knowledge deficit related to *C. trachomatis* infection.

Plan: Obtain prescription for broad-spectrum antibiotic. Teach to take acetaminophen for pain and fever, drink 2 L of fluid per day, and get additional rest. Teach to abstain from intercourse until treatment is complete. Assess knowledge level of safer sexual practices and provide accurate information. Report results to public health department and initiate partner notification process. Allow time for her to express her feelings and role play the words she will use when talking with partner.

Critical Thinking Challenge

- What are the differences between the APRN and RN roles?
- What nursing diagnoses might be appropriate given the new medical diagnosis?
- How will the effects on Teresa, her family, and her partner be assessed? What specific questions would the nurse ask?

Collaborating With the Interprofessional Team

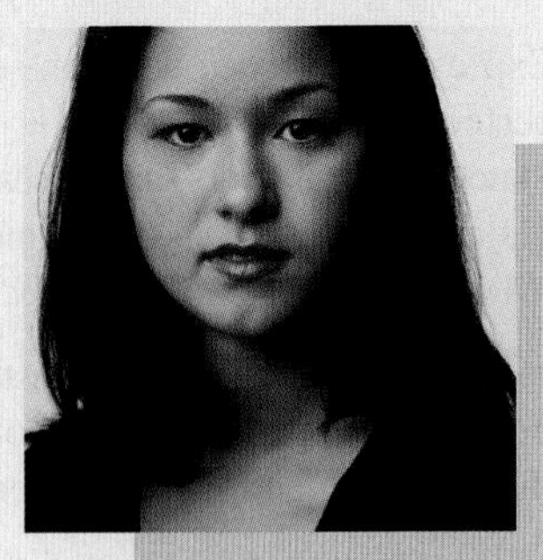

Teresa Nguyen will need to have further teaching based on her new diagnosis. Unfortunately, the nurse assesses that Teresa does not have coverage to pay for the prescription. The following conversation illustrates how the nurse might communicate with the pharmacy to solve this problem.

Teresa has been experiencing symptoms of vaginal secretions and pelvic pain. She is febrile and concerned about the risk for an STI.

Situation: "Hi, I'm Linda in the clinic. I have a patient who does not have money to pay for her prescription."

Background: "She hasn't been here before and was just diagnosed with PID and chlamydia infection. The nurse practitioner has prescribed an antibiotic and acetaminophen for symptoms."

Assessment: "She needs to get started on antibiotics soon; I would like her to have them before she leaves today."

Recommendations: "Do you have any programs that she would be eligible for free or reduced price prescriptions?"

Critical Thinking Challenge

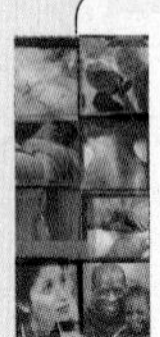

- What additional issues should be assessed when considering her future care?
- What questions will the nurse use to assess Teresa's knowledge of PID and chlamydia?
- What will be the top three priorities of assessment and teaching?

Pulling It All Together

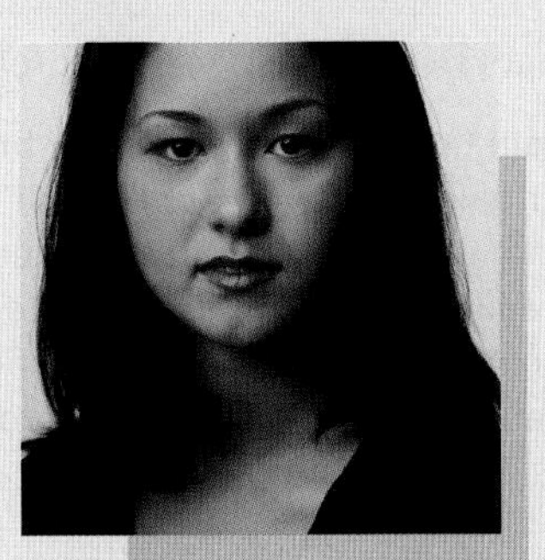

The nurse uses assessment data to formulate a nursing care plan with patient outcomes and interventions. Outcomes are specific to the patient, realistic to achieve, measurable, and have a time frame for completion. After interventions are completed, the nurse reevaluates and documents the findings in the chart to show progress toward the patient outcome. The nurse uses critical thinking and judgment to continue or revise the diagnosis, outcomes, or interventions. This is often in the form of a care plan or case note similar to the one below.

(case study continues on page 767)

Nursing Diagnosis	Patient Outcomes	Nursing Interventions	Rationale	Evaluation
Anxiety related to effects on sexual relationships and family processes	Patient states that she feels prepared to discuss situation with partner. Patient identifies one person with whom she feels comfortable sharing her concerns.	Rehearse words to use when telling partner about infection. Discuss which family or friends she would feel comfortable talking with. Offer assistance and time for processing the issues.	Practicing in advance can reduce anxiety. Talking about her concerns is therapeutic. During the initial crisis, the nurse can provide therapeutic communication.	Expressing anger at boyfriend and feeling betrayed. Able to state she feels prepared to notify partner. Has a sister who is very supportive that she can talk with. Given phone number to clinic if she has questions or needs to talk more.

Applying Your Knowledge

Using the previous steps of diagnostic reasoning, organizing, and prioritizing, consider all the case study findings woven throughout this chapter for Teresa Nguyen. When answering the following questions, begin drawing conclusions and see how the pieces of assessment must work together to create an environment for personalized, appropriate, and accurate care.

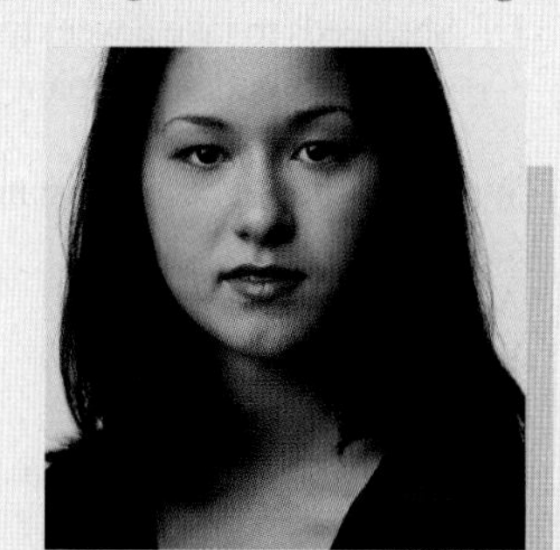

- What are some causes of vaginal discharge?
- What are the implications of Teresa's presenting condition for her boyfriend?
- What cultural considerations should the nurse incorporate into the care provided for Teresa?
- What lifestyle factors might be contributing to Teresa's present condition?
- What recommendations for screening and follow-up would the nurse suggest for Teresa?
- How will the nurse evaluate whether the assessment has been accurate and complete?

Key Points

- Examination of the female genitalia provides opportunities for free communication, exchange of information, and education between patient and nurse.
- Women have ongoing needs and concerns throughout the lifespan.
- Evidence-based research and protocols are the driving forces for health promotion and disease prevention.
- A genital examination does not have to cause anxiety or pain; through empathetic exchange and respect, the nurse can make it a positive experience.
- Adolescents struggle with issues of self-esteem demonstrated by experimentation with drugs, sex, and risk-taking behaviors. Nurses can attend to the physiological and psychological needs of an adolescent girl during this annual visit.
- Older women represent a great portion of the female population. As the average lifespan becomes greater, nurses must stay current with newer screening, therapeutics, and interventions that allow the greatest quality of life.

Review Questions

1. The nurse is taking a menstrual history. What would be an appropriate question to ask?
   A. Do you have any history of cancer in your family?
   B. Do you ever skip periods?
   C. Do you use condoms during intercourse?
   D. How many sexual partners have you had?

2. The nurse is inspecting the urethra and the Skene glands. She knows these are a part of what area?
   A. Mons pubis
   B. Vulva
   C. Posterior fourchette
   D. Vestibule

3. An annual Pap smear is recommended to screen for what condition?
   A. Cervical cancer
   B. Ovarian cancer
   C. Endometrial cancer
   D. Vaginal cancer

4. After completing a history on a 45-year-old patient, the nurse suspects the patient may have uterine fibroids. What information might have led her to this conclusion?
   A. History of STIs
   B. History of multiple births
   C. Vaginal discharge
   D. Heavier than usual menstrual periods

5. The practitioner has decided to place the patient on isotretinoin for her acne problems. The nurse is preparing to counsel the patient. What is the most important information she needs to tell the patient?
   A. She needs to take the medication daily and avoid missing a dose.
   B. She should not take this medication with antibiotics.
   C. She needs to use two forms of birth control or abstain from sex 1 month before, during, and 1 month after taking this medication.
   D. She needs to take a weekly pregnancy test to make sure she hasn't gotten pregnant while on this medication.

6. Which of the following organisms is associated with salpingitis?
   A. *Trichinella spiralis*
   B. *Chlamydia trachomatis*
   C. *Candida albicans*
   D. *Condyloma acuminatum*

7. The nurse is preparing the patient for her genital examination. What position will the nurse assist the patient into for a comfortable genital examination?
   A. Semi-Fowler
   B. Prone with her knees bent
   C. Supine with her knees bent
   D. Semi-lithotomy

8. One of the guests at a health promotion fair asks the nurse, "What is the greatest killer of women?" The nurse knows by current evidence that it is
   A. cardiovascular disease.
   B. lung cancer.
   C. breast cancer.
   D. osteoporosis.

9. The nurse practitioner is assessing a patient with frequent candidiasis. The test that the nurse will order for this patient is
   A. cultures for chlamydia.
   B. a blood test for glucose.
   C. a blood test for syphilis.
   D. a vaginal ultrasound.

10. Upon inspection, the nurse sees flesh-colored lesions surrounding the anal area. These lesions most likely indicate
   A. hemorrhoids.
   B. herpes simplex II.
   C. AIDS.
   D. *C. acuminatum* infection.

The Jensen suite offers these additional resources to enhance learning and facilitate understanding of this chapter:

- thePoint online resources, http://thepoint.lww.com/Jensen2e
- *Laboratory Manual for Nursing Health Assessment: A Best Practice Approach*
- *Pocket Guide for Nursing Health Assessment: A Best Practice Approach*
- *Lippincott DocuCare*, an electronic health record simulation software, http://thepoint.lww.com/docucare
- *Adaptive Learning | Powered by PrepU*, http://thepoint.lww.com/prepu

References

American Cancer Society. (2014). *Cancer facts and statistics*. Retrieved from http://www.cancer.org/research/cancerfactsstatistics/index

American Congress of Obstetricians and Gynecologists (ACOG). (2012). *Ob-gyns recommend women wait 3 to 5 years between Pap tests.* Retrieved from http://www.acog.org/About_ACOG/News_Room/News_Releases/2012/Ob-Gyns_Recommend_Women_Wait_3_to_5_Years_Between_Pap_Tests

Boardman, C. H. (2014). *Cervical cancer clinical presentation.* Retrieved from http://emedicine.medscape.com/article/253513-clinical#a0256

Bulechek, G. M., Butcher, H. K., Dochterman, J. M., & Wagner, C. M. (2013). *Nursing interventions classification (NIC)* (6th ed.). St. Louis, MO: Mosby.

Centers for Disease Control & Prevention. (2013). *Human papillomavirus (HPV) ACIP vaccine recommendations.* Retrieved on from http://www.cdc.gov/vaccines/hcp/acip-recs/vacc-specific/hpv.html

Chandra, A., Mosher, W. D., Copen, C., and Sionean, C. (2011). *Sexual behavior, sexual attraction, and sexual identity in the United States: Data from the 2006–2008 National Survey of Family Growth.* (National Health Statistics Reports No. 36) Hyattsville, MD: National Center for Health Statistics. Retrieved on from http://www.ncbi.nlm.nih.gov/pubmed/21560887

Frits, M. A., & Speroff, L. (2012). *Clinical gynecologic endocrinology and infertility* (8th ed.). Philadelphia, PA: Lippincott Williams & Wilkins.

Guttmacher Institute. (2014). American teen's sexual and reproductive health. Retrieved from http://www.guttmacher.org/pubs/FB-ATSRH.html

Hildebrand, J. S. (2013). Recreational physical activity and leisure-time sitting in relation to postmenopausal breast cancer risk. *Cancer Epidemiology, Biomarkers, and Prevention, 22*(10), 1906–1912.

Hocking, J. S., Vodstrcil, L. A., Huston, W. M., Timms, P., Chen, M. Y., Worthington, K., . . . Tabrizi, S. N. (2013). A cohort study of *Chlamydia trachomatis* treatment failure in women: A study protocol. *BMC Infectious Diseases, 13*, 379. doi:10.1186/1471-2334-13-379

Lucidi, R. S. (2013). *Polycystic ovarian syndrome workup*. Retrieved from http://emedicine.medscape.com/article/256806-workup

Marshall, W. A., & Tanner, J. M. (1969). Variations in pattern of pubertal changes in girls. *Archives of Disease in Childhood, 44*(235), 291–303.

Office on Women's Health. (2014). *Minority women's health.* Retrieved from http://womenshealth.gov/minority-health/index.html

Moorhead, S., Johnson, M., Maas, M. L., & Swanson, E. (2013). *Nursing outcomes classification (NOC): Measurement of health outcomes* (5th ed.). St. Louis, MO: Elsevier.

NANDA International (2012). *Nursing Diagnoses: Definitions and classification 2012-2014* (9th ed.). Oxford, United Kingdom: Wiley-Blackwell.

National Cancer Institute (NCI). (2014). *Genetics of breast and ovarian cancer*. Retrieved from http://www.cancer.gov/cancertopics/pdq/genetics/breast-and-ovarian/healthprofessional

National Heart, Lung, and Blood Institute (NHLBI). (2011). *Who is at risk for heart disease?* Retrieved from http://www.nhlbi.nih.gov/health/health-topics/topics/hdw/atrisk.html

National Institute for Health and Clinical Excellence (NICE). (2013). *Fertility: Assessment and treatment for people with fertility problems. NICE clinical guideline 156.* Retrieved from http://www.nice.org.uk/nicemedia/live/14078/62769/62769.pdf

National Osteoporosis Foundation (NOF). (n.d.). *Making a diagnosis.* Retrieved from http://nof.org/articles/8

Panay, N., Hamoda, H., Arya, R., & Savvas, M. (2013). The 2013 British Menopause Society & Women's Health Concern recommendations on hormone replacement therapy. *Menopause International, 19*(2), 59–68. doi: 10.1177/1754045313489645

Rogers, R. G., & Fashokun, T. B. (2014). *An overview of the epidemiology, risk factors, clinical manifestations, and management of pelvic organ prolapse in women.* Retrieved from http://www.uptodate.com/contents/an-overview-of-the-epidemiology-risk-factors-clinical-manifestations-and-management-of-pelvic-organ-prolapse-in-women

Sobel, J. D. (2013). *Patient information: Vaginal yeast infections: (beyond the basics).* Retrieved from http://www.uptodate.com/contents/vaginal-yeast-infection-beyond-the-basics

Troisi, R., Hyer, M., Hatch, E. E., Titus-Ernstoff, L., Palmer, J. R., Strohsnitter, W. C., . . . R. N. (2013). Medical conditions among adult offspring prenatally exposed to diethylstilbestrol. *Epidemiology, 24*(3), 430–438. doi: 10.1097/EDE.0b013e318289bdf7

U.S. Census Bureau. (2014). *The older population: 2010.* Retrieved from http://quickfacts.census.gov/qfd/states/00000.html

U.S. Department of Health and Human Services (USDHHS). (2013). *Healthy people 2020: Topics & objectives—objectives A-Z.* Retrieved from http://www.healthypeople.gov/2020/topicsobjectives2020/

U.S. Food and Drug Administration (FDA). (2010). *iPLEDGE information.* Retrieved from http://www.fda.gov/drugs/ drugsafety/postmarketdrugsafetyinformationforpatientsandproviders/ucm094307.htm

Tables of Abnormal Findings

TABLE 24.3 Common Infections

Condition and Presentation	Physical Examination and Wet Mount Findings	Diagnostic Follow-up
Candidiasis 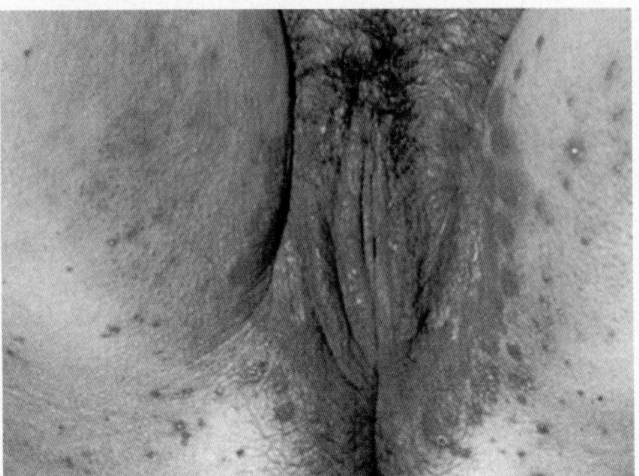 The patient reports vulvovaginal and possibly rectal pruritus and dyspareunia. Vaginal secretions can be thick or thin.	*Examination:* Vulvovaginal edema, erythema, and excoriation; thick white secretions, sometimes only along inner vaginal walls *Wet Mount:* Pseudohyphae, occasional budding yeast	If chronic infection, needs assessment of serum glucose levels to rule out diabetes mellitus and possibly also HIV testing (seen often in immunocompromised patients)
Bacterial Vaginosis 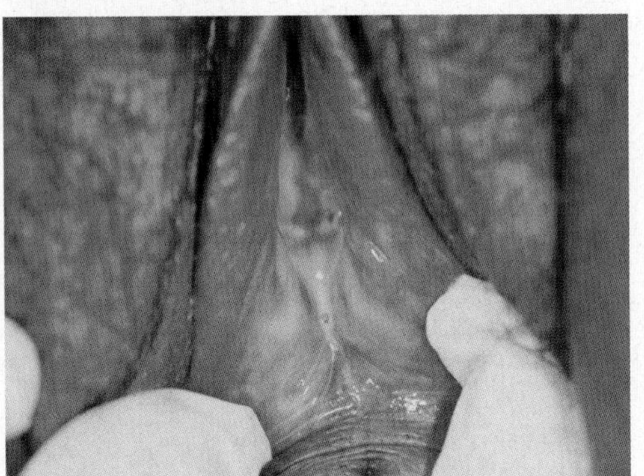 Signs and symptoms include vaginal secretions with a strong "fishy" odor and vaginal itching or burning.	*Examination:* Creamy white to gray secretions that coats the vaginal walls *Wet Mount:* Positive findings of clue cells on microscopy; possibly WBCs present as well	Positive amine (fishy odor) when secretion is mixed with KOH pH greater than 4.5 Gram stain
Chlamydia 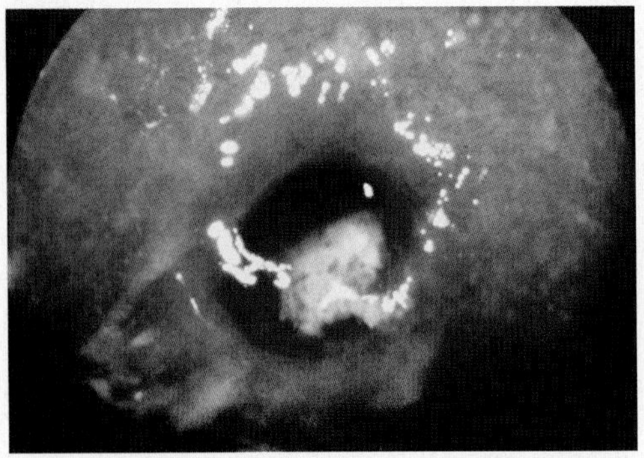 Often asymptomatic, although occasionally clear or white secretions are present. The patient reports dyspareunia, bleeding after intercourse, or both.	*Examination:* Changes in the cervical condition—reddened, mucopurulent from os, may bleed easily; possibly pain with pelvic examination *Wet Mount:* Increased WBCs and red blood cells (RBCs) on slide	DNA probe for CT and GC Serology for syphilis HIV testing Hepatitis B and C testing

(table continues on page 771)

TABLE 24.3 Common Infections *(continued)*

Condition and Presentation	Physical Examination and Wet Mount Findings	Diagnostic Follow-up
Gonorrhea 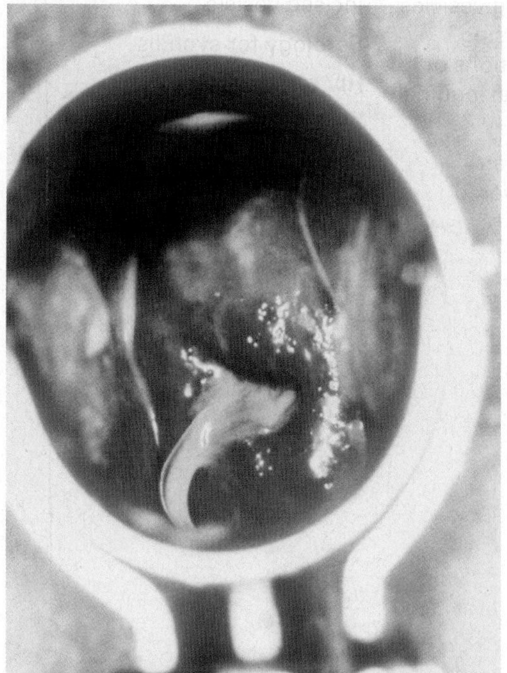 Vaginal secretions are yellow. The patient reports pain with urination (dysuria) and dyspareunia.	*Examination:* Purulent discharge from the cervix; tenderness or pain with the pelvic examination *Wet Mount:* Gram stain shows intracellular diplococci	Same testing as for chlamydia
Trichomoniasis 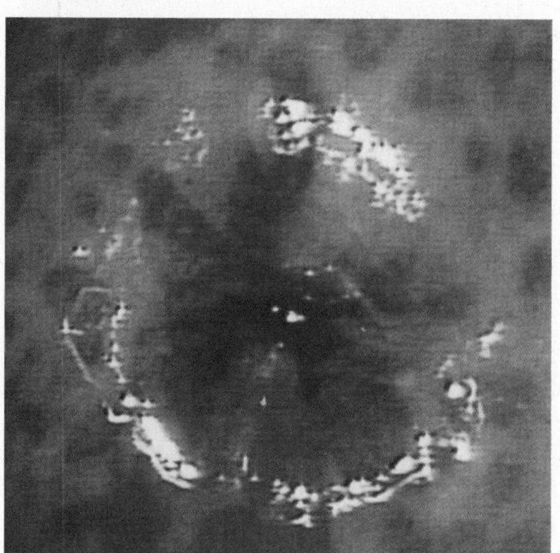 The patient has vaginal pruritus, thin or thick vaginal secretions, a foul vaginal odor, and occasionally dysuria.	*Examination:* Purulent yellow-to-green frothy discharge with foul odor; pain on pelvic examination; cervical redness (strawberry looking) and contact bleeding *Wet Mount:* Motile organisms greater than 10 WBCs per high powered microscopy	Cultures for CT, GC Serology for syphilis HIV testing UA

(table continues on page 772)

TABLE 24.3 Common Infections *(continued)*

Condition and Presentation	Physical Examination and Wet Mount Findings	Diagnostic Follow-up
Herpes Simplex Type 2 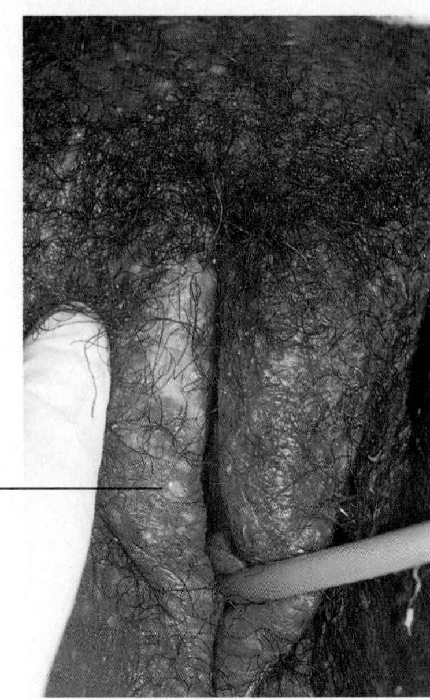 The patient reports vulvar or vaginal pain, flulike symptoms (e.g., chills, fever), and sores on the vulva or in the genital region.	*Examination:* Scattered vesicles along labia or matching vesicles on labia reflecting "kissing" lesions; surface ulcerations or crusted healing lesions; inguinal lymphadenopathy *Wet Mount:* Greater than 10 WBCs per high-powered microscopy	Viral culture from freshly incised vesicle Serology for syphilis HIV testing
Condyloma Acuminatum 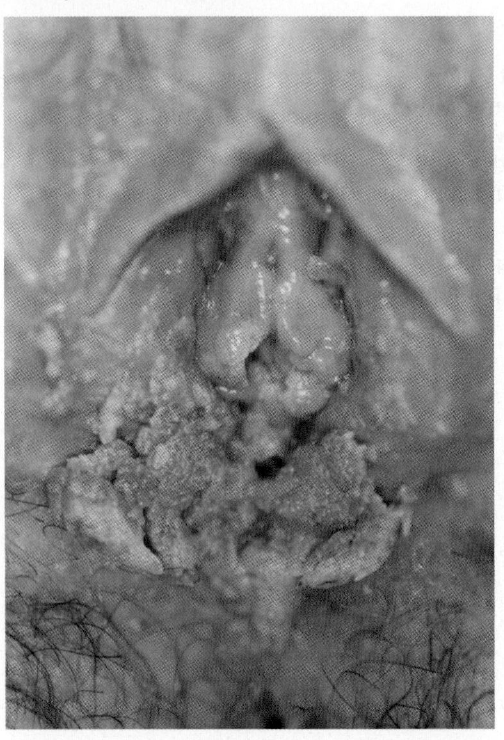 Common reports include vulvar or vaginal itching, vaginal secretions, and growths along the vagina or rectum.	*Examination:* Fleshy pink or grey papilloma or wartlike projections at vulva, vagina, or anus *Wet Mount:* Direct visualization	Application of 5% acetic acid (white vinegar) enhances visibility

TABLE 24.4 Abnormalities of the External Genitalia

Problems with the external genitalia can be isolated or part of another infectious process involving the internal genitalia. Below are some examples of external findings.

Condition and Appearance	Presentation and Description
Pediculosis Pubis (Crab Lice) 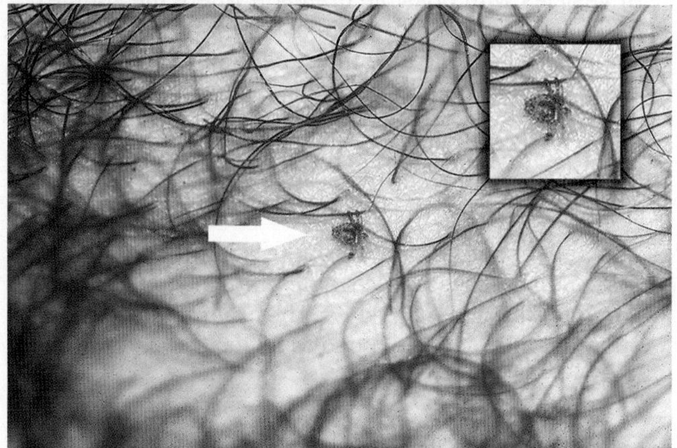	The patient presents with mild-to-severe itching, especially in the mons pubis and perineum. The external genitalia are excoriated based on the amount of itching. Tiny spots of blood may be seen on the underwear. Infestation of lice possible not only on the underwear but also around the pubis. Nits, which are the louse's eggs, normally adhere to the pubic hair; they can appear as small dark specks or may be translucent.
Urethral Caruncle 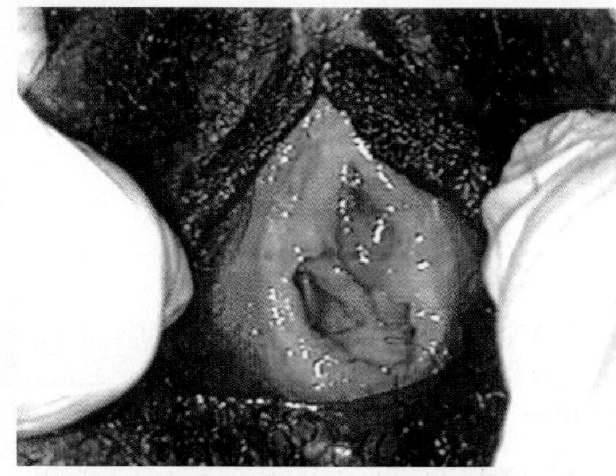	The affected patient usually has dysuria, **hematuria**, or frequently no response to antibiotics given for UTI. This condition is seen primarily in postmenopausal women. The caruncle develops from **ectropion** of the posterior urethral wall, which commonly develops as the vaginal tissue atrophies.
Chancre 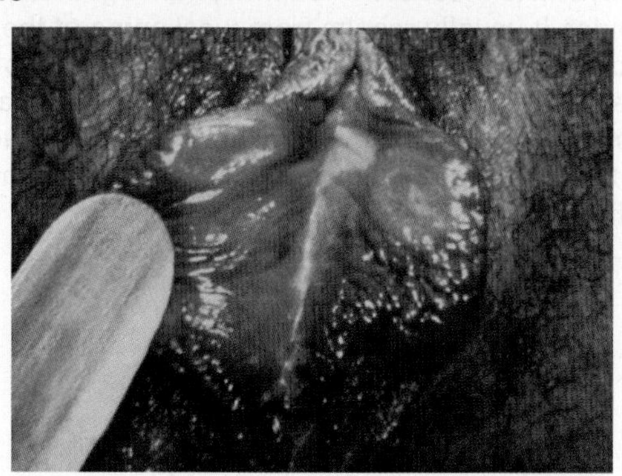	Seen in primary syphilis, this 1-cm (about ½ in.) buttonlike papule forms at the area of inoculation. This painless lesion with raised borders has a center filled with serous exudate. Present for 10–90 days.

(table continues on page 774)

TABLE 24.4 Abnormalities of the External Genitalia *(continued)*

Condition and Appearance	Presentation and Description
Contact Dermatitis 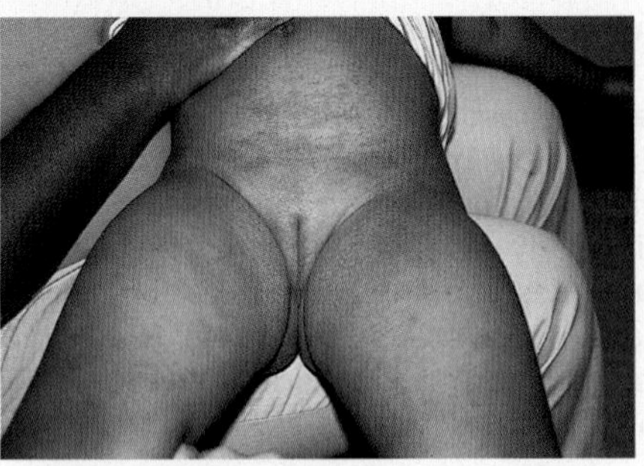	The patient has acute symptoms of external itching or burning, which may extend to the inner thigh. The perineum may be erythematous and possibly excoriated. Occasionally, the perineum has localized wheals or vesicles with possible drainage where the source of the inflammation came in contact with it. Scented sanitary pads can cause this type of inflammatory response, which will appear in the shape of the pad.
Abscess of the Bartholin Gland 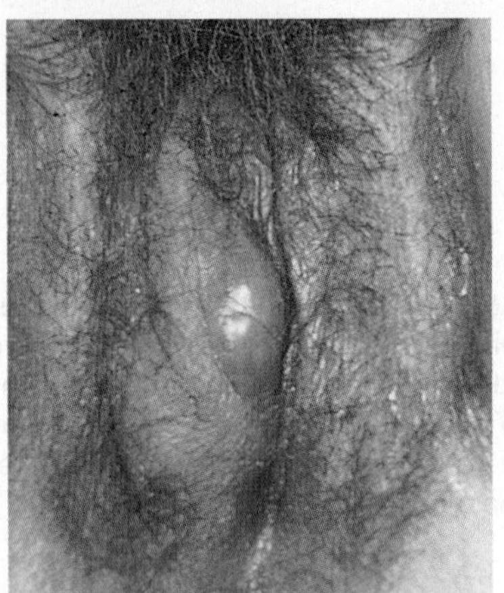	The patient has pain or tenderness in the Bartholin area. Some abscesses develop gradually but usually very quickly within 2–3 days. They may rupture spontaneously or may need to be incised and drained.

TABLE 24.5 Pelvic Organ Prolapse Conditions

Condition	Description
Cystocele 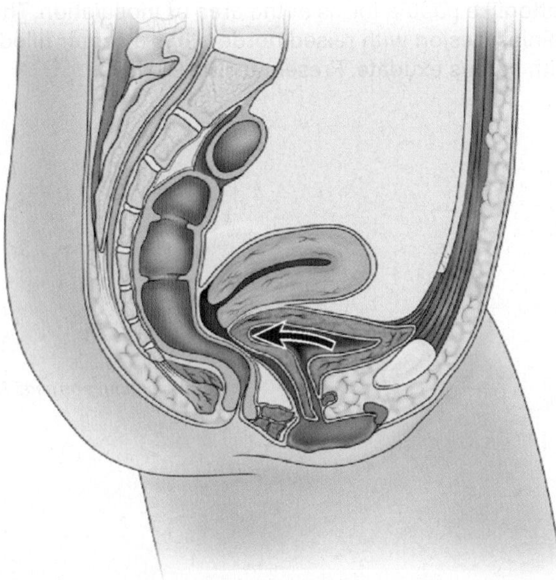	Protrusion of the bladder into the anterior vaginal canal and beyond is most common in women aged 40 years and older. It usually results from weakening of the supporting pelvic tissues. To evaluate this condition, the patient needs to be examined while standing as well as while lying down. The patient may have such symptoms as stress incontinence, urge incontinence, and discomfort with intercourse.

(table continues on page 775)

TABLE 24.5 Pelvic Organ Prolapse Conditions *(continued)*

Condition	Description
Rectocele 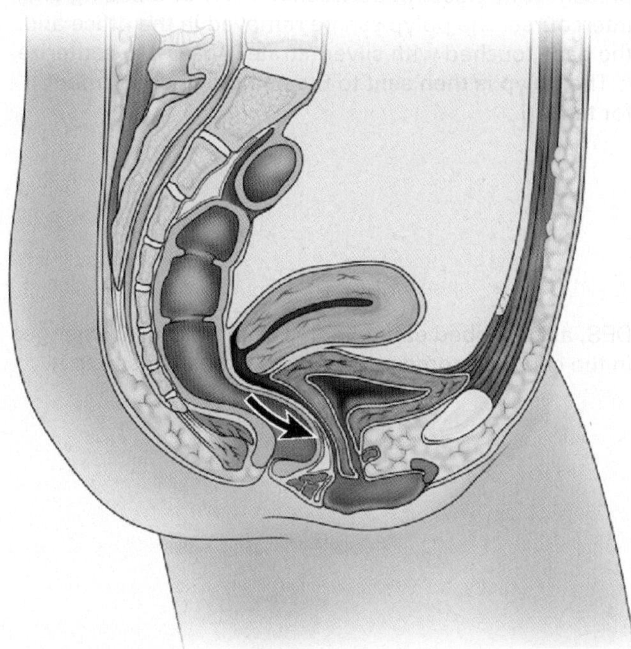	Prolapse of the rectum into the posterior vaginal wall may result from a lack of pelvic tissue support, which commonly follows lengthy vaginal labors and births. The patient has difficulty with bowel movements, pain with intercourse, and rectal pressure.
Uterine Prolapse 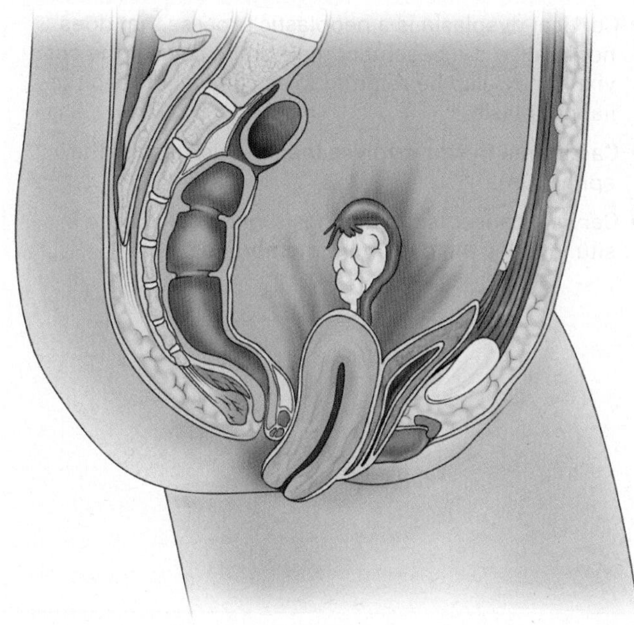	Descent of the uterus into the vagina and beyond results from pelvic relaxation and gradual weakening of uterine ligaments supporting the uterus. It may be a consequence of multiple vaginal births or an enlarging uterus. The patient presents with low pressure, fecal impaction, and vaginal and uterine irritation.

TABLE 24.6 Abnormalities of the Cervix

Cervical Polyps

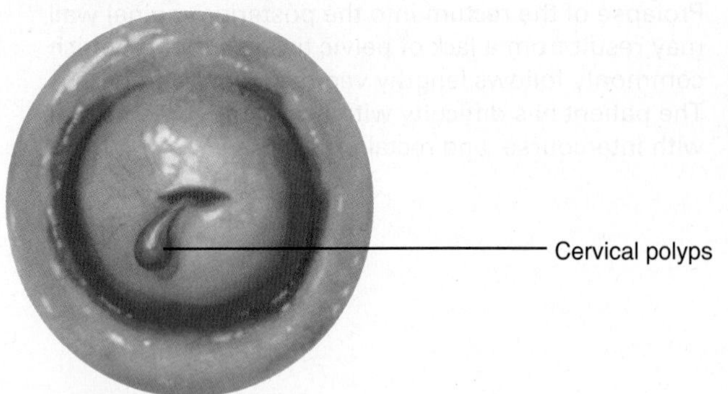

Polyps are 2–5 cm (¾–2 in.) red lesions that sit at or protrude from the cervical os. Some polyps are pedunculated (stalklike). Most are benign. The patient may present with bleeding between menses or bleeding after intercourse. The polyp can be removed in the office and the base touched with silver nitrate ($AgNO_3$) to cauterize it. The polyp is then sent to the pathology department for testing.

DES Syndrome

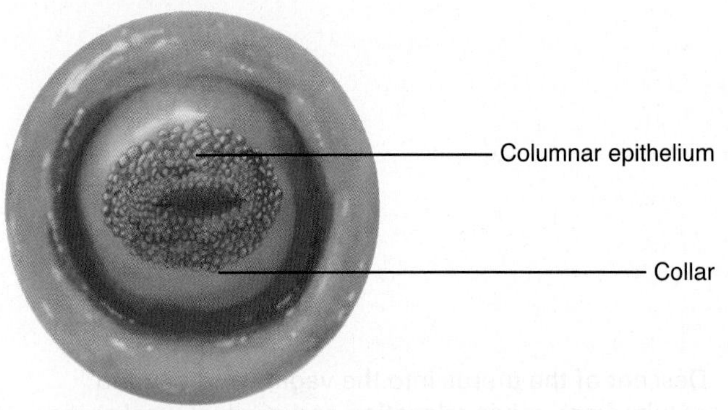

DES, as described earlier in this chapter, caused changes in the cervix in some women who were exposed to it.

Cervical Dysplasia, Carcinoma In Situ, and Cervical Cancer

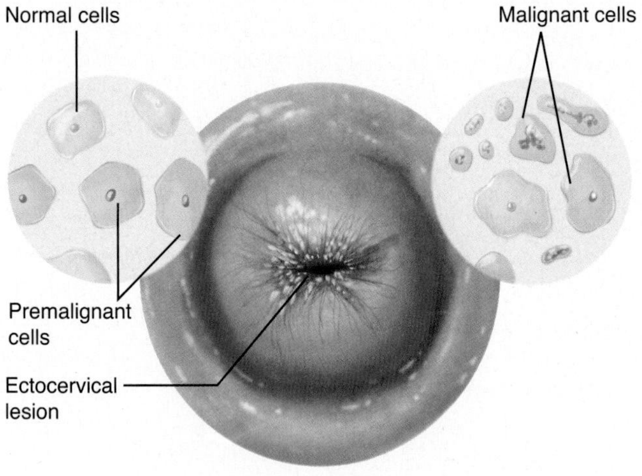

- Cervical dysplasia is a neoplastic process that does not involve the basement membrane cells of the cervix. It may also be referred to as cervical intraepithelial neoplasia.
- Carcinoma in situ involves the full thickness of the epithelium.
- Cervical cancer is the diagnosis when carcinoma in situ invades the basement membrane.

TABLE 24.7 Abnormalities of the Internal Reproductive Organs

Endometriosis

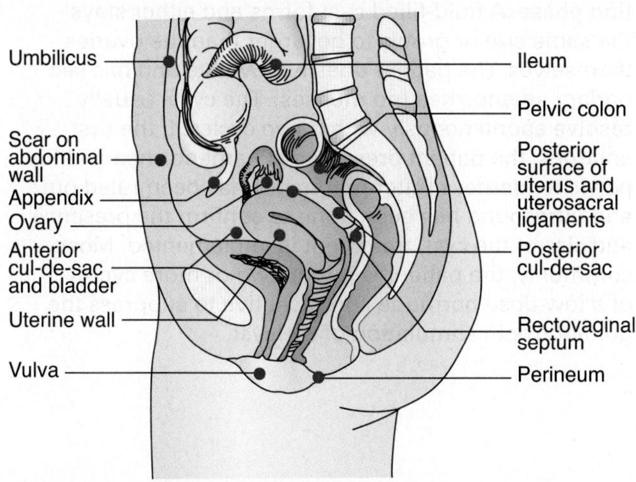

Endometrial tissue is found outside the uterus because of a retrograde flow of menstrual fluid into the peritoneal cavity. This tissue adheres to other organs and causes pelvic pain, dyspareunia, dysmenorrhea, and, in many patients, infertility. Treatments range from drug therapy to surgical removal.

Leiomyoma: Uterine Fibroids

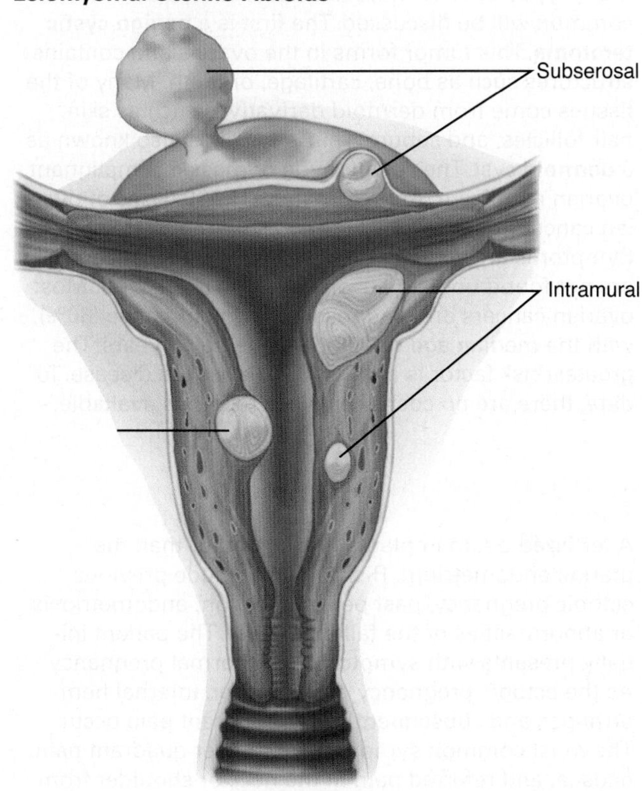

This benign (in 99% of cases) condition of the uterus and uterine walls appears as single or multiple tumors within the wall of the uterus, often extending from it on stalks (pedunculations). Fibroids are suspected when a patient presents with heavy menstrual flows, irregular bleeding, or pelvic pressure. Many women with fibroids are asymptomatic. Symptoms guide intervention, which usually involves surgery. If a woman is considering pregnancy and has fibroids greater than 8 cm (about 3 in.), surgical removal before pregnancy is often advised. Uterine fibroids are estrogen sensitive, which means they often enlarge with exposure to estrogen. Fibroids occur in 25% of Caucasian women and 50% of African American women.

(table continues on page 778)

TABLE 24.7 Abnormalities of the Internal Reproductive Organs *(continued)*

Fluctuant Ovarian Cyst

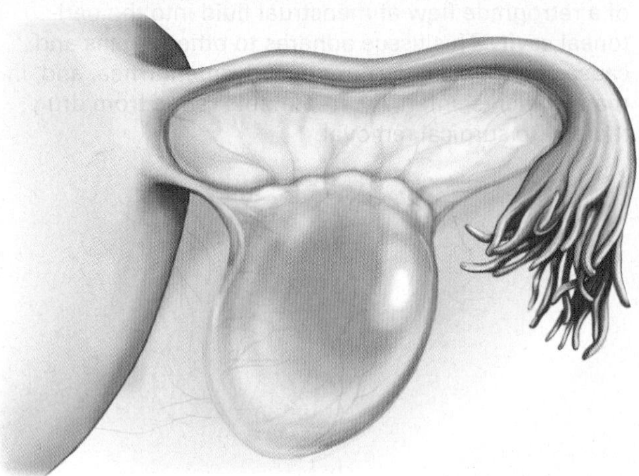

The ovarian follicle fails to rupture during the maturation phase. A fluid-filled cyst forms and either stays the same size or grows to be larger than the ovaries themselves. The patient does not ovulate and has secondary amenorrhea (no menses). The cysts usually resolve spontaneously within two cycles. If the cyst enlarges, the patient presents with amenorrhea and low pelvic tenderness. After pregnancy has been ruled out and ultrasound has been done to confirm the presence and size of the cyst, treatment is implemented. Most commonly, the patient is put on two or more cycles of a low-dose hormone contraceptive to suppress the gonadotropin stimulation of the cyst.

Solid Ovarian Mass

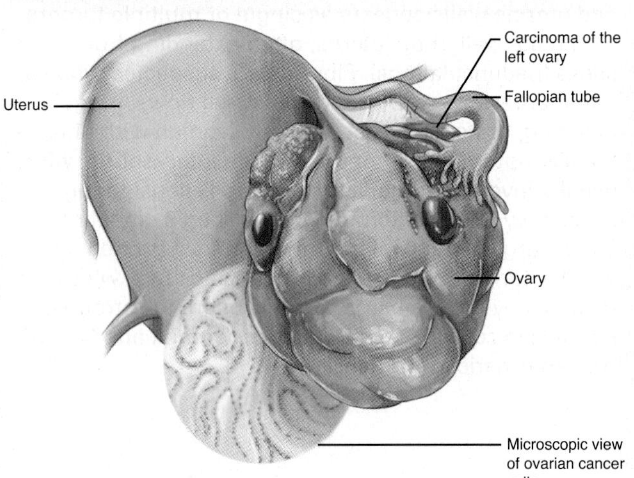

Many types of solid masses exist, but the two most common will be discussed. The first is a **benign cystic teratoma**. This tumor forms in the ovaries and contains structures such as bone, cartilage, or teeth. Many of the tissues come from dermoid derivatives such as skin, hair follicles, and sebum. This is why it is also known as a **dermoid** cyst. The second type of mass is a malignant ovarian neoplasm. Approximately 21,000 cases of ovarian cancer are diagnosed each year in the United States. Symptoms are so vague that many ovarian cancers are not found until an advanced stage is reached. Most ovarian cancers are diagnosed after menopause (80%), with the median age of diagnosis being 62 years. The greatest risk factor is a family history of the disease. To date, there are no cost-effective screenings available.

Ectopic Pregnancy

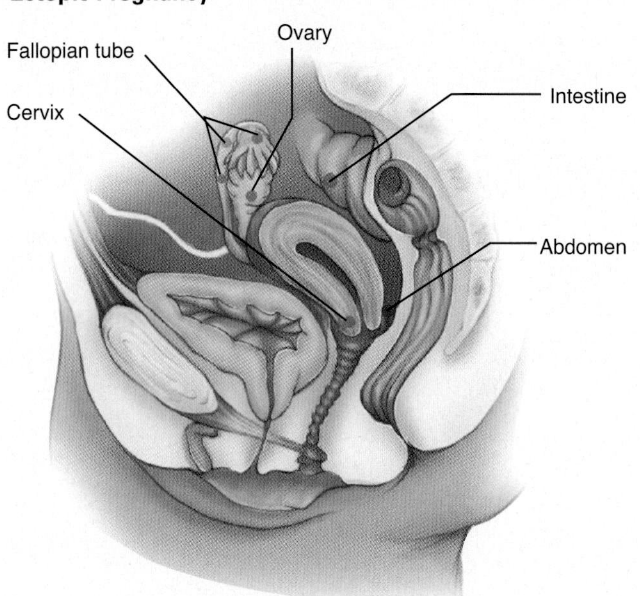

A fertilized ovum implants in a site other than the uterine endometrium. Risk factors include previous ectopic pregnancy, past pelvic infection, endometriosis, or abnormalities of the fallopian tube. The patient initially presents with symptoms of a normal pregnancy. As the ectopic pregnancy grows larger, internal hemorrhages and subsequent lower quadrant pain occur. The most common symptoms are lower quadrant pain, nausea, and referred pain in the neck or shoulder from blood beneath the diaphragm. If hemorrhage is severe, the patient is at risk for shock.

(table continues on page 779)

TABLE 24.7 Abnormalities of the Internal Reproductive Organs *(continued)*

Acute Salpingitis

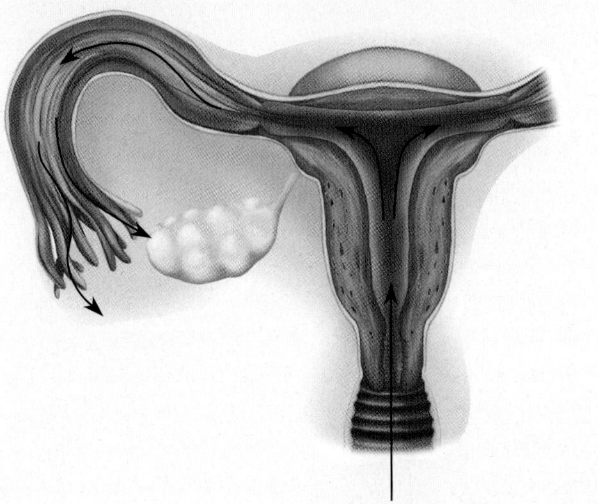

The most common cause of fallopian tube disease, salpingitis is also referred to as PID. Infection spreads throughout the uterus and up into the tubes. The tubes become swollen and rupture. Scarring can occur even when treatment has been implemented; potential for subsequent infertility is high. *C. trachomatis* and *Neisseria gonorrhoeae* are the most common organisms that cause salpingitis. Chronic infections with either of these organisms can lead to tubal occlusion or obstruction. The patient presents with pain in the lower quadrant, chills, fever, dysuria, pyuria, and often vaginal discharge.

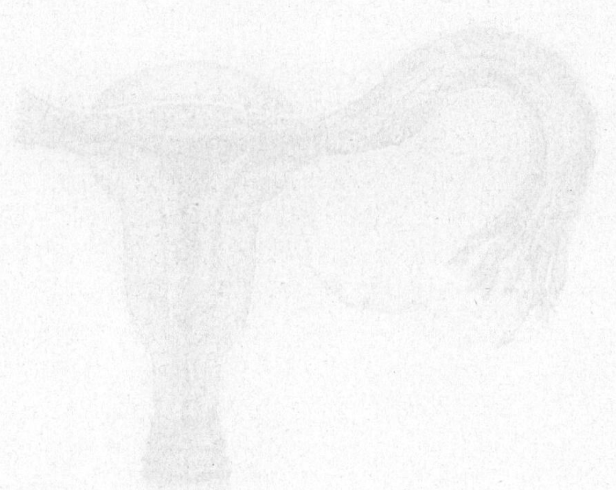

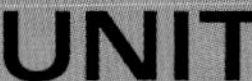

UNIT 4

Special Populations and Foci

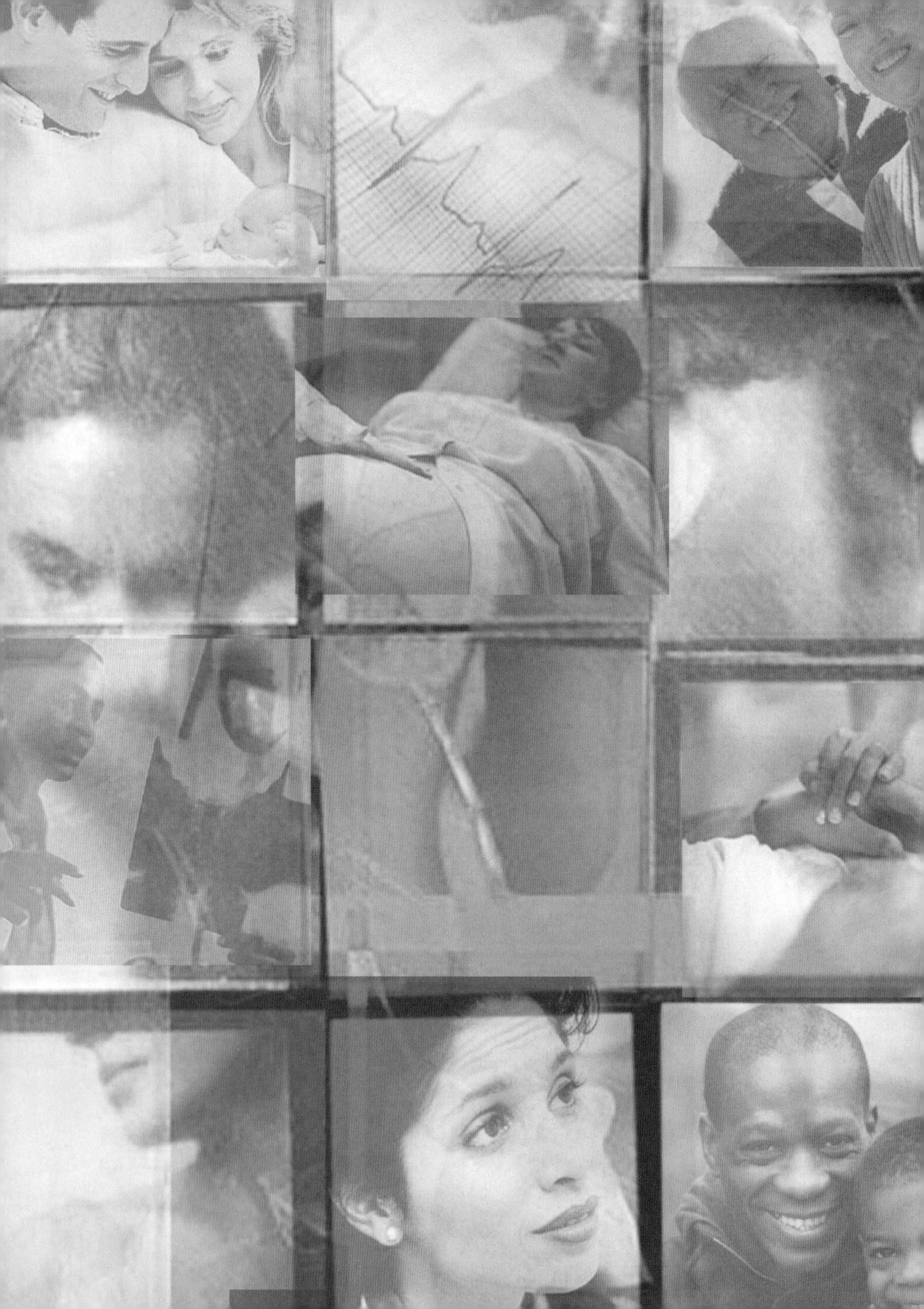

25

Pregnant Women

Learning Objectives

1 Demonstrate knowledge of anatomy and physiology related to pregnancy.

2 Describe how preexisting conditions affect or may be exacerbated by pregnancy.

3 Identify important topics for health promotion and risk reduction related to pregnancy.

4 Collect subjective data related to the pregnant woman.

5 Collect objective data related to the pregnant woman using physical examination techniques.

6 Identify expected and unexpected findings related to the pregnant woman.

7 Analyze subjective and objective data from the assessment of the pregnant woman and consider initial interventions.

8 Obtain history information from the pregnant woman and document accurately, using appropriate terminology.

9 Consider age, culture, family structure, and risk factors of the pregnant woman in order to individualize the assessment.

10 Identify nursing diagnoses and initiate a nursing plan of care based on findings from the assessment of the pregnant woman.

*M*ichelle Sherman, a 21-year-old Native American, is visiting the clinic following a positive home pregnancy test result. She is accompanied by her male partner and their 22-month-old son. Ms. Sherman, 1.65 m (5 ft 4 in.) tall, is concerned because she has not yet lost all the weight she gained during her first pregnancy and is starting this pregnancy at 93 kg (205 lb). She reports that she quit smoking during her last pregnancy but resumed smoking a half pack each day after the baby was born to manage the high stress of being a new mother. She thinks her last menstrual period was 6 weeks ago and reports that it was lighter than usual.

- What physical assessment data is the nurse responsible for gathering and assessing?
- What additional history does the nurse need to gather from Michelle today?
- What health promotion needs does Michelle have today?
- What findings would indicate that Michelle's condition is stable, urgent, or represents an emergency?
- What factors does the nurse need to consider to individualize Michelle's care?
- How will the nurse evaluate the success of health promotion and risk reduction for Michelle?

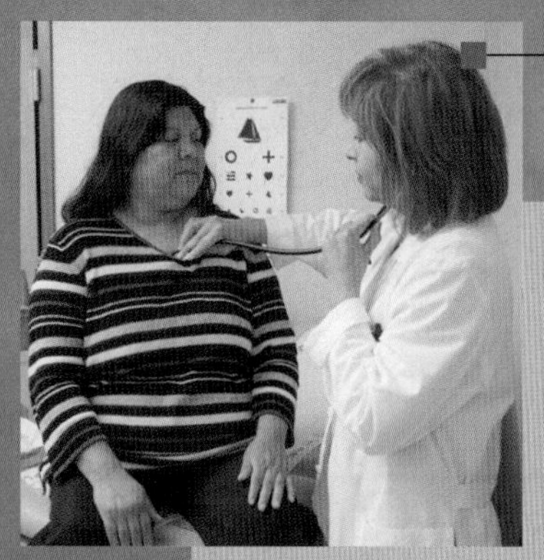

This chapter is based on the premise that pregnancy is not an illness. Rather, it is a healthy state of being and a normal life experience for most women. Typically, pregnancy, labor, childbirth, and postpartum recovery are uneventful and need only health promotion and risk-reduction interventions. For some patients, however, serious and even life-threatening problems can occur. Therefore, nurses must be able to distinguish expected findings from abnormal variations to identify conditions that require further attention.

This chapter describes expected anatomical and physiological changes of pregnancy as well as expected variations based on age, risk factors, and environment. It considers how cultural differences and family dynamics can affect care during pregnancy. It also details the nurse's role in obstetric care, including symptoms common to pregnancy and abnormal findings.

Structure and Function

Preconception

Preconception refers to the 3 months immediately before a pregnancy. However, because half of pregnancies are unplanned, sexually active women of childbearing age are potentially in the preconception phase at all times unless they have undergone surgical or physiological menopause (Bowen & Bickley, 2010).

The left and right ovaries typically ovulate in alternate cycles. Either ovary releases one egg into the fallopian tube approximately 14 days before the next menstrual period is expected (Fig. 25.1). After the release of the egg, the corpus luteum formed in the ovary begins to produce progesterone, which maintains the endometrial lining of the uterus in preparation for fertilization and implantation. Without sufficient progesterone, the endometrial lining will shed and menstruation will begin.

A sperm meets the egg in the fallopian tube, where fertilization occurs. Cilia in the fallopian tube assist the fertilized egg (zygote) toward the uterus. Factors that can delay progression of the zygote to the uterus include cigarette smoking and inflammation of the fallopian tube (salpingitis), most commonly caused by chlamydia or gonorrhea. Women with a history of these sexually transmitted infections (STIs), pelvic inflammatory disease (PID), or smoking are at increased risk for tubal pregnancy, which occurs when the zygote implants in the fallopian tube rather than the uterus (see Chapter 24).

> **SAFETY ALERT**
>
> *Ectopic pregnancy occurs when the embryo implants outside of the uterus. A large majority of ectopic pregnancies occur in the fallopian tube (i.e., tubal pregnancy). However, they can occur in other locations, such as the ovary, abdominal cavity, and cervix. Signs of this potentially life-threatening condition include severe lower abdominal pain on one side and vaginal bleeding. Confirmation of ectopic pregnancy is considered an obstetrical emergency requiring hospitalization and termination of the pregnancy to save the mother's life. Sometimes removal of the ruptured fallopian tube is required to control hemorrhage.*

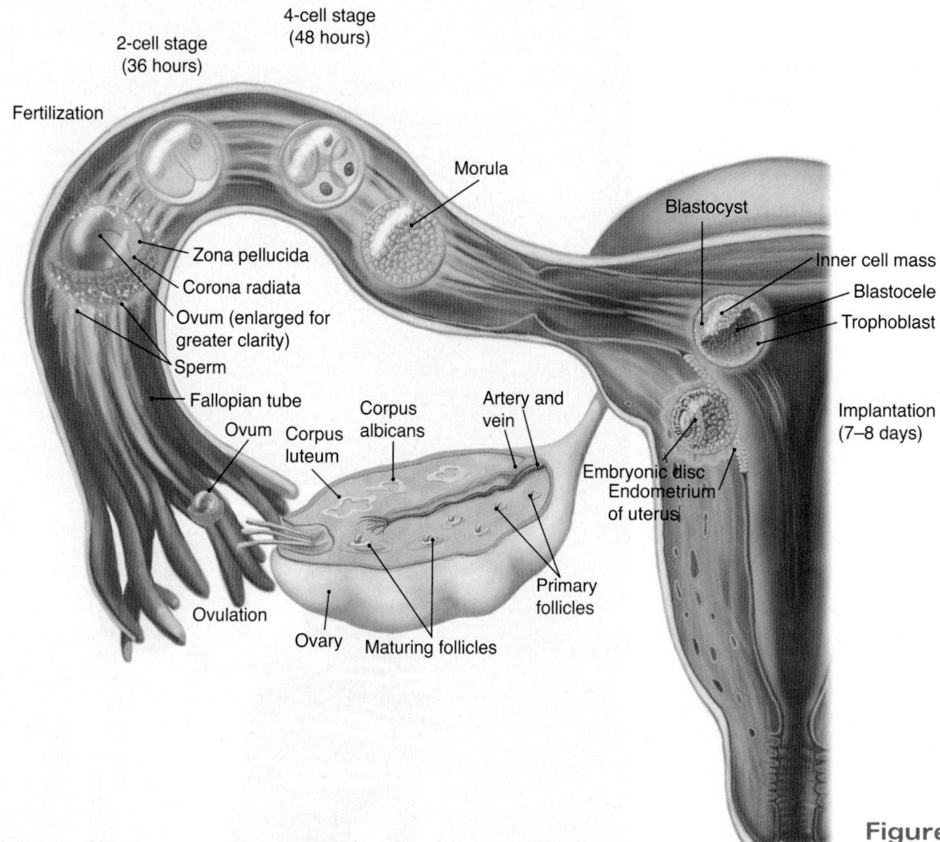

Figure 25.1 Follicular development and release.

First Trimester (0 to 13 weeks)

The zygote travels from the fallopian tube and implants in the upper portion (fundus) of the uterine lining, occasionally with a resulting small bleed. Typically, the process from ovulation to implantation takes approximately 10 to 14 days, so implantation bleeding, if present, usually occurs around the same time a woman expects her menstrual period. Vaginal bleeding after implantation is a potential concern that requires investigation.

After implantation, the outer layer of the developing embryo (trophoblast) produces human chorionic gonadotropin (hCG). Pregnancy tests (both urine and blood) measure levels of this hormone, whose presence validates the existence of a pregnancy and initiates a feedback loop that preserves the corpus luteum. The corpus luteum produces progesterone, which sustains the uterine lining until the placenta is mature enough to take over. The most accurate way to evaluate normal progression of early pregnancy is by checking levels of hCG and progesterone.

Clinical Significance

Women who bleed vaginally in early pregnancy may worry that they are miscarrying. Serum levels of hCG that increase approximately 50%–66% in 48 hours are reassuring (Cunningham et al., 2009). Even hCG levels that increase more slowly may indicate a normal pregnancy. If hCG levels are falling or the progesterone level is not increasing, or both, miscarriage is likely. Abnormally high hCG levels may be an indicator of an abnormal pregnancy and requires further investigation.

In weeks 2 to 8 after conception (a period known as the embryonic stage), all major fetal organs are formed. Therefore, it is very important for women to avoid **teratogens** during this time. This can be difficult because many women are not yet aware of the pregnancy. Teratogens are substances or infections that can cause malformations in the embryo or fetus. Examples of teratogens include x-rays and other radiation; hyperthermia; obesity; diabetes mellitus; infectious agents such as those causing syphilis and toxoplasmosis; rubella vaccine; toxic metals and polychlorinated biphenyls (PCBs); alcohol, tobacco, marijuana, and illicit drugs; and certain prescription medications such as benzodiazepines, phenobarbital, tetracycline, thalidomide, diethylstilbestrol (DES), and isotretinoin (Accutane). The U.S. Food and Drug Administration assigns all drugs a Pregnancy Category rating of A, B, C, D, or X to indicate fetal risk during pregnancy (Hale, 2012).

Between 25% and 50% of conceptions do not result in a viable pregnancy. Eighty percent of miscarriages (spontaneous abortions) occur during the first trimester. More than half of these miscarriages are the result of chromosomal abnormalities; another 40% have abnormal development of the egg just after fertilization, sometimes characterized as a "blighted ovum" or "chemical pregnancy."

The ready availability of home pregnancy tests promotes earlier detection of pregnancy than in generations past, when many women were unaware of the existence of a pregnancy at the time of miscarriage. Now, women may begin to attach to the fetus before it is clear that the pregnancy is viable. Most first-trimester miscarriages cannot be prevented, either by mother or clinician; nevertheless, women commonly wonder if they could have done something to prevent the miscarriage. Reassurance from nurses that early miscarriages are not preventable can help women experiencing the loss of a desired pregnancy to grieve and heal from their loss. In almost one third of cases, the woman may not experience feelings of loss, owing to personal beliefs or because the pregnancy was unwanted. Repeated miscarriage is cause for further investigation by the health care provider to rule out underlying conditions.

The rate of miscarriage drops dramatically after the first trimester. By 12 weeks' gestation, the placenta has grown sufficiently to take over production of progesterone and the corpus luteum is reabsorbed. Most women who have had morning sickness start feeling better after the placenta takes over progesterone production.

Second Trimester (13 to 26 weeks)

During the second trimester, fetal growth is significant. The fetus begins this trimester 3-in. long and weighing less than 30 g (1 oz). By the end of the second trimester, the fetus is about 15-in. long and weighs more than 1 kg (about 2 ¼ lb). Major organs develop sufficiently to provide the possibility of survival outside of the uterus. Delivery at this early gestation (22 to 26 weeks) requires significant interventions by neonatal intensive care providers to afford the best chance of survival with the fewest long-term health and developmental problems. Before 22 weeks' gestation, the fetus is not considered viable at this time in the developed world.

At the beginning of the second trimester, the maternal uterus is large enough to extend beyond the pelvic bone into the abdomen. Many health care providers perform a fetal survey by ultrasound at 20 weeks' gestation, or about halfway through the pregnancy. By this time, the fetus is large and developed enough so that all major organs are visible on ultrasound, including the sex organs that indicate gender. In some cases, functionality of organs (e.g., cardiac output) can also be assessed (Fig. 25.2). In addition, if ultrasound identifies certain abnormalities, preparations can be made to improve fetal chances for survival at birth. If the fetal anomaly is incompatible with life or presents great risk to the mother, parents may be faced with the possibility of a medical termination of the pregnancy.

The fetal survey also indicates placement, functional grade, and size of the placenta. At week 20, it is not uncommon for the placenta to be close to the **cervical os** (opening) or "low lying." Usually, as the uterus continues to expand, the placenta moves away from the os. If the placenta actually covers the os at the end of the pregnancy (a condition known as **placenta previa**), safe vaginal birth is not possible, so that a cesarean delivery is planned.

Grading of the placenta is related to how much calcification is present in the tissue. While normal in the third trimester, calcifications in early pregnancy indicate the placenta is aging too quickly, impairing nutrient exchange in placental tissue. If the placenta is aged or too small early in pregnancy, the fetus may need to be delivered early because the placenta may not be able to support expected third-trimester growth.

Two milestones for the healthy first-time mother (primipara) occur at about 20 weeks. The fundus of the uterus reaches the

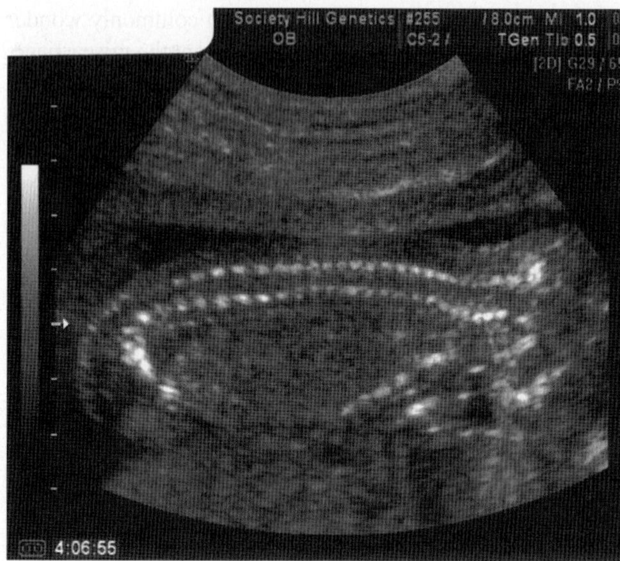

Figure 25.2 Ultrasound fetal scanning, focusing on spinal development, which, in this case, is progressing normally.

umbilicus, and she begins to "show." She also clearly feels fetal movements. In the 2 weeks leading up to the 20-week mark, she may feel "flutters" that seem like gas bubbles. By 20 weeks, however, most women feel definite kicks or "**quickening**." If a woman does not sense fetal movement by this time, her idea about when conception took place may be incorrect. If the placenta has implanted on the anterior surface of the uterus, the sensation of fetal movements may be somewhat dampened. The mother with an anterior placenta will feel the kicks more distinctly when the fetus grows big enough to kick the anterior abdomen around the edges of the placenta, usually at about 22 weeks.

Unless a cesarean delivery is required, it makes no difference where the placenta implants as long as it does not cover the cervical opening (os). The anterior abdomen has more sensory nerves than the posterior, so it is much easier to feels kicks in the front. The anterior placenta blunts the force of the fetal kicks on the anterior sensory nerves.

Third Trimester (26 to 40 weeks)

During the third trimester, the fetus gains weight at a rapid pace, but, proportionally, not as rapidly as during the second trimester. It begins the trimester weighing about 1 kg (2 lb, roughly) and at birth averages about 3 ½ kg (7 ½ lb) in the United States (with a range for healthy term newborns of 2 ¾ to 4 kg (6 to 9 lb). In the first two trimesters, most fetal growth is in the head and skeleton. During the third trimester, fetal organs grow and mature, muscles increase in size and strength, and a protective fat layer forms to assist with temperature control after birth. Fetal skin thickens and forms a more protective barrier than during the second trimester. During the last 4 weeks of pregnancy, the mother transfers immunoglobulin G (IgG) antibodies to the fetus; these antibodies assist in the formation of the fetal immune system. Integration of the nervous and muscular functions proceeds rapidly during the third trimester.

The amniotic fluid surrounding the fetus is manufactured between the chorion and amnion. It moves into the amniotic sac via osmosis. Near term, a normal fetus swallows nearly half the amniotic fluid volume each 24 hours; insoluble debris in the fluid is removed and stored as meconium (fetal stool) before the fluid is returned to the amniotic sac through fetal urine. The level of amniotic fluid present, known as the amniotic fluid index (AFI), is determined by ultrasound examination.

> **Clinical Significance**
>
> Several factors can contribute to excess fluid collection in the amniotic sac, known as **polyhydramnios**. Some common causes include maternal diabetes mellitus, malformations of the fetal central nervous system or gastrointestinal (GI) tract, chromosomal anomalies, isoimmunization, infection, and multifetal gestation. Approximately half of all cases of polyhydramnios are idiopathic. A deficiency of amniotic fluid is known as **oligohydramnios**. Common causes include postterm pregnancy, fetal urinary obstruction, renal agenesis, maternal hypertension, preeclampsia, and uteroplacental insufficiency. Oligohydramnios may result in poor fetal prognosis and perinatal complications. (Cunningham et al., 2009).

A key task of the third trimester is maturation of the fetal lungs. Growth factors found in amniotic fluid promote growth and differentiation of lung tissue. With normal amniotic fluid volume, functionality of the lungs depends on their ability to form surfactant, which prevents collapse of the alveoli during expiration of breath. If a fetus must be delivered between 28 and 34 weeks' gestation, a glucocorticosteroid injection (betamethasone or dexamethasone) is given to the mother at least 48 hours before delivery if possible. This steroid functions to promote formation of surfactant in the fetus.

Determining Weeks of Gestation

Human pregnancies last an *average* of 266 days after fertilization. By convention, pregnancies are dated from the first day of menstruation in a 28-day cycle, so 14 days are added (for a total of 280 days from the last menstrual period [**LMP**]) to calculate the "due date," or estimated date of delivery (**EDD**). Establishing an accurate EDD is one of the most important assessments for the pregnant woman. Critical decisions about management of preterm complications or postdate induction depend on the **gestational age** (number of weeks of maturity) of the fetus, calculated from the EDD.

Due date may be estimated by using the **Nagele rule**, which says to subtract 3 months from the first day of the LMP and add 7 days to the result. Then correct the year if necessary. Thus, a woman whose LMP began April 17, 2014 would have an EDD of January 24, 2015. Another way to calculate EDD is with a pregnancy wheel (Fig. 25.3), which is turned to line up the LMP on the inner wheel with the corresponding EDD on the outer wheel. The marker on the inner wheel then aligns with the probable date of delivery, which corresponds to a 40-week pregnancy (i.e., 38 weeks since conception).

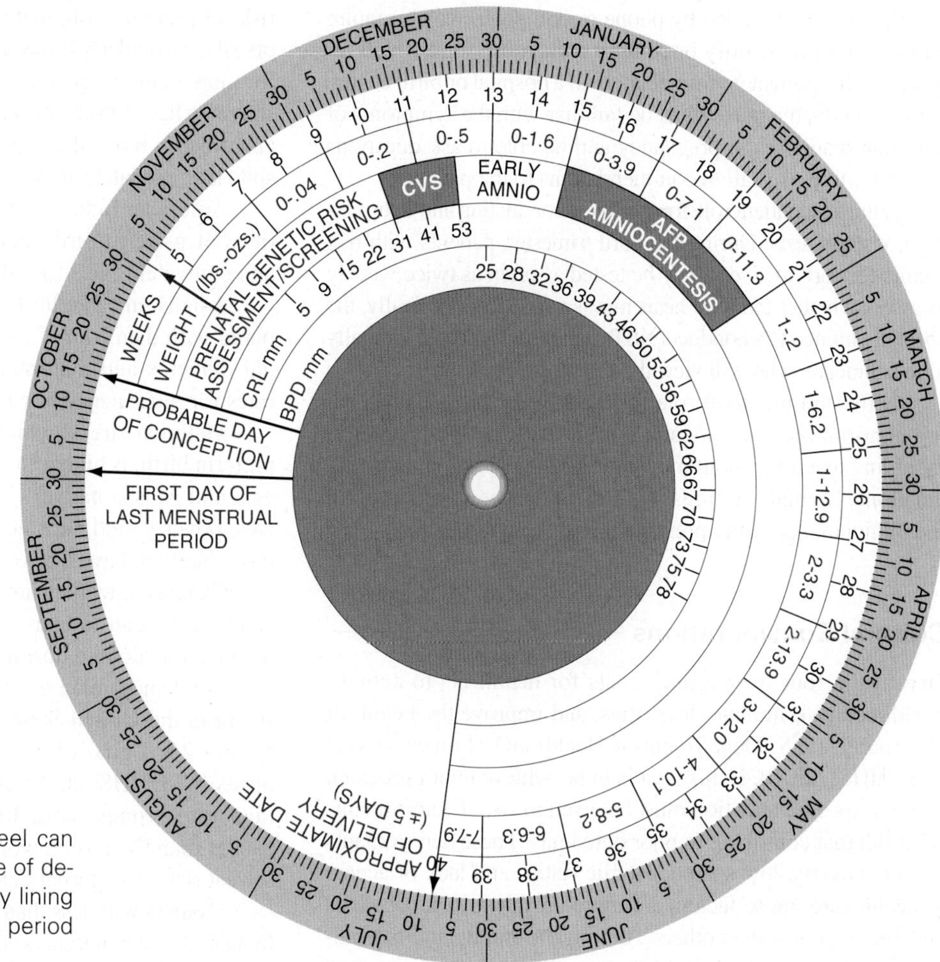

Figure 25.3 A pregnancy wheel can be used to find the estimated date of delivery (EDD) on the outer wheel by lining up the date of the last menstrual period (LMP) on the inner wheel.

Both the Nagele rule and the pregnancy wheel are less accurate in women who have an irregular menstrual cycle, in pregnancies that occur during breastfeeding or amenorrhea, and in women who are taking oral contraceptives. Normal variations in length of pregnancy also exist within certain ethnic groups and individuals. Thus, the EDD is only an approximation. The nurse plays an important role in establishing a probable due date by asking detailed questions to ensure that all pertinent facts are considered, including menstrual history and contraception methods.

Early ultrasound (in the first trimester) is the most accurate method of dating a pregnancy. With ultrasound, the practitioner uses measurements of the fetus to calculate the gestational age.

> **Clinical Significance**
>
> Inducing labor too soon can result in premature birth, prolonged labor, and complications such as cesarean delivery, chorioamnionitis, and hemorrhage. Failing to induce a postterm fetus can result in postmaturity syndrome or even stillbirth. The nurse can help prevent difficulties by explaining at the first visit that a baby born before 37 weeks is too early and that one born after 42 weeks is late. Babies born anytime during the 5-week window (i.e., 37–42 weeks) are considered full term.

Role of the Registered Nurse in the Outpatient Setting

Health care for most women who are pregnant occurs in an outpatient setting in which a registered nurse (RN) may be responsible for conducting the intake interview. Associated tasks include dating the pregnancy, taking a very detailed history, obtaining consent for prenatal testing, arranging for referrals if needed, and educating the patient about the practice. An intake visit typically lasts 60 to 90 minutes and gives the patient an idea of how the clinician will care for her. A caring, nonjudgmental, open attitude from the nurse will not only reassure the patient but also increase the chances that she will reveal personal information that may improve her prenatal care. Development of a trusting relationship requires that the nurse use his or her best communication skills at a time when a patient usually has many questions, and sometimes fears.

Another outpatient role for RNs is triage. Pregnant patients are understandably worried about events they think might be abnormal. It is impossible for busy clinicians to see a patient each time she has a concern; therefore, the nurse may handle many questions from pregnant women over the telephone or, increasingly, through secure e-mail. The nurse must know which concerns can be handled by phone or computer, which require an office visit to identify or confirm a diagnosis, and which require that the patient go immediately to a hospital or birth center. Consequently, the nurse must be familiar with the symptoms of common diagnoses in pregnancy and be able to ask questions necessary to make safe recommendations to the patient.

A third outpatient role for the RN is conducting and interpreting nonstress tests. During the third trimester, patients with risk factors for early delivery may be tested as often as twice weekly to assess whether the fetal heart rate is reassuring. Typically, the specially trained RN conducts NSTs and reports findings verbally to the clinician, who will view the monitoring strip later.

A fourth outpatient role for the RN is education regarding abnormal test results and options for treating problems, including teaching about medications and recommended vaccinations. In many settings, the RN, under the supervision of the clinician, sends the prescription to the pharmacy.

Cultural Considerations

One of the four overarching goals for health is "to achieve health equity, eliminate disparities, and improve the health of all groups" (U.S. Department of Health and Human Service [USDHHS], 2010). If this goal is to be achieved with pregnant women, specific attention must be given to social determinants of health that contribute to poor outcomes. These determinants include poverty, low socioeconomic status, and lack of access to health care; these factors are more prevalent in some racial and ethnic groups than others. Although mortality and morbidity rates have decreased modestly overall as a result of increased emphasis on nutrition, exercise, and prenatal care for all women, racial and socioeconomic disparities are greater than ever.

Late or inadequate prenatal care is more common among mothers younger than 20 years old, African American women, Hispanic women, and those who did not graduate from high school. Inadequate prenatal care is associated with increased risk of premature delivery, stillbirth, and neonatal death. Women who receive no prenatal care at all are at high risk for negative pregnancy outcomes and are more likely to be non-Caucasian. In contrast, Caucasian women and Asian/Pacific islanders are most likely to receive early prenatal care (Partridge, Balaya, Holcroft & Abenahim, 2012).

Although congenital or chromosomal disorders are the leading causes of infant mortality in most racial and ethnic groups, preterm birth and extremely low birth weight are the most common causes of infant death in African American and Puerto Rican mothers.

African American women are twice as likely as Caucasian women to deliver prematurely or suffer fetal death. In fact, African American women are also at increased risk for multiple negative outcomes compared with other races, including fetal growth restriction, primary cesarean delivery, maternal death, maternal hypertensive disorders, maternal diabetes, and maternal obesity (Bryant, Worjoloh, Caughey & Washington, 2010).

The most consistent racial/ethnic difference in congenital birth defects appears to be a higher rate of neural tube defects in Hispanic women. In addition, Hispanic mothers are at increased risk for preterm birth, maternal diabetes mellitus, and maternal obesity, particularly if they have been living in the United States for more than one generation. Foreign-born mothers have been shown to have lower infant mortality and fewer low birth weight and preterm births than their U.S.-born racial counterparts, despite later prenatal care and less education (Bryant, et al., 2010).

American Indian and Alaska native women have higher rates of preterm birth, maternal diabetes, maternal obesity, and equivalent rates for other negative outcomes.

Asians and Pacific Islanders have the lowest risk compared with data from Caucasians, with higher rates of maternal diabetes and maternal obesity, but lower or equivalent rates for other negative outcomes (Bryant et al., 2010).

Maternal stress, which has been shown to contribute to preterm birth, is higher in African Americans, American Indians, and Alaska native women owing to factors such as racism, poverty, and chronic stressors. These same groups are more likely to have inadequate weight gain during pregnancy.

Caucasian women are more likely to use tobacco. Caucasians, American Indians, and Alaska natives are more likely to consume alcohol during pregnancy.

Pregnancy-related maternal mortality, although rare, is rising in the United States and is still far above the *Healthy People 2010* goal of 3.3 maternal deaths per 100,000 live births (USDHHS, 2010). African American women are more than three times more likely to die of pregnancy-related causes than Caucasian women are. Hispanic women have the lowest risk of maternal death (Walker & Chesnut, 2009).

Mothers with less than a high school education have much higher rates of maternal death, smoking, and infant death, including deaths attributed to sudden infant death syndrome (SIDS). Less educated mothers also have lower rates of early prenatal care, attendance at childbirth classes, and breastfeeding.

Asians and Pacific Islanders have the highest rate of breastfeeding to 6 months (more than 50%), whereas African American women have the lowest rate of breastfeeding. Education also contributes strongly to breastfeeding, with college-educated mothers most likely to breastfeed their infants (Walker & Chesnut, 2009).

Urgent Assessment

Some conditions in pregnancy require immediate attention from a clinician, immediate hospitalization, or both.

In an ectopic pregnancy, the fertilized egg is implanted in the fallopian tubes or the abdominal cavity. This can occur in 2% of pregnancies (Bowen & Bickley, 2010). Ectopic pregnancy is an obstetrical emergency because if the fallopian tube ruptures, the woman may die from internal bleeding before surgery can be performed.

Another example of a condition requiring immediate attention is pyelonephritis, which occurs when a urinary tract infection is not treated promptly. Because the immune system does not fight infections as well during pregnancy, a bladder infection can quickly become a kidney infection, which is characterized by severe flank pain and a fever above 38°C (100.4°F). Although the nonpregnant patient with pyelonephritis is often treated on an outpatient basis, during pregnancy pyelonephritis require intravenous antibiotics immediately to prevent generalized sepsis, which is potentially fatal (Bowen & Bickley, 2010).

Any nonhospitalized patient with vaginal hemorrhage, defined as soaking a menstrual pad in less than 30 minutes, should be referred immediately to the nearest emergency department for evaluation and treatment. In addition, any woman who has lost enough blood to be symptomatic (e.g., light-headed, dizzy, cold, confused, diaphoretic, anxious) should be referred immediately for emergency care. Possible causes of bleeding include placenta previa (placenta over the cervical os), **abruptio placentae** or **placental abruption** (separation of the placenta from the uterus), and disseminated intravascular coagulation (painful bright red bleeding with excessive clotting) (Bowen & Bickley, 2010).

Pain in the calf with redness and edema of the leg may indicate a deep vein thrombosis. This requires immediate treatment to prevent a pulmonary embolism (see Chapter 16).

Abdominal conditions requiring emergency attention include appendicitis, cholecystitis/cholelithiasis, pancreatitis, bowel obstruction (especially during the third trimester), and ovarian tumors.

Gestational hypertension (preeclampsia) is a blood pressure higher than 140/90 with or without edema and with or without proteinuria. Treatment is required to prevent progression to eclampsia (in which seizures and coma may occur). Delivery of the infant results in rapid recovery from eclampsia.

Preterm labor is another acute situation that requires immediate care. If a woman is having regular painful contractions before 37 weeks, (more than six in 1 hour) she should be seen immediately for evaluation, preferably in an acute care setting with appropriate nursery facilities for preterm delivery.

Finally, if the mother reports a significant decrease in fetal movement, she should be evaluated by a professional to determine fetal well-being.

> **Clinical Significance**
>
> One way for mothers to determine whether the baby is moving normally is to perform daily "kick counts" starting at 26–28 weeks. The nurse often educates the patient using instructions like those in Box 25.1.

BOX 25.1 Kick Count Instructions for the Pregnant Woman

Kick Counts: Instructions on Counting Your Baby's Movement

A simple way to check your baby's well-being is to pay attention to how much your baby is moving. Most babies move at least ten (10) times within two hours.

Count your baby's movements once a day, at the same time each day:

- Lie on your left side and focus on your baby's movements: rolls, kicks or flutters.
- Use the chart below to record the **number of minutes** it takes to feel your baby move ten (10) times.
- You may stop counting after your baby has moved ten (10) times.
- Do this once a day at approximately the same time each day. (Babies' activity levels are usually higher in the evening after dinner.)

If your baby does not move at least ten (10) times in two (2) hours or if there is a sudden decrease in movement, call your doctor.

Daily Kick Counts

Record the number of minutes it takes to feel your baby move 10 times.
Start on the day of the week closest to your current week of pregnancy (weeks of gestation).

Daily Kick Counts by Week of Pregnancy

Days	27	28	29	30	31	32	33	34	35	36	37	38	39	40	41	42
Monday																
Tuesday																
Wednesday																
Thursday																
Friday																
Saturday																
Sunday																

Remember: if your baby does not move at least ten (10) times in two (2) hours or if there is a sudden decrease in movement, call your doctor.

Produced by the Center for Patient and Community Education in association with the Women and Children's Center at California Pacific Medical Center. Date: 3/06. Funded by: A generous donation from the Mr. and Mrs. Arthur A. Ciocca Foundation.

Note: This information is not meant to replace any information or personal medical advice which you get directly from your doctor(s). If you have any questions about this information, such as the risks or benefits of the treatment listed, please ask your doctor(s).

Subjective Data

Assessment of Risk Factors

As discussed earlier, the nurse gathers basic information during the intake interview, such as medical and obstetrical history and personal history that might affect the pregnancy. The nurse asks about current difficulties, family medical history, age, gender, ethnicity, occupation, level of education, medications and supplements, and additional risk factors. Knowledge of factors such as poverty, homelessness, and domestic violence, access to emergency care, transportation, environment, stress, sexual orientation, and family support helps identify topics for health promotion teaching.

History and Risk Factors	Rationale
Personal History ***Age.*** What is your date of birth? What is your age?	Pregnant teens have increased nutritional requirements because they, too, are still growing. In addition, their pelvises may not be fully developed. Pregnant teens are at increased risk for complications, especially preeclampsia, probably because of inadequate nutrient intake. Mothers of advanced maternal age are those who will be 35 years or older at the EDD. They are at increased risk for miscarriage and genetic anomalies and may have increased preexisting health problems (e.g., fibroids, advanced endometriosis, chronic hypertension).
Culture. With what ethnic group do you identify? Do you have a religious preference?	Many cultures or religions have important childbirth rituals, which may influence the role of the baby's father during labor, preferred anesthesia for surgery, handling of the newborn, or required or prohibited foods and activities during the postpartum period. These rituals often prescribe specific behavior for coping with the pain of labor and birth that may include silence, loud screaming, breathing techniques, prayer, or prohibition of medications or epidural anesthesia. Some cultures may consider the violation of such norms as potentially harmful for mother or baby. Some genetic diseases or pregnancy complications (e.g., cystic fibrosis, Tay-Sachs disease, sickle cell disease, gestational diabetes, hypertension) are more prevalent in certain ethnic groups (National Coalition for Health Professional Education in Genetics, 2013).
Pregnancy History. What previous miscarriages, terminations, or pregnancies have you had?	Document each pregnancy (including miscarriages and terminations) by date, length of gestation, length of labor, type of delivery (vaginal, forceps/vacuum, or cesarean), type of anesthesia and any adverse reaction, sex and weight of the infant, and any complications. Past patterns can suggest possible current issues. When documenting pregnancies, **gravida** (number of pregnancies) and **para** (number of deliveries) are the appropriate terms to use. Para is further described in the P-T-A-L format (*p*reterm, *t*erm, *a*bortion, *l*iving children).

Clinical Significance

Examples of religious or cultural beliefs that can affect the care of women who are pregnant are as follows:

- Jehovah's Witnesses accept no blood products, even to save the life of mother or baby.
- Women from many parts of Africa are victims of female genital mutilation (FGM), also known as female circumcision. Although the World Health Organization (WHO) (2013) and the United Nations have resolved to stop FGM (UNICEF, 2013), social pressures persist to continue the practice of removing the clitoris, and/or labia, or narrowing of the vaginal opening of girls age 8–15 years.
- Jewish mothers may refuse cesarean operation for a first-born son.

(table continues on page 791)

History and Risk Factors	Rationale
Pap Smears. Have you had any abnormal Pap smears in the past?	Patients with past abnormalities may have a recurrence with pregnancy. Those who have had surgery to remove abnormal cells may have scar tissue that needs to be removed during labor to permit vaginal birth.
STIs. Have you had any past STIs?	Verify that prior STIs were treated according to protocol. Assess risk of reexposure because many STIs are potentially harmful to the fetus.
Breast History. Have you had any breast reductions or implants? Any abnormal mammogram results? What are your feelings, questions, or concerns about breastfeeding?	Document augmentation or reduction surgeries and whether an attempt was made to preserve ability to breastfeed. Document any other breast health issues (discharge, abscesses) and type of nipple (everted, flat, inverted). Document any past difficulties with breastfeeding. Refer to a lactation consultant as needed.
Infertility. Have you had any difficulties with infertility?	If it was difficult for the woman to conceive or maintain the pregnancy, fully document her history, including any medication that she took and what, if any, type of assisted reproduction was used. In vitro pregnancies have a somewhat higher risk than spontaneous pregnancies of multiple gestation and fetal loss.
Psychological Issues. Are you currently coping with depression, anxiety, bipolar disorder, obsessive compulsive disorder, or eating disorders? Have you experienced postpartum depression or birth trauma stress disorders in the past?	Patients with a history of these psychiatric conditions are at risk for exacerbations during pregnancy and postpartum. Document past diagnosis, treatment, and medications. Medications should be evaluated for safety in pregnancy and lactation.
Headaches. Have you had headaches or migraines?	Only acetaminophen is recommended during pregnancy, so patients with frequent headaches may need to change their medication, especially in the third trimester. Those with frequent migraines are at somewhat increased risk for postpartum stroke. Persistent headaches, especially accompanied by visual changes, may be a sign of preeclampsia.
Allergies. Do you have any allergies to any medications or foods, or to latex? What is your reaction?	Note both the allergen and reaction to it. Although health care providers minimize medications prescribed during pregnancy and labor, some conditions common in pregnancy (i.e., urinary tract infections, group B streptococcus infection) are treated with antibiotics to which a patient may be allergic. Latex allergy presents a significant danger to the patient while in outpatient or inpatient settings.
Vaccination History. May I see your vaccination records? Have you had recommended influenza, rubella, varicella, and pertussis vaccines?	Document immunization records and titers for rubella and varicella. Both may present serious dangers to the fetus if the mother contracts the virus during pregnancy. The Tdap (tetanus, diphtheria, adult pertussis) vaccine is now recommended at 27–36 weeks' gestation during each pregnancy, even if the mother has previously had this vaccine. If the patient declines, Tdap may be given immediately postpartum (ACOG, 2013); this is primarily to protect the newborn from pertussis exposure.

(table continues on page 792)

History and Risk Factors	Rationale
Violence. Has someone ever, or is anyone now, hurting you verbally, physically, or sexually? Are you fearful of anyone that you live with?	Because violence is so common for so many people, you should routinely ask all patients about violent experiences—in the past and currently. (See Chapter 9.) In the initial interview, it is common for patients to minimize their experience with violence and abuse. Nevertheless, pregnancy and labor can elicit painful memories or cause overprotective behavior. In severe cases, a patient may experience flashbacks or psychotic episodes during labor or breastfeeding. Also, pregnancy is a time when domestic violence increases.
Support System. What type of social support system do you have?	Patients without a stable support system are at risk for poor nutrition, domestic violence, poor housing, and increased stress. Some patients achieve stability in marriage, others with a supportive family or partner.
Personal Habits. Do you use tobacco, alcohol, or other drugs?	Pregnancy is a time when patients are more likely to discontinue habits known to be harmful for their child. Your role as the nurse is to provide support and cessation resources to patients who want them.
Recent Immigration. How long have you lived in this country?	Immigrants may have been exposed to infections that can harm them or the fetus. A refugee may have had inadequate nutrition when her bony pelvis was forming, resulting in a small or misshapen pelvis. Even with better nutrition in this country, she may be at increased risk for cephalopelvic disproportion, which would require cesarean surgery for a safe delivery. Immigrants from certain areas may have had FGM.
Access to Care. Do you have any financial or transportation concerns? Are you able to come to appointments?	Patients with no access to medical care before pregnancy are less likely to have had a preconception visit to address any issues that might affect the pregnancy. Financial or transportation concerns may result in late or inadequate prenatal care. In some areas, public assistance with transportation to medical appointments is available.
Medications and Supplements	
Contraception. What type of contraception have you used? When did you last use it?	If the patient was using hormonal contraceptives within three cycles of conception, it is sometimes difficult to pinpoint the date of ovulation. Even if a woman is pregnant, she may have withdrawal bleeding at the usual time if she continues taking her birth control pills. If her conception date is unclear, ultrasound dating in the first trimester is recommended. Document whether the pregnancy occurred as a result of contraception failure (e.g., posttubal ligation or while an intrauterine device [IUD] was in place). This may be a good time to discuss postpartum contraception.
Family History	
Do you have a family history of diabetes, hypertension, twins, or genetic illnesses?	Positive family history of these findings may increase the patient's risk for them.

Risk Reduction and Health Promotion

Health goals for maternal, infant, and child health include improving the quality of life and reducing morbidity and mortality. The first of these goals is to "reduce the rate of all infant deaths within one year" of birth. The second is to "reduce the total number of preterm births" (USDHHS, 2010) (Table 25.1). Much work is needed to improve the health of pregnant women, fetuses, and newborns in the United States. The nurse who is aware of these national health objectives can significantly contribute to achieving these goals by educating both pregnant and nonpregnant patients.

The most effective way to promote individual health in the pregnant patient is to educate her regarding relevant aspects of her pregnancy and health. You can assess education needs as part of the intake interview and continue with each successive visit. You can evaluate the patient's knowledge level about various topics, including nutrition, plans for labor pain management, childbirth classes, breastfeeding, induction of labor, and surgical delivery indications. The patient can then ask questions and receive accurate information about risks and benefits to aid her in decisions about her labor and birth experience.

Topics for health promotion include the following (Bowen & Bickley, 2010):

- Prevention of gestational diabetes
- Promotion of good nutrition and oral health
- Promotion of healthy lifestyle habits
- Promotion of mental health and safety
- Prenatal and breastfeeding classes
- Follow-up visits and prenatal monitoring

Pregnant women who exercise and eat a well-balanced diet will be less likely to gain extensive weight or develop gestational diabetes. Screening for gestational diabetes should begin in the preconception phase, continue in the first trimester, and again between 24 and 28 weeks. You should begin nutritional health assessment and teaching in the preconception phase if possible, with a particular emphasis on including folate from foods and folic acid supplements. Counsel women who are underweight to increase intake during pregnancy. Keep in mind that women who are obese and those who gain more than recommended are at risk for complications such as an especially large infant and a late birth.

As part of health promotion, it is important to discuss the dangers of smoking, caffeine, alcohol consumption, and the use of recreational drugs. Smoking is linked to an increased number of spontaneous abortions and perinatal mortality, complications during labor, placenta previa, abruptio placentae, preterm delivery, low-birth-weight infants, babies with cleft lip or palate, and an increased rate of sudden infant death syndrome (Bowen & Bickley, 2010). Alcohol increases the risk for mental retardation, heart anomalies, intrauterine growth restriction, and fetal alcohol syndrome. Excessive caffeine intake increases risk for intrauterine growth restriction and low birth weight (Sengpiel et al., 2013). Street and recreational drug use can cause a variety of congenital anomalies and withdrawal symptoms.

It is also important to discuss unprotected sex, which can lead to STIs that may be transmitted to the fetus. Mental health is another important consideration: promotion of mental health of the mother increases a feeling of well-being and reduces stress, anxiety, and depression.

Common Symptoms

Common complaints of pregnancy are bothersome, but not dangerous, for either mother or fetus. Supportive care is normally all that is required. The nurse responsible for triage of pregnancy-related telephone calls can make an enormous difference in how a patient views her own competence as a mother, in how much trust she has in her health care provider and the staff where she plans to give birth (home, hospital, or birth center), and in how well she will tolerate labor.

Use of sound therapeutic communication is especially important during pregnancy because a pregnant woman is understandably concerned not only about her own health but also about the health of the fetus. What may seem like a common complaint of pregnancy to an experienced nurse may seem much more ominous to the pregnant patient. Often, simple reassurance by the nurse is all the mother needs.

Common Symptoms in Pregnancy

- Fatigue
- Morning sickness
- Round ligament of uterus pain
- Increased vaginal discharge
- Urinary frequency
- Breast tenderness or discharge
- Periumbilical pain in the second trimester
- Fetal hiccups
- Braxton Hicks contractions

TABLE 25.1 Priority Objectives for Obstetric Care

Priority Objectives for Obstetric Care
Reduce the rate of fetal and infant deaths.
Reduce the rate of maternal mortality, illness, and complications due to pregnancy, labor, and delivery.
Reduce cesarean births among low-risk (full term, singleton, and vertex presentation) women.
Reduce low birth weight (LBW), very low birth weight (VLBW), and preterm births
Increase the proportion of pregnant women who receive early and adequate prenatal care.
Increase abstinence from alcohol, cigarettes, and illicit drugs among pregnant women.
Increase the proportion of pregnant women who attend a series of prepared childbirth classes.
Increase the proportion of mothers who achieve a recommended weight gain during their pregnancies.

From U.S. Department of Health and Human Services. (2010). *Healthy People 2020: Maternal, infant, and child health objectives.* Retrieved from http://healthypeople.gov/2020/topicsobjectives2020/objectiveslist.aspx?topicId=26

Signs/Symptoms	Rationale/Abnormal Findings
Morning Sickness Have you been experiencing any nausea, vomiting, or other physical symptoms with this pregnancy? • Is there a particular time of day in which you have physical symptoms? • Does anything help relieve symptoms? • Does anything seem to make symptoms worse? **SAFETY ALERT** *Persistent uncontrollable morning sickness is known as* ***hyperemesis gravidarum****. Excessive vomiting results in weight loss of greater than 5% of body weight, dehydration, and electrolyte imbalance. Patients with this condition may require intravenous (IV) fluids or even hospitalization to stabilize fluid and electrolyte balance. Sometimes, medications such as serotonin antagonists (Zofran), antihistamines (Dramamine, Benadryl), or antidopaminergic agents (Promethazine) are prescribed for such cases. Untreated hyperemesis gravidarum can be fatal.*	It is unknown why some women with normal pregnancies have morning sickness. This condition is thought to be associated with high hormone levels, but it is also influenced by diet and emotions. Anxious patients seem to be at risk, as are those who have deficient water or vitamin B intake in early pregnancy. Provide the patient with strategies to manage symptoms. After the woman can keep down sips of water, advise her to eat small meals and to try the BRAT diet—*b*ananas, *r*ice, *a*pplesauce, and *t*oast—starting with one bite and increasing intake by an additional bite every 15 minutes as long as no emesis occurs. Other strategies include eating dry crackers before rising from bed in the morning, sucking on hard candies or pregnancy lollipops, lemon or ginger in water or tea, vitamin B_6, and relaxation techniques. For most patients, nausea and vomiting do not require medical intervention.
Round Ligament of Uterus Pain • Have you experienced pains or other sensations in your lower abdomen? • If so, describe how they feel and how long they last. • Does any movement or activity seem to trigger the pains? • How often do they occur? **SAFETY ALERT** *Appendicitis, pyelonephritis, ectopic pregnancy, and miscarriage can also present with abdominal pain. With these conditions, pain is more constant, increasing in severity, and may be accompanied by vomiting, diarrhea, fever, or vaginal bleeding.*	In the first trimester, sharp pains in the lower abdomen, known as **round ligament pain**, are common. These pains, which are usually very short (less than 5 seconds) and which have a stabbing quality, are caused by stretching of the round and broad ligaments that support the growing uterus. They are not repetitive but are often associated with positional changes or, later, with fetal movements. NOTE: Abdominal pain during pregnancy can have many causes, some of which are potentially dangerous.
Increased Vaginal Discharge • Have you noticed any increase in vaginal discharge with this pregnancy? • If so, describe the quantity and quality. • Does it have a particular odor or color? • Do you have any itching, burning, or discomfort associated with it?	It is normal for women who are pregnant to have increased clear vaginal discharge from increased estrogen production. Patients describe this discharge as typical but increased in quantity. If the discharge is thick or any color other than clear, or has a foul odor, this may be a sign of a vaginal infection or STI. Infections during pregnancy should be diagnosed and treated promptly because some can affect the fetus. Patients who report such symptoms need evaluation by a health care provider.
Increased Urination • Have you noticed a need to urinate more frequently with this pregnancy? • How much water are you drinking every day? • How often do you urinate? • Is urination accompanied by any pain or pressure? • Have you noticed any blood in your urine?	Increased urination in pregnancy is common, as a result of the relaxation of the urinary system due to increased progesterone. This is one reason why it is important for the woman to drink 2 L/day of water. If urinary frequency is accompanied by suprapubic pressure, dysuria, hematuria, or flank pain, she may have a urinary tract infection (UTI), which requires prompt treatment.

(table continues on page 795)

Signs/Symptoms	Rationale/Abnormal Findings
Clinical Significance Patients suffering from urinary frequency are often reluctant to increase water intake. Nevertheless, doing so helps prevent UTIs and constipation and reduces morning sickness. Fiber intake is also important, especially in later pregnancy when the growing fetus compresses the intestines, increasing transit time through the colon.	
Breast Tenderness and Discharge • Have you noticed any change in the size of your breasts? • Have you experienced any breast pain or feelings of fullness? • Have you noticed any nipple discharge? If so, please describe it.	Some patients can feel breast changes even before the pregnancy test is positive. Rapid growth of alveoli, addition of a fat layer, and construction of the duct system for breastfeeding can result in feelings of fullness or even pain. Teach the patient to use a supportive properly fitted bra and to take acetaminophen if necessary for pain relief. Later in pregnancy, the patient may notice nipple discharge. This is almost always colostrum leaking in preparation for birth, but the nurse instructs the patient to mention the discharge when she sees the clinician. The clinician should evaluate to verify that discharge is not from infection or a tumor.
Periumbilical Pain • Have you experienced any pain or pressure around your umbilicus? • If so, does any movement or activity trigger the pain?	About halfway through pregnancy, women commonly feel a stretching pain all around the umbilicus. The pain is similar to round ligament pain, which usually subsides by the end of the first trimester. These second-trimester pains are similar in origin, resulting from additional ligaments stretching as the uterus accommodates the growing fetus.
Fetal Hiccups and Other Spasms • Do you notice regular fetal movements? • Do you think that the fetus might be having hiccups?	By the third trimester, the patient may be aware of fetal hiccups, which tend to resolve as the fetus's neurological system matures. Mothers sometimes report that it feels as if the fetus is having a seizure; this is only rarely the case. Usually, the sensation is due to hypersensitivity of the fetus to external stimuli. Such symptoms typically resolve near term. The nurse can provide reassurance to the mother that these movements are normal. This is also an opportunity for the nurse to educate the mother about performing daily kick counts (see Box 25.1).
Braxton Hicks Contractions • Have you experienced any irregular contractions or cramping with this pregnancy? • If so, how often do they occur and how long do they last? • How painful are these contractions? • Is there anything you do that resolves the contractions?	**Braxton Hicks contractions** prepare the body for labor. They are usually irregular in frequency and duration, with fewer than five in 1 hour. They are also short (less than 30 seconds) but may be painful. These contractions may begin as early as the second trimester, especially for patients who have had babies before but are more common in the third trimester. They often resolve with positional changes, a hot shower, hydration, or relaxation. They are to be differentiated from preterm labor contractions, which are regular, do not resolve with comfort measures, occur more frequently than six in 1 hour, get longer and stronger over time, and result in cervical change.

Therapeutic Dialogue: Collecting Subjective Data

Michelle calls the hospital on a Sunday when she is at 30 weeks' gestation and says she is afraid she is in labor, but that she knows it is too early for the baby to come. The nurse uses techniques of therapeutic dialogue to gain more information.

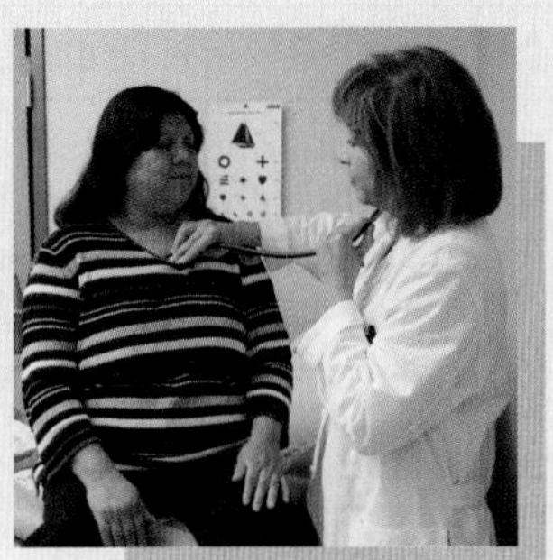

Nurse: Tell me more about what has happened so far and how you are feeling.

Michelle: Well, I am cramping.

Nurse: How long have you been cramping?

Michelle: They have been coming all day.

Nurse: Have you been timing them?

Michelle: Not really, but it seems like every few minutes, and they hurt!

Nurse: I'm sorry. Could you tell me when one is starting?

Michelle: Well, one is starting now.

Nurse: Can you tell me where you are feeling it and what it feels like?

Michelle: All over my tummy, and it feels kind of like menstrual cramps.

Nurse: Can you tell me when it's over? It's over now? Ok, then that lasted about 20 seconds. Let me know if you feel another one.

Michelle: Should I be worried? It's too early to have the baby. Will my baby be OK?

Nurse: We'd like to see you as soon as you can get a ride, just to be sure, but you are not telling me anything that makes me sure that something is wrong. So far, everything you are saying could happen in a normal pregnancy. We will do some tests so that we know everything is OK. When could you get here?

Critical Thinking Challenge

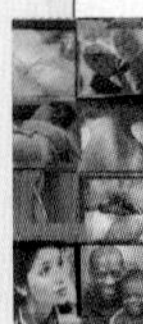

- How does the nurse show concern and avoid false reassurance?
- Why does the nurse assess social issues such as transportation?
- What knowledge base is important for a nurse to have to perform a complete assessment?

Objective Data

A physician or nurse practitioner usually conducts the initial full physical assessment with a pelvic examination at the first or second visit. Ideally, this happens during the first trimester.

Patients with normal pregnancies typically have office visits once a month for the first two trimesters, then every other week until the last month, and then every week until delivery. This results in a total of approximately 14 visits for low-risk pregnancies.

If this is the patient's first assessment, the nurse explains the procedures, showing instruments that will be used, and answers any questions. If the provider is male, a female RN may be asked to stay in the room during examination to serve as a chaperone. The RN may hand instruments and specimen containers to the health care provider during the examination. He or she also performs assessments and teaching related to nutrition and changes in the skin, breast, abdomen, urine, and vaginal secretions.

For the healthy woman, examination includes the following:

- General survey and vital signs (urinalysis or urine culture as indicated)
- Nutrition (including weight gain, need for iron supplementation)
- Skin integrity (document piercings, tattoos, scars, wounds, or lesions)
- Head (abnormal bumps, lesions, or infestations)
- Eyes (visual acuity, pupils equal, round, reactive to light and accommodation [PERRLA])
- Ears (hearing acuity, language barrier)
- Nose and mouth (lesions, bleeding, oral/dental health)
- Neck (for size, smoothness, placement of the thyroid)
- Breasts and axillae (abnormal lumps or lesions)
- Lung fields
- Heart sounds (mild systolic ejection murmurs are common in normal pregnancies)
- Peripheral vascular system (varicosities, edema)
- Abdomen (scars, striae, fundal height, fetal heart tones [FHT] [past 10 weeks], Leopold maneuvers)
- Reflexes, neurological system (see Chapter 22) (preeclampsia symptoms)
- External genitalia (lesions, infection, FGM)
- Pelvic examination with a speculum (vagina, cervix, wet mount, Pap smear, human papillomavirus, STIs; see Chapter 24)
- Uterus and adnexa (ovaries) with a bimanual examination (see Chapter 24)
- Pelvis (pelvimetry; see description later in this chapter)
- Rectum (for hemorrhoids; see Chapter 24)

Specific areas to be assessed may differ depending on the gestational age of the fetus. All areas need not necessarily be assessed at every visit; the initial assessment will understandably be more comprehensive than subsequent assessments.

Equipment

- Stethoscope
- Blood pressure cuff/sphygmomanometer
- Thermometer
- Scale
- Reflex hammer
- Fetal Doppler sonometer
- Metric measuring tape
- Urine collection cup and dipsticks
- Speculum, light, and swabs for pelvic exam (if indicated)
- Gown and drape for privacy

Comprehensive Physical Examination

Technique and Normal Findings	Abnormal Findings
General Survey and Vital Signs Document weight, blood pressure, other vital signs, and pain level. Test urine for glucose and protein using dipstick if indicated and chart the findings. Send a urine sample for culture if indicated. While collecting data, ask the patient how she is doing. Elicit a description of any difficulties she may be having and document them carefully.	Poor grooming or flat affect may indicate depression, abuse, or lack of resources; a social services referral may be indicated. Abnormal specific gravity of urine may indicate dehydration. Glucosuria can be normal in pregnancy but could also indicate gestational diabetes. Blood pressure (BP) elevated above 140/90 could be an indicator of chronic hypertension. Proteinuria 1+ or greater may indicate **preeclampsia** and thus requires a provider's attention. Other signs of preeclampsia include significantly increased blood pressure over baseline, visual changes, epigastric pain, sudden edema, hyperreflexia, and headache. Counsel patients who feel dizzy, especially when changing positions rapidly, to sit down to avoid possible syncope, falling, or both. Check for postural hypotension (see Chapter 5). Other possible causes of dizziness include dehydration, anemia, edema of the inner ear, and hypoglycemia.
Nutrition Most women gain very little weight (if any) in the first trimester. Typical gains are less than 7 lb, partly because of morning sickness for those who have it. In addition, not much structural change is necessary for the woman to accommodate the fetus and uterus, which are still small enough to fit behind the pubic bone. A simple rule of thumb for a woman of normal prepregnant weight is that she will gain about 10 lb by 20 weeks and about 1 lb/week for the remaining 20 weeks, for a total of 25–30 lb (Table 25.2).	Call excessive or inadequate weight gain to the attention of the health care provider. Women who are overweight prepregnancy, mothers of multiples, and teens will have different nutritional and weight gain requirements depending on their individual situation.

(table continues on page 798)

Technique and Normal Findings (continued)	Abnormal Findings (continued)

TABLE 25.2 Weight Distribution in the Pregnant Woman

Weight gained during pregnancy is distributed approximately as follows:

Tissues and Fluids	Average at Term: Grams	Average at Term: Pounds/Ounces
Fetus	3,400 g	7 lb/8 oz
Placenta	650 g	1 lb/7 oz
Amniotic fluid	800 g	1 lb/12 oz
Uterus enlargement	970 g	2 lb/2 oz
Breasts	405 g	1 lb/14.3 oz
Blood (excess volume)	1,450 g	3 lb/3 oz
Extravascular fluid volume increase	1,480 g	3 lb/4 oz
Maternal stores (fat)	3,345 g	7 lb/6 oz
Total	12,500 g	27 lb/8 oz

Iron Supplementation

In the third trimester, rate of iron transfer from mother to fetus increases. The amount of iron required for a healthy pregnancy is not usually available from the woman's prepregnant iron stores and a healthy diet. FDA-approved prenatal vitamins provide the extra iron required to maintain health during pregnancy.

Women whose initial iron stores are low or who do not obtain sufficient iron during pregnancy become anemic. Women with anemia at the time of childbirth are at increased risk for transfusion, especially if they have a cesarean delivery, because average blood loss for a cesarean birth is twice that for a vaginal delivery.

Clinical Significance

Mothers with a scheduled cesarean delivery or those at risk for postpartum hemorrhage (e.g., multiple gestation) need teaching about eating iron-rich foods, taking prenatal vitamins daily, and using any prescribed iron supplements as directed. Iron is not as well absorbed when taken with dairy (calcium) as with citrus (vitamin C). The nurse should also include teaching about prevention of constipation and hemorrhoids for patients taking increased supplements of iron.

(table continues on page 799)

Technique and Normal Findings (continued)	Abnormal Findings (continued)
Skin Increased melanization in the first trimester may lead to **linea nigra** (a hyperpigmented line between the symphysis pubis and the top of the fundus) and **melasma** (mask of pregnancy—a blotchy hyperpigmented area on the cheeks, nose, and forehead (Figs. 25.4 and 25.5). Changes during pregnancy are primarily attributable to the increasing fetus, uterus, and amniotic fluid volume. As the abdomen continues to grow, the woman may develop **striae gravidarum** (see Fig. 25.4). Striae may also appear on the enlarging thighs and breasts. Linea nigra may darken further and terminal hairs may appear on the abdomen. 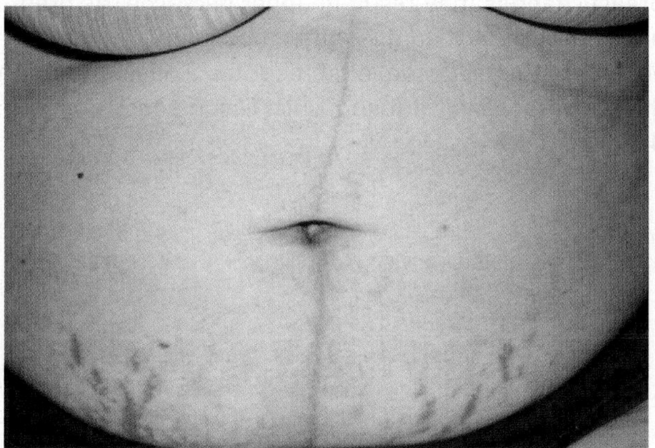 **Figure 25.4** Evident linea nigra and striae. 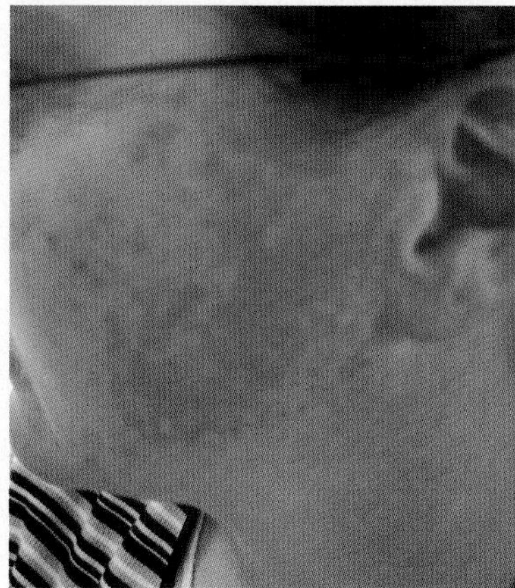 **Figure 25-5** Melasma evident on the cheeks.	Hyperpigmentation may be a source of psychological distress and may add to body image disturbance. Reassure the woman that these changes are temporary, and will fade during the postpartum period. **PUPPP** (*p*ruritic *u*rticarial *p*apules and *p*laques of *p*regnancy) is the most common skin rash found in pregnant women. Normally occurring around 35 weeks' gestation, PUPPP is characterized by an itchy red rash or welts on the abdomen that may spread to the armpits, chest, legs, and face. There is no known cause or danger to mother or baby other than discomfort for the mother resulting from itching. PUPPP is more common in primigravidas, mothers of boys, and mothers of multiples. Treatment is usually limited to topical preparations. PUPPP usually resolves during the early postpartum period (Cunningham et al., 2009).
Head Assess for abnormal lumps, lesions, or infestations.	Pesticides used to treat infestations such as head lice can be teratogens.
Eyes and Ears Assess visual and hearing acuity. Assess for a language barrier and the need for an interpreter.	Visually impaired women and those for whom English is a second language will require an interpreter for all legal consents and health education. Visual changes such as blurry vision or spots may indicate preeclampsia.

(table continues on page 800)

Technique and Normal Findings (continued)	Abnormal Findings (continued)
Nose and Mouth Capillaries with lax walls proliferate because of increased production of progesterone by the placenta.	Epistaxis (nosebleed) or bleeding gums is a common result of increased progesterone. Some women have nonpathological cervical spotting when a capillary breaks.
Assess for oral health.	Some evidence suggests that poor periodontal health contributes to preterm labor (Pagano, 2014).
Neck Assess for size, smoothness, and placement of the thyroid.	Hypothyroidism can negatively affect fetal development and may result in low milk production.
Breasts First trimester changes include increased breast size and sensitivity. Areolae may darken, Montgomery (areolar) glands may become more prominent, and nipples may be more erectile. As the pregnancy progresses, the nipples may enlarge (Fig. 25.6).	Breast changes may result in upper backache. As pregnancy progresses, some women notice the growth of accessory breast tissue, often near the axillae. Although the appearance is troubling, such tissue poses no danger.

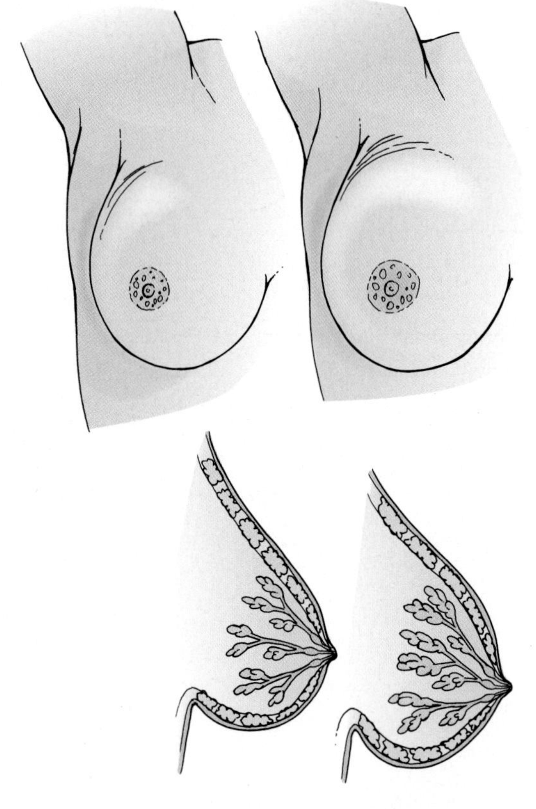

Figure 25.6 Comparison of the breasts in the nonpregnant versus pregnant states.

(table continues on page 801)

Technique and Normal Findings (continued)	Abnormal Findings (continued)
Lungs Although respiratory rate changes very little during pregnancy, tidal volume, minute ventilation, and blood flow through the lungs increase dramatically to meet the increased oxygen needs of both fetus and mother. The ability of the lungs to expand is limited by the growing fetus and uterus.	Toward the end of the second trimester, the pregnant woman may experience dyspnea with exertion.
Heart The maternal circulatory system changes significantly during the second trimester. Blood volume and cardiac output increase by about 40%; however, hematocrit falls. Increased work for the heart leads to a 10–15 beat increase in maternal heart rate.	The pregnant woman may experience palpitations. A systolic ejection murmur is common in pregnancy, beginning as early as 28 weeks.
Cardiac output decreases when the woman is supine because the weight of the fetus impedes venous return; it increases when she is in lateral positions. Sitting and standing also decreases venous return from the extremities.	Decrease in cardiac output may result in dependent edema. In the arms, it may lead to carpal tunnel syndrome when edematous tissues impinge on the nerve bodies.
Peripheral Vascular System Decreased peripheral vascular resistance results in a somewhat lower blood pressure during the second trimester. Optimal circulation to the placenta (and fetus) is achieved in the left lateral position, but right lateral is also acceptable for sleeping after the woman is past 20 weeks.	As blood volume increases and the growing fetus impedes venous return, pressure on valves in the legs and labia can result in their failure. Varicose veins form or worsen. Standing for long periods of time increases the risk of varicosities. Spider veins may appear late in pregnancy but usually disappear after delivery. You can help prevent these problems by teaching the woman ways to promote venous return. Examples include avoiding constrictive clothing or socks, elevating the arms and legs whenever possible, and sleeping on her side with a pillow between the knees.
Abdomen Palpate the abdomen using the side of your hand in the center of the abdomen at the umbilicus. Move downward toward the feet until your hands meet the fundus of the uterus (usually palpable from 12 weeks). Measure fundal height from the symphysis with a centimeter measuring tape, and assess for consistency with dates. From 20 weeks' gestation on, the fundal height should equal the gestation age in weeks (Fig. 25.7). Muscles of the abdominal wall may separate (**diastasis recti**) and not return to normal approximation until several weeks after childbirth.	

(table continues on page 802)

Technique and Normal Findings (continued)	Abnormal Findings (continued)
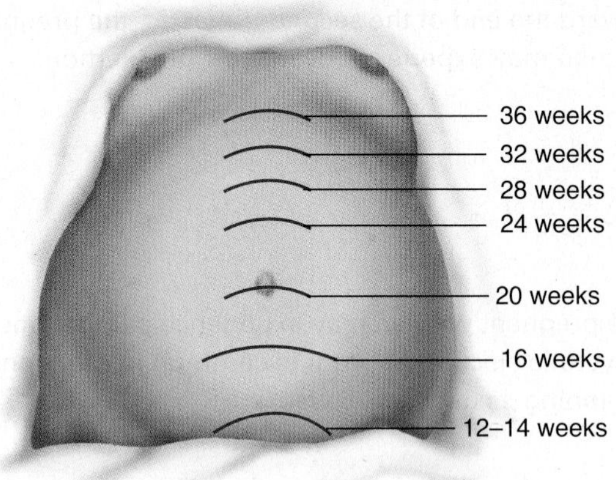 **Figure 25.7** Growth in fundal height over the three trimesters of pregnancy.	
By the end of pregnancy, the uterus will have stretched and grown from its nonpregnant 40–70 g to 1,100 g (1.5–2.5 oz to 39 oz), a more than 15-fold increase.	Supporting ligaments also stretch, which can lead to sharp round ligament pain as soon as the first trimester.
Smooth muscles (i.e., those of the intestines and kidneys) relax and dilate as a result of increased circulating progesterone levels.	Smooth muscle relaxation can result in stasis, causing constipation and UTIs.
During the third trimester, the growing uterus mechanically displaces the intestines, resulting in slowed movement of contents through the colon.	Gastric reflux is common during the third trimester, as sphincter tone decreases and gastric pressures increase from displacement of the stomach. Over-the-counter (OTC) antacids can usually relieve infrequent heartburn. For severe cases, use of OTC H2 blockers (e.g., ranitidine [Zantac]) is more efficacious.
The gallbladder does not contract as well as usual during pregnancy.	Retained bile salts can increase risk of gallstones. Stasis of bile salts can also occur in the liver, causing **pruritus gravidarum**, which produces a rash with intense itching, often along the striae of the abdomen. The itching resolves soon after delivery, after normal circulation of bile salts is restored.
Doppler Sonography. By 10–12 weeks, it is common to be able to auscultate the fetal heartbeat with a Doppler sonometer (Fig. 25.8). Ultrasonic gel is placed on the instrument's transducer, which is then placed with some pressure on the woman's abdomen. In the first trimester, the fetal heartbeat usually is audible just above the symphysis. If the uterus is palpable above the pubic bone, the heartbeat may be heard higher in the abdomen as well.	For overweight women, it may take until 14 weeks to hear the baby's heartbeat with a Doppler sonometer. Morbidly obese women may need serial ultrasounds to monitor fetal well-being.

(table continues on page 803)

Technique and Normal Findings (continued)	Abnormal Findings (continued)
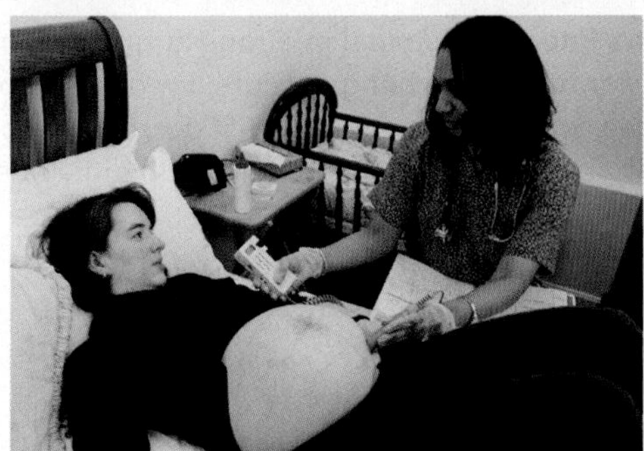 Figure 25.8 Assessing the fetal heart rate through use of Doppler ultrasound. As pregnancy progresses, the experienced RN can palpate the fetal back, which feels firm and smooth. Usually, it is easiest to hear the fetal heart by placing the instrument on the fetal back because the bony skeleton transmits sound well. For sonograms that do not give a digital readout of fetal heart rate, the number of beats is usually counted for 15 seconds and then multiplied by 4 to obtain a rate per minute. Normal fetal heart rate = 110–160 beats/min. Chart both the rate and location on the abdomen where the heartbeat was heard. Document any palpable contractions.	
Leopold maneuvers. Perform Leopold maneuvers for fetal position (see later in this chapter under Laboratory and Diagnostic Tests). Note any scars to the abdomen, especially previous surgical scars.	
Reflexes/Neurological System Assess patellar reflexes using reflex hammer.	Hyperreflexia can be a symptom of preeclampsia.
Musculoskeletal System With fetal growth, the maternal center of gravity changes, so the woman is at increased risk for falls. Pregnant women should not lift anything heavier than 9 kg (about 20 lb) and should use good body mechanics when doing it. At the end of pregnancy, there are noticeable changes in the musculoskeletal system. The modest increase in pelvic diameter that results from the relaxation of the cartilage allows the fetus to engage in the pelvis in preparation for childbirth.	Backaches are common during the second and third trimesters, partly from lumbar lordosis of pregnancy, and partly from poor back support when lifting or sleeping. Increased weight from the fetus and breast tissue, with the accompanying change in the center of gravity, places increased strain on the abdominal muscles. Teach the pregnant woman exercises to strengthen her abdominal muscles (pelvic tilts), and suggest a support band, which may provide some relief. Increased levels of relaxin loosen the cartilage between the pelvic bones, resulting in the characteristic "waddling" gait of the third trimester.
External Genitalia The woman may notice frequent urination and increased vaginal secretions. Document any varicosities, lesions, signs of STI, and details of FGM.	Varicosities of the labia occur in 10% of pregnancies but typically resolve in the postpartum period. Symptoms may include pain, pruritus, and dyspareunia. Some STIs may preclude vaginal delivery (e.g., herpes simplex virus).

(table continues on page 804)

Technique and Normal Findings (continued)	Abnormal Findings (continued)
As the woman's abdomen grows, couples may worry about the advisability of sexual relations. In the first trimester, before the uterus is very large, this is less likely to be a psychological and practical concern. Couples with normal pregnancies benefit from being reassured that sexual relations do not hurt the fetus, which is well protected, and that receptors for any oxytocin produced with orgasm are inactive until pregnancy ends. Couples may find that certain positions for intercourse are more comfortable than others, and women can be encouraged to try new positions.	Women's interest in sexual relations during pregnancy varies. For many, no change occurs; for others, libido increases, whereas for still others it decreases, possibly from fatigue, depression, or relationship difficulties that surface during pregnancy.
Pelvic (Speculum) Examination Examine the vagina and cervix using a speculum as detailed in Chapter 24. Chadwick sign (a bluish discoloration of the vaginal wall and cervix) may be present; it is a presumptive sign of pregnancy. Note the vaginal discharge. Note any scarring of the cervix or vagina and whether the cervix appears open.	Unusual color or odor of vaginal discharge may indicate STI or bacterial vaginosis. A friable cervix bleeds easily when touched and may indicate infection. Prepare a wet mount or cultures as indicated. Scarring may be present from lacerations in a previous birth. An open cervix early in pregnancy is suspicious for impending miscarriage.
Uterus and Ovaries Palpate using bimanual technique (see Chapter 24). Note the size and position of the uterus. Document the position, effacement, dilation, and consistency of the cervix and also the station of the presenting part, if palpable.	
Pelvis Pelvimetry is a specialty technique used by advanced practitioners in which measurements of the bones of the pelvis are used to estimate favorability of the pelvis for vaginal delivery.	
Rectum Assess for hemorrhoids (see Chapter 24).	Straining during bowel movements can cause painful itchy hemorrhoids. The best way to prevent hemorrhoids is by increasing exercise and intake of fiber and water.

Critical Thinking

Laboratory and Diagnostic Testing

The nurse should be familiar with common laboratory tests administered during pregnancy and the significance of abnormal findings. The clinic will have protocols (either written or verbal) about how abnormal findings are treated. It is common for the nurse to explain findings to the mother and also the proposed treatment. Table 25.3 lists and describes common laboratory tests performed throughout pregnancy.

Advanced Assessments

Beyond the basic assessment, pregnant women may require advanced assessment techniques. These must be performed by a specially trained RN. Results should be shared with the maternity care provider. Two common advanced assessments are described below: the nonstress test and Leopold maneuvers.

Nonstress Test

During the second or third trimester (after 23 weeks), the patient may be scheduled for a **nonstress test (NST)** in conjunction with her prenatal visit. The purpose of the NST is to assess fetal well-being. If the patient is scheduled for an NST, the nurse will conduct the test using the electronic fetal monitor (Fig. 25.9). The nurse puts the patient in a comfortable position, places the tocodynamometer on the fundus to measure uterine contractions, and places the ultrasound monitor where the fetal heart can be heard in order to measure its rate (FHR). The nurse checks periodically to make sure that the sensors are tracing accurately and that the mother is still comfortable.

A reactive NST is indicative of a healthy fetus. If the monitoring strip is nonreactive, the nurse may offer the mother a position change or a drink of cold water or juice to stimulate the fetus. The fetal response helps to distinguish a true nonreactive

TABLE 25.3 **Laboratory Tests Performed During Pregnancy**

Test	Rationale	Example of Plan/Treatment
Blood type and antibody screen	If the mother suffers from hemorrhage during or after labor, the blood bank will need her blood type to cross-match units for emergency transfusion.	Mothers with Rh negative blood are given RhoGAM at approximately 28 weeks' gestation or in cases of abdominal trauma or miscarriage. This is to prevent isoimmunization of the mother, which can endanger future pregnancies.
Complete blood count	Detects anemia, thalassemia, thrombocytopenia, and infection	Anemia may be treated with iron supplementation or iron-rich foods. Thalassemias may require referral to specialists because the condition poses some risks to the fetus. Patients with low-platelet levels are at risk for hemorrhage or disseminated intravascular coagulation and may not be candidates for epidurals. White blood cell (WBC) counts are usually elevated in pregnancy; they may be as high as 12,000/mm^3 prenatally, and during labor they may rise as high as 30,000/mm^3. WBCs in excess of these numbers suggest a potential infection.
Serology (Syphilis test developed by the Venereal Disease Research Laboratory of the U.S. Public Health Service [VDRL] and another test for sypilis called the rapid plasma reagin test [RPR])	Syphilis crosses the placental barrier to the fetus.	A positive test result is usually verified by additional testing, and if those results also are positive, the mother is treated with antibiotics.
Hepatitis B surface antigen (HBsAg)	Hepatitis can be transmitted from the mother to the fetus.	Newborns of positive mothers are given an HBIG (IgG antibodies) injection and are immunized against hepatitis B shortly after birth.
HIV	HIV can be transmitted from the mother to the fetus.	Administration of antiretroviral medications to the HIV-positive mother during pregnancy and labor significantly reduces the risk of transmission of the virus to the baby. HIV-positive mothers should not breastfeed.
Rubella titer	Maternal infection with rubella during pregnancy (especially the first 2 months) can cause congenital heart malformations, intrauterine growth restriction, cataracts, and deafness in the fetus.	Patients without sufficient titers to protect them from infection cannot be vaccinated during pregnancy because the vaccine is a live virus. However, they can be vaccinated promptly after delivery.
Triple or quad screen	Maternal blood drawn between 15 and 20 weeks; includes alpha-fetoprotein (aFP), hCG, and unconjugated estriol in the triple screen; the quadruple screen also includes inhibin A. These tests screen for Down syndrome and other trisomies, neural tube defects, gastroschisis, and other fetal abnormalities (Ricci, 2013).	This test has a high false-positive rate; further testing is required for a definitive diagnosis. Test accuracy depends on accurately dating the pregnancy. Ultrasound can usually clarify dating issues and also help with identifying any abnormalities. Amniocentesis is offered if the ultrasound does not reveal any dating problems.
Nuchal translucency	This screening is done via ultrasound at 11–14 weeks. This allows for early detection and diagnosis of fetal chromosomal and structural anomalies.	Increased nuchal translucency is associated with trisomy 21, 18, and 13, as well as diaphragmatic hernia, cardiac defects, and fetal skeletal and neurological anomalies (Ricci, 2013).

(table continues on page 806)

TABLE 25.3 **Laboratory Tests Performed During Pregnancy** *(continued)*		
Test	**Rationale**	**Example of Plan/Treatment**
50-g glucose challenge	Maternal blood is drawn exactly 1 hour after the woman ingests a glucose drink. The test used to screen for (gestational) diabetes at 24–28 weeks, when maternal glucose metabolism changes. It may be done earlier for those at high risk for diabetes (obese patients or those with extensive family history of the disease). Patient does not need to fast prior to the test. Uncontrolled diabetes during pregnancy can result in macrosomia, difficult delivery, neonatal hypoglycemia, perinatal morbidity and mortality, and a host of other complications.	Patients with an elevated glucose level (above 130 mg/dl) are given a 3-hour glucose tolerance test to confirm gestational diabetes (ACOG, 2011). These women are referred to a dietician for diabetes counseling and education about blood glucose monitoring. With strict diet control, many patients can control their blood glucose level; however, some will require oral medication or insulin injections to protect the fetus from glucose overload.
Group B Streptococcus (GBS)	Mothers with urine cultures positive for GBS are called "colonizers" and are at increased risk for fetal infection. Colonizers are treated with oral antibiotics immediately and given IV antibiotics during labor for the current and all future pregnancies. For other mothers, a swab of the vagina and rectum is collected at 35–37 weeks (or sooner if prematurity is a risk). If the mother is GBS-positive, the infant could be infected during prolonged rupture of membranes or a vaginal birth. If the infant is infected, serious complications (e.g., GBS sepsis, pneumonia) can occur in the infant, which have a high rate of mortality.	Protection for the infant is most efficacious when antibiotics are administered at least 4 hours prior to delivery, so positive mothers are encouraged to notify their providers early in labor.

From Siddique, J., Lantos, J., VanderWeele, T., & Lauderdale, D. (2012). Screening tests during prenatal care: Does practice follow the evidence? *Maternal and Child Health Journal, 16*, 51–59. doi: 10.1007/s10995-010-0723-3

test from a normal fetal sleep cycle. The nurse reports any sign of fetal distress to the primary care provider immediately.

Leopold Maneuvers

Leopold maneuvers are designed to estimate the position of the fetus. First, the nurse palpates the fundus of the uterus to determine whether it contains the head or the buttocks. The head moves independently of the torso, but the buttocks do not (Fig. 25.10A). Second, the fetal back is located by holding the fetus firmly on one side while the other is palpated and then the procedure is reversed. The back feels firm and smooth; the opposite side contains "small parts" (arms and legs) that feel irregular (Fig. 25.10B). Third, palpating just above the symphysis pubis identifies the presenting part. It should be the part opposite that found in the fundus (Fig. 25.10C). Fourth and finally, the fetal head is palpated to determine whether it is flexed or deflexed. If it is properly flexed, a protrusion (the brow) will be palpated on the opposite side of the fetal back. If the head is deflexed, the protrusion (the occiput) will be palpated on the same side as the back

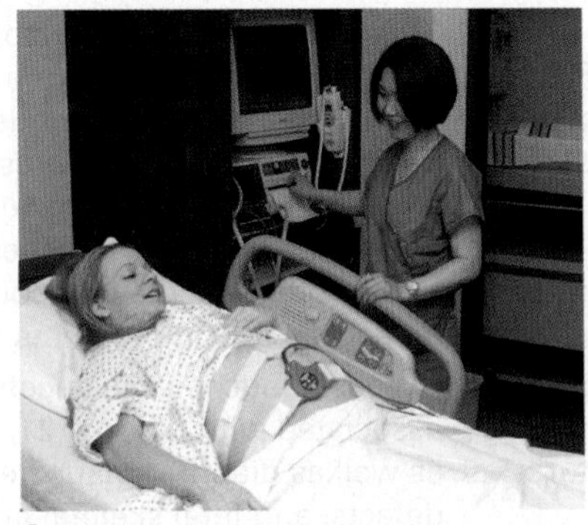
A

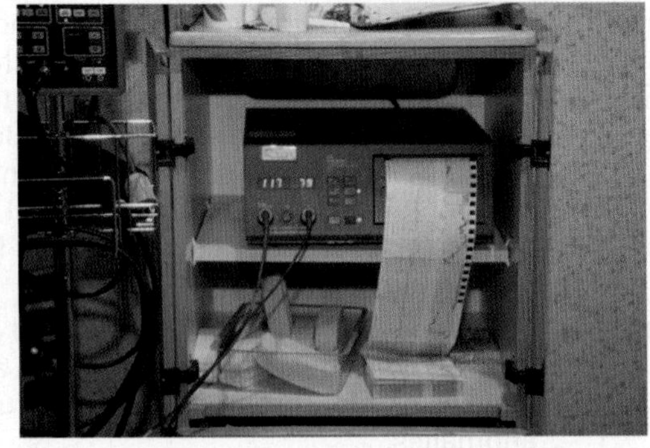
B

Figure 25.9 Nonstress testing. **A.** The nurse is observing external fetal monitoring of the patient. **B.** A reactive strip.

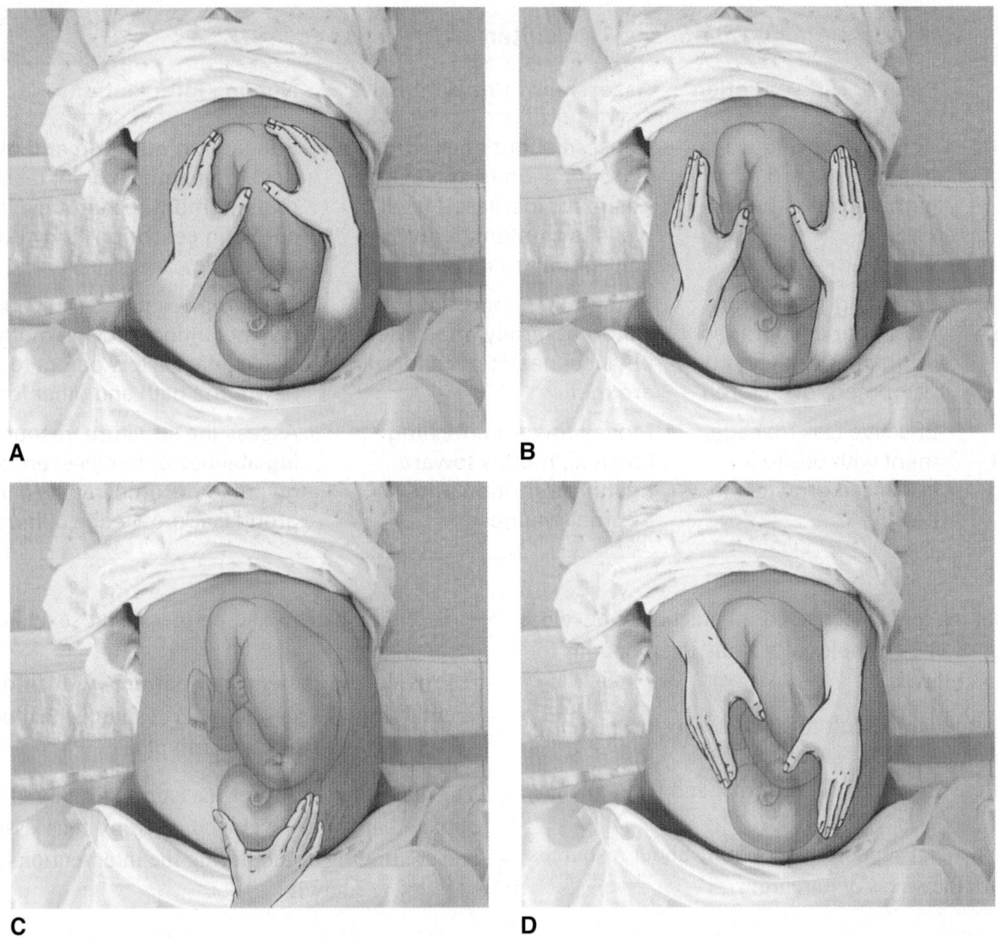

Figure 25.10 Leopold maneuvers. **A.** First maneuver. **B.** Second maneuver. **C.** Third maneuver. **D.** Fourth maneuver.

(Fig. 25.10D). Experienced practitioners usually only need to use the first and second maneuvers to locate the fetal heart rate and verify that the presenting part is the head.

Specialized Advanced Assessments: Abnormal Findings

Several disorders are specific to pregnancy, which require specialized care from a perinatologist or maternal-fetal medicine specialist. Because of the high-risk nature of these pregnancies, it is appropriate for the nurse practitioner (NP) or certified nurse midwife (CNM) to refer such patients to a higher level of care. Thorough and accurate assessment of disorders by the RN, NP, or CNM provide the best chance for early referral, intervention, and treatment, preventing negative outcomes for mother and baby. Common high-risk disorders of pregnancy are listed in Table 25.5 at the end of the chapter.

Diagnostic Reasoning

Nursing Diagnosis, Outcomes, and Interventions

When formulating a nursing diagnosis, it is important to use critical thinking to cluster data and identify patterns that fit together. Nursing diagnoses commonly used in the care of pregnant women include *Health-seeking behaviors*, *Readiness for enhanced parenting*, and *Readiness for enhanced family coping*. Table 25.4 provides a comparison of nursing diagnoses, abnormal findings, and interventions commonly related to pregnancy (NANDA International, 2009).

Nurses use assessment information to identify physical, developmental, and psychological outcomes for patients. Examples of some outcomes related to pregnancy include the following:

- Verbalizes decreased anxiety about the health of her fetus and herself
- Verbalizes improved family dynamics
- Shows appropriate weight gain patterns per trimester
- Reports increasing acceptance of changes in body image
- Demonstrates knowledge for self-management
- Seeks clarification of information about pregnancy and birth
- Reports signs and symptoms of complications
- Describes appropriate measures taken to relieve physical discomforts
- Develops a realistic birth plan
- Affirms desire to improve parenting skills
- Performs tasks needed for change
- States positive effects of changes made

After the outcomes have been established, nursing care is implemented to improve the status of the patient. The nurse

TABLE 25.4 Common Nursing Diagnoses Associated With Pregnancy

Diagnosis	Point of Differentiation	Assessment Characteristics	Nursing Interventions
Health-seeking behaviors	Actively seeking ways to move toward a higher level of health	Concern about environmental conditions on health status, desire for increased level of wellness, unfamiliarity with community resources	Educate on nutrition and overeating, develop exercise plan; teach stress management techniques. Instruct in smoking cessation; provide health screening.
Readiness for enhanced parenting	Providing an environment that encourages optimal growth and development of children	Emotional support of children, family attachment, physical needs of children are met	Use family-centered care, encourage positive parenting, provide mother-to-infant skin contact, allow parent to assist in newborn's bath and other forms of care.
Readiness for enhanced family coping	Effective task management with desire for enhanced growth and health	Moves toward enriching lifestyle, moves toward health promotion and optimal wellness	Assess the structure, resources, and coping abilities of families; encourage caregivers to become involved in support groups; acknowledge cultural influences.

uses critical thinking and evidence-based practice to develop the interventions. Some examples of nursing interventions for pregnancy are as follows:

- Assess the influence of cultural beliefs on the patient's perception of parenting.
- Teach the patient about normal maternal and fetal changes in pregnancy.
- Provide psychosocial support and teaching about resources for coping with the stress of parenting.
- Teach the patient and partner about sexual changes during pregnancy.
- Provide the patient and partner with information about childbirth classes and other resources that will aid them in creating a satisfactory birth plan.

The nurse then evaluates the care according to the patient outcomes that were developed, thereby reassessing the patient and continuing or modifying the interventions as appropriate. (Ackley & Ladwig, 2011).

Progress Note: Analyzing Findings

Michelle Sherman, a 21-year-old Native American, is visiting the clinic following a positive result using a home pregnancy test. She is accompanied by her male partner and their 22-month-old son. Michelle calls the hospital on a Sunday at 30 weeks' gestation and says she is afraid she is in labor, but that she knows it is too early for the baby to come.

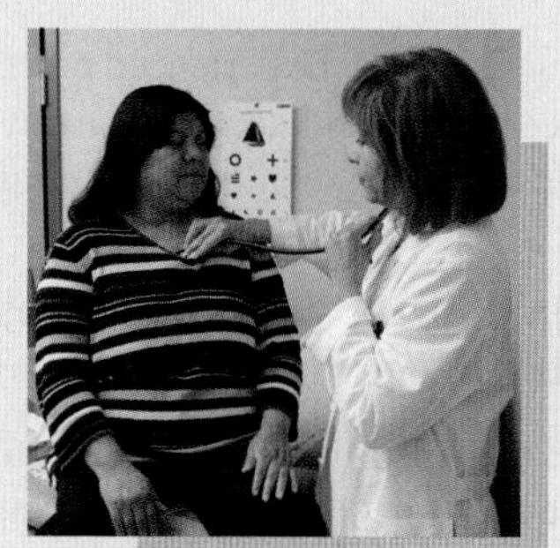

Subjective: Well, I am cramping. They have been coming all day. They are all over my tummy, and it feels kind of like menstrual cramps. They last about 20 seconds.

Objective: General exam unremarkable; pt well-nourished and groomed. Vital signs: T = 36.6°C (97.3°F), P = 71, R = 16, BP = 112/69. Lungs clear to auscultation bilaterally, HR regular; S1 and S2 audible with no extra heart sounds. Breasts tender with everted nipples. Dipstick urine negative. No vaginal discharge or lesions are noted. An ultrasound was done to confirm intrauterine pregnancy and dates. One fetus visible in the uterus. Penicillin (PCN) allergy.

Analysis: Pt to lab for blood draw; routine prenatal labs. Pt and partner happy about pregnancy. Physical exam WNL. Braxton-Hicks contractions present.

(case study continues on page 809)

Plan: Ultrasound today to confirm dates. Prenatal vitamins. Reviewed relief measures for nausea and warning signs for miscarriage. Return visit in 4 weeks. Provide reassurance that contractions are within normal limits. Michelle needs counseling regarding her diet, a diary to record everything she eats, a blood glucose monitor and instructions on its use, testing strips and lancets for the monitor, and a schedule for testing her blood glucose levels: fasting and 1-hour postprandial.

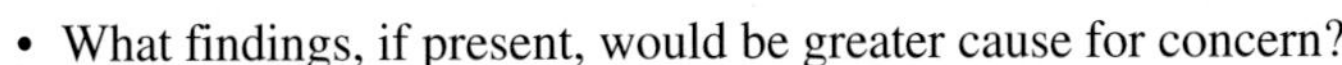

Critical Thinking Questions:

- What findings, if present, would be greater cause for concern?
- How can the nurse provide education and continued support for Michelle?
- What additional referrals and interventions are indicated?

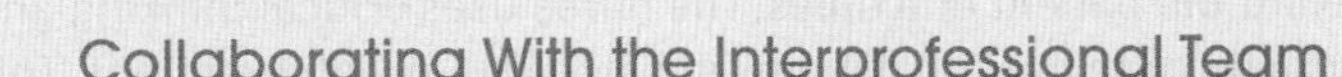

Collaborating With the Interprofessional Team

Michelle is tested for gestational diabetes at her prenatal visit because she is obese (body mass index [BMI] is 40.8). Further testing is done with a 3-hour glucose tolerance test. Results confirm that Michelle has gestational diabetes. The nurse also notes that recommended weight gain for Michelle is 15 lb or less for the pregnancy, but Michelle has already gained 26 lb (weight at last visit was 100 kg [221 lb]).

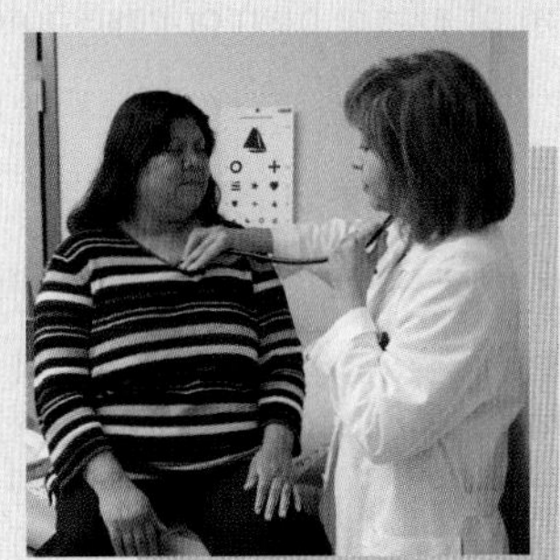

After the practitioner reviews laboratory values and determines the plan of care, the nurse calls Michelle to report the findings and conveys the recommendation that Michelle see a diabetes educator for nutritional counseling.

Below is the initial conversation between the nurse and the diabetes educator. The nurse uses SBAR to organize information for the educator.

Situation: "Michelle is a 21-year-old Native American. She is 30 weeks pregnant by LMP dates and ultrasound. Michelle did not pass her 3-hour glucose tolerance test today."

Background: "Michelle had a prepregnancy BMI of 40.8 so was given a 1-hour glucose test at her first visit, which was normal (122 mg/dl). Both her mother and her sister have Type 2 diabetes. So far, Michelle has gained about 12 kg (26 lb) since her initial visit."

Assessment: "Michelle has gestational diabetes and is at risk for Type 2 diabetes postpregnancy as evidenced by abnormal glucose test results and obesity."

Recommendation: "Michelle needs immediate counseling regarding her diet, a diary to record everything she eats, a blood glucose monitor and instructions on its use, testing strips and lancets for the monitor, and a schedule for testing her blood glucose levels: fasting and 1-hour postprandial. Goal glucose levels are 60–90 mg/dl fasting and 120 mg/dl or less at 1-hour postprandial. If Michelle cannot control her diabetes with diet or does not keep her follow-up visits with the diabetes educator, please let us know."

Evaluation: The educator answers Michelle's questions about the potential effects of diabetes on her and the fetus. The educator also explains that Michelle should be retested when the baby is 6 weeks old to ensure that Michelle has not developed Type 2 diabetes. The practitioner will review Michelle's recorded glucose values at her next prenatal visit. If diet is insufficient to control her glucose levels, insulin may be ordered.

(case study continues on page 810)

Critical Thinking Challenge

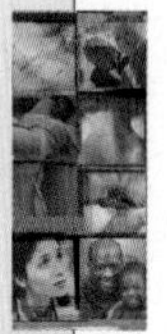

- What additional assessments should the nurse perform related to the diabetes?
- Why did the nurse choose a food diary as the assessment tool?
- How might Michelle's cultural background and age affect her perceptions of her gestational diabetes diagnosis?

Pulling It All Together

The nurse uses assessment data to formulate a nursing care plan with patient outcomes and interventions for Michelle. Outcomes are specific to the patient, realistic to achieve, measurable, and have a time frame for meeting them (Ackley & Ladwig, 2011). The interventions are actions that the nurse performs based on evidence and practice guidelines. After these interventions are completed, the nurse reevaluates Michelle and documents the findings in the chart to show progress toward the patient outcomes. The nurse uses critical thinking and judgment to continue or revise the diagnosis, outcomes, or interventions. This is often in the form of a care plan or case note similar to the one below.

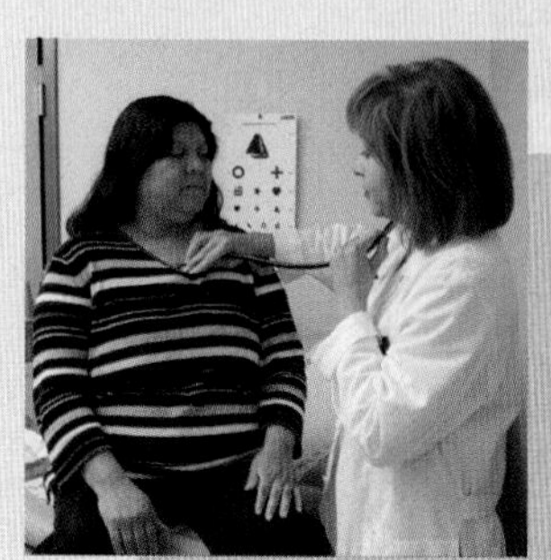

Nursing Diagnosis	Patient Outcomes	Nursing Interventions	Rationale	Evaluation
Health-seeking behaviors related to pregnancy	Patient will limit weight gain to around 7 kg (16 lb)	Assess the role that stress plays in overeating. Use nutritional guidelines to plan a diet high in protein, fiber, fruits, and vegetables.	People who eat under stress are more likely to gain weight and have elevated insulin and cortisol levels.	Goal has not been met. Patient has gained almost 12 kg (26 lb). Discuss changes that patient is willing and able to make in her diet. Refer to diabetes educator.

Applying Your Knowledge

Using the previous steps of diagnostic reasoning, organizing, and prioritizing, consider all the case study findings woven throughout this chapter. When answering the following questions, begin drawing conclusions and see how the pieces of assessment must work together to create an environment for personalized, appropriate, and accurate care.

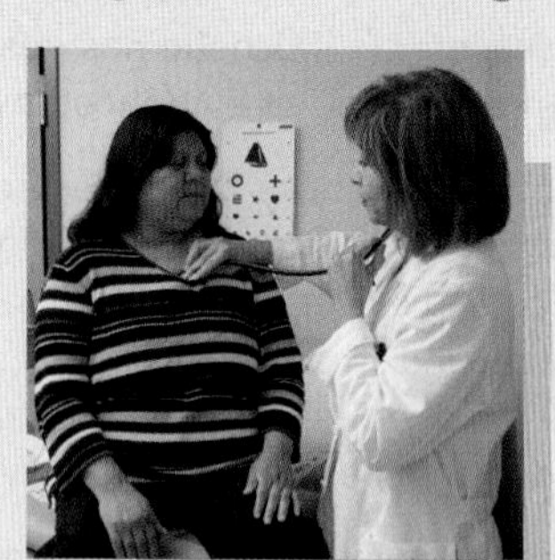

- What physical assessment data is the nurse responsible for gathering and assessing?
- What additional history does the nurse need to gather from Michelle today?
- What health promotion needs does Michelle have today? (Application)
- What findings would indicate that Michelle's condition is stable, urgent, or an emergency?
- What factors does the nurse need to consider to individualize Michelle's care?
- How will the nurse evaluate the success of health promotion and risk reduction for Michelle?

Key Points

- The due date is calculated using the Nagele rule. Subtract 3 months from the first day of the LMP and add 7 days or about a 40-week pregnancy.
- The role of the RN includes conducting the intake interview, performing triage, gathering preliminary data, conducting NSTs, and educating patients and families.
- Urgent conditions of pregnancy include ectopic pregnancy, pyelonephritis, preeclampsia, hemorrhage, and preterm labor.
- Health promotion issues for women who are pregnant include physical activity, recommended weight gain, avoidance of tobacco, prenatal vitamins, and breastfeeding.
- Some cultures and religions have important rituals related to birth. It is the nurse's responsibility to be aware of these and accommodate them whenever possible.
- Common symptoms of pregnancy include fatigue, morning sickness, round ligament pain, increased vaginal discharge, urinary frequency, breast tenderness, backaches, periumbilical pain, fetal hiccups, and Braxton Hicks contractions.
- A woman of average weight should gain 2 to 4 ½ kg (5 to 10 lb) in the first half of the pregnancy and about 1 lb a week for the remaining 20 weeks, for a total of 25 to 30 lb.
- Increased skin melanization occurs during pregnancy, resulting in linea nigra or melasma.
- In women of average weight, the fetal heartbeat may be heard with a Doppler sonometer by 10 to 12 weeks of gestation.
- Breast changes include enlargement, increased sensitivity, darkened areola, more prominent Montgomery glands, and more erect nipples.
- Signs of preeclampsia include elevated blood pressure, sudden edema, headache, visual changes, epigastric pain, and proteinuria.
- As the abdomen enlarges, the pregnant woman may develop striae gravidarum and linea nigra.
- Women may experience dyspnea toward the end of pregnancy as the growing fetus limits the ability of the lungs to expand.
- Cardiovascular changes of pregnancy include lower hematocrit, weight gain, elevated pulse, edema, and varicosities.
- Gastric reflux is common in pregnancy because of displacement of the stomach by the growing uterus.
- Musculoskeletal changes of pregnancy include relaxed cartilage, lower back pressure, and a waddling gait.
- Nursing diagnoses commonly related to pregnancy include *Health-seeking behaviors*, *Readiness for enhanced parenting*, and *Readiness for enhanced family coping*.

Review Questions

1. Michelle says that her last normal menstrual period was June 15. Using the Nagele rule, her EDD is
   A. September 8.
   B. March 8.
   C. March 22.
   D. January 22.

2. Michelle's fundal height measures 28 cm (11 in.). You expect the gestational age to be
   A. 20 weeks.
   B. 14 weeks
   C. 28 weeks
   D. 30 weeks.

3. A normal fetal heart rate as auscultated with a Doppler sonometer is
   A. 90 beats/min.
   B. 120 beats/min.
   C. 100 beats/min.
   D. 180 beats/min.

4. Which of the following conditions would be the highest priority to contact the health care provider about?
   A. Striae gravidarum
   B. Varicosities of the labia
   C. Contractions before 37 weeks
   D. Prominent Montgomery glands

5. A patient calls the provider's office to schedule an appointment because a home pregnancy test was positive. The nurse knows that the test identified the presence of which of the following in the urine?
   A. Estrogen
   B. Progesterone
   C. hCG
   D. Follicle-stimulating hormone

6. Which of the following symptoms is NOT an indicator of preeclampsia?
   A. Uncontrolled vomiting
   B. Headache
   C. Epigastric pain
   D. Hyperreflexia

7. The nurse is performing patient teaching about *normal* changes during late pregnancy. These include which of the following?
   A. Dark cloudy urine
   B. Waddling gait
   C. Vaginal bleeding
   D. Sudden edema

8. The nurse is caring for a patient who is admitted to the hospital with a possible ectopic pregnancy. Which of the following nursing actions is the priority?
   A. Monitoring daily weight
   B. Assessing for edema
   C. Monitoring the temperature
   D. Monitoring the blood pressure

9. The nurse assesses for possible complications of pregnancy. Which of these prompts referral to a perinatal specialist?
   A. Gastric reflux
   B. Previous cesarean procedure
   C. Oligohydramnios
   D. Anemia

10. A patient comes into the clinic for a scheduled NST when the nurse notes that the FHR tracing is nonreactive. Which of the following actions would be appropriate for the nurse to do *first*?
   A. Document the findings.
   B. Notify the provider.
   C. Change the mother's position.
   D. Instruct the patient to return to the clinic in 1 week for reevaluation of the fetal heart rate.

The Jensen suite offers these additional resources to enhance learning and facilitate understanding of this chapter:

- thePoint online resources, http://thepoint.lww.com/Jensen2e
- *Laboratory Manual for Nursing Health Assessment: A Best Practice Approach*
- *Pocket Guide for Nursing Health Assessment: A Best Practice Approach*
- *Lippincott DocuCare,* an electronic health record simulation software, http://thepoint.lww.com/docucare
- *Adaptive Learning | Powered by PrepU*, http://thepoint.lww.com/prepu

References

Ackley, B., & Ladwig, G. (2011). *Nursing diagnosis handbook: An evidence-based guide to planning care* (9th ed.). St. Louis, MO: Mosby.

American College of Obstetricians and Gynecologists (ACOG). (2011). Committee opinion no. 504: Screening and diagnosis of gestational diabetes mellitus. *Obstetrics and Gynecology, 118,* 751–753. doi: 10.1097/AOG.0b013e3182310cc3

American College of Obstetricians and Gynecologists (ACOG). (2013). ACOG Committee opinion no. 566: Update on immunization and pregnancy: Tetanus, diphtheria, and pertussis vaccination. *Obstetrics and Gynecology, 121,* 1411–1414. doi: 10.1097/01.AOG.0000431054.33593.e3

Bowen A., & Bickley, L. S. (2010). Assessing the woman who is pregnant. In T. S. Stephen, D. L. Skillen, R. A. Day, & L. S. Bickley (eds.). *Canadian Bates' guide to health assessment for nurses* (1st ed.). Philadelphia, PA: Lippincott Williams & Wilkins.

Bryant, A. S., Worjoloh A., Caughey A. B., & Washington, A. E. (2010). Racial and ethnic disparities in obstetric outcomes and care: Prevalence and determinants. *American Journal of Obstetrics and Gynecology, 202*(4), 335–343. doi: 10.1016/j.ajog.2009.10.864

Cunningham, F., Leveno, K., Bloom, S., Hauth, J., Rouse, D., & Spong, C. (2009). *Williams obstetrics* (23rd ed.). New York, NY: McGraw-Hill Professional.

Hale, T. (2012). *Medications and mother's milk: A manual of lactational pharmacology* (15th ed.) Amarillo, TX: Hale Publishing.

NANDA International. (2009). *Nursing diagnoses 2009–2011: Definitions and classifications*. West Sussex, United Kingdom: John Wiley & Sons.

National Coalition for Professional Education in Genetics. (2013). Family history for prenatal providers. In *Pregnancy health profile: A genetic risk assessment and screening tool.* Retrieved from http://www.nchpeg.org

Pagano, T. (2014). Understanding preterm labor and birth—the basics. Retrieved from http://www.webmd.com/baby/understanding-preterm-labor-birth-basics

Partridge, S., Balaya, J., Holcroft, C., & Abenahim, H. A. (2012). Inadequate prenatal care utilization and risks of infant mortality and poor birth outcome: A retrospective analysis of 28,729,765 U.S. deliveries over 8 years. *American Journal of Perinatology, 29*(10), 787–793. doi: 10.1055/s-0032-1316439

Ricci, S. (2013). Essentials of maternity, newborn, and women's health nursing (3rd ed.). Philadelphia, PA: Lippincott Williams &Wilkins.

Sengpiel, V., Elind, E., Bacelis, J., Nilsson, S., Grove, J., Myhre, R., . . . Brantsaeter, A. L. (2013). Maternal caffeine intake during pregnancy is associated with birth weight but not with gestational length: Results from a large prospective observational cohort study. *BMC Medicine,* 11, 42. doi: 10.1186/1741-7015-11-42

Siddique, J., Lantos, J., VanderWeele, T., & Lauderdale, D. (2012). Screening tests during prenatal care: Does practice follow the evidence? *Maternal and Child Health Journal, 16,* 51–59. doi: 10.1007/s10995-010-0723-3

United Nations Children's Fund. (2013). *Female genital mutilation/cutting: A statistical overview and exploration of the dynamics of change.* New York, NY: Author.

U.S. Department of Health and Human Services. (2010). *Healthy People 2020: Maternal, infant, and child health objectives.* Retrieved from http://healthypeople.gov/2020/topicsobjectives2020/objectiveslist.aspx?topicId=26

Walker, L. O. & Chesnut, L. W. (2009). Identifying health disparities and social inequities affecting childbearing women and infants. *Journal of Obstetric, Gynecologic, and Neonatal Nursing, 39*(3), 328–338. doi: 10.1111/j.1552-6909.2010.01144.x

World Health Organization. (2013). *Media centre fact sheet 241: Female genital mutilation.* Retrieved from http://www.who.int/mediacentre/factsheets/fs241

TABLE 25.5 Common High-Risk Disorders of Pregnancy

Preeclampsia
Pregnancy-specific syndrome; occurs in 3.9% of all pregnancies (Cunningham et al., 2009). Etiology unknown. Rarely occurs prior to 20 weeks' gestation. Greatly increases risk of maternal mortality and morbidity.

Predisposing factors: previous preeclampsia, multiple gestation, diabetes, obesity, age 35 years or older, African American race.

Symptoms include hypertension (compared with findings at baseline), proteinuria, headache, epigastric pain, visual changes, edema, and elevated liver enzyme levels.

Untreated preeclampsia progresses to eclampsia, characterized by seizures and vasospasm. Can cause infarcts of the placenta, endangering life of mother and baby.

HELLP Syndrome
*H*emolysis, *E*levated *L*iver enzymes, and *L*ow *P*latelets. A serious variant of preeclampsia; can be fatal to mother and baby. Requires immediate treatment, including delivery of baby.

Preterm Labor
Labor prior to 37 weeks' gestation, resulting in shortening or dilation of the cervix and engagement of the presenting part. Precedes preterm delivery. About 40%–45% of preterm births result from preterm labor (Cunningham et al., 2009).

Predisposing factors: Premature rupture of membranes, periodontal disease, chronic stress, previous preterm delivery, African American race, age less than 18 or greater than 35 years, chronic hypertension, low socioeconomic status, inadequate weight gain, multiple gestation, smoking, strenuous work, uterine or urinary tract infections.

Intrauterine Growth Restriction (IUGR)
Associated with increased morbidity and mortality of infant.

Predisposing factors: hypertension, late or no prenatal care, malnutrition, violence or abuse, preeclampsia, chronic stress, placental malformation, viral infections, multiple gestation, smoking, alcohol use, chromosomal or congenital anomalies of the fetus.

Polyhydramnios
Greater than 2,000 ml of amniotic fluid.

May be idiopathic or due to maternal diabetes, neural tube defects, fetal anomalies of the central nervous system or gastrointestinal tract, chromosomal deviations (Ricci, 2013).

Increases risk for maternal hemorrhage, placental abruption, fetal malpresentation, cord prolapse, and preterm labor.

Oligohydramnios
Less than 500 ml of amniotic fluid.

Associated with uteroplacental insufficiency and fetal renal anomalies (Ricci, 2013).

May result in poor fetal outcomes, including pulmonary hypoplasia, musculoskeletal malformations, cord compression/fetal distress.

Psychological Illness

Depression increases risk for low birth weight and preterm birth.

Medications used to treat psychological illness may not be safe for use in pregnancy.

26

Newborns and Infants

Learning Objectives

1 Demonstrate knowledge of anatomy and physiology of the newborn and infant.

2 List critical components of an acute assessment of the newborn and infant.

3 Identify important topics for health promotion and risk reduction related to the newborn and infant.

4 Collect subjective data related to the newborn and infant.

5 Collect objective data related to the newborn and infant using physical examination techniques.

6 Identify expected and unexpected findings related to the newborn/infant assessment.

7 Analyze subjective and objective data from assessment of the newborn and infant and consider initial interventions.

8 Document and communicate data from the newborn/infant assessment using appropriate terminology and principles of recording.

9 Consider age, condition, gender, and culture of the patient to individualize the newborn/infant assessment.

10 Identify nursing diagnoses and initiate a plan of care based on findings from the newborn/infant assessment.

Keri Meadows, who is a 1-month-old infant, is visiting the clinic today for her well-child checkup and hepatitis B immunization. She was born at term and has had no health problems. Her mother is breastfeeding her; they have adjusted well.

Keri is the first child in a two-parent family. The mother is a nurse who plans on returning to work in 2 months; the father is an accountant. Paternal grandparents live in the area and provide child care 1 day a week.

You will gain more information about Keri as you progress through this chapter. As you study the content and features, consider Keri's case and its relationship to what you are learning. Begin thinking about the following points:

- What is the expected growth for an infant each week for the first 6 months?
- Why is vitamin D supplementation important in a breastfeeding baby?
- What would you teach Mrs. Meadows to observe in Keri to know that she is "getting enough breast milk"?
- What factors could contribute to a slowed growth pattern in a newborn or an infant?
- What health promotion teaching would be important to discuss with Mrs. Meadows as Keri grows?
- How would you evaluate whether Mrs. Meadows is confident and comfortable in her knowledge of infant feeding and growth?

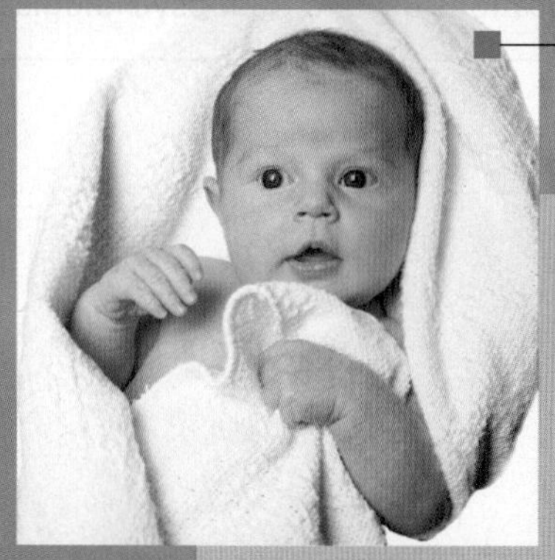

Infancy encompasses the first 12 months of life. A newborn (neonate) is an infant 28 days old or younger. This chapter examines health assessment of newborns and infants. It discusses important past and present health history and pertinent findings of the physical examination.

Because infants are preverbal and totally reliant on parents or guardians, the nurse must develop excellent observation skills and involve parents in assessment and care planning. For ease of comprehension, the term "parents" is used throughout this chapter to indicate one or both parents or a guardian.

Structure and Function

When assessing the individual child's physical, motor, and language development, it is important to determine whether the child is progressing steadily in these areas. Using rigid timetables to measure the child's development is not helpful and does not provide an accurate assessment. Milestones serve only as guidelines so that developmental delays can be identified early and appropriate interventions instituted.

Chapter 8 explores physical growth, motor, and language development milestones in detail. A brief review is presented in the following paragraphs.

Physical Growth

Physical growth and development that began in utero continue rapidly after birth. In fact, during the first year of life, the growth rate is more accelerated than at any other time in childhood.

Normal weight range for a full-term newborn is 2.5 to 3.3 kg (about 5 lb 8 oz to 8 lb 13 oz). Average length is 48 to 53 cm (19 to 21 in.). Most infants gain approximately 500 g to 1 kg/month (about 1 to 2 lb/month), double their birth weight by 4 to 6 months, and triple their birth weight by 1 year. By the end of the 12th month, most infants have increased their length by approximately 50% (Centers for Disease Control and Prevention [CDC], 2013). To determine the growth percentiles, weight and length (or height) should be plotted on the appropriate growth chart at each well-child visit and as indicated at interval visits.

Motor Development

Motor development refers to changes in the newborn's ability to control body movements. Motor development progresses in predictable patterns: cephalocaudally, central to distal, and gross to fine. For example, the infant develops head control before walking, can roll over before intentionally grabbing a toy, and can swat at a mobile before manipulating an object. Nurses assess newborn and infant motor development using standardized developmental screening tools. An example is the Denver II, which is described in more detail in the next chapter.

Language Development

Speech development begins with vocalizations and babbling. The infant learns language through listening, watching, and interacting with the environment. The spectrum of normal language development is wide. Language, psychosocial, and cognitive development of the infant are discussed in more detail in Chapter 8.

Cultural Considerations

Many families use home remedies to treat certain conditions. Ask the family if there are any home remedies their family finds helpful. If the parent describes a harmful practice (e.g., giving the infant a bottle of water with honey), then respectfully educate about possible consequences. Follow up by negotiating with the parent for a healthier way to meet the particular need that fits the family's culture.

Urgent Assessment

Urgent assessment of the newborn is performed immediately after birth. Because the newborn must adapt rapidly to life outside the womb, the nurse must quickly make several key assessments. The American Academy of Pediatrics (AAP), in collaboration with the American Heart Association (AHA), outlines critical components of the initial assessment in the Neonatal Resuscitation Program. The ABCs of resuscitation—airway, breathing, and circulation—are the same for infants as for adults; however, the assessments and interventions are modified to accommodate the infant's unique anatomical and physiological characteristics.

Immediately after birth, you must ask three key assessment questions about the newborn's health (American Academy of Pediatrics [AAP] & American Heart Association [AHA], 2011):

1. Was the newborn born at term gestation (37 weeks or greater)?
2. Is the newborn breathing or crying?
3. Does the newborn have good muscle tone?

If the answer to all questions is "Yes," then the newborn is adapting well and may be dried and placed skin-to-skin and receive care from the mother. If the answer to even one of these questions is "No," however, the baby needs stabilization resuscitation and should be placed under a preheated radiant warmer. (See the *Textbook of Neonatal Resuscitation* [AAP & AHA, 2011] for further information on neonatal resuscitation.)

Respiratory distress is common immediately after birth because of a poor transition from fetal to newborn life. Most emergency situations for the newborn involve respiratory decompensation. Signs of newborn respiratory distress include increased respiratory and heart rates, nasal flaring, intercostal/substernal retractions, grunting, and cyanosis. The first sign of respiratory distress in a newborn is often tachypnea, which is defined as a sustained respiratory rate of more than 60 breaths per minute. Moderate respiratory distress includes nasal flaring, retractions of the chest wall, grunting that was auscultated using a stethoscope, cyanosis on room air, and abnormal blood gas values. Severe distress is indicated by increasing work of breathing, deep retractions, grunting, and central cyanosis. Urgent assessment of the infant is the same as for a small child.

> **SAFETY ALERT**
> *Respiratory distress in the newborn and infant often progresses rapidly to severe distress, requiring positive pressure or mechanical ventilation. Nurses must intervene early at the first sign of distress to avert an emergency resuscitation, if possible.*

Subjective Data

Assessment of Risk Factors

History and Risk Factors	Rationale
Current Problems	
• What brings you to the clinic today?	This question elicits the presenting issue in a parent's own words.
• When was your baby last known to be well? (*Alternatively*: When was your baby last acting normal?)	These questions help identify how long any illness has been present and establishes normal state of health.
• How and when did the problem begin? What was the baby's health immediately before you noticed symptoms? • Has the infant been around anyone who has been not feeling well? • How has the illness progressed? • What symptoms does your baby have? In what order did they appear? • Does anything seem to make the symptoms better or worse? • What treatments or medications (including over-the-counter [OTC] and herbals) have you given? • Has your baby received medical attention for this illness before?	Questioning is designed to understand the course and progress of the present illness.
Family History	
Tell me a little bit about your family and your home.	This broad question helps you understand the socio-economic situation, living conditions, other family members, and the background and education level of the parents. Follow up with questions to obtain desired information if the broader question fails to elicit enough detail. Conversely, ask questions to gently refocus parents if they provide too much extra detail.
Personal History (Infant)	
• Were there any unusual circumstances or health problems during the pregnancy? • What was the duration of your pregnancy, type of labor and delivery, and type of anesthesia used for labor? • What was the Apgar score? Did the newborn require any resuscitation? • How much did he/she weigh? • Did the newborn spend any time in the neonatal intensive care unit (NICU) or did he/she go home with you? • Has your baby had any infections, illnesses, hospitalizations, or surgeries since birth? • How often has your baby had well-child checkups?	These questions help elicit the obstetrical and birth history to identify risk factors.

(table continues on page 817)

History and Risk Factors	Rationale
Medications and Supplements What medications is the infant taking (OTC preparations and vitamins)? Are immunizations up to date?	These questions help determine past medical history.
Family History Tell me a little bit about your family and your home.	This broad question may help you understand the socioeconomic situation, living conditions, other family members, and background and education of the parents. Follow up with questions to obtain desired information if the broader question fails to provide enough detail. Conversely, ask questions to gently refocus parents if they provide too much extra detail.
Risk Factors • Does your baby sleep on his/her back? • Does your infant sleep in his/her own bed? Own room? • Does your baby fall asleep with a bottle? • Have you childproofed your home for choking hazards. • Have you secured poisons? • Do you have a car seat approved for infants? Is it in the back seat? Rear-facing? • Have you learned cardiopulmonary resuscitation (CPR)? • Has your baby had any accidents or injuries?	These questions help identify risk factors and promote health. After you complete the assessment, you can perform patient teaching.

Risk Reduction and Health Promotion

Many health objectives apply to newborns and infants. Health promotion for parents of newborns and infants focuses on prevention, early detection of illness and developmental delays, and early intervention to optimize outcomes. As a nurse, you can help parents understand the importance of laying a foundation of healthy living and lifestyle choices that will allow the infant achieve his or her potential.

Health goals for newborns and infants and their families are as follows:

- Reduce the proportion of families that experience difficulties or delays in obtaining health care.
- Reduce hospitalization rates for pediatric asthma, uncontrolled diabetes mellitus, and immunization-preventable pneumonia and influenza.
- Reduce vaccine-preventable diseases.
- Reduce deaths caused by poisonings.
- Reduce deaths caused by suffocation and sudden infant death syndrome (SIDS).
- Increase the percentage of healthy full-term infants who are put down to sleep on their backs.
- Increase use of child restraints.
- Reduce residential fire deaths.
- Reduce occurrences of drowning.
- Reduce maltreatment and fatalities of children subsequent to maltreatment.
- Ensure appropriate newborn bloodspot screening, follow-up testing, and referral to services.
- Increase the proportion of mothers who breastfeed.
- Reduce growth retardation among low-income children younger than 5 years of age.
- Reduce the proportion of children and adolescents who have dental caries in their primary and permanent teeth.
- Reduce the proportion of nonsmokers exposed to environmental tobacco smoke.

U.S. Department of Health & Human Services (2013)

Infants should have regular examinations with a pediatrician or another health care professional with specialized pediatric training, such as an advanced practice registered nurse. Ideally, parents schedule an initial visit before the baby is born. At this visit, the primary care provider obtains family and prenatal history, gives anticipatory guidance, inquires about the chosen feeding method, and encourages breastfeeding.

After birth, the AAP recommends well-child visits at 3 to 5 days of age, by 1 month, and then at 2, 4, 6, 9, and 12 months. This frequency gives the primary care provider an opportunity to identify potential developmental delays and other health problems, continue anticipatory guidance, and give immunizations on schedule.

As the nurse, you will need to perform a risk assessment to plan for care and teaching. Anticipatory guidance for parents of newborns and infants focuses on safety. Parents require anticipatory guidance to avert preventable injury and illness. Most unexpected deaths during infancy are related to injury, SIDS, respiratory arrest, or near-drowning. The leading cause of injury-related death for infants is choking and suffocation (AHA, 2014). Major teaching topics include safe sleep habits, choking prevention, normal crying, immunization schedules, child safety car seats, CPR training for parents, poison control, breastfeeding, and preventing baby bottle tooth decay.

Safe Sleep Habits

Establishing safe sleep habits for infants helps prevent SIDS. The infant should not sleep on the same bed in which an adult is sleeping. The AAP recommends a separate but nearby cool sleeping environment. Infants should always be placed on their backs to sleep (Fig. 26.1). The mattress should be firm. Pillows, soft toys, excessive blankets, and bedding should not be in the crib when the infant is asleep. It is too easy for the infant's tiny face to be covered inadvertently and for the infant to be smothered. Pacifier use during sleep has been associated with a reduction in SIDS after breastfeeding is well established at approximately 1 month of age (AAP, 2012a).

Choking

Choking is the number one cause of unintentional deaths in infants (AHA, 2014). To prevent choking, parents should remain vigilant about the environment and remove choking hazards. Advise parents to get down on their hands and knees and survey the environment from the infant's perspective. Any small object within the infant's reach is a possible choking hazard. Anything that can fit in the infant's mouth or be inhaled should be removed from the infant's reach. Examples include balloons, toys with small parts, safety pins, small balls, broken crayons, coins, and so on.

Certain foods can increase the risk for choking. Firm or round foods, such as hot dogs, seeds, grapes, and raw carrots and apples, should be cooked or chopped into tiny pieces before serving to an infant or a very young child. See Chapter 27 for further discussion regarding safeguarding the home for small children.

Cardiopulmonary Resuscitation Training for Parents

Inquire if the parents know CPR. Traditionally, NICUs teach parents infant CPR before discharge because these infants are at higher risk than healthy infants are for respiratory and cardiac arrest. Nevertheless, it is important for all parents and babysitters to know CPR. Many communities offer CPR classes for nominal fees. Another resource is *Infant CPR Anytime* (AHA, 2014). This self-directed learning kit, developed by the AAP in coordination with the AHA, contains a manikin for practicing CPR and a video demonstrating CPR that the learner can view and review, as needed.

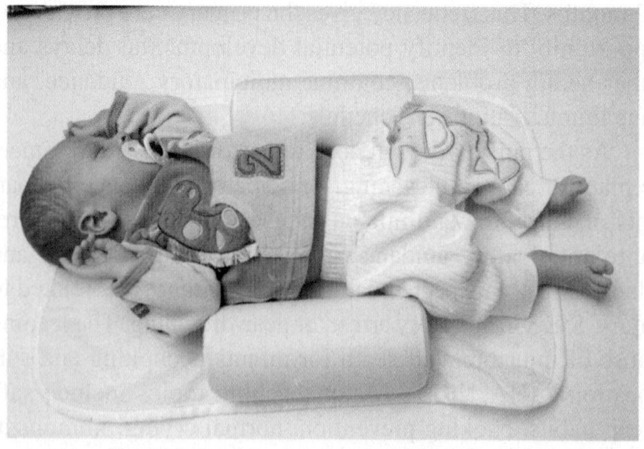

Figure 26.1 Placement of the infant on his back for sleep is a key prevention measure for sudden infant death syndrome.

Immunization Schedules

Newborns and infants need vaccines to protect them from diseases that can have serious consequences, such as seizures, brain damage, blindness, and even death. The CDC, the AAP, and the American Academy of Family Physicians collaborate to provide a schedule of immunizations recommended for infants and children.

Because immunizations are normally administered in conjunction with routine checkups, determine whether parents are keeping regularly scheduled appointments. Next, check the immunization record. The initial record is typically provided to parents before the newborn is discharged home when the first immunization is given. If the record is not up-to-date, ask the parents whether they are familiar with the immunization schedule. Provide a schedule, if needed, and help the parents determine where they can go to have the infant immunized.

Parents should be informed that it is important for their infant to receive vaccines at the ages and times recommended to ensure the highest level of protection against vaccine-preventable diseases. A catch-up schedule is available on the AAP Web site for the infant who misses an immunization or gets behind schedule.

> **SAFETY ALERT**
>
> *Many parents are concerned about the safety of vaccines, and a few physicians do not subscribe to current scientific evidence about, and recommendations for, vaccination. However, the evidence supports the safety of currently recommended vaccines. The diseases for which vaccines are protective can cause serious harm and even death. Encourage concerned parents to explore the evidence from the CDC and AAP.*

Child Safety Car Seat

It is important to ask the parents how the infant is secured when riding in the car. Is a car seat used? If so, is the restraint approved for use by infants? Is the restraint secured in the front or the back seat? General guidelines recommend a rear-facing seat until 2 years of age. Children 2 years of age or older who have outgrown the rear-facing weight or height limit should use a forward-facing car seat. Anytime an infant or a child younger than 4 years of age is in the car, the child should be restrained in a car seat for safety (Fig. 26.2). More detailed recommendations are listed on the AAP Web site. The article "Car Safety Seats: A Guide for Families 2014" available on the AAP Web site can be printed and given to parents for reference.

Poison Control

Ask the parents how they have secured medications, cleaning compounds, and other chemicals in the home. It is important to explain that safety locks should be placed on cabinets

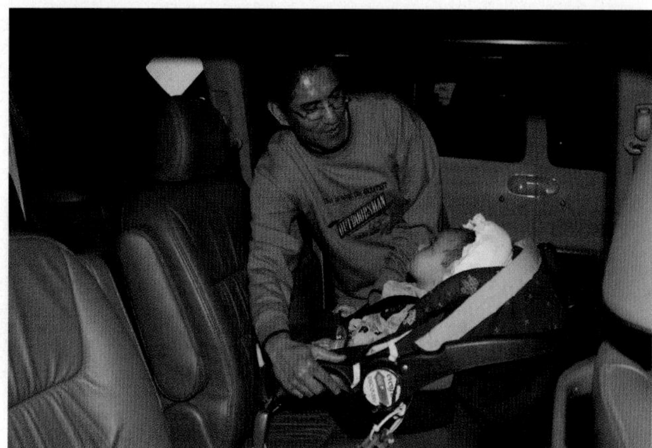

Figure 26.2 Infants should be in an appropriate-sized car seat in the back seat of the vehicle.

located close to the floor and that it is wise to put medication and other toxic chemicals in high locked cabinets. Ask whether emergency numbers are posted near all phones in the home and included on the parents' cell phones. The toll-free poison control number 1-800-222-1222 should be included in the list of emergency numbers.

Breastfeeding

Ask the mother if she is breastfeeding. If she is, determine how it has been going and how long she plans to continue. If the mother has already returned to work, ask whether she feels comfortable pumping her breasts at work and whether she has access to a private place where she can do this. Many companies are becoming "breastfeeding-friendly" work sites, providing private spaces and adequate time for pumping and refrigeration for pumped breast milk. Alternately, some employers allow the baby to be brought to the workplace or the woman to go home to feed the infant.

Breast milk is the best food for the growing infant. For the first 6 months, it is the only food that the infant needs, followed by continued breastfeeding as other food is introduced. Ideally, every baby should be breastfed for the first year of life or longer as mutually desired by mother and infant (AAP, 2012a). Iron-fortified infant formula is an acceptable alternative for mothers who cannot or choose not to breastfeed. Caution the parents that whole cow's milk is not an appropriate food for children younger than 1 year of age.

> *SAFETY ALERT*
>
> *Honey should not be given to infants. It is a known reservoir for the bacterium that causes botulism. The spores the bacteria produce make a toxin that can cause infant botulism, a serious form of food poisoning. The toxin affects the infant's neurological system and can lead to death.*

The breastfeeding mother's increased daily energy need of 500 kcal/day can be met by a modest increase in a well-balanced diet. There is no routine recommendation for maternal supplementation during lactation (AAP, 2012a). However, many providers recommend continued use of prenatal vitamins during lactation. The current recommendation for all breastfeeding infants is to provide vitamin D supplementation (AAP, 2012a).

Formula Feeding

Ensure that parents who chose to use commercially prepared formula have sufficient safety information. Commercial formula is designed to meet the basic nutritional needs of infants for their first year of life, in combination with solid foods from 6 to 12 months of age.

The AAP recommends that iron-fortified formulas be used for infants. These formulas are considered acceptable nutrition substitutes when breastfeeding is not chosen or not possible. Formulas are typically available in forms that include ready-to-feed liquid concentrate and also as a powder. For optimal infant health, formula must be prepared and stored according to package directions. Parents should be cautioned to read labels carefully for expiration dates and for preparation and storage instructions. Municipal water supplies are generally considered safe for mixing formula and washing bottles and nipples. It is recommended that water be drawn from the cold tap and allowed to run for 30 seconds to decrease lead and other substances. If well water is used, the water should be tested to ensure that it does not contain high levels of nitrate or lead. Well water should be boiled for 1 to 2 minutes and cooled before mixing with formula and supplies should be boiled for 5 minutes after washing. Bottled water can also be used for formula preparation.).

> *SAFETY ALERT*
>
> *Microwaving a bottle of formula or breast milk should be avoided. Hot spots can develop, or hot steam may escape from the nipple hole, which may burn the infant.*

> *SAFETY ALERT*
>
> *Parents may be tempted to use cow's milk before 1 year of age or to add extra water to formula. Parents should be cautioned that this can harm the infant by causing illness such as water intoxication, malnutrition, or anemia. Parents should also be advised not to add cereal or medications to bottles.*

Tooth Decay

Ask parents about the infant's daily intake of sugar, especially frequent consumption of sugary drinks and snacks (e.g., soft drinks, punch, juice). Ask whether the infant is ever allowed to go to sleep with a bottle of milk, formula, juice, or other sugary drink. This practice can lead to a condition known as **baby bottle tooth decay**. The sugar sticks to the primary teeth and coats them. Bacteria in the mouth break down the sugars to use for food. As this breakdown occurs, the bacteria produce acids that attack the teeth and cause decay.

Some parents may not understand why the primary teeth are important. Unlike adult tooth decay, baby bottle tooth decay is most pronounced on the upper front teeth and is highly visible while the child's self-image is forming. In addition, if the primary teeth experience significant decay, they may require extraction. Because the primary teeth serve as placeholders for the secondary teeth, if they are lost too early, the secondary teeth may come in excessively crooked.

The AAP recommends that the first dental visit should occur at or near 1 year of age. The nurse should assess fluoride intake to avoid risk of dental carries from insufficient or excessive fluoride.

Common Symptoms

Common Newborn and Infant Symptoms

- Respiratory complaints and/or distress
- Fever
- Skin conditions
- Gastrointestinal distress
- Crying/irritability

Signs/Symptoms	Rationale/Abnormal Findings
Respiratory Complaints/Distress Has your baby had trouble breathing? Have you noticed any wheezing? Have there been any episodes in which he/she turned blue? Has your baby had a stuffy or runny nose? Does he/she have frequent colds? Is there an associated cough or sneezing? Is there any sputum production or secretions? If so, how much? Have you noticed any wheezing? What has been the infant's temperature pattern? Are immunizations up-to-date?	It is important to determine associated symptoms and to identify severity and possible causation. This knowledge will guide the focused assessment.
Fever In addition to the respiratory questions above, ask the following: • What has been the infant's temperature pattern? • Has he/she been exposed to anyone sick? • Has he/she traveled with the family recently? If so, where? • Has the infant been pulling on one or both ears? • *If bottle feeding*: When feeding the baby, do you hold the bottle or prop it? • Have you noticed any change in eating or behavior patterns, such as irritability or difficulty rousing? • Has your baby demonstrated any abnormal posturing? • Has your infant had any periods when he/she stopped breathing momentarily (apnea)? • Is there an unusual odor to the urine? • Does there seem to be any pain associated with urination? • What, if any, treatments or medications have been given?	Fever is associated frequently with infection, which can range in severity from mild to life-threatening. This line of questioning helps reveal risk factors for infection as well as possible causes. The primary care provider needs to determine whether the fever likely has a respiratory origin (hence the respiratory questions). Could it be an ear infection (pulling on the ears) or urinary tract infection? Are there symptoms of meningitis (posturing), or is a blood infection likely? Although you will not make a final medical diagnosis, these data will guide the nursing assessment and care planning (Ward, 2013).
Skin Conditions • When did the rash or hives begin? On what part of the body did it begin? Has it spread? If so, where? • Have you noticed the infant scratching? Has there been any oozing, unusual odor, or pus-type material associated with lesions? Has there been crusting or erosion? • Has there been a recent change in laundry detergents, soaps, or shampoos? • Has there been a change in the texture or luster of the hair or nails? • Is there an associated temperature elevation?	These questions help pinpoint possible causes. Many skin conditions have predictable patterns of spread, parts of the body affected, and associated symptoms, such as pruritus (itching). It is important to differentiate if symptoms are localized versus systemic or if there might be an infectious versus an allergic origin.

(table continues on page 821)

Signs/Symptoms	Rationale/Abnormal Findings
Gastrointestinal Distress • Has there been vomiting? Is it projectile? What color, and how much vomitus has there been? • When was the last bowel movement? Describe the stool pattern and consistency. Has the stool been watery or unusually hard? What is the color and amount? • When was the last time your infant had something to drink? Eat? • Have you noticed a yellowish color to your infant's skin? • Does the child seem to be in pain? Has there been a fever?	Gastrointestinal symptoms can be associated with a wide range of conditions. In addition, infants can become dehydrated very quickly in the presence of vomiting or diarrhea.
Crying/Irritability • What are the circumstances of crying? Is there a pattern to the crying? Have you found a way to calm the infant? • Tell me about the infant's eating patterns. • When was the last bowel movement? Has the pattern of bowel movements changed? How many wet diapers in a day? • What has been the infant's temperature? • Has the infant been exposed to anyone who was sick? Are any other friends or family members currently ill? If so, what is the illness? • What is the infant's activity level?	Crying and irritability are nonspecific symptoms implicated in conditions that range in severity from minor to life-threatening. It is important to identify associated symptoms because this will guide the primary care provider's choice of diagnostic tests (Simon, 2009).

Therapeutic Dialogue: Collecting Subjective Data

The nurse's role in subjective data collection is to gather information to improve the patient's health status and to help determine the cause of the current symptoms. Remember Keri, who was introduced at the beginning of this chapter. This 1-month-old infant is visiting the clinic today for her well-child checkup and hepatitis B immunization.

The nurse uses professional communication techniques to gather subjective data from the mother, Diane Meadows.

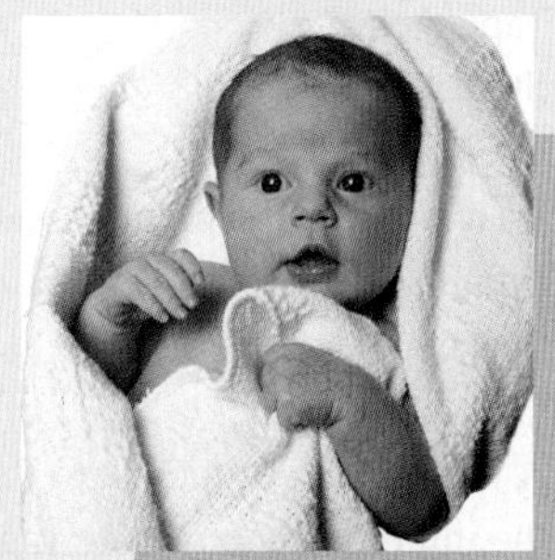

Nurse: Good morning, Mrs. Meadows. I am Keri's nurse for today. I see you have Keri wrapped up snugly for the cold weather we're having!

Mrs. Meadows: Yes, it's cold out.

Nurse: I will be asking you a few questions as part of the comprehensive assessment today and I will be performing a physical examination of Keri. Before we get started, do you have any concerns or questions you would like to discuss today?

Mrs. Meadows: No, but I'll ask if I have any.

Nurse: Great. Now during the first few weeks of life, the parents and baby are getting to know one another and establishing routines. What is Keri's routine at home?

Mrs. Meadows: She goes to bed around 8: 30 PM and wakes up around 8 AM but is up twice during the night. During the day, she nurses every 2–3 hours. Do you think that she's getting enough milk?

(table continues on page 822)

Nurse: It looks like Keri is growing nicely. That usually means that she is getting plenty of milk. Please tell me about your breastfeeding experience. (Waits for Mrs. Meadows to describe her experience.) How frequently is Keri nursing? Is Keri having any problems latching on?

Critical Thinking Challenge

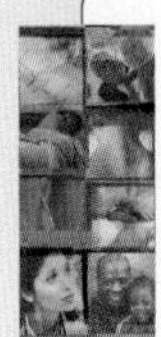

- What strategies does the nurse use to gather and share information?
- What techniques might the nurse use to normalize the experience of a new parent and open the door for therapeutic communication?
- What feelings might the nurse explore related to breastfeeding and attachment?

Objective Data

After completing subjective data collection with the parent holding the infant, collect equipment and prepare for the objective assessment. Well-child assessments include head-to-toe physical examinations, but the order is altered for infants, saving the least comfortable portions for last.

Equipment

Equipment that should be readily available includes the following:

- Tape measure
- Stethoscope
- Thermometer
- Watch or clock with a second hand
- Infant scale
- Otoscope
- Ophthalmoscope
- A pacifier, if acceptable to the parent, may help keep the infant from crying during the examination.

Preparation

The examination should be performed in a warm well-lit area. The environment should be comfortable, free from drafts, and quiet. There should be a place for both parent and nurse to sit while obtaining the history and performing parts of the examination that can be completed with the infant on the parent's lap.

After washing your hands, ensure that the parent and infant are comfortable. Introduce yourself and explain what the parent can expect. Commenting on positive features of the infant may help put the parent at ease. Engage the baby with friendly conversation while the parent continues to hold him or her. Sit at eye level and do not tower above the family, a stance that may be viewed as threatening. It may be helpful to have a soft toy to offer the infant while you obtain the health history from the parent.

Warm your hands by placing them in warm water before touching the infant. This can be accomplished in conjunction with washing the hands just before the examination. Likewise, warm the stethoscope with your hands before placing it on the infant's skin. If the infant is older, let him or her hold the stethoscope and demonstrate listening to the heart on the parent to prepare the infant for what to expect. These measures can decrease the infant's stress during the examination.

Comprehensive Physical Assessment

Physical assessment skills of observation, palpation, and auscultation are frequently used during the examination. The physical examination typically is not completed in a head-to-toe fashion, as for adults. Order varies depending on the infant's developmental level, temperament, and individual needs. Nevertheless, the approach should be systematic to minimize the omission of parts of the examination.

Physical assessment generally begins by observation of general appearance, overall skin color, level of activity, breathing pattern, posture, and tone. The most invasive techniques (i.e., assessment of tonsils, uvula, and ears) generally should be done at the end. If the infant is asleep or quietly alert, then count the respirations and listen to the heart, lungs, and abdomen before performing other parts of the examination that may disturb the infant and cause crying, which will disrupt your ability to hear clearly.

Two comprehensive assessments specific to newborns are the **Apgar score assessment** and the initial newborn assessment (including gestational age and reflexes). The Apgar score is a widely used rapid assessment of a newborn's health and well-being at birth and is one of the first newborn assessments the nurse makes. A complete head-to-toe assessment of the newborn occurs sometime after the first hour or after a breastfeeding attempt has occurred and is similar to that for older infants. Uninterrupted mother/infant skin-to-skin contact for the first hour after birth is recommended; therefore, all nonessential assessment tasks should be delayed until after this bonding time has occurred.

Gestational age is established by incorporating both obstetric and initial neurological findings of the newborn.

Technique and Normal Findings	Abnormal Findings
Apgar Score (Newborn) The Apgar score consists of five physiological components. Each component is assigned a score of 0, 1, or 2 for a possible total score of 10 (Table 26.1). The score is calculated at 1 minute and again at 5 minutes of life. It is not used to guide resuscitation efforts; resuscitation, if needed, is typically begun well before the 1-minute Apgar is scored. *A score of 7–10 indicates a vigorous newborn adapting well to the extrauterine environment.*	If the 5-minute score is less than 7, continue to score every 5 minutes up to 20 minutes until the score is above 7, the newborn is intubated, or the newborn is transferred to the nursery. A score of 4–6 indicates the newborn is moderately depressed, and 0–3 indicates severe respiratory depression and requires observation and care in a NICU.
Gestational Age (Newborn) During pregnancy, gestational age is calculated from the date of the last menstrual period or by results of an early sonogram. After birth, physical characteristics and neuromuscular assessment are performed at initial physical examination to evaluate gestational age. The New Ballard Score Maturational Assessment of Gestational Age tool (Fig. 26.3), commonly used in newborn nurseries, is most accurate if used between 10 and 36 hours of age. The examination is separated into two parts: neuromuscular maturity assessment and physical maturity assessment. *The New Ballard score ranges from −1 to 4 or 5 for each criterion. Possible totals range from −10 to 50, or a gestational range of 20–44 weeks. An increase in the score by 5 increases the age by 2 weeks.* Scores from both sections are added together to determine gestational age.	The New Ballard Score includes extremely premature newborns and has been refined to improve accuracy in more mature newborns.
General Survey Begin the general survey, keeping in mind the age of the infant in months and the correlated expected development. Continue to collect data through observation during the entire visit. The healthy infant has good muscle tone, a symmetrical appearance, and appears well. Respirations are unlabored with no signs of acute distress. Notice interactions between the infant and parent. If stranger anxiety is present, perform as much of the examination as possible with the infant on the parent's lap. The parent picks up on cues from the infant. The infant appears alert and engaged in the environment, unless sleeping. A normal variant is stranger anxiety that begins around 9 months.	The infant appears listless and uninterested in interaction. The parent pays little attention to the infant and does not pick up on cues, such as stress or readiness for interaction. Make note of any unusual odors. Certain diseases, such as phenylketonuria, maple syrup urine disease, and diabetic acidosis, are associated with characteristic odors (see Table 26.5 at the end of this chapter). Poor hygiene or inappropriate dress for the weather should alert you to watch for other signs of neglect.

(table continues on page 824)

TABLE 26.1 Apgar Scoring System

	0	1	2
Heart rate	Absent	Slow; below 100 beats/min	More than 100 beats/min
Respiratory effort	Absent	Slow or irregular	Good crying
Muscle tone	Limp	Some flexion of extremities	Active motion
Reflex irritability (response to catheter in nostril)	No response	Grimace, frown	Cough or sneeze
Color	Blue or pale	Body pink, extremities blue	Completely pink

NEUROMUSCULAR MATURITY

NEUROMUSCULAR MATURITY SIGN	SCORE −1	0	1	2	3	4	5	RECORD SCORE HERE
POSTURE								
SQUARE WINDOW (Wrist)	>90°	90°	60°	45°	30°	0°		
ARM RECOIL		180°	140°–180°	110°–140°	90°–110°	<90°		
POPLITEAL ANGLE	180°	160°	140°	120°	100°	90°	<90°	
SCARF SIGN								
HEEL TO EAR								
							TOTAL NEUROMUSCULAR MATURITY SCORE	

SCORE

Neuromuscular ____

Physical ____

Total ____

MATURITY RATING

Score	Weeks
−10	20
−5	22
0	24
5	26
10	28
15	30
20	32
25	34
30	36
35	38
40	40
45	42
50	44

PHYSICAL MATURITY

PHYSICAL MATURITY SIGN	SCORE −1	0	1	2	3	4	5	RECORD SCORE HERE
SKIN	sticky, friable, transparent	gelatinous, red, translucent	smooth, pink, visible veins	superficial peeling and/or rash, few veins	cracking pale areas, rare veins	parchment, deep cracking, no vessels	leathery, cracked, wrinkled	
LANUGO	none	sparse	abundant	thinning	bald areas	mostly bald		
PLANTAR SURFACE	heel-toe 40–50 mm: −1 <40 mm: −2	>50 mm no crease	faint red marks	anterior transverse crease only	creases ant. 2/3	creases over entire sole		
BREAST	impercep-tible	barely perceptible	flat areola no bud	stippled areola 1–2 mm bud	raised areola 3–4 mm bud	full areola 5–10 mm bud		
EYE-EAR	lids fused loosely: −1 tightly: −2	lids open pinna flat stays folded	sl. curved pinna; soft; slow recoil	well-curved pinna; soft but ready recoil	formed and firm instant recoil	thick cartilage, ear stiff		
GENITALS (Male)	scrotum flat, smooth	scrotum empty, faint rugae	testes in upper canal, rare rugae	testes descending, few rugae	testes down, good rugae	testes pendulous, deep rugae		
GENITALS (Female)	clitoris prominent and labia flat	prominent clitoris and small labia minora	prominent clitoris and enlarging minora	majora and minora equally prominent	majora large, minora small	majora cover clitoris and minora		
							TOTAL PHYSICAL MATURITY SCORE	

Figure 26.3 New Ballard Score Maturational Assessment of Gestational Age tool for use in screening newborns.

Technique and Normal Findings (continued)	Abnormal Findings (continued)
Vital Signs Axillary temperature measurement is appropriate for the newborn. After the first month of life, either axillary or tympanic temperatures are appropriate. First bath is delayed until temperature is stable. Temperature is taken again after the first bath. *Range of normal is the same as for adults: 36.5°–37°C (97.7°–98.6°F).*	Both elevated and decreased temperatures can signal infection in the newborn because the regulatory mechanisms are not fully mature. The newborn may cool during bathing and cannot shiver to raise heat.

(table continues on page 825)

Technique and Normal Findings (continued)	Abnormal Findings (continued)
Apical pulse and respiratory rate should be measured for a full minute each with the infant at rest. *Normal pulse range for the newborn is 110–160 beats/min, decreasing slightly to 80–140 beats/min for infants older than 1 month of age. Respiratory rate is 30–60 beats/min for newborns and 22–35 beats/min for infants.*	Tachycardia, bradycardia, tachypnea, and bradypnea are abnormal findings at rest. These terms describe findings that fall above or below the ranges listed.
Blood pressures are not measured routinely in the infant. If the blood pressures are taken, measure pressures in all four extremities. Make sure that the cuff fits appropriately. *Normal systolic pressures are 50–70 mm Hg for newborns and 70–100 mm Hg for infants older than 1 month of age.*	A difference between upper and lower extremity blood pressures may indicate coarctation of the aorta.
Pain Assess for pain (see Chapter 6). *The infant appears comfortable and not excessively irritable.*	Because the infant is preverbal, ask the parent to help interpret pain signals. Newborns cry indiscriminately when in pain. It may help to systematically eliminate other causes of crying, such as hunger or a soiled diaper.
Measurements Weigh the infant in supine position using an infant scale that is calibrated regularly. Place a protective covering on it, zero the scale, and then position the infant with your hands just above, but not touching, to prevent a fall (Fig. 26.4). 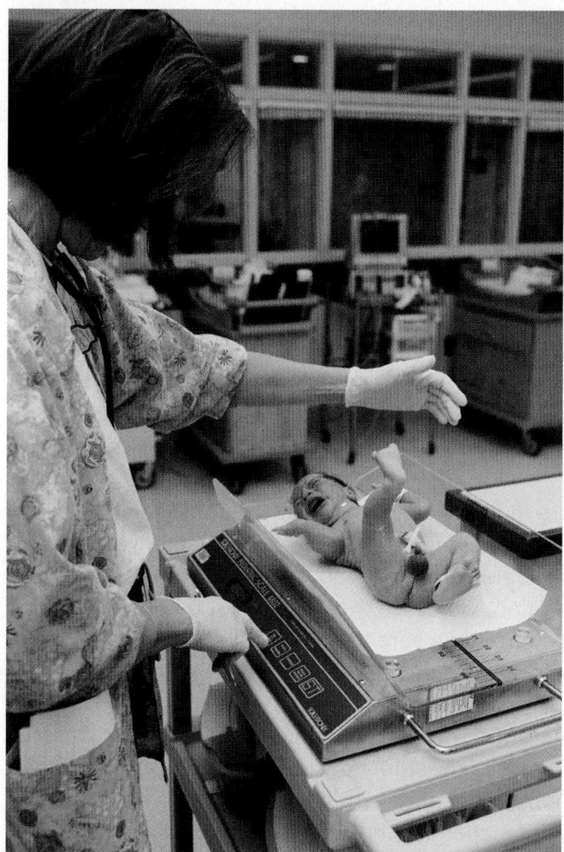 **Figure 26.4** Weighing the newborn.	When plotting measurements for premature infants, use the corrected age for comparison instead of the chronological age for at least the first 24 months. For example, if the infant was born at 30 weeks' gestation, the birth was 10 weeks before term (40 minus 10). So at 12 weeks (3 months) chronological or postnatal age, the infant's corrected age would be 2 weeks (12 minus 10). Length varies depending upon heredity. A small head may indicate microcephaly, whereas a large head may be from hydrocephalus or increased intracranial pressure. A small chest circumference may be from prematurity. **Clinical Significance** One measurement in time is not a basis for determining appropriate growth. Only by comparing measurements over time can growth delays be documented, because each infant grows as an individual influenced by genetics and environment.

(table continues on page 826)

Technique and Normal Findings (continued)	Abnormal Findings (continued)
Use the tape measure and carefully measure from the crown of the head to the heel. You may find it helpful to place the infant on the examination table and then use a pencil to place a mark at the infant's crown and another mark at the infant's heel (with the hip and knee extended). Use the tape measure to measure the length between the two markings. If done properly, this will give you an accurate measurement of length (Fig. 26.5). Plot the measurements on a standardized growth chart. *In general, the measurements are above the 10th percentile and below the 90th percentile.* Compare measurements with those taken during previous visits to ensure that the infant is gaining height and weight at a steady pace.	

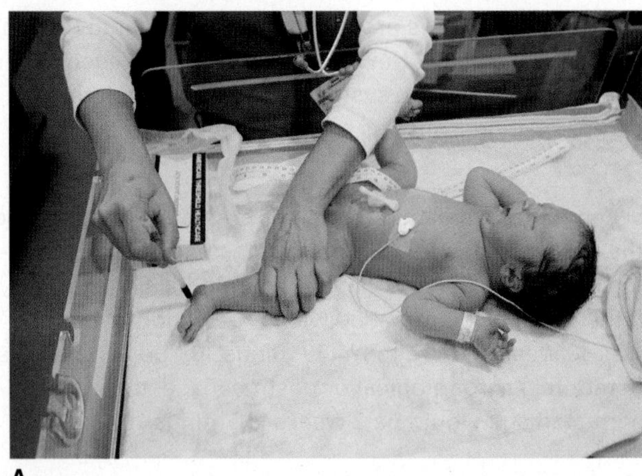

A

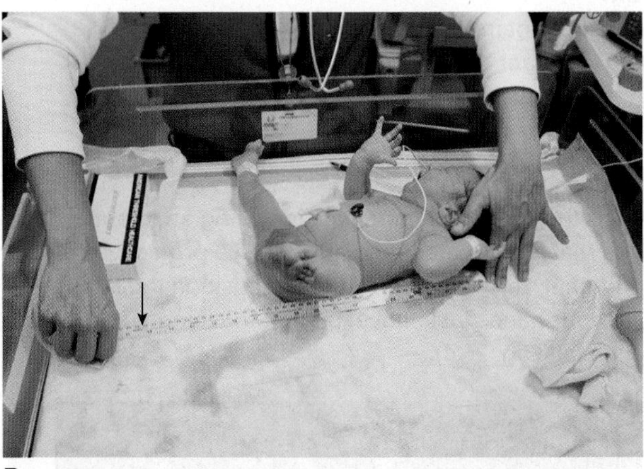

B

Figure 26.5 **A.** Marking the foot placement of the newborn with a pen. **B.** Using the tape measure to measure the length between the head and foot to arrive at an accurate length measurement.

Nutrition Inspect the general condition of the skin, hair, and nails. *A well-nourished infant has soft, supple skin and shiny hair.* Ask about urination and bowel movements. *On average, the infant getting enough to eat wets a diaper four to six times per day and has regular bowel movements that are soft and not watery.*	An indication that the infant is not eating enough is parental reports of fussing, crying, and not seeming satisfied after feeding. Other indications of inadequate nutrition include sallow skin tone with poor turgor, dry brittle hair and nails, losing weight or falling behind on growth charts compared with measurements from previous visits, and consuming less than 100 kcal/kg/day.
If the infant is bottlefeeding, ask the parent how many ounces per feeding and how many feedings per day. The infant is consuming approximately 100 kcal/kg/day. For example, if the infant weighs 4.5 kg (10 lb), then he or she should be eating approximately 450 kcal/day. Formulas for term infants contain 20 kcal/oz. Therefore, the infant in this example should be consuming 22–23 oz/day (4.5 kg × 100 kcal/kg/day ÷ 20 kcal/oz = 22.5 oz). If the parent is having difficulty determining intake and there is a question as to adequacy, ask the parent to keep a diary of the infant's intake for the next 3 days and report back.	Failure to thrive is described as weight that falls below the 5th percentile for the child's age (Rabinowitz et al., 2014). Evaluate for inadequate calorie intake, inadequate absorption, increased metabolism, or defective use of food sources. Be sure to differentiate inadequate intake from signs of acute dehydration, which include decreased skin turgor, sunken anterior fontanelle, dry mucous membranes, no tears, and an acutely ill appearance. Ask the parent to describe how infant formula is prepared in the home; improperly prepared formula is an important cause of inadequate nutrition. Safety issues related to infant formula preparation can be found on the U.S. Food and Drug Administration (FDA, 2014) Web site.

(table continues on page 827)

Technique and Normal Findings (continued)	Abnormal Findings (continued)
Mental Status In infants, mental status is determined by observing sleep states and behavior throughout the examination. Observe for developmentally appropriate behavior. *For example, an alert 1-month-old infant engages with the eyes when face-to-face with the parent or nurse and responds to the voice by turning toward the sound or by tracking with the eyes. An older infant reaches for an object the parent or examiner offers.* *During the first month or two, crying is a normal response to handling and undressing during a physical examination. Crying should stop with gentle rocking in the arms or while holding the infant against the shoulder. As the infant matures, the infant may smile and interact with you, as long as your movements are not sudden or threatening and your voice maintains a calm and reassuring quality.*	Interaction between infant and parent does not seem synergistic. The older infant is excessively clingy or does not warm up to the examiner after a period of interaction. Excessive irritability and inconsolable crying may be early signs of a change in mental status. Later signs may be a high-pitched cry, lethargy, or listlessness. **SAFETY ALERT** *If the infant cannot be aroused or does not move evasively when prodded during an examination, he or she is showing signs of a severe change in mental status. This infant needs immediate medical attention.*
Violence It is prudent to assess the parent for signs of domestic violence because children living in violent situations are much more likely to suffer abuse than children in households uncomplicated by violence (Giardino, Giardino, & Moles, 2014). *Normal parental findings include a relaxed, confident demeanor with appropriate affect, good grooming, and appropriate interaction with and concern for the infant. Normal infant findings include appropriate grooming and dress, no injuries, and willingness to engage with the parent and the nurse.*	Signs that should raise the index of suspicion for child abuse and neglect are listed in Table 26.6 at the end of the chapter. **Clinical Significance** Of all age groups, infants are the most likely to be abused. Shaken baby syndrome is the most common and severe form of infant abuse. A common trigger for shaking/abuse is inconsolable infant crying. More information is available through the National Center on Shaken Baby Syndrome (2014). Too often, health care providers do not suspect or report suspected abuse. Long-term psychological and emotional sequelae from abuse are cumulative (National Institute of Neurological Disorders and Stroke, 2013). When you report suspected abuse and thereby prevent future episodes, you have made a significant difference in a child's lifelong health.
Skin, Hair, and Nails Inspect newborn's entire body, including skin, skinfolds, scalp, hair, and nails. At birth, a newborn may be covered in vernix caseosa—a pasty, creamy cheeselike material—or this substance may appear only in skinfolds, the groin, or the axillae. Vernix develops in utero and serves as a protective coating; after 37 weeks' gestation, it gradually decreases. Skin color, birth marks, rashes, lesions, texture, and turgor should be noted. Shortly after birth, cyanosis of the hands, feet, and perioral area **(acrocyanosis)** are common findings that typically resolves in 24–48 hours (Fig. 26.6).	Generalized central cyanosis may be initially seen at the time of birth, when the newborn transitions from fetal to newborn circulation. Central cyanosis beyond the first few minutes after birth is an abnormal finding requiring immediate medical attention. Changes in color may be an initial sign of illness such as sepsis, cardiopulmonary problems, or hematologic disorders. Pallor or pale mucous membranes may indicate anemia.

(table continues on page 828)

Technique and Normal Findings (continued)	Abnormal Findings (continued)
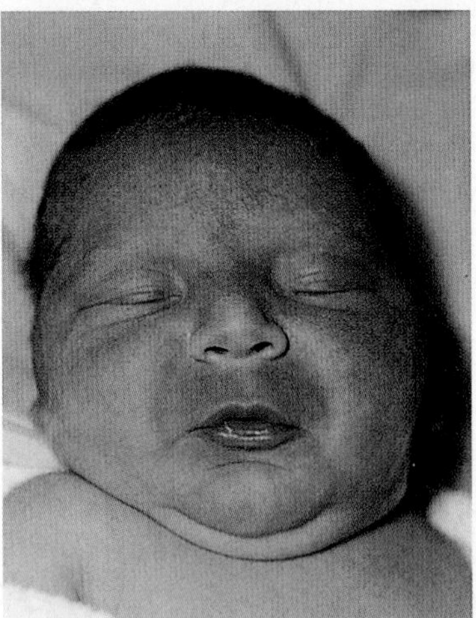 **Figure 26.6** Acrocyanosis in a newborn can show on lips, hands, and feet.	
Marked bruising of the face, often accompanied by petechiae, can occur during a difficult or precipitous delivery; this facial appearance can be mistaken for cyanosis. A quick color and skin assessment of rest of the body will make the diagnosis obvious. Bruising resolves within several days.	Localized petechiae may be present due to pressure during birth; widespread petechiae requires further evaluation.
Skin pigmentation depends on ethnicity and deepens over time. When the parents' skin tone is dark, the overall skin tone of the infant will typically be much lighter than the parents' at birth. Assessment of skin color changes is more difficult in African American and Asian newborns. If the tongue and mucus membranes of the mouth are pink, central cyanosis is not present.	Yellow, jaundiced skin tones require further investigation. Jaundice results from the inability of the newborn's immature liver to conjugate bilirubin. Accurate prediction of bilirubin levels is not possible through examination and requires further testing. Elevated bilirubin levels may be toxic to the growing brain.
Healthy infant skin is soft, not excessively dry, and supple. It snaps quickly back to original shape after gentle pinching. It is free of rashes, lesions, bruising, and edema. Normal skin variants (e.g., ***mongolian spots****, macular stains, spider nevi) are illustrated in Table 26.2.* Hair is soft and shiny. (Some infants shed hair in the first 2 months of life.) Nails are soft, of an appropriate length, and not growing inward. They are securely attached to the nail beds, which are pink (unless the child is dark-skinned).	Investigate and describe any rashes, lesions, or bruising. Note whether rashes or lesions are macular, patchy, petechial, or vesicular. Is there excoriation from scratching? Does the skin seem sensitive to touch? Is edema present? Are any nails lifting off the nail bed? Are nails dry and brittle? Areas of inflammation around nails with nails poking into the skin suggest ingrown nails. Poor elasticity and tenting of the skin when lightly pinched over the calf muscles and on the abdomen are associated with dehydration. Periorbital edema has various causes, such as crying, allergies, renal disease, or hypothyroidism. Dependent edema may occur with renal or cardiac disease. Multiple bruises in varied stages of healing, well-demarcated lesions, or bilateral burns may indicate physical abuse. See Table 26.7 at the end of this chapter for abnormal skin conditions.

(table continues on page 830)

TABLE 26.2 Normal Skin Variants in Newborns and Infants

Mongolian Spots

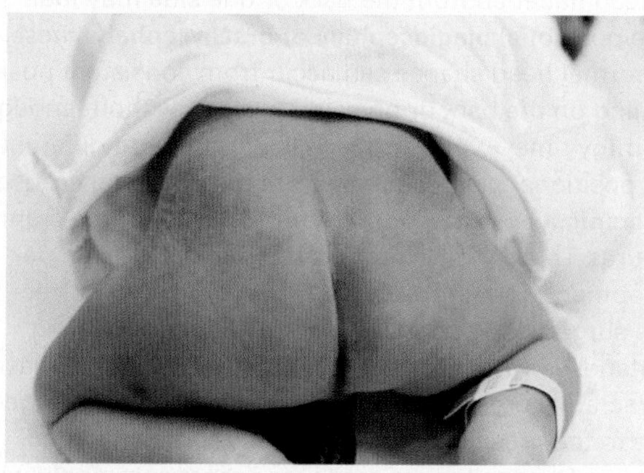

These bluish pigmented area(s) on the lower back or buttocks are common in infants of Asian, African, or Hispanic descent.

Macular Stains

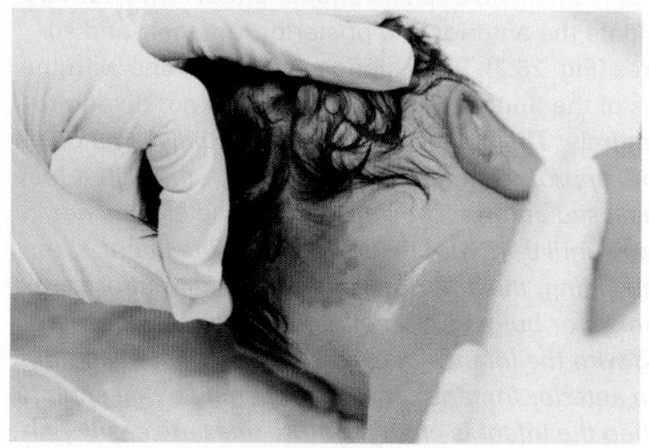

Also known as "stork bites," these capillary malformations appear on the eyelid(s), between the eyebrows, or on the nape of the neck. They tend to fade within 1 or 2 years.

Spider Nevus

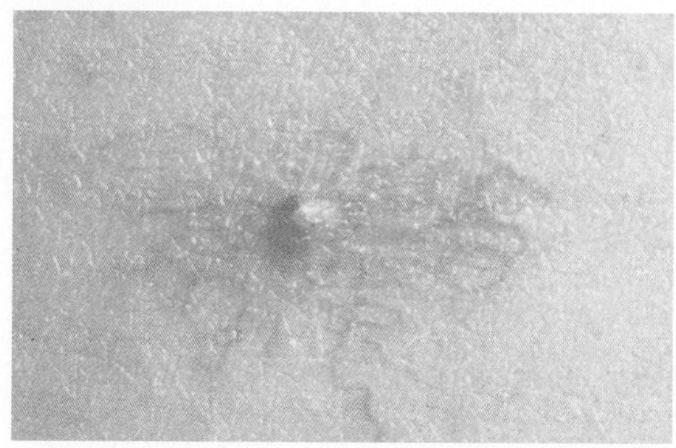

This benign lesion has a central arteriole from which thin-walled vessels radiate outward like spider legs. The lesion blanches when compressed.

Milia

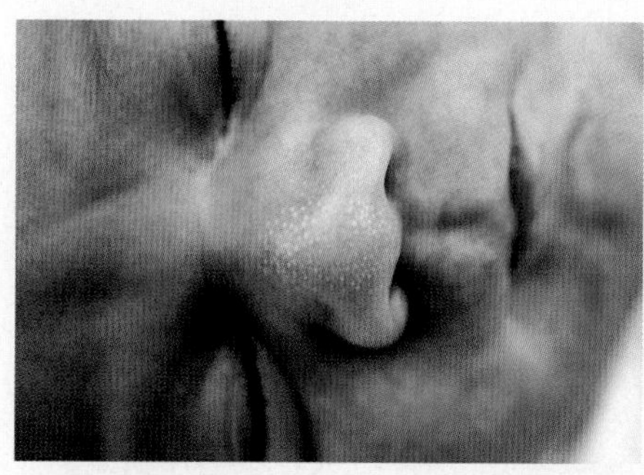

They occur when dead skin cells become trapped in small pockets at the surface of the skin or mouth. They are quite common in newborn infants.

Erythema Toxicum

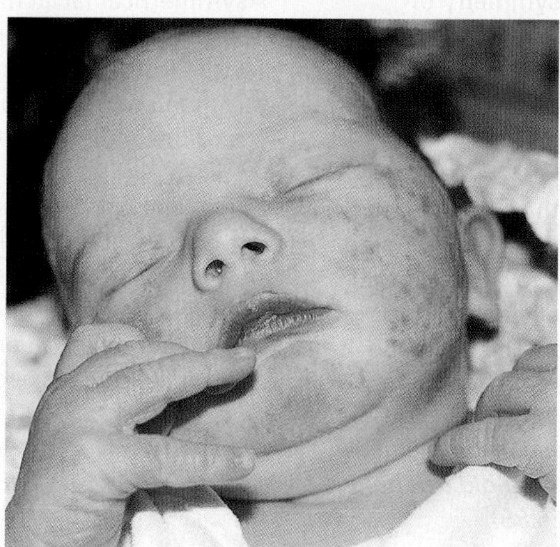

Normal variation with blotchy red spots on the skin and overlying white or yellow papules or pustules. Usually resolves in 2 weeks.

Technique and Normal Findings (continued)	Abnormal Findings (continued)
Head and Neck Assess the head size and shape. Check for symmetry. Palpate the anterior and posterior fontanels and sutures (Fig. 26.7). Trace along each suture line with the tips of the fingers to ensure they have not fused prematurely. *The posterior fontanelle usually is palpable until approximately 3 months of age, although it may be closed at birth. The anterior fontanelle does not close until 9–18 months of age. With the infant at rest and sitting, the anterior fontanelle is flat rather than sunken or bulging. Sometimes, pulsations correlating with the infant's pulse can be felt while palpating the anterior fontanel. The fontanel may bulge slightly when the infant is crying. Suture lines are easily palpable.* ***Craniotabes****, soft areas on the skull palpated along the suture line, are normal in infants, particularly those born prematurely.* 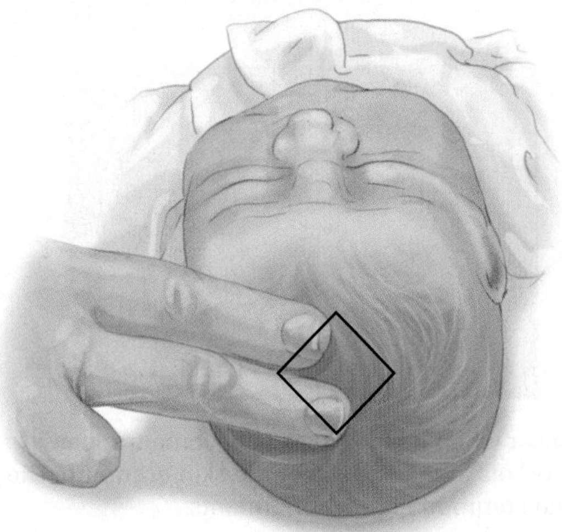 **Figure 26.7** Assessing the fontanelles and sutures.	A head flattened from the back or one side may indicate positional **plagiocephaly** or **brachycephaly**; these abnormal head shapes can occur from consistent positioning on the back or one side to sleep without enough "tummy time" while awake. It is important to differentiate positional plagiocephaly from plagiocephaly caused by **craniosynostosis**, or premature closure of the cranial sutures. This condition can lead to impaired brain development if several sutures are involved and corrective surgery is not done in a timely fashion. Bulging fontanelles with the infant at rest are a sign of increased intracranial pressure or **hydrocephalus**—head enlarged due to the presence of increased cerebrospinal fluid. Sunken fontanelles are associated most commonly with acute dehydration.
Observe the infant's face. Look for symmetry of movement.	Asymmetrical facial movements may indicate Bell palsy or a more serious heart condition. Bell palsy sometimes results from traumatic birth or delivery assisted by instrumentation (e.g., forceps). Bell palsy typically fades over time, although it may sometimes persist.
Check range of motion by rotating the head toward the right shoulder and then the left and then bending the neck so that the right ear moves toward the right shoulder and the left ear toward the left shoulder. The neck has full range of motion. Head lag and head control correlate with expected development. *For example, there is significant head lag in the newborn (Fig. 26.8A), whereas the 4-month-old can hold the head up without support (Fig. 26.8B).*	Persistence of head lag beyond the fourth month is a sign of developmental delay. Limited range of motion of the neck is associated with meningeal irritation. Webbing on the sides of the neck may indicate a congenital anomaly. An enlarged thyroid gland with a bruit is a sign of thyrotoxicosis.

(table continues on page 831)

Technique and Normal Findings (continued)	Abnormal Findings (continued)

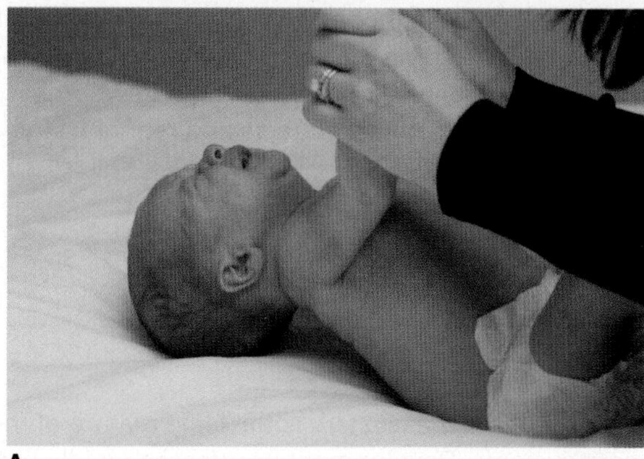
A

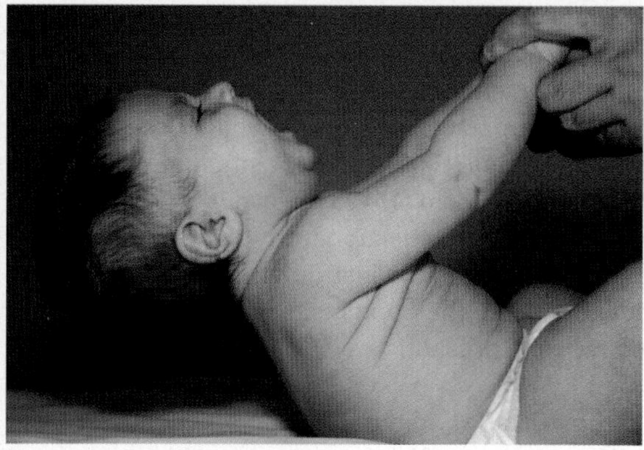
B

Figure 26.8 Head lag. **A.** The newborn has significant head lag. **B.** By 4 months of age, head lag has decreased noticeably.

Technique and Normal Findings (continued)	Abnormal Findings (continued)
Inspect and palpate the trachea. The trachea is midline and no swelling or masses are palpable. Auscultate for any bruits. No bruits are present. Palpate the clavicles in the newborn. The clavicles are smooth with no pain or crepitus. Palpate the following lymph node chains: preauricular (in front of the ear), suboccipital, parotid, submaxillary, submental, anterior and posterior cervical, epitrochlear (the area surrounding the elbow), and inguinal. Any palpable lymph nodes are small, mobile, and nontender.	A deviated trachea should be reported to the primary care provider. Crepitation over the clavicles in a newborn immediately after birth may indicate a fracture. By 3 weeks of age, a small lump may be palpated on the bone following a clavicle fracture. Treatment usually is not indicated.
Eyes Look for symmetry. Assess spacing of the eyes. Inspect the lids for proper placement and observe the general slant of the palpebral fissures. Inspect the inside lining of lids (palpebral conjunctivae), bulbar conjunctivae, sclerae, and corneae. Eyes are parallel and centered in the face. Ptosis is absent. Sclerae are clear and white.	Upward or downward slanting or small palpebral fissures can be normal; however, these findings are associated with some congenital conditions, such as fetal alcohol syndrome. Eyes too close together, too far apart, or positioned asymmetrically can occur with chromosomal abnormalities or illnesses. Exophthalmos is rare during infancy; its presence may indicate thyrotoxicosis. An eyelid that droops (ptosis) may indicate oculomotor nerve (cranial nerve III) impairment. It is important to correct any misalignment before age 4–6 years to prevent visual loss.
Assess ocular alignment to detect strabismus using the corneal light reflex test or cover test. *Some strabismus is normal in the first few months of life; eyes may transiently appear crossed or divergent. This is particularly noticeable when the infant is falling asleep or waking from sleep. If movements are transient, it is a normal finding.* Assess pupils for shape, size, and movement. Pupils are round, equal, and clear. Test their reaction to light by quickly shining a light source toward the eye and then removing it. The pupils are equal and reactive to light.	Abnormalities include asymmetrical pupils, pupils that respond sluggishly, and pupils that are "blown" or pinpoint. If dysconjugate eye movement is fixed (one eye is always out or always in), further evaluation is needed.

(table continues on page 832)

Technique and Normal Findings (continued)	Abnormal Findings (continued)
Use an ophthalmoscope to obtain the red reflex. Ensure that you have a +1 or =2 diopter lens. With the infant lying on the examination table or sitting in the parent's lap, approach from the side while looking into the ophthalmoscope. Shine the light into the eye from approximately 40–50 cm (15–26 in.) away. If you do not visualize a red/orange reflection from the eye, make small adjustments with the instrument until you see the red reflex. Repeat in the opposite eye. A red reflex is present.	If the red reflex cannot be elicited in the newborn, the infant needs a complete eye examination by an ophthalmologist. Absence of the red reflex in newborns is associated with congenital cataracts and retinoblastoma.
Observe the infant for light perception and ability to fix on and follow a target. *Newborns are sensitive to light and often keep their eyes closed for long periods. They have a limited ability to focus, but by 3 months, they can follow objects.* An infant with any abnormal findings during the eye assessment should be referred to an advanced practitioner for further testing.	At birth, the visual system is the least mature of the sensory systems. Development progresses rapidly over the first 6 months and reaches adult level by age 4–5 years. It is thought that visual acuity is sharpest at the distance from an infant being held in the mother's arms to the mother's face.
Ears Assess ear placement. Ears are symmetrical. *The top of the pinna lies just above an imaginary line from the inner canthus of the eye through the outer canthus and continuing past the ear.* Skin tags on the ears are a normal finding. Reassure the parent that these are easily removed if desired for cosmetic reasons.	Ears that fall below the imaginary line are low-set and may indicate chromosomal abnormalities. It may be helpful to note whether either parent has low-set ears; if so, then the low-set ears may be an inherited normal variant. One ear that is significantly smaller than the other or has extra ridges and pits may be associated with middle ear abnormalities or congenital kidney disorders. See Table 26.8 at the end of the chapter for ear shapes associated with Down syndrome and Turner syndrome (Ranweiler, 2009).
At the end of the examination, use the pneumatic otoscope to visualize the tympanic membranes and to check the eardrums if otitis media is suspected. Test the pneumatic otoscope before each use to ensure no leaks are present. Squeeze the bulb, then place the tip against your fingertip and release the bulb. Suction on the fingertip confirms the integrity of the system.	Otitis media is common in infants. Early diagnosis and intervention result in the best outcomes. It is important to ensure that every sick infant is examined using an otoscope (Rennie, van Wyk, Lee, & Toma, 2012).
Ask the parent to hold the infant with the body facing the parent. Then the parent should wrap one arm around the infant to draw the body close and pin down the arms. The other arm should hold the infant's head against the parent's chest. Hold the bulb in one hand, and then use that hand to pull the pinna up and back. Gently insert the otoscope approximately 6 mm (¼ in.) into the ear canal. Visualize the tympanic membrane and light reflex. The tympanic membrane is convex, intact, and translucent and allows visualization of the short process of the malleus. The cone of light is visible in the anterior inferior quadrant.	**SAFETY ALERT** *Always brace the hand holding the otoscope against the infant's face so that if the infant moves, the otoscope moves with him or her to avoid injuring the tympanic membrane.*

(table continues on page 833)

Technique and Normal Findings (continued)	Abnormal Findings (continued)
Gently squeeze the bulb to blow a puff of air into the ear canal. ■ The tympanic membrane responds by moving.	If movement is diminished or absent, suspect otitis media. Other conditions that can diminish movement include perforation (in only one ear) or tympanosclerosis.
Screening for hearing acuity in infants and young children includes evaluation of developmental milestones, such as the Moro reflex in neonates.	Abnormal findings include lack of Moro reflex, inability to localize sound, or lack of understandable language by 24 months.
Nose, Mouth, and Throat Inspect the nose. ■ It is in the midline of the face with symmetrical nares. The philtrum below the nose is fully formed (i.e., not flat), and the nasolabial folds are symmetrical.	Nasal flaring is a sign of respiratory distress. A flattened nasal bridge and macroglossia (enlarged tongue) are associated with chromosomal abnormalities. A flat philtrum and thin upper lip are associated with fetal alcohol syndrome. A deviated uvula or a uvula with a cleft (rare) and inflamed tonsils should be noted.
The best way to check patency is to hold a small mirror or specimen slide that has been chilled under the nose. Condensation on the glass is evidence of patency. ■ The nares are patent bilaterally.	A tight frenulum (**ankyloglossia**) may make latching or breastfeeding difficult. Depending on the severity, a frenotomy may be indicated.
Inspect the lips, mouth, and throat. Throat examination should be deferred to the end of the assessment, unless the infant cries. The uvula can easily be visualized when the infant is crying. ■ The lips are symmetrical and fully formed.	
Young infants may have a white nodule on the upper lip. Sometimes referred to as a sucking blister, this is harmless. ■ The tongue is of normal size, moves freely, and does not get in the way of feeding. The mucous membranes of the mouth, nose, and throat are moist and pink.	
Thorax and Lungs Breathing movements are best observed in the abdomen from pronounced diaphragmatic excursion in the infant. ■ The thorax is symmetrical. Chest expansion is equal bilaterally.	An asymmetrical chest wall, an expanded anterior–posterior diameter (pigeon breast), or a funnel shape (depressed sternum) are abnormal findings. Retractions anywhere on the chest wall are a sign of respiratory distress. Wheezes, crackles, and grunting are always abnormal, as are absent or diminished breath sounds.
Observe the infant's breathing pattern. ■ There are no signs of distress or use of accessory muscles. Auscultate all lobes of the lungs from the front and back and under the arms on both sides. *Breath sounds are equal bilaterally and typically louder and more bronchial than in adults. Inspiration is slightly longer than expiration. The normal rate of respirations is 40–60 breaths/min.* Count respirations for an entire minute. Periodic breathing (periods of rapid breathing followed by slow breathing) is a normal breathing pattern in infants, but it can lead to errors in rate assessment if the interval is short (e.g., 15 seconds multiplied by 4) to obtain the minute rate.	Grunting is a sign of respiratory distress. It frequently occurs in combination with nasal flaring and intercostal or subcostal retractions; it is associated with increased work of breathing.
Assess oxygenation. *Pink nail beds with crisp, circumoral cyanosis can be normal, especially when the infant is crying, as long as the lips and tongue remain pink.*	**Central cyanosis** (blueness in the center portions of the torso or of the lips, tongue, or oral mucous membranes) is a sign of poor oxygenation. Congenital heart disease is a possible cause.

(table continues on page 834)

Technique and Normal Findings (continued)	Abnormal Findings (continued)
	Clinical Significance If the infant is very pale and anemia is suspected, it is prudent to check the oxygen saturation. This is because it takes at least 5 g (less than ¼ oz) of reduced hemoglobin to produce the characteristic blueness of cyanosis. Anemic infants often do not have enough hemoglobin to exhibit cyanosis, even though they have very low oxygen saturation levels.
Heart and Neck Vessels Palpate the point of maximum impulse (PMI). Auscultate the heart; inspect and auscultate the neck vessels. *The PMI may be difficult to palpate in the infant.* ■ The heart rhythm is regular with a single S1 and a split S2. *Some murmurs are nonpathological—typically they are soft and nonspecific in character.* ■ The neck vessels are nondistended without bruits.	Tachycardia at rest, persistent bradycardia, and clubbing should not be present. Abnormal findings suggestive of a cardiac defect include a single S2, ejection clicks, and some murmurs, particularly loud harsh ones. If central cyanosis is present, evaluation of preductal and postductal oxygenation saturation is in order. Measure and compare readings in both upper extremities and one lower extremity. Oxygen saturation lower than 90% is abnormal, as are disparate readings between the upper and lower extremities. Infants with central cyanosis need a full cardiac evaluation by a cardiologist.
Peripheral Vascular Note the character and quality of the brachial and femoral pulses. Compare left to right and upper with lower. ■ All pulses are equal; pulse rate matches apical heart rate.	Weak thready pulses indicate low cardiac output. Bounding pulses are associated with conditions characterized by right-to-left shunts (e.g., patent ductus arteriosus). Palpable pulses in the upper extremities in correlation with diminished pulses in the lower extremities may indicate coarctation of the aorta or an interrupted aortic arch.
Breasts Observe the nipples. ■ The areolae are full and the nipple bud well formed. *It is normal for both male and female newborns to have swollen breasts that may even leak a watery fluid. The lingering effects of maternal hormones cause this.*	Check for any supernumerary (extra) nipples. These are usually found below the normal nipples and may not be recognized as nipples because they are usually small and not well formed. Although the condition is fairly common and usually benign, the number and location of the extra nipples should be documented. Reassure the parent that these nipples will not develop at puberty. See Table 26.8 for abnormalities related to Klinefelter syndrome.
Abdomen Inspect the abdomen. ■ It is cylindrical, protrudes slightly, and moves in synchrony with the diaphragm. *Superficial veins may be visible in fair-skinned infants.* ■ The umbilical area is clean without discharge, bulging areas, or scarring. Auscultate bowel sounds. ■ Bowel sounds are heard in all four quadrants.	A dull sound when percussing above the symphysis pubis may indicate a distended bladder. If abdominal distention is present, evaluate for a fluid wave. Note the size, shape, position, and mobility of any masses. Palpable kidneys indicate enlargement and should prompt further investigation by the primary care provider.

(table continues on page 835)

Technique and Normal Findings (continued)	Abnormal Findings (continued)
Bowel sounds may be softer immediately after the infant has eaten. Percuss the abdomen. *Dullness noted in the right upper quadrant helps outline the lower edges of the liver. Tympany is normal over an air-filled stomach and bowel.*	Loud, grumbling sounds may indicate hunger. Bowel sounds heard in the chest can indicate a diaphragmatic hernia.
Palpate the abdomen. *The abdomen is soft, without rigidity, tenderness, or masses.* *The lower margins of the liver can be palpated from 1 to 2 cm (about ½–¾ in.) below the right costal margin. The tip of the spleen may be palpable in the left upper quadrant.* Try to locate the kidneys using deep palpation in both upper quadrants. Be sure to palpate for hernias in the umbilical and inguinal regions. *Normally, the kidneys cannot be palpated and no hernias are present.*	The abdomen may be distended and firm with genitourinary masses or malformation. Gastrointestinal obstruction and imperforate anus are also the causes of a firm abdomen.
Back Inspect, then palpate along the length of the spine. There are no dimples or tufts of hair. Spine is closed, midline, straight, and without any bulge. Many newborns have an increased amount of hair covering the lower back and sacrum; this is common in newborns with increased skin pigmentation.	Sacral dimples, tufts of hair, and skin tags on the spinal area are potential indicators of spinal dysraphism and may require further evaluation. Dimpling or tufts of hair on the spine may indicate spina bifida occulta.
Musculoskeletal System, Extremities, and Joints By this point in the examination, you have had many opportunities to observe for symmetry of movement and strength of the musculoskeletal system. Note the shape and appearance of the hands, palms, fingers, feet, and toes. *Most newborns have two major creases on the palm.* Although bony deformities occur, positional deformities due to in utero position are more common and will resolve as the infant has full range of motion. The ankles have full range of motion, and feet return to a neutral position without assistance.	Throughout the examination, note any asymmetrical movements. Crepitus with joint movement or any limitation of movement is abnormal. In talipes varus (clubfoot), one or both feet are plantar flexed and turn abnormally inward. In talipes valgus, seen less commonly, the foot or feet turn outward. In a bony deformity, the position is rigid. A single transverse palmar crease is associated with Down syndrome and other genetic disorders; however, it can also be a normal inherited family trait.
Feet are flat before the infant begins walking.	Polydactyly is the presence of an extra digit that may be fully formed or may be attached only by a thin fleshy stalk. It is often an isolated finding and is an inherited disorder.
Perform the **Ortolani and Barlow maneuvers** to check for signs of hip dislocation. (Note that the maneuvers are performed in sequence, Barlow directly after Ortolani, while maintaining the hand position, as described below.) Looking for asymmetry between major creases in the thighs is another way to assess for hip dysplasia. ***Ortolani Maneuver.*** Position the infant supine on the examining table. With the baby's legs together, flex the knees and hips 90 degrees. Then, with your middle fingers over the greater trochanters and thumbs on the inner thighs, abduct the hips while applying upward pressure (Fig. 26.9A). No clicking or clunking sounds are heard.	Signs of congenital hip dislocation include positive results to the Ortolani and Barlow maneuvers and asymmetrical thigh and gluteal folds. Infants with talipes varus, talipes valgus, or hip dislocation should be referred to an orthopedist for evaluation and treatment.

(table continues on page 836)

Technique and Normal Findings (continued)	Abnormal Findings (continued)
Barlow Maneuver. Maintain your hold and the 90 degrees flexion; apply downward pressure while adducting the hips (Fig. 26.9B). The head of the femur remains in the acetabulum.	

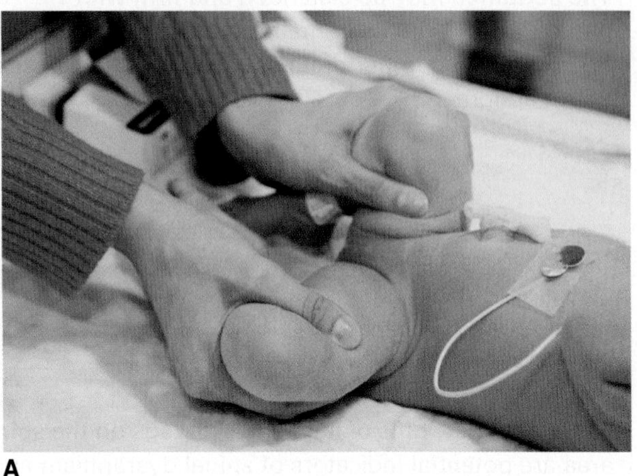

A

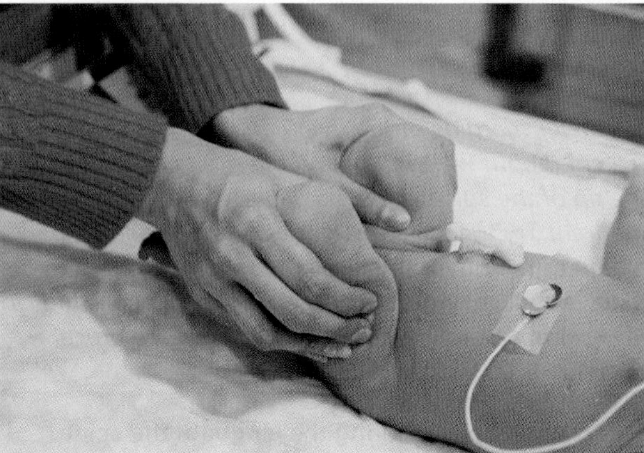

B

Figure 26.9 **A.** Ortolani maneuver. **B.** Barlow maneuver.

Neurological System

The assessments described earlier will provide clues about the status of the infant's nervous system and cranial nerve function. You will have had the opportunity to observe motor function (muscle size, symmetry, strength, tone, and movement), developmental maturation, and reaction to touch. You can assess tone from observing the posture and activity of the infant when undisturbed and when being handled.

The infant does not feel floppy when held. The infant blinks when a bright light is shone in the eyes and when a loud noise, such as a hand clap, is produced close by.

Signs of neurological dysfunction include persistence of newborn reflexes (see earlier discussion) past the time they normally disappear, involuntary movements, and abnormal posturing. Opisthotonos (Fig. 26.10) is usually the result of meningeal irritation that occurs with meningitis. Failure to blink when a bright light is shone in the eyes may be a sign of blindness, whereas absence of a blink on production of a loud noise may denote deafness. Further evaluation is indicated in both instances.

Clinical Significance

Infants can experience cerebral palsy despite having no risk factors. When the condition is identified early and therapy initiated promptly, long-term functioning is optimized. Watch for signs of neuromuscular dysfunction, such as hand preference before 1 year of age, bilateral fist clenching after 3 months of age, and involuntary or abnormal movements.

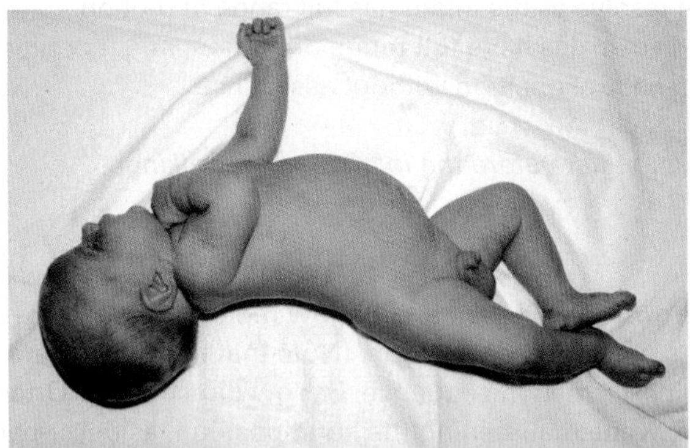

Figure 26.10 Opisthotonos, an indicator of meningitis.

Reflexes

Developmental reflexes are present at birth in the healthy term newborn. Evaluation of newborn reflexes gives information about neurological status. Assess rooting, suck, Moro (startle), Galant (trunk incurvation), stepping, grasp (can be elicited in both hands and feet), tonic neck, and Babinski reflexes (see Table 26.3).

Diminished reflexes indicate the possibility of neurological or developmental deficits.

(table continues on page 837)

TABLE 26.3 Newborn Reflexes

Rooting

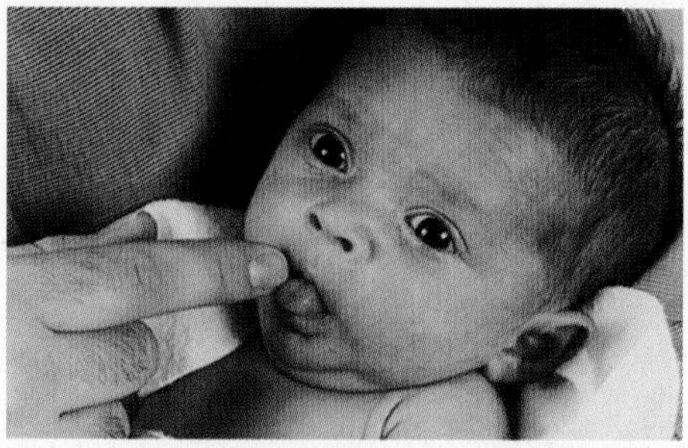

Gently stroke the cheek. The newborn turns toward the stimulus and opens the mouth. This reflex disappears at 3–4 months of age, although it may persist longer. Absence indicates a neurological disorder.

Moro (Startle)

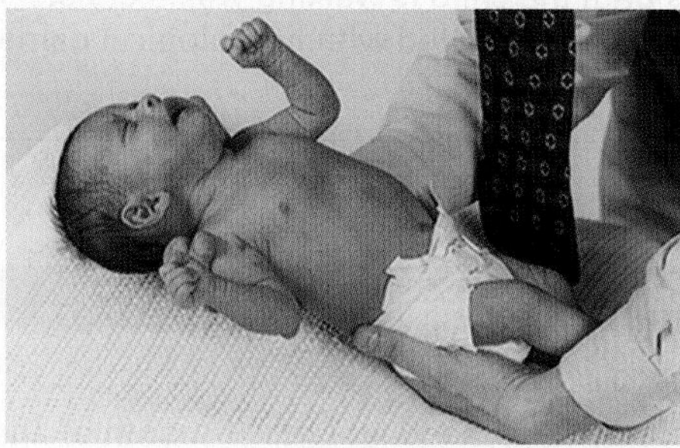

The Moro reflex occurs when the infant is startled or feels like he or she is falling. Sudden noise also can stimulate the reflex, verifying that the infant can hear. Bring the infant to a sitting position. Support the upper body and head with one hand; flex the chest. Suddenly, let the head and shoulders drop a few inches while releasing the arms. The arms and legs extend symmetrically. The arms return toward midline with the hand open and the thumb and index finger forming a "C."

The Moro reflex disappears by 4–6 months of age. Its absence or weakness points to an *upper motor neuron lesion*. An asymmetrical Moro occurs with *brachial plexus injury*.

Galant (Trunk Incurvation)

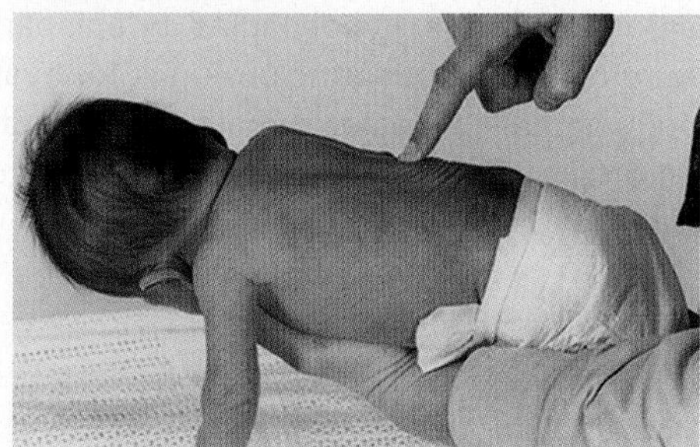

Place the newborn in ventral suspension. Stroke the skin on one side of the back. The trunk and hips should swing toward the side of the stimulus. The Galant reflex is normally present for the first 4–8 weeks of life. Its absence may indicate *spinal cord lesions*.

Suck

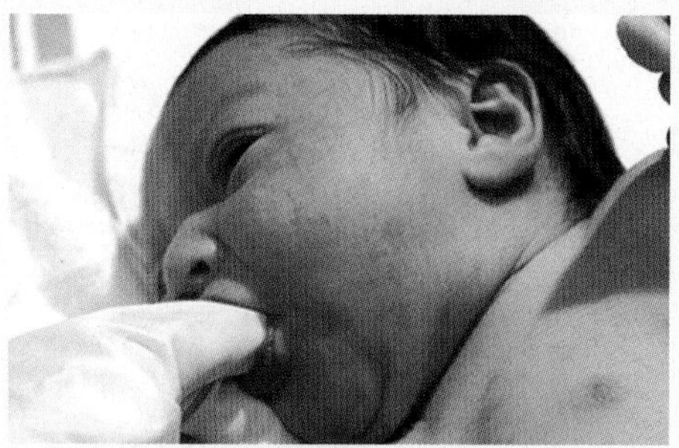

Place a gloved finger in the newborn's mouth. He or she should vigorously suck. The reflex may persist during infancy. A weak or absent reflex indicates a developmental or neurological disorder.

Tonic Neck

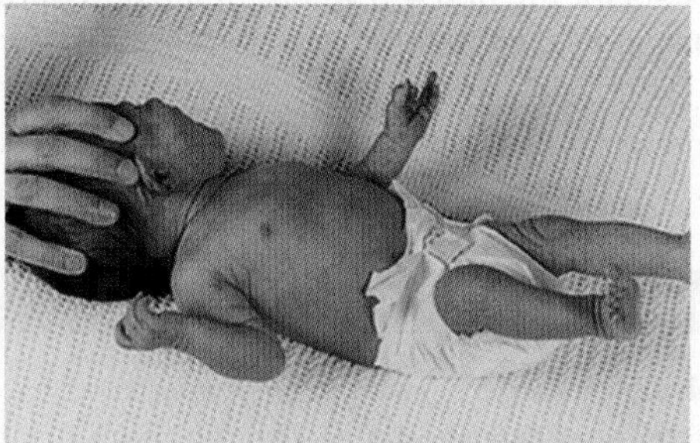

Turn the head of the supine infant to one side. The arm and leg extend on the side to which the face is pointed. The contralateral arm and leg flex, forming the classic fencer position. Repeat by turning the head to the other side—the position will reverse. This reflex is strongest at 2 months and disappears by 6 months. If still present at 9 months (an indicator of neurological damage), the infant will not be able to support weight to crawl.

Palmar Grasp

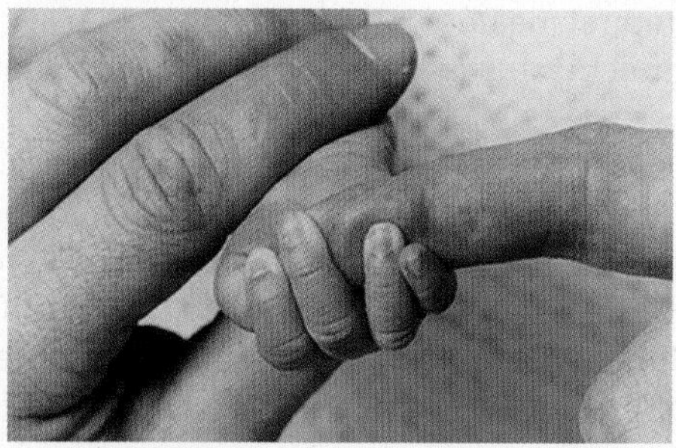

Place your finger in the newborn's palm; the infant's fingers will firmly grasp your finger. This reflex is strongest between 1 and 2 months of age. Persistence after 3 months of age indicates a *neurological disorder*.

(table continues on page 838)

TABLE 26.3 **Newborn Reflexes** *(continued)*

Stepping

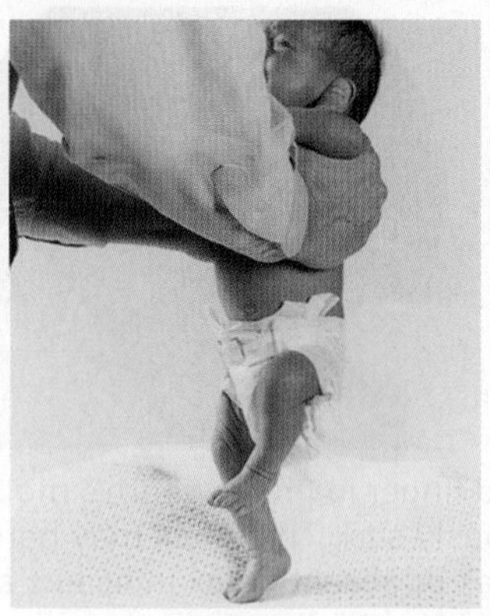

Hold the infant upright. Allow the soles to touch a flat surface. The legs flex and extend in a walking pattern. This reflex exists for the first 4–8 weeks of life and persists with neurological conditions (e.g., cerebral palsy).

Babinski

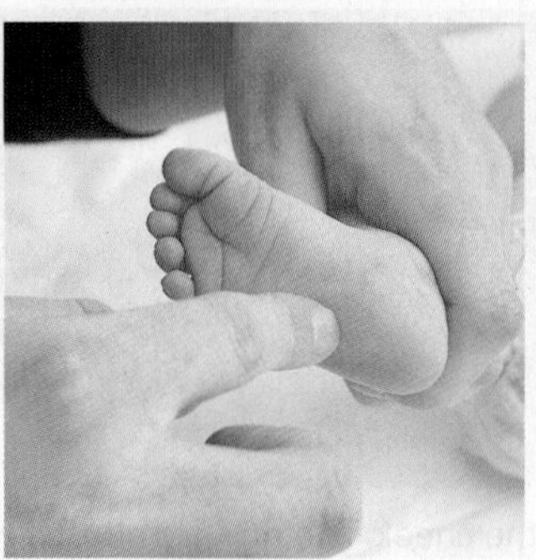

Stroke one side of the infant's foot upward from the heel and across the ball of the foot. The infant responds by hyperextending the toes: the great toe flexes toward the top of the foot and the other toes fan outward. This reflex lasts until the child is walking well. Persistence after age 2 years is associated with neurological damage (e.g., cerebral palsy).

Technique and Normal Findings (continued)	Abnormal Findings (continued)
Genitalia	
Female. Inspect the genitalia. *The labia majora cover the vestibule. The newborn girl may have an enlarged clitoris and labia, and the parent may have noticed a few drops of blood in the diaper.* These findings result from lingering effects of maternal hormones and should not be present after the first few weeks of life. Increased pigmentation over the labia in African American infants is normal. Both skin color of the parents and maternal hormones in utero affect the pigment tones; wide variation is normal. Gently part the labia and observe the structures of the vestibule. Inspect the vaginal opening. The genital area is clean and free from foul odors.	Redness, swelling, bleeding (after 1 month of age), or torn tissue may indicate sexual abuse. The law mandates the reporting of signs of abuse to child protective services. When the hymen completely covers the vagina, the infant has an imperforate hymen, which requires minor surgery before puberty to allow exit of menstrual flow. Other abnormal findings include labial adhesions/fusion, lesions, and foul-smelling discharge. If a foul smell is noted, check for a foreign body in the vagina. This is done by placing a gloved finger in the rectum to palpate along the vaginal wall. If an object is located, use a gentle milking motion to gradually work the object out.
Male. Inspect the penis. Note cleanliness and placement of the urethral meatus. Urethral meatus is at the top of the glans penis and midline. For the uncircumcised penis, you will need to partially retract the foreskin to observe the meatus. Do not forcibly retract the foreskin. Evaluate the scrotum for size, color, and symmetry. The amount of pigment in the scrotum can vary depending on ethnicity of the parents. Testes are descended bilaterally; the area is free of edema, masses, and lesions.	Meatal stenosis, an inadequate urethral opening, or a malpositioned meatus, hypospadias, or epispadias should be referred to a pediatric urologist for evaluation. Note whether the testes remain undescended; this condition requires evaluation if it persists into the toddler stage.

(table continues on page 839)

Technique and Normal Findings (continued)	Abnormal Findings (continued)
Anus and Rectum Inspect the anus. Use the little finger of a gloved hand to palpate it. The anus is well formed with no redness or bleeding. The muscle contracts with light pressure to the area. Rectal examination is not done routinely unless evidence of irritation, bleeding, or other symptoms is present.	Investigate redness, bleeding, or other signs of irritation for possible cause (e.g., sexual abuse, fissures). Small white worms indicate a pinworm infection.

Cultural Considerations

The length and weight of the newborn and infant vary according to heritage, so ranges outside of usual may be normal for some patients. Mongolian spotting is more common in infants of African American, Asian, and Native American origin.

Critical Thinking

You will have gleaned a wealth of data throughout the examination. With the first observations of the infant and parent, you begin to understand the child's emotional, musculoskeletal, neurological, and nutritional status as well as developmental level. As the examination progresses, additional details add to your understanding, so that by the end, you are ready to prepare the care plan. An approach that cultivates rapport with the infant and parent from the beginning and throughout the examination will facilitate the parent's willingness to collaborate with you. Such involvement will help to ensure that the plan is culturally appropriate, which increases the likelihood that the family will follow the plan.

You should now have enough data to communicate a concise yet thorough description of the infant's health status. This information, when reported to the primary care provider, helps to guide diagnostic testing and subsequent medical diagnoses. In this way, you help to streamline the infant's care and increase the likelihood of timely and accurate diagnoses.

Laboratory and Diagnostic Testing

Newborn screening tests look for developmental, genetic, and metabolic disorders. This allows interventions to be undertaken before symptoms develop. Many of these diseases are rare but can be treated if caught early. The types of newborn screening tests that are done vary from state to state. Most states require three to eight tests and the most thorough screening assesses for about 40 disorders. All states screen for congenital hypothyroidism, galactosemia, and phenylketonuria (PKU). In addition to the newborn screening blood tests, a hearing screen is recommended for all newborns.

Diagnostic Reasoning

Nursing Diagnoses, Outcomes, and Interventions

When formulating a nursing diagnosis, it is important to use critical thinking to cluster data and identify patterns. You will compare these clusters of data with the defining characteristics (abnormal findings) for the diagnosis to ensure the most accurate labeling and appropriate interventions. Table 26.4

TABLE 26.4 Common Nursing Diagnoses Associated With Newborns and Infants

Diagnosis	Point of Differentiation	Assessment Characteristics	Nursing Interventions
Neonatal jaundice	Yellow-orange tint of the skin resulting from accumulation of unconjugated bilirubin	Bilirubin high for age in hours or days (plotted on a nomogram), yellow-orange skin, yellow sclera	Encourage prompt early feeding to stimulate stooling and removal of bilirubin. Administer phototherapy as ordered.*
Effective breastfeeding	Mother and infant display proficient nursing behaviors	Appropriate weight for age, eagerness of infant to nurse, infant content after feeding	Facilitate skin-to-skin contact. Give positive feedback and encouragement. Refer to lactation consultant for assistance, if desired.
Ineffective thermoregulation	Difficulty maintaining normal temperature, easily becomes hypothermic in the newborn period; when ill during infancy, may become hypothermic or spike a very high temperature	Cool skin, cyanotic nail beds, pallor, piloerection, temperature below normal range; newborns do not shiver, which contributes to the hypothermia	Monitor temperature every 1–4 hours. Keep room temperature warm. Keep newborn's head covered. Use blankets.

*Collaborative interventions.

compares nursing diagnoses, abnormal findings, and interventions commonly related to newborn and infant assessment (NANDA International, 2012).

You use assessment information to identify patient outcomes. Some outcomes may be related to newborn or infant problems that need to be addressed, such as the following:

- Bilirubin is normal for age when plotted on a nomogram.
- Infant is gaining weight with normal pattern of growth.
- Temperature is 36.5° to 37.2°C (97.7° to 99°F) (Moorhead, Johnson, Maas, & Swanson, 2013).

After outcomes have been established, you implement care to improve the status of the patient. You use critical thinking and evidence-based practice to develop the interventions. Some examples of nursing interventions for newborn care are as follows:

- Protect the infant's eyes to prevent overexposure to phototherapy.
- Use valid and reliable tools to measure breastfeeding performance.
- Perform Apgar score after birth (Bulechek, Butcher, Dochterman, & Wagner, 2013).

Progress Note: Analyzing Findings

Remember Keri Meadows, whose case has been outlined throughout this chapter. Two and a half months after the 1-month appointment, Keri's mother calls the office to state that Keri is losing weight. It is necessary for her to return to the clinic so that health care providers can reassess the infant and document findings. The following nursing note illustrates how subjective and objective data are collected and analyzed and how nursing interventions are developed.

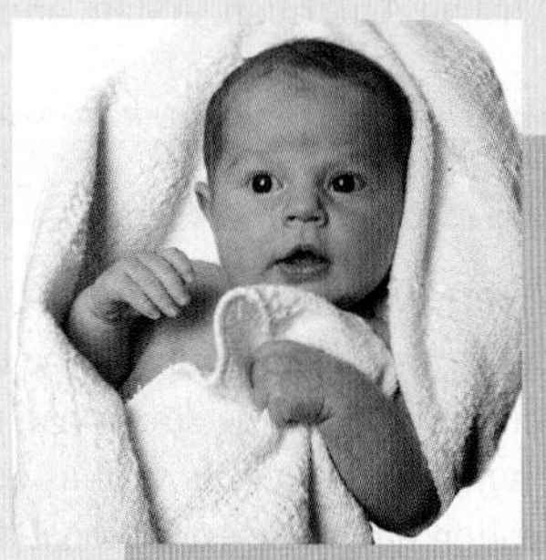

Subjective: Mother says that she is extremely frustrated with breastfeeding. At first, it went well, but now that she is back at work full time, she feels that she isn't making enough milk. Keri has been "fussy"; her weight has dropped by 500 g (1.2 lb).

Objective: Keri is irritable. Abdomen is soft and nondistended. T 37°C (98.6°F), P 138 beats/min, R 40 breaths/min. Mucous membranes are slightly dry, fontanelles sunken. Mother states Keri is stooling twice per day but notes that diapers sometimes have dark urine. She changes five to six diapers per day. Weight is 5.4 kg (12 lb), had been about 6 kg (13.2 lb) at previous visit, so it has dropped by 5%.

Analysis: Ineffective breastfeeding related to changes in family schedule, new stressors, compromised milk production

Plan: Encourage mother to drink 2 L/day (about 64 oz) of fluid and get proper nutrition. Teach mother about pumping at work to keep milk supply. She does not want to supplement with formula. Provide pamphlet about how to manage breastfeeding while working. Provide Web address where patient can obtain more information and post questions for other working mothers to answer. Make referral to a lactation specialist.

Critical Thinking Challenge

- How will the nurse assess the infant's other body systems that the weight loss might be affecting?
- What psychosocial issues might the nurse assess for this family?
- What other nursing diagnoses might be considered based on the data?

Collaborating With the Interprofessional Team

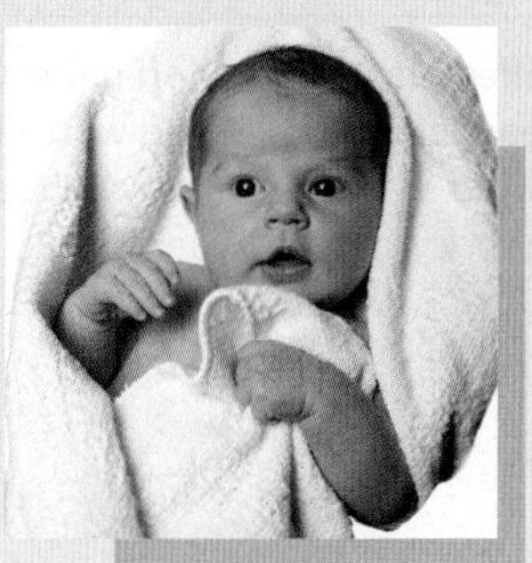

Results that might trigger a consult with a lactation specialist include pain while breastfeeding, a newborn who is wetting fewer than six diapers a day, a newborn having fewer than two bowel movements per day, a baby who is not gaining weight, or a baby who is not swallowing after milk is ejected.

Keri and her mother have been experiencing many of the problems outlined above; therefore, a consult is indicated. The following conversation illustrates how the nurse might organize the data and make recommendations about the patient's situation.

Situation: "Hi, I'm Jan, a nurse in the outpatient clinic in primary care. We saw patient Keri Meadows and her mother today."

Background: "Keri is 3½ months old. Her mother, Diane, brought her to the office because she was concerned about her weight loss. She recently returned to work and is having difficulty with her milk production. She is also very frustrated. I think that it would be nice to give her some extra attention with this change. The baby is also somewhat irritable and not getting enough fluid or calories."

Assessment: Ineffective breastfeeding

Recommendations: "I think that a 1-hour appointment would be helpful. She was successful before but needs some help with some strategies to improve her milk supply. I've already given her a pamphlet and access to a Web site."

Critical Thinking Challenge

- How might the nurse assess the relationship between Diane and Keri?
- What are some other things that the nurse might want to assess?
- How does a team of nurses work together to coordinate care?

Pulling It All Together

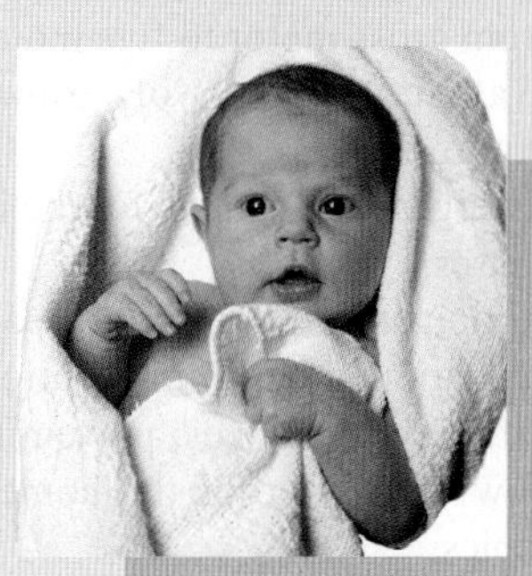

The nurse uses assessment data to formulate a nursing care plan with patient outcomes and interventions for Keri and her mother. Outcomes are specific to the patient, realistic, and measurable and have a time frame for completion. Interventions are actions that the nurse performs, based on evidence and practice guidelines. After completion of interventions, the nurse reevaluates Keri and documents the findings in the chart to show progress toward the patient outcome. The nurse uses critical thinking and judgment to continue or revise the diagnosis, outcomes, or interventions. This is often in the form of a care plan or case note similar to the following:

(case study continues on page 842)

Nursing Diagnosis	Patient Outcomes	Nursing Interventions	Rationale	Evaluation
Ineffective breastfeeding related to return to work	Keri gains weight and wets six or more diapers per day.	Refer to lactation specialist. Encourage mother to drink 2 L (about 64 oz) of water per day and attend to appropriate nutrition.	Lactation specialist has the expertise and allotted time to provide personal support. Calories and fluids are necessary for milk production.	Patient seen by lactation specialist and stated that she was very helpful in getting her milk supply up. Will continue to pump at work and keep fluids at around 2 L (about 64 oz) per day.

Applying Your Knowledge

Using your knowledge of the nursing process and critical thinking, consider all the case study findings woven throughout this chapter. When answering the following questions, begin drawing conclusions and see how the pieces of assessment must work together to create an environment for personalized, appropriate, and accurate care.

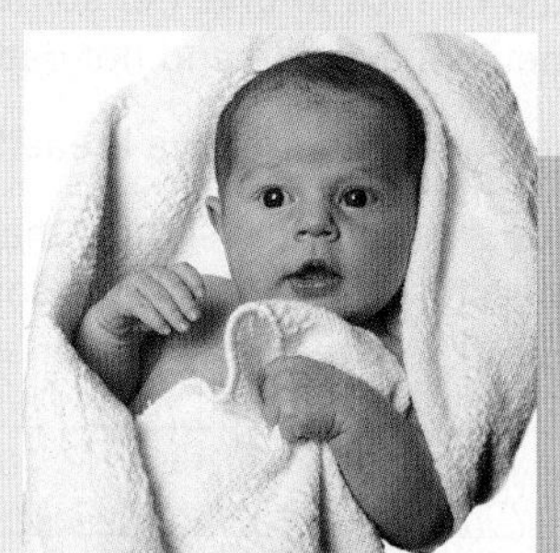

- What is the expected growth for an infant each week for the first 6 months?
- Why is vitamin D supplementation important in a breastfeeding baby?
- What would you teach Mrs. Meadows to observe in Keri to know that she is "getting enough breast milk"?
- What factors could contribute to a slowed growth pattern in a newborn or an infant?
- What health promotion teaching would be important to discuss with Mrs. Meadows as Keri grows?
- How would you evaluate whether Mrs. Meadows is confident and comfortable in her knowledge of infant feeding and growth?

Key Points

- The infant's growth and development progress in predictable ways: cephalocaudally, from central to distal, and from gross motor to fine motor control. It is important to evaluate patterns of growth and document steady progress.
- Emergency situations for the infant often have respiratory causes.
- Anticipatory guidance for parents of the infant includes education about immunization schedules, breastfeeding, safe sleep practices, preventing baby bottle tooth decay, how to childproof the home, and other general safety topics.
- Infants commonly present with respiratory symptoms, fever, skin disorders, gastrointestinal distress, and crying. Interview questions for these symptoms should elicit information regarding severity and possible causation.
- Key assessments immediately after birth are vital signs, including respiratory status, gestational age, and reflexes including muscle tone.
- Performing a physical examination on an infant requires you to be flexible about the order and timing of specific assessments based on the developmental stage and the unique needs of the infant.
- Many assessment techniques are unique to the infant or newborn, such as Apgar scoring, evaluating reflexes, performing gestational age assessment, and maneuvers to identify congenital hip dislocation. Other techniques require adaptation to accommodate the infant's unique anatomical and developmental needs. Examples include use of the ophthalmoscope and otoscope and examination of the throat.
- You can glean a wealth of information about the infant's development and the mental, psychosocial, neurological, musculoskeletal, and nutritional status by carefully

observing the infant's appearance, behavior, activity levels, and interaction with parents throughout the examination.

- Because infants are the age group most likely to be abused, screening for and identifying signs of child abuse and neglect are important ways you can make a difference in long-term outcomes.
- A thorough skin assessment also reveals information about the infant's nutrition and hydration status, cardiac and respiratory function, and renal and lymphatic systems.
- Positional plagiocephaly and brachycephaly must be distinguished from craniosynostosis, which can lead to impaired brain development if not caught and treated early.
- Many abnormal findings in infants result from chromosomal defects or are acquired congenital conditions resulting from environmental conditions (e.g., fetal alcohol syndrome).

Review Questions

1. A mother brings her 6-month-old infant to the clinic for a routine evaluation. At birth, the term infant weighed 3.5 kg (7 lb, 12 oz) and was 51 cm (20 in.) long. He now weighs 4.6 kg (10 lb, 2 oz). Which assessments are *most* important for you to do next?
   A. Obtain a thorough obstetrical and neonatal history and say, "I'm very worried that the baby hasn't gained more weight. What are you feeding him?"
   B. Measure head and chest circumference and length, then plot current weight, length, and head and chest circumferences on standardized growth charts.
   C. Review the immunization history, administer the Denver II assessment, and ask the mother if she has noticed any unusual patterns or behaviors.
   D. Screen for domestic violence and focus on the neurological, cardiac, and abdominal portions of the physical examination.

2. You are evaluating the growth pattern of a 5-month-old infant born at 27 weeks' gestation. Which of the following actions will yield the most accurate assessment of growth for this infant?
   A. Calculate how many kilocalories per day the infant is consuming, evaluate his bowel movement pattern, plot his measurements, and compare with the last two visits.
   B. Determine whether he has gained at least 2.2 kg (5 lb) since birth, because infants should gain 500 g to 1 kg (1 to 2 lb) per month in the first 6 months.
   C. Plot the weight and length on a standardized growth chart for a 7-week-old infant and compare with birth measurements and measurements on previous visits.
   D. Plot the weight and length on a standardized growth chart for a 12-week-old infant and compare with birth measurements and measurements on previous visits.

3. The nurse is assessing a 2-month-old infant whose mother brought her to the emergency department because the baby wasn't eating well and she "just looks sick." Which of the following assessment findings is most worrisome?
   A. Stiff neck with an arched back
   B. Circumoral cyanosis noted when crying
   C. PMI not palpable, anterior fontanel bulges slightly when crying
   D. T 36.4°C (97.5°F), heart rate (HR) 160 beats/min, respiratory rate (RR) 38 breaths/min

4. You are triaging infants who have presented to the emergency department on a Friday night. Which infant should you take in for treatment *first*?
   A. A 2-week-old infant whose mother reports, "She just won't stop crying. I'm so worried." The cry is medium pitch; T 37°C (99°F), HR 160 beats/min, RR 50 breaths/min; abdomen moves with each breath.
   B. A 6-week-old infant whose father reports, "He's vomited several times and he won't take his bottle." T 36°C (96.8°F), HR 70 beats/min, RR 20 breaths/min. His lips are white. He is limp.
   C. A 5-month-old infant with a stuffy nose who has been unusually fussy and has had three loose stools in the last 8 hours. T 37.6°C (99.8°F), HR 140 beats/min, RR 45 breaths/min while crying.
   D. An 8-month-old infant whose parents report he choked on a bean at dinner. The bean came out after five back pats. He turns blue around his mouth when he cries. T 37°C (98.6°F), HR 130 beats/min, RR 30 breaths/min.

5. You evaluate all the following children one morning in the clinic. Which should you refer for further assessment?
   A. A 6-week-old boy whose parents recently immigrated from Thailand; his head lags when pulled up by his arms; he has several dark spots that look like bruises on his lower back and buttocks.
   B. A 4-week-old African American girl whose liver margins are barely palpable along the right costal margin; her kidneys are easily palpable: her ears look "funny."
   C. A 4-month-old Caucasian boy with loud breath sounds throughout the lung fields; auscultation of the heart reveals a split S2.
   D. A 9-month-old Latina who is fussy; her tympanic membrane is pearly gray and moves during pneumatic otoscopy.

6. You are teaching a parenting class, and the parents are sharing baby pictures. Which picture indicates that the parent may need additional education?
   A. Baby is playing peek-a-boo in his car seat, which is installed in the middle part of the rear seat.
   B. Daddy is brushing his son's two front teeth while baby is splashing in the bathtub.
   C. Baby (10 months old) is in his high chair feeding himself banana cut in small pieces.
   D. Baby is sleeping supine in her crib, no pillow, one blanket, bottle lying beside baby and a tiny dribble of milk at the corner of her mouth.

7. An infant has a new onset of rash but otherwise seems well. Which interview question is *best* when trying to pinpoint a possible cause?
   A. "Was there a prolonged NICU stay?"
   B. "What treatments have you given her for the rash?"
   C. "Has anything changed lately, such as shampoos, soaps, or laundry detergent?"
   D. "How many diapers is she wetting per day, and what is the stool pattern?"

8. Which of the following activities *best* facilitates anticipatory guidance?
   A. Becoming very proficient in interviewing and performing the physical examination
   B. Doing as much of the examination as possible with the infant in the parents' lap
   C. Recognizing and reporting signs of physical abuse and neglect
   D. Encouraging parents to make an appointment with the pediatrician before the baby is born

9. Which of the following infants has the most signs that point to possible abuse?
   A. History of a long NICU stay for extreme prematurity; does not respond to loud clapping
   B. Positive Ortolani and Barlow maneuver results; one leg looks shorter than the other
   C. Small baby with large areas of denuded skin on his face and torso
   D. When baby cries, mother says, "Shut up already." Baby has a foul odor and looks dirty.

10. Which of the following 6-month-old infants has the most markers for a possible genetic disorder?
   A. Has large ears, is in the 95th percentile for weight and height, babbles
   B. Has large scaly plaques on face and torso, red reflex is absent in one eye, posterior fontanelle has closed
   C. Has significant head lag, one ear is small and malformed, nipples are unusually close together
   D. Sits up alone, cranial sutures are palpable, back of the head is flat

The Jensen suite offers these additional resources to enhance learning and facilitate understanding of this chapter:

- thePoint online resource, http://thepoint.lww.com/Jensen2e
- *Laboratory Manual for Nursing Health Assessment: A Best Practice Approach*
- *Pocket Guide for Nursing Health Assessment: A Best Practice Approach*
- *Lippincott DocuCare,* an electronic health record simulation software, http://thepoint.lww.com/docucare
- *Adaptive Learning | Powered by PrepU,* http://thepoint.lww.com/prepu

References

American Academy of Pediatrics. (2012a). Breastfeeding and the use of human milk. *Pediatrics*. Advance online publication. doi:10.1542/peds.2011-3552

American Academy of Pediatrics. (2012b). *Kids and vitamin D deficiency*. Retrieved on March 18 2014 from http://www.aap.org/en-us/about-the-aap/aap-press-room/pages/Kids-and-Vitamin-D-Deficiency.aspx.

American Academy of Pediatrics. (2014). *Car seats: Information for families 2014*. Retrieved from http://www.healthychildren.org/English/safety-prevention/on-the-go/pages/Car-Safety-Seats-Information-for-Families.aspx

American Academy of Pediatrics Committee on Nutrition. (2009). *Textbook of Neonatal Resuscitation* (6th ed.) Elk Grove Village, IL: Author.

American Academy of Pediatrics & American Heart Association. (2011). *Textbook of neonatal resuscitation* (6th ed.). Elk Grove Village, IL: American Academy of Pediatrics.

American Heart Association. (2014). *Fact sheet: Infant CPR anytime*. Retrieved from http://www.heart.org/HEARTORG/CPRAndECC/CommunityCPRandFirstAid/CommunityProducts/Infant-CPR-Anytime_UCM_428979_Article.jsp

Bulechek, G. M., Butcher, H. K., Dochterman, J. M., & Wagner, C. M. (2013). *Nursing interventions classification (NIC)* (6th ed.). St. Louis, MO: Mosby.

Centers for Disease Control and Prevention. (2013). *Use and interpretation of the CDC growth charts*. Retrieved on from http://www.cdc.gov/nccdphp/dnpa/growthcharts/guide.htm

Gelfer, P., Cameron, R., Masters, K., & Kennedy, K. A. (2013). Integrating "back to sleep" recommendations into neonatal ICU practice. *Pediatrics*. Advance online publication. doi:10.1542/peds.2012-185

Giardino, A. P., Giardino, E. R., & Moles, R. L. (2014). *Physical child abuse*. Retrieved from http://emedicine.medscape.com/article/915664-overview

Hurme, T., Alanko, S., Anttila, P., Juven, T., & Svedstrom, E. (2008). Risk factors for physical child abuse in infants and toddlers. *European Journal of Pediatric Surgery, 18*(6), 287–291.

Kemp, A. M., Dunstan, F., Harrison, S., Morris, S., Mann, M., Rolfe, K. I., . . . Maguire, S. (2009). Patterns of skeletal fractures in child abuse: Systematic review. *Child: Care, Health and Development, 35*(1), 141–142.

Moorhead, S., Johnson, M., Maas, M. L., & Swanson, E. (2013). *Nursing outcomes classification (NOC): Measurement of health outcomes* (5th ed.). St. Louis, MO: Elsevier.

NANDA International. (2012). *Nursing diagnoses: Definitions and classification 2012–2014* (9th ed.). Oxford, United Kingdom: Wiley-Blackwell.

National Center on Shaken Baby Syndrome. (2014). *Preventing shaken baby syndrome*. Retrieved from http://www.cdc.gov/concussion/pdf/preventing_sbs_508-a.pdf

National Institute of Neurological Disorders and Stroke. (2013). *Traumatic brain injury: Hope through research*. Retrieved from http://www.ninds.nih.gov/disorders/tbi/detail_tbi.htm

Nelson, K. E., & Williams, C. M. (2013). *Infectious disease epidemiology: Theory and practice* (3rd ed.). Sudbury, MA: Jones and Bartlett.

Rabinowitz, S. S., Rogers, G., Unnikrishnan, N., Mascarenhas, M. R., Windle, M. L., Bhatia, J., . . . Mehta, M. (2014). *Nutritional considerations in failure to thrive*. Retrieved from http://emedicine.medscape.com/article/985007-overview

Ranweiler, R. (2009). Assessment and care of the newborn with Down syndrome. *Advances in Neonatal Care, 9*(1), 17–24.

Rennie, C. E., van Wyk, F. C., Lee, M. S. W., & Toma, A. G. (2012). *Pneumatic otoscope examination*. Retrieved from http://emedicine.medscape.com/article/1348950

Simon, H. K. (2009). *Pediatrics, crying child*. Retrieved from http://emedicine.medscape.com/article/800964

U.S. Department of Health & Human Services. (2013). *2020 Topics & objectives – Objectives A–Z*. Retrieved from http://www.healthypeople.gov/2020/topicsobjectives2020/

U.S. Food and Drug Administration. (2014). *Infant formula guidance documents & regulatory information*. Retrieved from http://www.fda.gov/food/guidanceregulation/guidancedocumentsregulatoryinformation/infantformula/default.htm

Waseem, M., Aslam, M., & Wilson, L. A. (2008). *Otitis media*. Retrieved from http://emedicine.medscape.com/article/994656

Ward, M. (2013). *Fever in children*. Retrieved from http://www.uptodate.com/contents/fever-in-children-beyond-the-basics

Tables of Abnormal Findings

TABLE 26.5 Infant Diseases With Characteristic Odors

Odor	Disease or Condition
Rotten or offensive odor from the nose or vagina	Retained foreign body (e.g., anything little hands can grasp and push into these body openings); poor hygiene
Musty odor	Phenylketonuria
Maple syrup odor to the urine	Maple syrup urine disease
Foul odor of umbilical area	Omphalitis
Noxious mouth odor	Ingestion of a chemical such as kerosene, bleach, glue, alcohol, or other substances

TABLE 26.6 Red Flags for Child Abuse

Category	Details
Reported history of injury	The story keeps changing or is inconsistent between partners or over time. Details of the trauma do not correlate with the type or extent of injury. No history of trauma is given.
Delay in treatment	A significant delay elapses between the time of injury and when the parent seeks treatment.
"Doctor shopping"	Parent changes physicians, health care facilities, or both, frequently.
Injuries consistent with abuse	Bruises appear on an infant before the infant is walking. Bruising or other injuries are in varied stages of healing. Multiple types of injuries appear. Injuries resemble an object, such as cigarette burns, burns in the shape of an iron, or loop marks. Grab or slap marks or human bite marks are visible. Evidence exists of immersion burns. These are usually well demarcated and bilateral (e.g., both hands or feet) or occur on the buttocks and feet.
Fractured bone	Any fracture in an infant who is not walking should raise the index of suspicion for abuse, unless there is a verifiable cause (e.g., motor vehicle collision, documented bone disorder predisposing to bone fragility).
Types of fractures associated with physical abuse	These include the following: • Multiple fractures • Fractured ribs (about 70% chance infant was abused) • Fractured humerus, especially midshaft and spiral/oblique (about 50% chance of abuse) • Skull fracture (about 30% chance of abuse) (Kemp et al., 2009)
Pattern of injury consistent with shaken baby syndrome	Signs include subdural hematoma, retinal hemorrhages, rib fractures, and bilateral bruising in the rib cage.
Injuries consistent with sexual abuse	Any of the following in the genital area, anus, or both indicates sexual abuse: • Bleeding • Bruising • Redness
Signs of neglect	Examples include poor hygiene, clothes inappropriate for the weather, evidence of tissue wasting, signs of poor nutrition, failure to gain weight, and untreated illness.

Data from Giardino, A. P., Giardino, E. R., & Moles, R. L. (2014). *Physical child abuse.* Retrieved from http://emedicine.medscape.com/article/915664-overview; Hurme, T., Alanko, S., Anttila, P., Juven, T., & Svedstrom, E. (2008). Risk factors for physical child abuse in infants and toddlers. *European Journal of Pediatric Surgery, 18*(6), 287–291; Magana, J., & Kaufhold, M. (2014). *Child abuse.* Retrieved from http://emedicine.medscape.com/article/800657

TABLE 26.7 Abnormal Skin Conditions in Newborns and Infants

Infections and Infestations

Pediculosis Capitis (Head Lice)

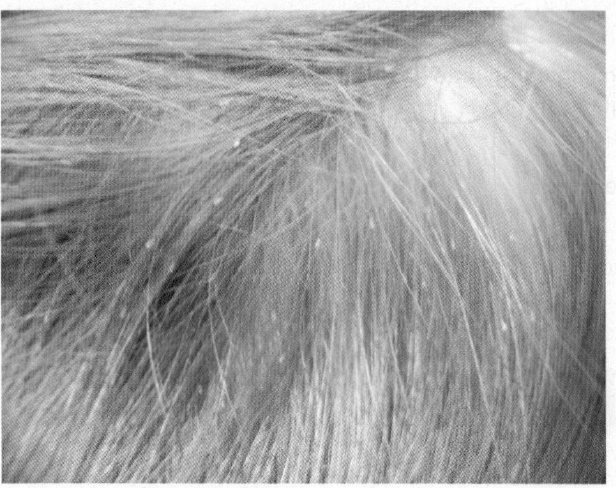

This highly contagious condition results from infestation with the human head louse, *Pediculus humanus capitis.* Lice spread easily among children through close personal contact and sharing hairbrushes and other belongings.

Tinea Corporis (Ringworm)

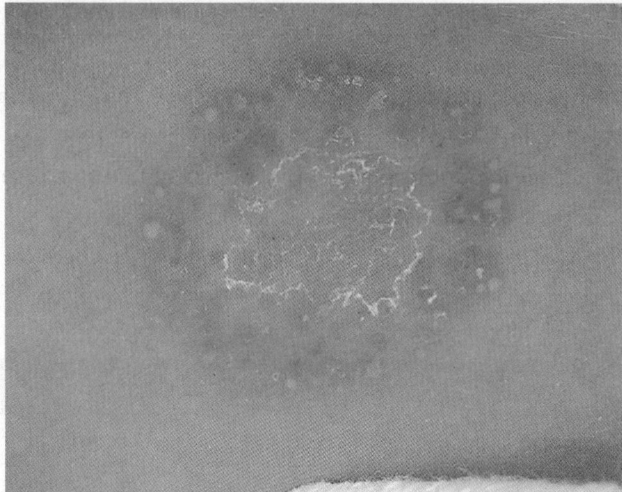

This fungal infection (dermatophytosis) is superficial. Because fungi prefer warm, moist environments, preventing ringworm involves keeping skin dry and avoiding contact with infectious material. Children are most likely to acquire the infection from an animal host, although human-to-human contact does occur as well.

Scabies

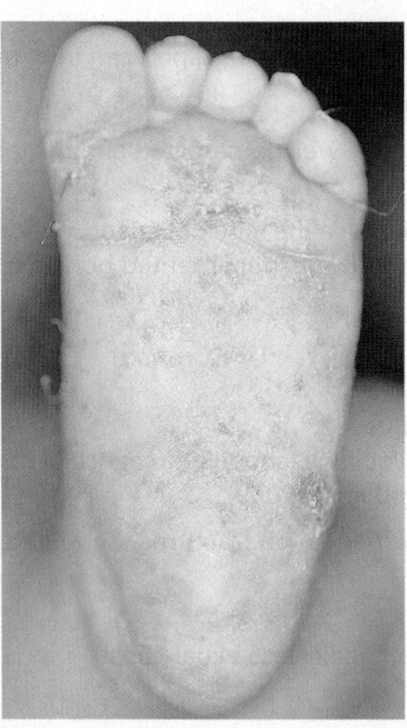

Scabies results from an allergic reaction to the *Sarcoptes scabiei* mite and its eggs. In infants, large blistering lesions and suppurative vesicles comprise the characteristic rash. The condition is highly contagious.

Staphylococcal Scalded Skin Syndrome

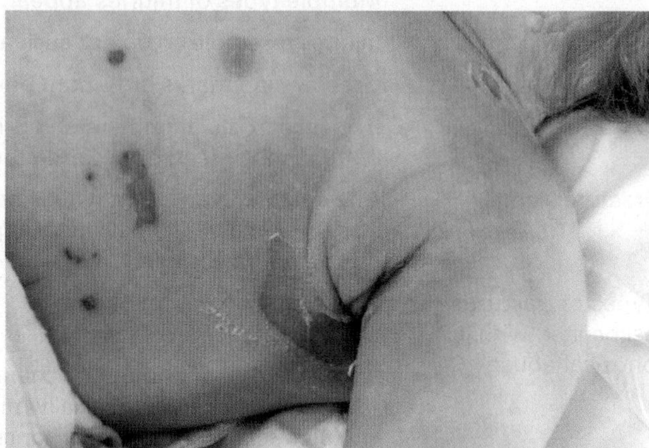

Acute exfoliation of the skin results from infection with a staphylococcal exotoxin. Pediatric populations are most susceptible to the condition, which usually heals within 2 weeks.

(table continues on page 847)

TABLE 26.7 Abnormal Skin Conditions in Newborns and Infants *(continued)*

Molluscum Contagiosum

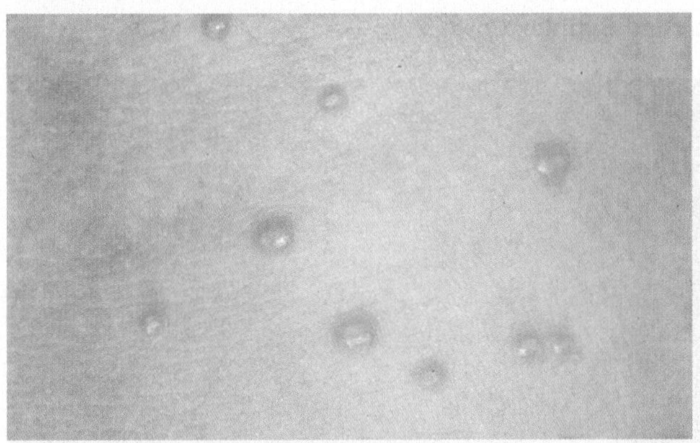

This virus spreads by direct contact; children with atopic dermatitis are especially vulnerable. The infection takes approximately 6–9 months to resolve.

Bullous Impetigo

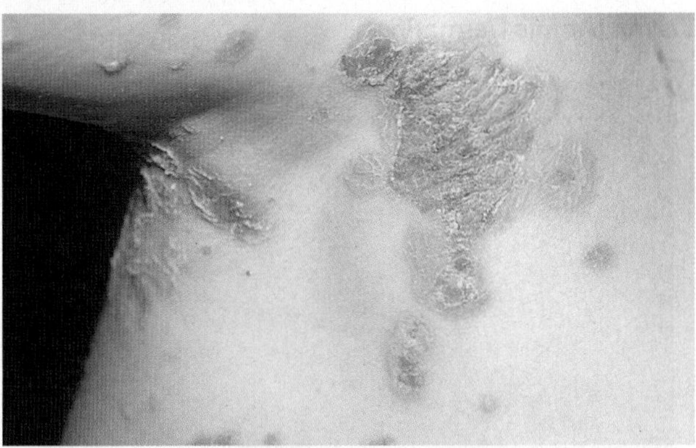

This common superficial staphylococcal infection is characterized by fluid-filled vesicles and blisters that easily rupture. It is a milder form of staphylococcal scalded skin syndrome.

Contact Dermatitis and Inflammatory and Allergy-Related Conditions

Intertrigo

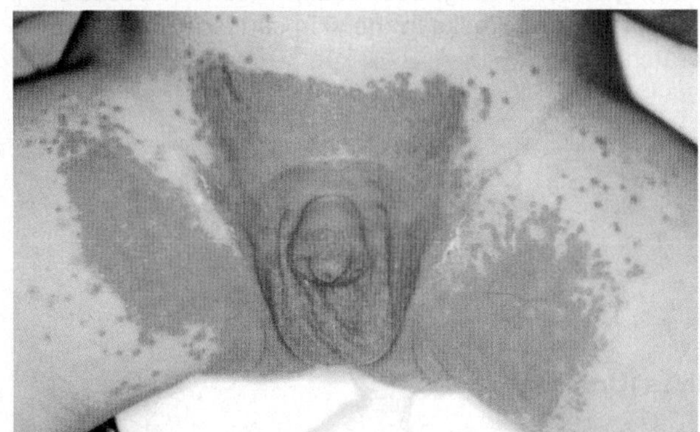

Inflammation of the skinfolds results from skin-on-skin friction. It can be a cause of diaper rash. Intertrigo frequently develops in obese people of older age groups as well.

Irritant Diaper Dermatitis

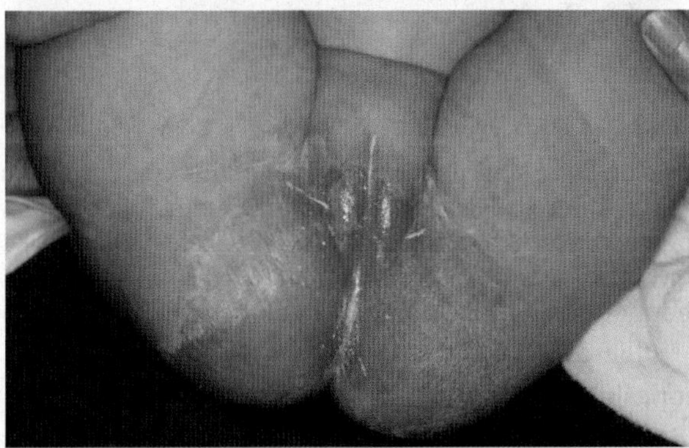

The typical "diaper rash" results from prolonged exposure of the affected areas to urine and stool. Aggravating factors include a diaper left on too long, a tight-fitting diaper, rubbing and chafing of the diaper, and diarrhea.

Candidal Diaper Dermatitis

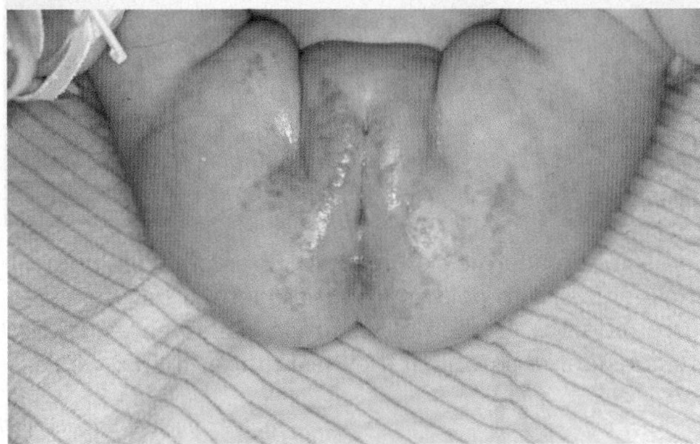

This type of diaper rash results from infection with *Candida albicans*, a fungus.

Allergic Contact Diaper Dermatitis

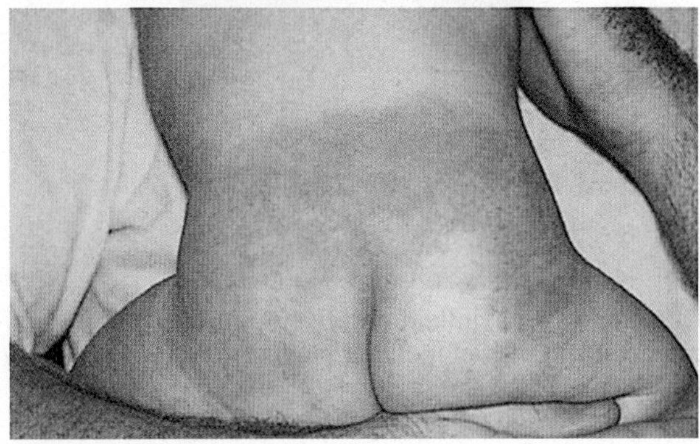

This type of diaper rash develops when the child's skin is in contact with an allergen.

(table continues on page 848)

TABLE 26.7 Abnormal Skin Conditions in Newborns and Infants *(continued)*

Contact Dermatitis and Inflammatory and Allergy-Related Conditions

Eczema (Atopic Dermatitis)

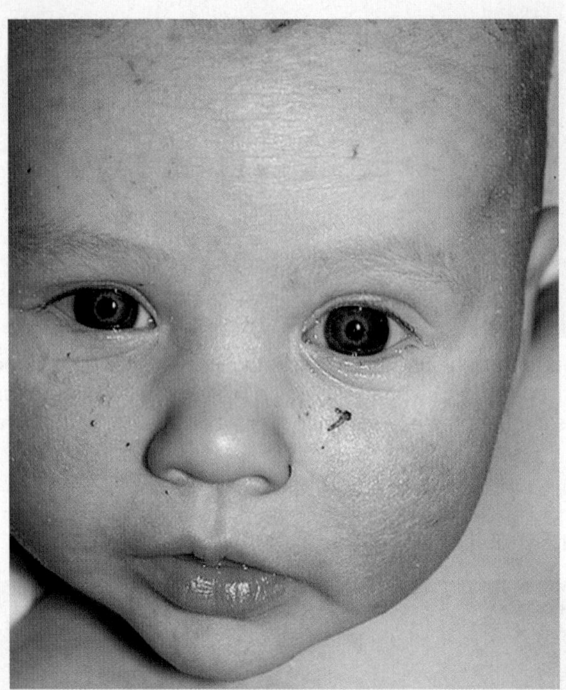

This skin condition usually appears in the first 6 months of life and typically resolves by age 5 years. It is characterized by dry, itchy, irritated skin. The exact cause is unknown, but a familial link and allergic component exist. Treatment, generally with topical corticosteroids, aims at controlling symptoms.

Lichen Simplex Chronicus

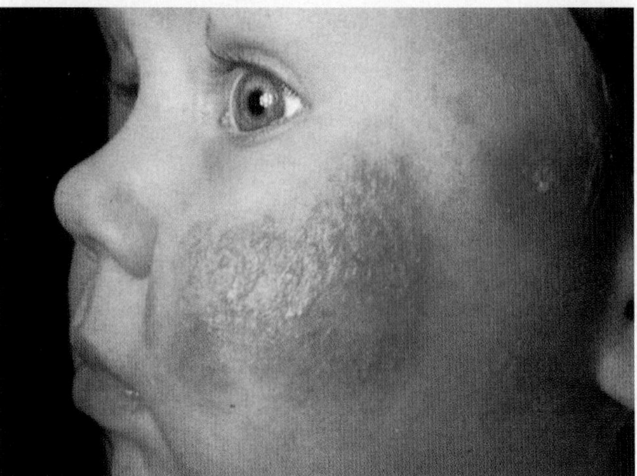

These discrete patches of eczema (thickened skin with scaling) result from irritation that follows repetitive rubbing or scratching. Secondary infections occasionally occur from breaks in the skin caused by excessive scratching.

Psoriasis

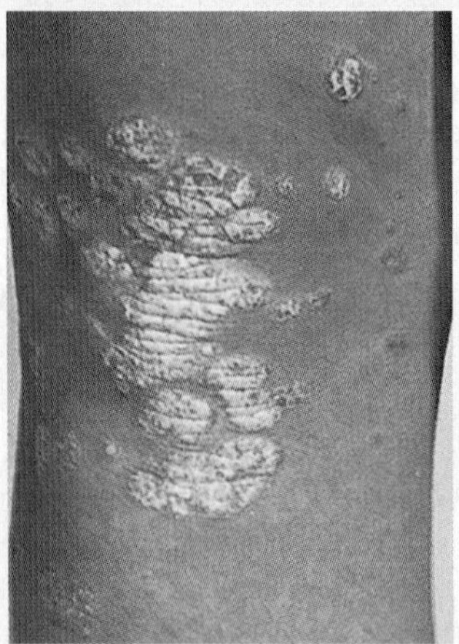

This proliferative, inflammatory autoimmune disease is characterized by well-defined plaques covered by silvery scales.

Hives (Urticaria)

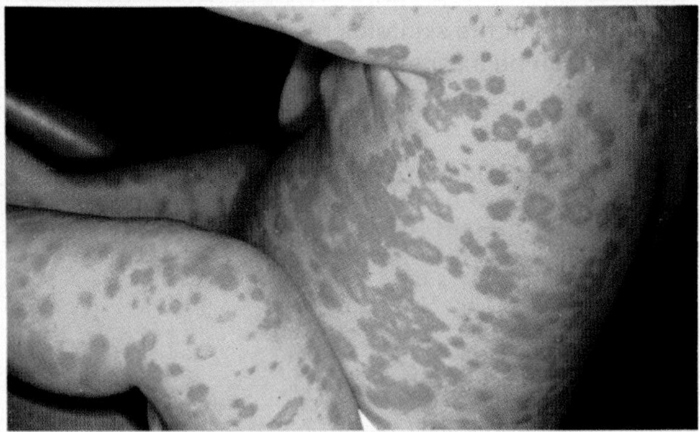

Hives are an allergic skin reaction characterized by pruritic plaques with pale centralized edematous wheals surrounded by erythematous areas, called flares. Hives are considered chronic if they last longer than 6 weeks.

(table continues on page 849)

TABLE 26.7 Abnormal Skin Conditions in Newborns and Infants *(continued)*

Skin Tumors/Hyperpigmented Lesions

Café Au Lait Spots

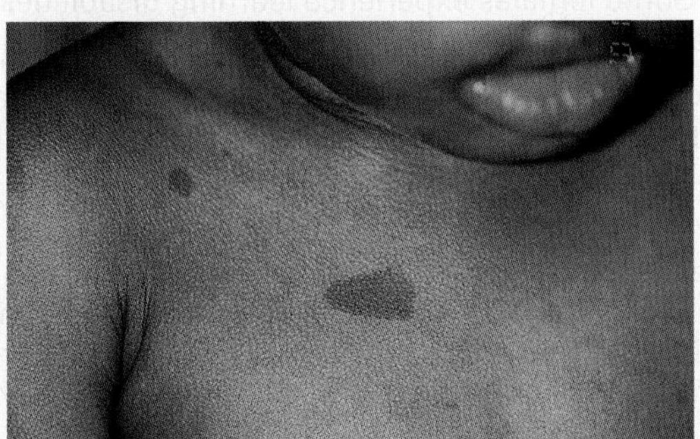

Spots start out as light-brown pigmented lesions during infancy. They grow and darken as the child grows. If these spots are noted during an examination, the infant needs medical evaluation to rule out neurofibromatosis. Cafe au lait spots may be the only sign of this inherited disorder; however, the child needs close medical observation throughout childhood because of the devastating sequelae of neurofibromatosis.

Port Wine Stains

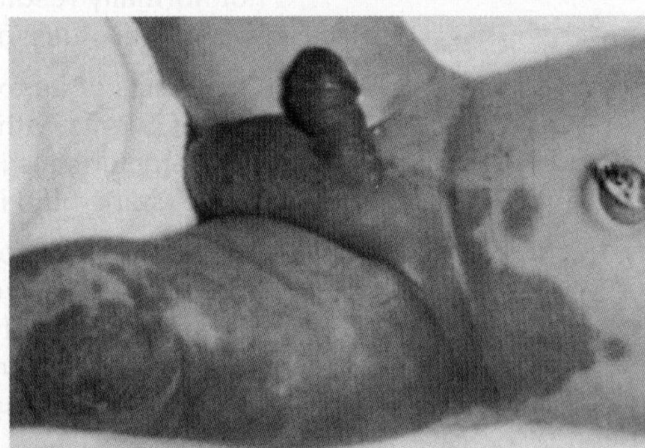

Also called *nevus flammeus*, these congenital capillary lesions are characterized by pink-to-purple or red patches anywhere on the body. The lesions can be disfiguring, particularly if they are large or on the face. Port wine stains grow proportionately with the child and often darken over time. Laser treatment is often effective.

From: Nelson, K. E., & Williams, C. M. (2013). *Infectious disease epidemiology: Theory and practice* (3rd ed.). Sudbury, MA: Jones and Bartlett.

TABLE 26.8 Genetic Disorders

Disorder	Description
Cystic fibrosis	This autosomal recessive disorder is most common in Caucasians. It is characterized by abnormal transport of chloride and sodium in exocrine tissues. The result is thick viscous secretions in the lungs, pancreas, liver, intestine, and reproductive tract. Pulmonary complications generally lead to early death. Average life expectancy is 30 years.
Down syndrome (trisomy 21)	An extra chromosome 21 leads to moderate-to-severe mental retardation and affects almost every organ system. Common dysmorphic features include microcephaly, brachycephaly, upslanting palpebral fissures, bilateral epicanthal folds, Brushfield spots, flat nasal bridge, pronounced curve on the ear helix, protruding tongue, and abnormally placed nipples. Low-set thumbs, inward curvature of the little fingers, a simian (single palmar) crease, and a wide space between the great and second toes are other characteristics. Generalized hypotonia is noted in infants.
Fragile X syndrome	This most common cause of inherited mental retardation results from extra genetic material on the X chromosome. Dysmorphic features in infants include a prominent forehead, long narrow face with a high arched palate, and large ears, jaw, and testes. Young children demonstrate delayed development, hyperactivity, and autistic behavior.
Klinefelter syndrome	A male inherits an extra X chromosome, with genotype XXY. The earlier the syndrome is diagnosed, the better the outcome; however, many patients are not diagnosed until adulthood, when infertility becomes apparent. Characteristics include enlarged breasts, sparse hair, small testes, and no sperm production.

(table continues on page 850)

TABLE 26.8 **Genetic Disorders** *(continued)*

Disorder	Description
Triple X syndrome	A female inherits an extra X chromosome, with genotype XXX. This condition does not normally result in infertility. Some females experience learning disabilities and social difficulties; others are affected so mildly that they are never diagnosed.
Trisomy 13	The effects of an extra chromosome 13 are so devastating that only approximately 18% of infants with it live more than 1 year. Survivors are severely retarded. Physical characteristics include microcephaly, microphthalmia (small eyes), cleft lip and palate, spina bifida, polydactyly, deafness, and heart defects.
Trisomy 18	An extra chromosome 18 severely affects all organ systems. Characteristics include profound retardation, microcephaly, prominent occiput, microphthalmia, epicanthal folds, short palpebral fissures, micrognathia (small jaw), ear malformations, and severe cardiac defects. Only approximately 10% of infants survive beyond 1 year of age.
Turner syndrome	Caused by a missing or partially missing X chromosome, this condition affects females only. Physical characteristics vary greatly, partly depending on how much X chromosome is missing. Characteristics include micrognathia, prominent ears, short neck with webbing, short fourth and fifth fingers, and heart and kidney defects. Incomplete sexual development and infertility are characteristics in adult women.

27

Children and Adolescents

Learning Objectives

1 Demonstrate knowledge of anatomy and physiology of each body system in the child or adolescent that may not be the same as in the adult.

2 Identify important topics for health promotion and risk reduction related to children and adolescents.

3 Collect subjective data related to children and adolescents from the child's and caregiver's perspectives.

4 Collect objective data related to children and adolescents using physical examination techniques.

5 Identify expected and unexpected findings related to children and adolescents.

6 Analyze subjective and objective data from the assessment of children and adolescents and consider initial interventions.

7 Document and communicate data from children and adolescents using appropriate terminology and principles of recording.

8 Consider age, condition, and culture of children and adolescents to individualize the assessment.

9 Identify nursing diagnoses and initiate a nursing plan of care based on findings from the assessment of children and adolescents.

Simon Chavez, a 4-year-old Hispanic boy, presents to the school-based health center for a preschool physical examination. Simon lives with his 20-year-old mother who stays home all day with him and his newborn sister. Simon's 21-year-old father is a delivery truck driver for a local grocery distributor; he leaves for work at 7 AM and returns most evenings by 5:30 PM, when he assists with care of the children.

Simon has not been in a structured preschool or day care environment. This September will be his first exposure to care and formalized instruction outside the home. He seems excited about his new opportunity and is willing to discuss the new school with the nurse. Simon has never been hospitalized, but he has been treated in the emergency department twice for coughing and wheezing. He also has had frequent ear infections; the last one was 3 weeks ago. He has never had surgery. He has no known allergies; his only medication is a daily multivitamin with iron.

You will acquire more information about Simon's present health status and past health history as you progress through this chapter. As you study the content and features, consider Simon's case and its relationship to what you are learning. Begin thinking about the following points:

- What health information and assessments are important for the toddler, preschooler, school-age child, and adolescent?
- How do assessment findings differ between the child and adult?
- What adaptations will you make when assessing a child?
- What factors could be contributing to Simon's language development?
- What recommendations for follow-up and future screening would you recommend for Simon?
- How would you evaluate Mrs. Chavez's ability to follow through with the recommendations on her return visit with Simon?

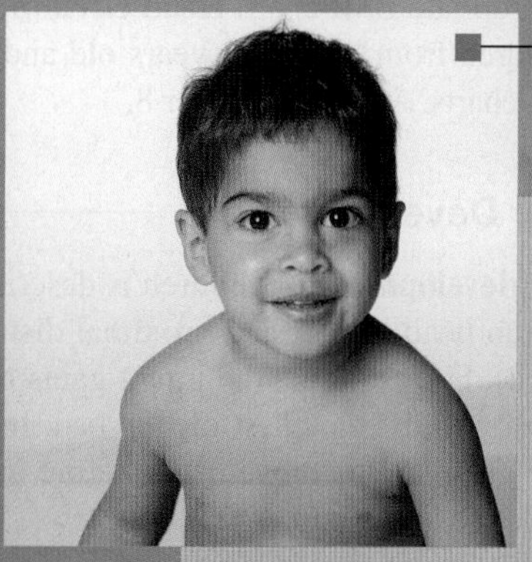

This chapter explores health assessment for children and adolescents. It highlights significant past and present health history along with related physical examination findings most pertinent to children and adolescents. Health care decision making for patients younger than 18 years of age resides with their parents or legal caregivers. Therefore, caring for children and adolescents requires that you involve both the parent/guardian and child/adolescent in assessment, diagnosis, planning, intervention, and evaluation.

Bright Futures is a national health promotion and disease prevention initiative that addresses children's health needs within the context of family and community (American Academy of Pediatrics [AAP], 2012). It acknowledges that a multitude of support people and agencies are necessary to raise healthy children and to build the necessary foundation for them to develop into productive adult citizens. Therefore, health assessment of the child or adolescent (Bright Futures/AAP, 2013) also includes assessing community support, environmental exposures, and potential opportunities for health promotion. Figure 27.1 delineates the Bright Futures/American Academy of Pediatrics Recommendations for Preventive Pediatric Health Care.

Structure and Function

Physical Growth

Although children grow and develop at varying rates, they do both at predictable times according to previously established normal ranges. Health care providers must evaluate a child's physical growth with the use of **standardized growth charts**. The growth charts for children 2 to 18 years of age were developed by the Centers for Disease Control and Prevention (CDC). The growth charts for children from birth to 2 years of age were developed by the World Health Organization (WHO, 2010) and are now recommended for children younger than 2 years of age worldwide. All charts can be downloaded from the Centers for Disease Control and Prevention Web site at http://www.cdc.gov/growthcharts/ (CDC, 2010).

Growth charts for boys and girls vary. Charts for children from birth to 2 years old are for heights measured while recumbent; charts for children 2 to 18 years of age are for children measured upright with a stadiometer. Children are weighed on a calibrated scale. For children older than 2 years of age, health care providers calculate and plot body mass index (BMI) on the appropriate BMI chart. **Head circumference** is measured on children from birth to 3 years old and plotted on similar growth charts. Also see Chapter 8.

Motor Development

Motor development of children is described as cephalocaudal (from head to toe) and proximal distal (from the center outward). For example, the infant gains head control before the ability to lift the chest off the bed. In addition, children master gross motor movements before attaining fine motor control. See also Chapter 8.

Refinement of motor activity and skills continues throughout childhood and adolescence. The Denver Developmental Screening Test II is discussed later in the Objective Data Collection section as a tool for evaluating motor development.

> **SAFETY ALERT**
> *Safety precautions in children change according to age group because of the variation in their developing motor abilities. For instance, covering electrical outlets is important after a child begins to be able to sit properly, whereas protecting the child from falls down stairs begins to matter more once the child can roll, crawl, or walk.*

Language

A child develops speech and speech sounds in a predictable manner. Evaluation of the child's initiation and continuance of sounds, as well as articulation, is critical throughout the early years.

At birth, the child cries. He or she then learns to coo and babble as well as how to gesture. By 10 to 15 months old, the child says the first word; by 18 months old, he or she has a vocabulary of approximately 50 words. Most children use two-word sentences by 2 years of age. By 3 years of age, their sentences are more complicated, and their speech is completely understandable to most people. See also Chapters 8 and 26.

A delay in **speech development** may signal a hearing loss or mental health concerns (e.g., autism). Bright Futures recommends screening for autism at 18 months and 2 years of age with a tool such as the Modified Checklist for Autism in Toddlers (M-CHAT) (Robins, Fein, & Barton, 1999) and with a structured developmental tool when the child is 2½ years old.

> **Clinical Significance**
> Children who babble at 4–6 months old and then stop babbling have an acquired hearing loss. Those who never babble may have a congenital hearing loss or a hearing loss acquired since birth.

Psychosocial and Cognitive Development

Psychosocial development and cognitive development related to, and influential on, the health of children and adolescents is discussed in detail in Chapter 8.

Cultural Considerations

Every child grows and develops in a family or care setting unique to that child, regardless of racial background. Health habits are not race related but defined culturally within the local community and family. Nevertheless, certain racial or ethnic groups are more prone than others to specific disorders or diseases. For instance, rates of obesity and Type 2 diabetes are higher among Hispanics and African Americans than among Caucasians.

Each child and family is unique; therefore, these **Recommendations for Preventive Pediatric Health Care** are designed for the care of children who are receiving competent parenting, have no manifestations of any important health problems, and are growing and developing in satisfactory fashion. **Additional visits may become necessary** if circumstances suggest variations from normal.

Developmental, psychosocial, and chronic disease issues for children and adolescents may require frequent counseling and treatment visits separate from preventive care visits.

These guidelines represent a consensus by the American Academy of Pediatrics (AAP) and Bright Futures. The AAP continues to emphasize the great importance of **continuity of care** in comprehensive health supervision and the need to avoid **fragmentation of care.**

The recommendations in this statement do not indicate an exclusive course of treatment or sta care. Variations, taking into account individual circumstances, may be appropriate.

	INFANCY								EARLY CHILDHOOD							MIDDLE CHILDHOOD						ADOLESCENCE								
AGE[1]	PRENATAL[2]	NEWBORN[3]	3–5 d[4]	By 1 mo	2 mo	4 mo	6 mo	9 mo	12 m	15 mo	18 mo	24 mo	30 mo	3 y	4 y	5 y	6 y	7 y	8 y	9 y	10 y	11 y	12 y	13 y	14 y	15 y	16 y	17 y	18 y	19 y
HISTORY																														
Initial/Interval	●	●	●	●	●	●	●	●	●	●	●	●	●	●	●	●	●	●	●	●	●	●	●	●	●	●	●	●	●	●
MEASUREMENTS																														
Length/Height and Weight		●	●	●	●	●	●	●	●	●	●	●	●	●	●	●	●	●	●	●	●	●	●	●	●	●	●	●	●	●
Head Circumference		●	●	●	●	●	●	●	●	●	●	●																		
Weight for Length		●	●	●	●	●	●	●	●	●	●																			
Body Mass Index												●	●	●	●	●	●	●	●	●	●	●	●	●	●	●	●	●	●	●
Blood Pressure[5]		★	★	★	★	★	★	★	★	★	★	★	★	●	●	●	●	●	●	●	●	●	●	●	●	●	●	●	●	●
SENSORY SCREENING																														
Vision		★	★	★	★	★	★	★	★	★	★	★	★	●[6]	●	●	●	★	●	★	●	★	●	★	★	●	★	★	●	★
Hearing		●[7]	★	★	★	★	★	★	★	★	★	★	★	★	●	●	●	★	●	★	●	★	★	★	★	★	★	★	★	★
DEVELOPMENTAL/BEHAVIORAL ASSESSMENT																														
Developmental Screening[8]								●			●		●																	
Autism Screening[9]											●	●																		
Developmental Surveillance[8]		●	●	●	●	●	●		●	●		●		●	●	●	●	●	●	●	●	●	●	●	●	●	●	●	●	●
Psychosocial/Behavioral Assessment		●	●	●	●	●	●	●	●	●	●	●	●	●	●	●	●	●	●	●	●	●	●	●	●	●	●	●	●	●
Alcohol and Drug Use Assessment																						★	★	★	★	★	★	★	★	★
PHYSICAL EXAMINATION[10]		●	●	●	●	●	●	●	●	●	●	●	●	●	●	●	●	●	●	●	●	●	●	●	●	●	●	●	●	●
PROCEDURES[11]																														
Newborn Metabolic/Hemoglobin Screening[12]		←—	●	——	—→																									
Immunization[13]		●	●	●	●	●	●	●	●	●	●	●	●	●	●	●	●	●	●	●	●	●	●	●	●	●	●	●	●	●
Hematocrit or Hemoglobin[14]						★			●		★	★		★	★	★	★	★	★	★	★	★	★	★	★	★	★	★	★	★
Lead Screening[15]							★	★	● or ★[16]		★	● or ★[16]		★	★	★	★													
Tuberculin Test[17]				★			★		★		★	★		★	★	★	★	★	★	★	★	★	★	★	★	★	★	★	★	★
Dyslipidemia Screening[18]												★			★		★		★		★	★	★	★	★	★	★	★	←—	——
STI Screening[19]																						★	★	★	★	★	★	★	★	★
Cervical Dysplasia Screening[20]																						★	★	★	★	★	★	★	★	★
ORAL HEALTH[21]							★	★	● or ★[21]		● or ★[21]	● or ★[21]	● or ★[21]	●[22]			●[22]													
ANTICIPATORY GUIDANCE[23]	●	●	●	●	●	●	●	●	●	●	●	●	●	●	●	●	●	●	●	●	●	●	●	●	●	●	●	●	●	●

1. If a child comes under care for the first time at any point on the schedule, or if any items are not accomplished at the suggested age, the schedule should be brought up to date at the earliest possible time.
2. A prenatal visit is recommended for parents who are at high risk, for first-time parents, and for those who request a conference. The prenatal visit should include anticipatory guidance, pertinent medical history, and a discussion of benefits of breastfeeding and planned method of feeding per AAP statement "The Prenatal Visit" (2001) [URL: http://aappolicy.aappublications.org/cgi/content/full/pediatrics;107/6/1456].
3. Every infant should have a newborn evaluation after birth, breastfeeding encouraged, and instruction and support offered.
4. Every infant should have an evaluation within 3 to 5 days of birth and within 48 to 72 hours after discharge from the hospital, to include evaluation for feeding and jaundice. Breastfeeding infants should receive formal breastfeeding evaluation, encouragement, and instruction as recommended in AAP statement "Breastfeeding and the Use of Human Milk" (2005) [URL: http://aappolicy.aappublications.org/cgi/content/full/pediatrics;115/2/496]. For newborns discharged in less than 48 hours after delivery, the infant must be examined within 48 hours of discharge per AAP statement "Hospital Stay for Healthy Term Newborns" (2004) [URL: http://aappolicy.aappublications.org/cgi/content/full/pediatrics;113/5/1434].
5. Blood pressure measurement in infants and children with specific risk conditions should be performed at visits before age 3 years.
6. If the patient is uncooperative, rescreen within 6 months per AAP statement "Eye Examination in Infants, Children, and Young Adults by Pediatricians" (2007) [URL: http://aappolicy.aappublications.org/cgi/content/full/pediatrics;111/4/902].
7. All newborns should be screened per AAP statement "Year 2000 Position Statement: Principles and Guidelines for Early Hearing Detection and Intervention Programs " (2000) [URL: http://aappolicy.aappublications.org/cgi/content/full/pediatrics;106/4/798]. Joint Committee on Infant Hearing. Year 2007 position statement: principles and guidelines for early hearing detection and intervention programs. *Pediatrics.* 2007;120:898–921.
8. AAP Council on Children With Disabilities, AAP Section on Developmental Behavioral Pediatrics, AAP Bright Futures Steering Committee, AAP Medical Home Initiatives for Children With Special Needs Project Advisory Committee. Identifying infants and young children with developmental disorders in the medical home: an algorithm for developmental surveillance and screening. *Pediatrics.* 2006;118:405–420 [URL: http://aappolicy.aappublications.org/cgi/content/full/pediatrics;118/1/405].
9. Gupta VB, Hyman SL, Johnson CP, et al. Identifying children with autism early? *Pediatrics.* 2007;119:152–153 [URL: http://pediatrics.aappublications.org/cgi/content/full/119/1/152].
10. At each visit, age-appropriate physical examination is essential, with infant totally unclothed, older child undressed and suitably draped.
11. These may be modified, depending on entry point into schedule and individual need.
12. Newborn metabolic and hemoglobinopathy screening should be done according to state law. Results should be reviewed at visits and appropriate retesting or referral done as needed.
13. Schedules per the Committee on Infectious Diseases, published annually in the January issue of *Pediatrics*. Every visit should be an opportunity to update and complete a child's immunizations.
14. See AAP *Pediatric Nutrition Handbook*, 5th Edition (2003) for a discussion of universal and selective screening options. See also Recommendations to prevent and control iron deficiency in the United States. *MMWR.* 1998;47(RR-3):1–36.
15. For children at risk of lead exposure, consult the AAP statement "Lead Exposure in Children: Prevention, Detection, and Management" (2005) [URL: http://aappolicy.aappublications.org/cgi/content/full/pediatrics;116/4/1036]. Additionally, screening should be done in accordance with state law where applicable.
16. Perform risk assessments or screens as appropriate, based on universal screening requirements for patients with Medicaid or high prevalence areas.
17. Tuberculosis testing per recommendations of the Committee on Infectious Diseases, published in the curr *Book: Report of the Committee on Infectious Diseases.* Testing should be done on recognition of high-risk
18. "Third Report of the National Cholesterol Education Program (NCEP) Expert Panel on Detection, Evaluatio of High Blood Cholesterol in Adults (Adult Treatment Panel III) Final Report" (2002) [URL: http://circ.ahajou content/full/106/25/3143] and "The Expert Committee Recommendations on the Assessment, Prevention, Child and Adolescent Overweight and Obesity." Supplement to *Pediatrics.* In press.
19. All sexually active patients should be screened for sexually transmitted infections (STIs).
20. All sexually active girls should have screening for cervical dysplasia as part of a pelvic examination beginn of onset of sexual activity or age 21 (whichever comes first).
21. Referral to dental home, if available. Otherwise, administer oral health risk assessment. If the primary wate cient in fluoride, consider oral fluoride supplementation.
22. At the visits for 3 years and 6 years of age, it should be determined whether the patient has a dental home does not have a dental home, a referral should be made to one. If the primary water source is deficient in oral fluoride supplementation.
23. Refer to the specific guidance by age as listed in Bright Futures Guidelines. (Hagan JF, Shaw JS, Duncan *Futures: Guidelines for Health Supervision of Infants, Children, and Adolescents.* 3rd ed. Elk Grove Village, Academy of Pediatrics; 2008.)

KEY

● = to be performed ★ = risk assessment to be performed, with appropriate action to follow, if positive ←—●—→ = range during which a service may be provided, with the symbol indicating the preferred age

Figure 27.1 Recommended intervals for health assessment of children and adolescents.

The norms of each family setting deserve assessment in regards to patterns of rest, activity, nutrition, illness intervention, health habits, and member roles. This includes who eats together, what is eaten, where food is obtained, who prepares food, and how food is prepared. These norms contribute to the health of the child and are important components of a nutritional assessment. Each area of assessment listed also contributes to or discourages the development of obesity. Some families do not prepare food at home and eat out most of the time; some families do not eat together; some eat in the front of the TV; some children eat only in their rooms; and some eat with grandparents. You will not be aware of the family's norms unless you ask about them. They are different for each family based not on race but on familial cultural norms.

Another example of cultural differences in families concerns activity levels. One family would never consider walking to the grocery store, even if it is just one block away. Another family would consider themselves lazy if they did not hike at least 3 miles every Saturday in the park close to their house.

Assessment of language development is difficult if the health care provider is not bilingual and the child speaks another language. If a language other than English is normally spoken in the home, language development may be delayed if the child is attempting to develop two languages at the same time. Such children will be bilingual, and language delay is not of concern if hearing is normal. Subjective assessment can be obtained by the registered nurse (RN) or the advanced practice registered nurse (APRN). The APRN, however, will know the interventions needed and the implications and consequences of the subjective information given.

Urgent Assessment

Children in physiological distress compensate with increased respiratory and heart rates. Physiological distress usually results from a respiratory disorder or significant blood loss. (Even children with a known congenital heart problem rarely present in acute distress from ischemic heart disease.) The additional work of breathing is evidenced in a distressed child by nasal flaring accompanied by supracostal, intercostal, and subcostal chest retractions (Fig. 27.2) or abdominal breathing. Administration of oxygen and support of the child's ability to breathe are the first interventions.

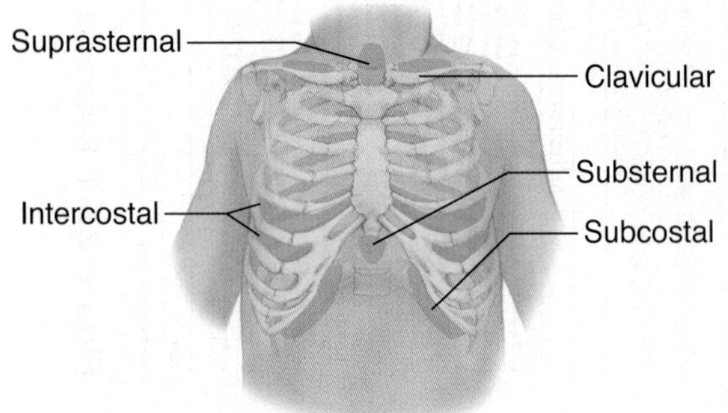

Figure 27.2 Sites of retractions.

The child being examined should remain sitting upright with the parent or in the parent's lap to promote optimal ventilation and to prevent the child from becoming upset because crying requires additional oxygen and respiratory effort. Supplemental oxygen can be delivered by the parent via a mask held in place over or close to the child's nose and mouth.

> **SAFETY ALERT**
> *Transfer to a tertiary care center is indicated for the child in distress. A child who cannot compensate for oxygen requirements may require mechanical ventilation. Other acute situations requiring transfer include trauma, head injury, meningitis, and acute abdomen (e.g., ruptured appendix).*

Subjective Data

When caring for a child, you should involve all interested adults who have a legal relationship with the child. If the parents and child have agreed to include other family members or friends in health care and have given written consent, you should also share information with those designated people. This situation is more common with very young children and with those who have a chronic condition requiring adaptations to everyday life.

As the child becomes an adolescent and begins to seek care for him or herself alone, sharing of information is less common. Legal consent for health care treatment is 18 years of age. Most states, however, permit contraception and treatment for sexually transmitted infections (STIs) at 13 years of age.

> **SAFETY ALERT**
> *Most states require patients to be of legal age of consent for the treatment of infections or other health problems, unless an adolescent has been deemed an emancipated minor by being married, being a parent, or having the appropriate legal documentation.*

Health assessment of a child or adolescent begins the moment that he or she enters the facility. You can learn a great deal by observing the patient's interactions with caregivers and health care providers. You can evaluate the pediatric patient's ability to communicate, along with movement capabilities, when transferring from one room to the next. Children and teens demonstrate many developmental skills during the screening process. Focused observation and purposeful interactions with children provide opportunities to assess children in a nonthreatening manner in the health care setting.

Assessment requires patience and skill to acquire health information from both cooperative and noncooperative children. The health assessment should not be traumatic for you or the patient. It is a time to learn about staying healthy and a chance for you to reinforce positive lifelong health habits.

Assessment of Risk Factors

History and Risk Factors	Rationale
Reason for Seeking Care Tell me why you came to the clinic today. *or* Why did you have to come to the hospital?	Obtain information about the reason for seeking care. Ask follow-up questions if the child has pain or discomfort.
Prenatal History Ask questions related to: • maternal health • medications • exposure to toxic substances, alcohol, or illicit drugs • birth history • birth weight • birth date/due date • labor and birth experience • Apgar scores at 1 and 5 minutes	Perinatal environment and exposures may affect the child's present health. Premature and small-for-gestational-age babies may have long-term sequelae if their transition to extrauterine life was difficult. If they experienced anoxia, long-term sequelae are possible.
Postnatal History • Did the baby go home with the mother from the hospital? • Were there any difficulties after getting home? • Did the baby have jaundice? If so, did he or she require treatment?	The postnatal period is the time just after birth; you can assume that the child's problems were limited if he or she went home with the mother 24–72 hours after birth. Extremely elevated postnatal bilirubin levels (greater than or equal to 25 mcg/dl) may be associated with neurological problems.
Developmental History • Did the child develop like other children? • At what age did he or she sit? Stand? Walk? • When was his or her first word? What was it? • When was the child toilet trained? Day? Night?	An accurate developmental history alerts you to possible delays requiring further intervention.
Personal History Has the child been hospitalized? Has the child had surgery? What were the problems? What were the outcomes?	Significant past health problems may be related to a present problem.
Medications and Supplements • Is the child taking any medications now? • Is the child taking any prescription medications? How? • Is the child taking any over-the-counter medications? How and how often?	All medications may affect the child's illness and also behavior. Medications taken together may interact. Children can be given too much or too little of an over-the-counter (OTC) drug (e.g., acetaminophen).
Family History Does anyone in your family have diabetes; hypertension; heart disease; elevated cholesterol levels; asthma; allergies; cancer; liver, kidney, or gastrointestinal problems; arthritis; or learning problems?	A positive response to any of these questions increases the child's risk as well and may signal a need for additional testing (e.g., serum cholesterol screening).
Has anyone in the family died before age 50 years?	Family history provides information about the seriousness of diseases reported above. Additionally, cardiac arrest of unknown origin may be associated with abnormal cardiac rhythms (e.g., prolonged Q-T interval); an electrocardiogram may be indicated.

(table continues on page 856)

History and Risk Factors	Rationale
Risk Factors ***Lead-risk Screening*** • Does your child live in or regularly visit a house or child care facility built before 1950? • Does your child live in or regularly visit a house or child care facility built before 1978 that is being or has recently (within the last 6 months) been renovated or remodeled? • Does your child have a brother, sister, or playmate who has or had lead poisoning?	"Yes" to any of these three questions requires health care providers to take a blood level on children from birth to 72 months old (and possibly beyond if at risk). Some toys may also contain lead (CDC, 2013a, 2013b).
Tuberculosis Screening • Is the child infected with HIV? • Is the child in close contact with people known or suspected to have tuberculosis (TB)? • Is the child in close contact with people known to be alcohol dependent or intravenous drug users? With people who reside in a long-term care facility, correctional or mental institution, nursing home/facility, or other long-term residential facility? • Is the child foreign-born and from a country with high TB prevalence? • Is the child from a medically underserved low-income population, including a high-risk racial or ethnic minority population? • Is the child/adolescent alcohol-dependent, an intravenous drug user, or a resident of a long-term-care facility, correctional or mental institution, nursing home/facility, or other long-term residential facility (CDC, 2012).	"Yes" to any of these questions requires the administration of a purified protein derivative tuberculin test to the patient.
Immunizations. Is the child current with immunizations?	**Immunization schedules** for children and adolescents can be found at the CDC (2014a) Web site, http://www.cdc.gov/vaccines/.
Car Safety. Does the child sit in an approved car seat? In the back seat? Does the adolescent always wear a seat belt (Fig. 27.3)?	A car seat is recommended for the newborn leaving the hospital and for all children for the first 4 years or until weighing at least 40 lb.

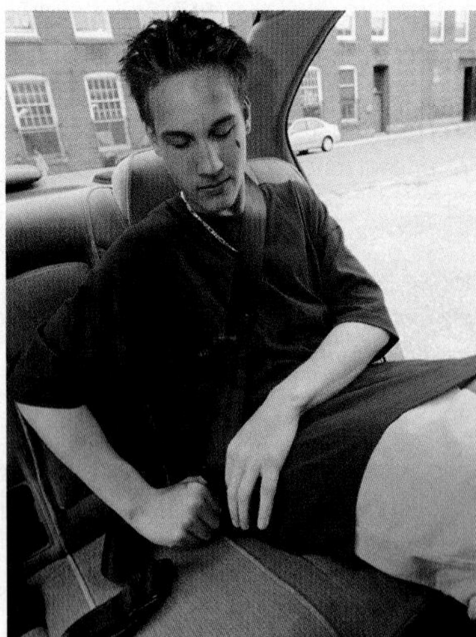

Figure 27.3 Adolescents need to understand the importance of the use of seat belts to optimize their protection whether as drivers or as passengers.

(table continues on page 857)

History and Risk Factors	Rationale
Poison Control. Are hazardous substances safely stored away from where the child can reach them?	The house and other environments where the child spends significant time should be childproofed by locking up cleaning supplies and keeping all medicines out of the child's reach. For a child suspected of ingesting a nonfood substance, the parent should call the Poison Help Line at 1-800-222-1222.
Safety in the Home. Is the child protected from falling down the stairs? From out of the windows? Are guns kept in the home? Are they secured?	Children need to be protected from falls from windows and down stairs. Guns should not be loaded; they should be locked up.
Fire Safety. Does your family have a fire escape plan?	Children need protection from burns related to open fire pits, campfires, grills, gas stoves, stovetop cooking of food, lighters of any kind, and matches.
Water Safety. Is the swimming pool secured by fencing? Ask whether the child can swim. Can the child swim to the side of the pool if he or she falls into the deep end?	Pools should have fences at least 6-ft high and entrance gates with locks at a level where only adults can reach them.
Outdoor Safety. Has your child been taught to safely cross streets when walking alone?	Child pedestrians are at risk for injury and need instruction about where and when to cross frequently traveled streets as well as where and how to walk down the street.
Does the child wear a helmet for high-risk activities?	Encourage the use of bike helmets when a child begins to ride a tricycle or a bicycle. Some states require bicycle helmets to be worn on state roads.
Does the child use sunscreen when outside?	Unprotected sun exposure increases risks for melanoma, basal cell carcinoma, and squamous cell carcinoma.
Drug and Alcohol Use. Ask the older child or adolescent • Have you or your friends used drugs, alcohol, or tobacco?	People between 12 and 20 years of age drink 11% of all alcohol consumed in the United States. More than 90% of this alcohol is consumed during binge drinking (CDC, 2014b).
Nutrition and Obesity. Describe what you eat on an average day.	Overweight and obesity have serious health consequences among children and adolescents, including a greater risk of high cholesterol, hypertension, and diabetes mellitus.
Violence and Suicide. Ask children and teens whether they feel threatened at school. Ask directly whether the patient has thought about hurting self or others.	Youth violence includes bullying, slapping, and hitting. Other physical threats include robbery, assault, and rape.
Contraception and Sexually Transmitted Infections. Ask adolescents • Do you engage in oral sex or are you sexually active?	Adolescents are more likely than adults to have multiple sexual partners and short-term relationships, to engage in unprotected intercourse, and to have partners at high risk for STIs (CDC, 2012).

Risk Reduction and Health Promotion

For children and adolescents, health-related patient teaching focuses on healthy lifestyle choices including nutrition and exercise. Teaching also includes information about the avoidance of unhealthy habits frequently acquired at early ages (e.g., tobacco use). Additional information includes safety and the importance of emotional health and positive interpersonal relationships. You can also incorporate assessment of school performance and its compatibility with stated life goals into the well-child health assessment.

Health promotion goals include the following:

- Increase the proportion of young children and adolescents who receive all vaccines that have been recommended for universal administration for at least the first 5 years of their lives.

- Reduce the proportion of children and adolescents who are overweight or obese.
- Reduce the proportion of children and adolescents who have dental caries in their primary or permanent teeth.
- Increase the proportion of children with mental health problems who receive treatment.
- Increase the proportion of adolescents who abstain from sexual intercourse or use condoms if currently sexually active.

(C.D.C., U.S.D.H.H.S., 2013)

Important education topics include immunizations, car safety, poison control, home safety, fire safety, water safety, outdoor safety, prevention of substance abuse, nutrition, prevention of obesity, and promotion of contraception and prevention of STIs.

Immunization Schedules

For children who have not received the full roster of recommended vaccines, encourage catch-up doses. Document administration and dates of vaccines and provide this information to caregivers/parents for their own records in addition to maintaining the health record at the place of regular health care.

Car Safety

Discuss with parents and children as appropriate the use of car seats, booster seats, and seat belts according to state laws. Car safety includes promoting car seats and booster seats for children from birth to 8 years of age and teaching adolescents about the dangers of drinking and driving.

Promoting Use of Car Seats and Belts. The infant seat should be in the back seat, facing backward, for at least the first year of the child's life. Depending on the construction of the car seat, it may be in the back seat facing backward until the child weighs 30 to 35 lb. A child may face forward after 1 year of age in some types of car seats. At 4 years of age (or at 40 lb), the child may switch from a car seat to a booster seat. The child should be seated and restrained with the automobile's seat belt in such a booster seat, which is designed for use until he or she is at least 49-in. tall (Fig. 27.4).

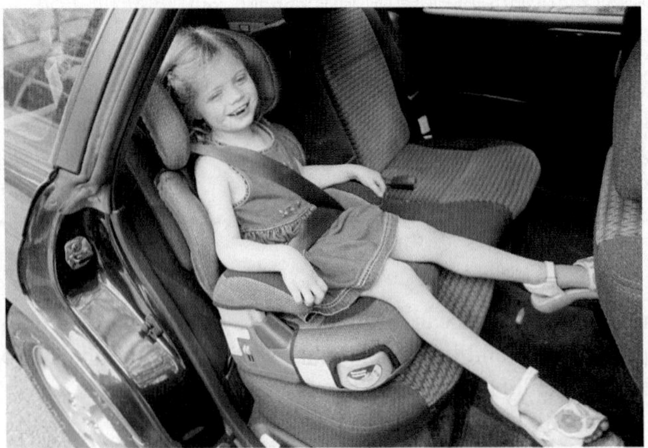

Figure 27.4 The booster seat requires the child to be restrained with a seat belt and also requires the seat to be in the back of the vehicle.

Children who have outgrown the booster seat should ride in the back with a seat belt fastened securely. A child may move to the front seat after 12 years of age if he or she is of adult size. Front air bags have been known to hurt younger and smaller children because of the force with which they are deployed. Although car seat and booster seat laws vary among states, the National Highway Traffic Safety Administration Web site (2013) is a good resource for more information about child safety restraint in cars.

Preventing Driving While Impaired. Discuss this topic by providing scenarios in which the adolescent has alternatives to riding with an impaired driver. Encourage the use of a designated driver if the teen is in a situation in which he or she anticipates drinking or drug use.

American Association of Poison Control Centers

The American Association of Poison Control Centers (AAPCC, n.d.) provides information needed for the home or hospital treatment of a child who has ingested a toxic substance. The Poison Help Line number is 1-800-222-1222. Recommendations might include use of ipecac syrup, activated charcoal, or both. Parents can buy these medications without a prescription; however, they should be used only when instructed to do so by the AAPCC. Currently, these medications are not recommended for home use because they have been used inappropriately in the past. The AAPCC provides telephone stickers or magnets with its emergency phone number to be posted on or near telephones.

Safety in the Home

Indications that a home that has been modified to optimize child safety include the following:

- Open windows have well-maintained screens.
- Additional bars or barriers protect low open windows that a toddler could reach and fall out of.
- Doors or gates block stairwells or open flight of steps.
- Any guns in the home are locked up and unavailable to children and adolescents.

Fire Safety

Children have a larger skin surface area than body weight. Burns on children make up a larger percentage of their surface area than on adults; therefore, burns are much more serious for children in terms of fluid replacement and potential for infection. Children and adolescents require protection against fire and must be taught the dangers of and significant respect for fire. The family should establish and discuss a family fire plan and escape routes from the house.

Water Safety

A young child who is unable to swim should always wear a life jacket when around a swimming pool or bodies of water. The necessity of a life jacket should continue until the adolescent can demonstrate strong swimming skills. Children should be encouraged to learn to swim and take swimming lessons to develop the ability to stay afloat in water that is deeper than they are tall.

Outdoor Safety

Outdoor safety includes safety while crossing streets; using helmets while riding tricycles, bicycles, or all-terrain vehicles; and using sunscreen.

Safe Street Crossing. Assess whether the child walks to school or other places such as parks or playgrounds alone. The safest route and safe street rules should be discussed with the child. Discuss walking facing traffic and crossing the street.

Helmet Use. Most states require helmets for riders of motorized vehicles on state roads. A child on an all-terrain motorized vehicle is encouraged to always wear a helmet. Helmets should also be worn during high-risk sports, such as football, hockey, baseball, skiing, and snowboarding. Head trauma secondary to accidents is a common childhood injury with long-term sequelae. Wearing bicycle helmets reduces the incidence of brain injury in children (Meehan, Lee, Fischer, & Mannix, 2013).

Use of Sunscreen. All children, no matter what their skin type or color, should apply sunscreen with a sun protection factor (SPF) of at least 15 when exposing skin to the sun or should be completely covered by clothing and wearing a wide-brimmed hat to prevent skin damage and skin cancer. Sunglasses that block both ultraviolet A (UVA) and ultraviolet B (UVB) light are also recommended to prevent the development of cataracts.

Prevention of Drug and Alcohol Use

Answer any questions the young person may have about drug and alcohol use. Counsel pediatric patients about the dangers of alcohol and drugs, emphasizing immediate over long-term risks. Also assess for mental health issues because drug-seeking behaviors often indicate an attempt to self-medicate for other problems. One potentially effective way to prevent young people from abusing substances is to explain how they interfere with the accomplishment of developmental tasks, which becomes difficult when the child or teen is impaired.

Nutrition and Prevention of Obesity

Discuss the child's BMI according to sex and age. It is important to provide nutritional and activity information early if the BMI is at or above the 85th percentile. The family should receive nutritional information from the U.S. Department of Agriculture ChooseMyPlate guidelines (2013) (see Chapter 7). Children aged 2 years and older should consume daily at least two servings of fruit; three servings of vegetables, with at least one third being dark green or orange; and six servings of grain products, with at least three being whole grains. Children aged 2 years and older should consume daily less than 10% of calories from saturated fat, no more than 30% of calories from total fat, and 2,400 mg or less of sodium; they also need to meet dietary recommendations for calcium.

You can ask questions and educate families about multivitamins with iron for high-risk patients as well as about food choices at school and how they can correlate with the guidance offered by ChooseMyPlate. Assess for engagement in vigorous physical activity and provide recommendations for appropriate activities. Young people need to exercise for at least 3 days/week for at least 20 minutes.

Mental Health Issues

Discuss actions to deal with threats at school, conflict resolution, and school resources available. Intervene immediately if a parent or child admits to concerns about hurting self or others. A patient or family member who describes a plan for suicide requires hospital admission for mental health concerns.

Promotion of Contraception and Sexually Transmitted Infection Prevention

Discuss abstinence, safe sex practices, and avoidance of high-risk behaviors with sexually active adolescents. Answer questions from all patients regarding sexuality and sexual health. Encourage nonsexual group activities and normalize the decision *not* to engage in sexual activity. For those adolescents who choose to continue sexual activity, encourage use of condoms.

You should also educate adolescents on the signs, symptoms, and consequences of untreated STIs. Urge immediate screening and treatment for symptoms and yearly examinations for sexually active adolescents even if they are asymptomatic. RN and APRN competence includes the assessment and education of known health risks to children and adolescents.

Common Symptoms

The symptoms listed below are common in children and adolescents; however, they are also common complaints of children attempting to avoid school. The pain goal is pain free (zero on the FACES pain scale) and elimination of the contributing symptom. Also, consider whether the situation represents acute illness that requires immediate attention.

Common Symptoms in Children and Adolescents

- Abdominal pain
- Headache
- Leg pain

Signs/Symptoms	Rationale/Unexpected Findings
Abdominal Pain • Can you point to where it hurts? • How bad is the pain?	Children usually cannot isolate abdominal pain to one specific area. If the child points to the right lower quadrant, appendicitis should be ruled out with abdominal scans.

(table continues on page 860)

Signs/Symptoms	Rationale/Unexpected Findings
• How long have you had this pain? • What does the pain feel like? (Cues may need to be added—e.g., sharp or dull.) • Does anything make your pain worse? • Does anything make your pain better? • Has your pain stopped you from going to school, playing sports, or other activities?	⚠ *SAFETY ALERT* *Acute intense pain with vomiting may indicate appendicitis. A child who stops activity or play because of pain requires additional evaluation. If rest relieves the pain, life-threatening concerns are usually not the problem.*
Headache • Can you point to where it hurts? • How bad is the pain? • How long have you had this pain? • What does the pain feel like? (Cues may need to be added—e.g., sharp or dull.) • Does anything make your pain worse? • Does anything make your pain better? • Has your pain stopped you from going to school, playing sports, or other activities?	For headaches, children usually cannot isolate to one specific area. ⚠ *SAFETY ALERT* *Acute, intense pain with vomiting may indicate a migraine or brain tumor. A child who cannot walk or who stops activity or play because of pain requires additional evaluation.*
Leg Pain • Can you point to where it hurts? • How bad is the pain? • How long have you had this pain? • What does the pain feel like? (Cues may need to be added—e.g., sharp or dull.) • Does anything make the pain worse? • Does anything make the pain better? • Has your pain stopped you from going to school, playing sports, or other activities?	For leg pain, children usually cannot isolate to one specific area. ⚠ *SAFETY ALERT* *If the child consistently limps, then fractures, dislocations, and bone tumors should be assessed before being ruled out.*

Therapeutic Dialogue: Collecting Subjective Data

Simon, introduced at the beginning of this chapter, is 4 years old and undergoing a preschool assessment. The nurse uses professional communication techniques to gather subjective data from Simon.

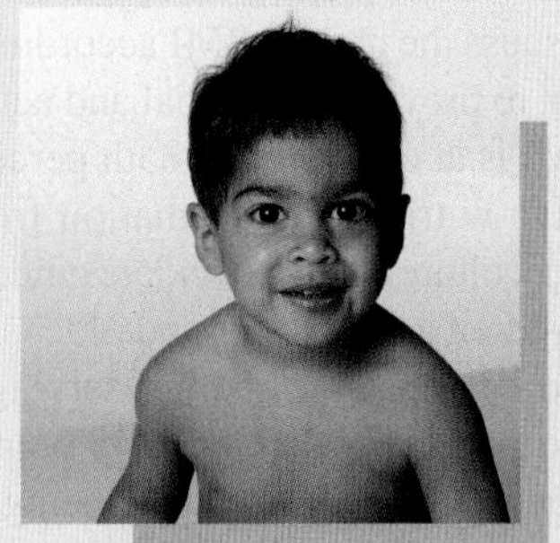

Nurse: It's nice to see you again, Simon and Mrs. Chavez. How are you today?

Mrs. Chavez: We are very well, thank you.

Nurse: Simon, how are you?

Simon: Chood.

(case study continues on page 861)

Nurse: (Leans in closer to hear speech clearly) So, Simon, why are you visiting the clinic?

Simon: I am choing to go to shool! (speech is somewhat garbled)

Nurse: Mrs. Chavez, is it difficult for you to understand Simon sometimes?

Mrs. Chavez: Yes, but I thought that it might be because he speaks both Spanish and English. His father's parents visit from Chile once a year. They bring him toys and candy that I don't approve of. I try to keep him healthy. He only watches TV an hour a day. He eats meat only once a day. He brushes his teeth every night and saw a dentist last year.

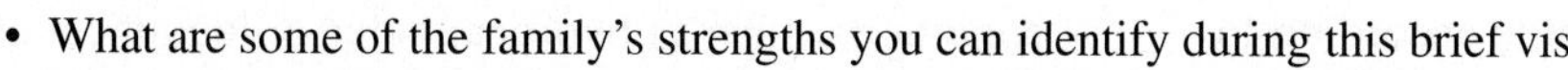
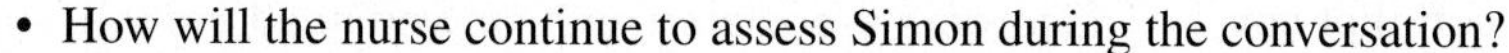

Critical Thinking Challenge

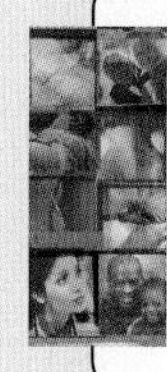

- What are some of the family's strengths you can identify during this brief visit?
- How will the nurse continue to assess Simon during the conversation?
- What risk factors might be identified? How will the nurse integrate health promotion?

Objective Data

Equipment

- Head-to-toe assessment equipment (see Chapter 5)
- Developmental screening test equipment
- Tape measure

Preparation

Ensure that the temperature in the examining room is comfortable and that seats are available for the health care provider, parent, and child. During the health interview, the child can be in the parent's lap or in his or her own chair. The toddler or very anxious small child can remain in the parent's lap for most of the physical examination. By age 3 years, most children enjoy the independence of climbing onto the examination table. Most 4 year olds are able to climb onto the examination table without difficulty if the initial screening process has not indicated trauma. While the child is climbing up, watch carefully and stay close to prevent a fall. Wash your hands before beginning the examination. The child is usually undressed at either the beginning of the examination or after assessment of the head and neck.

The examination of the child will start at the head and end at the toes. If, however, you anticipate that the child will become upset, listen to heart sounds first and then breath sounds. This is best done while the child is sitting on the parent's lap. Wipe the stethoscope with alcohol then warm the stethoscope with your hand.

Children, and most specifically young adolescents, want to be reassured that everything evaluated is normal. They may frequently mention what seems to be a minor concern to the health professionals. To gain trust, it is important to evaluate or intervene for all stated concerns.

Denver Developmental Screening Test

The **Denver Developmental Screening Test II** (DDST-II) (Frankenburg, Dodds, Archer, Shapiro, & Bresnick, 1992) is one of several standardized developmental screening tests used in the examination of the child and required for early and periodic screening and developmental testing. The DDST-II is considered the standard criterion for the developmental evaluation of children aged 1 month to 6 years. It evaluates four developmental areas of interest: personal/social, language, fine motor/adaptive, and gross motor.

During screening with the DDST-II, the examiner asks questions of the parent, but the child also performs certain tasks. Toys and blocks provided with the screening tool assist in standardizing the assessment (Fig. 27.5). The DDST-II and accompanying required materials to perform it can be purchased at http:// www.denverii.com/DenverII.html. A standardized evaluation such as the DDST-II is recommended over a nonstandard checklist of behaviors or skills; such a checklist is without validity or reliability and is thus difficult to interpret or to use in planning interventions.

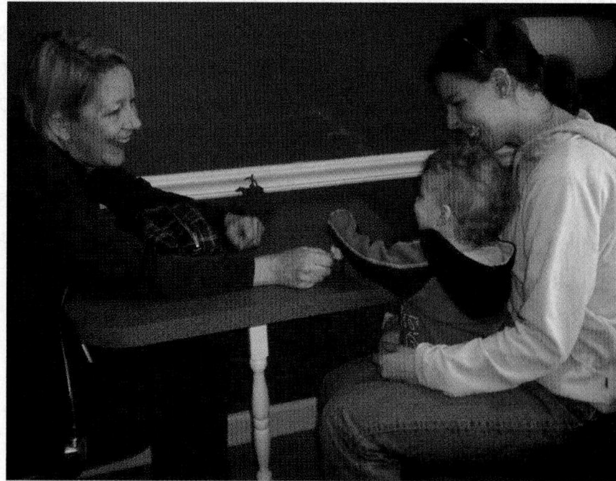

Figure 27.5 The nurse uses special toys and blocks to conduct the Denver Developmental Screening Test II (DDST-II).

Comprehensive Physical Assessment

Technique and Normal Findings	Abnormal Findings
Vital Signs Measure the patient's height, weight, heart rate, respiratory rate, temperature, and blood pressure. Measure head circumference (Fig. 27.6). Plot height and weight on the appropriate growth charts; calculate BMI. At 3 years of age, begin routine blood pressure measurement with a cuff and sphygmomanometer if the newborn's blood pressure was recorded in the nursery as within normal limits in all extremities. Assessment of blood pressure includes the percentile according to height and sex. Choose a blood pressure cuff that covers 80% of the child's upper arm. *Charts for blood pressure norms are found on the National Heart, Lung and Blood Institute's (2004) Web site* (http://www.nhlbi.nih.gov/health/public/heart/hbp/bp_child_pocket/bp_child_pocket.pdf) *and on* <thePoint>. 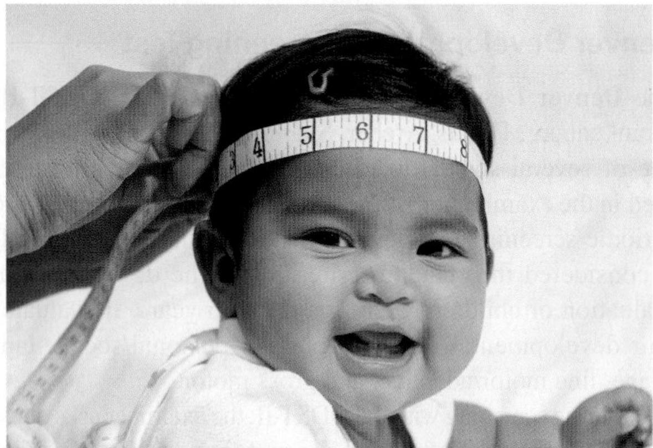 **Figure 27.6** Measure head circumference up to age 3 years.	Any blood pressure over the 90th percentile is considered borderline hypertensive and requires follow-up. The 90th percentile is 1.3 SD, 95th percentile is 1.6 SD, and the 99th percentile is 2.3 SD over the mean. Measuring head circumference, especially during the first 3 years, may identify neurological abnormalities as well as malnutrition. Identification of abnormal growth patterns can lead to early diagnosis of treatable conditions, such as hydrocephalus or identification of disorders associated with slowed head growth, such as Rett syndrome (Bright Futures/AAP, 2013).
General Survey Observe the child's demeanor. Look for signs of distress, discomfort, or anxiety. Note attentiveness and affect. *A 4-year-old child is generally talkative and engaged in the visit and can answer simple questions about self and concerns.* Listen for speech difficulties. *By 2 years of age, the child uses two-word sentences; by 3 years of age, a child should speak in more complicated sentences with speech that is understandable 75% or more of the time* (Drumwright, Drexler, VanNatta, Camp, & Frankenburg, 1973).	The interview provides an opportunity to assess the child's cognitive processing and ability to understand. Flat affect, no eye contact, and clinging to the caregiver may indicate further evaluation to assess for autism and other psychiatric concerns.
Observe for range of motion and musculoskeletal symmetry and coordination. Range of motion is full with 4–5+/5 strength symmetrically.	Asymmetry of movement and lack of coordination should be further evaluated.

(table continues on page 863)

Technique and Normal Findings (continued)	Abnormal Findings (continued)

Skin, Hair, and Nails

Inspect and palpate the skin, hair, and nails.

Skin is smooth and dry. Hair is smooth and evenly distributed. Nails are smooth and without clubbing.

Note any absence or overgrowth of nails. Dimpling, ripples, or discoloration in nails can be signs of trauma or fungus. There should be no unusual moles or hyperpigmented areas.

Eccrine glands begin to function by 2–18 days of life but become fully functional at adolescence. Apocrine glands do not become active until puberty.

Note acne in adolescent patients. With a gloved hand, palpate any rash or skin complaints to determine elevation and size of papules, nodules, or cysts.

Assess for burns. Use the Lund and Browder burn estimation chart (Fig. 27.7).

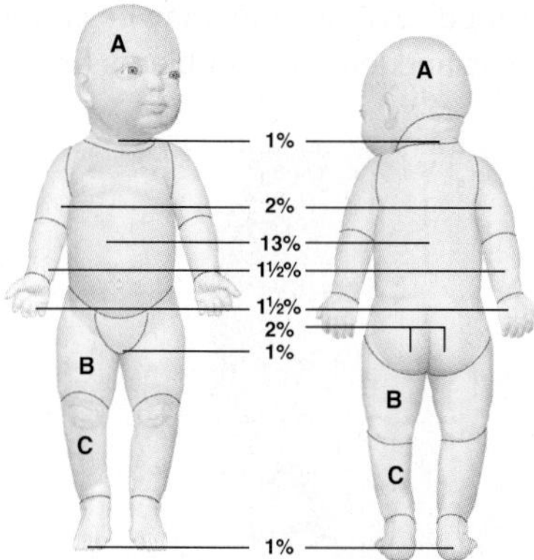

Figure 27.7 The Lund and Browder burn estimation chart commonly used in pediatric populations.

In a burn assessment, the relative percentage of body surface areas (% BSA) is affected by growth:

	0 yr	1 yr	5 yr	10 yr	15 yr
A – ½ of head	9 ½	8 ½	6 ½	5 ½	4 ½
B – ½ of 1 upper leg	2 ¾	3 ¼	4	4 ¼	4 ½
C – ½ of 1 lower leg	2 ½	2 ½	2 ¾	3	3 ¼

Head and Neck

Inspect the head and neck; observe range of motion of the neck.

The head and neck are symmetrical with full range of motion (ROM) in neck.

Palpate the head and neck. *Anterior and posterior cervical nodes may be palpable but not enlarged and are also nontender.* Palpate the head for nodules or pain due to infectious processes or trauma.

No nodule or tenderness is noted on the head.

Limited neck ROM requires further evaluation for possible meningitis or torticollis. Tender swollen lymph nodes of the neck and back of the head may indicate an infection. Lymph nodes are frequently palpable in children but they should be small, cylindrical, movable, and nontender. The lymphatic system grows exponentially between 6 and 12 years and reaches adult size around 12 years. Therefore, tonsils frequently look large at this time but will appear smaller as the head and neck grow throughout adolescence.

Palpate fontanelles of head on children up to 2 years old. *The anterior fontanelle closes by 18 months of age, the posterior fontanelle by 6 months of age.*

Eyes and Vision

Inspect the eyes. Test pupils for reaction.

The eyes have pupils equal, round, reactive to light and accommodation (PERRLA). Extraocular movements (EOMs) are at 180 degrees. Corneal light reflexes (CLR) are equal. No deviation is found during the cover and alternate cover tests. Funduscopic examination reveals a distinct disc with no vessel nicking.

Assessment of accommodation is difficult in young children. Unequal and nonreactive pupils may signify increased intracranial pressure. Unequal EOMs or CLR may indicate esotropia or exotropia. Deviation with the cover test demonstrates an esophoria or exophoria, depending on direction. All these findings require further evaluation. By 3 years of age, most children are cooperative enough for you to obtain a quick glimpse of the retina.

(table continues on page 864)

Technique and Normal Findings (continued)	Abnormal Findings (continued)
Assess distance vision using a screening test based on developmental stage (Table 27.1). *Normal findings in toddlers are 20/200 bilaterally. Normal visual acuity in preschoolers is 20/40, improving to 20/30 or better by 4 years old. By 5–6 years old, normal visual acuity should approximate that of adults (20/20 in both eyes).*	
Screen for color blindness in patients 4–8 years old.	
Ears and Hearing Inspect the ears. Ears have a formed pinna, the top of which touches an imaginary straight line through both pupils (Fig. 27.8).	Ear deformities are connected to kidney problems because organogenesis for both ears and kidneys occurs about the same time in utero. Evaluate renal function if the ears appear malformed. Low-set ears may be correlated with cognitive deficits and learning problems (Fig. 27.8B).

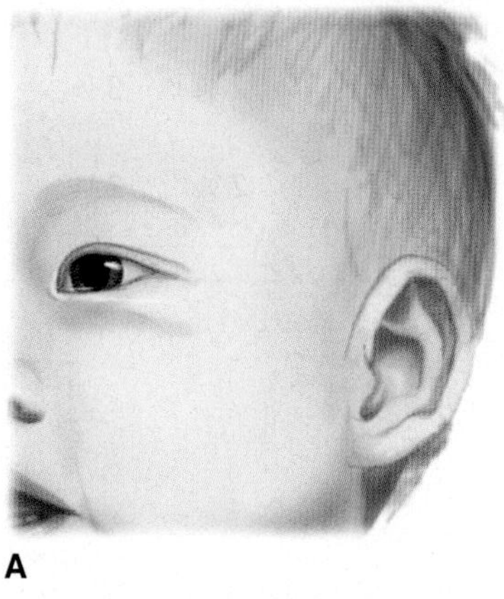

A

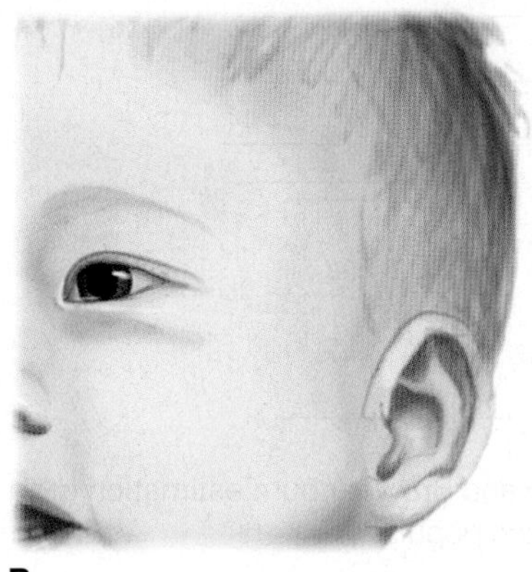

B

Figure 27.8 **A.** Normal positioning of the eyes in relation to the upper portion of the ears. **B.** Ear position that is set much lower than the outer canthus of the eye may indicate genetic abnormalities or other health problems.

As head shape changes, visualization of the tympanic membrane requires alterations in technique. In the child younger than 1 year, pull the pinna down and toward the face to straighten out the ear canal and promote visualization of the tympanic membrane. In the child 1–2 years of age, pull straight back on the pinna to straighten the ear canal for visualization of the tympanic membrane. After 2–3 years of age, pull up and back on the top of the pinna to visualize the tympanic membrane. Once you have visualized the membrane, use the pneumatic bulb to test for movement of the tympanic membrane. The tympanic membrane is gray and nonerythematous with the light reflex and landmarks visualized.	Suspect infection if the tympanic membrane is erythematous or yellow, if drainage is present in the canal, or if mobility is limited. **Clinical Significance** Children are prone to frequent cases of otitis media because the eustachian tube is more horizontal than in adults. This is one reason why a child should never be put to bed with a bottle. Formula can pool in the back of the throat and ascend the eustachian tubes, contributing to otitis media. As the head grows and its shape changes, the eustachian tubes become more vertical and the child is less prone to otitis media.
Mobility is demonstrated with pneumoscopy. Palpate the pinna for tenderness and nodules. The tympanic membrane is mobile; no tenderness or nodules are found on the pinna.	Tenderness with manipulation of the pinna may indicate otitis externa. Swollen erythematous turbinates may indicate infection. Pale swollen turbinates may indicate allergic rhinitis and seasonal allergies.

(table continues on page 866)

TABLE 27.1 Eye Screening Guidelines

The American Academy of Pediatrics Section on Ophthalmology, in cooperation with the American Association for Pediatric Ophthalmology and Strabismus and the American Academy of Ophthalmology, has developed these vision screening guidelines to be used by physicians, nurses, educational institutions, public health departments, and other professionals who perform vision evaluation services. These guidelines represent one of the most sensitive techniques for the detection of eye abnormalities in children.

From Birth to 3 Years of Age, Perform the Following:	*For Children 3 Years of Age and Older Perform the Following:*
1. Ocular history	*Numbers 1 through 6 at left, plus:*
2. Vision assessment	7. Age-appropriate visual acuity measurement
3. External inspection of the eyes and lids	8. Attempt at ophthalmoscopy
4. Ocular motility assessment	
5. Pupil examination	
6. Red reflex examination	

Children Ages 3–5 Years

Function	*Recommended Tests*	*Referral Criteria*	*Comments*
Distance visual acuity	Snellen letters Snellen numbers Tumbling E HOTV letters Picture tests	1. Fewer than 4 of 6 correct on 6-m (20 ft) line with either eye tested at 3 m (10 ft) monocularly (i.e., less than 10/20 or 20/40) or 2. Two-line difference between eyes, even within the passing range (i.e., 10/12.5 and 10/20 or 20/25 and 20/40)	1. Tests are listed in decreasing order of cognitive difficulty; the highest test that the child is capable of performing should be used; in general, the tumbling E or the HOTV test should be used for children 3–5 years of age and Snellen letters or numbers for children ages 6 years and older. 2. Testing distance of 3 m (10 ft) is recommended for all visual acuity tests. 3. A line of figures is preferred over single figures. 4. The nontested eye should be covered by an occluder held by the examiner or by an adhesive occluder patch applied to eye; the examiner must ensure that it is not possible to peek with the nontested eye.
Ocular alignment	Cross cover test at 3 m (10 ft) Random dot E stereo test at 40 cm (about 16 in.) Simultaneous red reflex test (Bruckner test)	Any asymmetry of pupil color, size, brightness	Direct ophthalmoscope used to view both red reflexes simultaneously in a darkened room from 60–90 cm (2–3 ft) away; detects asymmetric refractive errors as well.
Ocular media clarity (e.g., cataracts, tumors)	Red reflex	White pupil, dark spots, absent reflex	Direct ophthalmoscope, darkened room. View eyes separately at 30–45 cm (12–18 in.); white reflex indicates possible retinoblastoma.

(table continues on page 866)

TABLE 27.1 **Eye Screening Guidelines** *(continued)*

Children 6 Years of Age and Older			
Function	***Recommended Tests***	***Referral Criteria***	***Comments***
Distance visual acuity	Snellen letters Snellen numbers Tumbling E HOTV letters Picture tests	1. Fewer than 4 of 6 correct on 4.5-m (15 ft) line with either eye tested at 3 m (10 ft) monocularly (i.e., less than 10/15 or 20/30) or 2. Two-line difference between eyes, even within the passing range (i.e., 10/10 and 10/15 or 20/20 and 20/30)	1. Tests are listed in decreasing order of cognitive difficulty; the highest test that the child is capable of performing should be used; in general, the tumbling E or the HOTV test should be used for children 3–5 years of age and Snellen letters or numbers for children ages 6 years and older. 2. Testing distance of 3 m (10 ft) is recommended for all visual acuity tests. 3. A line of figures is preferred over single figures. 4. The nontested eye should be covered by an occluder held by the examiner or by an adhesive occluder patch applied to eye; the examiner must ensure that it is not possible to peek with the nontested eye.
Ocular alignment	Cross cover test at 3 m (10 ft) Random dot E stereo test at 40 cm (about 16 in.) Simultaneous red reflex test (Bruckner test)	Any asymmetry of pupil color, size, brightness	Direct ophthalmoscope used to view both red reflexes simultaneously in a darkened room from 60–90 cm (2–3 ft) away; detects asymmetric refractive errors as well.
Ocular media clarity (e.g., cataracts, tumors)	Red reflex	White pupil, dark spots, absent reflex	Direct ophthalmoscope, darkened room. View eyes separately at 30–45 cm (12–18 in.); white reflex indicates possible retinoblastoma.

Adapted from Committee on Practice and Ambulatory Medicine Section on Ophthalmology, American Association of Certified Orthoptists, American Association for Pediatric Ophthalmology and Strabismus and American Academy of Ophthalmology. (2003 and reaffirmed in 2007). Policy statement: Eye examination in infants, children, and young adults by pediatricians. *Pediatrics, 111*(4), 902–907. Retrieved from http://pediatrics.aappublications.org/content/111/4/902.full.pdf

Technique and Normal Findings (continued)	**Abnormal Findings** (continued)
Screening for hearing acuity in infants and young children includes evaluation of developmental milestones, such as the Moro reflex in neonates. If development is delayed or if caregivers are concerned, a pediatric audiologist should perform a formal pediatric evaluation. Refer to Table 27.2 for a list and description of audiologic tests appropriate for children of various ages.	Abnormal findings include lack of Moro reflex, inability to localize sound, and lack of understandable language by 24 months of age.

(table continues on page 868)

TABLE 27.2 Audiologic Tests for Infants and Children					
Developmental Age of Child	**Auditory Test/Average Time**	**Type of Measurement**	**Test Procedures**	**Advantages**	**Limitations**
All ages	Evoked otoacoustic emissions test (OAEs), 10-minute test	Physiological test specifically measuring cochlear (outer hair cell) response to presentation of a stimulus	Small probe containing a sensitive microphone is placed in the ear canal for stimulus delivery and response detection	Ear-specific results; not dependent on whether patient is asleep or awake; quick test time	Infant or child must be relatively inactive during the test; not a true test of hearing because it does not assess cortical processing of sound
Birth to 9 months	Auditory brainstem response (ABR), 15-minute test	Electrophysiologic measurement of activity in auditory nerve and brainstem pathways	Placement of electrodes on child's head detects auditory stimuli presented through earphones one ear at a time	Ear-specific results; responses not dependent on patient cooperation	Infant or child must remain quiet during the test; not a true test of hearing because it does not assess cortical processing of sound
9 months–2.5 years	Conditioned orienting response (COR) or visual reinforcement audiometry (VRA), 30-minute test	Behavioral tests measuring responses of the child to speech and frequency-specific stimuli presented through speakers	Both techniques condition the child to associate speech or frequency-specific sound with a reinforcement stimulus (e.g., lighted toy); VRA requires a sound-treated room	Assesses auditory perception of child	Only assesses hearing of the better ear; not ear-specific; cannot rule out a unilateral hearing loss
2.5–4 years	Play audiometry, 30-minute test	Behavioral test measuring auditory thresholds in response to speech and frequency-specific stimuli presented through earphones, bone vibrator, or both	Child is conditioned to put a peg in a pegboard or drop a block in a box when stimulus tone is heard	Ear-specific results; assesses auditory perception of child	Attention span of child may limit the amount of information obtained
4 years to adolescence	Conventional audiometry, 30-minute test	Behavioral test measuring auditory thresholds in response to speech and frequency-specific stimuli presented through earphones, bone vibrator, or both	Patient is instructed to raise his or her hand when stimulus is heard	Ear-specific results; assesses auditory perception of patient	Depends on the level of understanding and cooperation of the child

Adapted from Bachmann, K. R., & Arvedson, J. C. (1998). Early identification and intervention for children who are hearing impaired. *Pediatric Review, 19,* 155–165, with permission; Cunningham, M. D., & Cox, E. O. (2003). Hearing assessment in infants and children: Recommendations beyond neonatal screening. *Pediatrics, 111*(2), 436–440.

Technique and Normal Findings (continued)	Abnormal Findings (continued)
Nose, Mouth, and Throat Inspect the nose, mouth, and throat. ■ The nose is midline, nares are patent, and turbinates are pink with unrestricted air passage.	Dental caries are the most common infectious disease in childhood. Poor dental health is associated with poor physical health. Note any missing teeth. Erythema and exudate may indicate an infectious process.
Note the number of deciduous and permanent teeth. ■ No caries are present.	
In the mouth, tonsils are present and between +1 and +4. ■ No erythema or exudate seen.	
Thorax and Lungs Inspect the thorax and lungs. ■ No increased work of breathing and retractions.	
Palpate the thorax. ■ No tenderness along intercostal spaces (ICSs).	
Percuss the thorax and lungs. ■ The lungs are resonant.	Pain along ribs may be indicative of injury or viral infection such as costochondritis.
Auscultate the thorax and lungs. ■ Breath sounds are clear in all lobes. No crackles, gurgles, or wheezes are noted.	**SAFETY ALERT** *Respiratory distress requires immediate intervention and oxygen.*
Percuss the lungs if pneumonia is suspected. To encourage the child to take deep breaths for an adequate assessment, you can ask the child to blow on a pinwheel so that the wheel spins.	Because the young child has a pliable skeletal system, the lung's functional reserve can be exhaled with a gentle chest squeeze. The next breath, then, is deeper and longer than the previous breath; this assists with a complete assessment. Lower airway diameters in children are approximately half that of adults, which contributes to increased wheezing and pneumonia. The left main stem bronchus comes off at a more acute angle than the right in children; therefore, if a child aspirates, generally, a foreign object is found located in the right bronchus.
Heart and Neck Vessels Inspect for visible pulses on the thorax. Palpate and auscultate the point of maximal intensity (PMI). *The PMI is at the midclavicular line (MCL) in infancy and moves slightly laterally with age to the 4th ICS just to the left of the MCL in children younger than 7 years of age, and then to the 5th ICS in children older than 7 years of age.* ■ No bounding PMI found.	A visible PMI may signify increased cardiac load and increased oxygen requirements. See Figure 27.9 for locations of heart sounds in a child.

(table continues on page 869)

Technique and Normal Findings (continued)	Abnormal Findings (continued)
	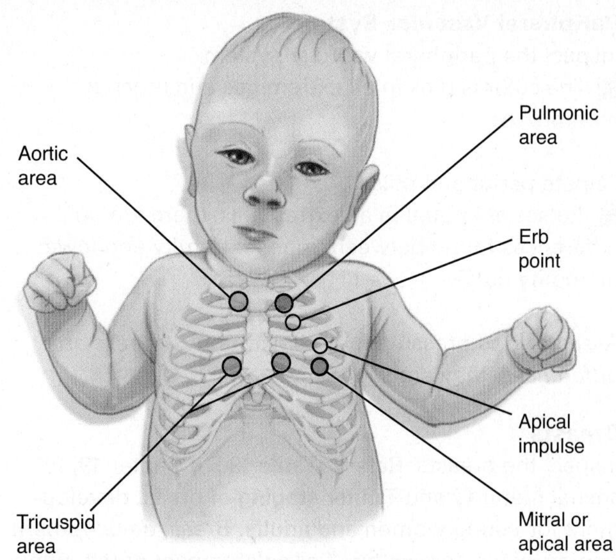 **Figure 27.9** Location of heart sounds in a young child. The heart moves lower as the child grows.
If heart enlargement is suspected, percussion can assist in determining size.	If a murmur is detected, description of the murmur should include the intensity (Grades 1 through 6), timing, duration, quality, pitch, PMI, and if (and to where) it radiates. Characteristics of **innocent heart murmurs** and abnormal murmurs are noted in Box 27.1.
Auscultate the heart in all six designated areas on the chest and back. Assess with the child in two positions: lying and/or sitting and/or standing. ■ Closure of the tricuspid and mitral valves (S1) and the pulmonic and aortic (S2) valves is clear, crisp, and single. No murmurs, rubs, or gallops found.	
Observe the jugular venous pulsations. ■ The neck vessels are not distended or flat.	

(table continues on page 870)

BOX 27.1 Characteristics of Innocent and Abnormal Heart Murmurs

Innocent Murmurs

Innocent murmurs are associated with normal first and second heart sounds (S1 and S2). They occur in systole (except for the venous hum). They are usually very brief, well localized, and heard near the left sternal border. On a scale from 1 to 6, these usually are graded 1 or 2 without a thrill. The intensity changes with position, usually decreasing when the child is standing. Innocent murmurs that may be auscultated in children are as follows:

- *Still murmur*: a vibratory functional murmur, louder in the supine position
- *Pulmonary flow murmur*: increased flow, louder in the supine position, accentuated by exercise, fever, excitement
- *Venous hum*: continuous, loudest when sitting

Abnormal Murmurs

A murmur that sounds like a breath sound or is harsh or blowing (of any degree of intensity) signifies regurgitation of blood and pathology. Factors that increase the likelihood of an abnormal murmur include the following:

Symptoms such as chest pain, squatting, fainting, tiring quickly, shortness of breath, or failure-to-thrive

- Family history of Marfan syndrome or sudden death in young (younger than 50 years old) family members
- Other congenital anomaly or syndrome (e.g., Down syndrome)
- Increased precordial activity
- Decreased femoral pulses
- Abnormal S2
- Clicks
- Loud or harsh murmur (more than Grade 2)
- Increased intensity of murmur when the patient stands

Data from Frank, J. E., & Jacobe, K. M. (2011). Evaluation and management of heart murmurs in children. *American Family Physician, 84*(7), 793–800. Retrieved from http://www.aafp.org/afp/2011/1001/p793.html

Technique and Normal Findings (continued)	Abnormal Findings (continued)
Peripheral Vascular System Inspect the peripheral vascular system. ■ The color is pink in all extremities and mucous membranes. Palpate peripheral pulses. ■ Pulses are equal in all extremities; there are no differences found between upper extremity and lower extremity pulses. Assess blood pressure in each extremity. *If there are differences, they are slight.*	Except in the immediate newborn period, cyanosis requires immediate intervention. **Coarctation of the aorta** can present with unequal pulses between the upper and lower extremities. After the aorta leaves the heart, if a narrowing of the vessel is found, then the lower extremities are not well oxygenated and pressure increases on the left side of the heart.
Breasts Inspect the breasts. Refer to Table 19.5 (Chapter 19) for sexual maturity and **Tanner staging** of breast development for young women and adults. *Breast development begins with a "breast bud" or enlargement of the areola followed by enlargement of breast tissue.*	Onset of pubertal changes before 8 years in girls and 9 years in boys may be too early and needs further evaluation.
Abdomen Inspect the abdomen. ■ No distension is noted. A protuberant abdomen is a common finding in toddlers (Fig. 27.10). Palpate the abdomen. ■ No masses or tenderness found. 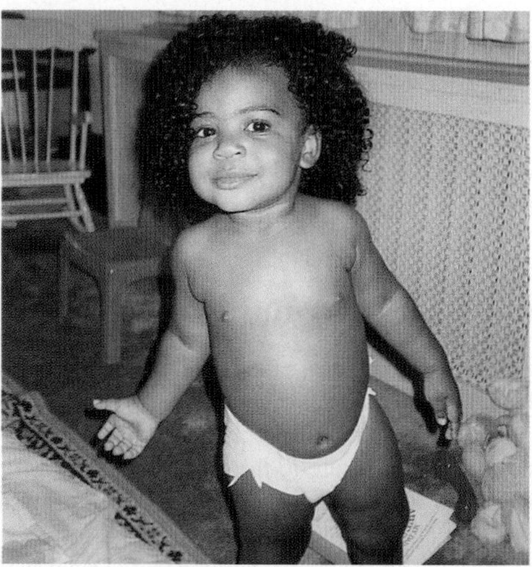 **Figure 27.10** Note the protuberant abdomen, common in toddlers. Percuss the abdomen. ■ No tenderness with percussion and tympany throughout. The abdomen has a normal hollow or tympanic sound. Percussion can assist in determining the size of the liver. *The liver is at the lower right costal margin.*	If distension is present, assess for tenderness and ascites; if these are present, further intervention is required. Palpation of the abdomen to assess for abdominal masses is important because Wilms tumors of the kidney occur in toddlers and early school-age children. The normally protuberant abdomen, however, may interfere with detection of these tumors until they are of significant size. Significant abdominal tenderness requires further evaluation for appendicitis, Crohn disease, ulcerative colitis, gastroenteritis, or other illnesses. Percussion can assist in determining the size of a palpable mass.

(table continues on page 871)

Technique and Normal Findings (continued)	Abnormal Findings (continued)
Musculoskeletal System Inspect the muscles and joints. Evaluation of scoliosis begins when the child can stand, but it is a focused part of the examination just prior to, and during, puberty. Observe ROM in all joints. Palpate the muscles and joints. *Normally, the spine is straight.* No joint tenderness is noted. ROM is full and symmetrical.	Limited ROM in any joint requires further evaluation. Joint tenderness with palpation should be further evaluated for trauma and infection. Screening for scoliosis usually occurs during the school health screening.
Neurological System Assess orientation. Observe for symmetry. Test deep tendon reflexes (DTRs) and evaluate for equality (Fig. 27.11). Ensure active movement and full strength in all extremities. *Older children are oriented to time and place.* Movements are symmetrical; DTRs are 2+. Strength is 4–5+.	Any noted asymmetry of gait, facial features, or movement needs further evaluation.
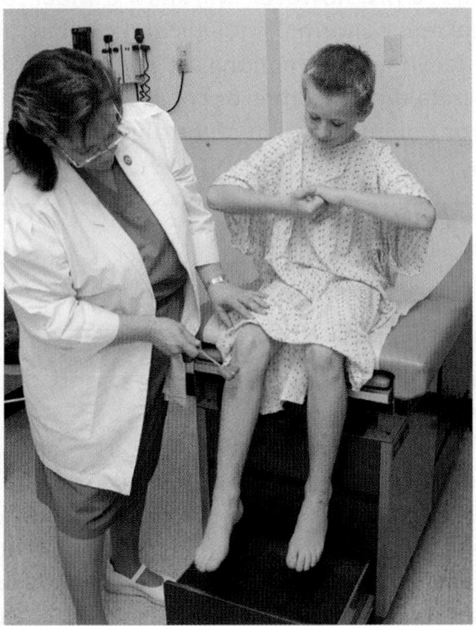 **Figure 27.11** Testing deep tendon reflexes in children.	
Assess developmental progress for age. The DDST-II is used for children 1 month to 6 years of age. For children older than 6 years of age, academic performance is noted. Scores are within norms for the age.	Confusion, unusual behaviors, delayed development progress, and poor academic performance need further assessment.
Male and Female Genitalia Inspect the genitalia. Refer to Tables 23.1 (Chapter 23) and 24.1 (Chapter 24) for sexual maturity and **Tanner staging** for females and males. The genitalia show no signs of erythema, discharge, or irritation.	Onset of pubertal changes before 8 years in girls and 9 years in boys may be too early and needs further evaluation. Visualization of the genitalia is recommended in a complete examination to detect early infections, trauma, or developmental concerns (e.g., labial adhesions in girls, undescended testicles [cryptorchidism] in boys) that require intervention.

(table continues on page 872)

Technique and Normal Findings (continued)	Abnormal Findings (continued)
Note whether the male is circumcised or uncircumcised with the urethra midline at the end of the glans. Palpate the male scrotum. ■ The testes are in the scrotal sac and are smooth with no nodules noted.	The testes descend into the scrotal sac by age 6 months. If surgical repair is required, it should ideally happen before 2 years of age to prevent decreased fertility. Hypospadias requires intervention; it is usually diagnosed and treated in infancy. Adolescent boys should be assessed for testicular nodules; if found, they must be evaluated to rule out testicular cancer. Other testicular abnormalities (e.g., hydrocele, varicocele, spermatocele) can be detected with testicular palpation.
Inspect the anus and rectum. ■ Skin on the anus and rectum is without irritation, erythema, or fissures.	Rectal irritation or fissures require further evaluation for constipation, worms, or sexual abuse. Objective assessment can be obtained by the RN with distinction made between normal and abnormal findings. Objective assessment can also be obtained by the APRN. The APRN, however, will know a wider range of normal and abnormal findings and will be able to determine when interventions are needed. The APRN can describe the outcomes or consequences of intervention or nonintervention of the abnormal objective findings.

Critical Thinking

Laboratory and Diagnostic Testing

No laboratory or diagnostic tests are recommended specifically for children and adolescents. Blood chemistry screening, hemoglobin (for anemia screening in patients aged 5 years or older), tuberculin skin screening (for children at average risk), and urinalysis are recommended when clinically indicated. The U.S. Preventive Services Task Force (USPSTF) states that screening for elevated blood lead levels is recommended only for symptomatic or at-risk children 1 to 5 years of age (USPSTF, n.d.).

Clinical Significance

A general hearing evaluation is required for children with speech difficulties before they are evaluated by a speech pathologist or undergo speech therapy.

In the primary care setting, vision screening is recommended for children younger than 4 years old. By age 5 years, vision screening is part of the preschool assessment. Assess car seat and seat belt use. Calculate the BMI as a screen for overweight and obesity. Screen sexually active women younger than 25 years of age for chlamydia (Institute for Clinical Systems Improvement [ICSI], 2013). Laboratory and diagnostic testing are performed by the RN. Laboratory and diagnostic testing is ordered and performed by the APRN.

Diagnostic Reasoning

Nursing Diagnoses, Outcomes, and Interventions

When formulating a nursing diagnosis, it is important to use critical thinking to cluster data and identify patterns. Compare these clusters with the defining characteristics (abnormal findings) for the diagnosis to ensure the most accurate labeling and appropriate interventions. Table 27.3 provides nursing diagnoses, points of differentiation, assessment characteristics, and nursing interventions commonly related to assessment of the child.

You use assessment information to identify patient outcomes. Some outcomes related to the child include the following:

- The family identifies health promotion systems.
- The child achieves developmental tasks on schedule for age.
- The family seeks information regarding health promotion.

After you have established outcomes, implement nursing care to improve the status of the child. Use critical thinking and evidence-based practice to develop the interventions. Some examples of nursing interventions for the child are as follows:

- Provide information about community support systems available to the family during times of stress.
- Identify conditions that contribute to altered growth and development.
- Provide information that contributes to an improved state of health.

TABLE 27.3 Common Nursing Diagnoses Associated With the Child or Adolescent

Diagnosis	Point of Differentiation	Assessment Characteristics	Nursing Interventions
Readiness for enhanced family processes	Pattern of family functioning that supports the well-being of family members	Activities support individual and family growth	Assess the family's coping abilities and stressors. Encourage attendance at community groups and classes. Assess cultural beliefs and norms.
Delayed growth and development	Child or teen shows significant deviations from norms of peers	Delays exist in the skills typically found with children of the same age	Assess the influence of cultural norms, values, and beliefs on the parent's perceptions of development.
Health-seeking behaviors	Actively seeking ways to change health habits to improve health level	Concern about current conditions, unfamiliarity with wellness community resources	Discuss benefits and barriers to staying healthy, environmental factors to health, stress placed on the family.

Progress Note: Analyzing Findings

Remember Simon Chavez, who is 4 years old and having a preschool assessment. Initial subjective and objective data collection is complete and the nurse has spent time reviewing the findings and other results. The following nursing note illustrates how subjective and objective data are collected and analyzed and nursing interventions are developed.

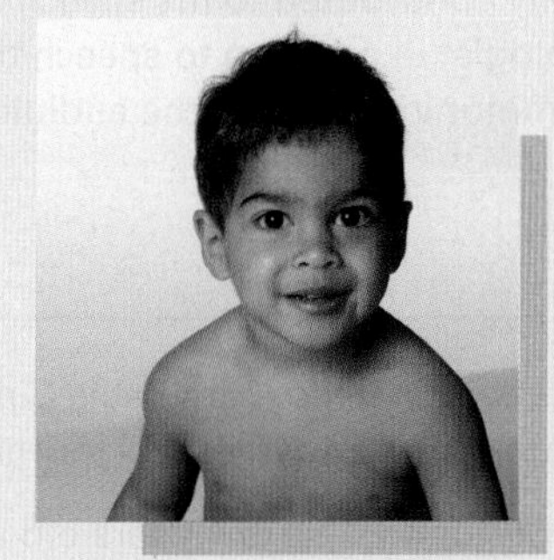

Subjective: Simon's mother reports that he has been very healthy. The family speaks Spanish at home but English at church and with his maternal grandparents. His paternal grandparents live in Chile and visit once a year. The family lives in a large Victorian home built in the 1920s; they are renovating the house on the weekends.

Objective: Cooperative 4-year-old child responds appropriately to questions and requests, generally pleasant. No complaints of pain, present discomfort, or health concerns. T 37°C (98.6°F), P 86 beats/min, R 20 breaths/min, BP 94/50 mm Hg left arm. Height 1 m, (3 ft, 3 3/8 in.). Weight 17.5 kg (38 ½ lb). BMI 16.3. Alert and cooperative; answers questions appropriately although difficult to understand at times. Knows what day it is and why he has come to the clinic for evaluation. Hearing = passed at 20 dB at 500, 1,000, 2,000, and 4,000 Hz. However, failed at 30 dB for 1,000, 2,000, and 4,000 Hz. Passed DDST in personal-social, fine motor, and gross motor areas. Failed language area.

Assessment: Disturbed sensory perception, auditory. Hearing impairment detected. Immunizations recommended for children 4–6 years of age needed. At risk for elevated blood lead level. Speech difficulties.

(case study continues on page 874)

Plan: Order blood lead level and refer for speech evaluation. Update immunizations. Provide information and handouts on nutrition, activity, limiting TV watching, reading, school readiness, immunizations, discipline, and safety. Refer to audiologist for further testing and treatment.

Critical Thinking Challenge

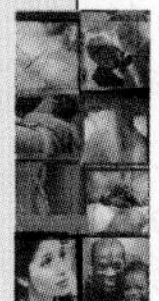

- How do the subjective and objective data fit together?
- What findings of Simon's are abnormal?
- How will the nurse evaluate if comprehensive and holistic care has been provided for Simon and his family?

Collaborating With the Interprofessional Team

Hearing screening is becoming increasingly common in the newborn period. Without such testing, the average age of detection of hearing impairment is 14 months (American Speech Language Hearing Association [ASHA], n.d.). If impairment is not detected until late in the preschool period, speech can be affected.

Simon's hearing loss was not detected until he was 4 years old; this delay has likely contributed to his speech difficulties. The nurse needs to refer Simon to an audiologist in addition to speech therapy. The information below illustrates the nurse's communication with the audiologist.

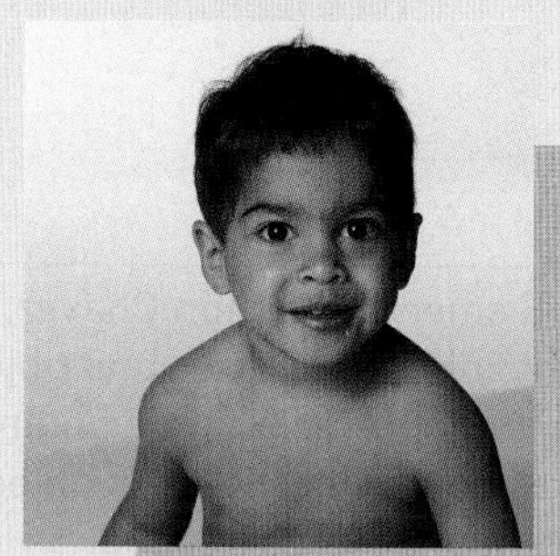

Situation: "Hello, I am Paula Singala, an advanced practice registered nurse. I saw Simon Chavez earlier this morning."

Background: "He is 4 years old and has some speech difficulties and hearing loss."

Assessment: "Simon passed his hearing test at 20 dB at 500; however, he failed at 30 dB for 1,000, 2,000, and 4,000 Hz."

Recommendations: "I would like you to evaluate him further."

Critical Thinking Challenge

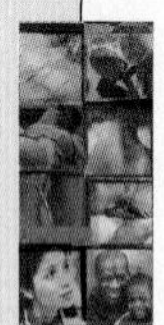

- Why might Simon be having hearing loss?
- What other things would you assess as the nurse?
- How might his ability to speak two languages affect his speech?

Pulling It All Together

The nurse uses assessment data to formulate a nursing care plan with patient outcomes and interventions for Simon. This includes a diagnosis, outcomes, and interventions, which the nurse uses critical thinking and judgment to continue or revise. This is often in the form of a care plan or case note similar to the one below.

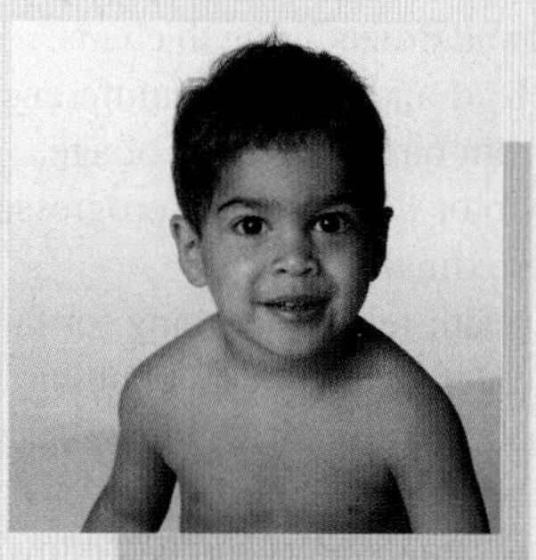

Nursing Diagnosis	Patient Outcomes	Nursing Interventions	Rationale	Evaluation
Disturbed sensory perception related to altered hearing	Patient uses assistive devices correctly. Speech becomes easier to understand.	Turn off TV and radio when communicating. Speak in lower tones if possible. Stand directly in front of the patient when talking.	Background noise interferes with hearing voices. The patient can use nonverbal cues, such as lip reading.	Patient obtained and is using hearing-assistive devices. Evaluate speech improvement at next visit.

Applying Your Knowledge

Using the previous steps of assessment and nursing process, consider all the case study findings presented in this chapter about Simon, who is undergoing a preschool physical examination. When answering the following questions, begin drawing conclusions and see how the pieces of assessment must work together to create an environment for personalized, appropriate, and accurate care. Consider Simon's case and answer the following questions.

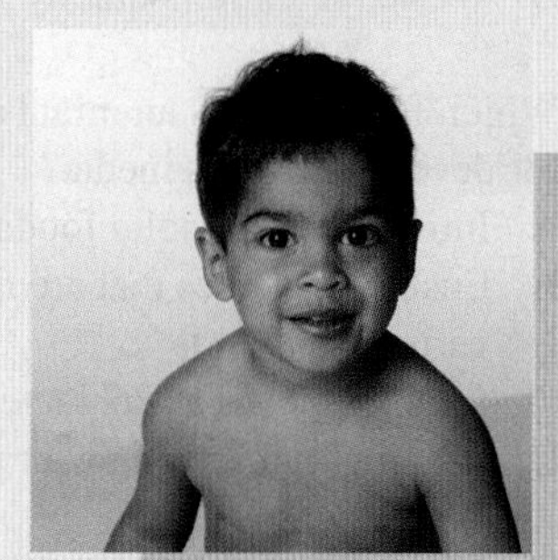

- What health information and assessments are important for the toddler, preschooler, school-age child, and adolescent?
- How do assessment findings differ between the child and adult?
- What adaptations will you make when assessing a child?
- What factors could be contributing to Simon's language development?
- What recommendations for follow-up and future screening would you recommend for Simon?
- How would you evaluate Mrs. Chavez's ability to follow through with the recommendations on her return visit with Simon?

Key Points

- Evaluation of a child's physical growth is performed with standardized growth charts.
- Head and chest circumferences are measured in children from birth to 3 years of age.
- Motor development progresses cephalocaudally and from proximal to distal.
- Health-related teaching for families with children and adolescents includes obtaining immunizations; using child safety car seats, window/stair guards, pool fences, life jackets, and bike helmets; keeping a safe distance from fire pits; crossing streets safely; following poison control measures; avoiding underage drinking and driving; using contraception; and taking measures for adequate nutrition and sunscreen.
- Most of the physical assessment of a toddler can be performed with the child sitting in the parent's lap.
- The DDST-II is the standard criterion for developmental evaluation of children ages 1 month to 6 years.
- In addition to objective assessment, the nurse also assesses physical growth; language; and psychosocial, cognitive, and developmental areas.
- Innocent murmurs occur in systole, are brief and well localized, and are usually heard near the left sternal border.

Review Questions

1. What is the best time to assess the respiratory rate of a young child?
   A. While the child is crying
   B. While the child is playing in the playroom
   C. Immediately after taking the child's blood pressure
   D. While the child is quietly sitting on the parent's lap

2. Which factor places an infant at greater risk than an adult for developing otitis media?
   A. Introduction of solid foods
   B. Eustachian tubes that are more horizontal (flat) than vertical and wide
   C. Immature cardiac sphincter
   D. Feeding in a semi-Fowler position

3. During assessment of a child's visual acuity, which finding may indicate myopia or nearsightedness?
   A. Holding a book close to the face
   B. Squinting
   C. Rapid eye movements
   D. Closing one eye

4. What is an easy way to determine whether a child has strabismus?
   A. Observe the red reflex.
   B. Check eyes for unequal pupil size.
   C. Shine the light in his or her eyes.
   D. Do a funduscopic examination.

5. All the following may be symptoms of a child experiencing lead poisoning **except**
   A. irritability.
   B. cardiomegaly.
   C. headaches.
   D. abdominal pain.

6. As soon as the child can stand, begin to measure the height in the upright position.
   A. True. Using the scale as soon as the child can stand next to it is fine.
   B. False. Measure the child standing starting between 2 and 3 years of age.
   C. It depends on when the child can stand independently.
   D. False. A child should always be measured in the recumbent position.

7. A child's head circumference is a measurement that should be obtained at every well-child visit until the child is 5 years old.
   A. True. This measurement is indicative of brain growth.
   B. False. One or two measurements are the standard of care.
   C. True. It will provide information on the child's readiness for kindergarten.
   D. False. The charts for head circumference norms end at 36 months of age.

8. You obtain a blood pressure reading of 110/70 mm Hg (left arm) in a 5-year-old boy. What would you do about this blood pressure?
   A. Call the physician immediately.
   B. Bring the child back to the clinic two more times to ensure accuracy of the assessment.
   C. Determine the blood pressure percentile based on age, sex, and height percentiles.
   D. It is normal; nothing needs to be done.

9. Health promotion for children should incorporate teaching about lifelong cardiovascular health, including which of the following?
   A. Information on good nutrition
   B. Information on the prevention of illnesses
   C. Information on exercise
   D. All of the above

10. Children are usually brought for health care visits by a parent. At about what age should you begin to question the child, rather than the parent, regarding presenting symptoms?
    A. 5 years of age
    B. 7 years of age
    C. 9 years of age
    D. 11 years of age

The Jensen suite offers these additional resources to enhance learning and facilitate understanding of this chapter:

- thePoint online resources, http://thepoint.lww.com/Jensen2e
- *Laboratory Manual for Nursing Health Assessment: A Best Practice Approach*
- *Pocket Guide for Nursing Health Assessment: A Best Practice Approach*
- *Lippincott DocuCare*, an electronic health record simulation software, http://thepoint.lww.com/docucare
- *Adaptive Learning | Powered by PrepU*, http://thepoint.lww.com/prepu

References

American Academy of Pediatrics (AAP). (2012). *Bright futures: Guidelines for health supervision of infants, children and adolescents.* Retrieved from http://brightfutures.aap.org/3rd_Edition_Guidelines_and_Pocket_Guide.html

American Association of Poison Control Centers (AAPCC). (n.d.). Retrieved from http://www.aapcc.org/

American Speech Language Hearing Association (ASHA). (n.d.). Hearing screening. Retrieved from http://www.asha.org/public/hearing/Hearing-Screening

Bright Futures/American Academy of Pediatrics (AAP). (2013). *Recommendations for preventative pediatric health care*. Retrieved from http://brightfutures.aap.org/pdfs/AAP%20Bright%20Futures%20Periodicity%20Sched%20101107.pdf

Centers for Disease Control and Prevention (CDC). (2010). *Growth Charts*. Retrieved from http://www.cdc.gov/growthcharts

Centers for Disease Control and Prevention (CDC). (2012). *TB in children in the United States*. Retrieved from http://www.cdc.gov/tb/topic/populations/TBinChildren/default.htm

Centers for Disease Control and Prevention (CDC). (2013a). *Lead prevention*. Retrieved from http://www.cdc.gov/nceh/lead/tips.htm

Centers for Disease Control and Prevention (CDC). (2013b). *Toys*. Retrieved from http://www.cdc.gov/nceh/lead/tips/toys.htm

Centers for Disease Control and Prevention (CDC). (2014a). *Vaccines and immunizations*. Retrieved from http://www.cdc.gov/vaccines

Centers for Disease Control and Prevention (CDC). (2014b). *Quick stats: Underage drinking*. Retrieved from http://www.cdc.gov/alcohol/quickstats/underage_drinking.htm

Committee on Practice and Ambulatory Medicine Section on Ophthalmology, American Association of Certified Orthoptists, American Association for Pediatric Ophthalmology and Strabismus and American Academy of Ophthalmology. (2003 and reaffirmed in 2007). Policy statement: Eye examination in infants, children, and young adults by pediatricians. *Pediatrics*, *111*(4), 902–907.

Drumwright, M. A., Drexler, H., VanNatta, P., Camp, B., & Frankenburg, W. K. (1973). Denver articulation screening exam. *Journal of Speech and Hearing Disorders*, *38*(3). Retrieved from http://denverii.com/denverii/

Frankenburg, W. K., Dodds, J., Archer, P., Shapiro, H., & Bresnick, B. (1992). The Denver II: A major revision and restandardization of the Denver developmental screening test. *Pediatrics*, *89*, 91–97. Retrieved from http://denverii.com/denverii

Frank, J. E., & Jacobe, K. M. (2011). Evaluation and management of heart murmurs in children. *American Family Physician, 84*(7), 793–800. Retrieved from http://www.aafp.org/afp/2011/1001/p793.html

Institute for Clinical Systems Improvement (ICSI). (2013). *Preventive services for children and adolescents*. Retrieved from https://www.icsi.org/guidelines__more/catalog_guidelines_and_more/catalog_guidelines/catalog_prevention__screening_guidelines/preventive_services_kids/

Meehan, W. P. III, Lee, L. K., Fischer, C. M., & Mannix, R. C. (2013). Bicycle helmet laws are associated with a lower fatality rate from bicycle–motor vehicle collisions. *The Journal of Pediatrics, 163*(3), 726–729.

National Heart, Lung, and Blood Institute (NHLBI). (2004). *Blood pressure tables for children and adolescents from the Fourth Report on the Diagnosis, Evaluation, and Treatment of High Blood Pressure in Children and Adolescents*. Retrieved from http://www.nhlbi.nih.gov/guidelines/hypertension/child_tbl.htm

National Highway Traffic Safety Administration (NHTSA). (2013). Retrieved from http://www.nhtsa.gov/

Robins, D. L., Fein, D., Barton, M. L. (1999). *M-CHAT tool and scoring*. Retrieved from https://www.m-chat.org/references.php

U.S. Department of Agriculture (USDA). (2013). ChooseMyPlate. Retrieved from http://www.choosemyplate.gov/

United States Department of Health and Human Services, Healthy People 2020. (2011). *Healthy people 2020*: *What are its goals?* Retrieved from http://healthypeople.gov/2020/topicsobjectives2020/default.aspx

U.S. Preventive Services Task Force (n.d.). *Child and Adolescent Recommendations*. Retrieved from http://www.uspreventiveservicestaskforce.org/tfchildcat.htm

World Health Organization (WHO). (2010). Growth charts from birth to 24 months. Retrieved from http://www.cdc.gov/growthcharts/who_charts.htm#The WHO Growth Charts

28

Older Adults

Learning Objectives

1 Demonstrate knowledge of normal changes in anatomy and physiology that occur with aging.

2 Identify important topics for health promotion and risk reduction in older adults.

3 Describe common signs and symptoms reported by older adults.

4 Collect subjective data using interviewing techniques that include adaptations based on age.

5 Collect objective data on the body systems using physical examination techniques and considering variations based on age.

6 Identify expected and unexpected findings related to the older adult.

7 Analyze subjective and objective data from the assessment of the older adult and consider initial interventions.

8 Document and communicate data from the older adult using appropriate terminology and principles of recording.

9 Consider age, condition, and culture of the older adult to individualize the assessment.

10 Identify nursing diagnoses and initiate a nursing plan of care based on findings from the assessment of the older adult.

Mr. Ralph Monroe is a 76-year-old man with a history of Parkinson disease. He has lived in a nursing home for the past 3 months because of functional limitations. He complains of "terrible constipation" and asks "What causes this?" His daily medications include carbidopa/levodopa (Sinemet) 25/250 four times before meals for Parkinson disease, vitamin E 400 IU for prevention of heart disease, calcium 600 mg with vitamin D 800 IU for bone health, and lisinopril (Zestril) 5 mg for his blood pressure.

You will gain more information about Mr. Monroe as you progress through this chapter. As you study the content and features, consider Mr. Monroe's case and its relationship to what you are learning. Begin thinking about the following points:

- How would you define primary and secondary aging?
- What is your rationale for using the Mini-Mental State Examination (MMSE) and a nutritional assessment tool with Mr. Monroe?
- What screening tests would you request for Mr. Monroe?
- What factors might contribute to Mr. Monroe's dislike of his roommate and other residents?
- What recommendations would you make about Mr. Monroe's requirements for immunizations?
- How would you evaluate your counseling regarding nutritional intake with Mr. Monroe?

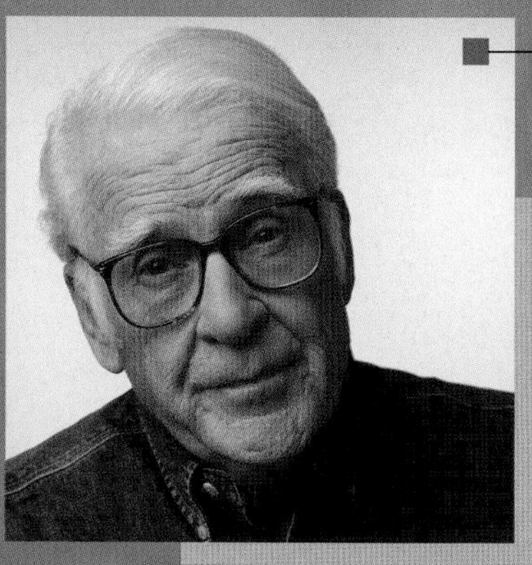

Conducting an accurate and complete assessment of an older adult is essential for the planning and management of care. **Geriatric** nursing experts identify the need for a comprehensive assessment of this population because elders often have a unique presentation of illness. In addition, many aspects of the lives of older adults can affect their health and ability to cope with chronic changes. An older adult's social situation, living situation, relationship with a caregiver, access to transportation, mobility, financial or economic situation, understanding, expectations, and cultural or religious views on disease can influence health as much as his or her health history, past medical diagnoses, understanding of medications, physical examination findings, and functional ability.

In recent years, U.S. life expectancy has increased to 78 years (Murphy, Jiaquan, & Kochanek, 2013). This increase in life expectancy, along with careful management of chronic diseases and prolonged periods of living with multiple chronic diseases, has changed the characteristics of the U.S. population of older adults.

As "baby boomers" (those born between 1946 and 1964) age into their 70s and 80s, we can expect to see increasing numbers of older adults in all health care settings. By 2030, in the United States 20% of the total population will be older than 65 (CDC, 2013). Canada, which is anticipating a similar demographic shift, expects the population of older adults to make up 25% of their population by the year 2051 (Madden & Wong, 2013).

This chapter begins with a review of physiological changes associated with aging and then moves to a discussion of best practices for conducting an interview with an older adult. It includes some common assessment tools used to identify risk for specific geriatric symptoms and tools in the context of physical examination findings. The normal aging process is separated from findings that represent unexpected changes commonly found in older adults. Previous chapters covered specific assessment considerations for older adults related to general survey, pain, nutrition/supplements/medications, developmental stages, mental status, social/spiritual/cultural concerns, and violence. Refer to Chapters 5 through 10 for more specific information on those subjects.

Structure and Function

Skin, Hair, and Nails

The epidermis thins with aging. The epithelium renews itself every 30 days, compared with every 20 days as in children and adults. This decreased activity of cells means that healing takes almost twice as long in the older adult. Other changes with aging include degeneration of the elastic fibers providing dermal support, a loss of collagen, and a loss of subcutaneous fat. The number of sweat glands and sebaceous glands decreases as a result of atrophy, and vascularity and capillary integrity of the skin layer are diminished. Nail beds become more rigid, thicker, and more brittle, with slowed growth.

A difference exists between normal aging processes and a lifelong cumulative exposure to sun. For example, fine wrinkling

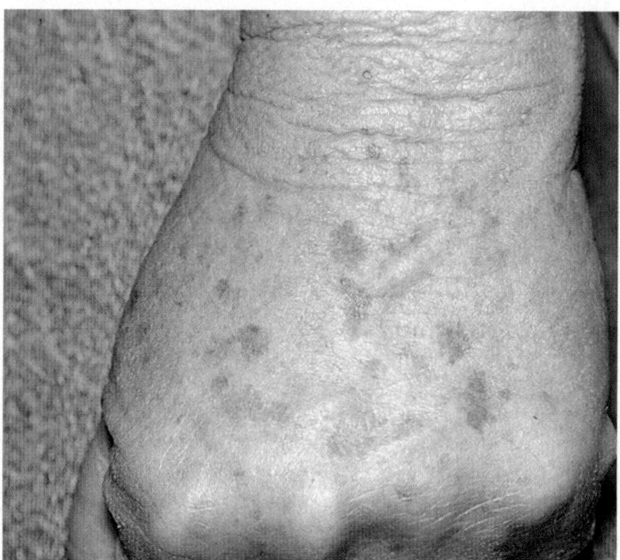

Figure 28.1 Solar lentigines, or "liver spots," are a common and expected skin finding in older adults.

of the skin is a normal part of aging, but coarse wrinkling is evidence of photoaging. Sun exposure also increases **solar lentigines** (age or liver spots, Fig. 28.1), mottled **dyspigmentation** areas, and **actinic keratoses**. Long-term smoking also alters skin by reducing dermal elastic fibers, reducing blood flow to the dermal layers, and slowing healing times for wounds.

Head and Neck

With aging, facial subcutaneous fat decreases, making the skeleton more pronounced. Skin may sag and wrinkle across the forehead, surrounding the eyes, at the tip of the nose, and on the cheeks, which alters facial appearance. Skin lesions are more likely, and careful assessment for possible cancers, especially in commonly sun-exposed areas, is important (Centers for Disease Control and Prevention [CDC], 2010; see Chapter 11).

Aging is associated with changes in thyroid hormones and thyroid function. Many medications commonly used in the older adult population are known to alter absorption and metabolism of thyroid hormones. Additionally, as people age, their need for thyroid replacement decreases. These factors, coupled with subtler symptoms of thyroid dysfunction, accentuate the need for detailed history and physical examination as well as frequent monitoring of thyroid levels. Untreated thyroid disease can cause cognitive impairments, depression, frailty, and increase the risk of coronary heart disease (Faggiano et al., 2011).

Eyes and Vision

Older adults have less fat in the orbital area, laxity of the orbital muscles, and decreased lid elasticity. They have fewer goblet cells that provide mucin, resulting in diminished lubrication for the eyes. Tear production decreases, which leads to dry eyes. Corneal sensitivity may diminish. Increased lipid deposits may be found at the periphery of the cornea around the iris. The ciliary body secretes less aqueous humor and the ciliary muscle may atrophy, compromising the ability to focus the lens. The lens becomes less elastic, larger, and denser with age and may become progressively yellowed and opaque. The iris loses some pigment, and the pupil shrinks progressively. Slowed pupillary responses lead to a difficulty in accommodating to changes in light, difficulty with night driving, and problems with glare (Brodie, 2010).

Ears and Hearing

Physiological changes to ears and hearing include a widening and lengthening of the auricle; coarse, wiry hair growth in the external ears (especially in men); narrowing of the auditory canal; and dry cerumen in the ear canal. The tympanic membrane in the middle ear becomes dull, less flexible, retracted, and turns gray. The organ of Corti atrophies, causing sensory hearing loss, and cochlear neurons are lost, causing neural hearing loss (Linton, Lach, Matteson, & McConnell, 2007). Changes to the inner ear can reduce the older adult's ability to discriminate sounds, especially in noisy conditions.

Nose, Mouth, and Throat

Because of an age-related loss of olfactory receptor neurons, older adults have a decreased sense of smell, which can start as early as the fourth decade of life. In addition, chronic medical conditions can alter the sense of smell. For example, older adults with Alzheimer disease or Parkinson disease may have difficulty with odor recognition. Olfactory dysfunction can significantly reduce food intake because smell and taste are important in the enjoyment of foods.

Tooth surfaces become worn with aging, which increases the risk of dental caries. Collagen and elasticity changes affect oral tissues, with mucosal thinning and smoothing of the tongue. Oral hygiene practices throughout the lifespan, however, greatly influence gum recession and tooth loss.

Many older adults experience changes in taste starting around 60 years of age. Changes in taste detection and sensation were originally thought to be linked to a loss of taste buds, which are replaced every 10 to 100 days; however, some studies have shown that healthy older adults do not lose taste buds. Researchers now believe that loss of taste sensation is more likely caused by medications, diseases, long-term smoking damage, and malnutrition. Older adults who regularly take medications or who have diseases that cause reduced saliva, or xerostomia, are more likely to have problems with taste.

Thorax and Lungs

Changes to connective tissue related to aging are evident throughout the respiratory system. The chest wall is less elastic and rigidity or lack of compliance limits chest expansion. Decreased respiratory muscle strength creates a less effective cough in older adults. Alveoli are thicker and fewer in older adult smokers, but the number of alveoli remains relatively constant in healthy older adults. Major changes in respiratory function are usually related to deconditioning and disease or damage from long-term smoking rather than to the aging process itself (Davies & Bolton, 2010).

Loss of alveolar elastic recoil produces approximately a 20% decrease in lung vital capacity (Davies & Bolton, 2010). Loss of alveolar surface area results in a smaller area being available for oxygen exchange, and more difficulties responding to hypoxic or hypercapnic episodes. Fewer cilia lining the airways results in less efficiency in clearing the lungs. Residual volume (the volume of air remaining in the lung after a maximal expiration) increases with age. The forced expiratory volume in 1 second (FEV_1)/forced vital capacity ratio declines.

Heart and Neck Vessels

Changes in connective and smooth muscle tissue affect the peripheral vessels and heart. Arterial walls are less elastic and stiffer. Subsequent decreased compliance affects blood pressure by increasing the afterload on the left ventricle. Systolic blood pressure increases, the left ventricle wall hypertrophies or thickens, and dependence on atrial contraction increases. Coronary artery blood flow decreases by about one third. The loss of atrial pacemaker cells and bundle of His fibers may decrease heart rate. Intrinsic cardiac contractile function diminishes, reducing cardiac output, stroke volume, and cardiac reserves (Bernhard & Laufer, 2008). Responsiveness to beta-adrenergic receptor stimulation and reactivity of baroreceptors and chemoreceptors decrease, whereas circulating catecholamines increase. Jugular venous pulsations increase with fluid volume excess and decrease with fluid volume deficit.

Peripheral Vascular System and Lymphatics

Calcification of the arteries, or arteriosclerosis, causes them to become more rigid (Fig. 28.2). Reduced arterial compliance results in increased systolic blood pressure. This is often compounded by the coexistence of atherosclerotic disease in the arteries supplying the brain, heart, and other vital organs. Incidence of peripheral arterial disease (PAD) increases dramatically in the seventh and eighth decades of life (Porth & Matfin, 2009). Patients with venous congestion may also develop edema from poor lymphatic drainage (see Chapter 18.)

Breasts and Lymphatics

Glandular breast tissue atrophies, becomes less dense, and is replaced by fat. As women age, glandular, alveolar, and lobular breast tissues decrease. After menopause, fat deposits replace glandular tissue, which continues to atrophy as a result of decreased secretion of ovarian hormones, estrogen, and progesterone. The inframammary ridge thickens, making this area easier to palpate. Suspensory ligaments relax, causing the breasts to sag and droop. Additionally, breasts shrink and lose elasticity. Nipples become smaller, flatter, and less erectile. Axillary hair also may stop growing. These changes are more apparent in the eighth and ninth decades of life. Women who have had mastectomies may develop lymphedema in the affected arm.

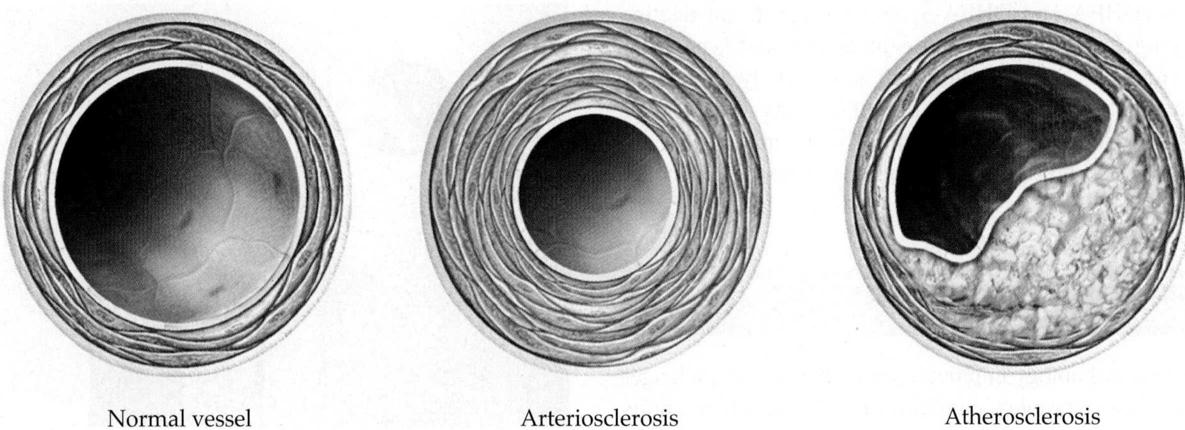

Figure 28.2 Arteriosclerosis (hardening of the arteries) develops as people age. It can eventually progress to atherosclerosis, which can cause life-threatening complications.

Abdomen, Metabolism, and Elimination

Although it was previously thought that parietal and chief cells in the stomach (also called zymogenic cells) decrease with aging, reducing hydrochloric acid and pepsin, some studies now show that older adults, in fact, have *increased* gastric acid secretion. Slowed peristalsis creates a delayed emptying of the stomach and delayed movement of food through the gastrointestinal system. Absorption of vitamin D, calcium, and zinc in the small intestine may be reduced (Elmadfa & Meyer, 2008). The number and size of hepatocytes decrease and hepatic blood flow is reduced. Metabolism of medications on the first pass through the liver decreases, leaving older adults at risk for higher circulating medication levels. Secretion of bicarbonate and enzymes in the pancreas decreases and the pancreatic duct becomes more dilated. The colonic transit rate is slower.

The size and function of the kidney decrease with age. Nephrons in the cortex of the kidneys are fewer, whereas abnormal glomeruli increase. The body responds to the sclerotic changes in the glomeruli by increasing the size of the remaining healthy glomeruli.

Older adults develop diverticular changes in the distal renal tubules. For older patients with vascular difficulties, the decrease in blood flow to glomerular units decreases glomerular filtration rate. These changes are reflected in a decrease in creatinine clearance and a loss of ability to conserve sodium. Older adults also experience a general reduction in peak bladder capacity and a weakening of the bladder muscles, which can lead to incomplete emptying of the bladder.

Musculoskeletal System

Older adults often lose height. Gradual compression of the spinal column is related to narrowing of intervertebral discs. Beginning at around age 30 years, bone absorption starts to exceed bone formation. In women, this bone loss accelerates in the decade immediately following menopause. Decreased lean body mass also occurs with aging. There is a loss of type II muscle (fast-twitch) fibers compared with type I muscle (slow-twitch, fatigue-resistant) fibers, which leads to muscle wasting. Regeneration of muscle tissues slows with age, but studies show that exercise can increase lean muscle mass even in frail older adults (Peterson, Rhea, Sen, & Gordon, 2010).

Neurological System

With aging, the number of neurons and glial cells gradually declines and these cells show structural changes. Nevertheless, current studies do not support the notion of extensive brain atrophy in normal aging. Atrophy is common in people with degenerative neurological diseases. The overall number of neuronal synapses decreases while lipofuscin granules in the nerve cells accumulate. There is increased production and accumulation of oxyradicals in all body systems.

Neurological changes worsen in people who have changes to those blood vessels that supply the nervous system (e.g., people with diabetes mellitus, smokers). Efficiency of the autonomic functions of the central nervous system decreases, so that recovery from stress becomes more difficult. Healthy older adults maintain cognitive function but retrieval speed for information slows. Speed of brain processing on tests of psychomotor performance shows slowing with age. Reaction times are slower but may be affected by other changes, including visual and musculoskeletal changes. Postural control, decreased vibratory sense, and decreased righting reflex ability may affect the balance of older adults (Linton et al., 2007).

Male and Female Genitourinary Systems

Age-related enlargement of the prostate can contribute to urinary retention or outlet obstruction. Genital hair thins. The vaginal mucosa thins and loses elasticity. Vaginal secretions diminish as estrogen levels lower with age (see Chapters 23 and 24 for the genital examination.)

Endocrine System

The pituitary gland decreases in size, weight, and vascularity. Secretion of growth hormone and circulating levels of insulin-like growth factor decreases. Plasma levels of the adrenal steroids (DHEA and DHEA-S) show a significant decline with aging. Prevalence of glucose intolerance and Type 2 diabetes increases. Older adults are more likely to have a decreased responsiveness to immunizations. Because of changes in the immune system, older adults may have more autoantibodies and risks for autoimmune diseases (Chahal & Drake, 2007).

Advance Care Planning

As medical technology improves, older adults are living longer with multiple complex comorbidities. Some older adults undergo lifesaving medical interventions without regard for quality of life. *Advance care planning (ACP)* is the term applied to the discussions between health care professionals and patients regarding their choices for future treatment. It gives patients and their families the opportunity to anticipate and discuss future health states and the treatments options they would like based on their cultural, religious, and personal views.

An advanced directive (AD) is the written expression of the patient's health care preference given specific circumstances, specifically those circumstances in which the patient is no longer able to make medical decisions due to incapacity. In 1991, The Patient Self-Determination Act was signed into law, mandating the recognition of patients' rights to make personal medical decisions and withhold life-sustaining treatments (Rushton, Kaylor, & Christopher, 2012).

Despite increased efforts by health care professionals, estimates indicate that less than 15% of older adults have completed an AD (Jones, Moss, & Harris-Kojetin, 2011). This places the burden of decision-making on family members and may lead to unwanted feeding tubes, ventilators, and other aggressive medical interventions. The Physician Orders for Life-Sustaining Treatment (POLST) form or Medical Orders for Life-Sustaining Treatment (MOLST) form is targeted at ill patients. Its use has become increasingly common in hospital and nursing home settings. It is a brief summary of the patient's preferences incorporated into medical orders and recorded on a two-sided, quick-reference form. The form reflects the patient's choices about cardiopulmonary resuscitation, the level and duration of emergent medical intervention, and the use of artificial nutrition and hydration (POLST, 2012).

In many facilities, nurses are responsible for initiating ACP discussions and reviewing POLST forms with their patients. The American Nurses Association (ANA) endorses the nurse's role in ACP and advocating for the patient's wishes regarding health care preferences (ANA, 1991). The nurse's position at the bedside puts her or him in a key position to have these very personal and intimate conversations.

Cultural Considerations

In many cultures, an older person would never be called by his or her first name at a first meeting and especially would not be addressed as "Sam" or "Nancy" by a younger stranger. You should establish a tone of respect for the older person at

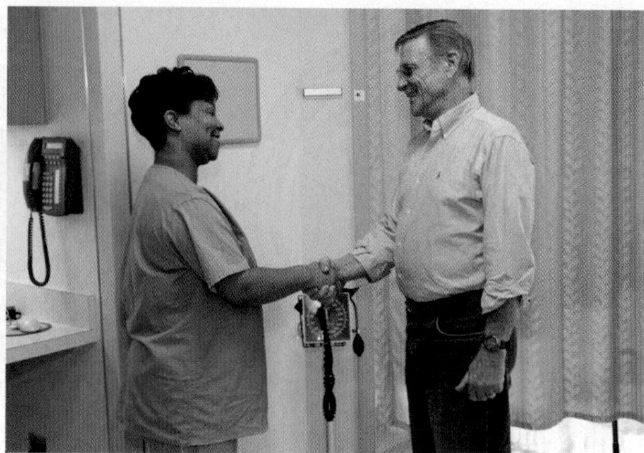

Figure 28.3 A respectful and pleasant introduction with an older patient can set the tone not just for the immediate health visit but also for the overall nurse–patient relationship.

the beginning of the interview by introducing yourself and then calling the patient by his or her formal name (Fig. 28.3). You can then clarify how the patient would like to be addressed in the interview.

Be aware and sensitive to the variations seen between and within different ethnic groups. Some areas to consider are the differences in the amount of personal space required for comfort and differences in eye contact and physical contact. For example, in some cultures eye contact is considered a sign of active listening, whereas in others it is disrespectful and may even be inappropriate between a male and female. Be mindful of ethnicity and culture during interactions with older adults and their families (McBride, 2012).

Urgent Assessment

Falls, especially if accompanied by fracture, are the most common reason for admission of older adults to emergency departments (Hastings, Whitson, Sloane, et al., 2014). Chronic conditions may be exacerbated in older adults; for example, chronic obstructive pulmonary disease (COPD) may worsen or congestive heart failure may be an acute condition. Infection, chest pain, abdominal pain, and delirium should be assessed and treated rapidly. Because older adults may not mount a successful immune response, infection may be present even in the absence of fever.

Subjective Data

Interviewing the Older Adult

Before interviewing the older adult, the nurse should set up the room and create an environment that facilitates hearing and understanding of communication. Although some acute situations do not allow for finding a quiet space, an environment that is calm and quiet is essential for conducting an interview with an older person. It is essential to reduce or eliminate background noise as much as possible when

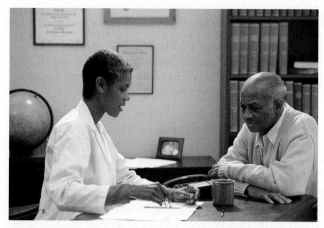

Figure 28.4 History taking with older adults needs to be at a slow and deliberate pace; it may need to be conducted over several visits for a comprehensive picture of the patient's health.

carrying on conversations. This includes turning off the television or radio in the patient's room and closing the door to reduce sounds of telephones, beepers, alarms, or pagers. In addition, cold or drafty environments are uncomfortable and can distract the older adult from the task at hand. The older adult needs to be warm and comfortable during the interview.

The interview of an older adult can take much longer than that for a younger healthier person. It might not be completed in one encounter. You need to allow additional time for an interview or health history (Lach & Smith, 2007; Fig. 28.4). Frail older adults may hesitate before answering questions; you should not rush in to fill the silence. You should respectfully address questions directly to the patient and allow time for his or her responses. It is disrespectful to ignore the patient and address all questions to the patient's family member. If the patient cannot provide information because of a cognitive deficit or another reason, the nurse may then address the family member with questions.

Consideration of the patient's educational level is critical and interview questions should match the older adult's knowledge level. It is not appropriate, for example, to ask an elderly patient with limited education, "Have you noticed any signs of cerebrovascular or neurological changes?" Instead, phrase questions in a way that might be better understood and that is specific to what is being asked—for example, "Have you ever noticed more clumsiness in one hand compared with in the other?" or "Has your speech been slurred or jumbled?"

When an older adult is hospitalized or more seriously ill, you should gather as much information as possible from previous records so that you can review and clarify findings with the patient rather than trying to gain all the information from the patient's memory (Lach & Smith, 2007). This helps the older person to conserve energy. If the older adult is acutely ill and fatigues easily, the nurse may need to return and complete the interview later.

Some older adults are reluctant to report symptoms that past health care professionals have dismissed or that they believe might be part of normal aging. For example, an older adult may avoid reporting knee pain because she has had the same pain for several years or believes that arthritis pain is expected in older people. It is best to use specific health screening questions to detect common complaints. Cues during the physical examination can help you complete some of the health history. For example, upon identifying three scars during examination of the abdomen, you might say, "During our interview you told me that you had your appendix removed when you were 7, but could you tell me about these other two scars?"

When interviewing older adults with limited physical or mental abilities, the interview may need to be conducted somewhat differently to gain the desired information. Box 28.1 presents suggestions for conducting interviews with hearing impaired or deaf older adults, visually impaired older adults, patients with forms of aphasia, and patients with cognitive impairments (e.g., Alzheimer disease and other dementias).

BOX 28.1 Conducting the Health Interview in Older Adults With Special Needs

Hearing-Impaired Older Adults

- Before starting the interview, check that a hearing aid is in place and turned on and has a working battery. It is helpful to have a pocket amplifier and earphones available if you cannot locate the patient's hearing aid.
- Seat yourself directly in front of the person, at eye level, so that he or she can observe your face for visual cues (Lach & Smith, 2007). Do not stand and talk down to a seated patient. If necessary, seat yourself on the bedside so that the patient can see you.
- Make certain that you have the patient's attention and are close enough to the person before you begin speaking.
- Hearing-impaired patients benefit from seeing your lips move, so keep your hands away from your face while talking.
- Speak normally or in a slightly louder fashion (i.e., if you are soft-spoken, you may need to speak a bit more boldly). Use a low-pitched, calm voice without shouting.
- If the person has difficulty understanding something, find a different way of saying the same thing rather than continually repeating the original words.
- If the person has more profound hearing impairment, be prepared to write questions or messages if necessary. Use pictures, illustrations, body language, or gestures to facilitate communication.
- Do not assume that the hearing-impaired older adult is unreliable or has dementia. Try to gain as much information as possible within the limitations of his or her hearing impairment.

Visually Impaired Older Adults

- If you are entering the room of a patient who is visually impaired, identify yourself and your intentions.
- Avoid shouting or speaking too loudly (not all visually impaired older patients are also hearing impaired).
- If the patient wears corrective lenses, make sure they are clean.
- Repeat or reflect the patient's responses to your questions a little more frequently during the interview if he or she cannot see your face for the usual visual cues that indicate understanding.
- When you speak, let the person know whom you are addressing, especially if you are directing that question to an adult child or colleague and not to the patient.

(box continues on page 884)

BOX 28.1 Conducting the Health Interview in Older Adults With Special Needs (continued)

- Ask what you can do to facilitate the interview—for example, increasing the light, placing yourself in a different spot, and describing where things are.
- Be sure to say the person's name and tell him or her what you are going to touch or do during the physical examination.
- Keep in mind that people categorized as legally blind may have some vision.
- When you complete your interview and examination, be sure to return items to their original location unless the person asks you to move them.

Older Adults With Aphasia

Patients who have experienced a stroke or another type of neurological injury or illness may have total or partial aphasia. Those with *expressive aphasia* may be able to partially or fully understand what you say but are unable to respond to your questions.

- Use patience and allow plenty of time to communicate.
- Let the patient know if you cannot understand what he or she is telling you.
- Allow the patient to try to complete thoughts, to struggle with words. Although it is recommended that you provide some words, avoid being too quick to guess what the person is trying to express.
- If possible, encourage the person to write the word he or she is trying to express and read it aloud. You may want to seek out a picture board or communication device provided by a speech therapist to better facilitate the discussion.
- Use gestures or pointing to objects if helpful in supplying words or adding meaning.

Patients With Alzheimer Disease or Related Disorders

Screening for Cognitive Impairment. As you conduct an interview with an older adult, you may find the patient has repeated the same story about three times within 20 minutes. This repetitive storytelling is often an indicator of cognitive impairment. Patients who repeat the same story as if you have not heard it before should be screened with the Mini-Mental State Examination (MMSE). If you conduct an MMSE early in the interview, you can better determine whether it is wise to continue to seek information from the patient.

Early-Stage Dementia. People in early stages of Alzheimer disease may be fairly accurate in their responses, especially about issues from early adulthood or childhood (remote memory). They are more likely to omit information about more recent issues (short-term memory).

Mild to Moderate Dementia. People with mild to moderate dementia who maintain language skills can still be accurate reporters of current symptoms and concerns. As dementia progresses, the patient may overestimate abilities to carry out self-care activities, instrumental activities of daily living (IADLs), or safe and independent medication management.

More Severe Dementia. People with MMSE scores of 11 or less are unlikely to be reliable reporters for your interview.

Interview Techniques

- When interviewing an older adult with known dementia, make sure that you approach from the front within the patient's line of vision.
- Provide the same respect that you would to any older patient. Introduce yourself, and greet the patient by formal name. Be sure to face the person as you interview.
- A quiet calm environment is essential. Avoid a heavy traffic area, an area with multiple conversations, or a very noisy place.
- A low-pitched, calm tone of voice tends to be heard well and sets the tone.
- Ask only one question at a time. Repeat key words if the person does not understand the first time.
- As much as possible maintain eye contact and provide respect of personal space (Miller, 2008).

Assessment of Risk Factors

As a nurse working with older adults, you should be familiar with instruments that have been developed to detect older adults' risk for the most common conditions or difficulties that accompany aging. These conditions or difficulties are often referred to as **geriatric syndromes** because of the interaction of multiple chronic diseases. Because these syndromes are common, you can play a key role in early detection or assessment of the problem so that interventions can be implemented (Linton et al., 2007). It is important to ask questions regarding family history, personal history, medications, and risk factors to detect the possibility of one or more of the following common syndromes seen in older adults:

- Nutritional changes
- Mobility impairments affecting activities of daily living (ADLs) and instrumental activities of daily living (IADLs)
- Fall risk
- Polypharmacy
- Skin breakdown

History and Risk Factors	Rationale
Personal History The reason for seeking care is a brief statement, usually in the patient's own words, about why he or she is making the visit. Ask, "Tell me why you came to the clinic today," or "What happened that brought you to the hospital?" Record this information in the subjective part of documentation or put the statement in quotes.	If a patient replies by giving a medical diagnosis such as "heart attack," encourage the patient to describe symptoms such as "shortness of breath and chest pain." If the patient is long-winded, it may be appropriate to summarize the reason for seeking care.

(table continues on page 885)

History and Risk Factors	Rationale
Nutritional Changes. There are many assessment tools used to screen older adults for nutritional deficiency. Registered dieticians in the hospital, facility, and community settings commonly perform nutritional screenings, but nurses should have basic knowledge of some of the more commonly used tests. The Malnutrition Universal Screening Tool (MUST) is one of the most commonly used tests, consisting of evaluation of the body mass index (BMI), history of unexplained weight loss, and illness. Once complete, a malnutrition risk of low, medium, or high is assigned. Two other tests, the Mini Nutritional Assessment (MNA) and the SCALES protocol (*S*adness, *C*holesterol, *A*lbumin, *L*oss of weight, *E*ating, and *S*hopping) were specifically designed for older patients. All of these tests are easy to perform and have been validated for clinic use (Ahmed & Haboubi, 2010).	Nutritional screening is an abbreviated assessment of risk factors that identify older adults who may require a more comprehensive nutritional assessment. The combination of physiological changes with aging, physical or mental health issues, medications, or functional losses can significantly increase risk for weight loss in older adults. Chapter 7 reviews components included in a comprehensive dietary and nutritional history. Poor nutritional status indicators are linked to longer hospital stays, poor wound healing, and poor health outcomes. Financial and transportation issues can limit an older adult's access to nutritional foods. Functional abilities or sensory losses can affect ability to physically prepare nutritious foods. Early cognitive losses that impair judgment, planning, foresight, or sequencing of complex tasks may reduce an older adult's ability to follow recipes or prepare complete meals. Recent weight loss can cause dentures to fit poorly and interfere with chewing. Medications can change tastes and interfere with appetite.
Mobility Level and Functional Abilities. The Katz Index of ADL (Katz, Ford, Moskowitz, Jackson, & Jaffe, 1963) was developed to quantify the degree of disability in a chronically ill population. Other measures of functional status include the Functional Independence Measure (FIM; Wright, 2000) and the Barthel Index (Mahoney & Barthel, 1965). The FIM is a more sensitive measure and has been most frequently used in research settings. It has several well-tested and validated versions for use, including the original in-person version, short-form version, telephone version, and proxy report version (Wright, 2000).	Many older adults define their health by their ability to perform self-care, which health care providers identify as functional abilities. Functional ability in an older adult can vary widely during his or her later years. Some older adults require complete assistance with care, whereas others are completely functionally independent. Ability to carry out daily activities can be affected by depression, motivation, cognitive status, medical conditions, or sensory losses. Nursing assessment of functional abilities is an essential component of a comprehensive assessment of an older adult and is included universally in every hospital, nursing home, and community-based comprehensive assessment form. Researchers who study interventions for chronic diseases in older adults often use a measurement of functional ability to gauge the effectiveness of intervention outcomes (Kane, Ouslander, Abrass, & Resnick, 2013).
When assessing an older adult returning to or living in the community, it is essential to identify his or her ability to manage IADLs (Lawton & Brody, 1969; Box 28.2). Abilities measured by the Lawton IADL scale include use of the telephone, finance management, shopping, laundry, housekeeping and food preparation, and use of transportation. Older adults who can manage these tasks are more likely to be able to live independently in the community. The Lawton IADL instrument has been designed for older adults to self-report their abilities in these important tasks.	Hospital discharge planners or community health nurses use the Lawton IADL instrument to identify appropriate matches of supportive services and family assistance that might allow an older adult to maintain independence in the community. Because the tool relies on accurate self-reporting by the elder, results can be misleading with cognitively impaired elders who lack insight into their functional losses. For example, an older woman with Alzheimer disease may believe she can manage the telephone but, in fact, cannot demonstrate how she would call for help or assistance if needed. For the patient with dementia, compare his or her perceived abilities with the report of a close family member when assessing IADLs.

(table continues on page 886)

BOX 28.2 Lawton Instrumental Activities of Daily Living

INSTRUCTIONS: Ask the patient to describe her/his functioning in each category; then complement the description with specific questions as needed.

Ability to Telephone

1. Operates telephone on own initiative: looks up and dials number, etc.
2. Answers telephone and dials a few well-known numbers.
3. Answers telephone but does not dial.
4. Does not use telephone at all.

Shopping

1. Takes care of all shopping needs independently.
2. Shops independently for small purchases.
3. Needs to be accompanied on any shopping trip.
4. Completely unable to shop.

Food Preparation

1. Plans, prepares, and serves adequate meals independently.
2. Prepares adequate meals if supplied with ingredients.
3. Heats and serves prepared meals or prepares meals but does not maintain adequate diet.
4. Needs to have meals prepared and served.

Housekeeping

1. Maintains house alone or with occasional assistance (e.g., heavy work done by domestic help).
2. Performs light daily tasks such as dishwashing and bed making.
3. Performs light daily tasks but cannot maintain acceptable level of cleanliness.
4. Needs help with all home maintenance tasks.
5. Does not participate in any housekeeping tasks.

Laundry

1. Does personal laundry completely.
2. Launders small items; rinses socks, stockings, and so on.
3. All laundry must be done by others.

Mode of Transportation

1. Travels independently on public transportation or drives own car.
2. Arranges own travel via taxi, but does not otherwise use public transportation.
3. Travels on public transportation when assisted or accompanied by another.
4. Travel limited to taxi, automobile, or ambulette, with assistance.
5. Does not travel at all.

Ability to Handle Finances

1. Manages financial matters independently (budgets, writes checks, pays rent and bills, goes to bank); collects and keeps track of income.
2. Manages day-to-day purchases but needs help with banking, major purchases, controlled spending, and so on.
3. Incapable of handling money.

Scoring: Circle one number for each domain. Total the numbers circled. The lower the score, the more independent the older adult is. Scores are only good for individual patients. It is useful to see the score comparison over time.

History and Risk Factors	Rationale
Risk for Falls. Ask the patient, "Have you ever fallen before? Do you have any dizziness?" Several fall risk assessment instruments assist health care providers in identifying those older adults most at risk. The Morse Fall Scale developed for hospitalized elders (Morse, Morse, & Tylko, 1989) is widely used in hospital settings and does not require major training of staff. Even modified, however, it does not include the risks posed by medications the elder is taking or potential environmental contributors (Tang, Chow, & Lin, 2014). Another assessment instrument designed for hospitals is the Hendrich II Fall Risk Model (Hendrich, Bender, & Nyhuis, 2003). This assessment tool measures intrinsic risk factors and does not include environmental factors. It does include higher risks for patients taking medications that might contribute to falling, although it limits this to two drug classes: seizure medications and benzodiazepines. The scale includes points for confusion or disorientation, depression, altered elimination, dizziness or vertigo, male sex, and medications.	More than one third of U.S. adults older than 65 years of age sustain a fall each year; of these, 20% have moderate to severe injuries, (Soriano, DeCherrie, & Thomas, 2007). Some of the more serious injuries include hip fractures and head injuries, both of which carry significant morbidity and mortality risk for the older adult.

(table continues on page 887)

History and Risk Factors	Rationale
Skin Breakdown. Identify risk for skin breakdown, which is especially important in hospitalized and inactive patients. Many health care facilities use the Braden scale, with interventions based on the total score (Bergstrom, Braden, Laguzza, & Holman, 1987). See Chapter 11.	The Braden scale scores patients from 1 to 4 in six subscales: sensory perception, moisture, activity, mobility, nutrition, and friction (Braden & Bergstrom, 1989). A score of 14–18 indicates a high risk for pressure ulcers.
Medications Ask the patient: • What medications are you taking? • What is the dose of medication that you take? • What is your schedule for taking your medications? • Do you understand why you are taking each of your medications?	Although older adults comprise only approximately 13% of the population, they consume more than 30% of prescription medications in the United States (Vincent & Velkoff, 2010). On average, older adults in the United States take three to eight medications daily, and that rate increases with age and with inpatient treatment in hospital and long-term care settings (Guay, 2010).
Ask the patient to bring in a bag of all medications that he or she has at home and to identify those currently being taken. If this is not possible, phrase questions about medications based on body system. For example, "Do you take any medications for your heart or blood pressure? Do you take any medications for pain?" This approach is also useful when asking about over-the-counter (OTC) medications. "Do you take any medicine from the drugstore to help you sleep? Do you take anything from the drugstore to help your stomach or bowels? Are you taking any vitamins or minerals?" Be sure to specifically ask how frequently the patient takes each OTC medication or supplement.	While examining the label of each medication, determine whether the patient is taking the drug as prescribed and whether he or she has medications that should not be used together because of interactions. Older adults with cognitive impairment may not take medications as scheduled even though they report that they do. You can identify accuracy by calculating how many days are between today's date and the refill date, noting how many pills the pharmacist included, and counting out the number of tablets left in the container to obtain an estimate of pills taken.
In addition to asking about herbal or nutritional supplements, ask if any alternative health care providers have recommended other kinds of treatments.	Older patients may believe, for example, that drinking Chinese herbs boiled into tea is not considered a medication or supplement.
Finally, it is wise to ask, "Do you take any medications belonging to other people, including medications prescribed to a spouse, caregiver, friend, or neighbor?"	It is not unusual for elders living in retirement communities to share medications.
In addition to finding out what particular medications the patient takes, identify how often and when he or she takes each drug: • Does your pattern of taking the medication follow the prescription on the bottle? If not, why not? • Are you experiencing adverse effects of the medication? If so, what kinds? • Do you take medications with food, water, or alcohol?	This important information allows you to identify how frequently the patient is missing doses or overdosing.
Older adults with limited education may not understand a question about a "history of substance abuse" but would understand direct questions such as • Do you take street drugs or drink alcohol? • Have you been treated in a rehabilitation facility?	
Family History Ask the patient about the health of close family members (i.e., parents, grandparents, siblings) to help identify those diseases for which patients may be at risk and to provide counseling and health teaching.	The following familial conditions are important to note: high blood pressure, coronary artery disease, high cholesterol, stroke, cancer, diabetes mellitus, obesity, alcohol or drug addiction, and mental illness.

Risk Reduction and Health Promotion

The health goals for the older adult include the following:

- Increase the proportion of older adults with chronic health conditions who have increased confidence in managing their conditions.
- Reduce the proportion of older adults who have moderate to severe functional limitations.
- Increase the proportion of older adults with reduced physical or cognitive function who engage in moderate to vigorous physical activity.
- Decrease the rate of pressure ulcer related hospitalization. (U.S. Department of Health and Human Services [USDHHS], 2013).
- Decrease the rate of emergency department visits for falls.

Teaching for older adults includes the use of sunscreen, adequate nutrition, management of polypharmacy, identification of elder abuse, and fall prevention. The following may be reported by the older adult: falls, urinary or fecal incontinence, mobility impairment, pain, vision or hearing changes, skin lesions, vascular disorders, sleep deprivation, depression, abuse, and cognitive changes.

Skin Cancers. Skin cancers increase with age and lifelong exposure to the sun. You should especially observe for skin cancer changes in older adults with the following risk factors: fair, freckling skin, light-colored eyes, red or blond hair, tendency to burn easily with sun exposure, male gender, and history of cigarette smoking. Teach patients to wear sunscreen at all times and recommend hats and clothing that covers the skin. Teach patients to do a skin assessment and observe for cancers. Basal cell carcinoma is a common form of skin cancer in older Caucasians.

Basal cell lesions in their early stage form a small, smooth, hemispherical, translucent papule covered by a thinned epidermis; they are most often located on the face, the bridge of the nose, the cheek, or below the eye. The papule gradually enlarges into a pearly nodule and has a central ulcerated lesion. Basal cell lesions can be locally invasive if not treated.

Squamous cell carcinoma usually starts as a hard, red, wartlike lesion with a raised or rolled gray-yellow edge that is located on a highly sun-exposed area. Look for these types of lesions on the auricle of the ear or the face and neck areas with the greatest sun exposure.

Malignant melanoma is a pigmented macule, papule, nodule, patch, or tumor with the ABCD warning signs (*A*symmetry, *B*order irregularity, *C*olor variegation, *D*iameter greater than 6 mm). This is a highly malignant form of cancer. Any suspicious lesions should be documented and the patient referred for follow-up. Refer to Chapter 11 for more information.

Nutrition. Older adults need added vitamin D because aging tends to impair vitamin D synthesis; smoking impairs it as well. Older adults are also at risk for folate deficiency, as are those with alcoholism, those who follow "fad" diets, and people of low socioeconomic status. Older adults also require special consideration during assessments of dietary requirements. They may compensate for diminished taste of sweet and salty foods by adding sugar and salt to their diet at a time when they are at increased risk for diabetes mellitus, hypertension, and heart disease. Their basal metabolic rate is declining concurrently with reductions in physical activity. When this occurs, caloric needs are significantly reduced. Older adults are also at increased risk for malnutrition as a result of social isolation. Eating alone is particularly problematic for people with reduced mobility, those receiving social assistance, or both. They may lack the resources required to maintain a nutritious and appealing diet. Poor dentition may also be an issue. Missing teeth, gum disease, or poorly fitting dentures can all detract from enjoying meals. Community programs are widely available and offer food services to people with disabilities or chronic illnesses who live in social isolation.

Medications. Older adults often have multiple chronic conditions and are thus prescribed multiple medications. This makes medication management, including assessment of patient knowledge and adherence to medication schedules, especially complex.

Safety. Assess for elder abuse and for safety in the home. The older adult may have stairs that present a risk for falling, cooking surfaces that can be a fire hazard, or electrical cords that can easily be tripped over. Teaching should focus on keeping cooking surfaces clean and having cords out of the normal path of walking. Rooms should also be well lit. For hospitalized patients, a bed alarm may be a good reminder to call for help.

Common Symptoms

The older adult may present with a confusing symptom or a group of symptoms because the classic presentation of common illnesses, such as burning with a urinary tract infection, does not consistently appear with older adults. For example, a change in mental status is one of the most common symptoms with acute illness in older adults but the source may be neurological, cardiac, or related to infection. Common nonspecific signs and symptoms in the older adult include confusion, self-neglect, falling, incontinence, apathy, anorexia, dyspnea, and fatigue. It takes an expert practitioner and diagnostician to track down the primary cause of presenting symptoms.

Common Symptoms in Older Adults

- Incontinence
- Sleep deprivation
- Pain
- Cognitive changes
- Depression
- Elder abuse

Signs/Symptoms	Rationale/Abnormal Findings
Incontinence • Have you ever leaked urine? • Have you ever lost control of your bladder?	There are three basic types of **incontinence** to assess: stress, urge, and functional. Incontinence is very common among hospitalized patients and those in long-term care. Risks include increasing age, caffeine intake, limited mobility, impaired cognition, diabetes mellitus, obesity, Parkinson disease, stroke, prostate difficulties, and use of medications such as diuretics.
Sleep Deprivation • What time do you turn off the lights? • How many awakenings do you have in a night? • Do you feel rested upon arising?	Insomnia may be either acute or chronic. It may include difficulty falling asleep or staying asleep or early morning wakening. Risk factors include female gender, increased age, medical or psychiatric illness, and shift work.
Pain • Do you have pain or discomfort? Where is it located? How long does it last? How intense is the pain? What makes it feel better? What makes it worse? Do you have a goal for your pain? • Has pain affected your ability to function normally? For example, has it affected your diet, sleep, or mood?	Chronic illnesses such as osteoarthritis or diabetic neuropathy increase the incidence of pain in the older adult. The patient may be hesitant to report pain because of fear of dependence or wanting to be a "good patient." Pain may affect normal functions.
Cognitive Status Assessment of cognitive status helps guide nursing care in various settings and can provide important information for discharge planning, patient and family education, interventions needed for safety, and general support. Some specific tips for performing cognitive assessments in older adults are found in Box 28.3.	The Mini-Cog is a short assessment test; the MMSE takes 10–15 minutes and is more thorough. Another screening tool that is gaining in popularity is the Montreal Cognitive Assessment, which offers different versions of the same test to limit possible learning effects with repeated administration (Ismail et al., 2013).
The MMSE is the one of the most widely used screening tools to detect cognitive impairment in older adults. It measures several areas of cognition: orientation (time and place); registration (ability to immediately register information); attention and calculation (ability to subtract sequential sevens); recall (short-term memory of three objects); language (ability to follow a three-step command), and visual–perceptual abilities (Folstein, Folstein, & McHugh, 1975). See Chapter 9.	**Clinical Significance** Suspicious patients with mild to moderate dementia have difficulty with time orientation questions. Avoid asking these questions first because they will highlight the patient's deficits and may make the patient more likely to refuse to answer the rest of the examination.
Normal findings are a score of 24–30.	Patients with **Parkinson disease** may have a slow retrieval time and very delayed responses.

(table continues on page 890)

BOX 28.3 Assessment of Cognitive Status

- Introduce the test. State "I am going to conduct a test of your thinking skills. This is a screening test and I want you to do your best."
- If a family member is present, it is wise to let him or her know that he or she is not allowed to answer for the older adult. Patients with mild dementia may look to a spouse or child to assist them with questions.
- If you detect that the patient is somewhat suspicious of your questions based on previous interactions, start with questions under the language section of the examination (i.e., "What is this?" point to your watch, and have him or her identify watch). Usually, these questions offer the patient some success in responses and allow you to complete more of the screening.
- Do not provide clues to answers. For example, when asking the orientation questions, simply say, "Can you tell me what month this is?" Do not say, "Well, we recently had our Thanksgiving break." If the patient is uncertain, simply restate the question. "Can you tell me the month?"
- Allow enough time for the patient to respond to the question that you have asked.
- Reassure the patient if he or she worries that the response might be incorrect. "It's OK if some of these are difficult for you." However, don't falsely tell patients that they are doing fine. Identify that this is simply a screening test and will help you better understand how to provide care for this patient.

Signs/Symptoms	Rationale/Abnormal Findings
Depression Although older adults are at risk for depression, the illness is not a normal or inevitable part of aging. To assess for depression, ask: • Do you struggle with depression? • Have you ever suffered from depression?	Depression may occur in older adults for various reasons. It is more common in people with multiple chronic health problems and in those who have recently suffered the loss of a spouse, friend, family member, or pet. Decisions about moving out of a family home because of increasing care needs may also lead to depressive symptoms.
The Geriatric Depression Scale (GDS) provides a brief screening for depressive symptoms. The longer 30-item version of the GDS asks about symptoms, self-image issues, and losses in a yes/no format. The short-form, 15-item GDS, also in a yes/no format, is used for patients with mild to moderate dementia (Yesavage, Brink, & Rose, 1982; Sheikh & Yesavage, 1986). Either version can be asked aloud (for visually impaired patients) or offered to the patient to read and complete privately. See Chapter 9.	On the short-form GDS, a score above 6 suggests depression and a score above 9 indicates depression.
If the screening examination reveals risk for or actual depression, assess for potential suicide risk. Mentally healthy older adults report that thoughts about death and suicide ideation are relatively rare. Chapter 9 discusses depression and suicide screening in more depth.	Factors that contribute to suicide in older adults include mental disorders (especially depression); physical illness; personality traits such as hostility, hopelessness, and inability to verbally express psychological pain and dependency on others; and recent life events and losses.
Elder Abuse Many older adults are vulnerable to abuse by family members. Abuse may continue because of nondetection by professionals, in part because elderly patients often do not report violence. If you notice injuries that could have been caused by abuse, question the patient: • Injuries like yours could have been caused by someone hurting you. Did someone hurt you?	Many abuse victims are isolated; some are ashamed and embarrassed or feel guilt and self-blame. In addition, some elders experience fear of reprisal, retribution from caregivers, or losing their home or independence. Others are pressured by relatives not to report.

Cultural Considerations

Additional Questions	Rationale/Abnormal Findings
• Do you have any food preferences? • What is your primary language? • Do you have any favorite activities? • Do you feel part of your community?	Many older adults prefer to experience environments similar to those they had in younger years. Based on assessment findings, the nurse may provide interventions, such as facilitating a Korean diet for a patient who prefers Korean food.

Therapeutic Dialogue: Collecting Subjective Data

Remember Mr. Monroe, introduced at the beginning of this chapter. This 76-year-old man with a history of Parkinson disease is complaining of constipation. The nurse uses professional communication techniques to gather subjective data from Mr. Monroe.

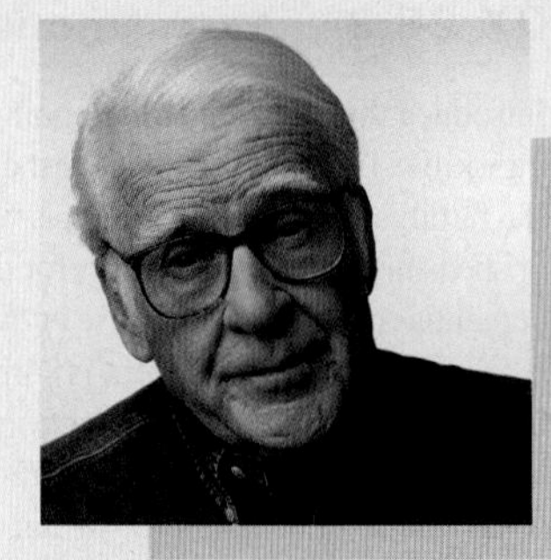

(case study continues on page 891)

Nurse: Hello, Mr. Monroe. How are you?

Mr. Monroe: Not so well. How about you?

Nurse: I'm OK. How do you feel about your new living situation?

Mr. Monroe: I don't like my roommate. He snores all night. I don't like the people here.

Nurse: I noticed that you have been taking the wheelchair to your meals. Why is that?

Mr. Monroe: The aides say that it's faster. I would rather take my walker on my own.

Nurse: We can talk with them. How about your eating?

Mr. Monroe: I drink 1–2 glasses of milk or juice at each meal. But I have trouble eating their food because my dentures don't fit (pause).

Nurse: (nods head, waits)

Mr. Monroe: I also would like to move my bowels before breakfast but I can't because I need help with zipping and buttoning my pants and the aides don't have time.

Critical Thinking Challenge

- What did the nurse do to obtain more information and provide a safe environment for the patient?
- What follow-up questions would you recommend?
- What additional assessments might the nurse make?

Objective Data

Equipment Needed

- Stethoscope
- Thermometer and blood pressure (BP) cuff or electronic vital signs monitor
- Watch or clock with a second hand
- Otoscope
- Ophthalmoscope

Preparation

After completing subjective data collection, collect equipment and prepare for the objective assessment. For a well assessment, perform a head-to-toe examination. If the patient is being seen for a particular complaint, the highest priority is assessment related to the patient's presenting problem.

When assessing an older adult, nurses need to allow extra time. The assessment may need to be broken into several sessions because older adults tend to fatigue easily.

It is important to rely on general observations and focus on the patient's functional abilities. Some older adults with major health conditions and numerous unexpected physical findings describe their health as "very good" because they can still carry out daily activities.

Documentation of unexpected findings is very important for this population because of their frequent transitions across health care settings. Excellent documentation can assist health care providers in a new setting to evaluate the patient's current examination findings and compare them with previous findings.

Comprehensive Physical Assessment

Technique and Normal Findings	Abnormal Findings
General Survey Observe expected changes that occur with aging. Assess for any decreasing abilities to function and care for self. Note any changes in mental status. *By the eighth or ninth decade, physical appearance changes, with sharper body contours and more angular facial features. Posture tends to have a general flexion and the patient's gait tends to have a wider base of support to compensate for diminished balance. Steps tend to be shorter and uneven. The patient may need to use the arms to help aid in balance.*	Poor hygiene and inappropriate dress may indicate decreased functional ability or may result from medications, infection, dehydration, or nutritional status. Inappropriate affect, inattentiveness, impaired memory, and inability to perform ADLs may indicate dementia from Alzheimer disease or another cause.

(table continues on page 892)

Technique and Normal Findings (continued)	Abnormal Findings (continued)
	SAFETY ALERT *In the frail older adult, confusion and changes in mentation from baseline are often the presenting symptom of underlying infections, dehydration, and electrolyte imbalances.*
Height and Weight An essential component of assessing nutritional status is an accurate measure of height and weight. If possible, measure height with the person standing erect without shoes against a wall.	**SAFETY ALERT** *Do not attempt to determine height when a frail older adult is standing on the weight scale. This creates a risk of falling because of the unsteadiness of the weight scale base.*
Height and weight are important components of the calculation for BMI. *BMI of 25–29 for older adults is linked to better health status and lower risks. This BMI is slightly higher than the recommended BMI for younger adults.*	BMI above 29 increases health risks for older adults. BMI of 24 or less also is associated with increased mortality.
Vital Signs ***Temperature.*** Assess temperature. *The temperature of older adults is at the lower end of the expected range. Mean body temperature for older adults is 36°–36.8°C (96.9°–98.3°F).*	Because of changes in the body's temperature regulatory mechanism and decreased subcutaneous fat, the aging adult is less likely to develop a fever but more likely to succumb to hypothermia. Temperatures within expected range for a younger adult may constitute fever in an older adult.
Pulse. Assess apical pulse for 1 minute. *The aging adult continues to have an expected range of 60–100 beats/min.*	Variation in rhythm may develop in some older adults. The radial artery may stiffen from peripheral vascular disease. A rigid artery does not indicate vascular disease elsewhere.
The pulse rate of older adults takes longer to rise to meet sudden increases in demand and longer to return to its resting state. Resting heart rate of older adults tends to be lower than for younger adults.	Heart sounds may be more difficult to assess and the point of maximum impulse (PMI) more difficult to palpate because of increased air space in the lungs, which increases the anteroposterior diameter of the chest.
Respirations. Assess respirations. *Decreased vital capacity and inspiratory volume can cause respirations to be shallower and more rapid than in younger adults, with an expected respiratory rate of 16–24 breaths/min. The respiratory rate of an older adult may be slightly higher than the usual 16–20.*	Aging causes the costal cartilage to become more rigid, decreasing chest expansion and vital capacity. Decreased efficiency of respiratory muscles results in breathlessness at lower activity levels. Respiratory rates greater than 24 are not normal and should be followed with further examination; look for cyanosis of the nail beds or the perioral area.
	SAFETY ALERT *In older adults with chronic lung disease or congestive heart failure, observe for generalized distress, confusion, or an impression that the patient is working hard to breathe. These symptoms may indicate decompensation.*

(table continues on page 893)

Technique and Normal Findings (continued)	Abnormal Findings (continued)
Pulse Oximetry. Assess pulse oximetry. Placement of the finger pulse oximetry probe can present a challenge in older adults. Sensors designed for the forehead or bridge of the nose may be indicated instead. Oxygen saturation is greater than 92%.	Peripheral vascular disease, decreased carbon dioxide levels, cold-induced vasoconstriction, and anemia may complicate assessment of oxygen saturation using a finger probe.
Skin, Hair, and Nails Inspect the skin, hair, and nails. The older adult's skin bruises and tears easily, exposing the patient to increased risk of wound infections. Examine skin carefully for breakdown, especially in the perineal area of older adults who are incontinent, and in any area that is at risk for pressure ulcers (see Chapter 11). Seborrheic keratoses are extremely common in older individuals. These dark brown pigmented lesions are waxy-appearing areas seen on the trunk of the body. They may appear on sun-exposed areas of the body. Photoaging findings of the skin include coarse wrinkles over sun-exposed areas, solar lentigines (age or liver spots) on the face, hands, forearms, upper chest, or back, and actinic keratosis. *There is increased wrinkling and skin is coarse in sun-exposed areas. Scalp hair is thin. The skin is less elastic and may be dry (although dryness of skin is more often linked to poor hydration status). It is common to note thinning of the epidermal layer, more pronounced in the eighth and ninth decades. Nail beds may have ridges. Toenails may become thickened.*	Nurses should be alert for bruising in various stages of healing that might indicate abuse. **Pressure ulcers** in the sacral and ischial areas, greater trochanteric area, or heels should be staged and interventions begun immediately. Patchy white scaly areas on the scalp or eyebrows are indicative of seborrhea, common in persons with Parkinson disease and usually treated with topical corticosteroids. Very thick, yellow, overgrown toenails are usually a sign of onychomycosis (tinea unguium), a fungal infection of the nail beds. These infected nails are difficult to treat and may eventually fall off, leaving a dry nail bed base. **Stasis dermatitis** is another common finding in older adults with a history of varicosities, phlebitis, and trauma. Lower extremities have a reddish-brown ruddy appearance and are usually edematous but are not inflamed or infected. Nurses often mistake stasis dermatitis for cellulitis, but the stasis changes do not respond to antibiotics. Stasis dermatitis may lead to leg ulcers on the lower shin area; these ulcers can become infected. Your assessment notes should include location, color and size of the area, size and depth of the ulcer (if present), presence of inflammation or warmth, and presence and severity of edema. Herpes zoster (shingles) is a painful red, vesicular or pustular rash that follows the distribution of a dermatome along the trunk or even into the legs. Older adults have a less vigorous immune response and are at risk for developing this rash, especially during times of illness or hospitalization. Prompt treatment is important to reduce postherpetic neuralgia pain.
Head and Neck Inspect the head and neck. Palpate the skull and hair. Palpate the sternocleidomastoid and trapezius muscles. Palpate the thyroid. The appearance is symmetrical. Facial expression is appropriate to the situation. The skull is smooth and there is no pain or mass. The hair is thin and gray. The thyroid is not enlarged.	A downward gaze with little eye contact may be a sign of depression. Any swelling, masses, or tumors are abnormal. Flat affect or facial tension may signify depression or anxiety. A patient who is extremely thin may have sunken hollows in his or her face. A patient with extremely thick structures may have thyroid problems. A goiter in the thyroid gland is also abnormal. Clicking or crepitus in the temporomandibular joint (TMJ) may be associated with jaw or neck pain. Note limitations in movement in the neck.

(table continues on page 894)

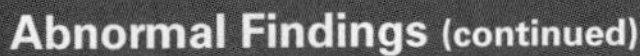

Technique and Normal Findings (continued)	Abnormal Findings (continued)
Eyes and Vision Inspect the eyes. *Senile ptosis or a sagging of the upper lid down across the eye, dry eyes that appear irritated and red, and a decrease in the corneal reflex may be present.* Test vision, pupillary reflex, and extraocular movements. *A smaller pupil size and a slower or sluggish papillary accommodation to light are expected. Also commonly seen is a grayish yellow ring surrounding the iris, called arcus senilis. Visual fields may be slightly diminished with confrontation but should not show unilateral differences.* Perform the ophthalmoscopic examination (see Chapter 13). *Retinal margins may be less distinct; drusen, yellow spots, may be on the macula.*	**Ectropion** (a turning of the lid outward) or **entropion** (a turning of the lid inward) may also be observed. Entropion can cause the eyelashes on the lower lid to scratch the corneal surface (Brodie, 2010; Fig. 28.5). Reduced visual fields, especially unilaterally, can be a sign of a stroke or central neurological lesion (refer to Chapter 13). Loss of vision can significantly affect daily functioning, including dressing, grooming, and ambulating safely. Older adults may have difficulty focusing properly or presbyopia, and may have difficulty with glare and accommodating to changes in light. Upward gaze is reduced because of muscle changes and laxity. Arcus senilis was thought to be an expected change of aging, but more recently has been linked to elevated lipid deposits.

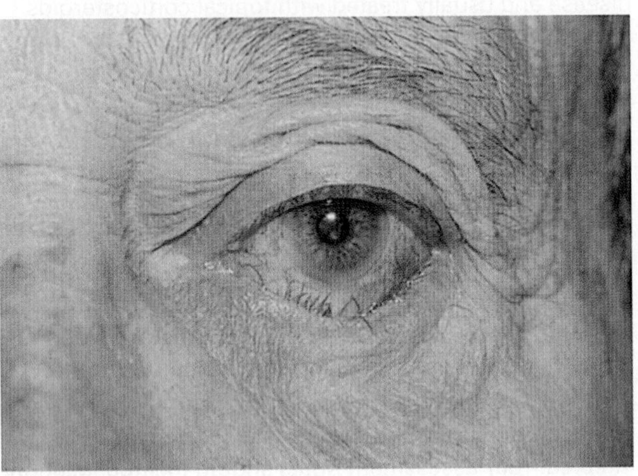

A

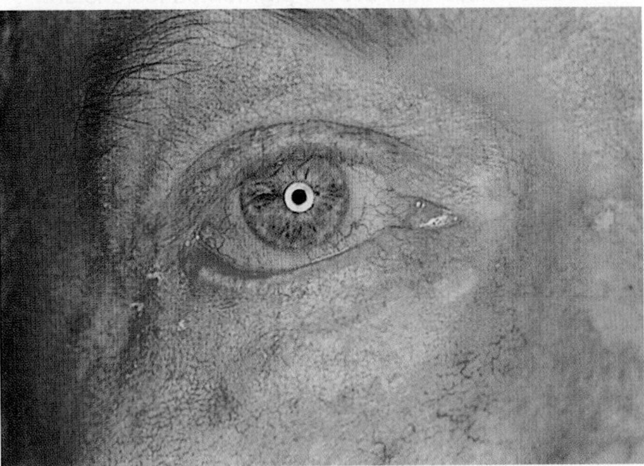

B

Figure 28.5 Eye findings in older adults. **A.** Entropion. **B.** Ectropion.

Technique and Normal Findings (continued)	Abnormal Findings (continued)
Ears and Hearing Inspect the ear for any lesions or changes to the auricle. No pain, masses, or lesions are present.	Ulcerated lesions on the auricle in older men with a history of sun exposure (e.g., golfers, outdoor workers, farmers) may represent squamous cell carcinoma and should be evaluated. Refer to Chapter 14.
Perform the otoscopic examination (see Chapter 14). *There may be a gray tympanic membrane or an ear canal that is narrowed or occluded with wax. The patient may have conductive hearing loss and will lateralize hearing to the ear occluded with wax on the Weber test or will hear bone conduction longer than air conduction in the ear occluded with wax on the Rinne test.*	Loss of hearing is found in 30% of people older than 65 years of age, and in 47% of those older than 75 years of age (National Institute of Deafness and Communication Disorders [NIDCD], 2010). High-frequency sounds are lost most commonly, so older adults may have difficulty hearing a female examiner with a high-pitched voice. Hearing loss can affect emotional health and functional abilities. Early treatment of the causes of conductive hearing loss or information on assistive devices is important.
Nose, Mouth, and Throat Inspect the nose, mouth, and throat. Test nasal patency (Fig. 28.6). *Deviation of the nasal septum is common in older adults.* Make note of the color and moisture of the mucosal membranes of the nose and oral cavity. These are pink to pinkish red and moist. The tongue is pinkish red, moist, and has no fissures.	

(table continues on page 895)

Technique and Normal Findings (continued)	Abnormal Findings (continued)
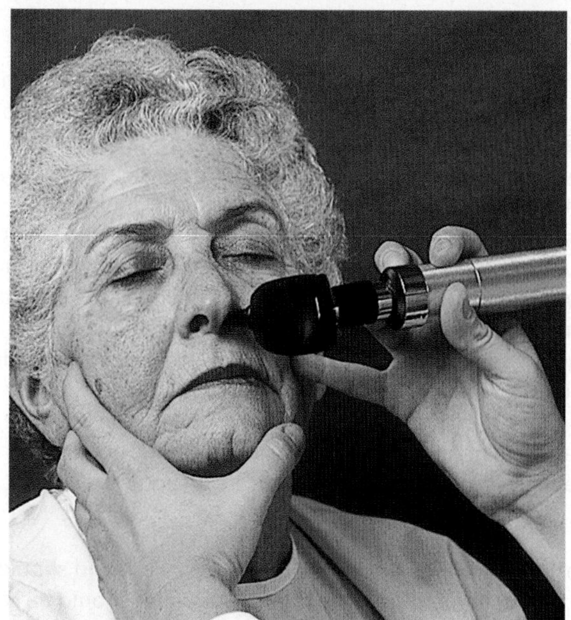 Figure 28.6 Assessing for nasal patency in the older adult. *A slightly dry oral mucosa is more common in older adults, but a fissured tongue is a sign of dehydration. Varicosities under the tongue are more common in older adults. The gag reflex is intact, although it may mildly diminish in frail older adults.*	Vasomotor rhinitis is common. Pale mucosal membranes can indicate anemia or malnutrition. Malodorous breath may indicate dental disease, poor dental hygiene, or underlying diseases. Poor dental condition, fractured teeth, or untreated dental caries should be referred to a dentist because these can markedly influence nutritional intake. A bright red tongue can indicate *vitamin C or B1 deficiency*. An overgrowth of white patchy plaque on the tongue may be related to poor dental hygiene or may be a fungal or yeast infection (oral candidiasis). Any signs of poor oral care may be indicative of forgetting to manage ADLs, a symptom of cognitive impairment. An absent or markedly diminished gag reflex can be found in patients who have had a stroke, long-standing alcoholism, or neurological disorders. Patients with diminished or absent gag reflexes are at risk for aspiration pneumonia (see Chapter 16).
Thorax and Lungs Inspect the chest. *The older adult may have an increased anteroposterior diameter related to rigidity of the chest wall.* Palpate the chest wall to test for tactile fremitus. Percuss the lungs. Chest wall is free of pain, swelling, or masses. Tactile fremitus is not increased; percussion is resonant. Auscultate breath sounds. *Older adults who can take good breaths should have normal breath sounds. Harsh rhonchi are sometimes found because of the difficulty of clearing materials from the lungs. Have the patient cough and then listen for breath sounds again. It is common for older adults to have some scattered fine crackles at the bases of their lungs.*	Increased fremitus or dullness with percussion, especially at the lung bases, can indicate fluid accumulation. Older adults with chronic lung disease have hyperresonance on examination. Older women may have kyphosis (curvature of the cervical or thoracic spine related to osteoporosis) that can affect your ability to hear lung sounds at the bases. You may need to listen at the lateral sides of the posterior wall to hear the breath sounds. Lung sounds may be difficult to hear with advanced lung disease or may sound diminished and tight. Listening after a nebulizer treatment may give a clearer picture. See Chapter 16.
Heart and Neck Vessels Auscultate heart sounds. *Pulse rates in the 50–60 range are common and often related to use of beta-blockers or other cardiac medications. Heart rate and rhythm are regular with no murmurs, rubs, or gallops. As older adults reach their 80s and 90s, murmurs are common, especially grade 2 systolic murmurs.* Observe neck vessels. No jugular venous distention is present.	**SAFETY ALERT** *Pulses greater than 100 are abnormal and should be taken seriously. Because of their poor cardiac reserves, older adults do not tolerate these pulse rates well for long periods.*

(table continues on page 896)

Technique and Normal Findings (continued)	Abnormal Findings (continued)
	Loud (grade 3 or greater) or harsh holosystolic murmurs suggest valvular (usually aortic) stenosis and can sometimes be heard radiating up to the neck. Loud murmurs that can be heard radiating from the apex to around the side of the chest wall are usually mitral valve in origin. Findings from the whole examination should be considered when a patient has a loud murmur; look specifically for lower extremity edema, abdominal distension, or other signs of fluid retention. In addition, perform a thorough respiratory examination to identify signs of congestive heart failure. Jugular venous distention is a sign of congestive heart failure. Arrhythmias, especially atrial fibrillation, are common in older adults but should be considered abnormal. Note whether this is an irregularly irregular rhythm and be concerned if the rate is greater than 100. Abdominal aortic pulsations that extend over a wide area indicate an aortic aneurysm.
Peripheral Vascular Palpate peripheral pulses. Pulses are 2–3 on a 4-point scale and symmetrical.	Absent peripheral pulses are of great concern and should be noted in the record. The primary provider should be contacted if this finding is new. It is more common in a person with a long history of smoking or in one who has diabetes; it can seriously interfere with wound healing. Vascular disease may be venous or arterial (see Chapter 18).
Breasts Palpate breasts. Because breast tissue loses density with age, masses or nodules are easier to feel. No masses or nodules are present.	Mastectomy scars should be noted and palpated.
Abdomen and Elimination Inspect, auscultate, palpate, and percuss the abdomen. Perform the rectal examination. *Take extra time to listen for bowel sounds in older adults with a history of constipation. Finding a mass of stool in the lower left quadrant is common. A flaccid or soft, distended abdomen is common but can be related to deconditioning and loss of muscle control. Bowel sounds may be slow but easy to hear. The rectal examination may show external hemorrhoids.*	A distended abdomen can signify excessive gas, stool, or fluid. Asymmetry or masses are important findings and may be signs of severe constipation or cancer. A rectal check should be performed for anyone with a lower abdominal mass. Patients with large amounts of abdominal ascites usually have liver disease or cancerous involvement of the liver. Hemorrhoids, internal or external, are common but should not be painful, fiery red, or inflamed. Fecal incontinence or involuntary passage of stool is abnormal in older adults. See Chapter 20.
Musculoskeletal System Measure height. *Loss of height of up to 6 in. can occur by 70–80 years of age.* Perform focused assessments of the bones, muscles, and joints as indicated. *Flexion and hyperextension of the neck are somewhat reduced. Likelihood of kyphosis of the spine is increased (more common in women than men). There may be a generalized decrease in strength and mildly decreased range of motion (ROM). Older adults with arthritis may have enlarged joints, especially at the knees and in the hands.* When possible, nurses should test the patient's ability to stand from a seated position, walk a short distance, and turn around. *Patients should be able to do this smoothly, without balance difficulties, stumbling, or assistance.*	Examination of ROM of the upper extremities is important, especially for hospitalized older adults. Limited abduction of the shoulder can be addressed immediately to prevent "frozen shoulder," a condition that commonly occurs during or after a hospital stay. Pain on palpation of the spine after a fall should raise concerns about possible compression fracture of the spine. Large nodules in the distal interphalangeal joints are Heberden nodes, whereas enlargements of the proximal interphalangeal joints are Bouchard nodes, common in patients with arthritis. Contractures of the hips and knees are abnormal but common in patients who spend much of their day in a wheelchair. These contractures change the structure of gait and balance, and place the patient at risk for further immobility. See Chapter 21.

(table continues on page 897)

Technique and Normal Findings (continued)	Abnormal Findings (continued)
Neurological System ***Cranial Nerves.*** Test cranial nerves. *Common expected findings in older adults include decreased upward gaze.*	Older adults who appear to have a blank or blunted affect may have depression, dementia, or Parkinson disease.
Balance and Coordination. Test balance and coordination. *There may be slowing of psychomotor finger–nose testing or finger-to-finger testing. Heel-to-toe walking may be impaired related to musculoskeletal conditions. Observation of gait with or without an assistive device shows smooth steps that may be widely based.* **SAFETY ALERT** *The Romberg test should only be done with a chair directly behind the patient and the examiner at the patient's side to assist if the patient begins to fall.*	Abnormal gait changes include difficulty initiating gait. A small, short, stepped gait that gradually becomes normal is a sign of Parkinson disease. A wide-based gait with a heel-to-toe foot slap to the floor is a sign of a cerebellar disorder; a gait in which the leg does not swing through smoothly, catches on the floor, drags, or stops next to the other foot is a sign of cerebrovascular disease. See Chapter 22.
Test sensation. *Peripheral sensation and proprioceptive (position) sense may diminish slightly with aging.*	**Clinical Significance** Unilateral findings on neurological examination are always important and may be evidence of a previous cerebrovascular accident.
Reflexes and Muscle Strength. Test reflexes and muscle strength. *Reflexes normally diminish with aging, and muscle strength against resistance may be slightly diminished in those with musculoskeletal conditions.*	Tremors are abnormal. If present, determine whether the tremor occurs only at rest and whether it involves only one limb, one side, or all extremities. Parkinson disease has a resting tremor that usually starts unilaterally and does not include the head and neck. Tremor of the hand or neck that is heard in changes in the voice or that occurs in the hand only when the person is initiating an action, is intentional or "essential" and has a very different treatment. Diminished grip strength or unilateral loss of strength against resistance is abnormal. Severely diminished or absent sensation or proprioception indicates peripheral neuropathy.
Genitourinary System Inspect genitals. *Thinning of genital hair and testicular or penile atrophy is common. Skin in the vaginal area may be thinned.*	Observe for a distended lower abdomen with resonant-to-dull percussion of fluid. A full bladder after recently voiding is a sign of **urinary retention**. Underwear smelling of urine, urine stains, or leaking urine indicates incontinence, which is common but not normal in older adults and should be treated. See Chapters 23 and 24.
Endocrine, Immunological, and Hematological Systems Evaluate laboratory data. *Older adults are likely to demonstrate decreased lean muscle and bone mass, increased fat mass and vasomotor symptoms, fatigue, depression, anemia, erectile dysfunction, decreased libido, and decline in immune function (Chahal & Drake, 2007).*	You may find that older adults do not mount a very high febrile response in the presence of infection. Total lymphocyte count may remain low despite infection.

Cultural Considerations

Common integumentary findings in African Americans include curly hair that tends to be coarser than in Caucasians because of an impaired ability of secreted sebum to travel along the hair shaft from the skin. Skin is commonly excessively dry, resulting in ashy dermatitis. Pityriasis rosea, a macular hyperpigmented viral dermatitis in Caucasians, commonly presents as papular, maroon-to-purplish lesions in African Americans.

Southeast Asian men have less body and facial hair than patients of other genetic heritages. Tattoos, body piercings, and other skin adornments are common in various Asian cultures. Skin discolorations from cupping or coining are commonly found. Henna tattoos are common in Arabic and Indian women.

Critical Thinking

Laboratory and Diagnostic Testing

The U.S. Preventive Services Task Force (2013) recommends the following screening as part of the well visit:

- Blood cholesterol levels
- Fecal occult blood test and/or sigmoidoscopy
- Mammogram for women 50 to 74 years of age every 2 years
- Papanicolaou (Pap) test (women) for those who have been sexually active and have a cervix

Routine testing of prostate-specific antigen (PSA) to screen for prostate cancer in men is debated because false positives are common.

Diagnostic Reasoning

Nursing Diagnosis, Outcomes, and Interventions

When formulating a nursing diagnosis, it is important to use critical thinking to cluster data and identify patterns that fit together. Compare these clusters with defining characteristics (abnormal findings) for the diagnosis to ensure the most accurate labeling and appropriate interventions. Table 28.1 provides a comparison of nursing diagnoses, abnormal findings, and interventions commonly related to the older adult assessment (NANDA International, 2012).

Use assessment information to identify patient outcomes (Moorhead, Johnson, Maas, & Swanson, 2013). Some outcomes related to the older adult are as follows:

- Patient maintains current weight.
- Patient has appropriate conversation that flows smoothly.
- Patient eats at least 75% of ordered meals.

After outcomes have been established, implement nursing care to improve the status of the older adult. Use critical thinking and evidence-based practice to develop interventions (Bulechek, Butcher, Dochterman, & Wagner, 2013). Some examples for older adult care are as follows:

- Provide between-meal snacks for smaller, more frequent meals.
- Locate and clean eyeglasses.
- Place hearing aid in patient's ear.
- Assess food preferences and obtain favorite foods.

TABLE 28.1 Common Nursing Diagnoses Associated With the Older Adult

Diagnosis	Point of Differentiation	Assessment Characteristics	Nursing Interventions
Adult failure to thrive	Progressive deterioration of functional abilities, physical skills, and cognition	Change in mood; decreased food intake at meals; neglect of home, finances, or other responsibilities	Assess for depression. Complete MMSE. Provide cues in the environment for food intake. Provide reality orientation. Encourage patients to reminisce and share life histories.
Disturbed sensory perception: visual or auditory	Change in stimuli	Reduced vision or hearing	Provide adequate lighting. Keep background noise low, such as turning off the TV when talking. Make sure that patient has devices such as eyeglasses or hearing aid.
Imbalanced nutrition: less than body requirements	Insufficient nutrient intake for metabolic needs	Nausea, vomiting, diarrhea; anorexia; lack of food; eating alone; reduced functional abilities for shopping, cooking, and cleaning	Note laboratory tests such as total protein, albumin, and prealbumin. Weigh patient daily. Monitor food intake and record the percentage of meal eaten.

MMSE, Mini-Mental State Examination.

Progress Note: Analyzing Findings

Mr. Monroe's difficulties have been outlined throughout this chapter. Initial subjective and objective data collection is complete and the nurse has spent time reviewing the findings and other results. The following nursing note illustrates how the nurse collects and analyzes subjective and objective data and develops nursing interventions.

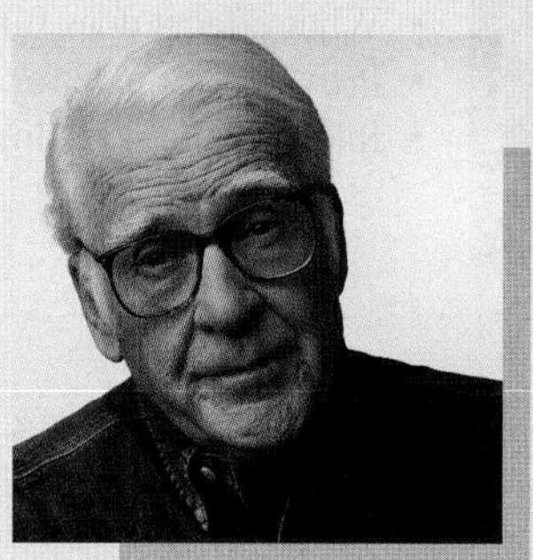

Subjective: A 76-year-old man, 10-yr history of Parkinson disease, mild dementia, seen for new constipation. Has large, hard, dry brown stool every fourth day. New admission to skilled care facility 3 months ago; "still adjusting"; does not like roommate. Can ambulate with walker. Takes wheelchair to meals "because it's faster." Ambulates in room. Fluids at meals 3–5 glasses milk or juice total, no additional water. Denies swallowing problems. Weight loss 16 lb over past year, dentures uncomfortable, prefers soft foods, no fresh fruit. Previous bowel movement (BM) after breakfast, states toilet not available before breakfast, needs help with pants zipping and buttoning. Medications: Sinemet 25/250 four times daily before meals, Vitamin E 400 IU daily, Calcium 600 mg with Vitamin D 800 IU daily, and Zestril 5mg daily.

Objective:

- Vitals: weight 156 lb (decreased 4 lb since admission), BP 104/60 mm Hg, P 76 beats/min, R 12 breaths/min, afebrile.
- General survey: Alert, conversant, thin man with resting tremor of hands bilaterally.
- Skin: dry, flaky, red raised areas on posterior scalp 3×5 cm.
- HEENT: dry oral mucosa, ill-fitting dentures, no oral sores or open areas, thyroid not enlarged, diminished gag reflex.
- Respiratory: no cough, clear to auscultation.
- Cardiac: S1, S2, RRR, no murmurs rubs or gallops.
- Abdomen: soft, nondistended, tender LLQ, with mass palpable. Approx. 4 cm diameter, BS + all 4 quads.
- Rectal: 2–3 cm external hemorrhoid, no fissures, sphincter tone within normal limits, large amount hard stool high in rectal vault.
- Neurological: Decreased blink; blunted affect; increased tone; rigidity in all extremities; short stepped gait with walker; steady, slow, difficulty rising and sitting.

Analysis: Constipation related to immobility, medications, dehydration related to disease processes and medications as evidenced by frequent use of wheelchair, limited walking, poor fiber intake, poor liquid intake, use of Sinemet, calcium, vitamin E, and Zestril (all potentially constipating medications).

Plan: *Goal*: Resident will have one bowel movement within 2–3 days without straining. *Interventions:* Ambulate to meals with walker three times daily. Increase fluids to more than 1.5 L every day. Offer 4–6 oz water at 10:00 AM, 2:00 PM, and 4:00 PM. Start fiber pudding 2 oz every day. Routinely schedule time for BM, find private bathroom near dining room.

Evaluate need for Zestril with primary health care provider. Evaluate need for multivitamin with iron and Vitamin E. Refer to dietician to increase dietary fiber. Refer to dentist for denture repair and refitting.

(case study continues on page 900)

Critical Thinking Challenge

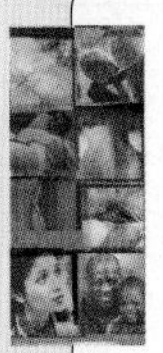

- What effects does functional status have on body systems?
- Provide rationale for the abnormal abdominal and rectal assessment findings.
- Interpret the neurological findings in the context of the patient's Parkinson disease.

Collaborating With the Interprofessional Team

In many facilities, nurses initiate referrals based on assessment findings. Results that might trigger a dental consult include chipped or loose teeth, dental caries, tooth pain, denture care, bad breath, snoring or sleep apnea, and dry mouth.

Mr. Monroe has been experiencing loose dentures stemming from weight loss; therefore, a dental consult is indicated. The following conversation illustrates how the nurse might organize data and make recommendations about the patient's situation.

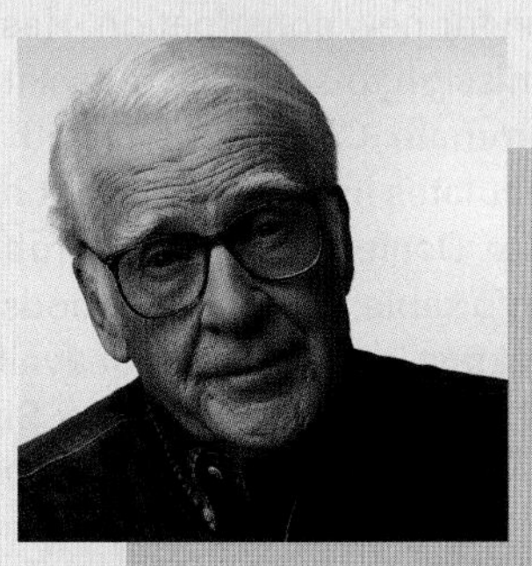

Situation: "Hello, I am Pat Jackson, the nurse practitioner who is caring for Mr. Ralph Monroe, date of birth 2-10-1938."

Background: "He was admitted 3 months ago with a loss of functional status related to Parkinson disease. He has been complaining of difficulty in chewing, and he has lost 4 lb."

Assessment: "I noticed that his oral mucosa is very dry. His dentures are loose and malfitting, although he has no oral sores or open areas."

Recommendations: "Would you have an opening to see him for denture fitting in the next week?"

Critical Thinking Challenge

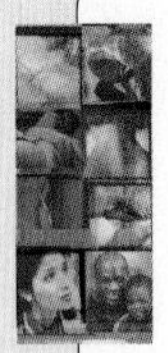

- How did the nurse prioritize which information to include and leave out in her report?
- What other assessments might be considered related to Mr. Monroe's nutrition?
- What nursing diagnoses are appropriate related to his mouth and dentures?

Pulling it All Together

The nurse uses assessment data to formulate a nursing care plan with patient outcomes and interventions for Ralph Monroe. Outcomes are specific to the patient, realistic to achieve, measurable, and have a time frame for completion. Interventions are based on evidence and practice guidelines. After their implementation the nurse reevaluates Mr. Monroe and documents findings in the chart to show progress. The nurse uses critical thinking and judgment to continue or revise the diagnosis, outcomes, and interventions.

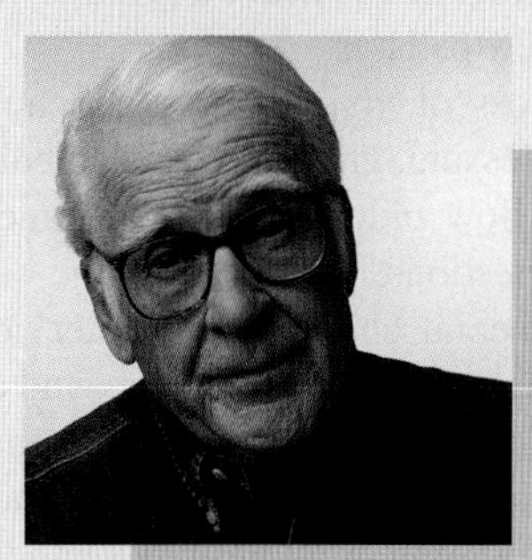

Nursing Diagnosis	Patient Outcomes	Nursing Interventions	Rationale	Evaluation
Constipation related to multiple medications, inactivity, and low fluid/bulk intake	Patient will have one BM in next 2–3 days without straining. Patient eliminates moderate amount of soft brown stool every 2 days.	Ambulate with walker tid. Offer fluids every 2 hours. Order fiber pudding with lunch. Schedule time for BM. Initiate diet consult.	Activity stimulates peristalsis. Fluids ensure that patient is well hydrated. Fiber increases bulk in the diet.	Patient had bowel movement of moderately hard brown stool. Will continue to monitor for improvement and re-establishment of regular patterns.

Applying Your Knowledge

Using the previous steps of diagnostic reasoning, organizing, and prioritizing, consider all the case study findings about Mr. Monroe woven throughout this chapter. When answering the following questions, begin drawing conclusions and see how the pieces of assessment must work together to create an environment for personalized, appropriate, and accurate care.

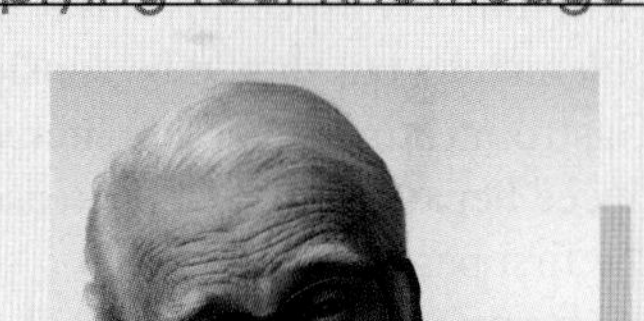

- How would you define primary and secondary aging?
- What is your rationale for using the Mini Mental Status Examination (MMSE) and a nutritional assessment tool with Mr. Monroe?
- What screening tests would you request for Mr. Monroe?
- What factors might contribute to Mr. Monroe's dislike of his roommate and other residents?
- What recommendations would you make about Mr. Monroe's requirements for immunizations?
- How would you evaluate your counseling regarding nutritional intake with Mr. Monroe?

Key Points

- Older adults heal more slowly because of slower growth of new cells.
- Loss of vision can significantly affect ADLs, including dressing, grooming, and ambulating safely.
- Allow older adults extra time to answer subjective data questions.
- Special challenges to interviewing older adults include hearing, visual, language, and cognitive impairments.
- Geriatric syndromes include nutritional changes, mobility impairment, falls, polypharmacy, and skin breakdown.
- Common problems of older adults include urinary incontinence, sleep problems, pain, cognitive changes, depression, and elder abuse.
- The skin of the older adult has increased wrinkling and is thinner, less elastic, and drier. Pressure ulcers in the sacral and ischial areas, greater trochanteric area, or heels should be staged and interventions begun immediately.
- Senile ptosis, dry or red eyes, smaller and slower pupillary responses, and difficulty with glare are common ocular findings.
- Loss of hearing is a common finding in the older adult.
- Unexpected findings in the mouth include pallor, malodorous breath, poor dentition, and candidiasis.
- The older adult has a less elastic chest wall, decreased respiratory muscle strength, loss of alveolar recoil, and increased residual volume.
- Arterial walls are less elastic and stiffer, causing increased systolic blood pressure, increased ventricular wall hypertrophy, decreased coronary blood flow, reduced cardiac output, and increased circulating catecholamines.
- Arrhythmias, especially atrial fibrillation, are common in older adults but should be considered abnormal.
- Gastrointestinal changes include slowed peristalsis, reduced hepatic flow, and decreased metabolism of drugs on the first pass.
- Common normal neurological findings include restricted upward gaze, slowed coordination, slowed gait, decreased reflexes, decreased strength, and impaired sensation.
- The older adult should be assessed for depression, dementia, Parkinson disease, and signs of cerebrovascular accident.
- Older adults often lose height and lean body mass.
- Large nodules in the distal interphalangeal joints are Heberden nodes. Enlargements of the proximal interphalangeal joints are Bouchard nodes, a common finding in association with arthritis.
- Kidney function decreases with age, causing a decreased glomerular filtration rate, decreased creatinine clearance, and inability to conserve sodium.
- Endocrine changes include decreased growth hormone, decreased adrenal hormones, decreased response of the immune system, and increased glucose intolerance.
- Common nursing diagnoses for older adults include Risk for falling, Risk for skin breakdown, Urinary incontinence, Altered sleep pattern, Confusion, Adult failure to thrive, Disturbed sensory perception, and Imbalanced nutrition.

Review Questions

1. Which of the following findings are considered an expected change in the skin in older adults?
   A. Solar lentigines (liver spots)
   B. Actinic keratoses
   C. Loss of subcutaneous fat
   D. Photoaging

2. Which of the following statements is true concerning changes in the older adult?
   A. The lens becomes smaller and less dense.
   B. The tympanic membrane becomes more flexible and retracted.
   C. Changes in the inner ear can interfere with sound discrimination.
   D. Increased pupillary responses lead to difficulty in light accommodation.

3. When speaking with a frail older adult, it is best to
   A. fill in silences to avoid discomfort.
   B. address all questions to the patient's family.
   C. rely on the patient's memory when gathering all information.
   D. ask questions using lay terms rather than medical terms.

4. The nurse assesses for geriatric syndromes, which are
   A. the interaction of multiple diagnoses that contribute to problems in the older adult.
   B. the exacerbation of chronic conditions such as congestive heart failure or chronic obstructive pulmonary disease.
   C. conditions in which older adults may not mount an immune response.
   D. decreases in growth hormones and steroids that reduce functional status.

5. Nutritional screening is an assessment of risk factors that
   A. indicate that the patient is at high nutritional risk.
   B. identify older adults who may require a more comprehensive assessment.
   C. calculate BMI and classify patients as obese versus malnourished.
   D. describe food frequency and microelements that may be lacking in the diet.

6. Which question or questions should you ask to assess medication use in the older adult living in the community? Select all that apply.
   A. "What medications are you taking?"
   B. "What is the schedule for your medications?
   C. "Do you understand why you are taking all of your medications?
   D. "What is the dose of the medication that you take?"

7. As part of the Mini Mental Status Examination, you ask the patient to immediately state three words. This is a measure of which of the following?
   A. Orientation
   B. Registration
   C. Recall
   D. Attention

8. Which of the following patients should the nurse see first?
   A. A patient with unilateral changes in vision
   B. A patient with ectropion of the lower lid
   C. A patient with presbyopia
   D. A patient with senile ptosis

9. You auscultate a loud murmur in an older adult patient. You should also assess for which of the following?
   A. Coarse rhonchi and purulent sputum
   B. Irregular heartbeat and pulse deficit
   C. Crackles in the lungs and leg edema
   D. Abdominal distention and liver tenderness

10. The patient has findings of cognitive decline, minimal to no intake of nutrition, and neglect of the home environment and finances. Which of the following is the appropriate nursing diagnosis?
   A. Disturbed sensory perception
   B. Impaired individual coping
   C. Imbalanced nutrition, less than body requirements
   D. Adult failure to thrive

The Jensen suite offers these additional resources to enhance learning and facilitate understanding of this chapter:

- thePoint online resources, http://thepoint.lww.com/Jensen2e
- *Laboratory Manual for Nursing Health Assessment: A Best Practice Approach*
- *Pocket Guide for Nursing Health Assessment: A Best Practice Approach*
- *Lippincott DocuCare*, an electronic health record simulation software, http://thepoint.lww.com/docucare
- *Adaptive Learning | Powered by PrepU*, http://thepoint.lww.com/prepu

References

Ahmed, T., & Haboubi, N. (2010). Assessment and management of nutrition in older people and its importance to health. *Clinical Interventions in Aging*, *5*, 207–216.

American Nurses Association (ANA). (1991). *Position statement: Nursing and the Patient Self-Determination Act*. Washington, DC: Author.

Bergstrom, N., Braden, B. J., Laguzza, A., & Holman, V. (1987). The Braden scale for preventing pressure sore risk. *Nursing Research*, *36*(4), 205–210.

Bernhard, D. & Laufer, G. (2008). The aging cardiomyocyte: A mini-review. *Gerontology*, *54*(1), 24–31.

Braden, B. J., & Bergstrom, N. (1989). Clinical utility of the Braden scale for predicting pressure sore risk. *Decubitus*, *2*(3), 44–51.

Brodie, S. E. (2010). Aging and disorders of the eye. In H.M. Fillit, K. Rockwood, & K. Woodhouse (Eds.), *Brocklehurst's textbook of geriatric medicine and gerontology* (7th ed., pp. 810–822). Philadelphia, PA: Saunders.

Bulechek, G. M., Butcher, H. K., Dochterman, J. M., & Wagner, C. M. (2013). *Nursing interventions classification (NIC)* (6th ed.). St. Louis, MO: Mosby.

Centers for Disease Control and Prevention (CDC). (2010). *Basic information about skin cancer*. Retrieved from http://www.cdc.gov/cancer/skin/basic_info/

Centers for Disease Control and Prevention (CDC). (2013). *The state of aging and health in America, 2013*. Atlanta, GA: Author. Retrieved from http://www.cdc.gov/features/agingandhealth/state_of_aging_and_health_in_america_2013.pdf

Chahal, H. S., & Drake, W. M. (2007). The endocrine system and aging. *Journal of Pathology*, *211*(2), 173–180.

Davies, G. A., & Bolton, C. E. (2010). Age related changes in the respiratory system. In H.M. Fillit, K. Rockwood, & K. Woodhouse (Eds.), *Brocklehurst's textbook of geriatric medicine and gerontology* (7th ed.). Philadelphia, PA: Saunders.

Elmadfa, I., & Meyer, A. L. (2008). Body composition, changing physiological functions and nutrient requirements of the elderly. *Annals of Nutrition and Metabolism*, *52*(Suppl 1), 2–5.

Faggiano, A., Del Prete, M., Marciello, F., Marotta, V., Ramundo, V., & Colao, A. (2011). Thyroid disease in elderly. *Minerva Endocrinologica*, *36*(3), 211–231.

Folstein, M. F., Folstein, S. E., & McHugh, P. R. (1975). "Mini-mental state": A practical method for grading the cognitive state of patients for the clinician. *Journal of Psychiatric Research*, *12*, 189–198.

Guay, D. R. P. (2010). The pharmacology of aging. In H.M. Fillit, K. Rockwood, & K. Woodhouse (Eds.), *Brocklehurst's textbook of geriatric medicine and gerontology* (7th ed.). Philadelphia, PA: Saunders.

Hastings, S. N., Whitson, H. E., Sloane, R., Landerman, L. R., Horney, C., Johnson, K. S. (2014). Using the past to predict the future: latent class analysis of patterns of health service use of older adults in the emergency department. *Journal of the American Geriatrics Society, 62*(4), 711–715..

Hendrich, A. L., Bender, P. S., & Nyhuis, A. (2003). Validation of the Hendrich II Fall Risk Model: A large concurrent case/control study of hospitalized patients. *Applied Nursing Research*, *16*, 9–21.

Ismail, Z., Mulsant, B. H., Herrmann, N., Rapoport, M., Nilsson, M., & Shulman, K. (2013). Canadian academy of geriatrics psychiatry survey of brief cognitive screening instruments. *Canadian Geriatrics Journal*, *16*(2), 54–60.

Jones, A. L., Moss, A. J., & Harris-Kojetin, L. D. (2011). Use of advance directives in long-term care populations (NCHS Data Brief No. 54). Retrieved from Centers for Disease Control and Prevention Web site: http://www.cdc.gov/nchs/data/databriefs/db54.htm

Kane, R. L., Ouslander, J. G., Abrass, I. B., & Resnick, B. (2013). *Essentials of clinical geriatrics* (7th ed.). New York, NY: McGraw-Hill.

Katz, S., Ford, A. B., Moskowitz, R. W., Jackson, B. A., & Jaffe, M. W. (1963). Studies of illness in the aged: The index of ADL: A standardized measure of biological and psychosocial functioning, *Journal of American Medical Association*, *185*, 94–101.

Lach, H. W., & Smith, C. M. (2007). Assessment: Focus on function. In A.D. Linton, H.W. Lach, M.A. Mattenson, & E.S. McConnell, *Matteson & McConnells' gerontological nursing concepts and practice* (3rd ed.). St. Louis, MO: Saunders-Elsevier.

Lawton, M. P., & Brody, E. M. (1969). Assessment of older people: Self-maintaining and instrumental activities of daily living. *Gerontologist*, *9*(3), 179–186.

Linton, A. D., Lach, H. W., Matteson, M. A., & McConnell, E. S. (2007). *Matteson & McConnells' gerontological nursing concepts and practice* (3rd ed.). St. Louis, MO: Saunders-Elsevier.

Madden, K. M. & Wong, R. Y. (2013). The health of geriatrics in Canada—more than meets the eye. *Canadian Geriatrics Journal*, *16*(1), 1–2.

Mahoney, F. I., & Barthel, D. W. (1965). Functional evaluation: The Barthel index. *Maryland State Medical Journal*, *14*, 61–65.

McBride, M. (2012). Ethnogeriatrics and cultural competence for nursing practice. Retrieved from http://consultgerirn.org/topics/ethnogeriatrics_and_cultural_competence_for_nursing_practice/want_to_know_more

Miller, C. A. (2008). Communication difficulties in hospitalized older adults with dementia. *American Journal of Nursing*, 108(3), 58–66.

Morse, J. M., Morse, R. M., & Tylko, S. J. (1989). Development of a scale to identify the fall-prone patient. *Canadian Journal on Aging*, *8*, 366–377.

Moorhead, S., Johnson, M., Maas, M. L., & Swanson, E. (2013). *Nursing outcomes classification (NOC): Measurement of health outcomes* (5th ed.). St. Louis, MO: Elsevier.

Murphy, S. L., Jiaquan, X., & Kochanek, K. D. (2013). Deaths: Final data for 2010. *National Vital Statistics Report*, *61*, 4. Retrieved from http://www.cdc.gov/nchs/data/nvsr/nvsr61/nvsr61_04.pdf

National Institute of Deafness and Communication Disorders (NIDCD) (2010). *Quick statistics.* Retrieved from http://www.nidcd.nih.gov/health/statistics/quick.htm

NANDA International (2012). *Nursing diagnoses: Definitions and classification 2012–2014* (9th ed.). Oxford, United Kingdom: Wiley-Blackwell.

Peterson, M. D., Rhea, M. R., Sen, A., & Gordon, P. M. (2010). Resistance exercises for musculoskeletal strength in older adults: A meta-analysis. *Ageing Research Reviews, 9*(3), 226–237.

POLST. (2012). Physician orders for life-sustaining treatment. Retrieved from http://www.polst.org

Porth, C. M., & Matfin, G. (2009). *Pathophysiology: Concepts of altered health states* (8th ed.). Philadelphia, PA: Lippincott Williams & Wilkins.

Rushton, C. H., Kaylor, B. D., & Christopher, M. (2012). Twenty years since Cruzan and the Patient Self-Determination Act: Opportunities for improving care at the end of life in critical care settings. *AACN Advanced Critial Care, 23*(1), 99–106.

Sheikh, J. I., & Yesavage, J. A. (1986). Geriatric Depression Scale (GDS): Recent findings and development of a shorter version. In T. L. Brink (Ed.), *Clinical gerontology: A guide to assessment and intervention*, (pp. 165–176). New York, NY: Haworth Press.

Soriano, T. A., DeCherrie, L. V., & Thomas, D. C. (2007). Falls in the community-dwelling older adult: A review for primary-care providers. *Clinical Interventions in Aging, 2*(4), 545–554.

Tang, W. S., Chow, Y. L., & Lin, S. K. S. (2014). The inter-rater reliability test of the modified Morse Fall Scale among patients ≥55 years old in an acute care hospital in Singapore. *International Journal of Nursing Practice, 20*(1), 32–38. doi: 10.1111/ijn.12111

U.S. Department of Health and Human Services (USDHHS). (2013). *2020 Topics & objectives: Older adults.* Retrieved from http://www.healthypeople.gov/2020/topicsobjectives2020/objectiveslist.aspx?topicId=31

U.S. Preventive Services Task Force (USPSTF). (2013). *Focus on Older Adults.* Retrieved from http://www.uspreventiveservicestaskforce.org/tfolderfocus.htm

Vincent, G. K., & Velkoff, V. A. (2010). The next four decades. The older population in the United States: 2010 to 2050. In *Current population reports* (pp. 25–1138). Washington, DC: U.S. Census Bureau.

Wright, J. (2000). *The FIM™. The center for outcome measurement in brain injury.* Retrieved from http://www.tbims.org/combi/FIM

Yesavage, J. A., Brink, T. L., & Rose, T. (1982). Development and validation of a geriatric depression screening scale: A preliminary report. *Journal of Psychiatric Research, 17*, 37–49.

UNIT

5

Putting It All Together

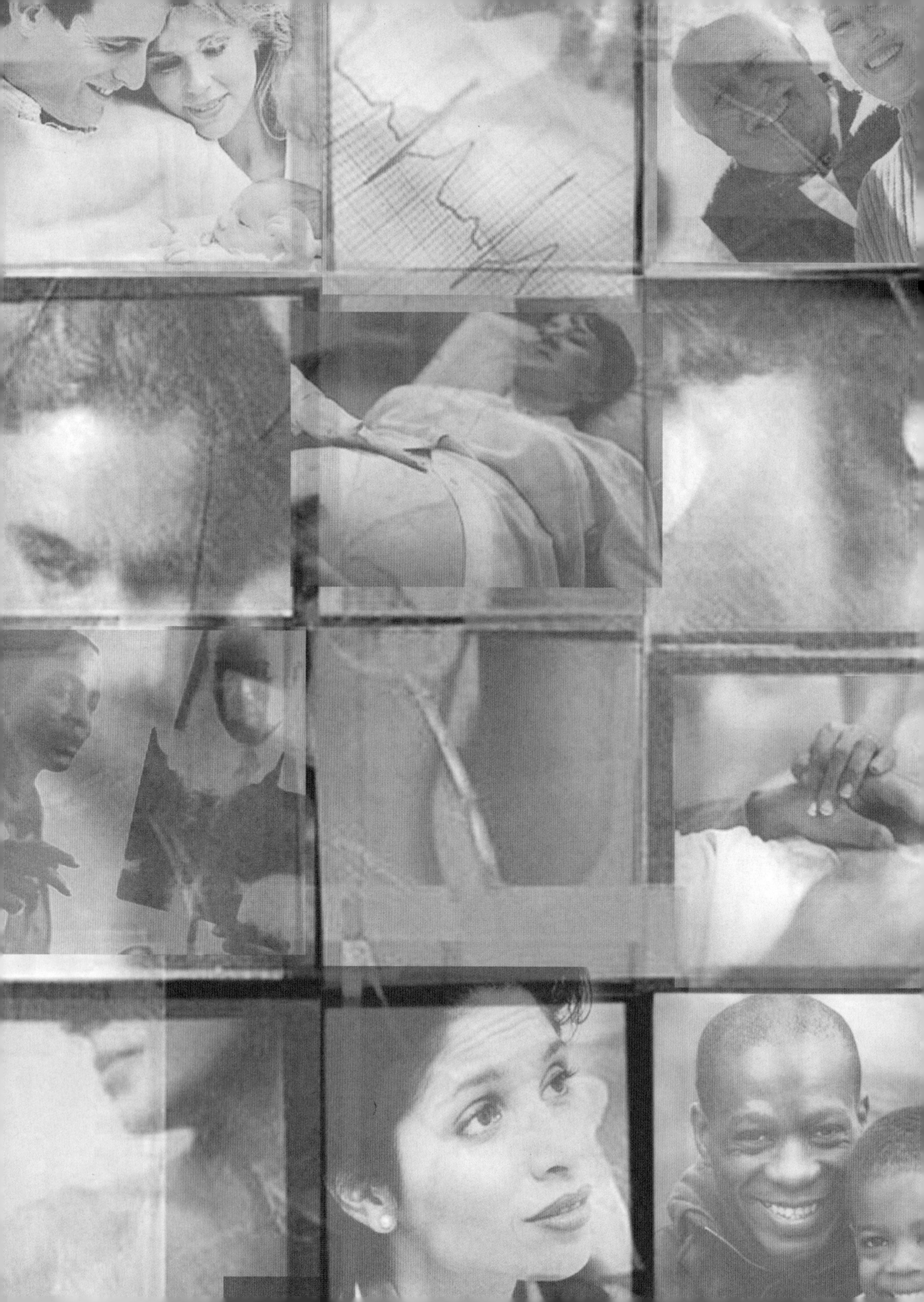

29

Assessment of the Hospitalized Adult

Learning Objectives

1. Demonstrate knowledge of anatomy and physiology related to the hospitalized adult patient.
2. Describe how preexisting conditions are affected by and affect the hospitalized adult patient.
3. Identify important topics for health promotion and risk reduction related to the hospitalized adult patient.
4. Collect subjective data related to the hospitalized adult patient.
5. Collect objective data related to the hospitalized adult patient using physical examination techniques.
6. Distinguish expected and abnormal findings related to the hospitalized adult patient.
7. Analyze subjective and objective data from the assessment of the hospitalized adult patient and consider initial interventions.
8. Document and communicate data from the hospitalized adult patient using appropriate terminology and principles of recording.
9. Consider age, condition, and culture of the hospitalized adult patient to individualize the assessment.
10. Identify nursing diagnoses and initiate a nursing plan of care based on findings from the assessment of the hospitalized adult patient.

Mr. Scott Kim, a 59-year-old man of Korean Japanese heritage, has been in an acute care unit since yesterday for a stroke. He is in the hospital for observation, evaluation, and rehabilitation. Current medications include an angiotensin-converting enzyme (ACE) inhibitor for high blood pressure and aspirin for antiplatelet properties. The nurse documented assessment findings last shift. Mr. Kim's temperature was 37.0°C (98.6°F) orally, pulse 92 beats/min, respirations 16 breaths/min, and blood pressure 152/78 mm Hg.

You will gain more information about Mr. Kim as you progress through this chapter. As you study the content and features, consider Mr. Kim's case and its relationship to what you are learning. Begin thinking about the following points:

- What are the major risk factors related to hospitalization?
- What admitting assessments are indicated given Mr. Kim's history?
- What items would you add to focus the assessment on Mr. Kim's problem?
- What complications might Mr. Kim develop that could trigger the need for an urgent assessment?
- What discharge planning interventions might you implement based on his condition?
- How will you evaluate whether those interventions are effective?

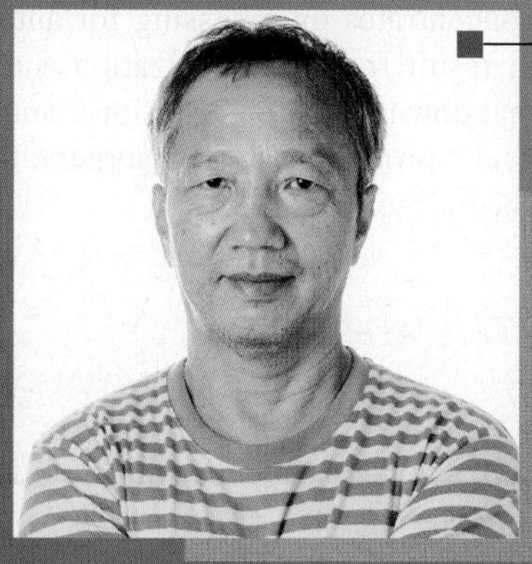

This chapter uses your previous experience in assessment to provide the structure for the assessment performed on the most acute and critically ill group of patients: those in the hospital setting. Because most hospital nurses are responsible for caring for more than one patient at a time, it is impractical to perform a complete assessment of each body system for each patient. Instead, the nurse streamlines and prioritizes the assessment to highlight the most important areas for the hospitalized patient, taking from 5 to 20 minutes per patient, depending on the acuteness and situation. Additional assessments are based on the patient's critical problems and anticipated complications that may result from those problems and interventions.

As you have learned about nursing health assessment, you have taken vital signs, assessed pain, gathered subjective data, collected objective data by body region, and clustered data. You have seen examples of how assessment data are analyzed in the nursing process to make a diagnosis, plan interventions, document and communicate findings, initiate interventions, and evaluate whether those interventions were effective. As you can see, assessment is the foundation for the care that is delivered to improve the health condition of your patient.

Clinical Significance

Assessment is one of the primary reasons that a patient is hospitalized. It is not uncommon that a patient is hospitalized entirely for observation.

Types of Hospital Assessments

The comprehensive admitting, shift, and focused assessments are important in establishing and maintaining documentation of current findings. As a hospital nurse, you perform a **comprehensive assessment** of the patient on admission. This assessment is more detailed and complete than shift and focused assessments, which evaluate progress toward a goal later in the stay. The **shift assessment** is performed at the beginning of the shift and includes an abbreviated exam, with emphasis on risk areas, such as auscultation of lungs and abdomen, and assessment of circulation and level of consciousness. The **focused assessment** concentrates on assessing for anticipated problems that can result from hospitalization, such as pneumonia, skin breakdown, falls, or infections, and those specific to the patient's problems, such as surgery, trauma, or specific medical condition.

SAFETY ALERT

As a nurse, you are continuously assessing patients. When there are signs of an emergency, acute, or urgent situation, you perform immediate assessments and interventions with a team of providers.

Subjective Data

Patient History

The history in a hospitalized patient includes detail on items that relate to safety, daily function, and basic needs. Although the basic care needs of a hospitalized patient may be delegated to other care providers, the registered nurse (RN) is responsible for proper delegation. The RN may delegate individual components of care but does not delegate the nursing process itself. The main functions of assessment, planning, evaluation, and nursing judgment cannot be delegated. For example, if the nurse delegates taking vital signs to a nursing assistant, he or she is responsible for making sure that the data is accurately collected and for following up if findings are abnormal.

SAFETY ALERT

*The RN uses critical thinking and professional judgment when following the **Five Rights of Delegation** to be sure that the delegation or assignment is*

1. *The right task*
2. *Under the right circumstances*
3. *To the right person*
4. *With the right directions and communication*
5. *Under the right supervision and evaluation*

(American Nurses Association & National Council of State Boards of Nursing [NCSBN], 2014)

The items included in assessment as part of the basic care activities include the following:

- Activities of daily living (ADLs) and assistive devices
- Sleep/rest
- Communication/speech, vision, and hearing
- Personal hygiene habits and routine

Clinical Significance

Basic care and comfort assessments are included in testing for RN licensure. They are considered basic client need **National Council Licensure Examination (NCLEX) competencies** (National Council of State Boards of Nursing, 2013).

Risk Reduction and Health Promotion

The Joint Commission (2014) has set **national safety goals** for hospital care. There are many associated assessments that need to be performed. You will learn more about these as you progress in your formal learning and continued knowledge in professional practice. The areas include the following:

- Adverse drug events (including medication reconciliation and high-alert medication safety)
- Catheter-associated urinary tract infections
- Central line–associated bloodstream infections
- Injuries from falls and immobility (including delirium)
- Pressure ulcers
- Surgical site infections

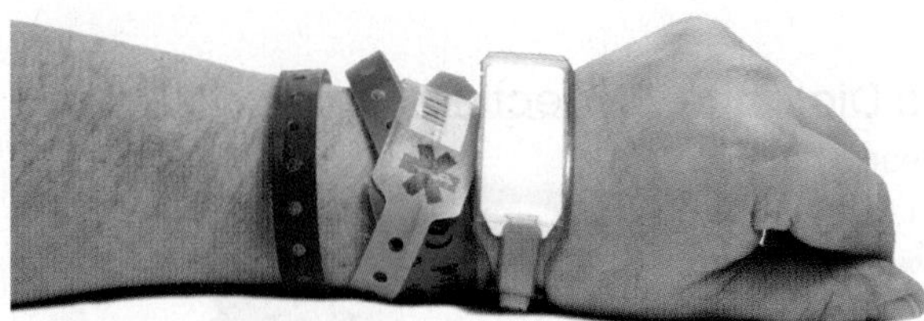

Figure. 29.1 Always use two identifiers and notice identification bands.

- Venous thromboembolism
- Ventilator-associated pneumonia

Additionally, The Joint Commission (2014) has set national safety interventions for hospital care. The interventions related to these safety standards that pertain to assessment are as follows:

- Identify patients correctly. Use **two patient identifiers**, such as name and date of birth, or bar code name bands before medication administration or blood transfusion (Fig. 29.1).
- Improve staff communication. Use written documentation, medical terminology, and SBAR (situation, background, assessment, recommendation) for verbal communication.
- Use alarms safely, especially to prevent those at risk for falls.
- Prevent infections.
  - Use the hand cleaning guidelines from the Centers for Disease Control and Prevention (CDC) or the World Health Organization (WHO). Set goals for improving hand cleaning. Use the goals to improve hand cleaning.
  - Use proven guidelines to prevent infections that are difficult to treat.
  - Use proven guidelines to prevent infection of the blood from central lines.
  - Use proven guidelines to prevent infection after surgery.
  - Use proven guidelines to prevent infections of the urinary tract that are caused by catheters.
- Identify patient safety risks.
- Prevent mistakes in surgery using a specific protocol for identification of correct surgical procedure, **time-outs** for procedures, and clear communication.

Clinical Significance

The main issues in quality hospital care include evidence-based medicine, quality assurance, medical ethics, and the reduction of medical error. Nurses working in hospitals are involved in processes that promote these activities on a daily basis.

Specialized Risk Assessments

Hospitalized patients have a specific risk for complications just based on the fact that they are in the hospital setting. Hospitalized patients are more at risk for complications of immobility, infection, and treatments such as wrong site surgeries or medication errors. Common causes of inpatient mortality for the hospitalized patient are listed in Box 29.1 (Agency for Healthcare Research and Policy [AHRQ], 2013c).

Nurses provide specific assessments related to these common complications to identify problems early so that they may be treated. As a nurse, you are responsible for these physiological NCLEX competencies as part of the RN scope of practice (NCSBN, 2013). These include assessment of the following:

- Skin breakdown
- Pain management
- Mobility: gait, strength, motor skills, immobility
- Eating, chewing, swallowing, aspiration, feeding tube tolerance
- Increased intracranial pressure (ICP), level of sedation
- Interactions between food and medications
- Edema and related signs and symptoms of dehydration
- Nutrition, calorie counts, body mass index, tube feedings
- Intake and output (I&O), emesis, diarrhea, fluid or electrolyte imbalance
- Elimination, bowel/urinary incontinence
- Response to medications
- Venous access devices, intravenous (IV) lines, invasive monitoring
- Responses to procedures and treatments
- Vascular perfusion, hypotension, decreased peripheral pulses, immobilized limb, postsurgical risks, diabetes, bleeding/hemorrhage
- Hemodynamics: sinus bradycardia, premature ventricular contractions (PVCs), ventricular tachycardia (VT), ventricular fibrillation (VF), medical emergencies
- Specific assessments: after procedures, high or low blood sugar, focused assessments, surgery, radiation, sepsis
- Therapeutic devices: chest tube, drainage tubes, wound drainage, continuous bladder irrigation (CBI), wound vacuum

BOX 29.1 Common Causes of Hospital Complications

- Pulmonary embolism or deep vein thrombosis
- Respiratory failure
- Sepsis
- Physiological and metabolic derangements
- Postoperative abdominopelvic wound dehiscence
- Hip fracture
- Postoperative hemorrhage or hematoma
- Pressure ulcer
- Selected infections due to medical care
- Iatrogenic (caused by medical procedure) pneumothorax
- Accidental puncture or laceration
- Foreign body left in during procedure
- Death among surgical inpatients with treatable serious complications (previously known as failure to rescue)
- Transfusion reaction (AB/Rh)

(A.H.R.Q., 2013c).

Clinical Significance

As an RN or advanced practice registered nurse practicing in the hospital setting, you have a specific and focused assessment to perform based on the patient's risk factors and primary problems. These risk factors and problems are often complex and require a high level of critical thinking. You must also evaluate the interventions provided for effectiveness and complications. For example, when a central line is placed, it can lead to pneumothorax, mortality, or a central line–associated bloodstream infection.

Therapeutic Dialogue: Collecting Subjective Data

Mr. Kim, introduced at the beginning of this chapter, is a 59-year-old man admitted after a stroke. The nurse uses professional communication techniques to gather subjective data from him. The following conversation is an example of how the nurse might gather data.

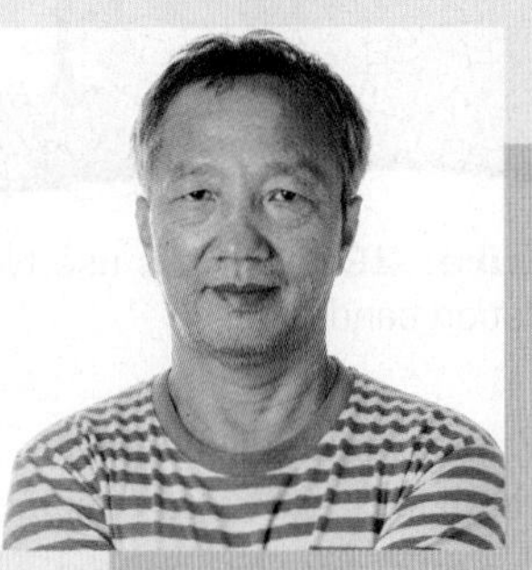

Nurse: Do you have a history of having high blood pressure?

Mr. Kim: Yes.

Nurse: Is this the medication that you are on at home?

Mr. Kim: Yes, but the doctor says that it's not working.

Nurse: Do you notice when your blood pressure gets high?

Mr. Kim: (Nods head). Yes, I get a headache.

Nurse: And did you get a headache with the stroke?

Mr. Kim: No, I was driving and then I couldn't see. I had to pull over and then I couldn't talk. I had to call 911.

Critical Thinking Challenge

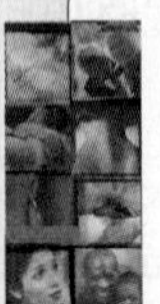

- How did the nurse link the medical issues to his current problem?
- What nursing considerations are you beginning to develop as you assess the patient?
- How will you further assess to determine teaching and rehabilitation needs?

Patient Satisfaction

Although their use is debated, **patient satisfaction** surveys provide measures of quality and may lead to improved patient outcomes (Manary, Boulding, Staelin, & Glickman, 2013). You can improve patient experiences by focusing on activities such as care coordination and patient engagement. Patient satisfaction–related interventions that pertain to assessment are as follows:

- Participate in **bedside handoff reports**. Bedside reports build the patient's trust, enhance teamwork, and protect safety.
- Practice **purposeful hourly rounding**. The nurse manager should round daily.
- Show respect. Protect confidentiality and privacy. Always introduce yourself and your role in care.
- Ask permission. If visitors are present, find out whether the patient wishes them to know information about his condition and treatment. Address the patient using the name he or she prefers.
- Use best communication practices. Ask open-ended questions and paraphrase patient responses to verify understanding

(Hospital Consumer Assessment of Healthcare Providers and Systems [HCAHPS], 2013).

Objective Data

Equipment

- Stethoscope
- Thermometer
- Watch with second hand
- Sphygmomanometer or vital signs machine
- Pulse oximeter

Preparation

Begin the general survey immediately when meeting the patient and continue it throughout the assessment. Perform a safety inspection of the hospitalized patient and environment immediately upon entering the room. You will often perform this assessment during the change-of-shift rounding or handoff procedure. The purpose is to assess the patient's immediate medical condition as well as potential hazards such as falls, impaired breathing, or complications from IV lines and intubation. The initial safety inspection includes the following steps:

- If the patient is awake, briefly introduce yourself and provide your name and contact information.
- Check that the patient's identification band includes two patient identifiers.
- Directly observe the patient for breathing, airway, skin color, signs of dyspnea, and airway secretions.
- Observe the patient while he or she is lying in bed, sitting in a chair, or moving around the room.
- Check that the lighting and call bell are within reach.
- Observe for cues of recent events (e.g., suctioning equipment, meals).
- Trace tubes to insertion site and check solutions and rates. Check IV fluids and tube feeding for accurate infusion. Check urinary catheter positioning.
- Check that equipment alarms are on, bed alarms are on, and restraints are in place, as necessary.

> **SAFETY ALERT**
> *This initial safety inspection as you come onto shift allows you to directly observe whether the patient has had his or her basic safety needs met. You need this information as you assume responsibility for the patient's care.*

Urgent Assessment

Acute and **urgent** situations such as the following warrant immediate attention and interventions:

- A respiratory rate lower than 8 or greater than 28 breaths/min
- An acute change in oxygen saturation below 90% despite oxygen administration
- A threatened airway
- Acute change in systolic blood pressure to less than 90 mm Hg or a sustained increase in diastolic blood pressure greater than 110 mm Hg
- Acute change in heart rate to fewer than 50 or greater than 120 beats/min
- New-onset chest pain or signs of acute myocardial infarction
- An acutely cold, cyanotic, or pulseless extremity
- Confusion, agitation, or delirium
- Unexplained lethargy or acute altered mental status
- Difficulty speaking or signs of acute stroke
- Acute change in pupillary response
- New seizure
- Temperature greater than 39.0°C (102.2°F)
- Uncontrolled pain
- Acute change in urine output less than 50 ml (about 1¾ oz) over 4 hours
- Acute bleeding
- Suspected severe sepsis

(AHRQ, 2013a)

Comprehensive Admitting Assessment

After any urgent needs have been addressed, you may then perform the initial **comprehensive hospital assessment** (Box 29.2). This includes collection of both subjective and objective data. Subjective assessment of risk factors, common symptoms, and health history are similar to that previously described; however, you may need to gather history from secondary sources such as the chart or relatives to avoid fatiguing the acutely ill patient. The general survey and vital signs are also similar. Risks for falling and skin breakdown are added because of the hospital environment.

Because a hospitalized patient is more often sicker than nonhospitalized patients, you prioritize which data to collect related to the presenting problems and perform a basic screening of other body systems. Use clinical judgment about which items to include and which to omit. Adapt assessment techniques to the individual patient situation. You will usually document the admitting assessment in a separate area of the patient chart, which may include input from other health care professionals.

The initial patient history and head-to-toe physical examination may take 30 to 45 minutes or longer to complete. Subsequent assessments are shorter because they focus on problem areas rather than the entire body. It is important to make this initial assessment comfortable and efficient for the patient. Adapt the assessment to the patient in a manner that is professional yet personal and individualized. Allow some time for documentation of findings and analysis of data. In addition to positive findings, it is essential to document absence of findings because, in the legal world, "if it's not documented, it's not done." For example, if the patient develops acute confusion, it is important to be able to look back in the chart and see "no confusion" to identify this change in status as significant. Additionally, it is especially important to assess for allergies, devices such as pacemakers, and adverse reactions to medications because this history may be difficult to obtain later if the patient's condition declines.

Be sure to allow time for validation of problems, mutual goal setting, and discussion of an action plan. This communicates to the patient that his or her concerns are well understood and helps to establish a trusting and lasting relationship, which in turn will make it more likely that the patient will agree to the action plan. Creating and maintaining an intimate and professional therapeutic relationship to make a difference in the outcomes is one of the most important and satisfying elements in the process. It is important to let the patient know that he or she should expect the highest quality care and that you will provide it (HCAHPS, 2013).

Shift and Focused Hospital Assessments

Because of the complications of immobility and being in a hospital environment, you perform a short shift assessment from head to toe at the beginning of each shift (Box 29.3). It includes those items that are relevant to all hospitalized

BOX 29.2 Admitting Assessment on the Hospitalized Patient

Perform safety checks. Wash hands.

Vital Signs

Temperature, pulse, respiration, blood pressure, oxygen saturation

Pain: location, duration, intensity, quality, aggravating and alleviating factors, pain goal and functional goals.

General Survey

Inspect overall skin color. Inspect skin and wounds head to toe.

Assess breathing effort, rate, rhythm and pattern, position to breathe.

Neurological Assessment

Assess level of consciousness, orientation, Glasgow Coma Scale if indicated.

Assess speech. Evaluate eye opening, hearing, and affect during conversation.

Head, Face, Eyes, Ears, Nose, Mouth, Throat Assessment

Assess face and eyes for symmetry; pupils equal, round, and reactive to light and accommodation (PERRLA).

Inspect mouth with light and tongue blade.

Anterior Thorax Asessment

Inspect chest shape; evaluate symmetry.

Auscultate breath sounds on anterior thorax.

Inspect precordium.

Assess heart rate, rhythm, murmurs, extra sounds.

Assess for cough; inspect sputum/secretions for amount, color, viscosity.

Upper Extremities Assessment

Evaluate skin turgor, color, condition, temperature, nails on upper extremities.

Inspect muscles and extremities for size and symmetry.

Observe range of motion of joints.

Palpate radial pulses bilaterally.

Assess capillary refill on both hands.

Perform hand grasp for muscle strength.

Abdominal Assessment

Inspect abdomen for distension.

Auscultate bowel sounds.

Palpate abdomen in all four quadrants for tenderness.

Posterior Thorax Asessment

Inspect chest shape.

Auscultate posterior thorax.

Evaluate risk for skin breakdown: sensory perception, moisture, activity, mobility, nutrition, friction, and shear.

Inspect back, pressure points, and heels for redness.

Inspect perineum for redness, integrity.

Lower Extremities Assessment

Evaluate skin turgor, color, condition, temperature, hair growth, varicosities, nails on lower extremities.

Test muscle strength of the feet and inspect muscles and extremities for size and symmetry.

Observe range of motion of joints.

Palpate dorsalis pedis pulses bilaterally.

Assess capillary refill on both feet.

Grade edema on ankle or shin.

Evaluate fall risk: history of falling, secondary diagnosis, ambulatory aid, IV therapy, gait, and mental status; ADLs, mobility.

Intake and Elimination Assessment

Evaluate swallowing, chewing, aspiration risk, special diet.

Evaluate fluid and nutritional intake, I&O.

Inspect and examine urine, stool, emesis, drains.

Assess IV lines, drainage, tubes, dressings, catheters, suction.

Psychosocial Assessment

Perform functional assessment: self-perception, role, sexuality, coping, values, and beliefs.

Assess pain or discomfort.

Evaluate discharge planning needs.

Assess for questions or further needs.

Wash hands when leaving.

BOX 29.3 Brief Shift Assessment of the Hospitalized Patient

Perform safety checks. Wash hands

Vital signs. Temperature, pulse, respiration, blood pressure, oxygen saturation. Pain (location, duration, intensity, quality, aggravating and alleviating factors, pain goal, and functional goal).

General survey. Inspect overall skin color (tone) head to toe and skin risk. Assess breathing effort, rate, rhythm.

Neurological assessment. Assess level of consciousness and mental status. Assess speech and evaluate hearing and affect during conversation or use Glasgow Coma Scale if patient is unconscious.

Head, face, eyes, ears, nose, mouth, throat assessment. Assess face and eyes for symmetry; pupils equal, round, and reactive to light and accommodation (PERRLA). Inspect lips and observe mouth.

Anterior thorax assessment. Inspect chest when auscultating breath sounds. Assess for cough; inspect sputum if present. Assess heart rate and rhythm.

Upper extremities assessment. Evaluate skin color, condition, temperature, nails, IV lines. Assess CMS and muscle strength. Inspect range of motion during movement.

Abdominal assessment. Inspect abdomen for distension. Auscultate bowel sounds. Palpate abdomen for tenderness.

Posterior thorax assessment. *(May perform later if patient is supine)* Inspect chest shape. Auscultate posterior thorax. Inspect back, pressure points, and heels for redness. With perineal care: Inspect perineum for redness and integrity.

Lower extremities assessment. Evaluate skin color, condition, temperature, nails. Assess CMS and muscle strength. Inspect range of motion during movement. Assess edema on ankle or shin.

Additional assessment based on the patient's problems. Assess pain or discomfort. Assess for questions or further needs.

Lines, tubes, dressings, bed alarms, restraints, other devices. Assess for correct solution, rate, patency, safety.

Evaluate fall risk. History of falling, secondary diagnosis, ambulatory aid, IV therapy, gait, and mental status; ADLS, mobility.

Wash hands when leaving.

patients, such as auscultating the heart and lungs. This assessment typically takes 5 to 10 minutes to provide a basis for comparison in the event of a sudden change in condition. This screening also enables you to identify the patient's immediate condition; need for immediate treatment, teaching, or discharge planning; and care priorities. You complete and document this assessment on the appropriate form, usually in a flow sheet format that allows for easy changes.

You also perform a focused assessment on each patient based on the admitting problems, integrating it into the head-to-toe shift assessment. This can take anywhere from an additional minute when assessing one or two items to 10 to 20 minutes for a more complete review of complex problems. Therefore, you must think critically about the information that needs to be collected. An abnormal finding or unexpected diagnosis triggers the need for a more complete and focused assessment. Use clinical judgment to determine which data are most important. Initially, as a beginning nurse, you may need to consult with a more experienced nurse about which items to assess, but with experience, typical patterns emerge. Adapt these assessments to the specific patients and practice area. By identifying trends of improving or declining status, treatment can be modified as necessary. You consult with other health care providers about the need for changes in the patient's orders or further diagnostic testing.

Additional Assessments for the Hospitalized Patient

Specific assessments must be performed for the hospitalized patient. These have been discussed in preceding chapters and include the following:

- **Injuries from falls and immobility.** Assess for falls. Use one of the tools described in the musculoskeletal chapter (see Chapter 21), such as the Hendrich II Fall Risk Model or the Morse Fall Scale. Items to consider include history of falling, medical diagnosis, use of ambulatory aids, presence of an IV/heparin lock, difficulty with gait/transferring, and impaired mental status (Fig. 29.2).
- **Pressure ulcers.** Use the Braden Scale or Norton Scale or another skin assessment tool according to hospital standard protocol. These are described in the skin assessment chapter (see Chapter 11) and include altered sensory perception, moisture, inactivity, immobility, poor nutrition, and friction/shear.
- **Venous thromboembolism.** Edema, pain or achiness, erythema, and warmth in the leg are common signs and symptoms of venous thromboembolism. Refer to peripheral vascular chapter for more information (Chapter 18).

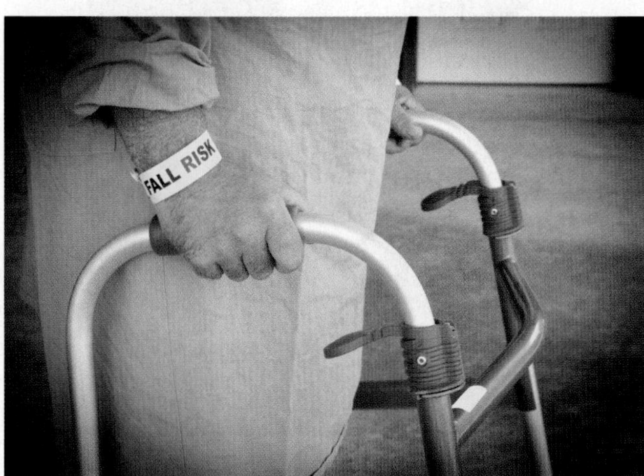

Figure 29.2 Identify the patient's fall risk. This patient is using a walker and wearing a fall-risk bracelet.

The following list provides a basic outline of some additional types of assessments that you will be expected to perform during your hospital experiences. (These will be covered more in depth in your medical surgical courses.)

- **Adverse drug events.** Preventive measures include medication reconciliation and high-alert medication safety. Make sure to always know and assess for the adverse effects of medications. Document the information in the patient's chart and notify the provider using the SBAR format if adverse effects are serious.
- **Catheter-associated urinary tract infections.** Signs and symptoms to assess for include fever (>38°C [104.8°F]), dysuria, urgency, suprapubic tenderness, frequency, costovertebral angle pain or tenderness, positive dipstick for leukocyte esterase and/or nitrite, pyuria, (urine specimen with white blood cell [WBC] count ≥10/mm^3), microorganisms seen on Gram stain, and positive urine culture of microorganisms (CDC, 2014).
- **Central line–associated bloodstream infections.** A central line–associated bloodstream infection is a laboratory-confirmed bloodstream infection where a central line was in place for more than 2 days on the date of the event (CDC, 2014). Fever (>38°C [100.4°F]), chills, or hypotension may be present.
- **Surgical site infections.** A surgical site infection is an infection that occurs within 30 to 90 days after the operative procedure, with purulent drainage from a deep incision; a deep incision that spontaneously dehisces or is deliberately opened; or an abscess that is detected on direct examination, during invasive procedure or by an imaging test. The patient has at least one of the following signs or symptoms: pain or tenderness, localized swelling, redness, or heat (CDC, 2014).
- **Ventilator-associated pneumonia.** Fever (>38°C [100.4°F]) and/or leukopenia (WBC count <4,000/mm^3) or leukocytosis (WBC count ≥12,000/mm^3.

  For adults aged 70 years or older: Altered mental status with no other recognized cause *and* at least **two** of the following:

  - New onset of purulent sputum or change in character of sputum, increased respiratory secretions, or increased suctioning requirements
  - New onset or worsening cough, dyspnea, or tachypnea

BOX 29.4 Severe Sepsis: Initial Recognition and Resuscitation

- Documented or suspected infection
- Heart rate greater than 90 beats/min
- Temperature less than 36°C (96.8°F) or greater than 38.3°C (101°F)
- Respiratory rate more than 20 breaths/min or $PaCO_2$ less than 32 mm Hg
- White blood cell count more than 12,000/mm^3 or less than 4,000 mm^3 or a left shift in the immaturation of granulocytes (bands) greater than 10%
- Altered mental status
- Systolic blood pressure less than 90 mm Hg or mean arterial pressure less than 70 mm Hg or a systolic blood pressure decrease of 40 mm Hg
- Blood glucose greater than 140 mg/dl in patients without diabetes
- Arterial hypoxemia (PaO_2/FiO_2) less than 300
- Acute oliguria (less than 0.5 ml/kg/hr for at least 2 hours)
- Creatinine increase greater than 0.5 mg/dl above baseline
- Coagulation abnormalities (INR greater than 1.5 or a PTT greater than 60 seconds)
- Ileus
- Thrombocytopenia (platelet count less than 100,000 μl)
- Hyperbilirubinemia (plasma total bilirubin greater than 2 mg/dl)
- Lactate greater than 2 mmol/L

Data from Dellinger, R. P., Levy, M. M., Rhodes, A., Annane, D., Gerlach, H., Opal, S. M., . . . Vincent, J. L. (2012). Surviving sepsis campaign: international guidelines for management of severe sepsis and septic shock: 2012. *Critical Care Medicine*, *41*(2), 580–637. doi:10.1097/CCM.0b013e31827e83af.

$PaCO_2$, partial pressure of carbon dioxide, arterial; PaO_2, partial pressure of oxygen, arterial; FiO_2, fraction of inspired oxygen; INR, international normalized ratio; PTT, partial thromboplastin time.

- Rales or bronchial breath sounds
- Worsening gas exchange, increased oxygen requirements, or increased ventilator demand (CDC, 2014)

- **Sepsis**. Recently recognized as a primary cause of mortality, early recognition and treatment of sepsis is a primary responsibility of the nurse. Criteria for sepsis are included in Box 29.4.

Lifespan Considerations: Older Adults

Geriatric medical patients have an increased risk of falls and associated fractures as well as delirium, nosocomial infections, and medication interactions. In addition, any elderly person, particularly a frail elderly person, experiences a great risk of deconditioning and loss of function during a hospital stay. Almost one quarter of older patients in the hospital are unable to return home and require nursing home placement—many simply because they have lost some basic ADL abilities during even a very short hospitalization (Palmer, 2014). Geriatric surgical patients in general are more at risk for major behavioral problems, pressure ulcers, and falls.

Geriatric trauma patients have twice the risk of developing the following complications as younger patients: abscess, wound infection, empyema, urinary tract infection, pneumonia, bacteremia, aspiration pneumonia, reduction/fixation failure, pressure ulcer, deep venous thrombosis, pneumothorax, and compartment syndrome (Min et al., 2013).

Because of these increased risks and the unique characteristics of the older adult patient, some hospitals have dedicated special units to the care of geriatric patients. Assessments should target the specific risk factors and unique characteristics of the older adult (Fig. 29.3).

Cultural Considerations

Generally, the quality indicators for hospitalized African Americans, Hispanics, and Asian Americans are not statistically worse than the quality indicators for hospitalized Caucasians. When Whites and minorities are admitted to the hospital for the same reason, or receive the same hospital procedure, they receive the same quality of care (Gaskin et al., 2013). However, minority patients often have poorer outcomes compared with Caucasians; this may be because minority patients tend to use specialists who have poorer clinical outcomes and primary care physicians who have less clinical training, compared with those used by Caucasian patients. Minorities also have more limited access to specialists. Elders in minority groups tend to develop complications following surgery more often. These complications include gastrointestinal (GI) bleeding or blood loss, respiratory compromise, renal dysfunction, delirium or psychosis, pneumothorax, shock, pneumonia, cardiac emergency, internal organ damage, postsurgical complication, wound infection, sepsis, and pressure ulcer (Brooks Carthon, Jarrín, Sloane, & Kutney-Lee, 2013). You should be aware of these health disparities and assess carefully for them.

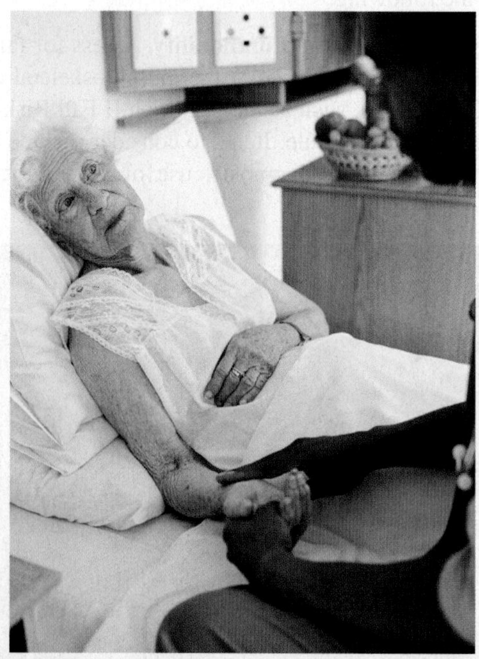

Figure 29.3 The older adult is at risk for complications of hospitalization. For instance, this bedridden patient is at risk for developing pneumonia.

Critical Thinking

Laboratory and Diagnostic Testing

The licensing examination for RNs includes several laboratory tests as essential knowledge (NCSBN, 2013). These include the following:

- Glucose monitoring for the hospitalized patient; hemoglobin A1C for longer term diabetic control
- Total cholesterol: for increased risk of stroke and cardiovascular disease
- Hematology: hematocrit and hemoglobin for bleeding and anemia; WBC count for infection (Fig. 29.4)
- Clotting factors: platelets, prothrombin time, partial thromboplastin time, activated partial thromboplastin time, international normalized ratio
- Chemistries: potassium, sodium electrolytes, blood urea nitrogen/creatinine for renal function

Additional diagnostic testing within the nursing scope of practice includes the following:

- Electrocardiogram (ECG) for ischemic cardiac changes
- Oxygen saturation and arterial blood gases (ABGs)

Diagnostic Reasoning

Nursing Diagnosis, Outcomes, and Interventions

When formulating a nursing diagnosis, you use critical thinking to cluster data and identify related patterns. You compare clusters with defining characteristics (abnormal findings) for the diagnosis to ensure the most accurate labeling and appropriate interventions (NANDA International, 2012). Note how the potential interventions often include assessments; this illustrates how the nursing process is interwoven and how assessment is a continuous part of nursing care. The most common nursing diagnoses for the hospitalized patient are listed in Box 29.5 (Scherb et al., 2011).

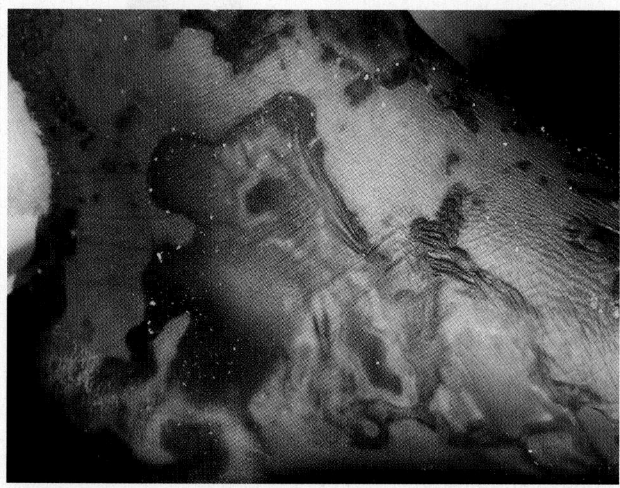

Fig. 29.4. The hospitalized patient is at risk for sepsis and disseminated intravascular coagulopathy.

BOX 29.5 Nursing Diagnoses for the Hospitalized Patient

Ineffective tissue perfusion: pulmonary, cardiac or cerebral
Acute pain
Impaired gas exchange
Risk for infection
Risk for impaired skin integrity
Risk for falls

Data from Scherb, C. A., Head, B. J., Maas, M. L., Swanson, E. A., Moorhead, S., Reed, D., . . . Kozel, M. (2011). Most frequent nursing diagnoses, nursing interventions, and nursing-sensitive patient outcomes of hospitalized older adults with heart failure: Part 1. *International Journal of Nursing Terminology Classification*, 22(1), 13–22. doi:10.1111/j.1744-618X.2010.01164.x

You use assessment information to identify patient outcomes. Some outcomes related to the hospitalized patient (Moorhead, Johnson, Maas, & Swanson, 2013) include the following:

- Pain level stabilized at patient goal
- Gas exchange with oxygen saturation greater than 92%
- Airway patent, breathing quiet, no dyspnea
- Sepsis score low risk, patient afebrile, WBC count within normal range
- Skin and mucous membranes intact; no redness, edema, or tenderness
- Patient maintains safety; no falls

After you have established outcomes, you can implement nursing care. Use critical thinking and evidence-based practice to develop interventions. Some examples of nursing interventions for hospital care (Bulechek, Butcher, Dochterman, & Wagner, 2013) are as follows:

- Assess pain every 4 hours and reassess 30 minutes after interventions.
- Assess oxygen and vital signs every 4 hours.
- Assess sepsis risk; evaluate laboratory test results every day and when needed.
- Assess Braden Scale and provide hygiene as needed every 8 hours.
- Perform **purposeful hourly rounding** with the five Ps (Box 29.6), no pass zone for bed alarms, and answer call bells immediately.

BOX 29.6 Scheduled Rounding Protocol ("Five Ps")

- **Pain:** Assess the patient's pain level. Provide pain medicine if needed.
- **Personal needs:** Offer help using the toilet, offer hydration, offer nutrition, empty commodes/urinals.
- **Position:** Help the patient get into a comfortable position or turn immobile patient to maintain skin integrity.
- **Placement:** Make sure patient's essential needs (e.g., call light, phone, reading material, toileting equipment) are within easy reach.
- **Prevent falls:** Ask patient/family to put on call light if patient needs to get out of bed.

Data from Agency for Healthcare Research and Quality. (2013c). *Inpatient quality indicators overview*. Retrieved from http://www.qualityindicators.ahrq.gov/Modules/iqi_resources.aspx

Progress Note: Analyzing Findings

The difficulties of Mr. Kim have been outlined throughout this chapter. Initial subjective and objective data collection is complete. The nurse is reviewing the findings and other results.

Mr. Kim is reassessed on the acute care unit using the neurological flow sheet. The following nursing note shows how the nurse clusters data to analyze the current condition and anticipate interventions.

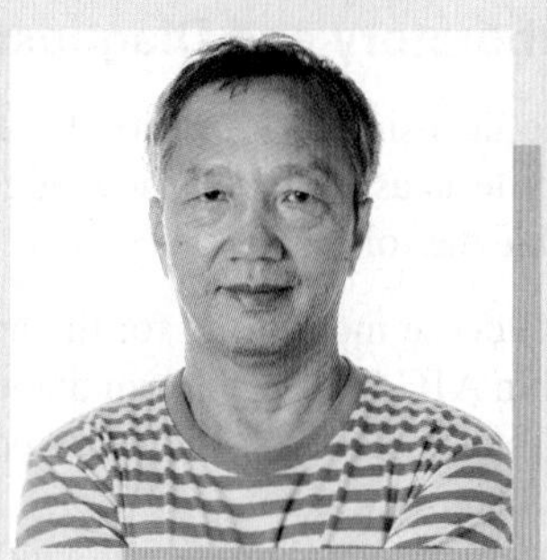

Subjective: A 59-year-old Korean Japanese man with a history of hypertension, high-sodium diet, high-stress lifestyle, and poor adherence to medications. Is alert; speech is comprehensible but slurred. Facial expression flat.

Objective: Remains hypertensive—see flow sheet for vital signs. Follows three-step commands. Pupils equal, round, and reactive to light and accommodation (PERRLA). Extraocular motions (EOM)s intact. Right ptosis and lower facial weakness, right tongue deviation. Muscle bulk symmetrical, tone slightly increased on right arm/leg. Strength 2/5 right arm, 5/5 left arm/leg, 3/5 right leg, 5/5 left leg. Circulation and sensation intact all four extremities. Gait weak, needs one-person assist.

Analysis: Findings consistent with right hemisphere stroke, no further progression. Risk for impaired cerebral perfusion. Risk for falls, dysphagia, and aspiration. Impaired physical mobility.

Plan: Frequent neurological assessment to monitor for stroke progression. Monitor blood pressure—currently not treated per stroke guidelines. Discuss in discharge planning rounds—patient may be unable to return to independent living. Evaluate safe ADLs performance with physical therapists and occupational therapists. Implement fall prevention plan; discuss speech pathology consult for swallowing evaluation before starting diet.

Collaborating With the Interprofessional Team

Mr. Kim needs discharge planning because of his recent stroke. Discharge planning is initiated upon the patient's admission. Most hospitals have teams of case managers or planning teams to facilitate transition out of the hospital as quickly as possible. The role of the team is to facilitate the following:

- Placement
- Teaching
- Equipment
- Continuity of care
- Resources

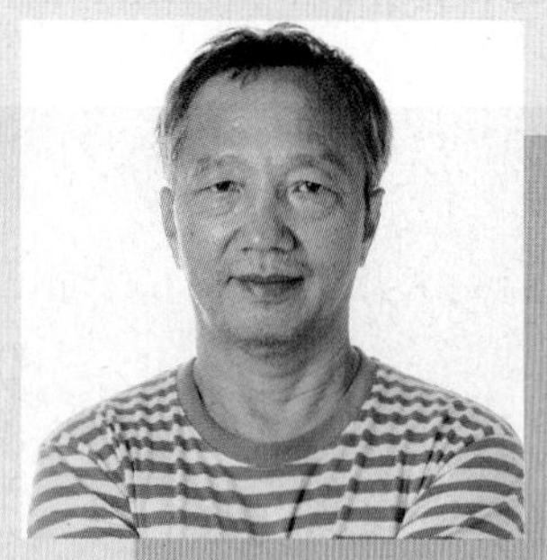

The nurse is presenting at discharge planning rounds during the shift. The following conversation illustrates how the nurse might organize data and make recommendations to the discharge team.

Situation: "Mr. Kim was admitted yesterday with a left-sided stroke."

Background: "He hasn't started a diet yet and has referrals in to physical therapy, occupational therapy, and speech therapy."

(case study continues on page 917)

Assessment: "He is employed as a computer technician. He was driving to work, stopped, and called 911 when he lost his vision. He will be discharged home and will need evaluations and recommendations for rehab before we decide when he will be discharged."

Recommendations: "He needs to be on nothing by mouth until speech therapy sees him to evaluate for aspiration. After physical therapy and occupational therapy see him, we'll know whether he can do outpatient therapies. His medications will need to be adjusted because he is still hypertensive. I think that he needs more teaching about medication management and evaluation of his medication regimen. We'll also need to do teaching on low-salt diet, stress management, and home management. Let's check in again tomorrow after further evaluations are completed and plan for discharge home in 2 days."

Critical Thinking Challenge

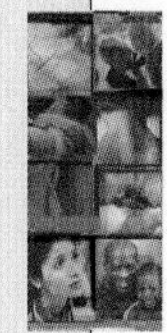

- Consider collected subjective data. Review the above report. What additional data might be helpful when planning for discharge?
- Consider the objective data. Is the organization logical? Is further information needed on his physical risks and needs?
- Critique the analysis and recommendations. How can the primary nurse best coordinate and collaborate assessments and planning with the discharge team?

Pulling It All Together

The nurse uses assessment data to formulate a nursing care plan with patient outcomes and interventions for Mr. Kim. Outcomes are specific to the patient, realistic to achieve, measurable, and have a time frame. After interventions are completed, the nurse will reevaluate Mr. Kim and document the findings to show progress toward outcomes. The nurse uses critical thinking and judgment to continue or revise the diagnosis, outcomes, or interventions. This is often in the form of a care plan or case note similar to the one below.

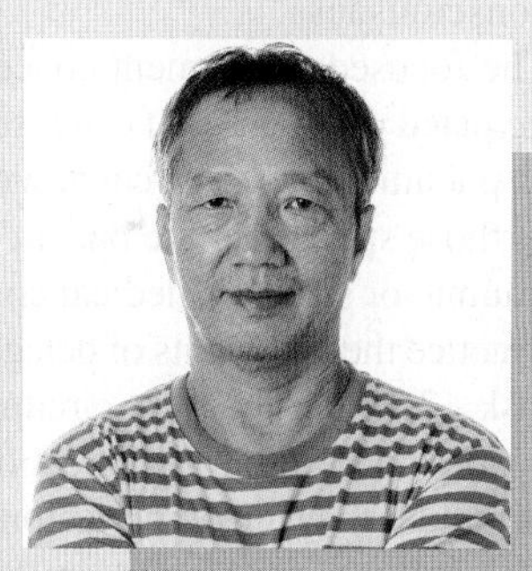

Nursing Diagnosis	Patient Outcomes	Nursing Interventions	Rationale	Evaluation
Knowledge deficit related to new diagnosis of stroke, medication management	Demonstrates measures to care for right side of body and keep it free from injury. States actions to prevent stroke.	Assess motor and neurological function every shift for extension or resolution of stroke. Assist with ADLs until strength returns. Provide education on diet, medications, home care, and return to work.	The initial priority is patient safety and injury prevention. Assess function to determine improvements or decline. Assist patient with ADLs until he can care for himself. Teach to promote health and prevent hospital readmission.	Needs assistance in two-handed tasks and one-person assist with transfers. Talk with wife about resources at home, preparing meals and shopping, driving, and return to work.

Applying Your Knowledge

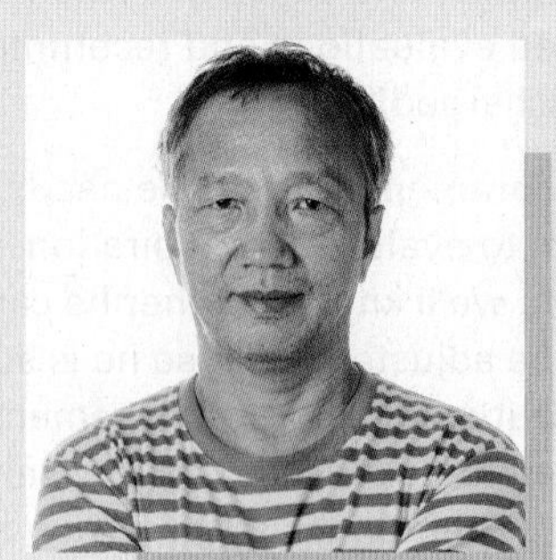

Using the previous steps of diagnostic reasoning, organizing, and prioritizing, consider the case study findings woven throughout this chapter. When answering the following questions, begin drawing conclusions and see how the pieces of assessment must work together to create an environment for personalized, appropriate, and accurate care. Note how assessment forms the foundation for accurate, individualized, and holistic nursing care.

- What are the major risk factors related to hospitalization?
- What admitting assessments are indicated given Mr. Kim's history?
- What items would you add to focus the assessment on Mr. Kim's problem?
- What complications might Mr. Kim develop that could trigger the need for an urgent assessment?
- What discharge planning interventions might you implement based on his condition?
- How will you evaluate whether those interventions are effective?

Key Points

- The comprehensive assessment is more detailed and complete than shift and focused assessments.
- The shift assessment is performed at the beginning of the shift and includes an abbreviated examination, with emphasis on risk areas, such as auscultation of lungs and abdomen and assessment of circulation and level of consciousness.
- The focused assessment concentrates on assessing for anticipated problems that can result from hospitalization, such as pneumonia, skin breakdown, falls, or infections, as well as those specific to the patient's problems, such as surgery, trauma, or specific medical condition.
- Practice the five rights of delegation, including: (1) the right task, (2) under the right circumstances, (3) to the right person, (4) with the right directions and communication, and (5) under the right supervision and evaluation
- The Institute for Healthcare Improvement (2014) national safety goals for hospital care include adverse drug events, catheter-associated urinary tract infections, central line–associated bloodstream infections (CLABSI), injuries from falls and immobility (including delirium), pressure ulcers, surgical site infections, venous thromboembolism, and ventilator-associated pneumonia.
- The Joint Commission (2014) interventions related to safety standards are as follows: Identify patients correctly. Improve staff communication. Use alarms safely. Prevent infections. Use the hand-cleaning guidelines. Identify patient safety risks. Prevent mistakes in surgery using a specific protocol for identification of correct surgical procedure, time-outs for procedures, and clear communication.
- Patient satisfaction surveys provide measures of quality and may lead to improved patient outcomes. Patient satisfaction–related interventions that pertain to assessment are as follows: Participate in bedside handoff reports. Practice hourly rounding. Show respect. Protect confidentiality and privacy.
- Always perform an initial safety inspection at the beginning of the shift.
- Identify acute and urgent situations including changes in vital signs and cognition.
- Assess for falls using one of the tools described in the musculoskeletal chapter, such as the Hendrich II Fall Risk Model or the Morse Fall Scale.
- Use the Braden Scale, Norton Scale, or another skin assessment tool according to hospital standard. These include altered sensory perception, moisture, inactivity, immobility, poor nutrition, and friction/shear.
- Edema, pain or achiness, erythema, and warmth in the leg are common signs and symptoms of venous thromboembolism.
- Recently recognized as a primary cause of mortality, early recognition and treatment of sepsis is a primary responsibility of the nurse.
- Provide purposeful hourly rounding: pain, personal needs, position, placement, and prevent falls.

Review Questions

1. Which of the phases of the nursing process is most foundational for delivery of care?
   A. Assessment
   B. Planning
   C. Diagnosis
   D. Evaluation

2. The nurse evaluates circulation, movement, and sensation on the right leg of a patient who was admitted with a tibia/fibula fracture. This type of assessment is considered a
   A. head-to-toe assessment.
   B. comprehensive assessment.
   C. emergency assessment.
   D. focused assessment.

3. Which of the following interventions is a lowest priority for patient safety during care?
   A. Use two patient identifiers such as name and date of birth.
   B. Provide documentation, medical terminology, and SBAR for verbal communication.
   C. Use alarms safely, especially to prevent harm to patients at risk for falls.
   D. Proceed with surgeries immediately with no time out,

4. Which of the following are interventions the nurse makes to prevent infections? Select all that apply.
   A. Use the hand cleaning guidelines from the CDC and WHO.
   B. Use proven guidelines to prevent infections that are difficult to treat.
   C. Use proven guidelines to prevent infection of the blood from corrupted central lines.
   D. Use proven guidelines to prevent infection after surgery.
   E. Use proven guidelines to prevent infections of the urinary tract that are caused by catheters.

5. Which of the following assessments is considered a basic care activity for the NCLEX licensing examination?
   A. Venous access devices, IV lines, invasive monitoring
   B. Personal hygiene habits, mobility routines
   C. Responses to procedures and treatments
   D. Vascular perfusion, hypotension, peripheral pulses

6. The nurse participates in bedside handoff reports, practices hourly rounding, introduces himself or herself, addresses the patient using the name he or she prefers, and paraphrases patient responses to verify understanding. These are interventions designed to
   A. improve patient safety.
   B. increase patient satisfaction.
   C. improve infection rates.
   D. increase efficient assessments.

7. The nurse enters the patient's room for the first time during the shift and directly observes the patient for breathing, airway, skin color, dyspnea, and airway secretions. This assessment is performed as part of a/an
   A. acute assessment.
   B. safety assessment.
   C. continuing assessment.
   D. comprehensive assessment.

8. The nurse enters a patient's room and initiates a rapid response call based on which of the following assessments? Select all that apply.
   A. An acute change in oxygen saturation less than 90% despite oxygen administration
   B. An acute change in systolic blood pressure to less than 90 mm Hg or a sustained increase in diastolic blood pressure greater than 110 mm Hg
   C. New-onset chest pain
   D. An acutely cold, cyanotic, or pulseless extremity
   E. An acute change in pupillary response

9. Which of the following interventions are common in the hospitalized patient? Select all that apply.
   A. Assess pain every 8 hours and reassess 2 hours after interventions.
   B. Assess oxygen and vital signs every day.
   C. Assess Braden Scale and provide skin hygiene as needed every 8 hours.
   D. Perform focused assessments every shift and as needed.
   E. Perform safety assessments every day.

10. The most common format for the comprehensive admitting assessment in the hospitalized adult is the
   A. head to toe.
   B. body systems.
   C. functional framework.
   D. systems framework.

The Jensen suite offers these additional resources to enhance learning and facilitate understanding of this chapter:

- thePoint online resources, http://thepoint.lww.com/Jensen2e
- *Laboratory Manual for Nursing Health Assessment: A Best Practice Approach*
- *Pocket Guide for Nursing Health Assessment: A Best Practice Approach*
- *Lippincott DocuCare*, an electronic health record simulation software, http://thepoint.lww.com/docucare
- *Adaptive Learning | Powered by PrepU*, http://thepoint.lww.com/prepu

References

Agency for Healthcare Research and Quality. (2013a). *Patient safety primers: Rapid response systems.* Retrieved from http://psnet.ahrq.gov/primer.aspx?primerID=4

Agency for Healthcare Research and Quality. (2013b). *Preventing falls in hospitals: A toolkit for improving quality of care.* Retrieved from http://www.ahrq.gov/professionals/systems/long-term-care/resources/injuries/fallpxtoolkit/fallpxtoolkit.pdf

Agency for Healthcare Research and Quality. (2013c). *Inpatient quality indicators overview.* Retrieved from http://www.qualityindicators.ahrq.gov/Modules/iqi_resources.aspx

American Nurses Association & National Council of State Boards of Nursing. (2014). *Joint statement on delegation.* Retrieved from https://www.ncsbn.org/Delegation_joint_statement_NCSBN-ANA.pdf

Brooks Carthon, J. M., Jarrín, O., Sloane, D., & Kutney-Lee, A. (2013). Variations in postoperative complications according to race, ethnicity, and sex in older adults. *Journal of the American Geriatric Society, 61*(9), 1499–1507. doi:10.1111/jgs.12419

Bulechek, G. M., Butcher, H. K., Dochterman, J. M., & Wagner, C. M. (2013). *Nursing interventions classification (NIC)* (6th ed.). St. Louis, MO: Mosby.

Centers for Disease Control and Prevention. (2014). *CDC/NHSN surveillance definitions for specific types of infections.* Retrieved from http://www.cdc.gov/nhsn/pdfs/pscmanual/17pscnosinfdef_current.pdf

Dellinger, R. P., Levy, M. M., Rhodes, A., Annane, D., Gerlach, H., Opal, S. M., . . . Vincent, J. L. (2012). Surviving sepsis campaign: International guidelines for management of severe sepsis and septic shock: 2012. *Critical Care Medicine, 41*(2), 580–637. doi:10.1097/CCM.0b013e31827e83af

Gaskin, D. J., Spencer, C. S., Richard, P., Anderson, G. F., Powe, N. R., & Laveist, T. A. (2013). Do hospitals provide lower-quality care to minorities than to whites? *Health Affairs, 27*(2), 518–527. doi:10.1377/hlthaff.27.2.518

Hospital Consumer Assessment of Healthcare Providers and Systems. (2013). *HCAHPS hospital survey*. Retrieved from http://www.hcahpsonline.org/home.aspx

The Joint Commission. (2014). Hospital: 2014 *National patient safety goals*. Retrieved from http://www.jointcommission.org/assets/1/6/HAP_NPSG_Chapter_2014.pdf

Manary, M. P., Boulding, W., Staelin, R., & Glickman, S. W. (2013). The patient experience and health outcomes. *New England Journal of Medicine, 368*, 201–203. doi:10.1056/NEJMp1211775

Min, L., Burruss, S., Morley, E., Mody L., Hiatt, J. R., Cryer, H., . . . Tillou, A. (2013). A simple clinical risk nomogram to predict mortality-associated geriatric complications in severely injured geriatric patients. *Trauma Acute Care Surgery, 74*(4), 1125–1132. doi:10.1097/TA.0b013e31828273a0.

Moorhead, S., Johnson, M., Maas, M. L., & Swanson, E. (2013). *Nursing outcomes classification (NOC): Measurement of health outcomes* (5th ed.). St. Louis, MO: Elsevier.

NANDA International. (2012). *Nursing diagnoses: Definitions and classification 2012–2014* (9th ed.). Oxford, United Kingdom: Wiley-Blackwell.

National Council of State Boards of Nursing. (2013). *2013 NCLEX-RN test plan*. Retrieved from https://www.ncsbn.org/2013_NCLEX_RN_Test_Plan.pdf

Palmer, R. M. (2014). *Caring for the hospitalized elderly: Current best practice and new horizons*. Retrieved from http://www.hospitalmedicine.org/AM/Template.cfm?Section=The_Hospitalist& Template=/CM/ContentDisplay.cfm&ContentFileID=1447

Scherb, C. A., Head B. J., Maas, M. L., Swanson, E. A., Moorhead, S., Reed, D., . . . Kozel, M. (2011). Most frequent nursing diagnoses, nursing interventions, and nursing-sensitive patient outcomes of hospitalized older adults with heart failure: Part 1. *International Journal of Nursing Terminology Classification, 22*(1), 13–22. doi:10.1111/j.1744-618X.2010.01164.x

30

Head-to-Toe Assessment of the Adult

Learning Objectives

1. Identify the rationale for a comprehensive screening or focused health assessment as appropriate to the patient situation and setting.
2. Collect subjective data, including history and risk assessment.
3. Identify teaching opportunities for health promotion and risk reduction.
4. Collect objective data by completing a head-to-toe physical assessment.
5. Individualize the health assessment, taking into consideration the condition, age, gender, and culture of the patient.
6. Identify normal and abnormal findings gathered from inspection, palpation, percussion, and auscultation during the head-to-toe assessment.
7. Document and communicate data using appropriate medical terminology.
8. Use subjective and objective data to analyze findings and plan interventions.
9. Use assessment findings to identify patterns and problems, set outcomes, and initiate a plan of care.

Dorothy Jane Suleri, 44 years old, is admitted with diarrhea, obesity, ulcerative colitis, abdominal pain, rosacea, fatigue, and anemia. Her current problem is bleeding related to the colitis, for which she uses prescribed medications. She has had three bloody stools today. She is married with two children, 15 and 13 years old. You will gain more information about Mrs. Suleri as you progress through this chapter. As you study the content and features, consider Mrs. Suleri's case and its relationship to what you are learning. Begin thinking about the following points: When is a focused health assessment used?

- Describe the differences among comprehensive, focused, and screening assessments.
- How will the nurse individualize the admitting history to focus it on Mrs. Suleri?
- How will the nurse focus the physical assessments considering Mrs. Suleri's diagnosis?
- How will the nurse use the assessment information to develop a plan of care?
- How will the nurse evaluate the effectiveness of the assessment?

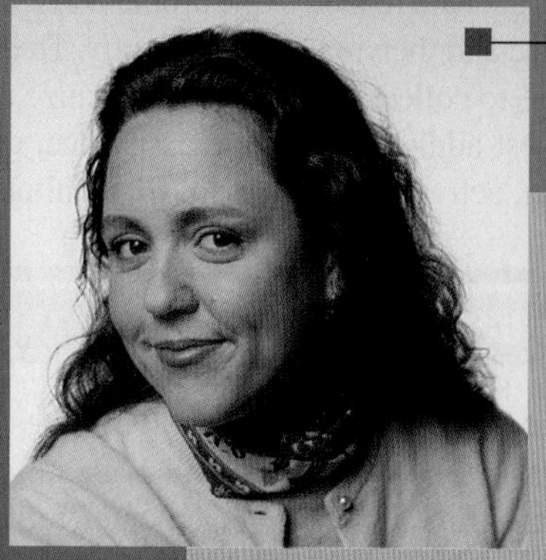

This chapter outlines a comprehensive assessment. As a beginning nurse, you learn the range of assessment skills, but the application of how and when to use these skills occurs in the clinical setting. You combine sensitive history taking with accurate and thorough physical assessment techniques by beginning with a firm foundation of evidence and scientific knowledge. With experience and support, patient assessment becomes an art. The most important thing is to develop a consistent, logical technique organized in a way comfortable for you but focused on the individual patient.

This chapter serves as a summary and synthesis of the individual body systems covered in previous chapters. No *new* information is presented, but in it, the information is collated in a head-to-toe pattern so that the examination is efficient and organized. The assessment is comprehensive and therefore lengthy; it may take 45 minutes to 1 hour to complete, even with repeated practice and expertise.

Findings help you form an overall impression of the patient and his or her condition. Complete subjective data are usually collected once and include information related to the patient's history and risk factors. You also collect objective data once, and then you collect focused data or, in the case of an acute or critically ill patient, you may want to repeat the head-to-toe examination. After gathering all data, you then reorganize them according to problem or diagnosis. You detect patterns and identify findings in associated systems. You analyze assessment data by using critical thinking to identify problems, and then you plan and evaluate care. Therefore, an accurate history (subjective data) and physical assessment (objective data) create an essential foundation for complete and individualized care.

Urgent Assessment

SAFETY ALERT

If skin color is cyanotic or pale, breathing is difficult, posture is strained, facial expression is anxious, and overall appearance indicates distress, focus on the immediate problem. Other cues that indicate an unstable condition in a patient are difficulty managing the airway; high or low respirations, pulse, or blood pressure; acute change in mental status; seizure; new onset of chest pain; or other concerns that heighten awareness.

In urgent cases, gather pertinent subjective and objective assessment data related to the problem to assist with identifying the cause and then intervene promptly. Treat the patient as you continue to collect, analyze, and prioritize data. You may need to request additional nursing assistance, contact the primary provider, activate a rapid response, or initiate a code team.

Subjective Data

Subjective data collection involves assessing present problems, taking health history, and evaluating risk factors. Give the patient time and encouragement to tell his or her story and experience of health or illness. Doing so provides an opportunity for the patient to express concerns; it often forms the foundation for a therapeutic relationship. If the patient is anxious, acknowledge that it is common for patients to feel uncomfortable at times; give the patient permission to disclose only information that he or she feels comfortable disclosing. Additionally, inform the patient that the information is confidential except in situations where there is concern about safety or harm.

If the patient is stable, you may perform the history first and then complete the physical examination. Alternatively, you may thread collection of subjective data throughout the physical examination (e.g., asking about cough when auscultating the lungs). After reviewing the patient chart, formulate a list of initial problems or topics to discuss, including health promotion and risk reduction assessment. You usually take the history with the patient clothed because most patients are more comfortable when covered.

Focused History

Begin with common chart items, such as demographic information, primary complaint(s), and a medication list, along with allergies. Review the chart before meeting the patient to avoid repetitive questions. Compare the medication list with home medications stated by the patient; you may suggest that the patient keep an accurate list of medications, drug allergies, and medical diagnosis if the patient has an extensive list. Additionally, validate the problem list and medications with the patient. If areas are inconsistent or unclear, obtain additional information, notify the primary care provider, and reconcile the differences.

Begin the patient interview with a focus on the primary problem and current symptoms. Ask about the reason for the visit and history of the present problem. Evaluate the reasons for the visit by asking, "Tell me why you came in today." At this point, obtain a history of the present illness by assessing pain or discomfort using the following parameters:

- Location: "Where does it hurt?"
- Duration: "When did it start? How long has it lasted?"
- Intensity: "On a scale of 1 to 10, how do you rate your pain?"
- Quality: "Tell me what it feels like."
- Alleviating/aggravating factors: "What makes it better? Worse?"
- Pain goal: "What level of pain is acceptable to you?"
- Functional goal: "What would you like to be able to do if you were not in pain?

Past Medical History

Assess past health history to provide context for how the current problem might be related. Assess findings considering the information previously reviewed in the chart. For example, you might say, "I'm going to ask you some questions about your health history. I noticed that your chart says that you have an allergy to ondansetron (Zofran). Tell me about that." This is a way of verifying information and obtaining further details. Some examples of categories for the past medical and family history include the following:

- **Assess for allergies.** Include iodine, shellfish, and latex. Also assess the patient's reaction including rash, hives, anaphylaxis, urticaria, pruritus, gastrointestinal upset, nausea, vomiting, or diarrhea. Validate answers with the information in the chart. Include reaction.
- **Obtain past history of illness.** Include medical, surgical, and obstetrical history.
- **Obtain list of medications.** Include over-the-counter (OTC) drugs, herbals, and supplements (medications listed in the chart and double checked and reconciled with patient).
- **Assess family history.** "What was the condition? Who had it? What is the family member's status now, deceased or alive and well?"
- **Assess childhood illnesses and immunizations.** Include influenza, pneumococcal, and purified protein derivative (PPD) (a tuberculosis [TB] test).
- **Obtain information on most recent screening assessments.** These include TB, vision or hearing screening, and mammograms.
- **Evaluate mental health and psychiatric history.** Medications may provide clues to mental health issues, such as antidepressants.

Review of Systems

Review the body systems using lay language focused on the following common areas. (As an alternative, the patient may complete a form.) Document findings using medical terminology (Fig. 30.1).

- **General survey:** Fever, chills, weight loss, weight gain, fatigue
- **Nutrition:** Nausea, loss of appetite, increase in appetite, vomiting, indigestion, problems swallowing or chewing

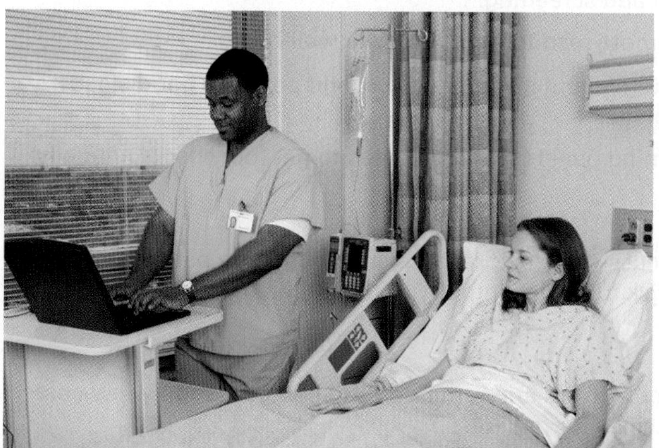

Figure 30.1 The nurse carefully documents findings from the health history in the patient's chart using medical terminology. (Photo by B. Proud)

- **Skin, hair, and nails:** Rash, itch, lesions, nails, hygiene, hair loss
- **Head and neck:** Headaches, dizziness, syncope, seizures, enlarged lymph nodes
- **Eyes:** Glasses, contacts, blurry vision, double vision, loss of vision, swelling, tearing up, dry eyes, date of last vision examination
- **Ears:** Hearing loss, pressure, earache
- **Nose, mouth, throat:** Congestion, sore throat, voice change, routine dental care, last dental visit
- **Thorax and lungs:** Shortness of breath, wheezing, cough
- **Heart:** Fast or slow pulse, heart murmur, chest pain, pounding or fluttering in chest, swelling in feet, rings tighter than usual
- **Peripheral vascular:** Cramping, pain, numbness in extremities
- **Breast:** Pain, tenderness, discharge, lump, date of last self-examination of breasts
- **Abdominal/gastrointestinal:** Frequency of bowel movements and description, bloody stool, diarrhea, constipation, soiling of clothes, hemorrhoids
- **Abdominal/genitourinary:** Frequency and description of urine, difficulty or burning with urination, blood in urine, urination during the night, urgency, increased frequency, wetting of clothes, feeling of incomplete emptying or dribbling
- **Musculoskeletal:** Mobility, pain, stiffness, spasm, tremor, gait, impaired balance, foreign bodies or implants
- **Neurological:** Headache, one-sided weakness, memory loss, confusion, speech pattern
- **Genitalia, female:** Vaginal discharge, pain with menstruation, excessive bleeding with menstruation, last menstrual period (LMP), is menstrual cycle regular or irregular, pain with sexual intercourse
- **Genitalia, male:** Discharge, pain, swelling, lumps, trauma, erectile dysfunction
- **Endocrine:** Excessive thirst, increased urination, hair loss, skin changes, hot flashes
- **Mental health:** Anxiety, depression, abnormal thoughts, difficulty sleeping. Remember the overall appearance and grooming of the patient can give clues about mental health.
- **Summary:** "How would you say that your health is in general?"

Psychosocial History

Assess psychosocial, spiritual, and cultural history; language of choice; and need for interpreter. You may ask, "Do you have any special religious, spiritual, or cultural needs? Would you like an interpreter?" Assess use of tobacco, alcohol, and recreational drugs by asking directly, "Do you use tobacco, alcohol, or other substances?" You may also find using current street names for recreational drugs helpful. Assess for safety and domestic violence by asking, "Because violence is so common in many people's lives, I ask all patients about it routinely. Are you in a relationship with a person who physically or sexually hurts or threatens you?"

Functional Health Status

As time allows and as the relationship is established, you also can obtain information about the patient's functional health status. For these questions, it is best to prioritize and ask one or two questions during the examination.

Activities of Daily Living

Assess the patient's ability to perform self-care activities, or **activities of daily living** (ADLs). These include behaviors such as eating, dressing, and grooming. Score these items based on whether the patient is totally independent, needs assistance from a person or device such as a cane, or is dependent on others.

Risk Reduction and Health Promotion

An important purpose of the health history is to gather information to promote health and provide health teaching. Health promotion activities focus on preventing disease, identifying problems early, and reducing complications of existing or established diagnoses. They also serve to reinforce existing healthy habits and encourage refinements to approaches the patient is already practicing. Promote patient education and healthy behaviors as they apply in the nursing process (Table 30.1).

Assessment of risk factors involves collecting comprehensive subjective data, including demographic information and other data from the chart, history of present problem, past health history, family history, review of systems, psychosocial history, functional status, ADLs, and growth/development. After collecting and analyzing all these data, you determine potential and actual risk factors for the patient and use this information to plan specific screening, health promotion, and patient teaching activities.

The U.S. Preventive Services Task Force (USPSTF, 2013) recommends that primary care providers discuss priority screening services with patients and offer them these services (Table 30.2). Screening and resulting teaching are primary prevention services that nurses offer as part of their professional responsibilities. You assess risk factors according to the individual's risks (e.g., injury in a teenager, genetic diseases in a pregnant woman). Cancer screening, dental caries prevention for preschoolers, Rh factor incompatibility screening for pregnant women, and behavioral counseling for a healthy diet are included as primary prevention activities. Cognitive and dementia screening for older adults and prevention of falls and fractures are more recent recommendations. These screenings are essential in maintaining high-level wellness.

Common Symptoms

In addition to the overall review of systems and general health promotion, focus your questions in a way that is specific to the patient's medical conditions—for example, ask about chest pain if the patient has a history of myocardial infarction. For questions related to the primary problems and concerns of the patient, refer to the system-specific chapters in this book.

TABLE 30.1 Health Goals for Primary Care

Goal	Patient Education Topics
Increase the proportion of patients appropriately counseled about health behaviors.	Review healthy diet, regular exercise, weight reduction, and recommended screenings.
Increase the proportion of patients who have a specific source of ongoing care.	Encourage patient to have regular visits for health promotion and screening.
Increase quality of life: physical, mental, and spiritual.	Promote resources to facilitate well-being.
Increase knowledge of sufficient sleep and treat sleep disorders to promote wellness.	Inquire about sleep practices, and promote good sleep hygiene.
Increase the proportion of adults with diabetes mellitus who have at least a foot examination at least annually.	Remind patients with diabetes to get foot checks annually.
Increase the proportion of HIV-infected adolescents and adults who receive testing, treatment, and prophylaxis consistent with current Public Health Service treatment guidelines.	Discuss safe-sex practices and encourage patients who are at risk to get testing.
Increase the proportion of adults who are vaccinated annually against influenza and who are ever vaccinated against pneumococcal disease.	Supply flyers and reminders for patients; supply low-cost vaccines for patients.

From U.S. Department of Health & Human Services. (n.d.) *Healthy people 2020: Topics and objectives.* Retrieved from http://healthypeople.gov/2020/topicsobjectives2020/default.aspx

TABLE 30.2 Screening and Health Promotion Activities From U.S. Preventive Services Task Force

Recommendation	Adults		Special Populations	
	Men	*Women*	*Pregnant Women*	*Children*
Alcohol abuse screening and behavioral counseling interventions; counseling to prevent tobacco use and tobacco-related disease	X	X	X	
Screening for asymptomatic bacteriuria; Rh (D) incompatibility screening			X	
Screening for breast cancer, and cervical cancer; screening for osteoporosis in postmenopausal women		X		
Prevention of dental caries in preschool children; screening for visual impairment in children younger than age 5 years				X
Depression screening; colorectal cancer screening; screening for Type 2 diabetes mellitus in adults; behavioral counseling in primary care to promote a healthy diet; screening for high blood pressure and lipid disorders; screening for obesity in adults	X	X		
Screening for gonorrhea, hepatitis B virus infection, syphilis infection, chlamydia infection; behavioral interventions to promote breastfeeding		X	X	
HIV screening	X	X	X	X

Data from U.S. Preventive Services Task Force. (2013). *Guide to clinical preventive services.* Retrieved from http://www.ahrq.gov/professionals/clinicians-providers/guidelines-recommendations/guide/index.html

Therapeutic Dialogue: Collecting Subjective Data

Mrs. Suleri, introduced at the beginning of this chapter, is a 44-year-old mother of two children. She was admitted with bloody diarrhea as the presenting complaint. The nurse uses professional communication techniques to gather subjective data from her.

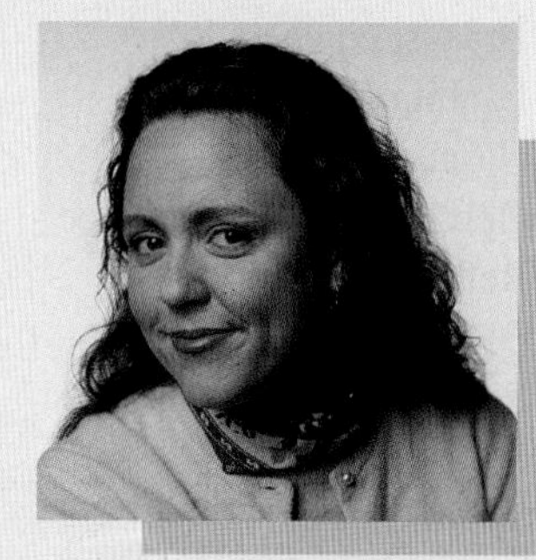

Nurse: How does your family depend upon you for things, and how are they coping with your illness?

Mrs. Suleri: Thanks for asking. Usually, I take the kids to soccer practice and ballet. My husband is a backup at home but he works late so this has been a stress on all of us. I've been so tired lately that I haven't been able to keep up.

Nurse: Do you generally feel rested and ready for activities after sleeping?

Mrs. Suleri: Not really, I'm exhausted (pause) and I barely can make it to work.

(case study continues on page 926)

Nurse: How is this hospital stay affecting your work?

Mrs. Suleri: I've been missing a lot.

Nurse: Because many people have financial concerns related to their hospital stay, I usually ask about that. Would you like to see a social worker about any financial concerns?

Mrs. Suleri: Actually I would. Talking with someone might put my mind at ease about paying for this.

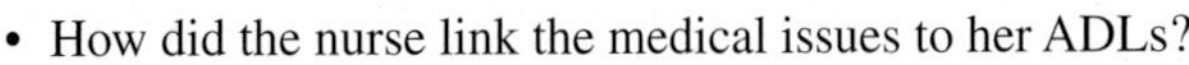

Critical Thinking Challenge

- How did the nurse link the medical issues to her ADLs?
- What nursing issues are you beginning to develop as you assess her?
- How might you ask the question about finances, which can be a sensitive subject?

Objective Data

Pulling together a smooth and organized physical assessment is challenging. You must practice and develop a pattern of assessment that eventually becomes automatic to avoid skipping or repeating items. You will organize sections of the assessment according to the body part being examined, even if they are related to different body systems. For example, while the patient stands, you assess sensory and motor neurological function, musculoskeletal range of motion, and peripheral vascular pulses.

Equipment

- Cotton swabs
- Drapes, gown
- Examining gloves
- Nasal speculum
- Ophthalmoscope/otoscope
- Reflex hammer
- Blood pressure cuff
- Scale with height measure
- Stethoscope
- Thermometer
- Tongue blade
- Watch with second hand
- Optional: vision charts

If specimens are needed:

- Vaginal speculum
- Lubricant
- Culture media
- Glass slides
- Potassium hydroxide
- Hemoccult testing cards and solution
- Papanicolaou smear spatula

Preparation

Following completion of the health history previously described, explain the process for the physical examination from head to toe and including auscultation of heart and lung sounds, auscultation and palpation of the abdomen, and screening for neuromuscular problems. Because some assessments may be uncomfortable (e.g., breast, gynecological), ask the patient for permission to perform them. Additionally, ask the patient whether he or she prefers to have a third person in the room or, if appropriate, a same-gender nurse. Explain that the patient will be draped and modesty will be a priority; only the body part being examined will be exposed.

Ask whether the patient would like to urinate because pressure during abdominal palpation may elicit the urge to void. Instruct the patient to change into a gown that ties in back. At this point, obtain the necessary equipment and leave the room so that the patient can change (Fig. 30.2). Instruct the patient to sit on the examination table after finishing undressing. Upon return, wash and warm the hands to avoid chilling the patient, and ask the patient about comfort level

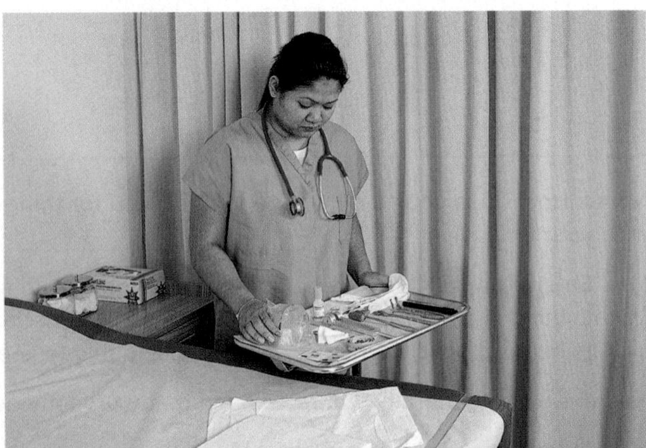

Figure 30.2 The nurse is setting up the examination room for a head-to-toe physical assessment.

and room temperature. If the patient is cold, offer an additional blanket. Encourage the patient to ask questions about the assessment techniques and findings.

Patients may be seen because of abnormal findings, so it is important to be honest when difficulties are present, such as, "Your blood pressure is a little high. We can talk more about that after we're finished." Instead of giving false reassurances, provide objective data. Nevertheless, avoid sharing conclusions before collecting all data because the initial problem list may change during the interaction. As you evaluate the response of the patient and family to actual or potential health problems, you are simultaneously performing assessments related to the direct care role.

Comprehensive Physical Assessment

The physical examination begins with height, weight, and vital signs if not previously obtained. Next is the head-to-toe assessment, during which you should strive to move efficiently and minimize the number of movements for the patient. You must consider how to remember each of the steps by combining items or developing cues to remember them. If you are a beginning nurse, a pocket guide might be helpful so that at the end you can review it for any forgotten items. Review the guide before leaving the patient's room so it will not be necessary to return to ask for more information. Reviewing findings with the patient at the end provides closure before leaving.

Technique and Normal Findings	Abnormal Findings
Wash hands or use gel. Wipe stethoscope.	
Vital Signs Obtain temperature. ☐ Average oral temperature is 36.5°–37.5°C (97.7°–99.5°F).	Hypothermia, hyperthermia
Obtain pulse. ☐ 60–100 beats/min. Heart rate and rhythm are regular.	Tachycardia, bradycardia, irregular rate. If irregular, take apical pulse (1 minute).
Obtain respirations. ☐ 12–20 breaths/min. Respirations are relaxed, smooth, effortless, and silent.	Bradypnea, tachypnea, hyperventilation, Cheyne-Stokes respiration, apnea
Obtain blood pressure. ☐ Systolic 100–120/diastolic 60–80 mm Hg. (Select appropriate cuff size.)	Hypertension, hypotension, auscultatory gap. Perform orthostatic blood pressure (BP) and pulse if indicated. BP that stays 120–139/80–89 mm Hg is considered prehypertension; above this level (140/90 mm Hg or higher) is high (hypertension) (American Heart Association, 2013).
Obtain oxygen saturation level. ☐ 92%–100%	Less than 92%
General Survey Inspect overall skin color. ☐ Skin is pink.	Pallor, jaundice, flushing, cyanosis (central vs. peripheral), erythema, ruddy, mottled
Evaluate breathing effort. ☐ No dyspnea.	Dyspnea, head of bed elevated, tripod position
Observe appearance. ☐ Patient appears stated age.	Appears older than stated age, appears acutely ill
Assess mood. ☐ Patient is calm, pleasant, and cooperative. Appropriate affect.	Flat or inappropriate affect, depression, elation, euphoria, anxiety, irritable, labile.
Observe nutritional status. ☐ Patient appears well nourished.	Appears poorly nourished, overweight, or obese (frail, robust)
Evaluate personal hygiene. ☐ Good personal hygiene.	Poor personal hygiene
Assess posture. ☐ Posture erect.	Slouching, bent to one side
Observe for physical deformities. ☐ No obvious physical deformities.	Obvious physical deformity present

(table continues on page 928)

Technique and Normal Findings (continued)	Abnormal Findings (continued)
Perform safety check. ☐ Call bell within reach; bedside stand positioned; identification band correct; intravenous (IV) lines, medications, tubes, and drains intact.	Unsafe environment; medications or IV fluids not verified.
Skin	
Inspect skin with each corresponding body area. Inspect color; check for rashes and lesions. ☐ Skin pink, no cyanosis. No telangiectasia, erythema, or papules.	Changes in skin pigmentation. If lesions, bruises, or rashes found, identify configuration and number. Note any infections (e.g., cellulitis). Note any infestations (e.g.,scabies, lice, fleas).
Palpate for moisture, temperature, texture, turgor, and edema. ☐ Skin warm, slightly dry, and intact. Good turgor on upper extremities; no edema, lesions, or tenderness.	Growths or tumors are abnormal. Describe any wounds or incisions including size, depth, color, exudate, and wound borders.
Head	
Evaluate facial structures. ☐ Symmetrical structures without edema, deformities, or lesions. Patent nares.	Asymmetrical, edema, deformities, ptosis, lesions Absence of "sniff"; deviated septum, polyps, drainage
Observe facial expression. ☐ Facial expression appropriate to situation.	Anxious facial grimace; facial droop, asymmetrical
Inspect skull, hair, and scalp. ☐ Skull intact; appropriate size, shape, and contour for gender and age. Straight hair with normal distribution. Hair supple and thick. Scalp pink and smooth without pests, flaking, lesions, or tenderness. Palpate cranium, temporal artery, and temporomandibular joint (TMJ). ☐ Normocephalic, head midline. Temporal artery 2–3+ bilaterally, nontender. TMJ moves freely, without crepitus or tenderness.	Facial asymmetry may indicate damage to facial nerve (cranial nerve [CN] VII) or a serious condition such as a stroke. Enlarged bones or tissues are associated with acromegaly. A puffy "moon" face is associated with Cushing syndrome. Increased facial hair in females may be a sign of Cushing syndrome or endocrinopathy. Periorbital edema is seen with congestive heart failure and hypothyroidism (myxedema).
Assess trigeminal nerve (CN V), motor strength and light touch, three facial branches. ☐ Strong contraction of muscles and senses light touch on forehead, cheek, and chin.	Decreased or dulled sensation, weakness, or asymmetrical movements are abnormal findings associated with CN V.
Assess CNs V and VII: Have patient squeeze eyes shut, wrinkle forehead, clench teeth, smile, and puff cheeks. ☐ Facial movements are strong and symmetrical.	A weak blink from facial weakness may result from paralysis of CN V or CN VII.
Inspect eyelids, eyelashes, and eyebrows. ☐ No ptosis, eyelid lag, discharge, or crusting. Even eyelash distribution. Eyebrows with hair loss on outer third.	Depressed or absent corneal response is common in contact lens wearers.
Mouth and Throat	
Inspect mouth with light and tongue blade. Inspect inside lips, buccal mucosa, gums, teeth, hard/soft palates, uvula, tonsils, pharynx, tongue, and floor of mouth (an advanced practice registered nurse [APRN] may use light from otoscope). ☐ Lips, mucosa, gums, and palates are pink and smooth. Floor of mouth intact, moist, and smooth. Pharynx pink, and intact. Tongue pink and rough. No lesions or tenderness. Teeth white and intact with good occlusion.	Lesions, sponginess, or edema; bleeding gums; missing or discolored teeth; malocclusion; inflammation or tenderness of ducts

(table continues on page 929)

Technique and Normal Findings (continued)	Abnormal Findings (continued)
Grade tonsils. *Tonsils 0–2+.* Pink with no discharge or lesions.	Swollen glands or tonsils (grade 3+ –4+)
Note mobility of uvula when patient says "ahh." Uvula at midline and rises symmetrically.	Uvula asymmetrical or enlarged.
Assess hypoglossal nerve (CN XII); look for symmetry of tongue when extended. Tongue at midline and extends symmetrically.	A tongue that deviates to one side is common with stroke.
Eyes Assess near and distant vision if appropriate. Reads newsprint accurately. Snellen test 20/20.	Less than 20/20 corrected. Vision blurred. Note use of glasses, contact lenses, or assistive devices.
Inspect conjunctiva and sclera. Pink, moist conjunctiva; white sclera.	Sclera yellow with jaundice. Conjunctiva pink with inflammation.
Inspect cornea, iris, and anterior chamber. *Cornea and lens are clear.* Assess oculomotor nerve (CN III), trochlear nerve (CN IV), and abducent nerve (CN VI) as well as extraocular movements (EOMs). EOMs intact, no nystagmus.	A narrow angle indicates glaucoma. Cloudiness of the lens may indicate cataract, which is associated with increased age, smoking, alcohol intake, and sunlight exposure. Risk factors for cataracts are primarily environmental.
Assess visual fields and peripheral vision. Visual fields equal to the examiner's.	
Darken room. Obtain light. Assess optic nerve (CN II). Pupils equal, round, and reactive to light and accommodation (PERRLA L 6–4, R 6–4).	Asymmetry, pinpoint, or "blown" pupils; describe measure of pupil and response to light.
Perform ophthalmoscopic examination: check red reflex, disc, vessels, and macula. Move to opposite side of patient. Red reflex symmetrical. Discs cream-colored with sharp margins. Retina pink. No hemorrhages or exudates; no arteriolar narrowing. Macula yellow.	Lack of red reflex may need urgent follow-up. If a white pupil reflex (leukocoria) is elicited, an urgent ophthalmological referral is required. Disease or trauma (e.g., retinoblastoma, hyphema, toxocariasis, retinal detachment) often causes a white pupil reflex. Blood vessels can be directly observed in the retina. Systemic diseases are often reflected in the blood vessels and can be directly observed in the eye.
Ears Turn on lights. Inspect ear alignment. Ears aligned properly.	Microtia, macrotia, edema, cartilage, *Pseudomonas* infection, carcinoma on auricle, cysts, and frostbite are abnormal findings.
Palpate auricle, lobe, and tragus. Ears are without lesions, crusting, masses, or tenderness.	
Change to otoscope head. Perform otoscopic examination of canal and tympanic membrane. Move to opposite side of patient. Canals with small amount of moist yellow cerumen. Tympanic membranes intact, gray, and translucent; light reflex and body landmarks present.	Redness, external swelling, and discharge indicate external otitis. Obstructed canal can be caused by either foreign body or cerumen buildup.
Assess vestibulocochlear nerve (CN VIII); hearing. Whispered words heard bilaterally.	Unable to repeat whispered words.

(table continues on page 930)

Technique and Normal Findings (continued)	Abnormal Findings (continued)
Obtain tuning fork. Perform Rinne test (on mastoid) if the patient has hearing loss. ■ Air conduction greater than bone conduction.	Bone conduction longer or the same as air conduction is evidence of conductive hearing loss.
Perform Weber test (at midline of skull) if patient has hearing loss. ■ No lateralization.	Unilateral identification of the sound indicates sensorineural loss in the ear that the patient did not hear the sound or had reduced perception.
Nose and Sinuses Inspect external nose. ■ Midline; no flaring or crusting.	Asymmetrical; swelling, or bruising may result from trauma or occur with lesions or growths.
Assess nostril patency. ■ Nostrils patent bilaterally.	Unable to sniff because of deviated septum or obstructed nostrils.
Perform otoscopic examination of mucosa, turbinates, and septum. ■ Nasal mucosa pink, intact; no polyps. No drainage. Turbinates and septum intact and symmetrical.	Inflammation of nasal mucosa may be present with viral or bacterial infection. With allergic rhinitis, nasal mucosa may be pale, bluish, or red.
Palpate frontal and maxillary sinuses. ■ No frontal or maxillary sinus tenderness.	Redness and swelling over the sinuses may represent acute infection, abscess, or mucocele.
Neck Inspect symmetry. ■ Neck symmetrical and moves freely without crepitus.	Neck asymmetrical or with crepitus.
Test flexion, extension, lateral bending, rotation, range of motion (ROM), and strength. ■ Full ROM; strength 4–5+ bilaterally.	Reduced neck ROM is less than 4+.
Palpate tracheal position midline. ■ Trachea at midline.	Deviated trachea.
Palpate carotid pulse. ■ Carotid pulse 2–3+ bilaterally.	Carotid pulses may be reduced as a result of carotid stenosis.
Inspect jugular veins. ■ No jugular venous distention (JVD).	Jugular veins may be either flat or distended.
Palpate preauricular, postauricular, occipital, and posterior cervical chains. ■ They are not palpable or tender.	Lymph nodes are not freely movable or are tender.
Palpate tonsillar, submandibular, submental, and anterior cervical chains. ■ They are not palpable or tender.	
Palpate supraclavicular nodes. ■ They are not palpable or tender.	
Neurological Assess mental status and level of consciousness. ■ Patient is alert. Eyes open spontaneously.	Agitated, asleep, lethargic, obtunded, restless, stuporous. Use Glasgow Coma Scale if reduced (eye opening, verbal, motor). Does not respond to stimuli or pain; decorticate rigidity, decerebrate rigidity, or no response to pain.
Assess orientation. ■ Oriented ×3.	Alert and oriented (A&O) ×2 (person and place). A&O ×1 (person), disoriented ×3. Can also assess orientation to situation (A&O ×4).

(table continues on page 931)

Technique and Normal Findings (continued)	Abnormal Findings (continued)
Assess ability to follow commands. ■ Patient follows directions.	Unable to follow commands, such as "squeeze my hand" or "sit up."
Evaluate short- and long-term memory. ■ Immediate, recent, and distant memory intact.	Immediate, recent, or distant memory impaired; describe specific details.
Assess speech. ■ Speech clear.	Speech difficult to understand.
Assess hearing. ■ Hears speech and responds appropriately.	Difficulty understanding spoken words. Hard of hearing. Note hearing aids or assistive devices.
Upper Extremities Evaluate circulation, movement, and sensation (CMS). Assess hands and joints. Evaluate nails on upper extremities. ■ CMS intact. Nails smooth without clubbing. Joints without swelling or deformity.	Decreased CMS, including color, temperature; capillary refill longer than 3 seconds; pulses; decreased movement; decreased sensation and paresthesia. Nails are breakable, cracking, inflamed, jagged, bitten, and clubbing.
Perform hand grasp for ROM and muscle strength. ■ 4–5+ muscle strength symmetrical.	Decreased ROM; swelling or nodules in joints. Muscle strength asymmetrical or 0–3+.
Musculoskeletal and Neurological. Perform finger-to-nose test if indicated. ■ Smooth and intact.	Ataxia is an unsteady movement with inability to touch the target. During rapidly alternating movements, lack of coordination is called adiadochokinesia.
Test rapid alternating movements if indicated. ■ Smooth and intact.	
Test stereognosis if indicated. ■ Patient identifies key or other object.	Inability to identify objects correctly (astereognosis) may result from damage to the sensory cortex caused by stroke.
Test graphesthesia if indicated. ■ Patient identifies the number 8.	Cortical sensory function may be compromised after a stroke.
Anterior Thorax Assess breathing effort, rate, rhythm, and pattern; position to breathe. ■ Breathes easily, with symmetrical expansion and contraction.	Dyspnea, orthopnea, paroxysmal nocturnal dyspnea. Rhythm regular; sitting straight upright or using tripod position to breathe.
Inspect chest shape and skin. ■ Anteroposterior (AP)-to-transverse ratio 1:2 symmetrical. Skin intact.	Barrel chest, funnel chest, pigeon chest, thoracic kyphoscoliosis
If patient is on an examination table, move in front of patient. Inspect costovertebral angle, configuration, and pulsations. ■ No pulsations visible. No dyspnea, retractions, or accessory muscle use.	
Auscultate breath sounds. ■ Bronchovesicular sounds midline, vesicular in lung periphery. Lung sounds clear.	Diminished or absent breath sounds; bronchial or bronchovesicular sounds in lung periphery. Describe adventitious sounds (crackles, gurgles, wheezes, stridor, pleural rub). Are they inspiratory or expiratory? Do they clear after coughing? Where specifically do you hear them?
Assess for cough; inspect sputum. ■ No cough or sputum.	Cough (brassy, harsh, loose, productive) present. Sputum (check color, consistency, amount) present.

(table continues on page 932)

Technique and Normal Findings (continued)	Abnormal Findings (continued)
Inspect precordium. ■ Point of maximal impulse (PMI) may be visible or absent.	PMI lateral to midclavicular line (MCL); heaves or thrills.
Assess heart rate, rhythm, murmurs, and extra sounds. ■ Heart rate and rhythm regular. No gallops, murmurs, or rubs.	Tachycardia, bradycardia, irregular rhythm, murmurs (systolic vs. diastolic), extra sounds (e.g., S3, S4, friction rub)
Auscultate heart with bell at apex and left sternal border with patient lying down. Auscultate heart with diaphragm in aortic, pulmonic, left sternal border, tricuspid, mitral with patient on left side. ■ Heart rate and rhythm regular; no murmurs, gallops, or rubs.	If rhythm is irregular, identify whether the irregularity has a pattern or is totally irregular. For example, every third beat missed would be a regular irregular rhythm. No detectable pattern is characteristic of atrial fibrillation, common in older adults. Murmurs, rubs, or gallops are abnormal in adults.
Palpate chest for fremitus, thrill, heaves, and PMI. ■ Tactile fremitus symmetrical; no thrill, heave, or lift. Cardiac impulse nonpalpable.	Asymmetrical fremitus may occur with unilateral disease (e.g., lung tumor). Thrills, heaves, and lifts indicate turbulence over a valve and are abnormal.
Percuss anterior chest from apex to base and sides. ■ Lung fields resonant with dullness over heart area.	Dull lung percussion indicates increased consolidation as with pneumonia.
Auscultate carotid artery. ■ No bruit.	Bruits over the carotid indicate carotid artery stenosis.
Female Breasts	
Inspect patient's breasts. Have patient raise up her arms, press her hands together, and lean forward. ■ No retraction or dimpling; symmetrical movement.	Retraction, dimpling, or discharge may indicate breast cancer.
Palpate breasts and nipple for discharge. ■ No lesions or masses; no discharge. Nontender.	
Palpate axillary nodes. ■ Axillary nodes not palpable, nontender.	Positive findings in nodes may indicate breast cancer, especially if immovable or tender.
Abdomen	
Inspect abdomen. ■ Abdomen symmetrical, rounded, or flat. Smooth, intact skin without lesions or rashes. Peristalsis and pulsations evident in thin patients. Flat, round umbilicus.	Scars, striae, ecchymosis, lesions, prominent dilated veins, rashes, marked pulsation; red, everted, enlarged, or tender umbilicus
Auscultate bowel sounds. ■ Bowel sounds present all quadrants.	Hypoactive, hyperactive, or absent bowel sounds
Auscultate aorta, renal, and femoral arteries with bell of stethoscope. ■ No bruit.	Venous hum, friction rub, or bruits are abnormal arterial sounds.
Percuss abdomen in all quadrants and for gastric bubble. ■ Abdomen tympanic in all quadrants. Gastric bubble percussed 6th left intercostal space (ICS) at MCL.	Abdomen dull or flat.
Percuss liver margin at right MCL. ■ Liver border above ribs at right MCL.	Liver margin palpable below ribs.
Percuss spleen. ■ Spleen percussed in 10th left ICS posterior to midaxillary line.	Spleen that deviates downward and medially

(table continues on page 933)

Technique and Normal Findings (continued)	Abnormal Findings (continued)
Palpate for abdominal tenderness and distention in all quadrants. ■ Nontender, soft.	Large masses, hard, tenderness with guarding or rigidity, rebound tenderness. Liver palpable more than one finger below costal border at right MCL.
Palpate liver, spleen, and kidneys. ■ Liver lower border less than one finger below costal border at right MCL. Spleen and kidneys nonpalpable.	
Palpate aorta, femoral pulses, and inguinal lymph nodes or hernias. ■ Aorta palpable, smooth. Femoral pulses 2–3+. No inguinal nodes or hernias.	An enlarged aorta (greater than 3 cm) or one with lateral pulsations that are palpable can indicate abdominal aortic aneurysm.
Evaluate swallowing, chewing, aspiration risk, special diet. ■ Eats greater than 75% of meal without difficulty.	Dysphagia, impaired chewing, impaired swallowing, medically prescribed diet, tube feedings, significant weight gain/loss
Ask about nausea, vomiting, and diarrhea. ■ No nausea, vomiting, or diarrhea.	Nausea, vomiting, constipation, or diarrhea. Describe characteristics of emesis (e.g., coffee grounds, bloody).
Inspect stool; record characteristics last bowel movement. Ask about passing flatus. ■ Last bowel movement within patient's normal; soft and brown. Passing flatus.	Dark stool may indicate presence of blood. If hemorrhoids are present, the stool may be normal but have bright red blood coating it.
Inspect urine color, character, and amount with voiding. ■ Urine clear, yellow, and more than 30 ml/hr.	Urine dark, bloody, red, visible sediment, cloudy, or less than 30 ml/hr.
Lower Extremities Inspect skin and toenails for symmetry, edema, veins, and lesions. ■ Toenails white and smooth. Skin intact, slightly pale, and symmetrical, without edema, varicose veins, or lesions.	Note areas of pressure on heels and whether they blanch under pressure. Lesions, ulcers, varicosities, edema. Mottled, ruddy, reddened, or flaky skin. Note indurations with infection or inflammation.
Palpate dorsalis pedis pulses bilaterally. Palpate popliteal pulse and posterior tibial pulse. ■ *Pulses 2–3+.*	Diminished or absent pulses. If present, obtain Doppler for assessment. Bounding (4+) pulses are also abnormal.
Assess capillary refill on both feet. ■ Brisk capillary refill (less than 3 seconds).	Capillary refill longer than 3 seconds
Inspect and palpate edema on ankle and shin. ■ No edema.	1+ barely perceptible (2 mm) 2+ moderate (4 mm) 3+ moderate (6 mm) 4+ severe (greater than 8 mm)
Palpate for tenderness and temperature. ■ Feet warm, no tenderness.	Tenderness to palpation, feet cool or cold.
Palpate lower extremities and joints from hips to toes. ■ No tenderness or swelling.	
Observe ROM of joints. ■ Full joint ROM.	Limited or reduced ROM.
Test muscle strength on feet; observe for symmetry. Test muscle strength in hips, knees, and ankles. ■ Strength 4–5+.	Strength 0–3+

(table continues on page 934)

Technique and Normal Findings (continued)	Abnormal Findings (continued)
Test sensation. ■ Appropriately identifies place when touched.	Loss of sensation
Obtain reflex hammer. Test deep tendon reflexes (DTRs)—patellar and Achilles—and Babinski reflex. ■ Patellar and Achilles DTRs 2+; Babinski negative.	If reflexes are 3–4+, they are brisker than normal. If they are 0–1+, they are diminished or absent. A positive Babinski sign indicates a poor neurological outcome.
Posterior Thorax Move behind patient. Palpate thyroid. ■ Thyroid borders palpable; no enlargement, nodules, or masses noted.	Thyroid enlargement or masses can be seen more easily when the patient swallows and while illuminating patient's neck with a tangential light.
Inspect skin, symmetry, configuration, and observe respirations. ■ Chest symmetrical, oval, without barrel chest. AP-to-transverse ratio 1:2. Respirations 20 breaths/min without dyspnea.	In barrel chest, which may accompany chronic obstructive pulmonary disease (COPD), the AP-to-transverse ratio approximates 1:1, giving the chest a round appearance.
Palpate spine and scapulae. ■ Spine straight, without scoliosis, kyphosis, or lordosis. Scapulae symmetrical.	Skeletal scoliosis and kyphosis can limit respiratory excursion. Asymmetry and paradoxical respirations occur in flail chest.
Assess tactile fremitus. ■ Tactile fremitus symmetrical.	Increased tactile fremitus over an area indicates increased consolidation.
Percuss posterior chest from apex to base to sides. ■ Lung fields resonant.	Dullness occurs with increased consolidation; hyperresonance occurs with hyperinflation as in COPD.
Test flank tenderness (kidney). ■ No tenderness to indirect percussion.	Kidney tenderness is present with urinary tract infection.
Auscultate breath sounds. ■ Breath sounds clear.	Coarse breath sounds are abnormal. Crackles, gurgles (rhonchi), and wheezing are abnormal adventitious sounds.
Inspect lower back and buttocks (redness, symmetry). ■ No redness, no skin breakdown.	Any redness, especially over pressure areas, is a concern.
Inspect spine. ■ Spine straight, skin intact.	Scoliosis, lordosis, and kyphosis are abnormal spine findings.
Gait and Balance/Fall Risk Evaluate fall risk: history of falling, secondary diagnosis, ambulatory aid, IV therapy, gait, and mental status. ■ Scores at low risk on fall scale.	Gait abnormalities include hesitancy, unsteadiness, staggering, reaching for external support, high stepping, foot scraping, inability to raise the foot completely off the floor, persistent toe or heel walking, excessive pointing of toes inward or outward, asymmetry of step height or length, limping, stooping, wavering, shuffling, waddling, excessive swinging of shoulders or pelvis, and slow or rapid speed.
Musculoskeletal and Neurological Perform heel-to-shin test for coordination. ■ Smooth, coordinated movement. Have patient stand. Note muscle strength and coordination when moving. ■ Moves easily in the environment.	The dominant side usually has slightly better coordination. Poor coordination may result from pain, injury, deformity, or cerebellar disorders. Coordination is often tested during assessment of the musculoskeletal system, but this is actually an assessment of the neurological system.
Observe spinal alignment, hip level, and gluteal and knee folds. ■ Spine straight, posture erect.	Scoliosis or low back pain may cause the patient to lean forward or to one side when standing or sitting.

(table continues on page 935)

Technique and Normal Findings (continued)	Abnormal Findings (continued)
Assess spine flexion, extension, lateral bending, and rotation. ■ Full ROM in spine.	
Ask patient to walk on heels and then toes and then to stand on one foot and then the other. ■ Good balance and coordination.	
Skin Breakdown Evaluate risk for skin breakdown: sensory perception, moisture, activity, mobility, nutrition, friction, and shear. ■ Scores at low risk for skin breakdown.	The Braden Scale scores patients from 1 to 4 in six subscales: sensory perception, moisture, activity, mobility, nutrition, and friction (Braden & Bergstrom, 1989). High scores place the patient at high risk.
Wounds, Drains, Devices Assess IV site, drainage, catheter, and suction. ■ Wound healing, drains intact, catheter draining well, suction on. IV site clean, dry, and without erythema or tenderness.	Pressure ulcers may be deep tissue, Stage I, Stage II, Stage III, Stage IV, or unstageable (Black, et al., 2007). Stages I and II are partial thickness into the dermis. Stages III and IV are full thickness. Wound drainage is classified as serous (clear), sanguineous (bloody), serosanguineous (mixed), fibrinous (sticky yellow), or purulent (pus). Note any signs or symptoms of infection.
Male Genitalia Obtain gloves and Hemoccult card. ■ No redness or discharge; skin intact. Palpate the scrotum for tenderness, lumps, and masses. ■ No tenderness, lumps, or masses. Assess for inguinal hernia. ■ No hernia.	Abnormal genital hair findings are no hair, patchy growth, or distribution in a female or triangular pattern with base over the pubis. Observe for infestations such as pediculosis, scabies, or other signs of parasites. Look for inflammation, lesions, or dermatitis. Candidiasis infections cause crusty, multiple, red, rounded erosions and pustules; this infection is associated with immunological deficiencies. Tinea cruris (commonly referred to as "jock itch") is a fungal infection present on the patient's groin and upper thighs. It appears with large, red, scaly patches that are extremely itchy. Tinea cruris rarely involves the scrotum.
Female Genitalia Obtain gloves, speculum, gel, and Hemoccult card. Inspect perineal and perianal areas. ■ No redness or tenderness; skin intact.	Symptoms of infection with herpes simplex virus 2 include vulvar or vaginal pain, flulike symptoms (e.g., chills, fever), sores on the vulva or genital region, scattered vesicles along the labia, matching vesicles on the labia reflecting "kissing" lesions, surface ulcerations or crusted healing lesions, and inguinal lymphadenopathy.
Insert speculum. Inspect cervix and vaginal walls. ■ Vaginal walls pink, no lesions. Cervix pink, round, no discharge.	
Obtain specimens. Remove speculum. ■ No infections; Pap test result negative.	
Perform bimanual examination of cervix, uterus, and adnexa. ■ No pain when moving the cervix, uterus midline; no enlargement, masses or tenderness. Adnexa and ovaries smooth; no masses or tenderness.	

(table continues on page 936)

Technique and Normal Findings (continued)	Abnormal Findings (continued)
Rectum Inspect perianal area. No redness or tenderness; skin intact.	Look for thrombosed hemorrhoids, rectal fissures, or hard stool. Hemorrhoids can be classified as external or internal. Hemorrhoids are usually caused by constant or excessive straining during defecation.
With lubricated finger, palpate rectal wall (and prostate in male). No hemorrhoids, fissures, lesions, masses, or tenderness. Rectal wall intact. Male: prostate smooth and round.	
Obtain stool sample to test for occult blood. Stool soft and brown.	
Closure • Summarize findings for patient. "Does this sound accurate?" • Assess room for safety (bedside table, lights, call light, toileting). "Do you have any concerns?" • Assess for questions or further needs. "Is there anything else I can do?" • Wash hands or use hand gel when leaving.	Summarizing findings provides closure and ensures accurate conclusions. Asking an open-ended question allows the patient to add any other information that might have been overlooked. Assessing for safety is of primary importance. Always assess the patient and environment for risks. Follow up on care planning and interventions for the next visit.

Documenting Case Study Findings

Mrs. Suleri's primary problem is related to the bleeding caused by ulcerative colitis. Other issues that can be clustered and further assessed include diarrhea from ulcerative colitis, pain from cramping, anemia from blood loss, fatigue resulting from anemia, and nutritional status related to obesity and dietary intake. Focusing on these problems, the nurse notes the following findings:

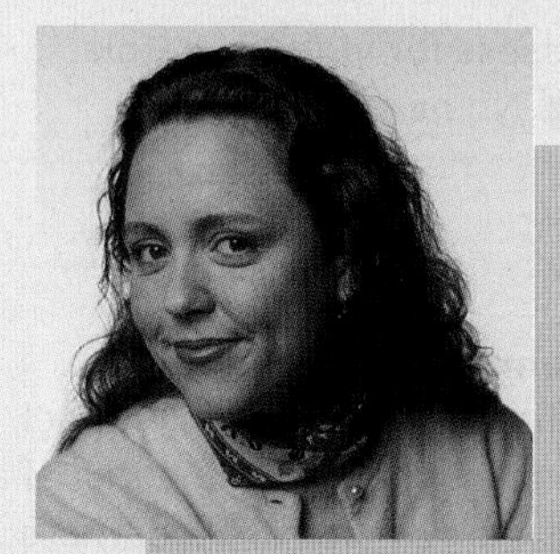

Inspection: Five dark-brown liquid stools over 12 hours totaling 500 ml. Hemoccult positive for blood. Reports abdominal pain primarily in lower quadrants. Rates pain as 5 on a 1–10 scale. Describes it as a cramping gnawing sensation that comes in waves but never completely goes away, rates it as 2/10 when best. Skin color pale, P 110 beats/min, BP 112/80 mm Hg, last hemoglobin 10 g/dl (low), and hematocrit 31% (low). Intake for past 12 hours 800 ml (27 oz) and output 860 ml (29 oz). Weight 92 kg (202.8 lb), down 1.5 kg (3.3 lb) from yesterday. Abdomen protuberant.

Auscultation: Bowel sounds hyperactive in all four quadrants.

Palpation: Abdomen soft but tender to light palpation. Facial grimace present, guarding abdomen.

Percussion: Abdomen tympanic.

Critical Thinking

Laboratory and Diagnostic Testing

Many patients in primary care settings and most hospitalized patients have a standard set of screening tests done to identify common problems. Electrolytes are measured to identify imbalances.

> ⚠ *SAFETY ALERT*
> *Serum potassium level may affect neural or cardiac cell conduction, leading to arrhythmias and potentially to cardiac arrest. Potassium must be maintained within normal limits and abnormalities must be corrected promptly.*

Any unexpectedly high or low serum sodium level can be a reflection of sodium intake but is more likely a reflection of having too much or too little water, therefore diluting or concentrating the sodium. Laboratory tests for red blood cells, hemoglobin, and hematocrit reflect the blood's oxygen-carrying capacity. Chest x-ray may be ordered for some patients to identify areas of infection, collapse, or fluid. Routine urinalysis may be ordered to identify whether an infection, blood, or sedimentation is present. Additional tests depend on the individual patient's problems. It is important to be able to recognize the significance of abnormal test results.

BOX 30.1 Nursing Diagnoses for Primary Care

- Health-seeking behaviors
- Risk for knowledge deficit
- Effective therapeutic regimen management
- Risk for impaired comfort
- Risk for injury

Diagnostic Reasoning

Nursing Diagnoses, Outcomes, and Interventions

Nursing diagnoses must be individualized to the patient and his or her current conditions. These include both actual diagnoses and those for which the patient is at risk. See Box 30.1.

Progress Note: Analyzing Findings

The nurse analyzes findings and synthesizes information to initiate a plan of care. The nursing thinking is shown in progress notes, in this case, using the SOAP format. The subjective and objective data are from the assessment that the nurse has performed. The analysis then leads to a preliminary plan of care.

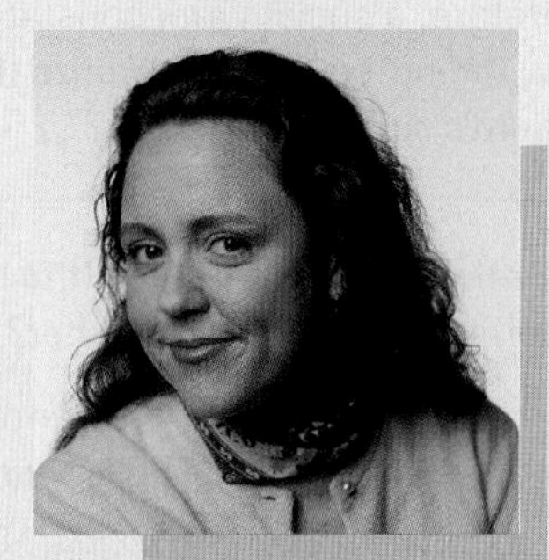

Subjective: "I've been having about 10 bloody stools a day and I'm just exhausted. This pain and cramping have just really gotten to me."

Objective: Reports abdominal pain primarily in lower quadrants. Rates pain as 5 on a 1–10 scale. Describes it as a cramping gnawing sensation that comes in waves but never completely goes away, rates it as 2/10 when best. Soaking in her bathtub and staying quiet seem to alleviate the pain. Stress, coffee, increased activity, and the end of the day make it worse. Hopes to achieve pain of 2/10 at peak and reduction in cramping. Functional goal is to return to normal activities at home, including cooking meals and transporting children, and also return to work. Concerned about financial issues. Facial grimace present, guarding abdomen.

Assessment: Pain related to ulcerative colitis exacerbation as evidenced by pain 5/10, facial grimace, and guarding. Risk for ineffective coping because of illness and financial concerns.

(case study continues on page 938)

Plan: Provide medication for pain as ordered. Teach relaxation techniques as a non-pharmacological pain measure. Limit mobility and provide rest. Allow periods of sleep at night. Assess foods that are preferred. Contact social work to evaluate need for additional resources.

Critical Thinking Challenge

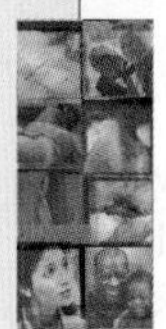

- What other assessment should be gathered based on the number of bloody stools?
- Are there other items that the nurse may want to assess based on the pain level?
- What other body systems might be affected based on the known assessments?

Collaborating With the Interprofessional Team

In many facilities, nurses initiate referrals based on assessment findings. Social workers help patients to cope with and solve issues related to family and personal problems. Some social workers help clients who face a disability, life-threatening disease, inadequate housing, unemployment, financial concern, or substance abuse. Social workers also assist families with domestic conflicts, such as child or spousal abuse. In the hospital setting, they assist with financial issues, patient placement, and funding for placements and resources after discharge.

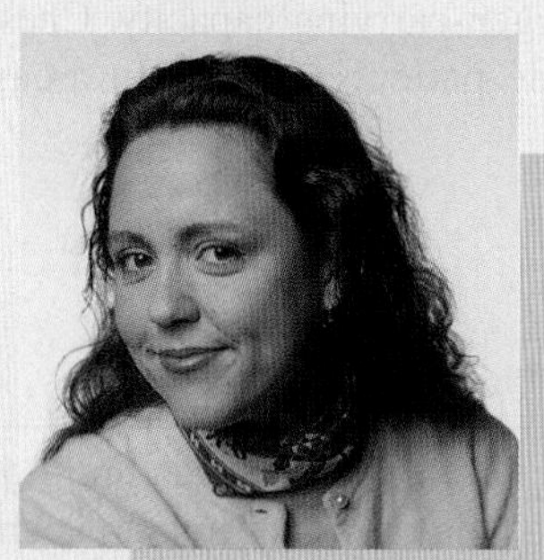

Mrs. Suleri has been experiencing many of the problems outlined above; therefore, a social work consult is indicated. The following conversation illustrates how the nurse might organize the data and make recommendations about the patient's situation.

Situation: "Hello, Margie" (the social worker for the unit). "I'm taking care of Mrs. Suleri today. Do you know her?" (Margie replies no.)

Background: "She is a 44-year-old woman who was admitted with bleeding related to her ulcerative colitis. She is married and has two children ages 15 and 13 years old."

Assessment: "She is currently employed but has been missing a lot of work because of her colitis. She's worried about caring for her family because she has two young teenagers. She also is worried about her finances and medical bills because her insurance only covers 80% of the hospital bill."

Recommendations: "Do you think that you would be able to see her in the next day or so to talk with her about resources?"

Critical Thinking Challenge

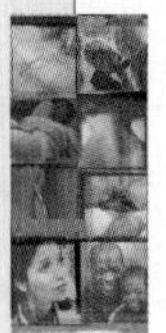

- What other assessments might the nurse make based on Mrs. Suleri's role in the family?
- How might her additional stressors be affecting her physiological health?
- What other nursing diagnoses might be considered regarding her psychological health?

Pulling It All Together

The nurse uses assessment data to formulate a nursing care plan with patient outcomes and interventions for Mrs. Suleri. Outcomes are specific to the patient, realistic to achieve, measurable, and have a time frame for meeting the outcome. The interventions are actions that the nurse performs, based on evidence and practice guidelines. After these interventions are completed, the nurse reevaluates Mrs. Suleri and documents the findings in the chart to show progress toward the patient outcome. The nurse uses critical thinking and judgment to continue or revise the diagnosis, outcomes, or interventions. This is often in the form of a care plan or case note similar to the one seen below.

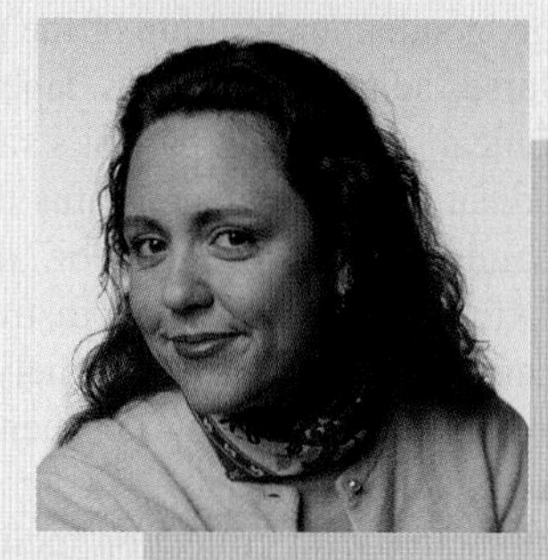

Nursing Diagnosis	Patient Outcomes	Nursing Interventions	Rationale	Evaluation
Fatigue related to anemia as evidenced by low hematocrit, hemoglobin; patient pale, tired	Patient will explain an energy conservation plan to offset effects of fatigue.	Assess severity of fatigue on a 0–10 scale. Evaluate adequacy of nutrition and sleep patterns. Collaborate with primary health care provider to treat anemia.	Fatigue is discomfort that can be rated using a numerical scale. A commonly suggested treatment is rest. Fatigue is related to the anemia from bleeding.	Patient stated that she has not been sleeping well because of cramping, pain, and frequent stools at night. Will plan to provide medication for diarrhea and sleeping tonight. Would like to have sign on the door asking to not be awakened. Taking 50% of meals at this time.

From NANDA International. (2012). *Nursing diagnoses: Definitions and classification 2012–2014* (9th ed.). Oxford, United Kingdom: Wiley-Blackwell; Bulechek, G. M., Butcher, H. K., Dochterman, J. M., & Wagner, C. M. (2013). *Nursing interventions classification (NIC)* (6th ed.). St. Louis, MO: Mosby; Moorhead, S., Johnson, M., Maas, M. L., & Swanson, E. (2013). *Nursing outcomes classification (NOC): Measurement of health outcomes* (5th ed.). St. Louis, MO: Elsevier.

Applying Your Knowledge

Using the previous steps of diagnostic reasoning, organizing, and prioritizing, consider all the case study findings woven throughout this chapter. When answering the following questions, begin drawing conclusions and see how the pieces of assessment must work together to create an environment for personalized, appropriate, and accurate care.

When is a focused health assessment used?

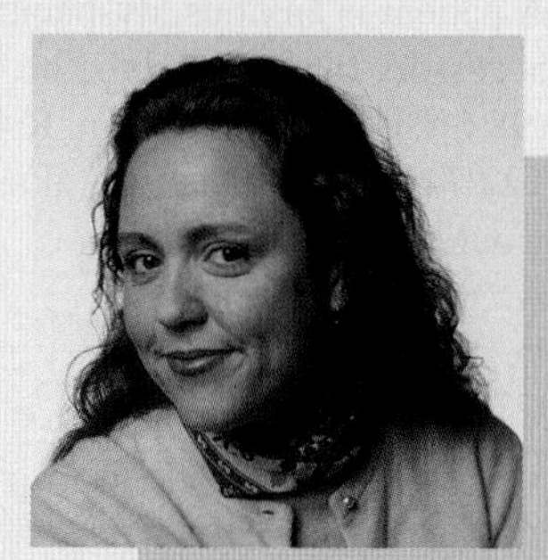

- Describe the differences among comprehensive, focused, and screening assessments.
- How will the nurse individualize the admitting history to focus it on Mrs. Suleri?
- How will the nurse focus the physical assessments considering Mrs. Suleri's diagnosis?
- How will the nurse use the assessment information to develop a plan of care?
- How will the nurse evaluate the effectiveness of the assessment?

Key Points

- Health assessment is individualized based on the condition, age, gender, and culture of the patient.
- Nurses adapt assessments depending on scope of practice, clinical setting, and patient's situation.
- Indications of unstable status that necessitate intervention include cyanosis or pallor, dyspnea, strained posture, anxious facial expression, distressed appearance, difficulty managing the airway, extremely high or low pulse or blood pressure, acute change in mental status, or new onset of chest pain.
- Subjective data collection includes health promotion, risk factors, history of present problem, past medical and family history, personal and social history, and assessment of common symptoms.
- Objective data collection is organized by body area, moving from head to toes for efficiency.
- Inspection, palpation, percussion, and auscultation are techniques used during the head-to-toe assessment.
- Nurses document and communicate assessment data using appropriate medical terminology.
- Assessment occurs during all phases of the nursing process.
- An accurate and complete health assessment is the foundation for appropriate holistic and individualized nursing care.

Review Questions

1. The nurse performs the first assessment on the hospitalized patient and documents it in the chart as the
   A. sporadic assessment.
   B. functional assessment.
   C. focused assessment.
   D. admitting assessment.

2. A patient is anxious, dyspneic, and pale and uses accessory muscles to breathe. Vital signs are T 37°C (98.6°F), P 126 beats/min, R 40 breaths/min, and BP 122/74 mm Hg. The type of assessment that the nurse would perform is a(n)
   A. acute assessment.
   B. general survey.
   C. health history.
   D. objective assessment.

3. The nurse assesses a patient presenting with nausea, vomiting, and diarrhea. In performing the focused assessment, the nurse uses the following techniques:
   A. Auscultate lungs, auscultate heart, auscultate abdomen.
   B. Evaluate for dehydration, assess skin turgor, auscultate lungs.
   C. Auscultate abdomen, palpate abdomen, evaluate for dehydration.
   D. Palpate abdomen, percuss abdomen, auscultate heart.

4. After receiving patient information from the previous-shift nurse and gathering data from the chart, the nurse will assess a group of four patients. Which one will the nurse assess first?
   A. A 32-year-old man with an open wound who is receiving antibiotics
   B. A 66-year-old woman 2 days postoperatively following ankle surgery
   C. A 45-year-old man with HIV and *Pneumocystis jiroveci* pneumonia with dyspnea
   D. An 88-year-old woman with confusion who had a stroke 4 days ago

5. The nurse gathers subjective data related to the history of the present problem. The following items are included:
   A. Onset, location, duration, character, aggravating/associated factors, relieving factors, temporal factors, severity
   B. Asymmetry, borders, color, diameter
   C. Heart rate, respiratory effort, response, color
   D. Eye opening, verbal response, motor response

6. The nurse usually performs a complete physical examination with elements in the following order:
   A. Face, heart, legs, arms
   B. Head, abdomen, lungs, legs
   C. Eyes, heart, abdomen, legs
   D. Ears, back, lungs, arms

7. A patient develops a sudden onset of acute chest pain. In addition to a complete description of the symptoms, what objective assessment is a priority?
   A. Pulse, blood pressure, peripheral pulses
   B. Heart sounds, rate, and rhythm
   C. Circulation, sensation, and movement
   D. Murmurs, rubs, and gallops

8. A 50-year-old patient is seen in the clinic for an annual physical examination and screening. The patient has no known health problems. This type of care is referred to as
   A. primary prevention.
   B. promotion prevention.
   C. tertiary prevention.
   D. healthy prevention.

9. The nurse assesses whether the patient outcome "Patient drinks 1 L every shift" has been met. This is called
   A. assessment.
   B. planning.
   C. implementation.
   D. evaluation.

10. Auscultation is one of the most important components of which body systems?
   A. Reproductive, neurological, integumentary
   B. Cardiovascular, pulmonary, gastrointestinal
   C. Pulmonary, gastrointestinal, neurological
   D. Gastrointestinal, neurological, reproductive

The Jensen suite offers these additional resources to enhance learning and facilitate understanding of this chapter:

- thePoint online resource, http://thepoint.lww.com/Jensen2e
- *Laboratory Manual for Nursing Health Assessment: A Best Practice Approach*
- *Pocket Guide for Nursing Health Assessment: A Best Practice Approach*
- *Lippincott DocuCare*, an electronic health record simulation software, http://thepoint.lww.com/docucare
- *Adaptive Learning | Powered by PrepU*, http://thepoint.lww.com/prepu

References

American Heart Association. (2013). *About high blood pressure*. Retrieved from http://www.heart.org/HEARTORG/Conditions/HighBloodPressure/AboutHighBloodPressure/About-High-Blood-Pressure_UCM_002050_Article.jsp#

Black, J., Baharestani, M., Cuddigan, J., Dorner, B., Edsberg, L., Langemo, D., . . . Ratliff, C. (2007). National Pressure Ulcer Advisory Panel's updated pressure ulcer staging system. *Dermatological Nursing*, *19*(4), 343–349.

Braden, B., & Bergstrom, M. (1989). Clinical utility of the Braden scale for predicting pressure sore risk. *Advances in Skin and Wound Care*, *2*(3), 44–51.

Bulechek, G. M., Butcher, H. K., Dochterman, J. M., & Wagner, C. M. (2013). *Nursing interventions classification (NIC)*, (6th ed.). St. Louis, MO: Mosby.

Moorhead, S., Johnson, M., Maas, M. L., & Swanson, E. (2013). *Nursing outcomes classification (NOC): Measurement of health outcomes* (5th ed.). St. Louis, MO: Elsevier.

NANDA-International. (2012). *Nursing diagnoses: Definitions and classification 2012–2014* (9th ed.). Oxford, United Kingdom: Wiley-Blackwell.

U.S. Department of Health & Human Services. (2013). *2020 Topics & objectives - Objectives A-Z*. Retrieved from http://www.healthypeople.gov/2020/topicsobjectives2020/

U.S. Preventive Services Task Force. (2013). *Guide to clinical preventive services*. Retrieved from http://www.ahrq.gov/professionals/clinicians-providers/guidelines-recommendations/guide/index.html

Appendix A

Key Terms and Definitions

Chapter 1, The Nurse's Role in Health Assessment

Advanced practice registered nurse (APRN): An umbrella term given to an RN who has achieved a bachelor's degree in nursing science (BSN), which includes educational and clinical practice requirements, as well as a minimum of a master's degree.

Advocacy: Nursing role that encompasses keeping patients safe, communicating their needs, identifying side effects of treatment and finding better options, and helping them to understand their diseases and treatments so they can optimize self-care.

Assessment: Gathering information about the health status of the patient, analyzing and synthesizing those data, making judgments about nursing interventions based on the findings, and evaluating patient care outcomes.

Body systems assessment: Assessment method in which a nurse examines the patient focused on a single system or clusters data related to that system together to identify issues.

CNM: Certified nurse midwife.

CNS: Clinical nurse specialist.

Collaborative problems: Problems that nurses monitor but require the expertise of other health care providers for intervention.

Communication: The use of words and behaviors to convey information.

Comprehensive assessment: An assessment that includes a complete health history and physical assessment; it is done annually on an outpatient basis, following admission to a hospital or long-term care facility, or every 8 hours for patients in intensive care.

Critical thinking: Thinking that requires specific knowledge, skills, and experience and is purposeful and outcome-directed (results-oriented); driven by patient, family, and community needs; based on the nursing process, evidence-based thinking, and the scientific method; guided by professional standards and codes of ethics; and constantly reevaluating, self-correcting, and striving to improve.

CRNA: Certified registered nurse anesthetist.

Cultural competence: The complex combination of knowledge, attitudes, and skills that a health care provider uses to deliver care that considers the total context of the patient's situation across cultural boundaries.

Diagnosis: Clustering of data that makes a judgment or statement about the patient's problem or condition.

Diagnostic reasoning: The process of gathering and clustering data to draw inferences and propose diagnoses.

Documentation: The recording of patient information.

Emergency assessment: An assessment that involves a life-threatening or unstable situation and that focuses on A—airway (with cervical spine protection if injury is suspected); B—breathing (rate and depth, use of accessory muscles); C—circulation (pulse rate and rhythm, skin color); D—disability (level of consciousness, pupils, movement); and E—exposure.

Evaluation: Judgment of the effectiveness of nursing care in meeting the patient's goals and outcomes based on the patient's responses to the interventions.

Evidence-based practice: Approach to patient care that minimizes intuition and personal experience and instead relies on research findings and high-grade scientific support.

Focused assessment: An assessment based on the patient's issues that can occur in all health care settings; it usually involves one or two body systems and is smaller in scope than the comprehensive assessment but more in depth on the specific issue(s).

Functional assessment: An assessment that focuses on the functional patterns that all humans share: health perception and health management, activity and exercise, nutrition and metabolism, elimination, sleep and rest, cognition and perception, self-perception and self-concept, roles and relationships, coping and stress tolerance, sexuality and reproduction, and values and beliefs.

Head-to-toe assessment: An assessment that organizes the collection of comprehensive physical data by proceeding through the entire body from head to toe.

Health assessment: Gathering information about the health status of the patient, analyzing and synthesizing those data, making judgments about nursing interventions based on the findings, and evaluating patient care outcomes.

Health history: Data relating to a patient's demographics, reason for seeking care, and present illness.

Healthy People: The national model for health promotion and risk reduction developed by the U.S. Department of Health & Human Services.

Illness: State in which patients experience objective signs and subjective symptoms of sickness, with subsequent disability.

NP: Nurse practitioner.

Objective data: Measurable findings from the health assessment, usually gathered in the physical examination.

Outcomes: More specific than goals; these are the realistic and measurable desired consequences of nursing interventions.

Planning care: Determining resources, targeting nursing interventions, and writing the plan of care.

Primary prevention: Strategies aimed at preventing health problems.

Priority setting: A professional nursing skill by which nurses organize activities and issues by focusing on the most important and immediate concerns first.

Research: The systematic gathering and analysis of information with the goal of informing nursing practice.

Risk reduction: Actions aimed at decreasing the likelihood that individuals or communities will experience health problems.

RN: Registered nurse.

Scholarship: Actions that systematically advance the teaching, research, and practice of nursing.

Secondary prevention: The early diagnosis of health problems and provision of treatment to prevent complications.

Subjective data: Findings from the health assessment that are based on patient experiences and perceptions. They are usually revealed during the interview and health history taking.

Tertiary prevention: Prevention of complications from an existing disease and promoting health to the highest level.

Urgent assessment: Appraisal of a life-threatening or unstable health situation.

Wellness: Process by which people maintain balance and direction in the most favorable environment.

Chapter 2, The Health History and Interview

Active listening: The ability to focus on patients and their perspectives.

Activities of daily living (ADLs): Self-care activities that include behaviors such as eating, dressing, and grooming.

Beginning phase: The phase of the interview process in which you introduce yourself, state the purpose of the interview, and try to put the patient at ease.

Caring: The demonstration of empathy for and connection with the patient. It also includes the ability to demonstrate emotional characteristics such as compassion, sensitivity, and patient-centeredness.

Clarification: A therapeutic communication technique that nurses use when a patient's word choice or ideas are unclear to better understand the meaning. For example, the nurse states, "Tell me what you mean by . . . ." Clarification prompts patients to identify other facts or give more information so that the nurse better understands.

Closed-ended (direct) questions: Questions that yield "yes" or "no" responses and are focused on obtaining facts. An example would be, "Do you have a family history of heart disease?"

Closing phase: The phase of the interview in which you summarize, elicit outstanding questions, and thank the patient for participating.

Communication etiquette: The code of conduct and good manners by which those engaged in communication show respect for others.

Elaboration (facilitation): Providing interview responses that encourage patients to say more and continue the conversation.

Empathy: The ability to perceive, reason, and communicate understanding of another person's feelings without criticism. It is being able to see and feel the situation from the patient's perspective, not your own.

False reassurance: Dismissing the patient's concerns in order to minimize uncomfortable feelings.

Focusing: A therapeutic communication technique used when patients are straying from a topic and need redirection. An example is, "We were talking about the reaction that you had to the penicillin. Tell me more about that reaction."

Functional health patterns: Gordon's (1987) approach to assessment that addresses each of the domains of a patient's quality of life and functional status.

Inaccurate historian: A patient who provides inconsistent or unreliable information.

Intercultural communication: The sender of an intended message belongs to one culture, whereas the receiver is from another. Cultural differences may exist related to group or ethnicity, region, age, degree of acculturation into Western society, or a combination of these factors.

Nonverbal communication: Form of communication including physical appearance, facial expression, posture and positioning in relation to the patient, gestures, eye contact, voice, and use of touch.

Nurse–patient relationship: The professionally intimate relationship that is built on communication within a specific setting.

Objective data: Data that are measurable and visible.

Open-ended questions: Questions that require patients to give more than "yes" or "no" answers. They are broad and provide responses in the patient's own words.

Preinteraction phase: The phase of the interview in which you collect data from various sources, including the medical record.

Primary data: Data that are collected directly from the patient.

Professional boundary: The practice of avoiding social, personal, or economic ties with a patient.

Reflection: Similar to restatement; however, instead of simply restating comments, the nurse summarizes the main themes of communication. The conversation may be longer, in which a patient discusses several elements related to a topic. The nurse listens carefully to the different thoughts expressed and attempts to identify their relationship. With this technique, patients gain a better understanding of the issues that underlie their thoughts, which helps to identify their feelings.

Reliable historian: A patient who provides accurate information that is comprehensive and consistent with existing records.

Restatement: A therapeutic communication technique by which the nurse makes a simple statement, usually using the words of the patient, to prompt the patient to elaborate. Restatement provides an opportunity for patients to further understand their communication.

Review of systems (ROS): A series of questions about all body systems that helps to reveal concerns as part of a comprehensive health assessment.

Secondary data: Data that are obtained from charts and the patient's family members.

Self-concept: An awareness of your own biases, values, personality, cultural background, and communication style.

Signs and symptoms: Objective (signs) and subjective (symptoms) data relating to a patient's health status.

Silence: Purposefully not speaking during an interview to allow patients time to gather their thoughts and provide accurate answers or to communicate nonverbal concern. Silence also gives patients a chance to decide how much information to disclose.

Subjective data: Sensations that the patient reports, which may not be perceived by observers.

Summarizing: Used at the end of the interview, during the closure phase, when the nurse reviews and condenses important information into two or three of the most important findings. Doing so helps ensure that the nurse has identified important information and lets the patient know that he or she has been heard accurately.

Sympathy: A nontherapeutic approach in which you claim to feel what the patient is feeling based on your own perception of the patient's experience.

Therapeutic communication: A basic tool that the nurse uses in a caring relationship with patients. In therapeutic communication, the interaction focuses on the patient and the patient's concerns. The nurse assists patients to work through feelings and explore options related to the situation, outcomes, and treatments.

Working phase: The phase of the interview process in which you collect data by asking specific questions.

Chapter 3, Physical Examination Techniques and Equipment

Auscultation: One of the techniques used for conducting a physical assessment by which the nurse listens for movements of air or fluid in the body.

Dull: A tone of a sound during physical assessment that is high in pitch, sounds like a thud, and is heard over the liver.

Flat: A tone of sound during physical assessment that is high in pitch, sounds dull, and is heard over bone.

Hand hygiene: Practices that include the use of alcohol-based hand rubs, handwashing, and use of gloves.

Inspection: A technique used in a physical assessment by which the nurse observes the patient for general appearance and any specific details related to the body system, region, or condition under examination.

Latex allergy: Hypersensitivity reaction that usually results from repeated exposures through skin contact or inhalation to proteins in natural rubber latex

Palpation: An assessment technique by which the nurse uses the hands to feel the firmness of body parts, such as the abdomen.

Percussion: An assessment technique by which the nurse uses tapping motions with the hands to produce sounds that indicate solid or air-filled spaces over the lungs and other areas.

Resonant: A tone of a sound during physical assessment that is very loud, hollow in quality, of long duration, and heard over healthy lungs.

Respiratory hygiene/cough etiquette: The expectation that patients and other people with symptoms of a respiratory infection will cover their mouths and noses with a tissue when coughing or sneezing.

Standard precautions: A set of guidelines from the Centers for Disease Control and Prevention that exist to help prevent disease transmission during contact with nonintact skin, mucous membranes, body substances, and bloodborne contacts (e.g., needlestick injury).

Tympanic: Refers to the membrane that separates the outer ear from the middle ear. It can also describe a loud, high-pitched, drumlike sound of moderate duration heard during the physical assessment.

Chapter 4, Documentation and Interdisciplinary Communication

Audit: Review of a health care facility by an agency or outside group to determine whether that facility is providing and documenting certain standards of care.

Batch charting: Waiting until end of shift or until all patients have been assessed to document findings from all of them.

Charting by exception: Use of predetermined standards and norms to record only significant assessment data.

Clinical pathway: A multidisciplinary tool that identifies a standard plan for a specific patient population.

Confidentiality: Keeping information private.

Flowsheet: Efficient and standardized form that assembles the collected information in a way that permits easy comparison among assessment data to detect trends or a sudden change in status.

Handoff: Transfer of care for a patient from one health care provider to another.

Meaningful use: An agency's ability to electronically transfer clinical information as the patient moves from one provider to another or one health care system to another.

Never event: A preventable error, treatment of which is not reimbursed by Medicare and Medicaid.

Point-of-care documentation: Occurs when nurses document assessment information as they gather it, often using a portable computer.

Progress note: An entry in the patient's record made by any member of the health care team.

Reporting: Occurs at handoffs, during patient rounds, during patient and family care conferences, and when calling or text-paging a provider to report a change in status or provide requested information.

Sentinel event: A serious, often life-threatening, error in health care.

Chapter 5, Vital Signs and General Survey

Afebrile: Condition of being without fever.

Apnea: The absence of spontaneous respirations for more than 10 seconds.

Asystole: The absence of a pulse.

Auscultatory gap: A period in which there are no Korotkoff sounds during auscultation.

Blood pressure: The measurement of the force exerted by the flow of blood against the arterial walls.

Bradycardia: A heart rate less than 60 beats/min.

Bradypnea: Persistent respiratory rate greater than 12 breaths/min.

Diastolic blood pressure: The lowest pressure in blood pressure, which occurs when the left ventricle relaxes between beats.

Doppler transducer: Handheld transducer that senses and amplifies blood pressure sounds.

Dyspnea: Difficulty breathing.

Eupnea: Normal respiratory rate, rhythm, and effort.

General survey: An assessment that begins with the first moment of the encounter with the patient and continues throughout the health history, during the physical examination, and with each subsequent interaction. It is the first component of the assessment, when the nurse makes mental notes of the patient's overall behavior, physical appearance, and mobility.

Hyperpnea: Resting respiration that is deeper and more rapid than normal.

Hypertension: A blood pressure greater than 140/90 mm Hg.

Hyperthermia: Temperature greater than 100°F (37.8°C).

Hyperventilation: Deep, rapid respirations.

Hypotension: Systolic blood pressure less than 90 mm Hg.

Hypothermia: Core temperature less than 95°F (35°C).

Hypoventilation: Shallow, slow respirations.

Mean arterial pressure: Blood pressure that is calculated by adding one third of the systolic blood pressure to two thirds of the diastolic blood pressure.

Orthostatic hypotension: When going from a supine or sitting position to a standing position, a drop in systolic blood pressure of 15 mm Hg or greater, drop in diastolic blood pressure of 10 mm Hg or greater, or increased heart rate.

Oxygen saturation: A relative measure of the amount of oxygen dissolved or carried in a given medium.

Pulse deficit: The difference that exists between apical and peripheral pulses.

Pulse oximetry: A noninvasive technique to measure oxygen saturation of arterial blood.

Pulse pressure: The difference between the systolic and diastolic blood pressures; reflects the stroke volume.

Sinus arrhythmia: .Pulse that speeds up during inspiration and slows down during expiration. It is a normal finding in children and some adults.

Sphygmomanometer: The instrument used to measure blood pressure.

Systolic blood pressure: Maximum pressure on the walls of the arteries with contraction of the left ventricle at the beginning of systole.

Tachycardia: A heart rate greater than 100 beats/min in an adult.

Tachypnea: A rapid, persistent respiratory rate greater than 20 breaths/min in an adult.

Vital signs: Important indicators of the patient's physiological status and response to the environment. They encompass temperature, pulse, respirations, and blood pressure.

Chapter 6, Pain Assessment

Acute pain: Pain that results from tissue damage, whether through injury or surgery.

Central sensitization: Excitatory process involving spinal nerves and produced by continued pain stimuli; it can persist even after peripheral stimulation is no longer present.

Chronic pain: Pain that lasts beyond the normal healing period and has no role.

Complex regional pain syndrome: A chronic neuropathic pain syndrome.

Cutaneous pain: Derives from the dermis, epidermis, and subcutaneous tissues. It is often burning or sharp, such as with a partial-thickness burn.

Gate control theory: The theory of pain with the widest acceptance; it posits that the body responds to a painful stimulus by either opening a neural gate to allow pain to be produced or creating a blocking effect at the synaptic junction to stop the pain.

Modulation: Inhibitory and facilitating input from the brain that eases or influences sensory transmission at the level of the spinal cord.

Neuronal plasticity: Ability of the nervous system to change or alter its function.

Neuronal windup: Enhanced response to pain stimulus produced by prolonged pain production.

Neuropathic pain: A condition that follows constant stimuli and sensitization, in which nonpainful touch or pressure becomes painful.

Nociception: The perception of pain by sensory receptors located throughout the body.

Nociceptors: Specialized peripheral A and C nerve fibers that carry the pain signal to the central nervous system.

Opioid hyperalgesia: An altered physiologic response to the pain stimulus in which repeated use of opioids causes a person to become more sensitive to pain.

OLDCARTS: A mnemonic for pain assessment (O: onset; L: location; D: duration; C: character; A: aggravating/relieving; R: radiation; T: timing; S: severity).

OPQRST: A mnemonic for pain assessment (O: onset; P: provocative or palliative; Q: quality; R: region and radiation; S: severity; T: timing).

Pain: An uncomfortable feeling transmitted along pain fibers to the central nervous system. One of the most common reasons patients seek help from health care professionals.

Perception: The impulses being transmitted to the higher areas of the brain are identified as pain.

Peripheral sensitization: Result of inflammatory process that creates hypersensitivity to touch or pressure.

Referred pain: Originates from a specific site, but the person experiencing it feels the pain at another site along the innervating spinal nerve.

Somatic pain: Originates from skin, muscles, bones, and joints. Patients usually describe somatic pain as sharp.

Transduction: Noxious stimuli create enough of an energy potential to cause a nerve impulse perceived by nociceptors (free nerve endings).

Transmission: The neuronal signal moves from the periphery to the spinal cord and up to the brain.

Visceral pain: Originates from abdominal organs and is often described as crampy or gnawing.

Windup: Enhanced response to pain stimulus produced by prolonged pain production.

Chapter 7, Nutrition Assessment

Adequate intake: The amount of a nutrient needed to keep the human healthy.

Albumin: A prime ingredient of blood oncotic pressure and a carrier protein for many body and pharmacological substances.

Body mass index: A guide for maintaining ideal weight for height. It is also used as a benchmark for obesity or protein-calorie malnutrition.

Cachexia: A highly catabolic state with accelerated muscle loss and a chronic inflammatory response. It is a distinct syndrome separate from anorexia with production of proinflammatory cytokines that contribute to breakdown of fat and muscle protein, causing loss of both muscle mass and fat stores.

Calorie count: A tool that counts every calorie a patient takes in during a 24-hour period.

Creatinine: A serum protein that is elevated with kidney disease.

Dysphagia: Difficulty swallowing; may be oral, pharyngeal, or esophageal in origin.

Electrolytes: Elements e.g., sodium, potassium) needed by the body to maintain functioning.

Food frequency questionnaire: A tool to identify the number of times a person eats a specific food in a designated period.

Food pathogens: Disease-causing microbes that live in the food supply.

Hydrogenation: The chemical processing of animal fats used by food manufacturers to extend the shelf life of products susceptible to rancidity, such as cookies and crackers.

Intake and output: Food and fluid taken into the body and urine expelled from the body.

Mid upper arm muscle circumference/mid upper arm muscle areas: Indicators of muscle and body protein reserves.

Percentage of ideal body weight: Calculation based on the ideal and current weight according to the formula: Percentage of ideal body weight = current weight/ideal weight × 100.

Percentage of usual body weight: Calculation following the formula: Percentage of usual body weight = current weight/usual weight × 100.

Percentage of weight change: Calculation following the formula: (Usual weight − present weight)/usual weight × 100.

Prealbumin: A circulating protein in the blood.

Primary nutrients: Nutrients essential for optimal body function: carbohydrates, proteins, fats, vitamins, minerals, water, and major electrolytes.

Three-day food diary: A diary kept by the patient that reviews 3 days worth of food intake.

Transferrin: A serum protein with a half-life of 9 days.

Triceps skinfold: A measurement of skinfold thickness. Not representative of adipose tissue throughout the body.

24-Hour recall: A tool used to quantify the amount of food taken in over a 24-hour time period.

Waist circumference: The measurement around the waist. An indicator of accumulated body fat in the abdomen; a high circumference places people at increased risk of obesity-related diseases and early mortality.

Weight-for-height calculations: Reference standards for height and weight.

Chapter 8, Assessment of Developmental Stages

Autonomy versus shame and doubt: Erikson's task for the toddler, who must master two simultaneous sets of social modalities: holding on and letting go.

Cognitive development: Qualitative changes in a person's thinking and intellectual skills. Begins at birth and continues until adulthood; the person uses experience to move from stage to stage as thinking becomes more sophisticated and complex in interaction with his or her environment.

Concrete operational: Piaget's stage of cognitive development that lasts from approximately ages 7 to 11 years, in which the child becomes capable of performing *operations*, or internalized sets of actions that people do mentally instead of physically. Examples of concrete operations include conservation and categorization.

Development: Qualitative changes in a person over time, particularly in the areas of motor skills, language, psychosocial skills, and cognition.

Ego integrity versus despair: Erikson's eighth and last stage, experienced during late adulthood. The major task is coming to terms with life choices.

Formal operational: The last stage in Piaget's cognitive theory; hallmarks include abstract reasoning and the ability to discuss theoretical concepts.

Generativity versus stagnation: The seventh stage in Erikson's model, faced by adults in middle age, in which the hallmark concern is feeling needed by others.

Growth: Quantitative physical changes in a person over time.

Identity versus role confusion: Erikson's task for adolescents, who begin to face adult tasks and roles and become concerned with how others evaluate them as compared with who they believe themselves to be.

Industry versus inferiority: Erikson's task for the school-age child, who must learn to use the tools that adults commonly use within the specific society or environment. As the child spends more time in the school culture, prepared by teachers for the literate world, the influence of other adults dilutes the role of parents in the child's life.

Initiative versus guilt: Erikson's task for the preschooler, who is actively engaged in making plans, setting goals, and accomplishing them.

Intimacy versus isolation: Erikson's sixth psychosocial task, occurring in early adulthood, in which the person who has successfully navigated the search for personal identity is willing to fuse with the identity of others.

Preoperational stage: The second stage of Piaget's cognitive model, which lasts from approximately ages 2 to 7 years, during which the child forms stable concepts, begins to develop mental reasoning, and constructs magical beliefs.

Psychosocial development: The individual's development in interaction with the immediate environment.

Sensorimotor: Piaget's first stage of cognition, experienced by infants and young toddlers.

Trust versus mistrust: Erikson's first task faced in infancy, in which the baby learns that physiologic regulation is linked to a caregiver's provision of comfort.

Chapter 9, Mental Health and Violence Assessment

ABCT: A method of organizing data from the objective assessment: **A** (appearance), **B** (behavior), **C** (cognitive function), and **T** (thought process).

Bullying: Verbal and physical violence common among school-age and adolescent populations. Behaviors can range from teasing to physical assault.

CAGE: An assessment tool for alcohol and substance abuse. Questions are Have you ever felt the need to Cut down on drinking? Have you ever felt Annoyed by criticism of drinking? Have you ever had Guilty feelings about drinking? Have you ever taken a drink first thing in the morning (Eye-opener)?

Child maltreatment: A wide range of abusive and neglectful behaviors toward children.

Delirium: Confusion that generally has an underlying medical cause and, once treated, resolves.

Dementia: Confusion caused by brain disease that is more common in older adults. It is usually a gradual process over months to years.

Elder abuse: Maltreatment of older adults in the form of abuse, neglect, financial exploitation, or abandonment. Abuse includes intentional actions by a caregiver or other person who stands in a trust relationship to a vulnerable elder that cause harm or create a serious risk to him or her. Examples include kicking, punching, slapping, or burning.

Family violence: All types of violent crime committed by an offender who is related to the victim either biologically or legally through marriage or adoption.

Geriatric Depression Scale: A tool to assess for risk of depression in older adults.

Hate crime: Crime in which a victim is selected based on a characteristic such as race, ethnicity, sexual orientation, age, and the like and for which the perpetrator provides evidence that hate prompted him or her to commit the crime.

HOPE: A tool to assess for spirituality.

Human trafficking: The recruitment, transportation, transfer, harboring, or receipt of people by threats, force, coercion, or deception.

Intimate partner violence: Behaviors between spouses or nonmarital partners involving threatened or actual physical or sexual violence, psychological/emotional abuse, and/or coercive tactics when there has been prior physical or sexual violence.

Mental status examination: As assessment to tell the mental state of the patient.

Mini-mental status examination: A tool to quickly assess level of cognitive function.

Punking: Verbal and physical violence, humiliation, and shaming, usually done in public or with an audience.

SAD PERSONAS: A mnemonic used to assess for risk of suicide.

Sexual violence: Forced sex in dating and marital relationships, gang rape, sexual harassment, inappropriate touching or molestation, sex with a patient, or forced prostitution and/or exposure to sexually explicit behavior.

Sibling violence: Violence between and among siblings.

War/combat violence: Witnessing the killing of human beings, including friends and fellow service people; intentionally killing and injuring other humans; and being intentionally injured or potentially killed by another human.

Youth violence: Violence in and around schools and neighborhoods.

Chapter 10, Assessment of Social, Cultural, and Spiritual Health

Alternative medicine: Therapies that are used instead of conventional treatments to restore health.

Asset mapping: A type of systematic community assessment framework in which community assessment data are clustered into building blocks.

Biomedical model: The model of health that views health as the absence of disease.

Community as Partner Assessment Model: Anderson and McFarlane's (2011) community assessment framework, which helps nurses assess the demographics of a community.

Complementary medicine: Therapies that are used with conventional medicine.

Complementary and alternative medicine (CAM) model: A model of health that is defined in terms of its relation to the biomedical model of health. Treatments are chosen instead of or alongside conventional treatments.

Cultural assessment: The systematic assessment of individuals, families, and communities regarding their health beliefs and values.

Cultural safety: The practice of analyzing power imbalances in order to provide quality nursing care for individuals from different ethnicities.

Culture: The shared, learned, and symbolic system of values, beliefs, and attitudes that shape and influence how people see and behave in the world.

Eudaimonistic model of health: The model of health emphasizing wholeness of the individual as being essential to maintaining good health.

Functional health model: Gordon's (2006) model of health in which people are considered healthy if they can fulfill their social roles by contributing to family and society in meaningful ways.

Functional health patterns: Gordon's (2006) categories of behaviors that occur over time and that constitute health.

Madeleine Leininger's theory and the Sunrise Model: A nursing model that identifies the relationships between cultural variables and health and highlights the nursing behaviors and skills necessary to carry out effective cultural assessment.

Primary and secondary characteristics of culture: The influences that shape worldview and the extent to which people identify with their culture of origin.

Primary, secondary, and potential building blocks: The community assets that are identified within the asset mapping framework of community assessment.

Roy's adaptation model: The model of health that conceptualizes health as the patient's ability to adapt, compensate, manage, and adjust to physiological–physical health-related setbacks.

Social assessment: The practice of identifying the social context that influences the patterns of health and illness for individuals, communities, and societies.

Spiritual assessment: The practice of collecting data relating to considerations such as the human soul and relationship with the divine.

Spirituality: Matters of the human soul, be it a state of mind, a state of being in the world, a journey of self-discovery, or a place outside the five senses.

Chapter 11, Skin, Hair, and Nails Assessment

ABCDEs of melanoma detection: **A**symmetry, **B**order irregularity, **C**olor, **D**iameter of more than 6 mm, **E**volution of lesion over time.

Abrasion: Wound caused by shear force or friction against the skin, removing several layers and exposing the dermis.

Abscess: A contained accumulation of pus within a tissue.

Avulsion: Ragged wound that occurs when trauma forces the skin to separate from underlying structures.

Blister: a fluid-filled bubble on the skin caused by friction, burning, or hypersensitivity.

Brawny: Skin that is dark and leathery.

Clubbing of the nails: Finding in the nails that indicates chronic hypoxia.

Coining: A practice among Southeast Asians in which a coin or other object is rubbed across the skin in a specific manner to treat various health concerns.

Cupping: A cultural practice involving the placement of a cup on the skin surface, applying heat to form a vacuum.

Cyanosis: Gray or blue skin color, indicating lack of oxygen.

Cyst: Skin lesion that is distinct and walled-off and which contains fluid or semisolid material.

Dysplastic nevus: An atypical mole.

Ecchymosis: Bruise or bruising.

Erythema: Redness.

Flushing: Turning red, as with fever.

Hematoma: A collection of blood under the skin usually resulting from blunt-force trauma.

Jaundice: Yellowish discoloration of the skin and conjunctiva caused by a buildup of bilirubin in the body.

Laceration: A superficial or deep skin tear, often requiring suturing to heal correctly.

Macule: Flat, distinct, colored area of skin that is less than 10 mm in diameter and does not include a change in skin texture or thickness.

Malar rash: Red macular lesions distributed over the forehead, cheeks, and chin, resembling the pattern of a butterfly.

Nodule: Solid palpable lesion greater than 1 cm in diameter, often with some depth.

Pallor: Paleness of the skin.

Papule: Raised, defined lesion of any color; less than 1 cm in diameter.

Petechiae: small reddish to purple macules or papules that can develop anywhere on the body in response to physical trauma.

Plaque: Raised, defined lesion of any color, greater than 1 cm in diameter.

Polyp: An abnormal growth of tissue originating on a mucous membrane.

Pressure ulcer: Loss of skin surface, extending into dermis, subcutaneous tissue, fascia, muscle, bone, or all of these.

Primary lesions: Reddened lesions that arise from previously normal skin and include maculae, papules, nodules, tumors, polyps, wheals, blisters, cysts, pustules, and abscesses. May be further described as nonelevated, elevated-solid, or fluid-filled.

Pruritus: Itching.

Puncture wound: Wound with greater depth than width caused by a sharp object piercing the skin.

Purpura: Red or purple skin discolorations that do not blanch when pressure is applied. They are caused by bleeding underneath the skin. Purpura measure 0.3 to 1.0 cm.

Pustule: Purulent fluid-filled raised lesion of any size.

Rubor: Redness of the skin, commonly as a result of inflammation.

Secondary lesions: Skin changes that appear following a primary lesion (e.g., formation of scar tissue, crusts from dried burn vesicles).

Skin self-examination: An examination of the skin that the patient himself or herself performs to identify potentially problematic lesions.

Tenting: A persistent pinch.

Tumor: An abnormal growth of tissue, whether malignant or benign.

Turgor: Skin's ability to change shape and return to normal (elasticity). Used to assess the status of fluid loss or dehydration in the body.

Uremic frost: Precipitation of renal urea and nitrogen waste products through sweat onto the skin.

Vesicle: Fluid-filled lesion less than 1 cm in diameter.

Vitiligo: Skin condition characterized by areas of no pigmentation.

Wheal: Raised, flesh-colored or reddened edematous papules or plaques, varying in size and shape.

Wound drainage: Classified as either serous (clear) or sanguineous (bloody).

Chapter 12, Head and Neck, Including Lymph Nodes and Vessels

Anterior triangle: Area of the neck between the sternocleidomastoid muscle and midline of the neck.

Cranium: The collective bones of the head. The term skull is used synonymously.

Lymph nodes: Small oval structures throughout the body that filter bacteria and viruses and help to fight infection. They normally range in size from very tiny (less than 1 mm) to more than 1 cm. Lymph nodes of the head and neck region are some of the most accessible to physical examination.

Mandible: Lower jaw.

Maxilla: Upper jaw.

Nasolabial folds: Slight prominence of tissue between the nose and lips; should be symmetrical upon inspection.

Posterior triangle: Area of the neck between the sternocleidomastoid muscle and trapezius muscles.

Salivary glands: Three pairs of glands that secrete saliva into the mouth: parotid, sublingual, and submandibular.

Sternocleidomastoid muscle: Large muscle attached to the sternum and clavicle inferiorly and mastoid process of the temporal bone superiorly. This muscle separates the anterior and posterior triangles of the neck.

Sutures: Flat joints between the bones of the skull. In the infant, these sutures are not calcified, allowing for skull bone and brain growth.

Trapezius muscle: Large muscle of the upper back and posterior neck connected to the occipital bone superiorly and spinous processes of the thoracic and 7th cervical vertebrae inferiorly and the shoulder.

Chapter 13, Eyes Assessment

Amblyopia (lazy eye): Condition in which the vision in one eye is reduced because the eye and brain are not working together. It is the most common cause of visual impairment in children.

Asthenopia: Eye strain.

Blepharitis: Inflammation of the margin of the eyelid.

Cardinal fields of gaze test: Assessment of the positions to which the eye may normally be moved by the extraocular muscles.

Cataract: Opacity of the crystalline lens of the eye, which obstructs the passage of light.

Chalazion: Cyst (meibomian gland lipogranuloma) in the eyelid resulting from inflammation of the meibomian gland.

Conjunctivitis: Inflammation or infection of the transparent membrane (conjunctiva) that lines the eyelid and part of the eyeball.

Corneal light reflex test: A clinical test that is used to screen for strabismus.

Cover test: A clinical assessment that is used to test for the presence and degree of ocular deviation.

Exophthalmos: Bulging of the eye anteriorly out of the orbit.

Floaters: Translucent specks that drift across the visual field; common in people older than 40 years of age and people who are nearsighted.

Glaucoma: Disease in which the optic nerve is damaged, leading to progressive, irreversible loss of vision. It is often, but not always, associated with increased pressure of the eye.

Hordeolum: Sty.

Hyperopia: Farsightedness.

Jaeger test: Acuity test for near vision.

Lacrimal apparatus: Physiologic system containing the orbital structures for production and drainage; consists of the lacrimal gland and its excretory ducts, lacrimal canaliculi, lacrimal sac, nasolacrimal duct, and nerve supply.

Limbus: Border between the cornea and sclera.

Macula: Structure lateral to the optic disc, the area with the greatest concentration of cones.

Macular degeneration: Disease that gradually causes loss of sharp central vision, needed for common daily tasks.

Myopia: Nearsightedness.

Palpebral fissure: Almond-shaped open space between the eyelids.

PERRLA: Acronym that stands for pupils equal, round, and reactive to light and accommodation.

Presbyopia: Considered a natural part of aging; a condition that results from loss of elasticity of the crystalline lens. As this happens, the ciliary muscles that bend and straighten the lens lose their power to accommodate.

Retinopathy: Damage to retinal blood vessels. The two most common causes are diabetes and hypertension.

Snellen test: Test using a Snellen chart to measure visual acuity.

Chapter 14, Ears Assessment

Acoustic neuroma: A type of vestibular tumor that results in sensorineural hearing loss.

Air conduction: Normal pathway by which sounds travel to the inner ear.

Audiogram: Test for auditory acuity conducted by an audiologist in a soundproof room.

Bone conduction: Pathway for sound transmission that bypasses the external ear and delivers sound waves/vibrations directly to the inner ear via the skull.

Bulb insufflator: A device that is attached to an otoscope for the purpose of observing tympanic membrane movement.

Cerumen: Waxy substance secreted by glands in the ear.

Cholesteatoma: An abnormal accumulation of squamous epithelium within the middle ear.

Conductive hearing loss: Hearing loss that results when sound wave transmission through the external or middle ear is disrupted.

Hemotympanum: Bleeding in the tympanic cavity of the middle ear.

Otalgia: Ear pain.

Otitis externa: Inflammation of the outer ear.

Otitis media: Inflammation of the middle ear.

Otorrhea: Ear drainage.

Otosclerosis: Common conductive hearing loss resulting from the slow fusion of any combination of the ossicles in the middle ear.

Presbycusis: Natural sensorineural loss.

Rinne test: Test conducted with a tuning fork to examine the differentiation between bone conduction (BC) and air conduction (AC).

Romberg test: A clinical test of equilibrium.

Sensorineural hearing loss: Hearing loss that results from a problem somewhere beyond the middle ear, from inner ear to auditory cortex.

Tinnitus: Perception of buzzing or ringing in one ear or both ears that does not correspond with an external sound.

Tympanic membrane rupture: The development of a hole or tear in the tympanic membrane.

Vertigo: Type of dizziness, where there is a feeling of motion when one is stationary.

Vestibular function: Proprioception and equilibrium.

Weber test: Use of a tuning fork to help to differentiate the cause of unilateral hearing loss.

Whisper test: Test in which an examiner whispers a sentence and asks the patient to repeat it to evaluate loss of high-frequency sounds.

Chapter 15, Nose, Sinuses, Mouth, and Throat

Angular cheilitis: Maceration of the skin at the corners of the mouth; caused by overclosure of the mouth.

Anosmia: Decreased smell.

Bifid uvula: Minor cleft of the posterior soft palate.

Choana: Opening of the nose.

Columella: Anatomical structure that divides the oval nares (nostrils).

Deviation of septum: Deflection of the center wall of the nose (septum).

Dysphagia: Difficulty swallowing.

Epistaxis: Nosebleed.

Fordyce granules: Small, isolated, white or yellow papules on the buccal mucosa, representing insignificant sebaceous cysts or salivary tissue.

Geographic tongue: Tongue appearance with creases, bends, and unusual appearance; tends to occur in people with allergic disease but has no significant pathology.

Gustatory rhinitis: Clear rhinorrhea stimulated by the smell and taste of food.

Halitosis: Bad breath.

Leukoplakia: White patches with well-defined borders found on the lips or gums.

Lingual frenulum: Anatomical structure that connects the base of the tongue to the floor of the mouth.

Ludwig angina: Swelling that results from infection in the floor of the mouth and pushes the tongue up and back. It can lead to eventual airway obstruction.

Oral candidiasis: White coating of the tongue. Also known as thrush.

Ostiomeatal complex: The collective middle turbinate and middle meatus area.

Peritonsillar abscess: Abscess in the anterior tonsillar pillar that may result from collection of fluid.

Petechiae: Small red spots under the skin resulting from blood that escapes the capillaries; may occur with trauma, infection, or decreased platelet counts.

Pharyngitis: Inflammation of the pharyngeal walls.

Polyps: Grapelike swollen nasal membranes; may appear white and glistening.

Scrotal tongue: Fissures that become inflamed with food or debris and appear in the tongue.

Smooth, glossy tongue: Tongue and buccal mucosa that appear smooth and shiny from papillary atrophy and thinning of the buccal mucosa.

Torus palatinus: Bony prominence in the middle of the hard palate.

Trismus: Inability to open the jaw.

Vermillion: Junction of the lip and facial skin.

Vestibule: Anatomical name for the nares; composed of skin and ciliated mucosa.

Xerostomia: Dry mouth.

Chapter 16, Thorax and Lung Assessment

Accessory muscles: The muscles used for inspiration.

Adventitious breath sounds: Abnormal breath sounds, such as crackles, wheezes, or rhonchi.

Anterior axillary lines: The regions that extend down from the top of the anterior axillary fold when the arms are at the sides.

Apex: The top of the lung fields.

Asymmetrical movements: Abnormal chest movements that indicate collapse or blockage of a significant portion of the lung.

Atelectasis: Airway collapse.

Barrel chest: Abnormal chest shape associated with COPD, chronic asthma, and aging.

Base: The bottom of the lung fields.

Bradypnea: Respiratory rate of less than 10 breaths/min.

Bronchophony: A transmitted voice sound that is clear and louder over dense areas.

Bronchial breath sounds: Loud, high-pitched breath sounds found over the trachea and larynx.

Bronchovesicular breath sounds: Breath sounds found centrally over major bronchi that have fewer alveoli.

Carina: The location where the trachea branches (bifurcates) into the right and left main stem bronchi.

Clubbing: An angle of 180 degrees or more of the fingers, indicating chronic hypoxia.

Coarse breath sounds: Bronchial or bronchovesicular sounds in the expected vesicular location, indicating airway thickening.

Costal angle: The angle between the ribs at the costal margins.

Crackles: Abnormal breath sounds caused by fluid-filled alveoli.

Crepitus: Crackling sensation with palpation.

Cyanosis: Bluish discoloration caused by hypoxia.

Diaphragmatic excursion: Distance that the diaphragm moves with inhalation.

Diminished or decreased breath sounds: Less audible breath sounds heard in areas of emphysema, atelectasis, or pleural effusion.

Dyspnea: Shortness of breath.

Effort or work of breathing: The amount of muscular activity necessary to achieve respiration.

Egophony: Abnormal voice sound that exists when the patient's "e e e" sounds like a loud "a a a."

Forced expiration: The use of the rectus abdominis and internal intercostal muscles, as in patients with COPD.

Guarding: Limitation of chest movement that may accompany pleuritic or postoperative pain.

Hemoptysis: Sputum with blood.

Intercostal bulging: Protrusion of the intercostal spaces, indicating the presence of trapped air.

Intercostal spaces: The spaces below each rib.

Midaxillary lines: The landmark reference lines that drop from the middle of the axilla running parallel between the anterior and posterior axillary lines.

Midclavicular lines: The landmark reference lines that run parallel to the midsternal line and extend down from each clavicle midway between the sternoclavicular and acromioclavicular joints.

Midscapular lines: The landmark reference lines that are parallel to the vertebral line and run vertically through the middle of each scapula.

Midsternal line: The landmark reference line that runs vertically down the center of the sternum.

Mucoid: Sputum that is clear or white.

Nasal flaring: A sign of respiratory distress, seen more often in children.

Orthopnea: Difficulty breathing when lying flat.

Pack years: Smoking history as measured by the number of years smoked × average number of packs per day.

Pallor: Very pale skin color.

Paroxysmal nocturnal dyspnea: Sudden onset of shortness of breath at night.

Pectus carinatum: Outward protrusion of the sternum, often referred to as pigeon chest.

Pectus excavatum: Sunken sternum, often referred to as funnel chest.

Posterior axillary lines: The landmark reference lines that run vertically along the posterior edge from the top of each axilla down to the lower thoracic area.

Pursed lip breathing: Exhalation through puckered lips, easing shortness of breath.

Purulent: Sputum cloudy with bacteria.

Respiratory distress: Difficulty breathing that is characterized by the use of accessory muscles; rapid, irregular breathing pattern; and O_2 saturation below 88%.

Retractions: Indentations in the supraclavicular fossa and intercostal spaces, indicating airflow resistance.

Rhonchi: Continuous, low-pitched, snoring sounds resulting from secretions moving around in airways.

Ruddy: A reddish-purple facial color due to increased red blood cells.

Sternal angle/angle of Louis/sternomanubrial angle: The ridge where the manubrium attaches to the sternum.

Stridor: A high-pitched crowing sound from the upper airway; results from tracheal or laryngeal spasm or constriction.

Tachypnea: A respiratory rate greater than 24 breaths/min.

Tactile fremitus: An assessment parameter that is tested to determine the density of lung tissue.

Tenacious mucous: Thick, sticky sputum that is difficult to expectorate.

Tripod: A posture adopted by patient in respiratory distress or with COPD, leaning forward on a stationary object such as a table or with their elbows on their knees.

Vertebral line: The reference landmark line that runs vertically down the center of the vertebral spinous processes.

Vesicular breath sounds: Soft, low-pitched sounds found over fine airways near the site of air exchange.

Wheezes: Continuous, high-pitched, musical sounds caused by air squeezing through narrowed airways.

Whispered pectoriloquy: The voice sounds that are evaluated by asking the patient to whisper "one-two-three" while listening to the chest, comparing sides.

Chapter 17, Heart and Neck Vessels Assessment

Afterload: Pressure in the great vessels.

Apex: The bottom of the heart.

Arrhythmias: Abnormal heart rhythms with early (premature), delayed, or irregular beats.

Bruit: Swooshing sound similar to the sound of the blood pressure.

Cardiac output: Amount of blood ejected from the left ventricle each minute.

Clicks: Abnormal heart sounds that occur during systole.

Contractility: The ability of the heart to shorten its muscle fibers, producing a contraction during systole.

Diastole: Ventricular relaxation.

Dyspnea on exertion: Shortness of breath with effort.

Erb point: The location on the chest where the valves are equally audible; the most effective site for taking an apical pulse.

Flat neck veins: Barely visible neck veins, even when lying flat.

Gallop: Common name for the heart sounds S3 and S4.

Hepatojugular reflex: A test in which the examiner presses gently on the liver to increase venous return. Pulsation increases for a few beats and then returns to normal less than 3 cm above the sternal angle.

Jugular venous distention: A condition associated with heart failure and fluid volume overload. The neck veins appear full, and the level of pulsation may be greater than 3 cm above the sternal angle.

Murmur: Abnormal heart sound that may result from intrinsic cardiovascular disease or circulatory disturbance. Murmurs in adults usually indicate disease.

Nocturia: Urinating during the night. A common symptom associated with redistribution of fluid from the legs to the core when lying. As the fluid shifts, the kidneys are better perfused, increasing urine production.

Orthopnea: Onset or worsening of dyspnea on assuming the supine position with improvement upon sitting up; most often seen in cardiac cases.

Palpitation: Rapid throbbing or fluttering of the heart; may be associated with arrhythmias.

Paroxysmal nocturnal dyspnea: Also known as cardiac asthma; sudden, severe shortness of breath at night that awakens a person from sleep, often with coughing and wheezing. It is most closely associated with congestive heart failure.

Point of maximal impulse: Point where the inferior tip of the heart may cause a pulsation.

Preload: Volume in the right atrium at the end of diastole.

Rub: Most important physical sign of acute pericarditis. It is triple phased during midsystole, middiastole, and presystole. The scratchy, leathery quality results from the parietal and visceral pleurae rubbing together. The sound increases on leaning forward and during exhalation. It is heard best in the 3rd left intercoastal space (ICS) at the sternal border.

Sinus arrhythmia: Normal variation in heart rate in which the rate increases at the peak of inspiration and slows at the peak of expiration.

Snap: Early diastolic sound associated with mitral stenosis.

Split heart sound: Audible heart sound that occurs when the valves close at slightly different times.

Stroke volume: How much blood is ejected with each beat or stroke.

Systole: Contraction of the ventricles.

Chapter 18, Peripheral Vascular and Lymphatic Assessment

Allen test: A test performed to assess the patency of the collateral circulation of the hands.

Ankle brachial index (ABI): A measure of the approximate degree of arterial occlusion in the lower extremities.

Arterial ulcer: A wound that results from decreased blood supply.

Atrophy: Reduction in muscle size that may result from arterial disease.

Auscultatory gap: Diminished or absent Korotkoff sounds during blood pressure measurement.

Axillary node: Lymph node which receives lymphatic flow from the arms.

Brownish discoloration: Pigmentation changes to the ankle area resulting from chronic venous disease.

D-dimer: Blood test used to assess for deep vein thrombosis and other disorders of coagulation.

Deep vein thrombosis (DVT): Clot that forms in a vein deep in the body; characterized by pain, edema, and warmth of an extremity.

Doppler stethoscope: Stethoscope that uses ultrasound to detect blood flow.

Ecchymosis: Bruising.

Edema: Swelling caused by fluid in the tissues.

Epitrochlear lymph node: One of the lymph nodes that receives lymphatic flow from the arms.

Erythema: Redness of the skin.

Homan sign: A test that was used in the past to assess for deep vein thrombosis.

Hypertrophic nail changes: Increase in the size of toenails or fingernails, resulting from decreased arterial blood supply.

Infraclavicular lymph node: One of the lymph nodes that receives lymphatic flow from the arms.

Inguinal lymph nodes: Nodes that receive most of the lymph that drains from the lower extremities.

Intermittent claudication (IC): Pain brought on by exertion and relieved by rest.

Lymphedema: Tissue enlargement resulting from the accumulation of lymph.

Pallor: Unusually light skin tone, often resulting from arterial insufficiency.

Peripheral arterial disease (PAD): Atherosclerosis in the peripheral arteries, causing their narrowing. Increases dramatically in the seventh and eighth decades of life.

Postthrombotic syndrome: Chronic pain and swelling at the site of an earlier DVT.

Pulmonary embolism (PE): Medical emergency in which a blood clot travels from the legs to the lungs.

Rest pain: Pain that awakens patients from sleep.

Rubor: Redness of the skin.

Six "Ps" of assessment: Signs and symptoms of arterial occlusion including pain, poikilothermia, paresthesia, paralysis, pallor, and pulselessness.

Turgor: The normal state of tension in skin cells, assessed to determine hydration status.

Ultrasonography: Noninvasive diagnostic test used to evaluate anatomical and hemodynamic functions.

Varicose veins: Dilated, elongated, and tortuous veins irrespective of size.

Venous thromboembolism (VTE): Medical emergency caused when a blood clot breaks loose and travels in the blood vessels.

Venous ulcer: Wound that results from inadequate return of blood from an extremity.

Wells Score System: Test used to assess an individual's risk for DVT.

Chapter 19, Breasts and Axillae Assessment

Breast abscess: A pocket of contained infection within the breast.

Breast Self-Examination (BSE): Inspection and palpation of the breasts by the woman herself.

Circular pattern: One of the commonly used patterns for performing breast palpation.

Clinical breast examination (CBE): Breast examination performed by a medical professional.

Colostrum: Milk precursor that is high in fat, protein, and antibodies.

Cyst: A fluid or semisolid sac.

Erythema: Redness of the skin resulting from inflammation.

Fibroadenoma: A well-defined, usually single (can be multiple), nontender, firm or rubbery, round or lobular breast mass.

Gynecomastia: Enlargement of the male breasts as a result of changing hormone levels.

Hyperpigmentation: Discoloration of the breast that can signify cancer.

Inframammary ridge: A firm transverse ridge of breast tissue.

Magnetic resonance imaging (MRI): A diagnostic test that can be used to detect and stage breast cancer and other breast abnormalities.

Mammography: A form of x-ray used to screen for breast abnormalities.

Mastitis: Infection of the breast tissue (often from a blocked duct) accompanied by swelling, warmth, and redness.

Menarche: The beginning of menstruation.

Paget disease: A form of cancer involving the nipple and areola.

Peau d'orange: Appearance of breast tissue that is caused by breast edema from blocked lymph drainage, indicating advanced cancer.

Premature thelarche: Isolated breast development in the absence of other hormone-dependent changes (e.g., menses, pubic hair) in girls younger than age 8 years.

Striae: Linear stretch marks.

Tanner staging: A scale for gauging breast development.

Transillumination: Test performed in a darkened room to differentiate between a solid and fluid-filled breast mass.

Ultrasound: A noninvasive test that produces a picture through high-frequency sound waves of the internal breast structures.

Vertical pattern: The technique for breast palpation that is currently recommended by the American Cancer Society.

Wedge pattern: A commonly used technique for breast palpation.

Chapter 20, Abdominal Assessment

Accessory organs: Liver, pancreas, and gallbladder.

Anorexia: Loss of appetite.

Ascites: Accumulation of fluid in the abdomen. It is found in patients with *cirrhosis* or primary or metastatic tumors of the liver.

Blumberg sign: Assessment technique elicited during abdominal assessment to check for *peritonitis*.

Borborygmi: Sounds made by a growling stomach.

Bruit: Auscultatory sound (swishing) that indicates turbulent blood flow from constriction or dilation of a tortuous vessel.

Constipation: Decrease in normal frequency of defecation with hard, dry stool.

Diarrhea: Passage of loose, unformed stools.

Dysphagia: Difficulty swallowing. May result from stress, esophageal stricture, gastroesophageal reflux disease (GERD), or tumor.

Friction rubs: Harsh, grating sounds on auscultation; occur in the right upper quadrant (RUQ) and left upper quadrant (LUQ) over the liver and spleen. Caused by tumors or inflammation of the underlying organs.

Iliopsoas muscle test: Right lower quadrant pain that occurs when placing pressure against a raised leg, suggesting appendicitis.

McBurney point: McBurney point is the name given to the point over the right side of the abdomen that is one third of the distance from the ASIS (anterior superior iliac spine) to the umbilicus. This point roughly corresponds to the most common location of the base of the appendix where it is attached to the cecum. Deep tenderness at McBurney point, known as McBurney sign, is a sign of acute appendicitis.

Murphy sign: A clinical test used to assess for cholecystitis; performed by palpating near the client's gallbladder during inhalation.

Obesity: Weight greater than 20% of ideal.

Odynophagia: Painful swallowing in the mouth or esophagus. It can occur with or without dysphagia.

Omentum: Large fold of peritoneum that hangs down and extends from the stomach to the posterior abdominal wall after associating with the transverse colon.

Parietal pain: Acute pain; results from inflammation of the peritoneum. It is usually severe and localized over the involved structure. Patients describe it as steady, aching, or sharp, especially with movement.

Peritoneum: Serous membrane that covers and holds the organs in place. It contains a parietal layer that lines the walls of the abdomen and a visceral layer that coats the outer surface of the organs.

Peritonitis: Inflammation of the lining of the abdominal cavity; symptoms include fever, nausea, and vomiting.

Rebound tenderness: Tenderness greater when the examiner quickly withdraws the hand from the point of the pain than when pressing slowly on the tender area.

Referred pain: Pain that occurs in distant sites innervated at approximately the same spinal level as the disordered structure.

Striae: Stretch marks.

Venous hum: A soft-pitched humming noise with a systolic and diastolic component, indicating partial obstruction of an artery and reduced blood flow to the organ.

Visceral pain: Pain that occurs when hollow organs are distended, stretched, or contract forcefully.

Chapter 21, Musculoskeletal Assessment

Abduction: Movement of a part away from the center of the body.

Acromion process: Anatomical feature on the shoulder blade (scapula), together with the coracoid process extending laterally over the shoulder joint.

Adduction: Movement of a part toward the center of the body.

Arthralgia: Pain in the joints.

Ataxia: Neurological finding of gross lack of coordination of muscle movements.

Atrophy: Wasting or shrinking of the muscle.

Ballottement: Sign that indicates increased fluid in the suprapatellar pouch over the patella at the knee joint.

Bouchard nodes: Hard, nontender bony growths or gelatinous cysts on the proximal interphalangeal joints. A sign of osteoarthritis.

Bursa: Fluid-filled sac in area of friction to cushion bones or ligaments that might rub against one another.

Circumduction: Circular motion that combines flexion, extension, abduction, and adduction.

Contracture: Shortening of tendons, fascia, or muscles; may result from injury or prolonged positioning. Once a contracture develops, it is difficult to stretch and may require surgery.

Crepitus: Medical term to describe the grating, crackling, or popping sounds and sensations experienced under the skin and joints.

Deviation: Lateral movement of the hand.

Diarthrotic joint: Freely movable joint.

Dorsiflexion: Bending the ankle so that the toes move toward the head.

Effusion: Synovial thickening.

Eversion: Sole of the foot is turned away from the other leg.

Extension: Movement of a joint whereby one part of the body is moved away from another. Increases the angle to a straight line or 0 degrees.

Fascia: Flat sheets that line and protect muscle fibers, attach muscle to bone, and provide structure for nerves, blood vessels, and lymphatics.

Flexion: Maneuver that decreases the angle between bones or brings bones together.

Goniometer: Scale used for measuring the angle at which a joint can flex or extend.

Heberden nodes: Hard, nontender bony growths on the distal intraphalangeal joint.

Hyperextension: Extension beyond the neutral position.

Inversion: Turning of a structure toward the opposite.

Kyphosis: Forward bending of the upper thoracic spine; may accompany osteoporosis, ankylosing spondylosis, and Paget disease.

Lordosis: Increased lumbar curvature.

Meniscus: Cartilage disc between bones to absorb shock and cushion joints.

Myalgia: Muscle pain.

Myositis: Inflammation of the muscles.

Olecranon process: Structure centered between the medial and the lateral epicondyles of the humerus.

Opposition: Moving the thumb to touch the little finger.

Plantar flexion: Pointing the toes downward toward the ground.

Polydactyly: Congenital anomaly in which humans have supernumerary fingers or toes.

Pronation: Turning a structure to face downward.

Protrusion: Pushing a structure forward.

Radiocarpal joint: Wrist joint.

Retraction: Returning a structure to neutral position.

Rotation: Turning of a joint around a longitudinal axis.

Scoliometer: Measuring device that may be used to obtain a measurement of the number of degrees that the spine is deviated in scoliosis.

Scoliosis: Lateral curvature of the spine.

Subluxation: Partial dislocation of a joint.

Supination: Turning a structure to face upward.

Syndactyly: Condition where two or more digits are fused together.

Chapter 22, Neurological Assessment

Abnormal plantar reflex: Great toe extends upward and the other toes fan out.

Adiadochokinesia: Lack of coordination during rapid alternating movements.

Aphasia: Impaired ability to interpret or use the symbols of language.

Astereognosis: Inability to identify objects correctly that may result from damage to the sensory cortex caused by stroke.

Ataxia: Unsteady, wavering movement with inability to touch the target.

Autonomic nervous system: Division of the nervous system that maintains involuntary functions of cardiac and smooth muscle and glands. It has two components: sympathetic (fight or flight) and parasympathetic (rest and digest).

Brain death: High cervical cord or extensive medulla damage. The brain is no longer showing electrical activity.

Broca area: Brain area that regulates verbal expression and writing ability.

Brudzinski sign: Resistance or pain in the neck and flexion in the hips or knees.

Clasp-knife spasticity: Resistance is strongest on initiation of the movement and "gives way" as the examiner slowly continues the movement. Type of hypertonicity noted in patients with Parkinson disease.

Clonus: Alternating flexion/extension movements (jerking) in response to a continuous muscle stretch.

Cogwheel rigidity: Seen in patients with Parkinson disease; manifested by a ratchet-like jerking noted in the extremity on passive movement.

Corneal reflex: Blinking in response to corneal stimulation by a cotton wisp.

Cushing response: Increased intracranial pressure.

Dermatome: Area of skin innervated by the afferent sensory fibers in the dorsal root of a spinal nerve.

Diplopia: Double vision.

Dysarthria: Deficits in speech articulation.

Dysphagia: Difficulty swallowing.

Expressive aphasia: Problems with speaking or finding words.

Extraocular movements: Movements of the eye.

Flaccid (atonic): Absolutely no resistance to movement.

Gag reflex: Reflex that is tested as an indicator for the client's risk of aspiration

Hypertonia: Increased resistance of the muscles to passive stretch.

Hypotonia: Muscle tone that seems decreased or "flabby."

Kernig sign: Resistance to straightening or pain radiating down the posterior leg.

Lead-pipe rigidity: State of stiffness and inflexibility that remains uniform throughout the range of passive movement; associated with diseases of the basal ganglia.

Nuchal rigidity: Rigidity in the neck.

Nystagmus: Rapid movement of the eye back and forth in the socket.

Paresthesia: Abnormal prickly or tingly sensations.

Peripheral nervous system (PNS): Part of the nervous system that resides or extends outside the CNS to serve the limbs and organs. Unlike the CNS, the PNS is not protected by bone, leaving it exposed to toxins and mechanical injuries. The peripheral nervous system is divided into the somatic nervous system and the autonomic nervous system.

Pronator drift: Drifting downward of the hand into pronation; a sign of weakness.

Pupillary reaction: Size (before and after light stimulus) and speed of the pupils' response to light.

Receptive aphasia: Difficulty understanding verbal communication.

Reflex arc: Neural pathway that mediates a reflex action. Involves a receptor-sensing organ, afferent sensory neuron, efferent motor neuron, and effector motor organ.

Rigidity: Steady, persistent resistance to passive stretch in both flexor and extensor muscle groups.

Romberg test: Neurological test to detect poor balance. The patient stands with feet together and arms at sides. The examiner notes any swaying. The patient is asked to close the eyes during the Romberg for additional testing.

Sensation: Reaction to a stimulus.

Spasticity: Muscular hypertonicity; disorder of the CNS in which certain muscles continually receive a message to tighten and contract; characterized by increased resistance to rapid passive stretch, especially in flexor muscle groups in the upper extremities, resulting from hyperexcitability of the stretch reflex.

Wernicke area: Area of the brain that integrates understanding of spoken and written words.

Chapter 23, Male Genitalia and Rectal Assessment

Benign prostatic hyperplasia: Nodular hyperplasia of the prostate; one of the most common conditions affecting men older than 40 years of age.

Catheter-acquired urinary tract infection (CAUTI): A hospital-acquired UTI that is solely attributable to the presence of a urinary catheter.

Epididymis: Elongated cordlike structure along the posterior border of the testis; its coiled duct provides for storage, transit, and maturation of spermatozoa and is continuous with the ductus deferens.

Epispadias: Condition when the urethral meatus is on the upper side of penis.

Erectile dysfunction: Failure to consistently maintain a sufficiently ridged erect penis to allow for sexual intercourse.

Glans: Sensitive bulbous structure at the distal end of the penis.

Hemorrhoids: Varicose veins of the anus that cause rectal itching, pain, or burning.

Hernia: Loop of intestine that prolapses through the inguinal wall or canal or abdominal musculature.

Hydrocele: A collection of serous in the tunica vaginalis surrounding the testis.

Hypospadias: Condition when the uretharal meatus is on the underside of penis.

Pilonidal cyst: A tender palpable cyst in the sacrococcygeal area.

Prepuce: In uncircumcised males, loose, hoodlike skin that covers the glans; also called *foreskin*.

Priapism: Long and painful erection.

Smegma: Thin, white, cheesy substance that develops between the foreskin and the glans.

Spermatocele: A benign scrotal mass or cyst that contains sperm.

Tanner's stages of maturation: Model used in the assessment of sexual development of preadolescent and adolescent males.

Testicular torsion: The twisting or rotation of the testes, resulting in acute ischemia.

Chapter 24, Female Genitalia and Rectal Assessment

Acanthosis nigricans: Areas of hyperpigmentation around the back of the neck and under arms.

Ambiguous genitalia: Congenital anomaly found in newborns in which hyperplasia of the adrenal glands causes excessive androgen production. The clitoris may look like a penis and the fusion of the labia resembles a scrotal sac. This emergent condition requires referral for diagnostic evaluation.

Amenorrhea: Absence of menstrual periods.

Bacterial vaginosis: Vaginal infections characterized by vaginal secretions that have a strong "fishy" odor and vaginal itching or burning.

BRCA1 and BRCA2 genes: Genes that are major risk factors for breast and ovarian cancer.

Chlamydia: A sexually transmitted infection (STI) that is currently the most common and frequently reported bacterial STI in the developed world.

Cystocele: Prolapse of the bladder into the vagina.

Diethylstilbestrol: A hormone formerly given to pregnant women to prevent miscarriages that is now known to be a risk factor for cancer.

Dysmenorrhea: Pain with menses.

Dyspareunia: Pain with intercourse.

Dysuria: Burning with urination.

Gonorrhea: STI indicated by yellow vaginal secretions, pain with urination (dysuria), and dyspareunia.

Gravida: The number of pregnancies a woman has had, including any current pregnancy.

Hirsutism: Increased hair along the abdomen and around the nipples.

HPV: Human papillomavirus.

HSV: Herpes simplex virus.

Libido: Sexual drive.

Menopause: Twelve consecutive months without menses; the cessation of fertility.

Nabothian cysts: Small, benign nodules on the cervix that resemble yellow pustules; common in women who have had vaginal births.

Papanicolaou smear: A cytological evaluation of the cells of the cervix to screen for precancerous cervical lesions.

Para: The number of births a woman has had after 20 weeks even if the fetus died at birth.

Pelvic organ prolapse: Descent of the uterus or bladder into the vagina.

Perimenopause: Irregularity of menstrual cycles and accompanying symptoms between 40 and 55 years of age and before actual cessation of menses.

Polycystic ovarian syndrome: A condition accompanied by obesity, acne, hirsutism, and acanthosis nigricans.

Rectocele: Prolapsed rectum.

Rectovaginal fistula: Opening between the vagina and the rectum allowing feces to enter the vagina.

Sexual harm: Any detrimental effect of a sexual nature.

Sexually transmitted infections (STIs): Any communicable disease that is communicated by sexual contact.

Tanner stages of maturation: A tool used in the assessment of physical development of preadolescent and adolescent females.

Trichomoniasis: An STI accompanied by characteristic odor and vaginal discharge.

Uterine prolapse: Descent of the uterus into the vagina and beyond resulting from pelvic relaxation and gradual weakening of uterine ligaments supporting the uterus.

Wet mount: A laboratory analysis of vaginal secretions for the identification of vaginal infections.

Chapter 25, Pregnant Women

Abruptio placentae: Separation of the placenta from the uterus.

Braxton Hicks contractions: Contractions that begin in the second trimester and prepare the body for labor. They are usually irregular in frequency and duration, with fewer than five in 1 hour. They are also short (<30 seconds) but may be painful.

Cervical os: The opening of the cervix.

Diastasis recti: Separation of the muscles of the abdominal wall.

EDD: Estimated date of delivery, or "due date."

Gestational age: Number of weeks of fetal maturity.

Gravida: Number of pregnancies.

Hyperemesis gravidarum: Severe morning sickness, which may cause dehydration and require hospitalization of the pregnant woman.

Leopold maneuvers: Technique for assessing fetal position by palpating the fundus.

Linea nigra: Hyperpigmented line between the symphysis pubis and the top of the uterine fundus of the pregnant woman.

LMP: Last menstrual period.

Melasma: (Also known as *chloasma* or *mask of pregnancy*) A blotchy hyperpigmented area on the cheeks, nose, and forehead.

Naegele rule: Method for calculating the due date of a pregnancy, by which the estimator subtracts 3 months from the first day of the last menstrual period (LMP) and adds 7 days, or about a 40-week pregnancy.

Nonstress test: Test to assess fetal well-being.

Oligohydramnios: Deficiency of amniotic fluid.

Para: Number of deliveries.

Placenta previa: A placenta that actually covers the os. Cesarean section is necessary or else mother and fetus can die from hemorrhage.

Placental abruption: Separation of the placenta from the uterine wall before the fetus is delivered. Life-threatening situation for both mother and fetus.

Polyhydramnios: Excess amniotic fluid.

Preeclampsia: Gestational hypertension with blood pressure greater than 140/90 mm Hg with or without edema and with or without proteinuria.

Pruritus gravidarum: A condition characterized by intense itching, which occurs in 1:300 pregnancies, beginning in the third trimester, first on the abdomen, later extending to the entire body surface.

PUPPP: Pruritic urticarial papules and plaques of pregnancy; the most common skin rash found in pregnant women.

Quickening: Maternal feeling of the fetus kicking and moving (usually at about 20 weeks of pregnancy).

Round ligament pain: Sharp pains in the lower abdomen of the pregnant woman caused by the stretching of ligaments.

Striae gravidarum: Stretch marks.

Teratogens: Substances or infections that can cause malformations in the embryo or fetus.

Chapter 26, Newborns and Infants

Acrocyanosis: Cyanosis of the hands, feet, and perioral area that typically resolves in 24 to 48 hours.

Ankyloglossia: A tight frenulum that may make latching or breastfeeding difficult.

Apgar score assessment: A rapid assessment tool used to determine a newborn's health.

Baby bottle tooth decay: A condition that develops from a child going to bed with a bottle. Sugar sticks to and coats the primary teeth. Bacteria in the mouth break down the sugars to use for food. As this breakdown occurs, the bacteria produce acids that attack the teeth and cause decay.

Barlow maneuver: A test for confirming a hip dislocation. Upon testing, the head of the femur comes out of the acetabulum.

Brachycephaly: Abnormal head shape caused by laying the infant on one side without enough "tummy" time while the child is awake.

Central cyanosis: Blueness in the center portions of the torso or of the lips, tongue, or oral mucous membranes; a sign of poor oxygenation.

Craniosynostosis: Premature closure of the cranial sutures.

Craniotabes: Soft areas on the skull felt along the suture line; normal in infants, particularly those born prematurely.

Hydrocephalus: Enlarged head from increased cerebrospinal fluid.

Mongolian spot: Bluish pigmented area(s) on the lower back or buttocks. Common in infants of Asian, African, or Hispanic descent.

Ortolani maneuver: Test for hip dislocation. The infant is positioned supine on the examining table. With the baby's legs together, the examiner flexes the knees and hips 90 degrees. Then, with the examiner's middle fingers over the greater trochanters and thumbs on the inner thighs, he or she abducts the baby's hips while applying upward pressure.

Plagiocephaly: Abnormal head shape from consistent positioning on the back or one side to sleep without enough "tummy time" while awake.

Chapter 27, Children and Adolescents

Coarctation of the aorta: A congenital defect in which the aorta is narrowed after leaving the heart.

Cognitive development: Development related to information processing, conceptual resources, perceptual skill, language learning, and other aspects of brain development.

Denver Developmental Screening Test II: One of several standardized developmental screening tests used in the examination of the child and required for early and periodic screening and developmental testing. Considered the gold standard.

Head circumference: Measurement of the circumference of the head at the largest point on the brow above the eyebrows.

Immunization schedule: Schedule developed by the Centers for Disease Control and Prevention (CDC) for giving immunizations.

Innocent heart murmur: Heart murmur with no accompanying signs or symptoms of heart disease. Common in children.

Motor development: Development of abilities that emerge in the same order and at approximately the same age. Includes skills related to movement, gross coordination, and fine coordination.

Psychosocial development: Progression of psychosocial growth from infancy through adulthood. Erikson's psychosocial theory is considered the gold standard.

Speech development: Development of the verbal means of communicating, which includes articulation, fluency, and voice. Development of use of the voice and physical elements of speaking to articulate the spoken language.

Standardized growth charts: Charts developed by the CDC to track the growth and weight of a child as it grows.

Tanner staging: Scale that defines physical measurements based on external primary and secondary sex characteristics (i.e., size of the breasts, genitalia, and development of pubic hair).

Chapter 28, Older Adults

Actinic keratoses: Skin lesions that appear as rough, scaly patches on the face, lips, ears, back of hands, forearms, scalp and neck. Cause is frequent or intense exposure to ultraviolet rays, typically from the sun.

Dyspigmentation: Disorder of pigmentation of the skin or hair.

Ectropion: An eyelid (typically the lower lid) that turns out, leaving the inner eyelid surface exposed and prone to irritation.

Entropion: An eyelid that turns inward so that eyelashes and skin rub against the eye surface, causing irritation and discomfort.

Geriatric: Relating to senior citizens/older adults; relating to the diagnosis, treatment; and prevention of illness in this age group.

Geriatric syndrome: The interaction of multiple chronic conditions and their treatments; very common in the elderly.

Incontinence: Loss of bladder or bowel control.

Mastectomy: Surgery to remove all breast tissue from a breast as a way to treat or prevent breast cancer.

Parkinson disease: Degenerative disorder of the central nervous system that often impairs the sufferer's motor skills, speech, and other functions.

Pressure ulcers: Areas of damaged skin and tissue that develop when sustained pressure cuts off circulation to vulnerable parts of the body.

Solar lentigines: Circumscribed area of a small blemish.

Stasis dermatitis: Skin changes in the leg resulting from "stasis" or blood pooling as a result of insufficient venous return; also called *varicose eczema.*

Urinary retention: Inability to urinate; a common complication of benign prostatic hypertrophy (also known as benign prostatic hyperplasia or BPH).

Chapter 29, Assessment of the Hospitalized Adult

Adverse drug event: An incident involving actual or potential harm to the patient resulting from medications

Bedside handoff reports: Communication between health professionals that is witnessed by the patient

Catheter associated urinary tract infection (CAUTI): Urinary tract infections that are attributable to the presence of an intermittent or indwelling urinary catheterization

Central line bloodstream infection (CLABSI): A laboratory-confirmed bloodstream infection where a central line was in place for more than 2 days on the date of the event Comprehensive assessment: An assessment that is more detailed and complete than shift and focused assessments; commonly performed on patients who are newly-admitted

Comprehensive hospital assessment: Assessment that includes collection of both subjective and objective data and is usually done at admission.

Five rights of delegation: Delegation that is characterized by the right task under the right circumstances to the right person with the right directions and communication and under the right supervision and evaluation.

Focused assessment: An assessment that concentrates on assessing for anticipated problems that can result from hospitalization

National safety goals: Specific aims that address major risks to patients as identified by the Institute for Healthcare Improvement

NCLEX competencies: Essential aspects of nursing care as identified by the National Council State Boards of Nursing

Patient satisfaction: The degree to which patients believe that they received safe, quality healthcare

Purposeful hourly rounding: Deliberately checking on a patient at least once per hour

Sepsis: Systemic infection

Shift assessment: The assessment performed at the beginning of the shift and including an abbreviated exam, with emphasis on risk areas

Surgical site infection (SSI): An infection occurs within 30 or 90 days after the operative procedure, with purulent drainage from the deep incision, or a deep incision that spontaneously dehisces or is deliberately opened, or an abscess that is detected on direct examination, during invasive procedure, or by or imaging test.

Time out: Deliberate collaboration by the surgical team in order to confirm the right patient, site and procedure

Two patient identifiers: The use of two independent sources for confirming a patient's identity

Urgent assessment: An assessment that is performed to address a serious and abrupt change in a patient's status

Ventilator associated pneumonia (VAP): Hospital-acquired pneumonia which occurs in patients who are receiving mechanical ventilation

Venous thromboembolism (VTE): A condition that includes both deep vein thrombosis and pulmonary embolism

Appendix B

Answers to Review Questions

Chapter 1: The Nurse's Role in Health Assessment

1. B. Advocate. Rationale: By voicing concerns about the patient, the nurse functions as an advocate to improve the quality of care.

2. C. Respect. Rationale: When nurses treat individuals, families, and communities to improve the disparities present in the health care system, they promote respect and social justice.

3. A. Ongoing professional responsibility. Rationale: Nurses continually learn and promote health as part of their ongoing professional responsibility.

4. A. Obtain subjective and objective data. Rationale: Health assessment is the method by which nurses gather subjective and objective data.

5. D. Nursing interventions. Rationale: Nursing interventions are actions taken by the nurse to promote health. They usually begin with a verb and have a time frame.

6. A. Health belief model. Rationale: The nurse will use the health belief model to assess the patient's perspective about the relationship between smoking and lung disease. Because of the patient's family experience, he may have some personal beliefs that influence his motivation to stop smoking, which the nurse must assess.

7. D. Using critical thinking. Rationale: Assessment provides a solid foundation for care, but it is only one step in the nursing process. Critical thinking is used in all phases of the nursing process.

8. C. Comprehensive. Rationale: Because surgery involves all body systems, it is important to perform a comprehensive assessment.

9. D. Examination of body systems. Rationale: In a comprehensive assessment, the nurse collects subjective and objective data. This includes a history of the current problem, medical history, and common symptoms, as well as a head-to-toe physical examination.

10. A. Functional framework. Rationale: It is based on the functional framework. In the medical model, the provider evaluates the medical diagnosis, such as myocardial infarction. The provider may order some diagnostic tests to evaluate the extent of damage. The nurse assesses the patient's response to the myocardial infarction, such as fluid retention or arrhythmias. Additionally, the nurse assesses functional abilities, such as coping, role performance, and activity tolerance.

Chapter 2: The Health History and Interview

1. A. subjective primary data. Rationale: Subjective data are open to interpretation; only the patient knows what they are. Objective data are measurable and visible signs, such as a facial grimace. Patients report primary data; nurses collect secondary data from other sources such as the family, chart, or staff. Pain is what the patient says it is.

2. C. working phase. Rationale: During the working phase, the nurse collects data. The preinteraction phase is when the nurse looks at the chart before talking with the patient. In the beginning, the nurse introduces self and at the closing summarizes.

3. D. "I'll stay with you." (gets a tissue). Rationale: Being present and using silence are effective tools in such circumstances. A is false reassurance, B is too personal, and C is giving unwanted advice.

4. C. inserting lines between parents to show marriage. Rationale: Lines between parents show marriages; a double slash through the line indicates divorce.

5. D. "You seem worried, but I need to ask a few questions." Rationale: This is an emergency assessment so it is important to gather the history. While acknowledging that the mother is worried, D also focuses the conversation back on the infant. Once the infant is stabilized, the nurse will have the opportunity to talk with the mother about her feelings.

6. D. values. Rationale: Values address important big concepts of life and death. Role addresses the daily duties or tasks. Assessment of self-perception focuses on how the patient thinks about himself or herself. Coping is in response to a stressor.

7. A. "How would you describe yourself?" Rationale: Assessment of self-perception focuses on how the patient thinks about himself or herself. Role addresses the daily duties or tasks. Values address important big concepts of life and death. Coping is in response to a stressor.

8. C. ADLs. Rationale: Activities of daily living (ADLs) are those things that a person needs to accomplish each day to care for the self.

9. C. sensory deficits, illness history, and lifestyle factors. Rationale: Includes items that are significant with aging. Pregnancies and OB history are pertinent to the pregnant female. Birth history, immunizations, and growth history are most important for children to identify the risk for problems, provide primary prevention, and assess for current problems. Religion and culture are assessed during the cultural assessment.

10. A. uses subjective data to analyze findings and intervene. Rationale: The nurse is using data from the assessment to analyze that nutrition is a risk for illness and intervenes with patient teaching.

Chapter 3: Physical Examination Techniques and Equipment

1. B. Hand hygiene. Rationale: Hand hygiene is the single most important intervention to prevent the spread of infection. Either handwashing or using hand gel between patients is acceptable.

2. A. are used on every patient because it is not always known whether a patient is infected. Rationale: Standard precautions are used with every patient to prevent exposure to potential viruses, bacteria, or fungi. Hand gel is ineffective against *Clostridium difficile*. Gowns, gloves, and masks are used only when there is potential contact with body secretions. Transmission-based precautions, including droplet, airborne, or contact precautions, are used with select groups of patients who have identified infections.

3. D. are more common in nurses and in frequently hospitalized patients. Rationale: Latex allergies are more common in nurses and frequently hospitalized patients. They may result in anaphylactic or less severe reactions (e.g., difficulty breathing, itching, hives). The only way to avoid latex reactions is to avoid exposure to latex, which may be present in some stethoscopes, equipment, and stoppers of some medication vials.

4. C. Gloves are worn during anticipated contact with body secretions. Rationale: Health care providers should wear gloves to prevent exposure when they are at risk of coming into contact with body secretions of patients. They protect patients by preventing nurses from transmitting infections from contaminated to cleaner areas. Generally, the area around the bed or examination table is considered most contaminated, whereas supply cupboards and computers are considered clean. Gloves should never be worn from the room into the hall.

5. D. Skin pink. Rationale: Inspection involves visual information.

6. B. Light palpation. Rationale: An overall impression of the abdomen is gained by lightly palpating for tenderness and firmness. Auscultation provides information about gastrointestinal motility. Percussion provides information about an air-filled versus a solid or fluid-filled cavity. Deep palpation is used to identify the location of organs, masses, or tumors.

7. C. abdomen. Rationale: Percussion sounds are hyperresonant (diseased lungs), resonant (normal lungs), tympanic (abdomen), dull (over organs), and flat (over bone).

8. A. Heart, lungs, and abdomen. Rationale: The nurse auscultates heart, breath, and abdominal sounds as part of the complete assessment. All these involve movement, which generates sounds.

9. C. The chestpiece of the stethoscope is sealed against the skin. Rationale: Earpieces always point toward the front, following the same position as the nose. Tubing should be short and thick to optimize sound transmission. The chestpiece should be completely on the patient's skin to diminish transmission of room noise and to optimize sounds from the patient. The diaphragm is used for high-frequency sounds (e.g., bowel sounds); the bell is used for low-frequency sounds.

10. A. A pediatric stethoscope is used for better contact. Rationale: A pediatric stethoscope is smaller than the adult size, allowing for the full diaphragm to be sealed on the patient's skin. The parent may wish to hold the child for security and comfort. If the room is full of toys, the child may prefer to play and be hesitant to be examined. The child is kept covered as much as possible to avoid chilling; when clothes are removed, the diaper usually partly covers the genitals to prevent the child from involuntarily urinating on the examiner.

Chapter 4: Documentation and Interdisciplinary Communication

1. A. Nurses can enter data by checking boxes and adding free full text. Rationale: Computerized records usually have boxes to click and choices to make so that nurses do not have to write the whole assessment each time. They also have room for adding free text. Computerization ensures that all entries are legible and time dated. It minimizes compliance issues because programs will not let nurses enter data until they have completed all required fields. This ensures a more complete assessment. Although implementing a computerized system is expensive and requires much planning and education, such systems significantly increase patient safety. Computerized provider order entry (CPOE) allows providers to enter all orders directly into the computer, electronically communicating orders to the laboratory, pharmacy, and nursing unit. Although there is no hard copy, the eMAR is still considered the legal record.

2. A. Failure to document completely; B. Inadequate admission assessment; C. Charting in advance; D. Bunch charting at the end of shift. Rationale: All are considered high-risk assessments for liability. Additionally, falsifying patient records, failure to record changes in patient condition, failure to document that the nurse notified the primary care provider when the patient's condition changed, and failure to follow agency's standards or policies on documentation are high risk.

3. C. To determine if staff members are providing and documenting standards of care. Rationale: Agencies usually perform audits to look at systems, not individuals, and to determine whether staff members are meeting the standard of care. Accrediting agencies, such as The Joint Commission or Department of Health, audit charts to make sure that an agency is meeting state or federal standards. They also may review charts for financial reimbursement, especially Medicare or Medicaid. The charts are used for learning in grand rounds, in conferences, and for individual students of the health professions. Researchers also use charts to gather retrospective data.

4. A. Communicate report with the next nurse during change of shift; B. Communicate with the primary provider about a patient's change in assessment. Rationale: The HIPAA Privacy Rule requires an agency to make reasonable efforts to limit use of, disclosure of, and requests for protected health information to the minimum necessary to accomplish the intended purpose. Because the purposes of A and B are for the benefit of the patient, these are acceptable. Consulting with the instructor is also appropriate, but the hall is an inappropriate location to do so. Talking with a colleague is also acceptable in the context of learning, such as a post conference. Elevators, cafeterias, and other public spaces are inappropriate locations because visitors and other patients may become anxious or fearful when overhearing details related to illness, procedures, and other health-related concerns.

5. D. Draw a single line through the error and initial. Rationale: The legal technique for correcting an error is to place a single line through it, write the word "error," and initial it. In a court of law, the court needs to see the underlying data, which were corrected. Also, the nurse must record the correct information.

6. A. All use the nursing process in some form to show nursing thinking. Rationale: Types of progress notes include narrative, SOAP, PIE, and focus notes. Nurses arrange narrative notes, which are the most loosely organized, by time or topic; they also usually cluster data and include some interventions in these notes as well. SOAP, PIE, and focus notes allow nurses to cluster data and reflect the critical thinking and diagnostic reasoning they used to plan and evaluate care. Case notes, care plans, or care maps may include patient outcomes or goals. They usually include an evaluation section near the outcomes. Usually, the assessment information focuses on the problem, and nurses write the complete head-to-toe information on an assessment flow sheet.

7. C. Allow an opportunity to ask and answer questions. Rationale: A standardized format such as SBAR for handoffs ensures that nurses present all important information predictably and clearly. Face-to-face verbal updates of current status and historical data with interactive questioning are recommended for handoffs. It is best for nurses to perform handoffs in areas with limited interruptions, although finding such a location can be challenging during this busy time. Nurses use "readback" policies to ensure that both parties agree and comprehend high-risk procedures or medications. Verbal handoffs do not replace required written documentation because written documentation serves as the legal record. By reporting in person, nurses can cross-monitor the handoffs of others.

8. B. Mr. Imami's lung sounds are decreased. Rationale: Assessment findings are subjective or objective data.

9. D. a focused assessment flow sheet. Rationale: The admission assessment is usually performed just once, upon admission to a facility. If the patient is unconscious or the data are incomplete, the nurse adds data to the admission assessment after 24 hours. Nurses use the plan of care to identify outcomes and direct future care, so that nursing care is consistent from shift to shift. Progress notes evaluate patient progress toward outcomes. A judgment is made about progressing or not progressing toward goals. Outcomes and interventions may be revised as needed, and a reassessment is made. The focused assessment would have information just on the neurological assessment, so that the treatment team could identify changes in the patient's status quickly. Nurses can incorporate data and trends into a plan of care and progress note to show how the assessment is a basis for interventions.

10. D. Contact the primary care provider and document the findings now. Rationale: This situation represents an acute emergency for which the nurse should take immediate action. Nurses communicate the assessment using the SBAR technique. Additionally, they document the findings in the chart. Nurses also note the interventions, such as pain medication, effectiveness, and assessment. They document that they contacted the primary care provider and the response. If the response was unacceptable, nurses may continue to call using the chain of command or may initiate a rapid response.

Chapter 5: Vital Signs and General Survey

1. B. BP. Rationale: In older adults, both the SBP and DBP increase due to increased stiffness of arterial walls. This finding is outside of the normal range. Temperature in the older adult tends to be at the lower range of normal.

2. Rate, rhythm, depth, and quality.

3. C. compare findings to previous findings and opposite extremity. Rationale: The popliteal pulse is often difficult to palpate. Comparing to previous findings and to the opposite extremity can assist to determine if any acute changes have occurred.

4. D. A 62-year-old woman who has had oral surgery. Rationale: Oral temperature measurement is contraindicated in patients who have altered mental status, those who are mouth breathers, those who have had recent oral intake or who have recently smoked, and those who have recently undergone oral surgery.

5. A. for a pulse deficit. Rationale: Assessing for a pulse deficit provides an indirect evaluation of the heart's ability to eject enough blood to produce a peripheral pulse. When a pulse deficit is present, the radial pulse is less than the apical pulse.

6. A. Obtaining a BP immediately after the patient has entered the room; B. Using a BP cuff 80% of the arm circumference; D. Pumping the cuff 10 mm Hg above the palpated systolic BP. Rationale: Common errors in blood pressure measurements can occur because of physical activity, incorrect cuff size, and placing the heart above or below heart level and failure to auscultate above an auscultatory gap. It is recommended to pump the cuff 20 to 30 mm Hg above the last sound.

7. D. exercise. Rationale: Exercise will increase heart rate due to increased metabolic demands. Sinus arrhythmia, a variation in pulse with respiration, is common among children. The pulse rate varies with respiration, speeding up during inspiration and slowing down during expiration.

8. A. tachycardia. Rationale: Tachycardia is a heart rate greater than 100 beats/min in an adult.

9. B. a period of silence heard between Korotkoff sounds. Rationale: The auscultatory gap is the period of no Korotkoff sounds during auscultation of a blood pressure. It is caused by stiffening of the arterioles and is common in the elderly and in those with chronic disease.

10. A. Disheveled appearance; B. Rapid speech; C. Lethargy. Rationale: The general survey provides valuable clues to the patient's overall status. Changes in appearance, speech, and alertness may indicate a change in mental status and require further evaluation. Asymmetrical movements may indicate a stroke and a specific change in neurological status.

Chapter 6: Pain Assessment

1. A. acute pain. Rationale: Acute pain is of short duration; chronic pain lasts more than 3 to 6 months. Neuropathic pain results from injury to a nerve related to trauma or diseases (e.g., diabetes). Complex regional pain syndrome can develop from acute pain, which is undertreated.

2. C. to point to the painful area. Rationale: Duration is how long a patient has had the pain. Patients identify intensity using a 0 to 10 scale, with 10 being the worst pain imaginable. Patients use adjectives to describe the quality of pain, such as burning, tingling, stabbing, crushing, or gnawing.

3. D. an aggravating factor. Rationale: An alleviating factor makes the pain better. The functional pain goal is set to determine the patient's desire for activities such as exercise, driving, cooking, or dressing. The quality and description include what the pain feels like (e.g., stabbing, throbbing).

4. B. Brief Pain Inventory. Rationale: The visual analogue scale (VAS) and Numeric Pain Intensity Scales are unidimensional, measuring intensity. Verbal descriptors measure pain intensity but with words instead of numbers. The Brief Pain Inventory (BPI) includes a pain intensity scale, a body diagram to locate the pain, a functional assessment, and questions about the efficacy of pain medications. Thus, the BPI is multidimensional.

5. A. Verbal description. Rationale: The McGill Pain Questionnaire consists of a set of verbal descriptors used to capture the sensory aspect of the pain experience, a VAS, and present pain intensity rating. The alleviating factors, functional status goal, and pain goals are elements assessed during the basic elements of a pain assessment.

6. B. Rubbing a body part. Rationale: Vocalizations, facial grimacing, bracing, rubbing, restlessness, and vocal complaints are behaviors in patients with dementia who cannot accurately express their pain. Sleep is interrupted and the patient may be anxious or restless.

7. B. Chronic pain. Rationale: Acute pain behaviors include increased pulse, respiration, and blood pressure; nausea; and reports of pain. Patients tend to describe neuropathic pain as tingling, burning, or numbness. Those with complex regional pain syndromes report high levels of pain and begin to experience loss of function, temperature sensitivity, swelling, or other skin changes, such as hair loss in the affected area.

8. A. Children. Rationale: FACES is most commonly used with children. A common scale for assessing pain in patients with dementia is the Pain Assessment in Advanced Dementia Scale (PAINAD), which includes breathing, negative vocalizations, facial expression, body language, and consolability. The Payen Behavioral Pain Scale is common for unconscious patients.

9. C. To establish the efficacy of medication. Rationale: Location means where the patient experiences pain; this is not expected to change in a reassessment. Duration is how long the patient experiences pain; the rationale for the 30- to 60-minute time frame for reassessment is to allow the pain medication to take effect. The pain goal is renegotiated upon admission, transfer to another location or facility, and with each shift in the initial assessment. The shorter pain reassessment is performed to assess the efficacy of treatment.

10. D. The nurse has difficulty accepting the patient's self-report as valid. Rationale: Nurses approach patient care with the influences of their education, cultural background, and family values. As much as they try to be open-minded and nonjudgmental, personal prejudices and biases can affect how nurses perceive the patient's self-report of pain. Nurses still have difficulty accepting the patient's report of pain as valid and credible.

Chapter 7: Nutrition Assessment

1. D. fluid and electrolyte function. Rationale: Water and sodium levels are indicators of fluid balance. Potassium levels must be maintained within a narrow range for proper electrolyte function.

2. A. carbohydrates, proteins, and fats. Rationale: Carbohydrates, proteins, and fats provide the energy necessary for cellular function. Folate, vitamin B_{12}, and iron are necessary for oxygenation and optimal hemoglobin and hematocrit counts. Vitamins A, D, E, and K are fat-soluble. Iron, zinc, and calcium are three important minerals.

3. C. Some supplements may interact with your medications. Rationale: St. John's wort reduces the effectiveness of oral contraceptives and medications prescribed for heart disease, depression, seizures, some cancers, and organ transplant rejection.

4. C. Food frequency questionnaire. Rationale: Food frequency questionnaires are used to assess the intake of certain required foods (e.g., calcium or folate intake in a pregnant woman). Such questionnaires evaluate the frequency with which a food is eaten over time, such as each day, each week, or each month. They are quick to use and often combined with the 24-hour food recall.

5. D. An eating plan that emphasizes fruits, vegetables, and whole grains. Rationale: MyPlate emphasizes the need to select foods from each of the five food groups to meet individual requirements for health while reducing fats, sugars, and sodium. Emphasis is on variety; increased intake of vegetables, fruits, lentils, and grains, particularly from plant sources; and meeting individual nutritional needs while avoiding either deficiencies or excesses in nutrient intake. The overall aim is to gradually promote healthier eating among Americans of all ages, lifestyles, classes, and cultures.

6. A. Provide additional high protein and calorie shakes. Rationale: Body mass index (BMI) is calculated as weight in kilograms divided by height in meters squared. BMI of 18.5 to 24.9 is considered healthy. BMI less than 18.5 is underweight, BMI of 25 to 29.9 is overweight, and BMI of 30 or greater is obese.

7. B. Imbalanced nutrition: more than body requirements. Rationale: Body mass index (BMI) is calculated as weight in kilograms divided by height in meters squared. BMI of 18.5 to 24.9 is considered healthy. BMI less than 18.5 is underweight, BMI of 25 to 29.9 is overweight, and BMI of 30 or greater is obese. The nursing diagnosis is more than body requirements for nutrition.

8. C. An 80-year-old widow who lives alone. Rationale: This patient has two risk factors. Others include having a disease, eating fewer than two meals per day, eating few fruits or vegetables, drinking excessive alcohol, having tooth or mouth problems, being poor, using three or more medications, experiencing unintentional weight loss, and lacking the physical capacity to shop/cook/eat independently.

9. D. Prealbumin. Rationale: Because of the long half-life (18 to 21 days) of albumin, this value is often not a good indicator of current nutritional status. Another circulating protein, prealbumin, has a half-life of 2 days. Although not as commonly ordered as albumin, the level of prealbumin is a better value for nutritional status because of its shorter half-life.

10. C. A 24-year-old woman who is attempting pregnancy. Rationale: Evidence shows that adequate intake of folate before conception and in the first trimester of pregnancy reduces the incidence of the neural tube defect known as spina bifida. The U.S. Public Health Service recommends that all women of childbearing age and capable of pregnancy consume 400 μg of synthetic folic acid daily from either foods or supplements.

Chapter 8: Assessment of Developmental Stages

1. C. concerned because Caitlyn should have tripled her birth weight by now. Rationale: Caitlyn should have tripled her birth weight by now.

2. A. concerned because Emily should have grown 25 to 30 cm (10 to 12 in.) by now. Rationale: Emily should have grown 25 to 30 cm (10 to 12 in.) by now. Her growth pattern indicates the need for a nutritional assessment.

3. B. 12.7 kg (28 lb). Rationale: Toddlers should quadruple their birth weight by age 2 years. All other answers should trigger the nurse to request or perform a nutritional assessment.

4. D. is at risk for developing a sense of shame and doubt because of her mother's behavior. Rationale: Erikson stressed the importance of a toddler being able to learn to be autonomous; doing things for Samantha that she can do for herself teaches her that she is not competent.

5. C. 1.37 m (54 in.). Rationale: School-age children should grow 5 cm (2 in.) per year, so in 4 years Oscar should have grown 20.3 cm (8 in.) (116.8 + 20.3 = 137.1 cm or 46 + 8 = 54 in.). He'll also gain 2.27 to 3.2 kg (5 to 7 lb) per year, so he'll have gained 9 to 12.7 kg (20 to 28 lb) as well. If he grows less than 2 in. per year, the nurse will need to do a nutritional assessment. If he's 1.57 m (62 in.), he'll need to talk to a basketball coach!

6. D. role confusion. Rationale: Erikson stated that the adolescent's task is to find an identity. Mallory is having difficulty with this task and is at risk for role confusion.

7. C. He will be less optimistic and more practical, considering the complexities of the situation. Rationale: Young adults, as opposed to adolescents, tend to think less optimistically, less logically, and more pragmatically about problems and their solutions. Steve must take a great many factors into account with the purchase of a home, and practical thinking will serve him well with the complexities of this situation.

8. B. Nell can expect to be slightly slower as she does cognitive tasks. Rationale: Nell can expect to be slightly slower as she does cognitive tasks. None of the other answers is a normal finding in a middle-aged adult.

9. A. His long-term memory will definitely be impaired. Rationale: Evidence shows that although episodic and semantic long-term memory may decrease slightly, episodic long-term memory may look impaired because of slower processing speed. Earl simply has more long-term memories to sort through than do younger people.

10. A. needs stimuli each day in short periods when she is awake. Rationale: Short periods of appropriate stimuli during wakefulness are essential for infant development.

Chapter 9: Mental Health and Violence Assessment

1. A. "These are questions that I ask all my patients." Rationale: This response makes the encounter seem normal. The other answers discount the importance of the questions, which might prevent the patient from further disclosing information.

2. D. the family member may be a perpetrator of abusive behavior, and thus the patient may be hesitant to honestly answer questions. Rationale: There are many reasons why a family member should not be used to interpret. Doing so changes the role and dynamics for the family member acting as the interpreter. In addition, if any legal matter arises, the interview would be considered unacceptable documentation. Family members can be used to help with educating patients, encouraging them to take medications, and encouraging them to perform self-care.

3. B. will cover both suicidal and parasuicidal thoughts. Rationale: This broad and general question opens the conversation, normalizes the response, and covers a wide variety of ways that patients may hurt themselves.

4. D. "Clothes disheveled." Rationale: General appearance and behavior represent objective data that the nurse obtains through observation. The other assessments are subjective data based on conversation with the patient.

5. C. uncoordinated. Rationale: Normal movements are voluntary, deliberate, coordinated, smooth, and even. Uncoordinated movements include akathisia, akinesia, dystonia, parkinsonism, tardive dyskinesia, and neuroleptic malignant syndrome.

6. C. Loudness. Rationale: The term "audible" refers to loudness. Characteristics of speech to evaluate include rate, rhythm, loudness, fluency, quantity, articulation, content, and pattern.

7. D. Geriatric Depression Scale. Rationale: The Geriatric Depression Scale would be used because the patient is a 90-year-old with a type of depression. MMSE is used to test cognition, CAGE is the alcohol assessment tool, and HOPE is the tool for spirituality.

8. A. Pleasant or appropriate to situation. Rationale: Abnormal moods are described as sad, tearful, depressed, angry, anxious, grandiose, and fearful.

9. C. divergent tactics. Rationale: The patient is attending to the nurse in this situation but is using distracting tactics, so the nurse does not get answers to the questions asked. The patient who perseverates repeats content. Those with auditory hallucinations may respond to voices rather than the nurse. Patients with an altered mood will be more focused on their mood than the nurse.

10. D. Adults, to assess for cognitive impairment. Rationale: The MMSE was developed for adults and, although tested in groups with a cultural focus, is valid for all adults.

11. C. move from general to specific questions. Rationale: Open-ended questions are more general and give the patient the freedom to disclose the situation without bias or judgment. It is best to start with open-ended questions and to follow-up with clarifying questions as the patient appears more comfortable and rapport is established.

12. B. Displaying mood and behavior changes. Rationale: Red flags include new onset or changes in behaviors, withdrawal, depression, agitation, hyperarousal, new displays of anger, noncompliance, sexualized behavior, bowel or bladder problems, sleep problems, and unexplained and/or curious injuries.

Chapter 10: Assessment of Social, Cultural, and Spiritual Health

1. D. be upheld in every health care setting. Rationale: The national standards should be used in all health care settings, public and private, and acute and outpatient.

2. A. alternative. Rationale: Therapies used with conventional medicine are often labeled *complementary*, whereas those used instead of conventional treatments are called *alternative*.

3. B. focus groups in multiple locations. Rationale: Assessment of the patient's health beliefs and practices, postpartum practices, and religious practices are individually based assessments. Focus groups are social assessments at the societal level.

4. C. provide a picture of the individual's culture-based health care needs. Rationale: Although the other answers may be important, they relate to the spiritual assessment more closely than to the cultural assessment.

5. B. determine which questions to ask. Rationale: Because the list of suggested transcultural assessment questions is extensive, nurses are not able for every patient to conduct a complete assessment on admission to inpatient or outpatient care. Instead, the nurse must determine which questions to ask based on the patient's symptoms, learning needs, and potential health effects of culturally based practices.

6. C. culture. Rationale: This is the common definition of culture.

7. A. spiritual distress. Rationale: *Spiritual distress* indicates a disruption in concepts by which the patient integrates the meaning of life into his or her world view. *Impaired social interaction* is related to an insufficient quantity or quality of social exchange. *Readiness for enhanced spiritual well-being* is appropriate when a patient is developing inner strengths to understand life's purpose and harmony with all. *Social isolation* is used when the patient is experiencing loneliness.

8. D. avoid making assumptions. Rationale: Making assumptions or generalizations about the patient's spiritual needs based on ethnic or religious affiliation is almost certain to be an oversimplification.

9. C. may affect patients' adherence to treatments. Rationale: For some patients, health care services may not be affordable or culturally relevant, especially when dietary habits and preferences are not considered when treatments are ordered. Other patients, because of the unequal distribution and underrepresentation of ethnic minorities in health care, may reluctantly decide, after traditional healing remedies prove unsuccessful, to seek conventional care from a health care provider who does not represent the patients' own culture.

10. D. Support and accommodate his preference. Rationale: A devout Muslim patient may request to turn his bed to face Mecca, change his hospital gown, and place a basin of water near his bed for ritualistic handwashing before praying. The health risks are minimal compared with the benefit of supporting his spiritual needs.

Chapter 11: Skin, Hair, and Nails Assessment

1. C. clubbing. Rationale: Chronic hypoxia decreases oxygenation of the distal extremities. Associated clubbing changes will be evident.

2. D. herpes zoster. Rationale: The lesions of herpes zoster are vesicular, warts and moles are benign papules, and acne lesions include papules as well as pustules.

3. B. *B*irthmark: recently changed in appearance. Rationale: The B in ABCD stands for irregular *b*order of the lesion.

4. A. Patch. Rationale: Patches are nonpalpable, defined lesions larger than 1.0 cm. Macules have the same characteristics of patches but are less than 1.0 cm. Papules are solid, raised, palpable lesions less than 1.0 cm. Plaques are papules larger than 1.0 cm.

5. C. pinch a fold of skin just below the midpoint of one of the clavicles and allow the skin to recoil to normal. Rationale: To assess turgor in an adult, the most reliable method is to pinch a fold of skin on the anterior chest, release, and observe for the skin to promptly recoil to its original state.

6. D. A mild sunburn is acceptable, and is tanning is attractive in a fair-skinned blonde. Rationale: Teaching the patient about the harmful effects of UVA and UVB exposure will help her understand the importance of sun protection. Sunscreens or sunblocks applied in time for the skin to fully absorb them afford the best protection. Avoiding the sun during the midday decreases exposure to intense and harmful UVA and UVB rays.

7. A. Varicella. Rationale: Varicella (chicken pox) is a highly contagious infectious disease. It occurs most frequently in children. It is characterized by single to multiple erythematous vesicles anywhere on the body. As the disease progresses, the vesicles progress into shallow ulcers covered with scabs. Measles is a rash of macules and papules. Herpes simplex is generally localized to one area of the body and consists of grouped vesicles on an erythematous base. Roseola is a macular and papular rash.

8. A. Satellite. Rationale: Single lesions in close proximity to a larger lesion are termed satellite lesions. Discrete distribution identifies lesions that are totally separate from one another. Confluent lesions are several lesions that have merged together, and zosteriform distribution identifies lesions, which follow a dermatomal pathway.

9. C. Keloid. Rationale: Keloid is an excessive accumulation of fibrin tissue in response to wound healing. Lichenifications are exaggerated skin lines as a result of chronic irritation or scratching. Crust is a dried secretion from a primary lesion, and a scale results from excessive proliferation of the upper epidermal skin layers without normal shedding of dead cells.

10. A. Thinning of the skin. Rationale: The skin layers thin with aging, resulting in decreased skin turgor. Thinned skin is subject to increased trauma from shearing or friction, which increases the risk for purpuric lesions. Nevertheless, such lesions are not a normal variant of aging skin. Hyperpigmented macules and papules (commonly seborrheic keratoses) are present on sun-damaged skin.

11. B. Pustule. Rationale: Pustules are palpable erythematous lesions containing pus or other infectious material. Papules are solid. Cysts can contain serous as well as infectious substances and extend into the deeper layers of skin. Vesicles are small, thin-roofed lesions containing clear serous fluid.

Chapter 12: Head and Neck, Including Lymph Nodes and Vessels

1. A. Document this finding as normal. Rationale: The thyroid gland is often not palpable. With no signs or symptoms of hypothyroidism or hyperthyroidism, a nonpalpable thyroid would be a normal finding.

2. A. preauricular nodes. Rationale: The preauricular are, as the name implies, in front of (or pre-) the ear (auricle). Occipital nodes are at the base of the skull posteriorly. Cervical nodes are in the neck and supraclavicular are above the clavicle.

3. B. Slightly obese female with periorbital edema and a flat facial expression, who complains of constipation, deceased appetite, and fatigue. Rationale: The patient with hypothyroidism would likely demonstrate clinical signs and symptoms of a low metabolic rate resulting from relative depletion of circulating thyroid hormone.

4. C. firm but movable and tender. Rationale: Infected lymph nodes are usually tender. Fixed, hard, or irregular nodes should be further evaluated as a sign of possible cancer.

5. D. dehydration. Rationale: When water is lost from subcutaneous tissues, the skin becomes less elastic. The result is "tenting," which results when the skin is pulled away from the body and released. This is a sign of possible dehydration.

6. C. turn his or her head against resistance. Rationale: The sternocleidomastoid muscles play an important role in turning the head from side to side. Asking the patient to turn the head against resistance is one way to determine that the strength of these muscles is symmetrical and equal.

7. D. "Please tilt your head slightly down and to one side." Rationale: During assessment of the thyroid, it is helpful for the patient to relax the sternocleidomastoid muscle by turning the head slightly and lowering it slightly toward the chin. This position makes it easier for the nurse to palpate each lobe of the thyroid.

8. A. Recognize that it is not common to palpate lymph nodes in this region but that they must be carefully evaluated. Rationale: Cancers of the lung, breast, and abdomen may metastasize to the lymph nodes and be first accessible during clinical assessment in the supraclavicular region.

9. B. hypothyroidism. Rationale: With hypothyroidism, TSH from the pituitary gland usually is increased. Because of decreased thyroid function, there is a decrease in circulating thyroid hormones as measured by T3 and T4 levels in the blood.

10. B. Cranial nerve V. Rationale: Cranial nerve (CN) V, the trigeminal nerve, is responsible for motor and sensory of the muscles of the face, forehead, cheeks, and chin. When CN V is damaged or diseased, the patient will exhibit asymmetry of these structures. It includes forehead, cheek, and chin assessment.

Chapter 13: Eyes Assessment

1. B. A 20-year-old man with sudden visual loss after playing football. Rationale: Sudden loss of vision is an emergency, especially following a potentially traumatic injury; this patient is at risk for retinal detachment. The 8-year-old girl may have conjunctivitis. The 52-year-old woman has symptoms of cataract, and the 77-year-old man has symptoms of macular degeneration.

2. A. Always wear eye protection for occupational exposures. Rationale: Two health goals are to (1) increase the proportion of public and private schools that require use of appropriate head, face, eye, and mouth protection for students participating in school-sponsored physical activities and (2) reduce occupational eye injury and increase the use of appropriate personal protective eyewear in recreational activities and hazardous situations around the home.

3. D. Floater. Rationale: A blind spot may be related to a problem of the optic nerve (CN II). Ptosis is usually related to stroke or paralysis in the eye area. A halo is seen in patients with glaucoma, lens opacities, and some drug toxicities.

4. C. Glaucoma and cataracts. Rationale: Glaucoma, cataracts, and macular degeneration are all more common in the elderly. Myopia is nearsightedness; with strabismus, a person cannot align both eyes simultaneously under normal conditions (cross eyes). Blepharitis is inflammation of the margin of the eyelid; chalazion is a cyst in the eyelid. Exophthalmos is anterior protrusion of the eyeball out of the socket; presbyopia is believed to be caused by the loss of elasticity of the crystalline lens.

5. B. Snellen chart. Rationale: The Allen chart is used to test near vision. Ishihara cards are used to test color blindness. Confrontation is a test for peripheral vision.

6. D. 20/100. Rationale: Normal refractive index is 20/20. Visual acuity for distance vision is documented in reference to what a person with normal vision can see standing 6 meters (20 feet) in front of the test (which is the numerator). The numerator is compared to what a person with normal visual acuity could read on that particular line (which is the denominator). Someone with 20/20 vision can read at 20 feet what a person with normal vision can read at 20 feet.

7. A. the loss in the ability of the eye to accommodate. Rationale: Loss of the ability to accommodate (contract the pupil for near vision) begins at around age 40 years, when many patients start using reading glasses. Unequal pupils usually are from a defect in efferent nervous pathways controlling the oculomotor nerve. Amblyopia (lazy eye) is used to describe a condition in which vision in one eye is reduced because the eye and brain do not work together correctly. Asthenopia (eye strain) develops after reading, computer work, or other visually tedious tasks.

8. C. confrontation test. Rationale: The corneal light reflex is a test for strabismus. The cover test is to assess the presence and amount of ocular deviation. The cardinal fields of gaze test is used to evaluate motor function in the eyes.

9. B. III, IV, and VI. Rationale: The cranial nerves for the eye include II, III, IV, and VI. The optic nerve is in the central nervous system, whereas cranial nerves III, IV, and VI control the muscles of the eye.

10. B. PERRLA. Rationale: The pupils are equal, round, and reactive to light and accommodation. This is abbreviated as PERRLA.

Chapter 14: Ears Assessment

1. A. hearing and equilibrium. Rationale: The ear has two primary functions: hearing and equilibrium. Perforations of the tympanic membrane are abnormal. Equilibrium means balance.

2. A. contains the malleus, incus, and stapes. Rationale: The malleus, incus, and stapes are in the middle ear. They conduct sound waves to the inner ear. The semicircular canals and vestibule provide the body with proprioception and equilibrium.

3. A. Using a loud or monotonous voice; B. Asking to repeat questions; C. Concentrating on lip movement; D. Leaning forward to hear. Rationale: All are correct. Additionally, the patient may lean forward with the "good" ear.

4. A. Frequent ear infections; C. Exposure to smoke. Rationale: Lack of immunizations and increased age are risk factors. Additionally, family history, some medications, loud noises, allergies, airplane travel, diving, and inappropriate cleaning of the ears are risk factors.

5. C. ringing in the ear. Rationale: Inability to hear well is hearing loss, loss of equilibrium is dizziness, and ear pain is described as otalgia.

6. A. Caucasian man older than 70 years. Rationale: Older adult men of European descent have the highest incidence, which may be related to previous occupational exposure.

7. D. Otoscopic assessment. Rationale: The nursing roles are similar, but the nurse practitioner also has developed expertise with the otoscopic assessment.

8. B. disturbed sensory perception. Rationale: The nursing diagnosis is *disturbed sensory perception*. It is further defined as visual (eye), auditory (ear), kinesthetic (movement), gustatory (taste), tactile (touch), or olfactory (smell).

9. D. Patient explains plan to accommodate hearing impairment. Rationale: A, B, and C are interventions. The outcomes are what the goals are for the patient.

10. A. Be current on immunizations; B. Avoid secondhand smoke; C. Clean only external ear. Rationale: The audiogram is recommended if screening reveals problems.

Chapter 15: Nose, Sinuses, Mouth, and Throat

1. C. Throat. Rationale: The throat is part of the upper gastrointestinal tract. The other answers reflect parts of the upper respiratory tract.

2. C. Kiesselbach plexus. Rationale: Kiesselbach plexus is a highly vascular area of the nose and a common site for bleeding.

3. A. Absorption of sublingual medications. Rationale: The sublingual palate is a good location for taking oral temperatures and for the absorption of sublingual medications.

4. D. quickly assessed and treated. Rationale: Acute airway obstruction is a life-threatening emergency that requires immediate treatment.

5. A. topical decongestant use, smoking, and allergies. Rationale: Risk factors specific to this area include topical decongestant use, smoking, inhaling substances and chemicals, allergies, and dust exposure.

6. B. nose symmetrical and midline. Rationale: Normal documentation of the assessment of the nose would include findings such as symmetrical, midline, without drainage, and proportional to facial features.

7. D. *C. albicans*. Rationale: Antibiotics alter the normal flora of the mouth and may cause overgrowth of the yeast that exists in the mouth, which is *Candida albicans*.

8. B. nasal trauma. Rationale: Nasal trauma is the most common cause of epistaxis in adolescents.

9. C. foreign body in nose. Rationale: The foreign body causes discharge; the most significant finding is that the drainage is unilateral. Most other processes involve both nares.

10. A. Illicit drug use. Rationale: Cocaine and inhaled substances irritate the nose and may cause perforation.

Chapter 16: Thorax and Lung Assessment

1. B. Airway patency. Rationale: Consider the ABCs. Airway always assumes priority.

2. A. Chest pain. Rationale: Chest pain is assumed to be heart pain and must be evaluated immediately. Ischemic heart pain, such as with a myocardial infarction, must be ruled out before considering another diagnosis.

3. A. Increased wheezing. Rationale: Wheezing is associated with the airway inflammation and narrowing that accompany asthma. Bronchial indicates secretions in the airway such as pneumonia. Increased respirations are expected with decreased oxygenation. Pulse oximetry less than 92% is cause for concern.

4. D. Emergency. Rationale: Stridor indicates upper airway obstruction and is considered an emergency. Because it is accompanied in this case by retractions and tachypnea, a rapid response may be indicated.

5. D. Excess fluid volume. Rationale: Patients with chronic obstructive pulmonary disease (COPD) often retain fluid because of the increased workload of the heart that the disease imposes. Fluid accumulates in the bases and peripheral parts of the lungs, leading to increased shortness of breath and weight gain.

6. C. Tobacco smoking. Rationale: Smoking is the most common cause of COPD. It is a risk that should be assessed; assistance with smoking cessation should be offered.

7. B. Dyspnea. Rationale: Shortness of breath is observed during the initial contact with the patient. This datum assists in determining the acuity of the problem. Chest pain will be assessed during the history; sputum and lung sounds are assessed during the physical assessment.

8. A. Shortness of breath; B. Decreased breath sounds; C. Decreased oxygen saturation; D. Increased tactile fremitus. Rationale: With atelectasis, the lung tissue has collapsed, which leads to less tissue for oxygenation. Consequently, the oxygen saturation is low, breath sounds are decreased, and the patient is short of breath. Because the tissue is consolidated, tactile fremitus is increased. The percussion sound might be dull, not hyperresonant, as a result of consolidation.

9. B. Vesicular breath sounds, O_2 saturation 96%, pink. Rationale: If bronchodilators are effective, assessment findings would indicate adequate gas exchange. Abnormal findings include wheezing, low oxygen saturation, pallor, bronchial breath sounds, erythema, crackles, and cyanosis.

10. B. a normal finding over the bronchi. Rationale: The trachea bifurcates at the second intercostal space (ICS), and bronchovesicular sounds are expected. Bronchial breath sounds are auscultated over the trachea; vesicular breath sounds are heard over the lung fields.

Chapter 17: Heart and Neck Vessels Assessment

1. A. It is a double pump with pulmonary and systemic elements. Rationale: The heart is a double pump with four chambers, four valves, and a conduction system that has a pacemaker originating in the atrium (sinoatrial [SA] node). Concepts of preload, afterload, and contractility are used when considering the effectiveness of the pumping.

2. C. systole. Rationale: The SA node depolarizes and the atria contract, which appears as the P wave on an electrocardiogram (ECG). After a brief pause at the atrioventricular (AV) junction, the impulse travels through the bundle of His, bundle branches, and Purkinje fibers. The muscle cells depolarize and contract, appearing as the QRS complex on the ECG. The end result is ventricular systole and ejection of blood to the lungs and body, producing the heartbeat.

3. A. S1 greater than S2. Rationale: Closure of the mitral and tricuspid valves at the beginning of systole produces the S1. This closure prevents backflow of blood from the ventricles into the atria. S1 is loudest over these valves, located in the fifth left ICS at the sternal border (tricuspid) and the fifth left ICS at the midclavicular line (mitral).

4. C. The highest level of jugular venous pulsation. Rationale: The nurse looks for fluid volume overload in the patient with congestive heart failure (CHF). An elevated jugular venous pulsation reflects fluid volume overload in the right heart.

5. D. Obtain a blood pressure reading. Rationale: Blood pressure serves as an indicator of hemodynamic stability in this acute situation. Although heart sounds will be auscultated, the highest priority is identifying the consequences of chest pain and cardiac ischemia. Abnormal heart sounds may or may not reflect ischemia; evaluating the pulse and blood pressure is a higher priority.

6. C. Discuss risk factors that the patient is interested in modifying. Rationale: Because multiple risk factors are apparent, the most effective strategy may be for the patient to identify those items that he or she would like to change. Presentation of many brochures is likely to overwhelm the patient; it is better to focus attention on one or two things that the patient is interested in modifying.

7. D. Fatigue, difficulty sleeping, dyspnea. Rationale: Men typically have chest pain, nausea, and diaphoresis. Weight gain, edema, and nocturia are typical symptoms of CHF. Dizziness, palpitations, and low pulse are common with arrhythmias.

8. A. Grade III decrescendo systolic murmur. Rationale: A medium loud murmur might be graded III or IV on a I to VI scale. A sound that softens is considered decrescendo. Murmurs between S1 and S2 are systolic; those between S2 and S1 are diastolic.

9. A. S3 gallop. Rationale: Because of the clinical situation, the nurse is concerned about the pump function with loss of muscle from the myocardial infarction. A systolic ejection click would be heard between S1 and S2. The split S2 is best heard over the aortic and pulmonic areas, not at the apex. The S4 gallop immediately precedes S1.

10. D. Excess fluid volume. Rationale: *Ineffective cardiac tissue perfusion* describes the lack of blood being supplied to the myocardium and relates to cardiac ischemia and chest pain. *Impaired gas exchange*, a respiratory diagnosis, focuses on the exchange of oxygen and carbon dioxide at the alveolar level. *Decreased cardiac output* relates to CHF and reduced circulation. Dyspnea from fluid in the lungs and edema and weight gain from fluid accumulation in the body support the most accurate labeling of *excess fluid volume*.

Chapter 18: Peripheral Vascular and Lymphatic Assessment

1. C. 1.0. Rationale: A normal ankle-brachial index (ABI) is 1.0 to 1.29. All other options represent problematic findings.

2. B. Raynaud disease. Rationale: Raynaud disease has an unknown etiology.

3. B. compares side to side. Rationale: Bilateral comparison is essential to accurate assessment of the peripheral vascular system.

4. C. pain. Rationale: The six "Ps" are pain, poikilothermia, paresthesia, paralysis, pallor, and pulselessness.

5. C. PAD. Rationale: Smoking is one of the most devastating risk factors for peripheral arterial disease (PAD).

6. B. PAD. Rationale: A weak pulse is most closely correlated with PAD.

7. A. Intermittent claudication. Rationale: Intermittent claudication is the appropriate terminology when a patient has pain that comes on with activity or exercise and goes away with rest.

8. D. Press the fingers in the edematous area evaluating for a remaining indentation after the nurse removes his or her fingers. Rationale: Swelling requires evaluation for pitting edema.

9. A. Nothing—this finding is normal. Rationale: The documentation reflects findings consistent with a normal lymph node.

10. B. How to assess her feet daily. Rationale: Meticulous foot care is essential for patients with diabetes to prevent complications of ulcers.

Chapter 19: Breasts and Axillae Assessment

1. B. Just after the menstrual period; C. On the 4th to 7th days of the menstrual cycle. Rationale: The breasts are least congested and smallest right after the menstrual period (or days 4 to 7 of the menstrual cycle).

2. D. carcinoma. Rationale: Gynecomastia is noninflammatory enlargement of male breast tissue. Paget disease may cause intraductal carcinoma, presenting with clear, yellow discharge and dry, scaling crusts that spread outward from the nipple to the areola.

3. A. testosterone deficiency. Rationale: Changes in testosterone levels promote breast growth. Lymphatic engorgement does not naturally accompany aging. Trauma may cause inflammation but not gynecomastia. Decreased activity level may occur with aging, but it does not affect the breast tissue.

4. C. A granular feel to the breast tissue. Rationale: In older women, secretion of estrogen and progesterone decreases, leading to atrophy of the glandular tissue and its replacement with fibrous connective tissue. This tissue feels granular. Axillary lymph nodes do not enlarge. Multiple large, firm lumps are a sign of benign breast disease (BBD), which occurs in patients 30 to 55 years. Areolae do not change in color.

5. B. where most breast tumors develop. Rationale: Most tumors occur in this region, which is called the tail of Spence.

6. C. cyclical breast changes are normal. Rationale: Breasts often change throughout the menstrual cycle, with corresponding variations in hormonal levels.

7. D. resolve after menopause. Rationale: BBD occurs most often in patients 30 to 55 years and decreases or resolves after menopause. It does not predispose someone to breast cancer and is not treated with hormone-replacement therapy (HRT).

8. A. a fibroadenoma. Rationale: A cyst is soft to firm, often tender, round, and mobile. Fibrocystic breast changes feel nodular and ropelike. Breast cancer is irregular, firm, and fixed.

9. A. Breast cancer. Rationale: B represents enlargement of the breasts common in teenage boys and elderly men. C is small tumors of the subareolar ducts. D is clear, milky white fluid that precedes milk production.

10. C. supine with arm over head. Rationale: A pillow should also be placed under the patient's shoulder on the side being assessed. The patient should be supine for the examination. B indicates the position for inspection. Placing the arm over the head stretches the skin and makes palpation easier.

Chapter 20: Abdominal Assessment

1. D. Auscultation, inspection, palpation, percussion. Rationale: For the abdomen, auscultation must be performed before percussion and palpation to prevent minimizing bowel sounds.

2. B. What was your bowel pattern before you noticed the change? Rationale: Determining the patient's bowel pattern before symptoms began is most valid in establishing the normal pattern.

3. A. Liver. Rationale: The spleen is normally found in the left upper quadrant (LUQ), under the ribs. An enlarged spleen would present as a mass between the midclavicular and midaxillary lines. The colon is in the lower quadrants. The kidney is located in the flank, posterior to the lower rib cage. It is percussed for tenderness and is not always palpable.

4. D. Tympany. Rationale: The small intestine and colon, which are hollow organs, are predominant over most of the abdominal cavity. The result is tympany as the percussion sound.

5. C. Percussion for CVA tenderness. Rationale: Fist percussion over the costovertebral angle (CVA) is the only technique listed that reflects a technique for assessing the kidney. The remaining techniques are used to assess peritoneal inflammation.

6. C. Right iliac artery. Rationale: The iliac arteries are located to the left and right of the midline of the abdomen, below the umbilicus. The aorta is midline, the renal artery is above the umbilicus, and the femoral artery is located in the groin.

7. B. By percussing the abdomen for shifting dullness. Rationale: Percussing elicits a change from tympany to dullness when the abdomen is in its most dependent position. Fat remains static.

8. A. Murphy sign. Rationale: The Murphy sign tests for gallbladder pain. The other signs test for peritoneal irritation in the lower quadrants.

9. D. Percussion along the left midaxillary line and gentle palpation. Rationale: Percussion is the best technique to estimate the size of the spleen; gentle palpation is necessary to reduce the risk of splenic rupture.

10. A. epigastric. Rationale: The epigastric region is located above the umbilicus and straddles the midline between the right and left upper quadrants.

Chapter 21: Musculoskeletal Assessment

1. B. Compare the swollen knee with the other knee. Rationale: The first thing to do is to compare one knee with the other for symmetry. All the other answers are procedures for assessing joints, which may be indicated but do not represent the first step that the nurse should take.

2. D. Phalen and Tinel tests. Rationale: Both Phalen and Tinel signs are specific findings with carpal tunnel syndrome. Based on Mrs. Johnson's occupation, she is at risk for this problem. Bulge and ballottement tests look for effusion in the knee joint. The McMurray test assesses for meniscus tears in the knee. The Thomas test is used to identify flexion contracture of the hip. The Drawer test is for knee injury and the Trendelenberg test is for hip disease.

3. A. Height, weight, and vital signs. Rationale: Nurses frequently delegate the taking of height, weight, and vital signs to unlicensed care providers. The other items are parts of assessment that cannot be delegated to unlicensed personnel.

4. C. Kyphosis. Rationale: Many older adults normally have an exaggerated forward curve of the thoracic spine, which may appear even more curved because of fat pad deposits.

5. C. spasticity. Rationale: Spasticity. A is lack of tone or strength, B is involuntary contractions of muscles, and D is involuntary twitching.

6. B. make a fist, spread and close fingers, and do finger–thumb opposition. Rationale: Finger movements are flexion, extension, abduction, and adduction. The fingers do not perform rotation or lateral flexion. Touching the finger to the nose is part of neurological assessment, not range-of-motion (ROM) testing. The wrist performs supination, pronation, and lateral deviation.

7. C. Allis sign. Rationale: A positive Allis sign indicates hip dysplasia in a newborn. Advanced practice nurses use ballottement to assess for fluid in joints. The Thomas test assesses for hip contractures and involves extending one leg and flexing the other. Genu varum, or bowleg, is when the knees do not meet when a person stands with the feet together.

8. B. 2/5. Rationale: Nurses can describe muscle strength by percentage, in terms, or on a scale from 0 to 5. For example, a nurse would describe inability to overcome gravity as 25%, poor, or 2/5, respectively. Nurses do not use "within normal limits" when documenting findings because it does not clearly identify the data that have been collected.

9. D. bend forward at the waist while you palpate the spine. Rationale: Checking the height of the iliac crest will provide information about scoliosis but will not differentiate functional from structural. With functional scoliosis, the spine straightens with bending. This problem usually is associated with uneven leg length.

10. A. Adduction. Rationale: Adduction of the hip may cause the artificial hip to dislocate. The other activities are not restricted.

11. C. Consume three servings of dairy products per day. Rationale: Weight-bearing exercise is necessary to maintain bone strength. Dark green leafy vegetables contain calcium, but one serving per day will not provide an adequate amount of calcium. Three servings of dairy products supply the 1,200 mg of calcium, which an adult needs daily for bone health.

Chapter 22: Neurological Assessment

1. B. verbal response, eye opening, and motor response. Rationale: The Glasgow Coma Scale (GCS) does not include pupillary response and sensation. Abnormalities of pupil reaction are associated with altered consciousness but may also result from peripheral nerve injury. Sensation cannot be assessed accurately if the patient has any difficulty with communication.

2. A. Decreased LOC and sluggish pupil. Rationale: Because increasing intracranial pressure is a global process, the findings are more general and less specific. Findings localized to the left or right side are more commonly associated with specific areas of the brain, as with a stroke.

3. D. Weakness in the left arm. Rationale: Weakness results from loss of motor function in the motor cortex of the brain. Tremors are associated with other diseases (e.g., Parkinson disease, multiple sclerosis). The deficit is on the opposite side of the body because the motor fibers cross, causing left-sided weakness.

4. B. High blood pressure, diet high in fat, and smoking. Rationale: A health history of diabetes mellitus, carotid artery disease, atrial fibrillation, and sickle cell disease places a person at risk for neurovascular disease. Additionally, the lifestyle choices of smoking, high-fat diet, obesity, and physical inactivity increase the person's risk for stroke.

5. D. Babinski sign. Rationale: The Babinski sign indicates pathologic hyperreflexia. A normal plantar reflex would result in toes curling downward to the same stimulus. The Cushing response refers to a pattern of changes in vital signs, not reflexes.

6. A. legs. Rationale: The level of injury in the spinal cord correlates with innervation on the skin according to the level of the dermatome. Innervation of the arm roughly correlates with C5 to T1. Innervation of the chest correlates with T1 to T8. Innervation of the abdomen corresponds with T9 to T12. Innervation of the legs corresponds with L1 to S1.

7. B. risk for injury. Rationale: Safety assumes priority because of the *risk for injury. Impaired memory* is also a likely diagnosis because of his forgetfulness. No data exist about *confusion*, so that is an area that needs further assessment. *Ineffective brain perfusion* is associated more with a stroke.

8. B. bowel/bladder incontinence. Rationale: Dizziness and difficulty swallowing are potential signs of cerebral rather than spinal cord lesions. Arm weakness from spine problems would indicate cervical injury (with associated neck rather than back pain). Bowel and bladder incontinence can occur with spinal cord injury at any level.

9. A. cluster headache. Rationale: Migraine headaches typically last 4 to 72 hours (if unsuccessfully treated) and are accompanied by at least one of the following: nausea, vomiting, phonophobia, or photophobia. Migraine auras, as opposed to lacrimation or nasal congestion, indicate either cortical or brainstem dysfunction. Tension headaches are typically mild or moderate, often bilateral, and described as "pressing" or "tightening" rather than sharp pain.

10. B. Altered mentation. Rationale: Mental status changes are the earliest (often initially subtle) indications of generalized hemispheric dysfunction and occur prior to the cranial nerve or brainstem compression required to produce the other listed signs.

Chapter 23: Male Genitalia and Rectal Assessment

1. D. Standing and leaning over the exam table, chest and shoulders resting on the table. Rationale: Standing is preferred because it allows for visualization of the anus and palpation of the rectum. If the patient cannot stand, the Sims position (A) is used.

2. D. Cremasteric reflex. Rationale: The superficial cremasteric reflex is created by stroking the upper thigh, which causes the ipsilateral testicle to rise. Absence of this reflex is seen in association with disorders of the pyramidal tract above the level of the first vertebra.

3. B. Personal history of cryptorchidism. Rationale: Cryptorchidism (undescended testicle at birth) is a risk factor for testicular cancer.

4. A. testicular torsion. Rationale: Testicular torsion required immediate surgical intervention to prevent strangulation of the testicle.

5. C. You note an impulse at the tip of your finger during hernia examination. Rationale: Indirect inguinal hernia presents with an impulse at the tip of the nurse's finger during hernia examination. All other answers represent normal findings.

6. C. Asymmetrical sac with left side lower than right side. Rationale: Elevation of the affected testicle will usually lessen pain in epididymitis. All other choices usually present with testicular torsion.

7. A. Teach testicular self-examination. Rationale: This age group is at high risk for testicular cancer; prostate cancer usually occurs later in life.

8. B. Varicocele. Rationale: Varicocele is a condition caused by abnormal dilation and tortuosity of the veins along the spermatic cord, often on the left side. Upon palpation, the varicocele feels like a bag of worms.

9. A. Benign prostatic hypertrophy (BPH). Rationale: As men age, fibromuscular structures of the prostate gland atrophy and are gradually replaced by collagen, which enlarges the gland. Consequences include nocturia, dribbling, and hesitancy when voiding.

10. D. Smegma under the foreskin. Rationale: Smegma is a thin, white, cheesy substance that may normally be present under the foreskin. Pediculosis is infestation with lice. Hypospadias occurs when the urethral meatus is on the ventral side of the penis. Yellow discharge indicates an infection.

11. D. Herpes simplex virus 2 (HSV-2). Rationale: Herpes presents with painful vesicles along the penis or on the glans.

Chapter 24: Female Genitalia and Rectal Assessment

1. B. Do you ever skip periods? Rationale: In a menstrual history, the nurse asks information related only to menstrual function. History of cancer in relatives is part of family history. Questions related to sex or sexually transmitted infections (STIs) are asked later in the history, after the nurse has established a trusting relationship.

2. D. Vestibule. Rationale: Within the vestibule lies the urethra at the upper middle area. The bilateral paraurethral Skene glands are at the seven- and five-o'clock positions, respectively.

3. A. Cervical cancer. Rationale: A Pap smear is a screening tool for detecting precancerous or cancerous cells of the cervix.

4. D. Heavier than usual menstrual periods. Rationale: Fibroids are suspected when a patient presents with heavy menstrual flow, irregular bleeding, pelvic pressure, or all of these symptoms.

5. C. She needs to use two forms of birth control or abstain from sex 1 month before, during, and 1 month after taking this medication. Rationale: Because of the severe teratogenic effects of this medication, anyone of childbearing age must either abstain from sex or use at least two forms of birth control during treatment and for 1 month before and 1 month after treatment.

6. B. *Chlamydia trachomatis*. Rationale: The most common organisms that cause salpingitis are *Chlamydia trachomatis* and *Neisseria gonorrhoeae*.

7. D. Semi-lithotomy. Rationale: The patient is placed in the semi-lithotomy position so that she has eye contact with the health care practitioner and can see what is going on.

8. A. cardiovascular disease. Rationale: Heart disease is the number one killer of women.

9. B. a blood test for glucose. Rationale: Frequent vaginal candidiasis can be a symptom of abnormal blood glucose levels.

10. D. *C. acuminatum* infection. Rationale: Condyloma present as fleshy white to gray-appearing lesions. These lesions can be individual or may cluster in groups.

Chapter 25: Pregnant Women

1. C. March 22. Rationale: The Nagele rule states that to determine EDD, subtract 3 months from the first day of the LMP and add 7 days to the result.

2. C. 28 weeks. Rationale: From 20 weeks' gestation on, the fundal height should equal the gestational age in weeks.

3. B. 120 beats/min. Rationale: Normal fetal heart rate is 110 to 160 beats/min, using any method (Doppler, electronic fetal monitor, or fetoscope).

4. C. Contractions before 37 weeks. Rationale: Contractions prior to 37 weeks are symptomatic of preterm labor and may lead to preterm birth and poor outcomes for the baby. Striae gravidarum, labial varicosities, and prominent Montgomery glands are all normal findings in pregnancy.

5. C. hCG. Rationale: After implantation, the outer layer of the developing embryo (trophoblast) produces human chorionic gonadotropin (hCG). Pregnancy tests (both urine and blood) measure levels of this hormone, whose presence validates the existence of a pregnancy and initiates a feedback loop that preserves the corpus luteum.

6. A. Uncontrolled vomiting. Rationale: Headache, epigastric pain, and hyperreflexia are typical symptoms of preeclampsia. Uncontrolled vomiting is the defining characteristic of hyperemesis gravidarum.

7. B. Waddling gait. Rationale: Increased levels of relaxin loosen the cartilage between the pelvic bones, resulting in the characteristic "waddling" walk of the third trimester. This is a normal change of pregnancy. Dark cloudy urine is not normal and suggests infection or renal impairment. Significant vaginal bleeding (more than scant spotting) is never normal in pregnancy before the start of labor. Sudden edema is abnormal and may indicate preeclampsia.

8. D. Monitoring the blood pressure. Rationale: A significant drop in blood pressure is an indicator of hemorrhage due to a ruptured ectopic pregnancy. Temperature, edema, and weight are important, but hemorrhage is the life-threatening concern.

9. C. Oligohydramnios. Rationale: Oligohydramnios is an insufficient level of amniotic fluid, which can result in poor fetal prognosis and perinatal complications. Gastric reflux and anemia are common features of pregnancy, which can be managed by a nurse practitioner, certified nurse midwife, or physician. A previous cesarean procedure does not increase risk significantly enough to demand the care of a specialist and can also be managed by an NP, CNM, or MD.

10. C. Change the mother's position. Rationale: A reactive NST is indicative of a healthy fetus. If the monitoring strip is nonreactive, the nurse may offer the mother a position change or a drink of cold water or juice to stimulate the fetus. The fetal response helps to distinguish a true nonreactive test from a normal fetal sleep cycle. If the position change is not effective, this is an indicator of fetal distress and should be reported to the provider immediately. Genuine fetal distress may indicate urgent delivery of the baby to prevent a poor outcome. Findings should be documented after the intervention is complete. It would be inappropriate to wait 1 week to intervene or reevaluate the fetal heart rate, as there is the possibility of fetal distress.

Chapter 26: Newborns and Infants

1. B. Measure head and chest circumference and length, then plot current weight, length, and head and chest circumferences on standardized growth charts. Rationale: First, the nurse needs to determine in what percentile the anthropometric measurements fall to compare findings with measurements from previous visits. It is important to establish the trend in the infant's physical growth pattern.

2. C. Plot the weight and length on a standardized growth chart for a 7-week-old infant and compare with birth measurements and measurements on previous visits. Rationale: This baby was born 13 weeks prematurely. At 5 months, he is now 20 months old. Subtract 13 from 20 to get 7 weeks, which is his corrected age.

3. A. Stiff neck with an arched back. Rationale: A stiff neck and arched back describe opisthotonos, which occurs with meningeal irritation. Meningitis will need to be ruled out.

4. B. A 6-week-old infant whose father reports, "He's vomited several times and he won't take his bottle." T 36°C (96.8°F), HR 70 beats/min, RR 20 breaths/min. His lips are white. He is limp. Rationale: This infant's vital signs are low; he is pale and limp. All these signs are very worrisome. Typically, heart and respiratory rates increase when an infant is stressed. By the time they start to fall, the infant is decompensating. Because he is pale (white lips), it is difficult to tell if he is cyanotic. The nurse needs to check his oxygen saturation.

5. B. A 4-week-old African American girl whose liver margins are barely palpable along the right costal margin; her kidneys are easily palpable: her ears look "funny." Rationale: Palpable kidneys mean they are enlarged. In addition, "funny-looking" ears could be another sign of kidney problems.

6. D. Baby is sleeping supine in her crib, no pillow, one blanket, bottle lying beside baby, and a tiny dribble of milk at the corner of her mouth. Rationale: Although it is good that the baby is on her back to sleep and doesn't have excess toys and things in her crib, the bottle in the crib and little dribble of milk indicate that the baby fell asleep while drinking formula. This practice can lead to baby bottle tooth decay.

7. C. "Has anything changed lately, such as shampoos, soaps, or laundry detergent?" Rationale: Because the baby is otherwise well, the condition may be allergic or irritant dermatitis. Asking about a change in shampoo, soap, or laundry detergent will focus the line of questioning toward trying to pinpoint any allergen or irritant. Although it is important to ask about treatments that have been given, this question is less likely to elicit information that will help determine the cause.

8. D. Encouraging parents to make an appointment with the pediatrician before the baby is born. Rationale: All the actions mentioned are good things to do; however, encouraging a prenatal visit to the pediatrician sets up the opportunity for parents to ask questions and for the pediatrician to help prepare the parents (anticipatory guidance) for the new baby.

9. D. When baby cries, mother says, "Shut up already." Baby has a foul odor and looks dirty. Rationale: The mother's response indicates an inability or unwillingness to respond to the baby's cues. The foul odor and uncleanliness signify possible neglect. A careful physical examination, with the nurse looking for other signs of abuse, is in order.

10. C. Has significant head lag, one ear is small and malformed, nipples are unusually close together. Rationale: This is the only answer choice with three markers that point to a possible genetic disorder. Large ears on a baby whose growth is in the 95th percentile on the growth chart is not a strong sign. Large scaly plaques are associated with psoriasis. An absent red reflex in one eye is abnormal but not a strong marker of a genetic disorder. Cranial sutures should be palpable; a head that is flat in the back is most likely from positional plagiocephaly related to sleeping on the back.

Chapter 27: Children and Adolescents

1. D. While the child is quietly sitting on the parent's lap. Rationale: Respirations are best determined while the child is sleeping or quietly awake. When a child is playing or upset, respirations may increase from activity or crying.

2. B. Eustachian tubes that are more horizontal (flat) than vertical and wide. Rationale: Infants have horizontal (flat) and wide Eustachian tubes, which make them more prone to otitis media. Feeding in a semi-Fowler position helps decrease the risk of otitis media because the infant is not flat. Introduction of solids does not influence the incidence of otitis media. An immature cardiac sphincter causes vomiting, not otitis media.

3. A. Holding a book close to the face. Rationale: A child with myopia can see things up close but not far away. Holding a book close is a common symptom of myopia. Squinting is more of a habit because children with myopia generally try to widen their eyes to see. Closing one eye is indicative of strabismus. Rapid eye movements are indicative of cataracts or complete blindness.

4. C. Shine the light in his or her eyes. Rationale: The corneal light reflex should be at the same spot on both eyes. Any deviation requires further evaluation for strabismus. Unequal pupil size is a congenital disorder of no consequence generally. The red reflex or funduscopic examination will not diagnose strabismus.

5. B. cardiomegaly. Rationale: Lead poisoning may be associated with all the symptoms except cardiomegaly. Lead is a heavy metal, a neurotoxin, and is not cardiotoxic.

6. B. False. Measure the child standing starting between 2 and 3 years of age. Rationale: The child should stand for height measurements between ages 2 to 3 years. Growth charts for children 2 to 20 years represent standing heights. Growth charts for children 0 to 3 years are recumbent heights.

7. D. False. The charts for head circumference norms end at 36 months. Rationale: There are no reference points after 36 months; however, if concern is noted, continued measurements are appropriate.

8. C. Determine the blood pressure percentile based on age, sex, and height percentiles. Rationale: This blood pressure may be normal, but the nurse cannot tell until it is evaluated against the blood pressure norms for children in the same age range.

9. D. All of the above. Rationale: Exercise and good nutrition with maintenance of an appropriate weight are important for cardiovascular health. By preventing illnesses with immunizations, pregnant women are not exposed to viral illnesses (e.g., rubella, rubeola) that may injure the developing fetal heart. Hand hygiene and avoidance of sick people may help decrease the spread of bacteria that could potentially injure the heart valves.

10. A. 5 years. Rationale: The nurse should begin to ask the child direct questions early to encourage self-care and to assist in establishing rapport. Of course, the information received from a child of any of the listed ages would be confirmed, refined, or denied by the parent.

Chapter 28: Older Adults

1. C. Loss of subcutaneous fat. Rationale: The skin normally thins and loses subcutaneous fat with aging, making it more susceptible to tears and breakdown.

2. C. Changes in the inner ear can interfere with sound discrimination. Rationale: As the older adult ages, sound discrimination is altered, making it difficult to hear voices when around a lot of background noise, such as a television.

3. D. ask questions using lay terms rather than medical terms. Rationale: The older adult needs more time to answer questions. It is best to talk directly with the patient and use the family as a resource as needed. Information from the chart can be validated with the patient, but it is best to gather information ahead of time to avoid asking unnecessary questions and fatiguing the patient.

4. A. the interaction of multiple diagnoses that contribute to problems in the older adult. Rationale: Although no agreement exists on which clusters of symptoms are geriatric syndromes, agreement exists that they are syndromes that involve multiple systems and diagnoses.

5. B. identify older adults who may require a more comprehensive assessment. Rationale: Although the DETERMINE is a screening tool, it is less reliable than other methods. Thus, more comprehensive assessment should be performed, which includes a calorie count, food diary, or food frequency questionnaire.

6. A. "What medications are you taking?"; B. "What is the schedule for your medications?"; C. "Do you understand why you are taking all of your medications?"; D. "What is the dose of the medication that you take?" Rationale: All of the above. It is best to have the patient demonstrate how he or she takes medications. The nurse can see which medications that the patient is taking correctly, those that he or she might be skipping, and those that he or she might be taking too much.

7. B. Registration. Rationale: Registration indicates that the brain has processed the information and that the patient has heard the information correctly. Recall is the ability to remember it at a later time.

8. A. A patient with unilateral changes in vision. Rationale: Unilateral changes in vision might indicate a stroke, which should be treated as an acute situation.

9. C. Crackles in the lungs and leg edema. Rationale: A loud murmur indicates that there may be backflow of blood through the valve (regurgitation) or difficulty with the blood moving forward over the valve (stenosis). Either of these conditions may result in symptoms of heart failure. Right heart failure causes leg edema; left heart failure causes pulmonary congestion.

10. D. Adult failure to thrive. Rationale: These findings are some defining characteristics of adult failure to thrive. Although some data may support the other diagnoses, this is the best diagnosis based on the symptoms.

Chapter 29: Assessment of the Hospitalized Adult

1. A. Assessment. Rationale: This assessment determines which diagnoses will be the focus of care, the interventions that will be initiated, and those that will be reevaluated. In this way, the assessments drive care, and the reassessments loop back into further assessments and revision of care planning.

2. D. Focused assessment. Rationale: The assessment focuses on the patient's problem and is usually combined with a screening assessment for common hospital complications.

3. D. Proceed with surgeries immediately with no time-out. Rationale: All surgeries must have a "time-out" period to avoid wrong site surgeries and other complications.

4. A. Use the hand-cleaning guidelines from the CDC and WHO; B. Use proven guidelines to prevent infections that are difficult to treat; C. Use proven guidelines to prevent infection of the blood from corrupted central lines; D. Use proven guidelines to prevent infection after surgery; E. Use proven guidelines to prevent infections of the urinary tract that are caused by catheters. Rationale: All of the above are practices recommended by the Institute for Healthcare Improvement and The Joint Commission on Accreditation of Healthcare Organizations.

5. B. Personal hygiene habits, mobility routines. Rationale: The other items are considered physiological dimensions and assessments will be included in foundations and medical surgical courses.

6. B. Increase patient satisfaction. Rationale: Patient satisfaction has been linked to improved outcomes and nurses are routinely involved in assessing this.

7. B. Safety assessment. Rationale: Safety inspections are routinely performed when initially coming on to shift to make sure that the patient is not in acute distress and is in no immediate danger of falling or injuring himself or herself.

8. A. An acute change in oxygen saturation less than 90% despite oxygen administration; B. An acute change in systolic blood pressure to less than 90 mm Hg or a sustained increase in diastolic blood pressure greater than 110 mm Hg; C. New-onset chest pain; D. An acutely cold, cyanotic, or pulseless extremity; D. An acute change in pupillary response. Rationale: All of the above are emergency situations and the nurse may need additional assistance to provide immediate interventions. Additional situations include unexplained lethargy, new seizure, temperature greater than 39.0°C (102.2°F), uncontrolled pain, acute change in urine output less than 50 ml (about 1¾ oz) over 4 hours and acute bleeding.

9. C. Assess Braden scale and provide skin hygiene as needed every 8 hours; D. Perform focused assessments every shift and as needed. Rationale: Pain is reassessed 30 minutes after an intervention; vital signs are assessed every 4 to 8 hours routinely, and safety inspections are performed at the beginning of the shift and whenever needed.

10. A. head to toe. Rationale: This format is efficient and comfortable for the patient. Focused assessments are usually integrated.

Chapter 30: Head-to-Toe Assessment of the Adult

1. D. admitting assessment. Rationale. When the patient is admitted to the hospital, a more complete admitting assessment gathers patient history, subjective data, and objective data. Assessments follow that focus on the problems identified.

2. A. acute assessment. Rationale: An acute assessment focuses on data related to the problem, so that interventions can be implemented early and the problem can be resolved. Both subjective and objective data are gathered in the acute assessment.

3. C. Auscultate abdomen, palpate abdomen, evaluate for dehydration. Rationale: With nausea, vomiting, and diarrhea, concern arises about fluid volume deficit and the potential for dehydration, which would be noted with poor skin turgor. The lungs are not grouped with the symptoms. Auscultating the heart is an option to determine heart rate, but increases in heart rate can be evaluated when vital signs are collected. The abdomen needs to be auscultated to evaluate for suspected hyperactive sounds from the increased peristalsis.

4. C. A 45-year-old man with HIV and *Pneumocystis jiroveci* pneumonia with dyspnea. Rationale: Assessments are prioritized by airway, breathing, and circulation, so the patient with shortness of breath should be seen first. The patients receiving antibiotics and 2 days postoperative are stable. The elderly female with confusion would most likely be seen second because she may be at risk for injury or falls.

5. A. Onset, location, duration, character, aggravating/associated factors, relieving factors, temporal factors, severity. Rationale: The OLDCARTS mnemonic may be used to describe history of the present problem. B is the warning signs for skin cancer; C is elements of the Apgar score; D is elements in the Glasgow Coma Scale.

6. C. Eyes, heart, abdomen, legs. Rationale: Moving from head to toe is most efficient for the nurse and conserves energy for the patient. Subjective data are usually collected first. The most sensitive areas (e.g., genitals) may be deferred until last.

7. A. Pulse, blood pressure, peripheral pulses. Rationale: The primary concern is the effect of cardiac ischemia on the patient. To know how well the heart is circulating blood, the nurse assesses blood pressure and peripheral pulses. Findings provide information about cardiac output. B and C provide data about the heart but not about its effectiveness; D is assessment of the periphery only.

8. A. primary prevention. Rationale: Primary prevention is screening and teaching that occur prior to disease. Secondary prevention focuses on preventing problems once disease is detected. Tertiary prevention addresses reducing complications from known disease.

9. D. evaluation. Rationale: Assessment occurs throughout different parts of the nursing process. When the intent of the assessment is to determine whether outcomes are met, this is referred to as evaluation.

10. B. Cardiovascular, pulmonary, gastrointestinal. Rationale: Auscultation plays a minimal role in the reproductive, neurological, and integumentary systems. Auscultation of the heart provides information on rate, rhythm, extra sounds, and murmurs. Auscultation of the lungs provides information on the underlying sound and adventitious sounds, which relate to pathology in the alveoli and airways. Gastrointestinal sounds may be absent, hypoactive, or hyperactive.

Illustration Credit List

CHAPTER 1
Figure 1.4: Photo by B. Proud.

CHAPTER 2
Case Figure: Photo by A. Powdrill, Getty Images®.
Figures 2.2A and 2.4: Photo by B. Proud.

CHAPTER 3
Figures 3.2, 3.4, 3.5, and 3.12: Photo by B. Proud.
Figure 3.3: Craven, R. F., Hirnle, C. J., & Jensen, S. (2013). *Fundamentals of nursing: Human health and function* (7th ed.). Philadelphia, PA: Lippincott Williams & Wilkins.

CHAPTER 4
Figure 4.1: Courtesy of Lippincott DocuCare, http://thepoint.lww.com/docucare.
Figures 4.3, 4.5, and 4.7: Photo by B. Proud.
Figure 4.4: Courtesy of Lippincott DocuCare, http://thepoint.lww.com/docucare.
Figure 4.6: Courtesy of Lippincott DocuCare, http://thepoint.lww.com/docucare.

CHAPTER 5
Figures 5.2, and 5.6: Photo by B. Proud.
Figure 5.3A and B: Lynn, P. (2011). *Taylor's clinical nursing skills: A nursing process approach* (3rd ed.). Philadelphia, PA: Lippincott Williams & Wilkins.
Figure 5.4A and B: Lynn, P. (2011). *Taylor's clinical nursing skills: A nursing process approach* (3rd ed.). Philadelphia, PA: Lippincott Williams & Wilkins.
Figure 5.5: Lynn, P. (2011). *Taylor's clinical nursing skills: A nursing process approach* (3rd ed.). Philadelphia, PA: Lippincott Williams & Wilkins.
Figure 5.7: Lynn, P. (2011). *Taylor's clinical nursing skills: A nursing process approach* (3rd ed.). Philadelphia, PA: Lippincott Williams & Wilkins.
Figures in Table 5.9: *Achondroplastic Dwarfism:* Sadler, T. (2003). *Langman's medical embryology* (9th ed. Image Bank). Baltimore, MD: Lippincott Williams & Wilkins; ***Acromegaly:*** McConnell, T.H. (2007). *The nature of disease pathology for the health professions*. Philadelphia, PA: Lippincott Williams & Wilkins; ***Gigantism:*** Gagel R. F., & McCutcheon, I. E. (1999). Images in clinical medicine. *New England Journal of Medicine, 340*, 524. Copyright © 2003. Massachusetts Medical Society; ***Obesity, Anorexia Nervosa:*** Biophoto Associates/Photo Researchers, Inc.

CHAPTER 6
Figure 6.6: Adapted from McCaffery, M., & Pasero, C. (1999). *Pain: Clinical manual* (2nd ed., p. 37). St. Louis, MO: C. V. Mosby.
Figure 6.7: Copyright © 1991, Charles S. Cleeland, PhD.
Figure 6.8: Hockenberry, M. J., & Wilson, D. (2009). *Wong's essentials of pediatric nursing* (8th ed.). St. Louis, MO: C. V. Mosby. Used with permission. Copyright Mosby.

CHAPTER 7
Figure 7.1: United States Department of Health and Human Services, MyPlate.gov.
Figure 7.2: http://www.bapen.org.uk/pdfs/must/must-full.pdf
Figure 7.3: From Baer, H. J., Blum, R. E., Rocket, H. R., Leppert, J., Gardner, J. D., Suitor, C. W., & Colditz, G. A. (2005). Use of a food frequency questionnaire in American Indian and Caucasian pregnant women: A validation study. *BMC Public Health, 5*, 135. Retrieved from http://www.biomedcentral.com/content/pdf/1471-2458-5-135.pdf
Figures in Table 7.4: *Alopecia*, *Bitot Spots*, *Magenta Tongue:* Ostler, H. B., Maibach, H. I., Hoke, A. W., & Schwab, I. R. (2004). *Diseases of the eye and skin: A color atlas*. Philadelphia, PA: Lippincott Williams & Wilkins; ***Follicular Keratosis:*** Tasman, W., & Jaeger, E. (2001). *The Wills eye hospital atlas of clinical ophthalmology* (2nd ed.). Philadelphia, PA: Lippincott Williams & Wilkins; ***Genu Varum:*** Courtesy of Shriners Hospitals for Children, Houston, TX.

CHAPTER 8
Figure 8.4: Jeffrey Greenberg/Photo Researchers, Inc.
Figure 8.5A: Bill Aron/Photo Researchers, Inc.
Figure 8.5B: Lawrence Migdale/Photo Researchers, Inc.

CHAPTER 10
Figure 10.1: Adapted from Andrews, M. M., & Boyle, J. S. (2008). *Transcultural concepts in nursing care* (5th ed.). Philadelphia, PA: Lippincott Williams & Wilkins.
Figure 10.2: Anderson, E. T., & McFarlane, J. (2011). *Community as partner: Theory and practice in nursing* (6th ed.). Philadelphia, PA: Lippincott Williams & Wilkins.

CHAPTER 11
Figures 11.4A and B and 11.7: Goodheart, H. P. (2008). *Goodheart's photoguide of common skin disorders* (3rd ed.). Philadelphia, PA: Lippincott Williams & Wilkins.
Fig. 11.5: Photo by B. Proud.
Fig 11.9: Courtesy of Philip Siu, MD.
Figures in Table 11.1: *A, C, D, E:* Goodheart, H. P. (2008). *Goodheart's photoguide of common skin disorders* (3rd ed.). Philadelphia, PA: Lippincott Williams & Wilkins; ***B:*** Courtesy of Art Huntley, M.D., University of California at Davis.
Figures in Table 11.8: *Pallor:* Shutterstock; ***Cyanosis and Fingernail Clubbing:*** Pillitteri, A. (2013). *Maternal and child health nursing: Care of the childbearing and childbearing family*. Philadelphia, PA: Lippincott Williams & Wilkins; ***Pigmented Macules:*** Robinson, H. B. G., & Miller, A. S. (1990). *Colby, Kerr, and Robinson's color atlas of oral pathology*. Philadelphia, PA: JB Lippincott; ***Hirsutism:*** Goodheart, H. P. (2008). *Goodheart's photoguide of common skin disorders* (3rd ed.). Philadelphia, PA: Lippincott Williams & Wilkins; ***Cushing Disease:*** Weber, J. R., & Kelley, J. H. (2009). *Health assessment in nursing* (4th ed.). Philadelphia, PA: Lippincott Williams & Wilkins; ***Pressure Ulcer:*** Goodheart, H. P. (2008). *Goodheart's photoguide of common skin disorders* (3rd ed.). Philadelphia, PA: Lippincott Williams & Wilkins; ***Café Au Lait Macules***: Fleisher, G. R., Ludwig, W., & Baskin, M. N. (2004). *Atlas of pediatric emergency medicine*. Philadelphia, PA: Lippincott Williams & Wilkins; ***Malar Rash:*** McConnell, T. H. (2007). *The nature of disease pathology for the health professions*. Philadelphia, PA: Lippincott Williams & Wilkins; ***Pallor of Fingers:***Craft, N., Fox, L. P., Goldsmith L. A., Papier, A., Birnbaum, R., Mercurio, M. G., . . . Tumeh, P. C. (2010). *VisualDx: Essential adult dermatology*. Philadelphia, PA: Lippincott Williams & Wilkins.
Figures in Table 11.9: *Macule, Patch, Papule, Plaque, Wheal, Lipoma, Vesicle, Bulla, Pustule, Cyst:* Goodheart, H. P. (2008). *Goodheart's photoguide of common skin disorders* (3rd ed.). Philadelphia, PA: Lippincott Williams & Wilkins.
Figures in Table 11.10: *Atrophy, Keloid, Scale, Lichenification, Excoriation, Erosion, Fissure:* Goodheart, H. P. (2008). *Goodheart's photoguide of common skin disorders* (3rd ed.). Philadelphia, PA: Lippincott Williams & Wilkins; ***Scar:*** Weber, J., & Kelley, J. (2003). *Health assessment in nursing* (2nd ed.). Philadelphia, PA: Lippincott Williams & Wilkins; ***Crust:*** McConnell, T. H. (2007). *The nature of disease pathology for the health professions*. Philadelphia, PA: Lippincott Williams & Wilkins.
Figures in Table 11.11: *Annular, Iris, Linear, Polymorphous, Serpiginous, Nummular, Umbilicated, Verruciform:* Goodheart, H. P. (2008). *Goodheart's photoguide of common skin disorders* (3rd ed.). Philadelphia, PA: Lippincott Williams & Wilkins; ***Filiform:*** Ostler, H. B., Maibach, H. I., Hoke, A. W., & Schwab, I. R. (2004). *Diseases of the eye and skin: a color atlas*. Philadelphia, PA: Lippincott Williams & Wilkins.
Figures Table 11.12: *Assymetrical, Diffuse, Discrete, Generalized, Grouped, Localized, Satellite, Symmetrical, Zosteriform:* Goodheart, H. P. (2008). *Goodheart's photoguide of common skin disorders* (3rd ed.). Philadelphia, PA: Lippincott Williams & Wilkins; ***Confluent:*** Bickley, L. S. (2009). *Bates' guide to physical examination and history taking* (10th ed.). Philadelphia, PA: Lippincott Williams & Wilkins.
Figures in Table 11.13: *Pustular Acne, Cystic Acne, Warts, Cellulitis, Impetigo, Herpes Simplex (Cold Sores), Pityriasis Rosea, Roseola, Candida, Tinea Corporis, Tinea Versicolor:* Goodheart, H. P. (2008). *Goodheart's photoguide of common skin disorders* (3rd ed.). Philadelphia, PA: Lippincott Williams & Wilkins; ***Measles (Rubeola):*** Stocker, J. T., Dehner, L. P., & Husain, A. N. (2011). *Stocker and Dehner's pediatric pathology*. Philadelphia, PA: Lippincott Williams and Wilkins.
Figures in Table 11.14: *Psoriasis, Eczema, Contact Dermatitis, Urticaria, Allegic Drug Reaction, Insect Bites, Seborrhea:* Goodheart, (2008). *Goodheart's photoguide of common skin disorders* (3rd ed.). Philadelphia, PA: Lippincott Williams & Wilkins.
Figures in Table 11.15: *Scabies, Ticks:* Goodheart, H. P. (2008). *Goodheart's*

Photoguide of common skin disorders (3rd ed.). Philadelphia, PA: Lippincott Williams & Wilkins; ***Lice (Pediculosis):*** Goodheart, H. P. (2003). *Goodheart's photoguide of common skin disorders* (2nd ed.). Philadelphia, PA: Lippincott Williams & Wilkins.

Figures in Table 11.16: *Moles or Nevi, Skin Tags, Lentigo, Actinic Keratosis, Basal Cell Carcinoma, Squamous Cell Carcinoma, Malignant Melanoma, Kaposi Sarcoma:* Goodheart, H. P. (2008). *Goodheart's photoguide of common skin disorders* (3rd ed.). Philadelphia, PA: Lippincott Williams & Wilkins; ***Lipoma:*** Lippincott Williams & Wilkins, Barakin Collection.

Figures in Table 11.17: *Hemangioma:* O'Doherty, N. (1979). *Atlas of the newborn.* Philadelphia, PA: JB Lippincott; ***Nevus Flammeus:*** From Sauer, G. C., & Hall, J. C. (1996). *Manual of skin diseases* (7th ed.). Philadelphia, PA: Lippincott-Raven; ***Venous Lake:*** Goodheart, H. P. (2008). *Goodheart's photoguide of common ski disorders* (3rd ed.). Philadelphia, PA: Lippincott Williams & Wilkins.

Figures in Table 11.18: *Petechiae:* McConnell, T. H. (2007). *The nature of disease pathology for the health professions.* Philadelphia, PA: Lippincott Williams & Wilkins; ***Purpura, Ecchymosis:*** Goodheart, H. P. (2008). *Goodheart's photoguide of common skin disorders* (3rd ed.). Philadelphia, PA: Lippincott Williams & Wilkins; ***Laceration, Puncture Wound:*** From Fleisher, G. R., Ludwig, S., & Baskin, M. N. (2004). *Atlas of pediatric emergency medicine.* Philadelphia: Lippincott Williams & Wilkins; ***Avulsion:*** Dr. P. Marazzi/Photo Researchers, Inc; ***Hematoma:*** Barankin Collection.

Figures in Table 11.19: National Pressure Ulcer Advisory Panel.

Figures in Table 11.20: *Venous Ulcer (Vascular), Arterial Ulcer (Vascular):* Nettina, S. M. (2001). *The Lippincott manual of nursing practice* (7th ed.). Philadelphia, PA: Lippincott Williams & Wilkins; ***Neuropathic Ulcer*** Goodheart, H. P. (2008). *Goodheart's photoguide of common skin disorders* (3rd ed.). Philadelphia, PA: Lippincott Williams & Wilkins.

Figures in Table 11.21: *Longitudinal Ridging, Onycholysis, Pitted Nails, Yellow Nails, Half-and-half Nails, Dark Longitudinal Streaks:* Goodheart, H. P. (2008). *Goodheart's photoguide of common skin disorders* (3rd ed.). Philadelphia, PA: Lippincott Williams & Wilkins; ***Koilonychia, Clubbing, Splinter Hemorrhages:*** Image provided by Steadman's; ***Beau Lines:*** Bickley, L. S. (2009). *Bates' guide to physical examination and history taking* (10th ed.). Philadelphia, PA: Lippincott Williams & Wilkins.

Figures in Table 11.22: *Alopecia Areata, Traction Alopecia, Trichotillomania:* Goodheart, H. P. (2008). *Goodheart's photoguide of common skin disorders* (3rd ed.). Philadelphia, PA: Lippincott Williams & Wilkins; ***Hirsutism:*** Image provided by Steadman's.

CHAPTER 12

Figures in Table 12.3: *Hydrocephalus, Fetal Alcohol Syndrome:* Gold, D. H., & Weingeist, T. A. (2001). *Color atlas of the eye in systemic disease.* Baltimore, MD: Lippincott Williams & Wilkins; ***Cretinism (Congenital Hypothyroidism):*** Centers for Disease Control and Prevention Public Health Image Library.

Figures in Table12.4: *Acromegaly:* Willis, M. C. (2002). *Medical terminology: A programmed learning approach to the language of health care.* Baltimore, MD: Lippincott Williams & Wilkins; ***Bell Palsy, Cerebral Vascular Accident (Stroke), Myxedema:*** Dr. P. Marazzi/Photo Researchers, Inc.; ***Cushing Syndrome:*** Ostler, H. B., Maibach, H. I., Hoke, A. W., & Schwab, I. R. (2004). *Diseases of the eye and skin: A color atlas.* Philadelphia, PA: Lippincott Williams & Wilkins; ***Scleroderma:*** Gold, D. H., & Weingeist, T. A. (2001). *Color atlas of the eye in systemic disease.* Baltimore, MD: Lippincott Williams & Wilkins; ***Goiter:*** Scott Camazine/Photo Researchers, Inc.

CHAPTER 13

Figures 13.15, 13.27, 13.28, and 13.29: Tasman, W., & Jaeger, E. (2001). *The Wills eye hospital atlas of clinical ophthalmology* (2nd ed.). Philadelphia, PA: Lippincott Williams & Wilkins.

Figures 13.17 and 13.30: Gold, D. H., & Weingeist, T. A. (2001). *Color atlas of the eye in systemic disease.* Baltimore, MD: Lippincott Williams & Wilkins.

Figure 13.19: Onofrey 3e Fig 3-24; retrieved from Vault

Figure 13.20: Courtesy of Terri Young, MD.

Figures 13.21, 13.22, and 13.24: Bickley, L. S. (2009). *Bates' guide to physical examination and history taking* (10th ed.). Philadelphia, PA: Lippincott Williams & Wilkins.

Figures in Table 13.5: *Nystagmus:* Bickley, L. S. (2009). *Bates' guide to physical examination and history taking* (10th ed.). Philadelphia, PA: Lippincott Williams & Wilkins; ***Esotropia:*** Courtesy of Dean John Bonsall, MD, FACS; ***Exotropia, Vertical Deviation***: Tasman, W., & Jaeger, E. (2001). *The Wills eye hospital atlas of clinical ophthalmology* (2nd ed.). Philadelphia, PA: Lippincott Williams & Wilkins.

Figures in Table 13.6: *Jaundice, Cataract:* Rubin, E., & Farber, J. L. (1999). *Pathology* (3rd ed.). Philadelphia, PA: Lippincott Williams & Wilkins; ***Iris Nevus, Blepharitis, Bacterial Conjunctivitis, Glaucoma, Amblyopia, Hordeolum (Sty):*** Tasman, W., & Jaeger, E. (2001). *The Wills eye hospital atlas of clinical ophthalmology* (2nd ed.). Philadelphia, PA: Lippincott Williams & Wilkins; ***Hyphema, Allergic Conjunctivitis:*** Fleisher, G. R., Ludwig, S., & Baskin, M. N. *Atlas of pediatric emergency medicine.* Philadelphia, PA: Lippincott Williams & Wilkins; ***Chalazion:*** Bickley, L. S. (2009). *Bates' guide to physical examination and history taking* (10th ed.). Philadelphia, PA: Lippincott Williams & Wilkins; ***Exophthalmos:*** Goodheart, H. P. (2008). *Photoguide of common skin disorders* (3rd ed.). Philadelphia, PA: Lippincott Williams & Wilkins; ***Osteogenesis Imperfecta:*** Ostler, H. B., Maibach, H. I., Hoke, A. W., & Schwab, I. R. (2004). *Diseases of the eye and skin: A color atlas.* Philadelphia, PA: Lippincott Williams & Wilkins.

Figures in Table 13.7: *Horner Syndrome, Miosis (Small Fixed Pupil), Adie Pupil, Mydriasis (Dilated Fixed Pupil), Oculomotor (CN III) Nerve Damage:* Tasman, W., & Jaeger, E. (2001). *The Wills eye hospital atlas of clinical ophthalmology.* (2nd ed.). Philadelphia, PA: Lippincott Williams & Wilkins; ***Keyhole Pupil (Coloboma):*** Courtesy of Brian Forbes, MDGold, D. H., & Weingeist, T. A. (2001). *Color atlas of the eye in systemic disease.* Baltimore, MD: Lippincott Williams & Wilkins.

Figures in Table 13.8: *AMD, Retinopathy, Retinitis Pigmentosa:* Tasman, W., & Jaeger, E. (2001). *The Wills eye hospital atlas of clinical ophthalmology* (2nd ed.). Philadelphia, PA: Lippincott Williams & Wilkins; ***Copper Wiring:*** McConnell, T.H. (2007). *The nature of disease pathology for the health professions.* Philadelphia, PA: Lippincott Williams & Wilkins.

CHAPTER 14

Figure 14.10: Moore, K. L., & Dalley, A. F. (1999). *Clinically oriented anatomy* (4th ed.). Baltimore, MD: Lippincott Williams & Wilkins.

Figure 14.11: Mills, S. E. (2007). *Histology for pathologists* (3rd ed.). Philadelphia, PA: Lippincott Williams & Wilkins.

Figures in Table 14.2: *Microtia:* Biophoto Associates/Photo Researchers, Inc.; ***Macrotia:*** Saturn Stills/Photo Researchers, Inc.; ***Edematous Ears, Cartilaginous* Staphylococcus *or* Pseudomonas *Infection:*** Ostler, H. B., Maibach, H. I., Hoke, A. W., & Schwab, I. R. (2004). *Diseases of the eye and skin: A color atlas.* Philadelphia, PA: Lippincott Williams & Wilkins; ***Carcinoma on Auricle:*** Goodheart, H. P. (2008). *Goodheart's photoguide of common skin disorders* (3rd ed.). Philadelphia, PA: Lippincott Williams & Wilkins; ***Cyst:*** Young, E. M., Jr., Newcomer, V. D., & Kligman, A. M. (1993). *Geriatric dermatology: Color atlas and practitioner's guide.* Philadelphia, PA: Lea & Febiger; ***Tophi:*** Weber, J., & Kelley, J. (2003). *Health assessment in nursing* (2nd ed.). Philadelphia, PA: Lippincott Williams & Wilkins.

Figures in Table 14.3: *TM Rupture:* Courtesy of Michael Hawke, MD, Toronto, Canada; ***Acute Otitis Media:*** Moore, K. L., & Dalley, A. F., II. (1999). *Clinically oriented anatomy* (4th ed.). Baltimore, MD: Lippincott Williams & Wilkins; ***Scarred TM:*** Weber, J., & Kelley, J. (2003). *Health assessment in nursing* (2nd ed.). Philadelphia, PA: Lippincott Williams & Wilkins; ***Foreign Body:*** Dr. P. Marazzi/Photo Researchers, Inc.

CHAPTER 15

Figure 15.1: Moore, K. L., & Dalley, A. F., II. (2008). *Clinically oriented anatomy* (6th ed.). Baltimore, MD: Lippincott Williams & Wilkins.

Figures 15.6 and 15.15: Bickley, L. S. (2009). *Bates' guide to physical examination and history taking* (10th ed.). Philadelphia, PA: Lippincott Williams & Wilkins.

Figure 15.7: Lippincott Williams & Wilkins. (2011). *Lippincott Williams & Wilkins' comprehensive dental assisting.* Philadelphia, PA: Author.

Figures 15.16, 15.20, and 15.24: Goodheart, H. P. (2008). *Goodheart's photoguide of common skin disorders* (3rd ed.). Philadelphia, PA: Lippincott Williams & Wilkins.

Figure 15.21: Fleisher, G. R., Ludwig, W., & Baskin, M. N. (2004). *Atlas of pediatric emergency medicine.* Philadelphia, PA: Lippincott Williams & Wilkins.

Figure 15.22: Chung Visual Diagnosis and Treatment in Pediatrics,

Figure 15.23: Courtesy of Seth Zwillenberg.

Figure 15.26: Robinson, H. B. G., & Miller, A. S. (1990). *Colby, Kerr, and Robinson's color atlas of oral pathology.* Philadelphia, PA: JB Lippincott.

Figures in Table 15.6: *Epistaxis (Nosebleed):* Ian Boddy/Photo Researchers, Inc.; ***Nasal Polyps:*** Handler, S. D., & Myer, C. M. (1998).

Atlas of ear, nose and throat disorders in children (p. 59). Ontario, Canada: BC Decker; ***Deviated Septum:*** Moore, K. L., & Dalley, A. F., II. (2008). *Clinically oriented anatomy* (6th ed.). Baltimore, MD: Lippincott Williams & Wilkins; ***Perforated Septum, Foreign Body:*** Dr. P. Marazzi/Photo Researchers, Inc.

Figures in Table 15.7: ***Cleft Lip/Palate:*** Rubin, E., & Farber, J. L. (1999). *Pathology* (3rd ed.). Philadelphia, PA: Lippincott Williams & Wilkins; ***Bifid Uvula:*** Courtesy of Paul S. Matz, MD; ***Acute Tonsillitis or Pharyngitis:*** BSIP/Photo Researchers, Inc.; ***Strep Throat:*** Centers for Disease Control and Prevention Public Health Image Library.

Figures in Table 15.8: ***Herpes Simplex Virus, Candidasis, Leukoplakia, Black Hairy Tongue, Carcinoma:*** Goodheart, H. P. (2008). *Goodheart's photoguide of common skin disorders* (3rd ed.). Philadelphia, PA: Lippincott Williams & Wilkins.

Figures in Table 15.9: ***Dental Caries:*** Langlais, R. P., & Miller, C. S. (1992). *Color atlas of common oral diseases*. Philadelphia, PA: Lea & Febiger; ***Gingival Hyperplasia:*** Courtesy of Dr. James Cottone; ***Ankyloglossia (Tongue-tie):*** Courtesy of Paul S. Matz, MD.

CHAPTER 16

Figure 16.1: Moore, K. L., & Dalley, A. F., II. (2008). *Clinically oriented anatomy* (6th ed.). Baltimore, MD: Lippincott Williams & Wilkins.

Figures 16.4, 16.5, 16.6, 16.7, and 16.8: Bickley, L. S. (2009). *Bates' guide to physical examination and history taking* (10th ed.). Philadelphia, PA: Lippincott Williams & Wilkins.

Figures 16.11, 16.12, 16.13, 16.14, and 16.15: Photos by B. Proud.

Figure 16.16: Bickley, L. S. (2009). *Bates' guide to physical examination and history taking* (10th ed.). Philadelphia, PA: Lippincott Williams & Wilkins.

CHAPTER 17

Figures 17.4 and 17.15: Photo by B. Proud.

Figure 17.13: Hogan-Quigley, B., Palm, M. L., & Bickley, L. S. (2012). *Bates' nursing guide to physical examination and history taking*. Philadelphia, PA: Lippincott Williams & Wilkins.

CHAPTER 18

Figures in Table 18.3: Acute arterial occlusion. (2001). In S. M. Nettina (Ed.), *The Lippincott manual of nursing practice* (7th ed.). Philadelphia, PA: Lippincott Williams & Wilkins; ***Abdominal Aortic Aneurysm:*** Moore, K. L., & Dalley, A. F., II. (2008). *Clinically oriented anatomy* (6th ed.). Baltimore, MD: Lippincott Williams & Wilkins; ***Raynaud Phenomenon and Raynaud Disease:*** Craft, N., Fox, L. P., Goldsmith, L. A., Papier, A., Birnbaum, R., Mercurio, M. G., . . . Tumeh, P. C. (2010). *VisualDx: Essential adult dermatology*. Philadelphia, PA: Lippincott Williams & Wilkins.

Figures in Table 18.4: ***Chronic Venous Insufficiency, Neuropathy:*** Marks, R. (1987). *Skin disease in old age*. Philadelphia, PA: JB Lippincott; ***Deep Vein Thrombosis:*** Dr. P. Marazzi/Photo Researchers, Inc.; ***Thrombophlebitis:*** Biophoto Associates/Photo Researchers, Inc.; ***Lymphedema:*** Rubin, E., & Farber, J. L. (1999). *Pathology* (3rd ed.). Philadelphia, PA: Lippincott Williams & Wilkins.

CHAPTER 19

Figures 19.2A and 19.3: Moore, K. L., & Dalley, A. F., II. (2008). *Clinically oriented anatomy* (6th ed.). Baltimore, MD: Lippincott Williams & Wilkins.

Figure 19.4: Courtesy of Esther K. Chung, MD.

Figures 19.6, 19.9A–D, 19.11, 19.12A–C, and 19.13: Photo by B. Proud.

Figure 19.7: Harris, J. R., Lippman, M. E., Morrow, M., & Osborne, C. K. (2014). *Diseases of the breast* (5th ed.). Philadelphia, PA: Lippincott Williams & Wilkins.

Figure 19.8A: Harris, J. R., Lippman, M. E., Morrow, M., & Osborne, C. K. (2014). *Diseases of the breast* (5th ed.). Philadelphia, PA: Lippincott Williams & Wilkins.

Figure 19.8B: Andolina, V., & Lilla, S. L. (2010). *Mammographic imaging* (3rd ed.). Philadelphia, PA: Lippincott Williams & Wilkins.

Figures 19.10 and 19.14: Mulholland, M. W., & Maier, R. V. (2006). *Greenfield's surgery: Scientific principles and practice* (4th ed.). Philadelphia, PA: Lippincott Williams & Wilkins.

Figures in Table 19.4: ***Carcinoma 1, Carcinoma 2:*** Mulholland, M. W., & Maier, R. V. (2006). *Greenfield's surgery: Scientific principles and practice* (4th ed.). Philadelphia, PA: Lippincott Williams & Wilkins; ***Paget Disease, Mastitis:*** Sweet, R. L., & Gibbs, R. S. (2005). *Atlas of infectious diseases of the female genital tract*. Philadelphia, PA: Lippincott Williams & Wilkins; ***Mastectomy:*** Steve Percival/Photo Researchers, Inc.; ***Gynecomastia:*** Courtesy of Christine Finck, MD.

CHAPTER 20

Figure 20.4: Gregory, D., Raymond-Seniuk, C., Patrick, L., & Stephen, T. (2015). *Fundamental: perspectives on the art and science of Canadian nursing*. Philadelphia, PA: Lippincott Williams & Wilkins.

Figures 20.7, 20.8, 20.9, 20.13, and 20.14: Photo by B. Proud.

Figures from Table 20.3: ***Acute Abdomen 1, Acute Abdomen 2, Abdominal Aortic Aneurysm:*** Photo by B. Proud; ***Appendicitis (Rovsing Sign), Acute Cholecystitis:*** Berg, D., & Worzala, K. (2006). *Atlas of adult physical diagnosis*. Philadelphia, PA: Lippincott Williams & Wilkins; ***Obturator Sign:*** Bickley, L. S. (2009). *Bates' guide to physical examination and history taking* (10th ed.). Philadelphia, PA: Lippincott Williams & Wilkins.

CHAPTER 21

Case Figure: Joe Sohm/Photo Researchers, Inc.

Figure 21.11: Oatis, C. A. (2004). *Kinesiology—The mechanics and pathomechanics of human movement*. Baltimore, MD: Lippincott Williams & Wilkins.

Figures 21.12 and 21.24: Bickley, L. S. (2009). *Bates' guide to physical examination and history taking* (10th ed.). Philadelphia, PA: Lippincott Williams & Wilkins.

Figures 21.23 and 21.25A, C, and D: Photo by B. Proud.

Figure 21.25B: Bickley, L. S., (2013). *Bates' guide to physical examination and history taking* (11th ed.). Philadelphia, PA: Lippincott Williams & Wilkins.

Figures 21.26A and B and 21.27A and B: Moore, K. L., & Dalley, A. F., II. (2008). *Clinically oriented anatomy* (6th ed.). Baltimore, MD: Lippincott Williams & Wilkins.

Figures from Table 21.8: ***Bulge Test:*** Bickley, L. S. (2009). *Bates' guide to physical examination and history taking* (10th ed.). Philadelphia, PA: Lippincott Williams & Wilkins; ***McMurray Test, Thomas Test, Lasègue Test, Drawer Sign, Trendelenburg Test:*** Berg, D., & Worzala, K. (2006). *Atlas of adult physical diagnosis*. Philadelphia, PA: Lippincott Williams & Wilkins.

Figures in Table 21.13: ***Atrophy, Joint Effusions, Epicondylitis:*** Bickley, L. S. (2009). *Bates' guide to physical examination and history taking* (10th ed.). Philadelphia, PA: Lippincott Williams & Wilkins; ***Joint Dislocation, Polydactyly, Swan Neck and Boutonnière Deformity, Syndactyly, Ulnar Deviation:*** Strickland, J. W., & Graham, T. J. (2005). *Master techniques in orthopedic surgery: The hand* (2nd ed.). Philadelphia, PA: Lippincott Williams & Wilkins; ***Long-Standing Rheumatoid Arthritis:*** Gold, D. H., & Weingeist, T. A. (2001). *Color atlas of the eye in systemic disease*. Baltimore, MD: Lippincott Williams & Wilkins; ***Rotator Cuff Tear, Bursitis, Dupuytren Contracture, Heberden and Bouchard Nodes, Carpal Tunnel Syndrome:*** Berg, D., & Worzala, K. (2006). *Atlas of adult physical diagnosis*. Philadelphia, PA: Lippincott Williams & Wilkins; ***Genu Valgum:*** Courtesy of Bettina Gyr, MD; ***Congenital Hip Dislocation:*** Bucholz, R. W., & Heckman, J. D. (2001). *Rockwood and Green's fractures in adults* (5th ed.). Philadelphia, PA: Lippincott Williams & Wilkins; ***Herniated Nucleus Pulposus:*** Daffner, R. H. (2007). *Clinical radiology the essentials* (3rd ed.). Philadelphia, PA: Lippincott Williams & Wilkins; ***Talipes Equinovarus:*** Courtesy of J. Adams; ***Acute Rheumatoid Arthritis:*** Image provided by Stedman's; ***Ankylosing Spondylitis:*** McConnell, T. H. (2007). *The nature of disease pathology for the health professions*. Philadelphia, PA: Lippincott Williams & Wilkins; ***Ganglion Cyst:*** Weber, J., & Kelley, J. (2003). *Health assessment in nursing* (2nd ed.). Philadelphia, PA: Lippincott Williams & Wilkins.

CHAPTER 22

Figure 22.1A: Porth, C. (2012). *Essentials of pathophysiology: Concepts of altered health states* (3rd ed.). Philadelphia, PA: Lippincott Williams & Wilkins.

Figure 22.4: Rhoades, R. A., & Bell, D. R. (2012). *Medical physiology* (7th ed.). Philadelphia, PA: Lippincott Williams & Wilkins.

Figures 22.13, 22.19, 22.22, and 22.23A–C: Bickley, L. S. (2009). *Bates' guide to physical examination and history taking* (10th ed.). Philadelphia, PA: Lippincott Williams & Wilkins.

Figure 22.18: Photo by B. Proud.

Figures from Table 22.9: ***Paralysis:*** Weber, J. R., & Kelley, J. H. (2013). *Health assessment in nursing* (5th ed.). Philadelphia, PA: Lippincott Williams & Wilkins; ***Dystonia:*** Fleisher, G. R., Ludwig, W., & Baskin, M. N. (2004). *Atlas of pediatric emergency medicine*. Philadelphia, PA: Lippincott Williams & Wilkins.

CHAPTER 23

Figure 23.2: Moore, K. L., & Dalley, A. F., II. (2008). *Clinically oriented anatomy* (6th ed.). Baltimore, MD: Lippincott Williams & Wilkins.

Figures 23.7, 23.8, 23.9, and 23.10 and Box 23.3: Photos by B. Proud.

Figures from Table 23.7: ***Scabies Infection, Syphilis:*** Goodheart, H. P. (2008). *Goodheart's photoguide of common skin disorders* (3rd ed.). Philadelphia, PA: Lippincott Williams & Wilkins; ***Chlamydia:*** Image from Rubin, E., & Farber, J. L. (1999). *Pathology* (3rd ed.). Philadelphia, PA: Lippincott Williams & Wilkins; ***Gonorrhea:*** Sanders, C. V., & Nesbitt, L. T. (1995). *The skin and infection*. Baltimore, MD: Lippincott Williams & Wilkins.

Figures from Table 23.8: ***Phimosis, Paraphimosis, Hypospadias:*** Courtesy of T. Ernesto Figueroa; ***Balanitis:*** Fleisher, G. R., Ludwig, S., & Baskin, M. N. (2004). *Atlas of pediatric emergency medicine*. Philadelphia, PA: Lippincott Williams & Wilkins; ***Epispadias:*** MacDonald, M. G., Mullett, M. D., & Seshia, M. M. K. (2005). *Avery's neonatology pathophysiology & management of the newborn* (6th ed.). Philadelphia, PA: Lippincott Williams & Wilkins.

Figures from Table 23.9: ***Rectal Polyp, Carcinoma of the Rectum and Anus:*** Mulholland, M. W., & Maier, R. V. (2006). *Greenfield's surgery: Scientific principles and practice* (4th ed.). Philadelphia, PA: Lippincott Williams & Wilkins.; ***Rectal Prolapse:*** Courtesy of Mary L. Brandt, MD; ***Prostatitis:*** Image from Rubin, E., & Farber, J. L. (1999). *Pathology* (3rd ed.). Philadelphia, PA: Lippincott Williams & Wilkins.

Figures from Table 23.11: ***Testicular Torsion, Varicocele:*** Courtesy of T. Ernesto Figueroa, MD.

CHAPTER 24

Equipment Box and Figures 24.6B, 24.7, 24.10, 24.13, 24.17, 24.19A, and 24.20A: Photo by B. Proud.

Figures 24.8, 24.15, and 24.16: Berg, D., & Worzala, K. (2006). *Atlas of adult physical diagnosis*. Philadelphia, PA: Lippincott Williams & Wilkins.

Figures from Table 24.3: ***Candidiasis:*** Goodheart, H. P. (2008). *Goodheart's photoguide of common skin disorders* (3rd ed.). Philadelphia, PA: Lippincott Williams & Wilkins; ***Bacterial Vaginosis, Chlamydia, Gonorrhea, Trichomoniasis, Condylomata Acuminatum:*** Sweet, R. L., & Gibbs, R. S. (2005). *Atlas of infectious diseases of the female genital tract*. Philadelphia, PA: Lippincott Williams & Wilkins.

Figures from Table 24.4: ***Chancre:*** Sweet, R. L., & Gibbs, R. S. (2005). *Atlas of infectious diseases of the female genital tract*. Philadelphia, PA: Lippincott Williams & Wilkins; ***Urethral Caruncle:*** Courtesy of Allan R. De Jong, MD; ***Contact Dermatitis:*** Courtesy of George A. Datto, III, MD; ***Pediculosis:*** Goodheart, H. P. (2008). *Goodheart's photoguide of common skin disorders* (3rd ed.). Philadelphia, PA: Lippincott Williams & Wilkins; ***Abscess of the Bartholin Gland:*** Weber, J. R., & Kelley, J. H. (2009). *Health assessment in nursing* (4th ed.). Philadelphia, PA: Lippincott Williams & Wilkins.

CHAPTER 25

Case Figure: Lawrence Migdale/Photo Researchers, Inc.

Figure 25.4: Goodheart, H. P. (2008). *Goodheart's photoguide of common skin disorders* (3rd ed.). Philadelphia, PA: Lippincott Williams & Wilkins.

CHAPTER 26

Figure 26.3: Ballard, J. L., Khoury, J. C., Wedig, K., Wang, L., Eilers-Walsman, B. L., Lipp, R. (1991). New Ballard score, expanded to include extremely premature infants. *J Pediatr, 119*, 417–423.

Figure 26.6: Bickley, L. S. (2013). *Bates' guide to physical examination and history taking* (11th ed.). Philadelphia, PA: Lippincott Williams & Wilkins.

Figure 26.10: MacDonald, M. G., Mullett, M. D., & Seshia, M. M. K. (2005). *Avery's neonatology pathophysiology & management of the newborn* (6th ed.). Philadelphia, PA: Lippincott Williams & Wilkins.

Figures from Table 26.2: ***Normal Variation:*** Weber, J. R., & Kelley, J. H. (2013). *Health assessment in nursing* (5th ed.). Philadelphia, PA: Lippincott Williams & Wilkins; ***Erythema Toxicum:*** Pillitteri, A. (2013). *Maternal and child health nursing: Care of the childbearing and childbearing family.* Philadelphia, PA: Lippincott Williams & Wilkins.

Figures from Table 26.7: ***Pediculosis Capitis:*** Courtesy of Hans B. Kersten, MD; ***Tinea Corporis, Scabies, Café Au Lait Spots:*** Fleisher, G. R., Ludwig, S., & Baskin, M. N. (2004). *Atlas of pediatric emergency medicine*. Philadelphia, PA: Lippincott Williams & Wilkins; ***Staphylococcal Scalded Skin Syndrome:*** Courtesy of Gary Marshall, MD; ***Molluscum Contagiosum, Bullous Impetigo, Allergic Contact Diaper Dermatitis, Eczema:*** Goodheart, H. P. (2008). *Goodheart's photoguide of common skin disorders* (3rd ed.). Philadelphia, PA: Lippincott Williams & Wilkins; ***Intertrigo, Lichen Simplex Chronicus:*** Sauer, G. C., & Hall, J. C. (1996). *Manual of skin diseases* (7thed.). Philadelphia, PA: Lippincott-Raven; ***Irritant Diaper Dermatitis, Candidal Diaper Dermatitis:*** Courtesy of Jan E. Drutz, MD.

Chapter 27

Figure 27.1: Bright Futures (2014). Recommendations for preventative pediatric health care. Retrieved from http://brightfutures.aap.org/pdfs/AAP_Bright_Futures_Periodicity_Sched_101107.pdf

Figure 27.6: Shutterstock.

Chapter 29

Figure 29.1: Shutterstock.

Figure 29.2: Shutterstock.

Figure 29.3: Eliopoulos, C. (2014). *Gerontological nursing* (8th ed.). Philadelphia, PA: Lippincott Williams & Wilkins.

Figure 29.4: Craft, N., Fox, L. P., Goldsmith L. A., Papier, A., Birnbaum, R., Mercurio, M. G., . . . Tumeh, P. C. (2010). *VisualDx: Essential adult dermatology*. Philadelphia, PA: Lippincott Williams & Wilkins.

Chapter 30

Figure 30.1: Taylor, C. R., Lillis, C., LeMone, P., & Lynn, P. (2011). *Fundamentals of nursing: The art and science of nursing care* (7th ed.). Philadelphia, PA: Lippincott Williams & Wilkins.

Index

Note: Page numbers followed by the letter *f* refer to figures; those followed by the letter *t* refer to tables.

D

E